FIFTH EDITION

Medical
BIOCHEMISTRY

JOHN W. BAYNES, PhD

Carolina Distinguished Professor Emeritus

Department of Pharmacology, Physiology and Neuroscience
University of South Carolina School of Medicine
Columbia, SC, USA

MAREK H. DOMINICZAK, MD, Dr Hab Med, FRCPath, FRCP (Glas)

Hon Professor of Clinical Biochemistry and Medical Humanities

College of Medical, Veterinary and Life Sciences
University of Glasgow
Glasgow, Scotland, UK

Docent in Laboratory Medicine

University of Turku
Turku, Finland

Consultant Biochemist

Clinical Biochemistry Service
National Health Service (NHS) Greater Glasgow and Clyde
Gartnavel General Hospital
Glasgow, Scotland, UK

ELSEVIER

ELSEVIER

First edition 1999
Second edition 2005
Third edition 2009
Fourth edition 2014
Fifth edition 2019

ISBN: 978-0-7020-7299-4

Content Strategist: Jeremy Bowes
Content Development Specialist: Nani Clansey
Project Manager: Beula Christopher
Design: Paula Catalano
Illustration Manager: Karen Giacomucci
Marketing Manager: Melissa Darling

your source for books,
journals and multimedia
in the health sciences
www.elsevierhealth.com

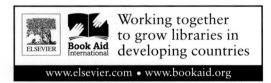

Working together
to grow libraries in
developing countries

www.elsevier.com • www.bookaid.org

The
publisher's
policy is to use
**paper manufactured
from sustainable forests**

Printed in China
Last digit is the print number: 9   8   7   6   5   4   3   2   1

FIFTH EDITION

Medical
BIOCHEMISTRY

3 0116 00570 9181

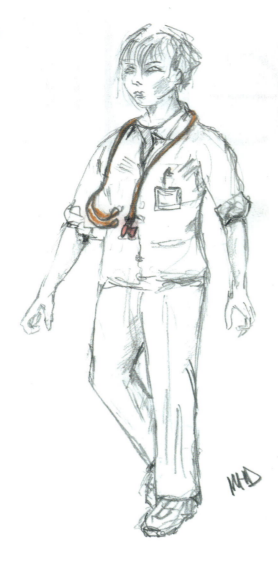

Caption: Resident2. Pencil on paper by Marek H. Dominiczak©

Your medical studies culminate in becoming a resident, where you will be in a position to help patients by solving clinical problems. This will require you to make decisions on diagnosis and treatment. The reason you learn basic science, including biochemistry, is to hone your clinical thinking so that these decisions are better.

We have placed this sketch by Marek Dominiczak here to remind ourselves that one should always see learning biochemistry in the context of this future role.

Contents

List of Contributors

Catherine N. Bagot, BSc, MBBS, MD, MRCP, FRCPath
Consultant Haematologist
Department of Haematology, Glasgow Royal Infirmary
Glasgow, Scotland, UK

John W. Baynes, PhD
Carolina Distinguished Professor Emeritus
Department of Pharmacology, Physiology and Neuroscience
University of South Carolina School of Medicine
Columbia, SC, USA

Hanna Bielarczyk, PhD
Assistant Professor and Chair
Department of Laboratory Medicine
Medical University of Gdańsk
Gdańsk, Poland

Iain Broom, DSc, MBChB, FRCPath, FRCP (Glas), FRCPE
Professor Emeritus of Metabolic Medicine
Aberdeen Centre for Energy Regulation and Obesity
University of Aberdeen
Aberdeen, Scotland, UK

Wayne E. Carver, PhD
Professor and Chair
Department of Cell Biology and Anatomy
University of South Carolina School of Medicine
Columbia, SC, USA

David Church, BMedSci (Hons), MSc, MRCP
Clinical Research Fellow
Honorary Specialty Registrar
University of Cambridge Metabolic Research Laboratories
Wellcome Trust-MRC Institute of Metabolic Science;
National Institute for Health Research Cambridge
Biomedical Research Centre;
Department of Clinical Biochemistry and Immunology
Addenbrooke's Hospital
Cambridge, UK

Marek H. Dominiczak, MD, Dr Hab Med, FRCPath, FRCP (Glas)
Hon Professor of Clinical Biochemistry and Medical
Humanities
College of Medical, Veterinary and Life Sciences
University of Glasgow
Glasgow, Scotland, UK;
Docent in Laboratory Medicine
University of Turku,
Turku, Finland;
Consultant Biochemist
Clinical Biochemistry Service
National Health Service (NHS) Greater Glasgow and Clyde
Gartnavel General Hospital
Glasgow, Scotland, UK

Alan D. Elbein, PhD (deceased)
Professor and Chair
Department of Biochemistry and Molecular Biology
University of Arkansas for Medical Sciences
Little Rock, AR, USA

Norma Frizzell, PhD
Associate Professor
Department of Pharmacology, Physiology and Neuroscience
University of South Carolina School of Medicine
Columbia, SC, USA

Junichi Fujii, PhD
Professor
Department of Biochemistry and Molecular Biology
Graduate School of Science,
Yamagata University
Yamagata, Japan

J. Alastair Gracie, PhD BSc (Hons)
Senior University Teacher
School of Medicine, Dentistry and Nursing
College of Medical, Veterinary and Life Sciences
University of Glasgow
Glasgow, Scotland, UK

Alejandro Gugliucci, MD, PhD
Professor of Biochemistry and Associate Dean
Touro University California College of Osteopathic Medicine
Vallejo, CA, USA

Margaret M. Harnett, PhD
Professor of Immune Signalling
Institute of Infection, Immunity and Inflammation
University of Glasgow
Glasgow, Scotland, UK

Simon J. R. Heales, PhD, FRCPath
Professor of Clinical Chemistry
Neurometabolic Unit, National Hospital
Queen Square and Laboratory Medicine
Great Ormond Street Hospital
London, UK

George M. Helmkamp, Jr., PhD
Emeritus Professor of Biochemistry
Department of Biochemistry and Molecular Biology
University of Kansas School of Medicine
Kansas City, KS, USA

Koichi Honke, MD, PhD
Professor of Biochemistry
Department of Biochemistry
Kochi University Medical School
Kochi, Japan

Edel M. Hyland, PhD
Lecturer in Biochemistry
School of Biological Sciences
Queen's University Belfast
Belfast, Northern Ireland, UK

Susan Johnston, BSc, MSc, FRCPath
Clinical Biochemist
Clinical Biochemistry Service
National Health Service (NHS) Greater Glasgow and Clyde
Glasgow, Scotland, UK

Alan F. Jones, MA, MB, BChir, DPhil, FRCP, FRCPath
Consultant Physician and Divisional Director
Heart of England NHS Foundation Trust
Bordesley Green East
Birmingham, UK

Fredrik Karpe, MD, PhD
Professor of Metabolic Medicine
Oxford Centre for Diabetes, Endocrinology and Metabolism
Radcliffe Department of Medicine
University of Oxford
Oxford, UK

Gur P. Kaushal, PhD
Professor of Medicine
University of Arkansas for Medical Sciences;
Research Career Scientist
Central Arkansas Veterans Healthcare System
Little Rock, AR, USA

Walter Kolch, MD
Professor, Director, Systems Biology Ireland
University College Dublin
Belfield, Dublin, Ireland

Matthew C. Kostek, PhD, FACSM, HFS
Associate Professor
Department of Physical Therapy
Duquesne University
Pittsburgh, PA, USA

Jennifer Logue, MBChB, MRCP, MD, FRCPath
Clinical Senior Lecturer and Honorary Consultant in Metabolic Medicine
Institute of Cardiovascular and Medical Sciences
University of Glasgow
Glasgow, Scotland, UK

Masatomo Maeda, PhD
Professor of Molecular Biology
Department of Molecular Biology
School of Pharmacy
Iwate Medical University
Iwate, Japan

Teresita Menini, MD, MS
Professor and Assistant Dean
Touro University California College of Osteopathic Medicine
Vallejo, CA, USA

Alison M. Michie, PhD
Reader in Molecular Lymphopoiesis
Institute of Cancer Sciences
University of Glasgow
Glasgow, Scotland, UK

Ryoji Nagai, PhD
Associate Professor
Laboratory of Food and Regulation Biology
School of Agriculture
Tokai University
Kumamoto, Japan

Jeffrey R. Patton, PhD
Associate Professor
Department of Pathology, Microbiology and Immunology
University of South Carolina School of Medicine
Columbia, SC, USA

Verica Paunovic, PhD
Research Associate
Institute of Microbiology and Immunology
School of Medicine
University of Belgrade
Belgrade, Serbia

Georgia Perona-Wright, PhD, MA, BA
Senior Lecturer
Institute of Infection, Immunity and Inflammation
College of Medical, Veterinary and Life Sciences
University of Glasgow
Glasgow, Scotland, UK

Andrew R. Pitt, PhD
Professor of Pharmaceutical Chemistry and Chemical
Biology
Life and Health Sciences
Aston University
Birmingham, UK

Simon Pope, PhD
Clinical Biochemist
Neurometabolic Unit
National Hospital
UCLH Foundation Trust
London, UK

Matthew Priest, MB, ChB, FRCP (Glas)
Consultant Gastroenterologist and Honorary Senior
Lecturer
NHS Greater Glasgow and Clyde and University of Glasgow
Glasgow, Scotland, UK

Allen B. Rawitch, PhD
Vice Chancellor Emeritus
Emeritus Professor of Biochemistry and Molecular Biology
University of Kansas Medical Center
Kansas City, KS, USA

Ian P. Salt, PhD
Senior Lecturer
Institute of Cardiovascular and Medical Sciences
University of Glasgow
Glasgow, Scotland, UK

Robert Semple, PhD, FRCP
Reader in Endocrinology and Metabolism
Wellcome Trust Senior Research Fellow in Clinical Science;
Honorary Consultant Physician
University of Cambridge Metabolic Research Laboratories
Wellcome Trust-MRC Institute of Metabolic Science;
National Institute for Health Research Cambridge
Biomedical Research Centre
Cambridge, UK

L. William Stillway, PhD
Emeritus Professor of Biochemistry and Molecular Biology
Department of Biochemistry and Molecular Biology
Medical University of South Carolina
Charleston, SC, USA

Mirosława Szczepańska-Konkel, PhD
Emeritus Professor of Clinical Chemistry
Department of Clinical Chemistry
Medical University of Gdańsk
Gdańsk, Poland

Andrzej Szutowicz, MD, PhD
Professor, Department of Laboratory Medicine
Medical University of Gdańsk
Gdańsk, Poland

Naoyuki Taniguchi, MD, PhD
Group Director, Systems Glycobiology Group
RIKEN Advanced Science Institute
Saitama, Japan

Yee Ping Teoh, FRCPATH, MRCP, MBBS
Consultant in Chemical Pathology
Biochemistry Department
Wrexham Maelor Hospital
Wrexham, UK

Robert W. Thornburg, PhD
Professor of Biochemistry
Department of Biochemistry, Biophysics and Molecular
Biology
Iowa State University
Ames, IA, USA

Acknowledgments

First of all, we wish to thank our contributors for sharing their expertise with us and for fitting the writing—again—into their busy research, teaching and clinical schedules. In the 5th edition, we are delighted to welcome new contributors: David Church, Edel Hyland, Susan Johnston, Simon Pope, Teresita Menini, and Georgia Perona-Wright.

As in the previous edition, we greatly value the excellent secretarial assistance of Jacky Gardiner in Glasgow.

Our inspiration to change and improve this text comes from the problems, questions, and decisions that arise in our everyday clinical practice, in the outpatient clinics, and on the hospital wards. We are grateful to all our clinical colleagues and doctors in training for their insight, discussions, and sharing of their clinical experience. We are also grateful to students and academics from universities around the world who continue to provide us with comments, suggestions, and criticisms. We acknowledge the contribution of scholars who participated in the writing of previous editions of Medical Biochemistry: Gary A Bannon, Graham Beastall, Robert Best, James A Carson, Alex Farrell (deceased), William D Fraser, Helen S Goodridge, D Margaret Hunt, Andrew Jamieson, W Stephen Kistler, Utkarsh V Kulkarni, Edward J Thompson, and A Michael Wallace (deceased).

Last but not least, the key to success of the whole project has been, of course, the Elsevier team. Our thanks go to Nani Clansey, Senior Development Editor, whose expertise and enthusiasm steered the project through; to Madelene Hyde, who formulated the strategy; to Jeremy Bowes for his contribution to the initial stages of this edition; and to Beula Christopher, who gave the book its final form.

To inspirational academics
Inquisitive students
And all those who want to be good doctors

Preface

Medical Biochemistry has now served the global medical student community for 19 years. In the 5th edition our aim remains, as before, to provide a biochemical foundation for the study of clinical medicine—with down-to-earth practical relevance.

Each edition has provided a snapshot of a constantly changing field. Perhaps the most exciting sign of progress is the ever-increasing relevance of basic science to the practice of medicine, expressed in new drugs targeting biochemical regulatory and metabolic pathways and in new concepts that both change and supplement our approaches to everyday clinical challenges.

Apart from describing the core of basic science, we continue to emphasize the contribution of biochemistry to the understanding of major global health problems such as diabetes mellitus, obesity, malnutrition, and atherosclerotic cardiovascular disease. As before, we remain convinced that the biochemistry of water, electrolyte, and acid–base balance is as important for future clinicians as are the key metabolic pathways and thus deserves more emphasis in the biochemistry curriculum.

In addition to substantial updates, we have changed the structure of the book, aiming to provide a clearer perspective on the entire field. The details of this reorganization are summarized in Chapter 1.

We have also updated literature and web references throughout the textbook. To facilitate familiarity with new terminologies and acronyms currently abundant in the scientific slang, in this edition we have provided an easily accessible list of abbreviations in each chapter. We have also expanded the index to provide more comprehensive access to topics discussed in the text.

We now have even more clinical cases throughout the book, plus additional cases in Appendix 2. We hope that these will strengthen the link between biochemistry and clinical medicine and provide a stronger foundation for clinical problem solving.

A question bank for self-assessment and many more resources are available at the Elsevier website, www.studentconsult.com, to which the reader is referred. There is also a companion publication, *Medical Biochemistry Flash Cards*, which provides a means for quick review.

As before, we welcome comments, criticisms, and suggestions from our readers. There is no better way to continue making this a better text.

Abbreviations

1,25(OH)$_2$D$_3$	1,25-dihydroxycholecalciferol, calcitriol	ALL	Acute lymphoblastic leukemia
1,3-BPG	1,3-bisphosphoglycerate	ALP	Alkaline phosphatase
17-OHP	17-hydroxyprogesterone	ALPS	Autoimmune lymphoproliferative syndrome
2,3-BPG	2,3-bisphosphoglycerate		
4E-BP1	eIF4E-binding protein 1	ALT	Alanine aminotransferase
5-ALA	5-aminolevulinate	AML	Acute myeloid leukemia
5-HIAA	5-hydroxyindoleacetic acid	AMPA	α-amino-3-hydroxy-5-methyl-4-isoxazolepropionic acid
5-HT	5-hydroxytryptamine, serotonin		
8-oxoG	8-oxo-2'-deoxyguanosine	AMPK	AMP-activated protein kinase; AMP-dependent protein kinase
α-MSH	Melanocortin		
A1AT	Alpha-1 antitrypsin	ANP	Atrial natriuretic peptide
AADC	Aromatic amino acid decarboxylase	AP-1	Activator protein-1
ABC	ATP binding cassette	APAF1	Apoptotic protease activating factor 1
ABCA1, ABCG5, G8, A1, G1, and G4	ATP-binding cassette transporters	APC	Anaphase-promoting complex
		APC	Antigen-presenting cell
Abl	Nonreceptor protein tyrosine kinase	apoA	Apolipoprotein A
ACAT	Acyl-CoA: acyl-cholesterol transferase	apoB	Apolipoprotein B
ACAT	Cholesterol acyltransferase	apoB100/apoB48	Apolipoprotein B
ACC1, ACC2	Acetyl-CoA carboxylase	apoC	Apolipoprotein C
ACD	Autophagic cell death (autophagy)	ApoE	Apolipoprotein E
ACE	Angiotensin-converting enzyme	APP	Amyloid precursor protein
Acetyl-CoA	Acetyl-coenzyme A	APRT	Adenosine phosphoribosyl transferase
ACh	Acetylcholine	APTT	Activated partial thromboplastin time
ACP	Acyl carrier protein	AQP	Aquaporin
ACTH	Adrenocorticotropic hormone	ARDS	Acute respiratory distress syndrome
AD	Alzheimer's disease	ARE	Antioxidant response element
ADA	American Diabetes Association	ASCVD	Atherosclerotic cardiovascular disease
ADAR	Adenosine deaminase acting on RNA	AST	Aspartate aminotransferase
ADH	Alcohol dehydrogenase	AT1, AT2	Angiotensin receptors
ADH	Antidiuretic hormone, vasopressin	ATCase	Aspartate transcarbamoylase
AE	Anion exchanger	ATF	Activation transcription factor
AFP	α-fetoprotein	ATG	Autophagy-related gene
AG	Anion gap	ATM	Ataxia-telangiectasia mutated, checkpoint kinase
AGE	Advanced glycation (glycoxidation) end products	ATP III	National Cholesterol Education Treatment Panel III
AGPAT2	Acylglycerol acyltransferase 2	ATP	Adenosine triphosphate
AHA	American Heart Association	ATR	Ataxia-telangiectasia Rad3–related checkpoint kinase, CHK1 and CHK2
AHF	Antihemophilic factor		
AI	Adequate Intake	AUC	Area under the curve
AIC	Acute intermittent porphyria	AVP	Arginine vasopressin
Akt	Protein kinase	AZT	Azidothymidine
ALD	Alcoholic liver disease	BAD	Bcl-2-associated death promoter
ALDH	Aldehyde dehydrogenase	Bak	Bcl-2 homologous antagonist/killer
ALE	Advanced lipoxidation end-products	BAX	Bcl-2-associated X protein

BBB	Blood–brain barrier
Bcl-2	B-cell lymphoma protein 2; Bcl-2 family members include prosurvival family members (Bcl-2, Bcl-xL, Bcl-W, Mcl-1); proapoptotic BAX/BAK family, and proapoptotic BH-3-only proteins (BIM, Bid, PUMA, NOXA, BAD, BIK)
BCR	B-cell receptor
BCR	Breakpoint cluster region
BH-3	Interacting-domain death agonist
BH4	Tetrahydrobiopterin
BMI	Body mass index
BMR	Basal metabolic rate
BNP	Brain natriuretic peptide
BrdU	Bromodeoxyuridine
Btk	A protein tyrosine kinase
BUN	Blood urea nitrogen
bw	Body weight
C1q, C1r, C1s, and C2–C9	Complement components
C3G	Guanyl nucleotide exchange factor
CA	Carbonic anhydrase
CAD	Carbamoyl phosphate synthetase-Aspartate transcarbamoylase-Dihydroorotase
CAH	Congenital adrenal hyperplasia
CAK	CDK-activating complex, composed of CDK7, cyclin H, and MAT1 (ménage a trois)
CaM	Calmodulin
cAMP	Adenosine 3′,5′-cyclic monophosphate
cAMP	Cyclic adenosine monophosphate
CAMS	Cell adhesion molecules
CAP	Cbl-associated protein
CAT	Catalase
CBG	Cortisol-binding globulin (also known as transcortin)
Cbl	Adaptor protein in insulin signaling pathway
CD	Cluster of differentiation system; cell surface molecules
CD4$^+$	T helper cells (T_H)
CD40L	CD40 ligand
CD8$^+$	Cytotoxic T lymphocyte (CTL)
CDG	Congenital disease of glycosylation
CDK	Cyclin-dependent kinase
CDKIs	Cyclin-dependent kinase inhibitory proteins
cDNA	Complementary DNA
CDP	Cytidine diphosphate
CDP-DAG	CDP-diacylglycerol
CE	Cholesterol ester
CEA	Carcinoembryonic antigen
CETP	Cholesterol ester transfer protein
CF	Cystic fibrosis
CFDA SE	Carboxy-fluoresceindiacetate succinimidyl ester
cFLIP	Modulator of FADD, Fas-associated death domain
CFTR	Cystic fibrosis transmembrane conductance regulator
CGD	Chronic granulomatous disease
CGH	Comparative genome hybridization
cGMP	Cyclic guanosine 3′5′-monophosphate
cGMP	Cyclic guanosine monophosphate
C_H	Constant heavy fragment; antigen-binding sequence domains
ChAT	Choline acetyltransferase
ChIP	Chromatin immunoprecipitation
ChIP-on-chip	Combination chromatin immunoprecipitation and microarray technology
ChIPseq	Combination chromatin immunoprecipitation and RNAseq technology
CHK1	CHK2, checkpoint kinases
CK	Creatine (phospho)kinase
CK-MB	MB fraction of creatine kinase
C_L	Constant light, fragment; antigen-binding sequence domains
CLL	Chronic lymphocytic leukemia
CLR	C-type lectin receptors
CMA	Chromosomal microarray analysis
CML	Chronic myeloid leukemia
CML	Ne-(carboxymethyl)lysine
CMP-NeuAc	CDP-neuraminic (sialic) acid
CMP-PA	Cytosine monophosphate-phosphatidic acid
CNS	Central nervous system
COAD	Chronic obstructive airway disease
CoA-SH	Acetyl-coenzyme A
COHb	Carboxyhemoglobin
COMT	Catecholamine-O-methyltransferase
CpG	Cystine-guanine dinucleotide
CPS	Carbamoyl phosphate synthetase
CPT-I, CPT-II	Carnitine palmitoyl transferase I and II
CRBP	Cytosolic retinol-binding proteins
CREB	cAMP response element-binding protein
CRH	Corticotropin-releasing hormone; Corticoliberin
cRNA	Complementary RNA
CRP	C-reactive protein
CSC	Cancer stem cell
CSF	Cerebrospinal fluid
CT	Computed (computerized) tomography scan
CT	Computerized tomography
CTD	C-terminal domain
CTL	Cytotoxic T lymphocytes (CD8$^+$ cells)
CTX	Carboxy-terminal telopeptide
Cyt a, b, c	Cytochrome a, cytochrome b, cytochrome c
DAG	Diacylglycerol

DAMPs	Damage-associated molecular patterns
DAPI	4'-6'-diamidino-2-phenylindole
DAT	Dopamine transporter
DC	Dendritic cell
DCCT	Diabetes Control and Complications Trial
DD	Death domain
DDI	Drug–drug interaction
DED	Death effector domain
DEXA	Dual-energy X-ray absorptiometry
DGAT	Diacylglycerol acyltransferase
DHAP	Dihydroxyacetone phosphate
DHEA	Dehydroepiandrosterone
DHEAS	Dehydroepiandrosterone sulfate
DHT	Dihydrotestosterone
DIC	Disseminated intravascular coagulation
DILI	Drug-induced liver injury
DISC	Death-inducing signaling complex
DIT	Diiodotyrosine
DLDH	Dihydrolipoyl dehydrogenase
DLTA	Dihydrolipoyl transacetylase
DMP	Dentin matrix protein
DNA	Deoxyribonucleic acid
DNL	De novo lipogenesis
DNP	Dinitrophenol
Dol	Dolichol
DPP-4	Dipeptidyl peptidase-4
DPPC	Dipalmitoylphosphatidylcholine
DRI	Dietary Reference Intakes
dsRNA	Double stranded RNA
DTI	Direct thrombin inhibitor
DVT	Deep vein thrombosis
E2F	Family of transcription factors
EAR	Estimated Average Requirement
EBNA1	The Epstein–Barr virus nuclear antigen 1
ECF	Extracellular fluid
ECM	Extracellular matrix
EDRF	Endothelium-derived relaxing factor (nitric oxide)
EDTA	Ethylenediaminetetraacetic acid
eEF	Eukaryotic elongation factor
EFA	Essential fatty acid
EGF	Epidermal growth factor
EGFR	Epidermal growth factor receptor
eGFR	Estimated glomerular filtration rate
eIF	Eukaryotic initiation factor
EMSA	Electrophoretic mobility shift assay
ENaC	Amiloride-sensitive calcium channel
ENaC	Epithelial sodium channel
eNOS	Endothelial nitric oxide synthase
EPA	Eicosapentaenoic acid
Epacs	Exchange proteins directly activated by cAMP
ER	Endoplasmic reticulum
ERAD	ER-associated degradation pathway
eRF	Eukaryotic releasing factor complex

ERK 1 and 2	Extracellular-signal regulated kinases; two isoforms of MEK kinase that activate MAPK
ESR	Erythrocyte sedimentation rate
ETC	Electron transport chain
FAD/FADH$_2$	Flavin adenine dinucleotide (oxidized/reduced)
FADD	Fas-associated death domain (Fas, death receptor, TNF family member)
FasL	Fas ligand
Fc	"Fragment constant" of immunoglobulin molecule
FcγR	Fc-γ receptor (receptor for immunoglobulin G)
FDB	Familial defective apolipoprotein B
FDPs	Fibrin degradation products
FGF	Fibroblast growth factor
FGFR3	Fibroblast growth factor receptor 3
FH	Familial hypercholesterolemia
FIRKO	Adipose tissue (fat) insulin receptor knockout
FISH	Fluorescence in situ hybridization
FMN	Flavin mononucleotide
FOXA2	Transcription factor, also known as HNF-3B
FOXO	Forkhead box O proteins; transcription factors belonging to the forkhead family (contain proteins designated FOXA to FOXR)
FOXP3	Transcription factor
FP	Flavoprotein
FRTA	Free radical theory of aging
Fru-1,6-BP	Fructose-1,6-bisphosphate
Fru-1,6-BPase	Fructose 1,6-biphosphatase
Fru-1,6-BPase	Fructose-1,6-bisphosphatase
Fru-1-P	Fructose-1-phosphate
Fru-2,6-BP	Fructose 2,6-biphosphate
Fru-2,6-BPase	Fructose-2,6-bisphosphatase
Fru-6-P	Fructose-6-phosphate
FSF	Fibrin-stabilizing factor
FSH	Follicle-stimulating hormone
fT3 and fT4	Free T3 and free T4
FVII	Factor VII
FXR	Farnesyl X receptor
Fyn	Nonreceptor protein tyrosine kinase
G0	Resting, or quiescent, phase
G1	Interval between M and S phases
G2	Interval between S and M phases
G6PDH	Glucose-6-phosphate dehydrogenase
GABA	γ-Aminobutyric acid
GAD	Glutamic acid decarboxylase
GAG	Glycosaminoglycan
Gal	Galactose
Gal-1-P	Galactose-1-phosphate
GALD-3-P	Glyceraldehyde-3-phosphate
GalNAc	N-acetylgalactosamine

GAPDH	Glyceraldehyde-3-phosphate dehydrogenase	HIV	Human immunodeficiency virus
GAPs	GTPase-activating protein	HLA	Human leukocyte antigen
GAS	Gamma interferon activation site	HLA-DR, HLA-DQ, HLA-DM and HLA-DP	MHC class II genes
GC-MS	Gas chromatography–mass spectrometry		
GCS	Glycine cleavage systems		
GDM	Gestational diabetes mellitus	HMDB	Human Metabolome Database
GDP-Fuc	Guanosine diphosphate fucose	HMG-CoA	3-hydroxy-3-methylglutaryl-CoA
GDP-Man	Guanosine diphosphate mannose	HMG-CoA	Hydroxymethylglutaryl-CoA
GFAP	Glial fibrillary acidic protein	HMGR	HMG-CoA reductase
GFR	Glomerular filtration rate	HMWK	High-molecular-weight kininogen
GGT	γ-glutamyl transpeptidase	HNE	Hydroxynonenal
GH	Growth hormone	HNF1A, HNF1B	Transcription factors
GHRH	Growth hormone–releasing hormone	hnRNA	Hetergeneous nuclear RNA
GI	Gastrointestinal (tract)	HPLC	High-performance liquid chromatography
GI	Glycemic index	HRE	Hormone response element
GIP	Gastric inhibitory peptide	HRG	Histidine-rich glycoprotein
GK	Glucokinase	HSP	Heat shock protein
Glc	Glucose	HSV	Herpes simplex virus
Glc-6-P	Glucose-6-phosphate	HTGL	Hepatic triglyceride lipase
Glc-6-Pase	Glucose-6-phosphatase	HVA	Homovanillic acid
GlcNAc	N-acetylglucosamine	IAP	Inhibitor of apoptosis gene family
GlcNH$_2$	Glucosamine	ICAM-1	Intercellular adhesion molecule 1 (CD54)
GlcUA	Glucuronic acid	ICF	Intracellular fluid
GLP-1	Glucagon-like peptide-1	IDDM	Insulin-dependent diabetes mellitus
GLUT	Glucose transporter	IDL	Intermediate-density lipoprotein(s)
Glycerol-3-P	Glycerol-3-phosphate	IdUA	Iduronic acid
GnRH	Gonadotropin-releasing hormone	IEF	Isoelectric focusing
GPCR	G-protein coupled receptor	IF	Intrinsic factor
GPI	Glycosylphosphatidylinositol anchor	IFCC	International Federation of Clinical Chemistry and Laboratory Medicine.
GPIb-IX, GPIIb-IIIa	Platelet membrane glycoprotein receptors		
GPx	Glutathione peroxidase	IFG	Impaired fasting glucose
Grb2	Growth factor receptor-bound protein 2, adapter molecule	IFN	Interferon (IFN-α, IFN-β, and IFNγ)
		Ig	Immunoglobulin
GSH	Glutathione (reduced)	Ig	Immunoglobulin (IgG, IgA, IgM, IgD, and IgE)
GSSG	Glutathione (oxidized)		
GTPase	Guanosine triphosphatase	IGF	Insulin-like growth factor
GWAS	Genome-wide association study	IGFBP	IGF-binding proteins
Hb	Hemoglobin	IgG	Immunoglobulin G
HbA	Adult (normal) hemoglobin	IGT	Impaired glucose tolerance
HbA$_{1c}$	Hemoglobin A$_{1c}$, glycated hemoglobin	Ihh	Indian hedgehog, a signaling protein
HbF	Fetal hemoglobin	IKK	NFκB kinase
HbS	Sickle Cell hemoglobin	IL	Interleukin (IL-1, IL-6, etc.)
hCG	Human chorionic gonadotrophin	IMAC	Immobilized metal affinity chromatography
HCL	Hairy cell leukemia		
hCS-A, hCS-B, hCS-L, and hGH-V	Human somatomammotropin (GH) genes	IMM	Inner mitochondrial membrane
		IMP	Inosine monophosphate
		IMS	Intermembrane space
HDL	High-density lipoprotein(s)	INR	International Normalized Ratio
HFE	Hereditary hemochromatosis protein	IP$_3$	Inositol 1,4,5-trisphosphate
HGF	Hepatocyte growth factor	IP$_3$	Inositol trisphosphate
hGH	Human growth hormone	IP$_3$	Inositol-1,4,5-trisphosphate
HGP	Human genome project	IPP	Isopentenyl diphosphate
HGPRT	Hypoxanthine-guanine phosphoribosyl transferase	IR	Insulin receptor
		IRE	Iron response element
HIT	Heparin-induced thrombocytopenia	IRES	Internal ribosomal entry site

IRI	Ischemic reperfusion injury		MDRD	Modification of diet in renal disease study
IRS	Insulin receptor substrate		MEK	Mitogen-activated protein kinase. A protein kinase that activates MAPK
ITAM/ITIM	Immunoreceptor tyrosine activation/inhibition motif		MET	Metabolic equivalent of task
IU	International unit		metHb	Methemoglobin (Fe^{+3})
JAK	Janus kinase		MetSO	Methionine sulfoxide
JAK/STAT	Janus kinase/signal transducer and activator of transcription		MGO	Methylglyoxal
			MHC	Major histocompatibility complex
JNK	C-Jun terminal kinase		miRNA	MicroRNA
kb	Kilobase		MIT	Monoiodotyrosine
KCC1	K^+ and Cl^- cotransporter		MMP	Matrix metalloproteinase
KCCT	Kaolin–cephalin clotting time, APTT		MMP	Mitochondrial membrane potential
KIP2	57-kDa inhibitor of cyclin–CDK complexes		MODY	Maturity-onset diabetes of the young
KIT	Tyrosine kinase 3 genes		MPO	Myeloperoxidase
KLF	Kruppel-like factor		MRI	Magnetic resonance imaging
K_m	Michaelis constant		MRM	Multiple reaction monitoring
LACI	Lipoprotein-associated coagulation inhibitor		mRNA	Messenger RNA
			MRP	Multidrug resistance-associated protein
LBBB	Left bundle branch block		MS	Mass spectrometry
LC3	Microtubule-associated protein light chain 3		MSH	Melanocyte stimulating hormone
			MSLP	Maximum lifespan potential
LCAT	Lecithin:cholesterol acyltransferase		mtDNA	Mitochondrial DNA
LC-MS	Liquid chromatography/mass spectrometry		MTHFR	5,10-methylenetetrahydrofolate reductase
LDH	Lactate dehydrogenase		mTOR	Mechanistic target of rapamycin; a serine/threonine protein kinase
LDL	Low-density lipoprotein(s)			
LFA-1	Lymphocyte function–associated antigen 1		mTORC-1 and mTORC-2	mTor complexes
LH	Luteinizing hormone			
LMWH	Low-molecular-weight heparin		mTORC	Mammalian target of rapamycin complex
lncRNA	Long non-coding RNA		MTP	Microsomal transfer protein
LPL	Lipoprotein lipase		MudPIT	Multidimensional protein identification technology
LPLAT	Lysophospholipid acyltransferase			
LPS	Lipopolysaccharide		MWCO	Molecular weight cut-off
LRP5	LDL-receptor-related protein 5		Myc	Transcription factor
LSC	Laser-scanning cytometry		N5MeTHF	5-methyl tetrahydrofolate
LT	Leukotriene		N^5-N^{10}-THF	N^5-N^{10}-tetrahydrofolate
LTA	Light transmission aggregometry		NAA	N-acetyl-l-aspartate
LXR	Liver X receptors		NABQI	N-acetyl benzoquinoneimine
M	Mitosis		NAC	N-acetylcysteine
MAC-1	Macrophage adhesion molecule 1		NAD^+/NADH	Nicotinamide adenine dinucleotide (oxidized/reduced)
MAG	Monoacylglycerol			
MALT	Mucosa-associated lymphoid tissues		$NADP^+$	Nicotinamide adenine dinucleotide phosphate
Man-6-P	Mannose-6-phosphate			
MAO	Monoamine oxidase		NADPH	Nicotinamide dinucleotide phosphate (reduced)
MAOI	Monoamine oxidase inhibitor			
MAPK	Mitogen-activated protein kinase		NAFLD	Nonalcoholic fatty liver disease
MAS	Angiotensin 1–7 receptor		NCC	Sodium–chloride co-transporter
Mb	Myoglobin		ncRNA	Non-coding RNA
MBL	Mannose-binding lectin		NEFA	Nonesterified fatty acid
MCH	Melanin-concentrating hormone		NeuAc	Neuraminic (sialic) acid
MCL	Mantle cell lymphoma		NFAT2	Transcription factor; nuclear factor of activated T cells-2
MCP	Multicatalytic protease			
MCP-1	Monocyte chemoattractant protein 1		NFκB	Nuclear factor kappa-light-chain-enhancer of activated B cell
M-CSF	Monocyte-colony stimulating factor			
MCV	Mean corpuscular volume		NGF	Nerve growth factor
MDA	Malondialdehyde		NGS	Next generation sequencing

NHE	Sodium/hydrogen exchanger	PET/MRI	Positron emission tomography/magnetic resonance imaging
NIDDM	Noninsulin-dependent diabetes mellitus	PFK	Phosphofructokinase
NK	Natural killer cells	PFK-2/Fru-2,6-BPase	Phosphofructokinase-2/fructose-2,6-bisphosphatase
NKCC1	Na^+ K^+ and $C\lambda^-$ cotransporter		
NKCC2	Sodium–potassium–chloride co-transporter	PG	Prostaglandins
NKH	Non-ketotic hyperglycinemia	PGE_2	Prostaglandin E_2
NLR	NOD-like receptor	PGI_2	Prostaglandin I_2
NMDA	N-methyl-d-aspartate	PH	Pleckstrin homology domains
NMR	Nuclear magnetic resonance	pI	Isoelectric point
NO	Nitric oxide	PI	Phosphatidylinositol
NOS	Nitric oxide synthase	PI	Propidium iodide
NPC1L1	Niemann–Pick C1-like protein.	PI3K	Phosphatidylinositol-3-kinase
NPY	Neuropeptide Y	PIP_2	Phosphatidylinositol 4,5- bisphosphate
nt	Nucleotide	PIP_3	Inositol 1, 4,5- bisphosphate
NTX	N-terminal (Amino-terminal) telopeptide	PIP_3	Phosphatidylinositol 3,4,5-trisphosphate
OAA	Oxaloacetate		
OGTT	Oral glucose tolerance test	PK	Protein kinase: PKA, PKC
OI	Osteogenesis imperfecta	PK	Pyruvate kinase
OMM	Outer mitochondrial membrane	PKA	Protein kinase A
ONDST	Overnight dexamethasone suppression test	PKC	Protein kinase C
OPG	Osteoprotegerin	PKU	Phenylketonuria
OSF-1	Osteoblast-stimulating factor 1	PL	Phospholipase: PLA_2, PLC, PLC-β, PLD
o-Tyr	Ortho-tyrosine	PLA2	Phospholipase A2
P1CP	Procollagen type 1 C-terminal peptide	PLC	Phospholipase C
P1NP	Procollagen type 1 N-terminal propeptide	PLP	Pyridox(am)ine-5′-phosphate oxidase
p38	Stress-activated protein kinase	PNH	Paroxysmal nocturnal hemoglobinuria
p53	Tumor-suppressor protein	PNPO	Pyridoxal phosphate
p62	Nucleoporin	PNS	Peripheral nervous system
PA	Phosphatidic acid	pO_2	Partial pressure of oxygen
PAF	Platelet-activating factor	POMC	Proopiomelanocortin
PAGE	Polyacrylamide gel electrophoresis	PP2A	Protein phosphatase-2A
PAI-1	Plasminogen activator inhibitor type 1	PPAR	Peroxisome proliferator-activated receptor
PAMP	Pathogen-associated molecular pattern	PPi	Pyrophosphate
PAPS	Phosphoadenosine-5′-phosphosulfate	Prot	Protein
PAR2	Protease-activated receptor 2	PRPP	Phosphoribosyl pyrophosphate
PBG	Porphobilinogen	PRR	Pattern-recognition receptors
PC	Phosphatidylcholine	PS	Phosphatidylserine
PC	Pyruvate carboxylase	PSA	Prostate-specific antigen
PCD	Programmed cell death	PT	Prothrombin time
PCI	Percutaneous coronary intervention	PTA	Plasma thromboplastin antecedent
pCO_2	Partial pressure of carbon dioxide	PTEN	Phosphatase and TENsin homologue
PCP	Phencyclidine	PTH	Parathyroid hormone
PCR	Polymerase chain reaction	PTK	Protein tyrosine kinase
PCSK9	Proprotein convertase subtilisin/kexin type 9	PTM	Posttranslational modification
		PTPase	Phosphotyrosine phosphatase
PDE	Phosphodiesterase	PUFA	Polyunsaturated fatty acid
PDGF	Platelet-derived growth factor	PXR	Pregnane X receptor
PDH	Pyruvate dehydrogenase	Q	Ubiquinone/ubiquinol
PDK1	Phosphoinositide-dependent kinase 1	RA	Rheumatoid arthritis
PE	Phosphatidylethanolamine	RABP	Retinoic acid–binding protein
PECAM-1	Platelet/cell-adhesion molecule 1 (CD31)	RAE	Retinol activity equivalent
PEM	Protein energy malnutrition	Raf	Family of serine/threonine kinases
PEP	Phosphoenolpyruvate	RANK	Receptor activator of nuclear factor NFκB
PEPCK	Phosphoenolpyruvate carboxykinase	RANKL	RANK ligand
PEST	ProGluSerThr degradation signal	Rap	Small GTPase

RAR	Retinoid acid receptor	SHBG	Sex hormone–binding globulin
Ras	A GTPase	Shc	Src-homology and collagen-like adapter proteins
Ras	Small monomeric G-protein; a GTPase		
Rb	Retinoblastoma protein	SHP	SH2 domain-containing phosphatase
RBC	Red blood cell	SIADH	Syndrome of inappropriate antidiuretic hormone secretion
RBP	Serum retinol-binding protein		
RDA	Recommended dietary allowance	sIg	Surface Ig
RER	Respiratory exchange rate	siRNA	Small interfering RNA
RER	Rough endoplasmic reticulum	SLE	Systemic lupus erythematosus
RFLP	Restriction fragment length polymorphism	SMPDB	Small Molecule Pathway Database
RGD	Arg-gly-asp recognition sequence	SNO-Hb	S-nitrosohemoglobin
Rheb	Ras homologue enriched in brain	snoRNA	Small ribonuclear RNA
Rho GEF	Rho GTPase guanine nucleotide exchange	snoRNP	Small ribonuclear protein comples
factor		SNP	Single nucleotide polymorphism
Rictor	mTORC-2 complex	SOD	Superoxide dismutase
RIP	Receptor-interacting protein	SOS	Son of Sevenless, guanine nucleotide exchange factor
RIP1	Serine/threonine kinase		
RISC	RNA-induced silencing complex	SPCA	Serum prothrombin conversion accelerator
RLR	RIG-1-like receptor	SpO_2	Peripheral capillary oxygen saturation
RMR	Resting metabolic rate	SR	Sarcoplasmic reticulum
RNA	Ribonucleic acid	Src	Homology and collagen domain protein, a nonreceptor PTK
RNApol	RNA polymerase		
RNAseq	Deep sequencing technology for transcriptome analysis	Src	A tyrosine kinase
		SRE	Sterol regulatory element
RNS	Reactive nitrogen species	SREBP	Sterol regulatory element-binding protein
ROS	Reactive oxygen species	SRP	Signal recognition particle
ROTEM	Rotational thromboelastometry	SSB	Sugar-sweetened beverage
RP-HPLC	Reversed phase HPLC	STAT1	Signal transducer and activator of transcription-1
rRNA	Ribosomal RNA		
RSK1	A kinase	STATs	Signal transducer and activators, transcription factors
rT3	Reverse T3		
RTA	Renal tubular acidosis	Succ-CoA	Succinyl-CoA
RXR	Retinoid X receptor	T1D	Type 1 diabetes mellitus
S	Substrate	T2D	Type 2 diabetes mellitus
S	Synthetic phase of interphase	T3	Triiodothyronine
S6K1	Ribosomal S6 kinase 1	T4	Thyroxine
SAC	Spindle assembly checkpoint	TAG, TG	Triacylglycerol, also known as triglyceride
SAM	S-adenosylmethionine	T-ALL	T lymphocyte–acute lymphoblastic leukemia
SCAP	SREBP-cleavage-activating protein		
SCD	Sickle cell disease	TBG	Thyroxine-binding globulin
SCD	Stearoyl-CoA desaturase	TC-10	A G-protein
SCFA	Short-chain fatty acid	TCA cycle	Tricarboxylic acid cycle
SCID	Severe combined immunodeficiency	TCA	Tricarboxylic acid cycle
SCIDS	Severe Combined Immunodeficiency Syndrome	TCI	Transcobalamin I
		TCII	Transcobalamin II
SDS	Sodium dodecylsulfate	TCR	T-cell receptor
SDS-PAGE	Sodium dodecylsulfate-polyacrylamide gel electrophoresis	TCT	Thrombin clotting time
		TdT	Terminal deoxynucleotidyl transferase
SECIS	Selenocysteine insertion sequence	TEG	Thromboelastography
SGLT	Na^+-coupled glucose transporter	TF	Transcription factor
SGLT-1	Sodium/glucose-linked transport-1 (a membrane transporter)	T_{FH}	T follicular helper cells
		TFIIH	General transcription factor
SGOT	Serum glutamate oxaloacetate transaminase	TFPI	Tissue factor pathway inhibitor
SGPT	Serum glutamate pyruvate transaminase	Tg	Thyroglobulin
SH2	Src-homology region 2	TG	Triacylglycerol (also triglyceride)

TGF-α	Transforming growth factor-alpha	UDP-Glc	Uridine diphosphate glucose
TGF-β	Transforming growth factor-beta	UDP-GlcNAc	Uridine diphosphate N-acetylglucosamine
T_H	T helper cells (CD4$^+$ T cells)	UDP-Xyl	Uridine diphosphate xylose
THF	Tetrahydrofolate	UFC	24-h urine free cortisol
THRB	Thyroid hormone receptor beta gene	UFH	Unfractionated heparin
TIM	Transporter in inner membrane	UKPDS	UK Prospective Diabetes Study
TIMP	Tissue inhibitor of MMPs	uPA	Urinary-type plasminogen activator
TKI	Tyrosine kinase inhibitor	UPR	Unfolded protein response
TLR	Toll-like receptor	UPS	Ubiquitin–proteasome system
T_{max}	Maximum rate of transport	URL	Upper reference limit
TNF	Tumor necrosis factor	UTR	Untranslated region
TNFR	Death receptor, TNF family member	UVRAG	UV radiation resistance–associated gene protein
TNF-α	Tumor necrosis factor α		
TOM	Transporter in outer membrane	Va/Q	The ratio of ventilation to perfusion
tPA	Tissue-type plasminogen activator	VAChT	Acetylcholine transporter
TPN	Total parenteral nutrition	VCAM-1	Vascular cell adhesion molecule 1
TPO	Thyroid peroxidase	VDCC	Voltage-dependent Ca^{2+}-channel
TPP	Thiamine pyrophosphate	VEGF	Vascular endothelial growth factor
TRADD	TNF-receptor-associated death domain	VIP	Vasoactive intestinal peptide
TRAFs	TNF-receptor-associated factors	VLDL	Very-low-density lipoprotein(s)
TRAIL	Death receptor, TNF family member	V_{max}	Maximum velocity
Tregs	T regulatory cells, suppressive T cells	VO$_2$	Oxygen consumption rate
TRH	Thyrotropin-releasing hormone, thyreoliberin	VP	Vasopressin; antidiuretic hormone
		VSMC	Vascular smooth muscle cell(s)
tRNA	Transfer RNA	vWF	Von Willebrand factor
TSC1/2	Tuberous sclerosis complex 1/2	WHO	World Health Organization
TSH	Thyroid-stimulating hormone	Wnt	A signaling pathway related to cell growth and proliferation; The pathway abbreviation relates to "Wingless-related integration site"
TSS	Transcriptional start site		
T-tubule	Transverse tubule		
TWEAK	Death receptor, TNF family member		
TX	Thromboxane	XP	Xeroderma pigmentosum
TXA$_2$	Thromboxane A$_2$	ZAP-70	PTK that is essential for antigen-dependent T-cell activation
UAS	Upstream activation sequence		
UCP	Uncoupling protein	ZF	Zona fasciculata
UDP-Gal	Uridine diphosphate galactose	ZG	Zona glomerulosa
UDP-GalNAc	Uridine diphosphate N-acetylgalactosamine	ZR	Zona reticularis

Introduction

John W. Baynes and Marek H. Dominiczak

BIOCHEMISTRY AND CLINICAL MEDICINE: INTRODUCTION AND OVERVIEW

Biochemistry is constantly changing

Research into the human **genome** and particularly gene regulation has been one of the main drivers of medical progress for some time now. A similar systemic approach has been applied to three other expanding fields: the study of the **transcriptome**, the **proteome**, and the **metabolome** (Fig. 1.1). From the biochemistry perspective, perhaps the most exciting development in the last few years has been the expansion of knowledge about proteins participating in the transfer of external metabolic signals to intracellular pathways and to and from the genome as well as the role of these networks in the regulation of cell division and growth (Fig. 1.2). This has also provided new insights into the pathogenesis of cancer and enabled new therapies for a range of diseases.

All these developments have changed the way we look at metabolism. **In addition to the strings of chemical reactions that have been the essence of biochemistry since its inception, we now recognize the sequences (cascades) of interacting signaling molecules that complement these reactions and are essential to their control.** This poses new challenges for the student of biochemistry, who needs to face a novel and complex protein terminology.

Familiarity with abbreviations and acronyms depicting signaling molecules and transcription factors is now necessary to gain a complete picture of metabolic pathways and their regulations.

Another dimension of new knowledge is the growing understanding of **links between metabolism and diseases that are related to nutrition, lifestyle, and environment**. Obesity, diabetes, atherosclerosis, and cardiovascular disease, on the one hand, and malnutrition and nutritional deficiencies, on the other, are major global health concerns.

Finally, the progress in **neurochemistry** is facilitating a better grasp of the science underpinning mental health problems.

Biochemistry has fuzzy borders

Biochemistry is not a discipline with clear borders. It links seamlessly to fields such as cell biology, anatomy, physiology, and pathology. In fact, it is not possible to understand or solve a clinical problem without crossing interdisciplinary borders. In this book, we cross these borders frequently, both in the text and in clinical boxes. The chapters covering **nutrition, water and electrolytes, acid–base balance,** and **specialized tissues** and their functions are fundamentally interdisciplinary and address several such crossover issues.

A textbook is a snapshot of rapidly changing knowledge

A doctor is constantly exposed to new developments in clinical medicine as he or she gains practical clinical experience. It is essential to integrate the new developments into everyday practice. What only a few years ago was theory and speculation is now a part of the toolkit used during ward rounds and in case conferences.

We wrote *Medical Biochemistry* because we are convinced that understanding biochemistry helps in the practice of medicine. The question we asked ourselves many times during the writing process was, "How could this piece of information improve your clinical reasoning?" Throughout the text, we highlight the clinical issues that a physician encounters at the bedside and link them to basic concepts. We believe that such an approach provides knowledge based on understanding and not only on facts - the essence of a cutting-edge education.

We believe that a textbook should provide a core education essential for a doctor in clinical practice but it should also flag emerging topics that are likely to become fundamental in the foreseeable future. Thus we continue to expand the

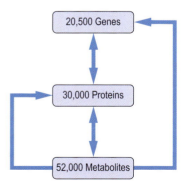

Fig. 1.1 **Human genes, proteins, and metabolites.** Data based on Human Genome Project, Human Proteome Map, and Human Metabolome Database (see websites) Numbers are approximate.

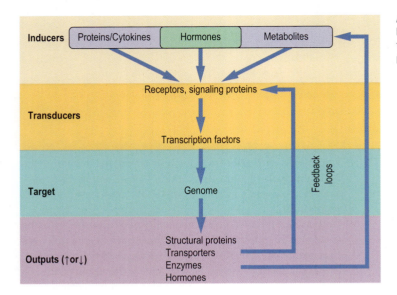

Fig. 1.2 **Integrated view of regulatory loops between signalling proteins, enzymes, genome, and metabolism.** Note that many signaling proteins are also enzymes. There are both protein and non-protein (metabolite-derived) hormones.

neurochemistry chapter and, especially, update the chapters on DNA, RNA, and the regulation of gene expression.

Keep in mind that *Medical Biochemistry* is not designed to be a review text or resource for preparation for multiple-choice exams. It is a resource for your clinical career. Our text is shorter than many of the heavy tomes in our discipline, and it focuses on explanation of key concepts and relationships that we hope you will retain in your recall memory and use in your future clinical practice.

Improvements in the fifth edition

This book has now served the global student community for 19 years. During preparation of the fifth edition, we sought to improve the quality of explanation of complex concepts. We also changed the narrative, dividing the book into several large thematic blocks.

We start with **Molecules and Cell**s and move on to **Metabolism,** the core of biochemistry. Then we address the **Molecular Basis of Inheritance**, discussing DNA, RNA, protein synthesis, regulation of gene expression, and the systemic approaches: genomics, proteomics, and metabolomics. We also expand our presentation of **Cellular Signaling and Growth** and their links to aging and cancer. We then focus on **Fuels and Nutrients,** discussing the gastrointestinal tract, glucose and lipoprotein absorption, and metabolism and linking the underlying biochemistry to major public health issues.

In the **Specialized Tissues and Their Function** section, we describe the tissue environment and address the function of the liver, muscle, and the brain. Here we also discuss metabolism of foreign substances, including therapeutic drugs. The last section, **Blood and Immunity,** describes the body defense mechanisms of hemostasis (blood coagulation) and the immune response and the impact of inflammation and

oxidative stress. Fig. 1.3 shows our Map of the Book and illustrates the integration of biochemical topics in a broader biological context.

In addition to providing core information, we also suggest directions for further study. The references and websites listed at the end of the chapters will expand on what has been learned, should you wish to look for more details. Further, through its **Student Consult** program, Elsevier provides links to expanded discussions in textbooks in anatomy, cell biology, microbiology, physiology, pharmacology, immunology, pathology, and clinical chemistry. These resources are conveniently hyperlinked to topics in biochemistry.

One studies biochemistry to understand the interplay of nutrition, metabolism, and genetics in health and disease: let's start here with the shortest possible overview of the field

The human organism is, on the one hand, a **tightly controlled, integrated, and self-contained** metabolic system. On the other hand, it is a system that is **open** and communicates with its environment. Despite these two seemingly contradictory characteristics, the body manages to maintain its internal environment for decades. We regularly top up our fuel (consume food) and water and take up oxygen from inspired air to use for oxidative metabolism (which is, in fact, a chain of low-temperature combustion reactions). We then use the energy generated from metabolism to perform work and maintain body temperature. We get rid of (exhale or excrete) carbon dioxide, water, and nitrogenous waste. The amount and quality of food we consume have a significant impact on our health - malnutrition, on the one hand, and obesity and diabetes, on the other, are currently major public health issues worldwide.

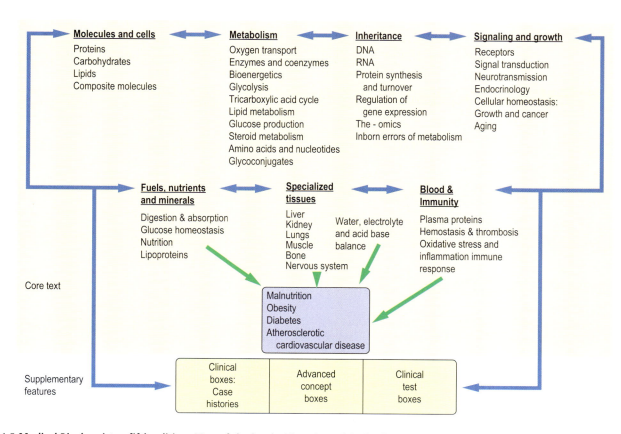

Fig. 1.3 *Medical Biochemistry*, **fifth edition: Map of the book.** All sections of the book are strongly interrelated. As you learn about metabolism, you'll gain the knowledge of the key inherited metabolic errors and their effects. Major contemporary health issues, such as diabetes mellitus, atherosclerosis, obesity, and malnutrition, are emphasized in relevant chapters. Throughout the book, you will find Clinical Boxes and Clinical Test Boxes, which integrate basic science with clinical practice, and Advanced Concept Boxes that expand on selected issues. Updated literature and web references will facilitate further study.

Proteins, carbohydrates, and lipids are the major structural components of the body

Proteins are building blocks and catalysts; as structural units, they form the "architectural" framework of tissues; as enzymes, together with helper molecules (**coenzymes** and **cofactors**), they catalyze biochemical reactions. Proteins also play a fundamental role in the transfer of information (**signaling**) at both the cell and the entire-organism level, processes that are essential for the function of DNA and the regulation of **gene expression**.

Carbohydrates and **lipids** as monomers or relatively simple polymers are our major **energy sources**. They can be stored in tissues as glycogen and triglycerides. However, carbohydrates can also be linked to both proteins and lipids, forming complex structures (glycoconjugates) essential for **cell-signaling systems** and processes such as cell **adhesion** and **immunity**. Lipids such as **cholesterol** and **phospholipids**, form the backbone of biological membranes.

Chemical variables, such as **pH, oxygen tension**, and **inorganic ion and buffer concentrations**, define the homeostatic environment in which metabolism takes place. Minute changes in this environment - for example, just a few degrees' change in body temperature - can be life-threatening.

Biological membranes partition metabolic pathways into different cellular compartments. Their water-impermeable structure is dotted with an array of "doors and gates" (membrane transporters) and "locks" that accept a variety of keys, including hormones and cytokines that initiate intracellular signaling cascades. They play a fundamental role in **ion** and **metabolite transport** and in **signal transduction**, both within individual cells and between cells. In fact, most of the body's energy is consumed to generate heat for homeotherms and to maintain ion and metabolite gradients across membranes. Cells throughout the body are critically dependent on **electrical and chemical potentials across membranes** for nerve transmission, muscle contraction, nutrient transport, and the maintenance of cell volume.

Carbohydrates and lipids are our primary sources of energy, but our nutritional requirements also include **amino acids** (components of proteins), **inorganic molecules**

(sodium, calcium, potassium, chloride, bicarbonate, phosphate, and others), and micronutrients - **vitamins** and **trace elements**.

Glucose (present in blood in a pure form and stored in the form of glycogen) is metabolized through **glycolysis,** a universal non-oxygen-requiring (anaerobic) pathway for energy production. It yields **pyruvate,** setting the stage for oxidative metabolism in the mitochondria. It also generates metabolites that are the starting points for the synthesis of **amino acids, proteins, lipids,** and **nucleic acids**.

Glucose is the most important fuel for the brain; therefore maintaining its concentration in plasma is essential for survival. Glucose homeostasis is regulated by the hormones that coordinate metabolic activities among cells and organs - primarily insulin and glucagon but also epinephrine and cortisol.

Oxygen is essential for energy production but can also be toxic

During aerobic metabolism, pyruvate, the end product of anaerobic glycolysis, is transformed into **acetyl coenzyme A (acetyl-CoA),** the common intermediate in the metabolism of carbohydrates, lipids, and amino acids. Acetyl-CoA enters the central metabolic engine of the cell, the **tricarboxylic acid (TCA) cycle** located in mitochondria. Acetyl-CoA is oxidized to **carbon dioxide** and reduces the important coenzymes **nicotinamide adenine dinucleotide (NAD$^+$)** and **flavin adenine dinucleotide (FAD)**. Reduction of these nucleotides captures the energy from fuel oxidation.

Most of the energy in biological systems is obtained by **oxidative phosphorylation**. This process involves oxygen consumption, or **respiration,** by which the organism oxidizes NADH and FADH$_2$ in the mitochondrial **electron transport chain (ETC)** to produce a hydrogen ion gradient across the inner mitochondrial membrane. The energy in this **electrochemical gradient** is then transformed into the chemical energy of **adenosine triphosphate (ATP)**. Biochemists call ATP the "common currency of metabolism" because it allows energy produced by fuel metabolism to be used for work, transport, and biosynthesis. Although oxygen is essential for aerobic metabolism, it can also cause **oxidative stress** and widespread tissue damage during **inflammation**. Powerful **antioxidant defenses** exist to protect cells and tissues from the damaging effects of reactive oxygen.

Metabolism continuously cycles between fasting and posteating modes

The direction of the main pathways of carbohydrate and lipid metabolism changes in response to food intake. In the fed state, the active pathways are **glycolysis, glycogen synthesis, lipogenesis,** and **protein synthesis,** rejuvenating tissues and storing the excess of metabolic fuel. In the fasting state, the direction of metabolism reverses: glycogen and lipid stores are degraded through **glycogenolysis** and **lipolysis,** providing a constant stream of **substrates for energy production.** As glycogen stores become depleted, proteins are sacrificed to make glucose through **gluconeogenesis,** guaranteeing a constant supply, while other biosynthetic pathways are slowed down. Common conditions such as **diabetes mellitus, obesity,** and atherosclerotic cardiovascular disease that are currently major public health issues result from impairment of fuel transport and metabolism.

Tissues perform specialized functions

Specialized tissue functions include muscle contraction; nerve conduction; bone formation; immune surveillance; hormonal signaling; maintenance of pH, fluid, and electrolyte balance; and detoxification of foreign substances. **Glycoconjugates** (glycoproteins, glycolipids, and proteoglycans) are needed for tissue organization and cell-to-cell communications. Recent progress in understanding cellular signaling systems has improved our insight into **cell growth** and **repair mechanisms**. Their time-dependent decline leads to **aging,** and their failure causes age-related diseases such as **neurodegenerative diseases** and **cancer.**

The genome underpins it all

The genome provides the mechanism for conservation and transfer of genetic information through regulation of the expression of constituent genes and control of protein synthesis. The synthesis of individual proteins is controlled by information encoded in **deoxyribonucleic acid (DNA)** and transcribed into **ribonucleic acid (RNA),** which is then translated into peptides that fold into **functional protein molecules.** The spectrum of expressed proteins and the control of their temporal expression during development, adaptation, and aging are responsible for our protein makeup, our **proteome. Epigenetics,** the study of gene regulation caused by modification of DNA function by means other than changes in its nucleotide sequence, provides deeper insight into the regulation of gene expression.

In the past decade, **bioinformatics,** genome-wide association studies, and epigenetics have provided truly fascinating insights into the complexity of genetic regulatory networks. Further, applications of **recombinant DNA** technology have revolutionized the work of clinical laboratories and have recently provided novel tools for editing the genome. The ability to scan the entire genome and the information obtained by **genomics, proteomics,** and **metabolomics** provide new insights into gene regulation, protein synthesis, and metabolism.

All of this is summarized in Fig. 1.4, a complex scheme that resembles the plan of the London Tube (see Further reading). Like the Tube, with its many stations, biochemistry is navigable with a good map; don't be intimidated by the many as-yet unfamiliar terms. Refer back to this figure as you progress in your studies, and you will notice how your understanding of biochemistry improves.

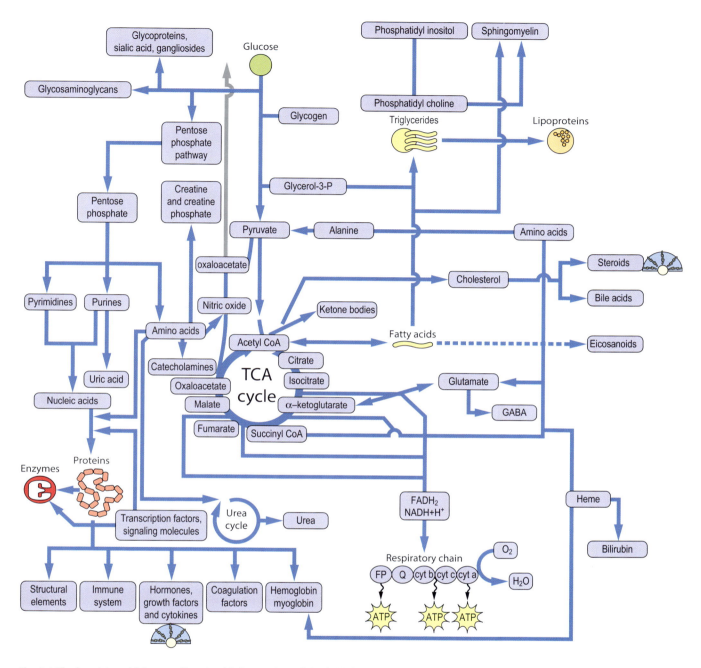

Fig. 1.4 **Biochemistry: All in one.** Here is a bird's-eye view of the field, focusing on metabolism and bioenergetics. It may help to structure your study or revision. Refer back to it as you study the following chapters, and see how your perspective on biochemistry broadens. ATP, adenosine triphosphate; cyt, cytochrome; FAD/FADH₂, flavin adenine dinucleotide (oxidized/reduced); FP, flavoprotein; GABA, γ-aminobutyric acid; glycerol-3-P, glycerol-3-phosphate; NAD⁺/NADH, nicotinamide adenine dinucleotide (oxidized/reduced); Q, ubiquinone/ubiquinol; TCA cucle, tricarboxylic acid cycle.

FURTHER READING

Atkins, P. (2013). *What is chemistry?* Oxford, UK: Oxford University Press.

Cooke, M., Irby, D. M., Sullivan, W., et al. (2006). American medical education 100 years after the Flexner Report. *New England Journal of Medicine, 355,* 1339–1344.

Dominiczak, M. H. (1998). Teaching and training laboratory professionals for the 21st century. *Clinical Chemistry and Laboratory Medicine, 36,* 133–136.

Dominiczak, M. H. (2012). Contribution of biochemistry to medicine: Medical biochemistry and clinical biochemistry. *UNESCO encyclopedia of life support systems (UNESCO-EOLSS).* Retrieved from http://www.eolss.net.sample-chapters/c17/e6-58-10-12.pdf.

Ludmerer, K. M. (2004). Learner-centered medical education. *New England Journal of Medicine, 351,* 1163–1164.

Transport for London. (n.d.). Tube map. Retrieved from http://www.tfl.gov.uk/assets/downloads/standard-tube-map.pdf.

RELEVANT WEBSITES

Human Metabolome Database (HMDB), version 3.6: http://www.hmdb.ca/
Human Proteome Map: http://www.humanproteomemap.org/
Overview of the Human Genome Project, NIH National Human Genome
Research Institute: https://www.genome.gov/12011238/an-overview-of-the
-human-genome-project/

ABBREVIATIONS

Acetyl-CoA	Acetyl-Coenzyme A
ATP	Adenosine triphosphate
Cyt a, b, c	Cytochrome a, cytochrome b, cytochrome c
DNA	Deoxyribonucleic acid
FAD/FADH$_2$	Flavin adenine dinucleotide (oxidized/reduced)
FP	Flavoprotein
GABA	γ-Aminobutyric acid
Glycerol-3-P	Glycerol-3-phosphate
NAD$^+$/NADH	Nicotinamide adenine dinucleotide (oxidized/reduced)
Q	Ubiquinone/ubiquinol
RNA	Ribonucleic acid
TCA cycle	Tricarboxylic acid cycle

Amino Acids and Proteins

Ryoji Nagai and Naoyuki Taniguchi

INTRODUCTION

Proteins are major structural and functional polymers in living systems

Proteins have a broad range of activities, including catalysis of metabolic reactions and transport of vitamins, minerals, oxygen, and fuels. Some proteins make up the structure of tissues; others function in nerve transmission, muscle contraction, and cell motility, with still others in blood clotting and immunologic defenses and as hormones and regulatory molecules. Proteins are synthesized as a sequence of amino acids linked together in a linear polyamide (polypeptide) structure, but they assume complex three-dimensional shapes in performing their functions. There are about 300 amino acids present in various animal, plant, and microbial systems, but **only 20 amino acids are coded by DNA to appear in proteins.** Many proteins also contain modified amino acids and accessory components, termed prosthetic groups. A range of chemical techniques is used to isolate and characterize proteins by a variety of criteria, including mass, charge, and three-dimensional structure. Proteomics is an emerging field that studies the full range of expression of proteins in a cell or organism and changes in protein expression in response to growth, hormones, stress, and aging.

AMINO ACIDS

Amino acids are the building blocks of proteins

Stereochemistry: Configuration at the α-carbon and D- and L-isomers

Each amino acid has a central carbon, called the α-carbon, to which four different groups are attached (Fig. 2.1):

▪ A basic amino group (–NH₂)
▪ An acidic carboxyl group (–COOH)
▪ A hydrogen atom (–H)
▪ A distinctive side chain (–R)

One of the 20 amino acids, proline, is not an α-amino acid but an α-imino acid (see following discussion). Except for glycine, all amino acids contain at least one asymmetric carbon atom (the α-carbon atom), giving two isomers that are optically active (i.e., they can rotate plane-polarized light). These isomers, referred to as **stereoisomers** or enantiomers, are said to be chiral, a word derived from the Greek word meaning "hand." Such isomers are nonsuperimposable mirror images and are analogous to left and right hands, as shown in Fig. 2.2. The two amino acid configurations are called D (for *dextro*, meaning "right") and L (for *levo*, meaning "left"). **All amino acids in proteins are of the L-configuration** because proteins are biosynthesized by enzymes that insert only L-amino acids into the peptide chains.

Classification of amino acids based on chemical structure of their side chains

The properties of each amino acid are dependent on its side chain (–R), which determines the structure and function of proteins and the electrical charge of the molecule. Knowledge of the properties of these side chains is important for understanding methods of analysis, purification, and identification of proteins. Amino acids with charged, polar, or hydrophilic side chains are usually exposed on the surface of proteins. The nonpolar hydrophobic residues are usually buried in the hydrophobic interior, or core, of a protein and are out of contact with water. The 20 amino acids in proteins encoded by DNA are listed in Table 2.1 and are classified according to their side chain functional groups.

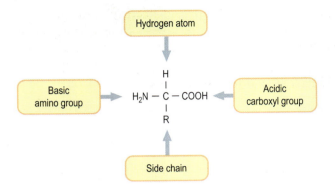

Fig. 2.1 **Structure of an amino acid.** Except for glycine, four different groups are attached to the α-carbon of an amino acid. Table 2.1 lists the structures of the R groups.

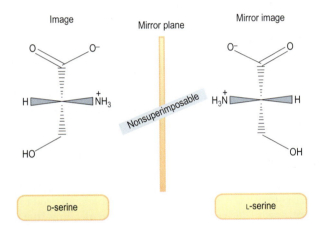

Fig. 2.2 **Enantiomers.** The mirror-image pair of amino acids. Each amino acid represents nonsuperimposable mirror images. The mirror-image stereoisomers are called enantiomers. Only the L-enantiomers are found in proteins.

Aliphatic amino acids

Alanine, valine, leucine, and isoleucine, referred to as aliphatic amino acids, have saturated hydrocarbons as side chains. Glycine, which has only a hydrogen side chain, is also included in this group. Alanine has a relatively simple structure, a side chain methyl group, whereas valine, leucine and isoleucine have isopropyl, sec- and iso-butyl groups. All of these amino acids are hydrophobic in nature.

Aromatic amino acids

Phenylalanine, tyrosine, and tryptophan have aromatic side chains

The nonpolar aliphatic and aromatic amino acids are normally buried in the protein core and are involved in hydrophobic interactions with one another. Tyrosine has a weakly acidic hydroxyl group and may be located on the surface of proteins.

Table 2.1 20 amino acids found in proteins*	
Amino acids	**Structure of R moiety**
Aliphatic amino acids	
glycine (Gly, **G**)	—H
alanine (Ala, **A**)	—CH₃
valine (Val, **V**)	
leucine (Leu, **L**)	
isoleucine (Ile, **I**)	
Sulfur-containing amino acids	
cysteine (Cys, **C**)	—CH₂—SH
methionine (Met, **M**)	—CH₂—CH₂—S—CH₃
Aromatic amino acids	
phenylalanine (Phe, **F**)	
tyrosine (Tyr, **Y**)	
tryptophan (Trp, **W**)	
Imino acid	
proline (Pro, **P**)	
Neutral amino acids	
serine (Ser, **S**)	—CH₂—OH
threonine (Thr, **T**)	
asparagine (Asn, **N**)	
glutamine (Gln, **Q**)	
Acidic amino acids	
aspartic acid (Asp, **D**)	–CH₂—COOH
glutamic acid (Glu, **E**)	—CH₂–CH₂—COOH
Basic amino acids	
histidine (His, **H**)	
lysine (Lys, **K**)	—CH₂—CH₂—CH₂—CH₂—NH₂
arginine (Arg, **R**)	

*The three-letter and single-letter abbreviations in common use are given in parentheses.

Reversible phosphorylation of the hydroxyl group of tyrosine in some enzymes is important in the regulation of metabolic pathways. **The aromatic amino acids are responsible for the ultraviolet absorption of most proteins, which have absorption maxima ~280 nm.** Tryptophan has a greater absorption in this region than phenylalanine or tyrosine. The molar absorption coefficient of a protein is useful in determining

the concentration of a protein in solution, based on spectrophotometry. Typical absorption spectra of aromatic amino acids and a protein are shown in Fig. 2.3.

Neutral polar amino acids

Neutral polar amino acids contain hydroxyl or amide side chain groups. Serine and threonine contain hydroxyl groups. These amino acids are sometimes found at the active sites of catalytic proteins, enzymes (Chapter 6). Reversible phosphorylation of peripheral serine and threonine residues of enzymes is also involved in regulation of energy metabolism and fuel storage in the body (Chapter 12). **Asparagine and glutamine have amide-bearing side chains. These are polar but uncharged under physiologic conditions.** Serine, threonine, and asparagine are the primary sites of linkage of sugars to proteins, forming glycoproteins (Chapter 17).

Acidic amino acids

Aspartic and glutamic acids contain carboxylic acids on their side chains and are ionized at pH 7 and, as a result, carry negative charges on their β- and γ-carboxyl groups, respectively. In the ionized state, these amino acids are referred to as aspartate and glutamate, respectively.

Basic amino acids

The side chains of lysine and arginine are fully protonated at neutral pH and, therefore, positively charged. Lysine contains

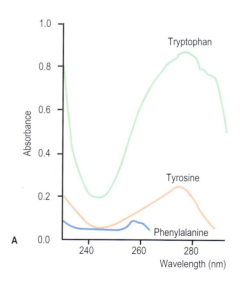
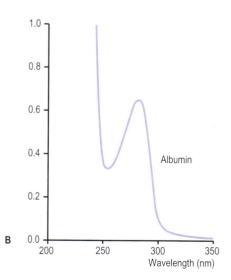

Fig. 2.3 **Ultraviolet absorption spectra of the aromatic amino acids and bovine serum albumin.** (A) Aromatic amino acids such as tryptophan, tyrosine, and phenylalanine have absorbance maxima at 260–280 nm. Each purified protein has a distinct molecular absorption coefficient at around 280 nm, depending on its content of aromatic amino acids. (B) A bovine serum albumin solution (1 mg dissolved in 1 mL of water) has an absorbance of 0.67 at 280 nm using a 1-cm cuvette. The absorption coefficient of proteins is often expressed as $E_{1\%}$ (10 mg/mL solution). For albumin, $E_{1\%}280_{nm} = 6.7$. Although proteins vary in their Trp, Tyr, and Phe content, measurements of absorbance at 280 nm are useful for estimating protein concentration in solutions.

Table 2.2 Summary of the functional groups of amino acids and their polarity

Amino acids	Functional group	Hydrophilic (polar) or hydrophobic (nonpolar)	Examples
acidic	carboxyl, −COOH	polar	Asp, Glu
basic	amine, −NH₂	polar	Lys
	imidazole	polar	His
	guanidino	polar	Arg
neutral	glycine, −H	nonpolar	Gly
	amides, −CONH₂	polar	Asn, Gln
	hydroxyl, −OH	polar	Ser, Thr,
	sulfhydryl, −SH	nonpolar	Cys
aliphatic	hydrocarbon	nonpolar	Ala, Val, Leu, Ile, Met, Pro
aromatic	C-rings	nonpolar	Phe, Trp, Tyr

a primary amino group (NH_2) attached to the terminal ε-carbon of the side chain. The ε-amino group of lysine has a $pK_a \approx 11$. Arginine is the most basic amino acid ($pK_a \approx 13$), and its **guanidine** group exists as a protonated guanidinium ion at pH 7.

Histidine ($pK_a \approx 6$) has an **imidazole** ring as the side chain and functions as a general acid–base catalyst in many enzymes. The protonated form of imidazole is called an imidazolium ion.

Sulfur-containing amino acids

Cysteine and its oxidized form, cystine, are sulfur-containing amino acids characterized by low polarity. Cysteine plays an important role in the stabilization of protein structure because it can participate in the formation of a disulfide bond with other cysteine residues to form cystine residues, crosslinking protein chains and stabilizing protein structure. Two regions of a single polypeptide chain, remote from each other in the sequence, may be covalently linked through a disulfide bond (intrachain disulfide bond). **Disulfide bonds** are also formed between two polypeptide chains (interchain disulfide bond), forming covalent protein dimers. These bonds can be reduced by enzymes or reducing agents, such as 2-mercaptoethanol or dithiothreitol, to form cysteine residues. Methionine is the third sulfur-containing amino acid and contains a nonpolar methyl thioether group in its side chain.

Proline, a cyclic imino acid

Proline is different from other amino acids in that its side chain **pyrrolidine ring** includes both the α-amino group and the α-carbon. This imino acid forces a "bend" in a polypeptide chain, sometimes causing abrupt changes in the direction of the chain.

Classification of amino acids based on the polarity of the amino acid side chains

Table 2.2 depicts the functional groups of amino acids and their polarity (hydrophilicity). Polar side chains can be involved in hydrogen bonding to water and to other polar groups and are usually located on the surface of the protein. Hydrophobic side chains contribute to protein folding by hydrophobic interactions and are located primarily in the core of the protein or on surfaces involved in interactions with other proteins.

Ionization state of an amino acid

Amino acids are amphoteric molecules - they have both basic and acidic groups

Monoamino and monocarboxylic acids are ionized in different ways in solution, depending on the solution's pH. At pH 7, the "zwitterion" $^+H_3N–CH_2–COO^-$ is the dominant species of glycine in solution, and the overall molecule is therefore electrically neutral. On titration to acidic pH, the α-amino and carboxyl groups are protonated, yielding the cation $^+H_3N–CH_2–COOH$, whereas titration with alkali yields the anionic $H_2N–CH_2–COO^-$ species:

$$^+H_3N\ CH_2\ COOH \underset{}{\overset{H^+}{\rightleftharpoons}} {}^+H_3N\ CH_2\ COO^- \underset{}{\overset{OH^-}{\rightleftharpoons}} H_2N\ CH_2\ COO^-$$

pK_a values for the α-amino and α-carboxyl groups and side chains of acidic and basic amino acids are shown in Table 2.3. The overall charge on a protein depends on the contribution from basic (positive charge) and acidic (negative charge) amino acids, but the actual charge on the protein varies with the pH of the solution. To understand how the side chains affect the charge on proteins, it is worth recalling the Henderson–Hasselbalch (H-H) equation.

Table 2.3 pK_a values for ionizable groups in proteins

Group	Acid (protonated form) (conjugate acid)	H$^+$ + base (unprotonated form) (conjugate base)	pK_a
terminal carboxyl residue (α-carboxyl)	$-$COOH (carboxylic acid)	$-$COO$^-$ + H$^+$ (carboxylate)	3.0–5.5
aspartic acid (β-carboxyl)	$-$COOH	$-$COO$^-$ + H$^+$	3.9
glutamic acid (γ-carboxyl)	$-$COOH	$-$COO$^-$ + H$^+$	4.3
histidine (imidazole)	HN⊕NH (imidazolium)	N NH + H$^+$ (imidazole)	6.0
terminal amino (α-amino)	$-$NH$_3^+$ (ammonium)	$-$NH$^+$ + H$^+$ (amine)	8.0
cysteine (sulfhydryl)	$-$SH (thiol)	$-$S$^-$ + H$^+$ (thiolate)	8.3
tyrosine (phenolic hydroxyl)	⬡—OH (phenol)	⬡—O$^-$ + H$^+$ (phenolate)	10.1
lysine (ε-amino)	$-$NH$_3^+$	$-$NH$_2$ + H$^+$	10.5
arginine (guanidino)	$-$NH═C(NH$_2$)(NH$_2$)⊕ (guanidinium)	$-$NH—C(NH$_2$)(NH$_2$) + H$^+$ (guanidino)	12.5

Actual pK_a values may vary by several pH units, depending on temperature, buffer, ligand binding, and especially neighboring functional groups in the protein.

Henderson–Hasselbalch equation and pK_a

The H-H equation describes the titration of an amino acid and can be used to predict the net charge and isoelectric point of a protein

The general dissociation of a weak acid, such as a carboxylic acid, is given by the following equation:

(1) $$HA \rightleftarrows H^+ + A^-$$

where HA is the protonated form (conjugate acid, or associated form), and A$^-$ is the unprotonated form (conjugate base, or dissociated form).

The dissociation constant (K_a) of a weak acid is defined as the equilibrium constant for the dissociation reaction (1) of the acid:

(2) $$K_a = \frac{[H^+][A^-]}{[HA]}$$

The hydrogen ion concentration [H$^+$] of a solution of a weak acid can then be calculated as follows. Eq. (2) can be rearranged to give

(3) $$[H^+] = K_a \times \frac{[HA]}{[A^-]}$$

Eq. (3) can be expressed in terms of a negative logarithm:

(4) $$-\log[H^+] = -\log K_a - \log\frac{[HA]}{[A^-]}$$

Because pH is the negative logarithm of [H$^+$] (i.e., $-\log[H^+]$), and pK_a equals the negative logarithm of the dissociation constant for a weak acid (i.e., $-\log K_a$), the Henderson–Hasselbalch Eq. (5) can be developed and used for analysis of acid–base equilibrium systems:

(5) $$pH = pK_a + \log\frac{[A^-]}{[HA]}$$

For a weak base, such as an amine, the dissociation reaction can be written as

(6) $$RNH_3^+ \rightleftarrows H^+ + RNH_2$$

and the Henderson–Hasselbalch equation becomes

(7) $$pH = pK_a + \log\frac{[RNH_2]}{[RNH_3^+]}$$

From Eqs. (5) and (7), it is apparent that the extent of protonation of acidic and basic functional groups, and therefore the net charge of an amino acid, will vary with the pK_a of the functional group and the pH of the solution. For alanine, which has two functional groups with pK_a = 2.4 and 9.8, respectively (Fig. 2.4), the net charge varies with pH, from +1 to −1. At a point intermediate between pK_{a1} and pK_{a2}, alanine has a net zero charge. This pH is called its isoelectric point, pI (Fig. 2.4).

BUFFERS

Amino acids and proteins are excellent buffers under physiological conditions

Buffers are solutions that minimize a change in [H⁺] (i.e., pH) on addition of acid or base. A buffer solution, containing a weak acid or weak base and a counter-ion, has maximal buffering capacity at its pK_a - that is, when the acidic and basic forms are present at equal concentrations. The acidic protonated form reacts with added base, and the basic unprotonated form neutralizes added acid, shown as follows for an amino compound:

$$RNH_3^+ + OH^- \rightleftharpoons RNH_2 + H_2O$$

$$RNH_2 + H^+ \rightleftharpoons RNH_3^+$$

An alanine solution (Fig. 2.4) has maximal buffering capacity at pH 2.4 and 9.8 - that is, at the pK_a of the carboxyl and amino groups, respectively. When dissolved in water, alanine exists as a dipolar ion, or **zwitterion**, in which the carboxyl group is unprotonated (–COO⁻) and the amino group is protonated (–NH₃⁺). The pH of the solution is 6.1, the pI (isoelectric point) halfway between the pK_a of the amino and carboxyl groups. The titration curve of alanine by NaOH (Fig. 2.4) illustrates that alanine has minimal buffering capacity at its pI and maximal buffering capacity at a pH equal to its pK_{a1} or pK_{a2}.

PEPTIDES AND PROTEINS

Primary structure of proteins

The primary structure of a protein is the linear sequence of its amino acids

In proteins, the carboxyl group of one amino acid is linked to the amino group of the next amino acid, forming an amide (peptide) bond; water is eliminated during the reaction (Fig. 2.5). The amino acid units in a peptide chain are referred to as amino acid residues. A peptide chain consisting of three amino acid residues is called a tripeptide - for example, glutathione in Fig. 2.6. By convention, the amino terminus (N-terminus) is taken as the first residue, and the sequence of amino acids is written from left to right. When writing the peptide sequence, one uses either the three-letter or the one-letter abbreviations for amino acids, such as Asp-Arg-Val-Tyr-Ile-His-Pro-Phe-His-Leu

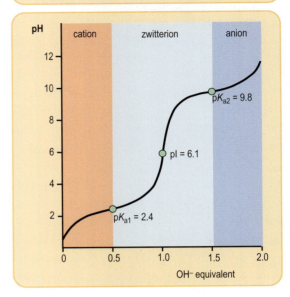

Fig. 2.4 **Titration of amino acid.** The curve shows the number of equivalents of NaOH consumed by alanine while titrating the solution from pH 0 to pH 12. Alanine contains two ionizable groups: an α-carboxyl group and an α-amino group. As NaOH is added, these two groups are titrated. The pK_a of the α-COOH group is 2.4, whereas that of the α-NH₃⁺ group is 9.8. At very low pH, the predominant ion species of alanine is the fully protonated, cationic form:

$$\left[\begin{array}{c} CH_3 \\ | \\ {}^+H_3N—CH—COOH \end{array} \right]$$

At the mid-point in the first stage of the titration (pH 2.4), equimolar concentrations of proton donor and proton acceptor species are present, providing good buffering power.

$$\left[\begin{array}{c} CH_3 \\ | \\ {}^+H_3N—CH—COOH \end{array} \right] \approx \left[\begin{array}{c} CH_3 \\ | \\ H_2N—CH—COO^- \end{array} \right]$$

At the mid-point in the overall titration (pH 6.1) the zwitterion is the predominant form of the amino acid in solution. The amino acid has a net zero charge at this pH - the negative charge of the carboxylate ion being neutralized by the positive charge of the ammonium group.

$$\left[\begin{array}{c} CH_3 \\ | \\ {}^+H_3N—CH—COO^- \\ \text{Zwitterion} \end{array} \right]$$

The second stage of the titration corresponds to the removal of a proton from the –NH₃⁺ group of alanine. The pH at the mid-point of this stage is 9.8, equal to the pK_a for the –NH₃⁺ group. The titration is complete at a pH of about 12, at which point the predominant form of alanine is the unprotonated, anionic form:

$$\left[\begin{array}{c} CH_3 \\ | \\ H_2N—CH—COO^- \end{array} \right]$$

The pH at which a molecule has no net charge is known as its isoelectric point, pI. For alanine, it is calculated as follows:

$$pI = \frac{pK_{a1} + pK_{a2}}{2} = \frac{(2.4 + 9.8)}{2} = 6.1$$

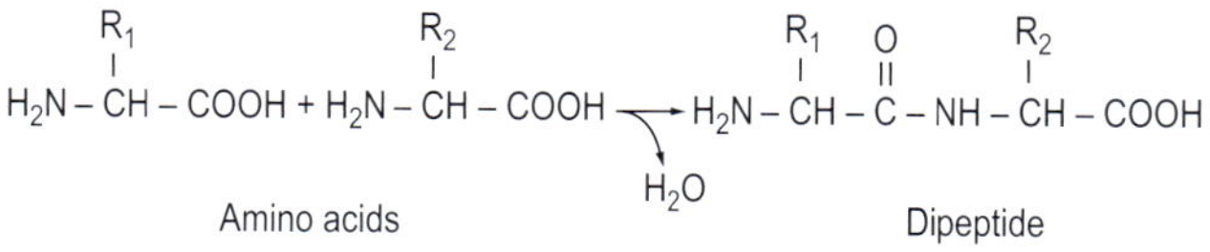

Fig. 2.5 **Structure of a peptide bond.**

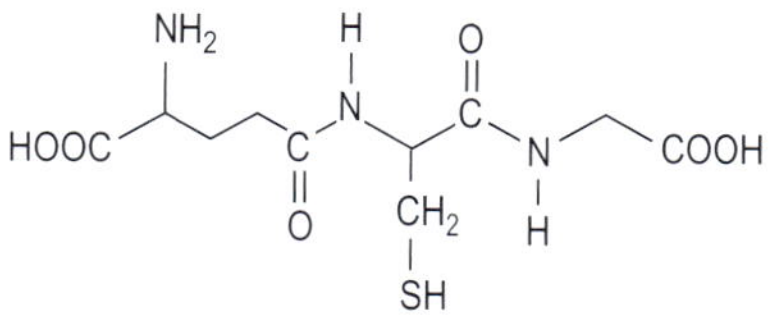

Fig. 2.6 **Structure of glutathione.**

ADVANCED CONCEPT BOX
GLUTATHIONE

Glutathione (GSH) is a tripeptide with the sequence γ-glutamyl-cysteinyl-glycine (Fig. 2.6). If the thiol group of the cysteine is oxidized, the disulfide GSSG is formed. GSH is the major peptide present in the cell. In the liver, the concentration of GSH is ~5 mmol/L. GSH plays a major role in the maintenance of cysteine residues in proteins in their reduced (sulfhydryl) forms and in antioxidant defenses (Chapter 42). The enzyme γ-glutamyl transpeptidase is involved in the metabolism of glutathione and is a plasma biomarker for some liver diseases, including hepatocellular carcinoma and alcoholic liver disease.

or D-R-V-Y-I-H-P-F-H-L (see Table 2.1); this peptide is angiotensin, a peptide hormone that affects blood pressure. The amino acid residue having a free amino group at one end of the peptide, Asp, is called the N-terminal amino acid (amino terminus), whereas the residue having a free carboxyl group at the other end, Leu, is called the C-terminal amino acid (carboxyl terminus). Proteins contain between 50 and 2000 amino acid residues. The mean molecular mass of an amino acid residue is about 110 dalton units (Da). Therefore the molecular mass of most proteins is between 5500 and 220,000 Da.

Amino acid side chains contribute both charge and hydrophobicity to proteins

The amino acid composition of a peptide chain has a profound effect on its physical and chemical properties. Proteins rich in aliphatic or aromatic amino groups are relatively insoluble in water and are likely to be found in cell membranes. Proteins rich in polar amino acids are more water soluble. Amides are neutral compounds, so the amide backbone of a protein, including the α-amino and α-carboxyl groups from which it is formed, does not contribute to the charge of the protein.

Instead, the charge on the protein is dependent primarily on the side chain functional groups of amino acids, plus a minor contribution from the amino and carboxyl groups of the terminal amino acids. Amino acids with side chain acidic (Glu, Asp) or basic (Lys, His, Arg) groups will confer charge and buffering capacity to a protein. The balance between acidic and basic side chains in a protein determines its **isoelectric point** (pI) and net charge in solution. Proteins rich in lysine and arginine are basic in solution and have a positive charge at neutral pH, whereas acidic proteins, rich in aspartate and glutamate, are acidic and have a negative charge. Because of their side chain functional groups, all proteins become more positively charged at acidic pH and more negatively charged at basic pH. Proteins are an important part of the buffering capacity of cells and biological fluids, including blood.

Secondary structure of proteins

The secondary structure of a protein is determined by hydrogen bond interactions between backbone carbonyl and amide groups

The secondary structure of a protein refers to the local structure of the polypeptide chain. This structure is determined by hydrogen bond interactions between the carbonyl oxygen group of one peptide bond and the amide hydrogen of another nearby peptide bond. There are two types of secondary structure: the α-helix and the β-pleated sheet.

The α-helix

The α-helix is a rodlike structure with the peptide chain tightly coiled and the side chains of amino acid residues extending outward from the axis of the spiral. Each amide carbonyl group is hydrogen-bonded to the amide hydrogen of a peptide bond that is four residues away along the same chain. There are, on average, 3.6 amino acid residues per turn of the helix, and the helix winds in a right-handed (clockwise) manner in almost all proteins (Fig. 2.7A).

The β-pleated sheet

If the H-bonds are formed laterally between peptide bonds, the polypeptide sequences become arrayed parallel or antiparallel to one another in what is commonly called a β-pleated sheet. The β-pleated sheet is an extended structure as opposed to the coiled α-helix. It is pleated because the carbon–carbon (C–C) bonds are tetrahedral and cannot exist in a planar configuration. If the polypeptide chains run in the same direction, they form a parallel β-sheet (Fig. 2.7B), but in the opposite direction, they form an antiparallel structure. The β-turn, or β-bend, refers to the segment in which the polypeptide abruptly reverses direction. Glycine (Gly) and proline (Pro) residues often occur in β-turns on the surface of globular proteins.

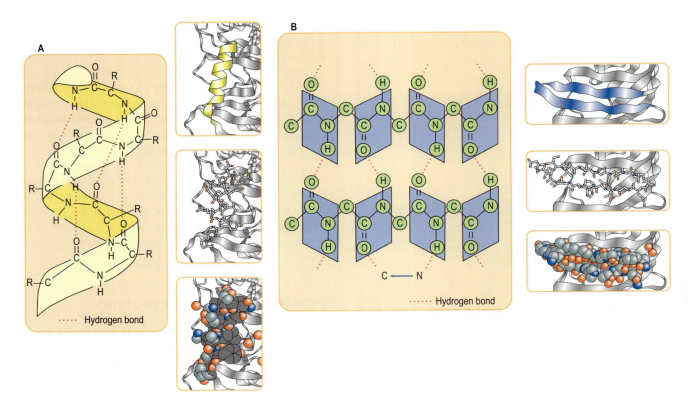

Fig. 2.7 **Protein secondary structural motifs.** (A) An α-helical secondary structure. Hydrogen bonds between "backbone" amide NH and C=O groups stabilize the α-helix. Hydrogen atoms of the OH, NH, or SH group (hydrogen donors) interact with electron pairs of the acceptor atoms such as O, N, or S. Even though the bonding energy is lower than that of covalent bonds, hydrogen bonds play a pivotal role in the stabilization of protein molecules. Ribbon, stick, and space-filling models are shown. R, side chain of amino acids that extend outward from the helix. (B) The parallel β-sheet secondary structure. In the β-conformation, the backbone of the polypeptide chain is extended into a zigzag structure. When the zigzag polypeptide chains are arranged side by side, they form a structure resembling a series of pleats. Ribbon, stick, and space-filling models are shown.

Tertiary structure of proteins

The tertiary structure of a protein is determined by interactions between side chain functional groups, including disulfide bonds, hydrogen bonds, salt bridges, and hydrophobic interactions

The three-dimensional, folded, and biologically active conformation of a protein is referred to as its tertiary structure. This structure reflects the overall shape of the molecule and generally consists of several smaller folded units termed **domains.**

The tertiary structure of a protein is stabilized by interactions between side chain functional groups: covalent disulfide bonds, hydrogen bonds, salt bridges, and hydrophobic interactions (Fig. 2.8). The side chains of tryptophan and arginine serve as hydrogen donors, whereas asparagine, glutamine, serine, and threonine can serve as both hydrogen donors and acceptors. Lysine, aspartic acid, glutamic acid, tyrosine, and histidine also can serve as both donors and acceptors in the formation of ion pairs (salt bridges). Two opposite-charged amino acids, such as glutamate with a γ-carboxyl group and lysine with

an ε-amino group, may form a salt bridge, primarily on the surface of proteins (see Fig. 2.8). Compounds such as urea and guanidine hydrochloride block these interactions and cause denaturation, or loss of secondary and tertiary structure, when present at high concentrations - for example, 8 mol/L urea. These reagents are called **denaturants** or **chaotropic agents.**

Quaternary structure of proteins

The quaternary structure of multisubunit proteins is determined by covalent and noncovalent interactions between the subunit surfaces

Quaternary structure refers to a complex, or an assembly, of two or more separate peptide chains that are held together by noncovalent or, in some cases, covalent interactions. In general, most proteins larger than 50 kDa consist of more than one chain and are referred to as dimeric, trimeric, or multimeric proteins. Many multisubunit proteins are composed of different kinds of **functional subunits, such as the regulatory and**

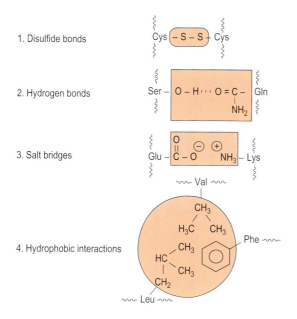

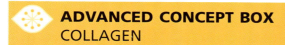

1. Disulfide bonds — Cys – S – S – Cys

2. Hydrogen bonds — Ser – O – H ⋯ O = C – Gln (NH₂)

3. Salt bridges — Glu – C – O ⊖ ⊕ NH₃ – Lys

4. Hydrophobic interactions — Val, Phe, Leu (CH₃ groups)

Fig. 2.8 **Elements of tertiary structure of proteins.** Examples of amino acid side chain interactions contributing to tertiary structure.

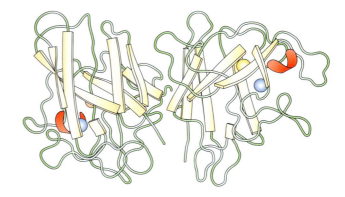

Fig. 2.9 **Three-dimensional structure of a dimeric protein.** Quaternary structure of Cu,Zn-superoxide dismutase from spinach. Cu,Zn-superoxide dismutase has a dimeric structure, with a monomer molecular mass of 16,000 Da. Each subunit consists of eight antiparallel β-sheets called a β-barrel structure, in analogy with geometric motifs found on Native American and Greek weaving and pottery. Red arc, short a-helix. Courtesy of Dr. Y. Kitagawa.

overview of the primary, secondary, tertiary, and quaternary structures of a tetrameric protein.

PURIFICATION AND CHARACTERIZATION OF PROTEINS

Protein purification is a multistep process, based on protein size, charge, solubility, and ligand binding

The complete characterization of a protein requires its purification and determination of its complete primary, secondary, and tertiary structure and, for a multimeric protein, its quaternary structure. To characterize a protein, it is first necessary to purify the protein by separating it from other components

catalytic subunits. Hemoglobin is a tetrameric protein (Chapter 5), and beef heart mitochondrial ATPase has 10 protomers (Chapter 8). The smallest unit is referred to as a monomer, or subunit. Fig. 2.9 illustrates the structure of the dimeric protein Cu,Zn-superoxide dismutase. Fig. 2.10 is an

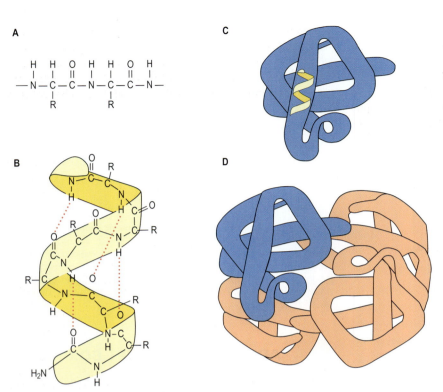

Fig. 2.10 **Primary, secondary, tertiary, and quaternary structures.** (A) The primary structure is composed of a linear sequence of amino acid residues of proteins. (B) The secondary structure indicates the local spatial arrangement of the polypeptide backbone yielding an extended α-helical or β-pleated sheet structure as depicted by the ribbon. Hydrogen bonds between the "backbone" amide NH and C=O groups stabilize the helix. (C) The tertiary structure illustrates the three-dimensional conformation of a subunit of the protein, and the quaternary structure (D) indicates the assembly of multiple polypeptide chains into an intact, tetrameric protein.

in complex biological mixtures. The source of the proteins is commonly blood or tissues or microbial cells such as bacteria and yeast. First, the cells or tissues are disrupted by grinding or homogenization in buffered isotonic solutions, commonly at physiologic pH and at 4°C to minimize protein denaturation during purification. The "crude extract" containing organelles such as nuclei, mitochondria, lysosomes, microsomes, and cytosolic fractions can then be fractionated by high-speed centrifugation, or ultracentrifugation. Proteins that are tightly bound to other biomolecules or membranes may be solubilized using organic solvent or detergent.

ADVANCED CONCEPT BOX
POSTTRANSLATIONAL MODIFICATIONS OF PROTEINS

Most proteins undergo some form of enzymatic modification after the synthesis of the peptide chain. The "posttranslational" modifications are performed by processing enzymes in the endoplasmic reticulum, Golgi apparatus, secretory granules, and extracellular space. The modifications include proteolytic cleavage, glycosylation, lipation, and phosphorylation. Mass spectrometry is a powerful tool for detecting such modifications based on differences in molecular mass (see Chapter 24).

Protein purification-precipitation

Protein purification is based on differences in a protein's solubility, size, charge, and binding properties

The solubility of a protein may be increased by the addition of salt at a low concentration (salting in) or decreased by high salt concentration (salting out). When ammonium sulfate, one of the most soluble salts, is added to a solution of a protein, some proteins precipitate at a given salt concentration, whereas others do not. Human serum immunoglobulins are precipitable by 33%–40% saturated $(NH_4)_2SO_4$, whereas albumin remains soluble. Saturated ammonium sulfate is about 4.1 mol/L. Most proteins will precipitate from an 80% saturated $(NH_4)_2SO_4$ solution.

Proteins may also be precipitated from solution by adjusting the pH. Proteins are generally least soluble at their isoelectric point (pI). At this pH, the protein has no net charge or charge–charge repulsion between subunits. Hydrophobic interactions between protein surfaces then lead to aggregation and precipitation of the protein.

Dialysis and ultrafiltration

Small molecules, such as salts, can be removed from protein solutions by dialysis or ultrafiltration

Dialysis is performed by adding the protein–salt solution to a semipermeable membrane tube (commonly a nitrocellulose or collodion membrane). When the tube is immersed in a dilute buffer solution, small molecules will pass through, but large protein molecules will be retained in the tube, depending on the pore size of the dialysis membrane. This procedure is particularly useful for removal of $(NH_4)_2SO_4$ or other salts during protein purification because the salts will interfere with the purification of proteins by ion-exchange chromatography (see following discussion). Fig. 2.11 illustrates the dialysis of proteins.

Ultrafiltration has largely replaced dialysis for purification of proteins. This technique uses pressure to force a solution through a semipermeable membrane of a defined, homogeneous pore size. By selecting the proper molecular-weight cut-off value (MWCO; pore size) for the filter, the membranes will allow solvent and lower-molecular-weight solutes to pass through the membrane, forming the filtrate, while retaining higher-molecular-weight proteins in the retentate solution. Ultrafiltration can be used to concentrate protein solutions or to accomplish dialysis by continuous replacement of buffer in the retentate compartment.

Gel filtration (molecular sieving)

Gel filtration chromatography separates proteins on the basis of size

Gel filtration, or gel-permeation, chromatography uses a column of insoluble but highly hydrated polymers, such as dextran, agarose, or polyacrylamide. Gel filtration chromatography

depends on the differential migration of dissolved solutes through gels that have pores of defined sizes. This technique is frequently used for protein purification and for desalting protein solutions. Fig. 2.12 describes the principle of gel filtration. There are commercially available gels made from polymer beads

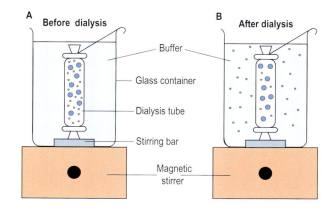

Fig. 2.11 **Dialysis of proteins.** Protein and low-molecular-mass compounds are separated by dialysis on the basis of size. (A) A protein solution with salts is placed in a dialysis tube in a beaker and dialyzed with stirring against an appropriate buffer. (B) The protein is retained in the dialysis tube, whereas salts will exchange through the membrane. By use of a large volume of external buffer, with occasional buffer replacement, the protein will eventually be exchanged into the external buffer solution.

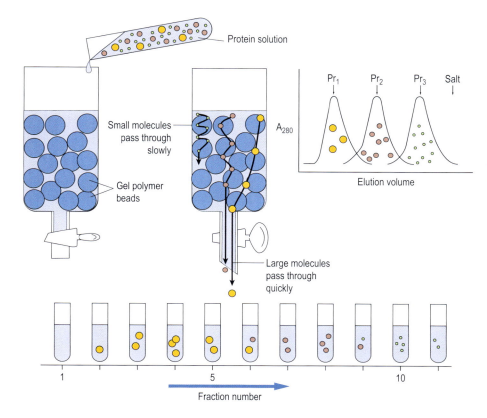

Fig. 2.12 **Fractionation of proteins by size: gel filtration chromatography of proteins.** Proteins with different molecular sizes are separated by gel filtration based on their relative size. The smaller the protein, the more readily it exchanges into polymer beads, whereas larger proteins may be completely excluded. Larger molecules flow more rapidly through this column, leading to fractionation on the basis of molecular size. The chromatogram on the right shows a theoretical fractionation of three proteins, Pr_1–Pr_3, of decreasing molecular weight.

designated as dextran (Sephadex series), polyacrylamide (Bio-Gel P series), and agarose (Sepharose series), respectively. The gels vary in pore size, and one can choose the gel filtration materials according to the molecular-weight-fractionation range desired.

Ion-exchange chromatography

Proteins bind to ion-exchange matrices based on charge–charge interactions

When a charged ion or molecule with one or more positive charges exchanges with another positively charged component bound to a negatively charged immobilized phase, the process is called cation exchange. The inverse process is called anion exchange. The cation exchanger, carboxymethylcellulose ($R–O–CH_2–COO^-$), and anion exchanger, diethylaminoethyl [(DEAE) cellulose [$R–O–C_2H_4–NH^+(C_2H_5)_2$], are frequently used for the purification of proteins. Consider purifying a protein mixture containing albumin and immunoglobulin. At pH 7.5, albumin, with a pI of 4.8, is negatively charged; immunoglobulin, with a pI ~8.0, is positively charged. If the mixture is applied to a DEAE-cellulose column at pH 7.0, the albumin sticks to the positively charged column, whereas the immunoglobulin passes through the column. Fig. 2.13 illustrates the principle of ion-exchange chromatography. As with gel-permeation chromatography, proteins can be separated from one another based on small differences in their

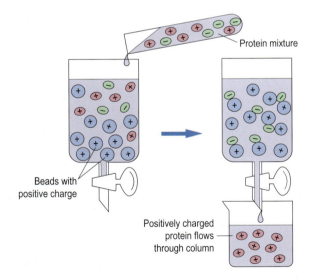

Fig. 2.13 **Fractionation of proteins by charge: ion-exchange chromatography.** Mixtures of proteins can be separated by ion-exchange chromatography according to their net charges. Beads that have positively charged groups attached are called anion exchangers, whereas those having negatively charged groups are cation exchangers. This figure depicts an anion-exchange column. Negatively charged protein binds to positively charged beads, and positively charged protein flows through the column.

pI. **Adsorbed proteins are commonly eluted with a gradient formed from two or more solutions with different pH and/or salt concentrations.** In this way, proteins are gradually eluted from the column and are separated based on their pI.

Affinity chromatography

Affinity chromatography purifies proteins based on ligand interactions

Affinity chromatography is a convenient and specific method for the purification of proteins. A porous chromatography column matrix is derivatized with a ligand that interacts with, or binds to, a specific protein in a complex mixture. The protein of interest will be selectively and specifically bound to the ligand, whereas the others wash through the column. The bound protein can then be eluted by a high salt concentration, by mild denaturation, or by a soluble form of the ligand or ligand analogs.

Determination of purity and molecular weight of proteins

Polyacrylamide gel electrophoresis in sodium dodecylsulfate can be used to separate proteins based on charge

Electrophoresis can be used for the separation of a wide variety of charged molecules, including amino acids, polypeptides, proteins, and DNA. When a current is applied to molecules in dilute buffers, those with a net negative charge at the selected pH migrate toward the anode, and those with a net positive charge migrate toward the cathode. A porous support, such as paper, cellulose acetate, or a polymeric gel, is commonly used to minimize diffusion and convection.

Like chromatography, electrophoresis may be used for preparative fractionation of proteins at physiologic pH. Different soluble proteins will move at different rates in the electrical field, depending on their charge-to-mass ratio. A denaturing detergent, sodium dodecylsulfate (SDS), is commonly used in a polyacrylamide gel electrophoresis (PAGE) system to separate and resolve protein subunits according to molecular weight. The protein preparation is usually treated with both SDS and a thiol reagent, such as β-mercaptoethanol, to reduce disulfide bonds. Because the binding of SDS is proportional to the length of the peptide chain, each protein molecule has the same mass-to-charge ratio, and the relative mobility of the protein in the polyacrylamide matrix is proportional to the molecular mass of the polypeptide chain. Varying the extent of crosslinking of the polyacrylamide gel provides selectivity for proteins of different molecular weights. A purified protein preparation can be readily analyzed for homogeneity on SDS-PAGE by staining with dyes, such as Coomassie Blue, or with a silver staining technique, as shown in Fig. 2.14.

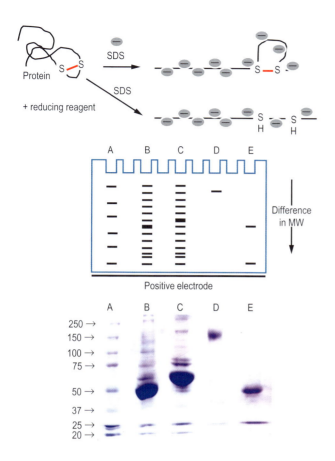

Fig. 2.14 **SDS-PAGE.** Sodium dodecylsulfate (SDS) polyacrylamide gel electrophoresis (PAGE) is used to separate proteins on the basis of their molecular weights. Larger molecules are retarded in the gel matrix, whereas the smaller ones move more rapidly. Lane A contains standard proteins with known molecular masses (indicated in kDa on the left). Lanes B, C, D, and E show results of SDS-PAGE analysis of a protein at various stages of purification: B, total protein isolate; C, ammonium sulfate precipitate; D, fraction from gel-permeation chromatography; E, purified protein from ion-exchange chromatography.

<table>
<tr><td>✿</td><td>**ADVANCED CONCEPT BOX**</td></tr>
</table>

HIGH-PERFORMANCE LIQUID CHROMATOGRAPHY (HPLC)

HPLC is a powerful chromatographic technique for high-resolution separation of proteins, peptides, and amino acids. The principle of the separation may be based on the charge, size, or hydrophobicity of proteins. The narrow columns are packed with a noncompressible matrix of fine silica beads coated with a thin layer of a stationary phase. A protein mixture is applied to the column and then the components are eluted by either isocratic or gradient chromatography. The eluates are monitored by ultraviolet absorption, refractive index, or fluorescence. This technique uses finely packed micron-size beads and requires high pressure for efficient elution, but it yields high-resolution separations.

Isoelectric focusing (IEF)

IEF resolves proteins based on their isoelectric point

IEF is conducted in a microchannel or gel containing a stabilized pH gradient, formed by ampholytes, which are zwitterionic species with a range of isoelectric points. When a charge is applied to the solution, the ampholytes self-organize into a stable pH gradient. A protein applied to the system will be either positively or negatively charged, depending on its amino acid composition and the ambient pH. Upon application of a current, the protein will move toward either the anode or cathode until it encounters that part of the system that corresponds to its pI, where the protein has no charge and will cease to migrate. **IEF is used in conjunction with SDS-PAGE for two-dimensional gel electrophoresis** (Fig. 2.15). This technique is particularly useful for the fractionation of complex mixtures of proteins for proteomic analysis.

ANALYSIS OF PROTEIN STRUCTURE

The typical steps in the purification of a protein are summarized in Fig. 2.16. Once purified, for the determination of its amino acid composition, a protein is subjected to hydrolysis, commonly in 6 mol/L HCl at 110°C in a sealed and evacuated tube for 24–48 h. Under these conditions, tryptophan, cysteine, and most of the cystine are destroyed, and glutamine and asparagine are quantitatively deaminated to give glutamate and aspartate, respectively. Recovery of serine and threonine is incomplete and decreases with increasing time of hydrolysis. Alternative hydrolysis procedures may be used for measurement of tryptophan, whereas cysteine and cystine may be converted to an acid-stable cysteic acid prior to hydrolysis.

Following hydrolysis, the free amino acids are separated on an automated amino acid analyzer using an ion-exchange column or, following pre-column derivatization with colored or fluorescent reagents, by reversed-phase high-performance (hydrophobic surface) liquid chromatography (RP-HPLC). Free amino acids fractionated by ion-exchange chromatography are detected by post-column reaction with a chromogenic or fluorogenic reagent, such as ninhydrin or dansyl chloride, Edman's reagent (see following discussion), or *o*-phthalaldehyde. These techniques allow the measurement of as little as 1 pmol of each amino acid. A typical elution pattern of amino acids in a purified protein is shown in Fig. 2.17.

Determination of the primary structure of proteins

Historically, analysis of protein sequence was carried out by chemical methods; today, both sequence analysis and protein identification are performed by mass spectrometry

Information on the primary sequence of a protein is essential for understanding its functional properties, the identification of

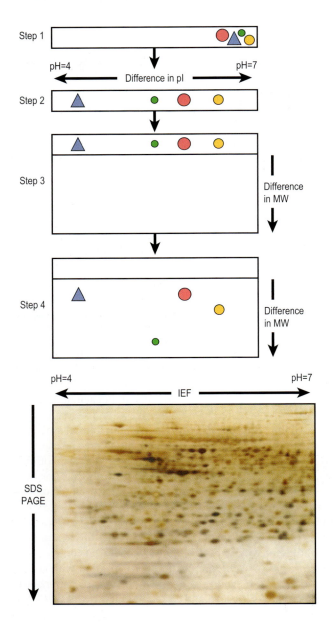

pH=4

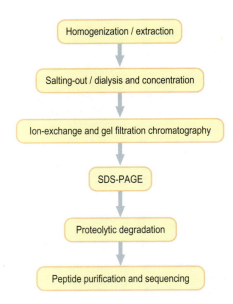

Fig. 2.16 **Strategy for protein purification.** Purification of a protein involves a sequence of steps in which contaminating proteins are removed based on differences in size, charge, and hydrophobicity. Purification is monitored by SDS-PAGE (see Fig. 2.14).

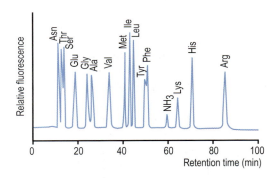

Fig. 2.15 **Two-dimensional gel electrophoresis.** (Top) **Step 1:** Sample containing proteins is applied to a cylindrical isoelectric-focusing gel within the pH gradient. **Step 2:** Each protein migrates to a position in the gel corresponding to its isoelectric point (pI). **Step 3:** The IEF gel is placed horizontally on the top of a slab gel. **Step 4:** The proteins are separated by SDS-PAGE according to their molecular weight. (Bottom) Typical example of 2D-PAGE. A rat liver homogenate was fractionated by 2D-PAGE, and proteins were detected by silver staining.

Fig. 2.17 **Chromatogram from an amino acid analysis by cation-exchange chromatography.** A protein hydrolysate is applied to the cation-exchange column in a dilute buffer at acidic pH (~3.0), at which all amino acids are positively charged. The amino acids are then eluted by a gradient of increasing pH and salt concentrations. The most anionic (acidic) amino acids elute first, followed by the neutral and basic amino acids. Amino acids are visualized by post-column reaction with a fluorogenic compound, such as o-phthalaldehyde.

the family to which the protein belongs, and the characterization of mutant proteins that cause disease. Because of the large size of proteins, they are typically cleaved by digestion by specific endoproteases, such as trypsin (Chapter 6), V8 protease, or lysyl endopeptidase, to obtain peptide fragments. Trypsin cleaves peptide bonds on the C-terminal side of arginine

and lysine residues, provided the next residue is not proline. Lysyl endopeptidase is also frequently used to cleave at the C-terminal side of lysine. Cleavage by chemical reagents such as cyanogen bromide is also useful; cyanogen bromide cleaves on the C-terminal side of methionine residues. Before cleavage, proteins with cysteine and cystine residues are reduced

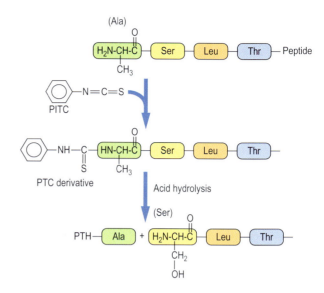

Fig. 2.18 **Steps in Edman degradation.** The Edman degradation method sequentially removes one residue at a time from the amino end of a peptide. Phenyl isothiocyanate (PITC) converts the N-terminal amino group of the immobilized peptide to a phenylthiocarbamyl (PTC) amino acid derivative in alkaline solution. Mild acid treatment removes the first amino acid as the phenylthiohydantoin (PTH) derivative, which is identified by HPLC.

ADVANCED CONCEPT BOX
THE PROTEOME

A proteome is defined as the full complement of proteins produced by a particular genome. Proteomics is defined as the qualitative and quantitative comparison of proteomes under different conditions. The proteome is tissue and cell specific, and it changes during development and in response to hormonal signaling and environmental stresses. In one approach to analyzing the proteome of a cell, proteins are extracted and subjected to two-dimensional (2D) polyacrylamide gel electrophoresis (2D-PAGE). Individual protein spots are identified by staining, then extracted and digested with proteases. Small peptides from such a gel are sequenced by mass spectrometry, permitting the identification of the protein. In 2D-differential gel electrophoresis (DIGE), two proteomes may be compared by labeling their proteins with different fluorescent dyes (e.g., red and green). The labeled proteins are mixed, then fractionated by 2D-PAGE (see Fig. 2.15). Proteins present in both proteomes will appear as yellow spots, whereas unique proteins will be red or green, respectively (see Chapter 24).

by 2-mercaptoethanol and then treated with iodoacetate to form carboxymethylcysteine residues. This avoids spontaneous formation of inter- or intramolecular disulfides during analyses.

The cleaved peptides are then subjected to RP-HPLC to purify the peptide fragments, then sequenced on an automated protein sequencer using the **Edman degradation** technique (Fig. 2.18). The sequence of overlapping peptides is then used to obtain the primary structure of the protein. The Edman degradation technique is largely of historical interest. Mass spectrometry is more commonly used today to obtain both the molecular mass and sequence of polypeptides simultaneously (Chapter 24). Both techniques can be applied directly to proteins or peptides recovered from SDS-PAGE or two-dimensional electrophoresis (IEF plus SDS-PAGE).

Protein sequencing and identification is currently done by electrospray ionization liquid chromatography tandem mass spectrometry (HPLC-ESI-MS/MS; Chapter 24). This technique is sufficiently sensitive that proteins separated by 2D-PAGE (Fig. 2.15) can be recovered from the gel for analysis. As little as 1 µg of protein can be digested with trypsin in situ, then extracted from the gel and identified based on the amino acid sequence of its peptides. This technique, and a complementary technique called matrix-assisted laser desorption ionization-time of flight (MALDI-TOF) MS/MS (Chapter 24), can be applied for determination of the molecular weight of intact proteins and for sequence analysis of peptides, leading to unambiguous identification of a protein.

Determination of the three-dimensional structure of proteins

X-ray crystallography and nuclear magnetic resonance (NMR) spectroscopy are usually used for determination of the three-dimensional structure of proteins

X-ray crystallography depends on the diffraction of X-rays by the electrons of the atoms constituting the molecule. However, because the X-ray diffraction caused by an individual molecule is weak, the protein must exist in the form of a well-ordered crystal, in which each molecule has the same conformation in a specific position and orientation on a three-dimensional lattice. Based on diffraction of a collimated beam of electrons, the distribution of the electron density, and thus the location of atoms, in the crystal can be calculated to determine the structure of the protein. For protein crystallization, the most frequently used method is the hanging drop method, which involves the use of a simple apparatus that permits a small portion of a protein solution (typically a 10-µL droplet containing 0.5–1.0 mg/protein) to evaporate gradually to reach the saturation point at which the protein begins to crystallize. NMR spectroscopy is commonly used for structural analysis of small organic compounds, but high-field NMR is also useful for determination of the structure of a protein in solution and complements information obtained by X-ray crystallography.

ADVANCED CONCEPT BOX
PROTEIN FOLDING

For proteins to function properly, they must fold into the correct shape, or conformation. Proteins have evolved so that one conformation is more favorable than all others: the native state. Numerous proteins assist other proteins in the folding process. These proteins, termed **chaperones,** include "heat shock" proteins, such as HSP 60 and HSP 70, and protein disulfide isomerases. A protein-folding disease is a disease that is associated with the abnormal conformation of a protein. This occurs in chronic, age-related diseases, such as Alzheimer's disease, amyotrophic lateral sclerosis, and Parkinson's disease. The accumulation of aggregates of misfolded protein contributes to the development of pathology in these diseases.

CLINICAL BOX
CREUTZFELDT–JAKOB DISEASE

A 56-year-old male cattle rancher presented with epileptic cramps and dementia and was diagnosed as having Creutzfeldt–Jakob disease, a human prion disease. The **prion diseases,** also known as transmissible spongiform encephalopathies, are neurodegenerative diseases that affect both humans and animals. This disease in sheep and goats is designated as scrapie and in cows as spongiform encephalopathy (mad cow disease). The diseases are characterized by the accumulation of an abnormal isoform of a host-encoded protein, prion protein-cellular form (PrPC), in affected brains.

Comment

Prions appear to be composed only of PrPSc (scrapie form) molecules, which are abnormal conformers of the normal, host-encoded protein. PrPC has a high α-helical content and is devoid of β-pleated sheets, whereas PrPSc has a high β-pleated sheet content. The conversion of PrPC into PrPSc involves a profound conformational change. The progression of infectious prion diseases appears to involve an interaction between PrPC and PrPSc that induces a conformational change of the α-helix-rich PrPC to the β-pleated sheet–rich conformer of PrPSc. PrPSc-derived prion disease may be genetic or infectious. The amino acid sequences of different mammalian PrPCs are similar, and the conformation of the protein is virtually the same in all mammalian species.

SUMMARY

- Proteins are macromolecules formed by polymerization of amino acids. There are 20 different α-L-amino acids in proteins, linked by peptide bonds. The side chains of the amino acids contribute charge, polarity, and hydrophobicity to proteins.

ACTIVE LEARNING

1. Mass spectrometry analysis of blood, urine, and tissues is now being applied for clinical diagnosis. Discuss the merits of this technique with respect to specificity, sensitivity, throughput, and breadth of analysis, including proteomic analysis for diagnostic purposes.
2. Review the importance of protein misfolding and deposition in tissues in age-related chronic diseases.

- The linear sequence of the amino acids constitutes the primary structure of the protein. Higher-order structures are formed by hydrogen bonds between backbone carbonyl and amide groups (secondary structure), by hydrophobic interactions, by salt bridges and covalent bonds between the side chains of amino acids (tertiary structure), and by noncovalent association of multiple polypeptide chains to form polymeric proteins (quaternary structure).
- Purification and characterization of proteins are essential for elucidating their structure and function. By taking advantage of differences in their solubility, size, charge, and ligand-binding properties, proteins can be purified to homogeneity using various chromatographic and electrophoretic techniques. The molecular mass and purity of a protein, and its subunit composition, can be determined by SDS-PAGE.
- Deciphering the primary and three-dimensional structures of a protein by chemical methods, mass spectrometry, X-ray crystallographic analysis, and NMR spectroscopy leads to an understanding of structure–function relationships in proteins.

FURTHER READING

Bada, J. L. (2013). New insights into prebiotic chemistry from Stanley Miller's spark discharge experiments. *Chemical Society Reviews, 42,* 2186–2196.

Chen, C., Huang, H., & Wu, C. H. (2017). Protein bioinformatics databases and resources. *Methods in Molecular Biology, 1558,* 3–39.

Dill, K. A., & MacCallum, J. L. (2012). The protein-folding problem, 50 years on. *Science, 338,* 1042–1046. Retrieved from http://science.sciencemag.org/content/338/6110/1042.full.

Elsila, J. E., Aponte, J. C., Blackmond, D. G., et al. (2016). Meteoritic amino acids: Diversity in compositions reflects parent body histories. *ACS Central Science, 22,* 370–379.

Faísca, P. F. (2015). Knotted proteins: A tangled tale of structural biology. *Computational and Structural Biotechnology Journal, 13,* 459–468.

Kaushik, S., & Cuervo, A. M. (2015). Proteostasis and aging. *Nature Medicine, 21,* 1406–1415.

Raoufinia, R., Mota, A., Keyhanvar, N., et al. (2016). Overview of albumin and its purification methods. *Advanced Pharmaceutical Bulletin, 6,* 495–507.

Rodgers, K. J. (2014). Non-protein amino acids and neurodegeneration: The enemy within. *Experimental Neurology, 253,* 192–196.

Watts, J. C., & Prusiner, S. B. (2017). β-Amyloid prions and the pathobiology of Alzheimer's disease. *Cold Spring Harbor Perspectives in Medicine.* Advance online publication. doi:10.1101/cshperspect.a023507.

RELEVANT WEBSITES

Protein Data Bank: http://www.rcsb.org

ABBREVIATIONS

GSH	Glutathione (reduced)
GSSG	Glutathione (oxidized)
IEF	Isoelectric focusing
HPLC	High performance (pressure) liquid chromatography
MWCO	Molecular weight cut-off
PAGE	Polyacrylamide gel electrophoresis
pI	Isoelectric point
RP-HPLC	Reversed phase HPLC
SDS	Sodium dodecylsulfate
SDS-PAGE	Sodium dodecylsulfate-polyacrylamide gel electrophoresis

3   Carbohydrates and Lipids

John W. Baynes

LEARNING OBJECTIVES

After reading this chapter, you should be able to:

- Describe the structure and nomenclature of carbohydrates.
- Identify the major carbohydrates in our bodies and in our diet.
- Distinguish between reducing and nonreducing sugars.
- Describe various types of glycosidic bonds in oligosaccharides and polysaccharides.
- Identify the major classes of lipids in our bodies and in our diet.
- Describe the types of bonds in lipids and their sensitivity to saponification.
- Outline the general features of the fluid mosaic model of the structure of biological membranes.

INTRODUCTION

Carbohydrates and lipids are major sources of energy and are stored in the body as glycogen and triglycerides (fat)

This short chapter, which is largely an overview of collegiate studies, describes the structure of carbohydrates and lipids found in the diet and in tissues. These two classes of compounds differ significantly in physical and chemical properties. Carbohydrates are hydrophilic; the smaller carbohydrates (sugars) are soluble in aqueous solution, whereas large polymers such as starch or cellulose form colloidal dispersions or are insoluble. Lipids vary in size but rarely exceed 2 kDa in molecular mass; they are insoluble in water but soluble in organic solvents. Both carbohydrates and lipids may be bound covalently or noncovalently to proteins (glycoproteins, glycolipids, lipoproteins) and have important structural and regulatory functions, which are elaborated in later chapters. This chapter ends with a description of the **fluid mosaic model** of biological membranes, which describes how protein, carbohydrates, and lipids are integrated into the structure of biological membranes that surround the cell and compartmentalize cellular functions.

CARBOHYDRATES

Nomenclature and structure of simple sugars

The classic definition of a carbohydrate is a polyhydroxy aldehyde, or ketone

The simplest carbohydrates, having two hydroxyl groups, are glyceraldehyde and dihydroxyacetone (Fig. 3.1). These three-carbon sugars are trioses; the suffix *-ose* designates a sugar. Glyceraldehyde is an **aldose**, and dihydroxyacetone is a **ketose** sugar. Prefixes and examples of longer-chain sugars are shown in Table 3.1.

Numbering of the carbons begins from the end containing the aldehyde, or ketone, functional group. Sugars are classified into the D or L family based on the configuration around the highest numbered asymmetric center (Fig. 3.2). In contrast to the L-amino acids, nearly all sugars found in the body have the D configuration.

An aldohexose, such as glucose, contains four asymmetric centers, so that there are 16 (2^4) possible stereoisomers, depending on whether each of the four carbons has the D or L configuration (see Fig. 3.2). Eight of these aldohexoses are D-sugars. Only three of these are found in significant amounts in the body: glucose (blood sugar) and mannose and galactose in the form of metabolic intermediates, or glycoconjugates (see Fig. 3.2). There are four possible D-ketohexoses; fructose (fruit sugar; see Fig. 3.2) is the only ketohexose present in significant concentration in our diet or in the body.

Because of their asymmetric centers, sugars are optically active compounds. The rotation of plane-polarized light may be dextrorotatory (+) or levorotatory (−). This designation is also commonly included in the name of the sugar; thus D(+)-glucose or D(−)-fructose indicates that the D form of glucose is dextrorotatory, whereas the D form of fructose is levorotatory.

Cyclization of sugars

Except for the trioses, sugars exist primarily in cyclic conformations. The linear sugar structures shown in Fig. 3.2 imply that aldose sugars have a chemically reactive, easily oxidizable, electrophilic, aldehyde residue. Aldehydes such as formaldehyde or glutaraldehyde react rapidly with amino groups in protein

Table 3.1 Classification of carbohydrates by length of the carbon chain

Number of carbons	Name	Examples in human biology
Three	Triose	Glyceraldehyde, dihydroxyacetone
Four	Tetrose	Erythrose
Five	Pentose	Ribose, ribulose,* xylose, xylulose,* deoxyribose
Six	Hexose	Glucose, mannose, galactose, fucose, fructose
Seven	Heptose	Sedoheptulose*
Eight	Octose	None
Nine	Nonose	Neuraminic (sialic) acid

*The syllable ul indicates that the sugar is a ketose; the formal name for fructose would be gluculose. As with fructose, the keto group is located at C-2 of the sugar, and the remaining carbons have the same geometry as the parent aldose sugar.

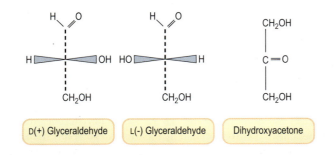

| D(+) Glyceraldehyde | L(-) Glyceraldehyde | Dihydroxyacetone |

Fig. 3.1 **Structures of the trioses: D- and L-glyceraldehyde (aldoses) and dihydroxyacetone (a ketose).**

to form Schiff base (imine) adducts and crosslinks during fixation of tissues. However, glucose is relatively resistant to oxidation and does not react rapidly with protein. As shown in Fig. 3.3, glucose exists largely in nonreactive, inert, cyclic hemiacetal conformations, 99.99% in aqueous solution at pH 7.4 and 37°C. Of all the D-sugars in the world, D-glucose exists to the greatest extent in these cyclic conformations, making it the least oxidizable and least reactive with protein. It has been proposed that the relative chemical inertness of glucose is the reason for its evolutionary selection as blood sugar.

When glucose cyclizes to a hemiacetal, it may form a **furanose** or **pyranose** ring structure, named after the five- and six-carbon cyclic ethers, furan and pyran (see Fig. 3.3). Note that the cyclization reaction creates a new asymmetric center at C-1, which is known as the **anomeric carbon**. The preferred conformation for glucose is the β-anomer (~65%), in which the hydroxyl group on C-1 is oriented equatorial to the ring. The β-anomer is the most stable form of glucose because all of the hydroxyl groups, which are bulkier than hydrogen, are oriented equatorially in the plane of the ring, minimizing steric interactions. The α- and β-anomers of glucose can be isolated in pure form by selective crystallization from aqueous and organic solvents. They have different optical rotations but equilibrate over a period of hours in aqueous solution to form the equilibrium mixture of 65 : 35 β:α anomers. These differences in structure may seem unimportant, but in fact, some metabolic pathways use one anomer but not the other, and vice versa. Similarly, although the fructopyranose conformations are the primary forms of fructose in aqueous solution, most of the fructose metabolism proceeds from the furanose conformation.

In addition to the basic sugar structures just discussed, a number of other common sugar structures are presented in Fig. 3.4. These sugars, deoxysugars, aminosugars, and sugar acids, are found primarily in oligomeric or polymeric structures in the body (e.g., ribose in RNA and deoxyribose in DNA), or they

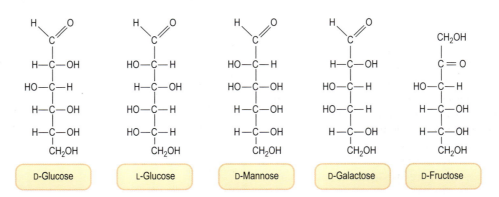

| D-Glucose | L-Glucose | D-Mannose | D-Galactose | D-Fructose |

Fig. 3.2 **Structures of hexoses: D- and L-glucose, D-mannose, D-galactose and D-fructose.** These linear projections of carbohydrate structures are known as Fischer projections. The D and L designations are based on the configuration at the highest numbered asymmetric center, C-5 in the case of hexoses. Note that L-glucose is the mirror image of D-glucose (i.e., the geometry at all of the asymmetric centers is reversed). Mannose is the C-2 epimer, and galactose the C-4 epimer, of glucose; epimers differ at only one stereogenic center.

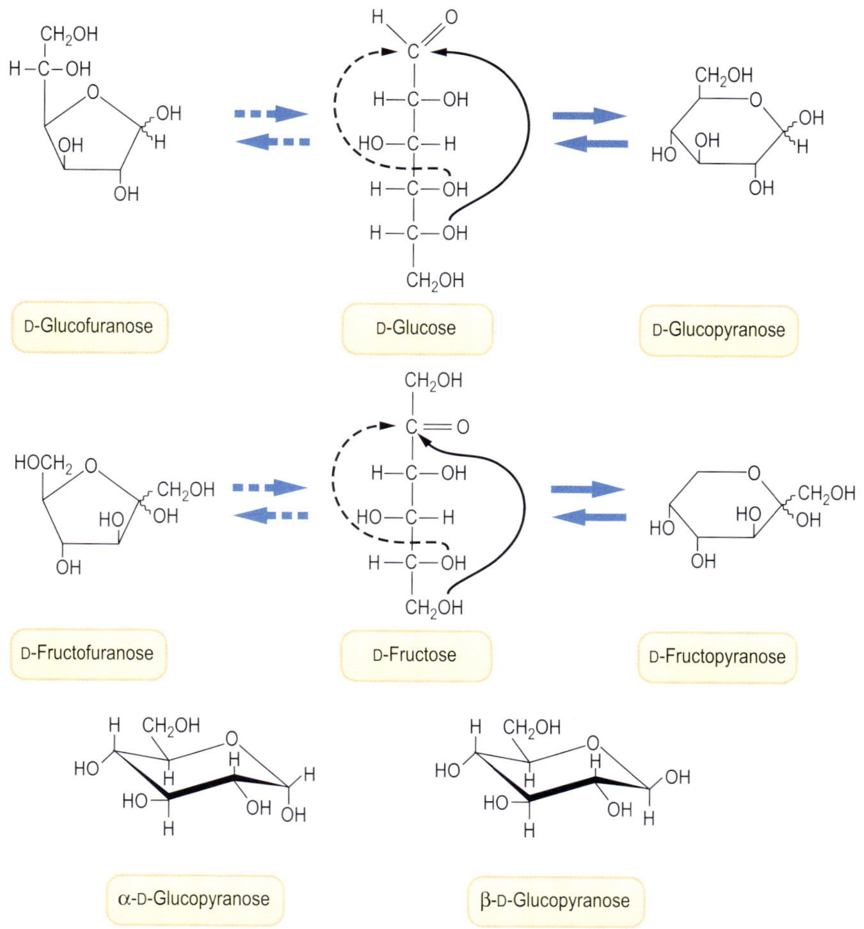

D-Glucofuranose   D-Glucose   D-Glucopyranose

D-Fructofuranose   D-Fructose   D-Fructopyranose

α-D-Glucopyranose   β-D-Glucopyranose

Fig. 3.3 **Linear and cyclic representations of glucose and fructose.** (Top) There are four cyclic conformations of glucose, in equilibrium with the linear form: α- and β-glucopyranose and α- and β-glucofuranose. The pyranose forms account for more than 99% of total glucose in solution. These cyclic structures are known as Haworth projections; by convention, groups to the right in Fischer projections are shown below the ring, and groups to the left are shown above the ring. The squiggly bonds to H and OH from C-1, the anomeric carbon, indicate indeterminate geometry and represent either the α or the β anomer. (Middle) The linear and cyclic forms of fructose. The ratio of pyranose:furanose forms of fructose in aqueous solution is ~3:1. The ratio shifts as a function of temperature, pH, salt concentration, and other factors. (Bottom) Stereochemical representations of the chair forms of α- and β-glucopyranose. The preferred structure in solution, β-glucopyranose, has all of the hydroxyl groups, including the anomeric hydroxyl group, in equatorial positions around the ring, minimizing steric interactions.

may be attached to proteins or lipids to form glycoconjugates (glycoproteins or glycolipids, respectively). **Glucose is the only sugar found to a significant extent as a free sugar (blood sugar) in the body**.

Disaccharides, oligosaccharides, and polysaccharides

Sugars are linked to one another by glycosidic bonds to form complex glycans

Carbohydrates are commonly linked to one another by glycosidic bonds to form disaccharides, trisaccharides, oligosaccharides, and polysaccharides. Polysaccharides composed of a single sugar are termed *homoglycans*, whereas those with complex compositions are termed *heteroglycans*. The name of the more complex structures includes not only the name of the component sugars but also the ring conformation of the sugars, the anomeric configuration of the linkage between sugars, the site of attachment of one sugar to another, and the nature of the atom involved in the linkage - usually an oxygen or O-glycosidic bond, sometimes a nitrogen or N-glycosidic bond. Fig. 3.5 shows the structure of several common disaccharides

in our diet: **lactose** (milk sugar); **sucrose** (table sugar); **maltose** and isomaltase (products of digestion of starch); cellobiose, which is obtained on hydrolysis of **cellulose**; and **hyaluronic acid**.

Differences in linkage of sugars make a big difference in metabolism and nutrition

Amylose, a component of **starch**, is an α-1→4-linked linear glucan, whereas **cellulose** is a β-1→4-linked linear glucan. These two polysaccharides differ only in the anomeric linkage between glucose subunits, but they are very different molecules. Starch forms a colloidal suspension in water, whereas cellulose is insoluble; starch is pasty, whereas cellulose is fibrous; starch is digestible, whereas cellulose is indigestible by humans; starch is a food, rich in calories, whereas cellulose is roughage.

LIPIDS

Lipids are found primarily in three compartments in the body: plasma, adipose tissue, and biological membranes

This introduction focuses on the structure of **fatty acids** (the simplest form of lipids, found primarily in plasma),

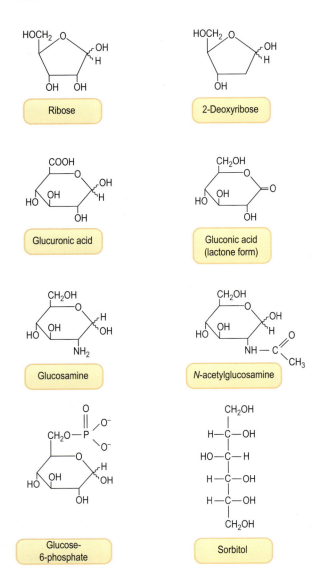

Fig. 3.4 **Examples of various types of sugars found in human tissues.** Ribose, the pentose sugar in ribonucleic acid (RNA); 2-deoxyribose, the deoxypentose in DNA; glucuronic acid, an acidic sugar formed by oxidation of C-6 of glucose; gluconic acid, an acidic sugar formed by oxidation of C-1 of glucose, shown in the δ-lactone form; glucosamine, an amino sugar; *N*-acetylglucosamine, an acetylated amino sugar; glucose-6-phosphate, a phosphate ester of glucose, an intermediate in glucose metabolism; sorbitol, a polyol formed on reduction of glucose.

triglycerides (the storage form of lipids, found primarily in adipose tissue), and **phospholipids** (the major class of membrane lipids in all cells). Steroids, such as cholesterol, and (glyco)sphingolipids are mentioned in the context of biological membranes, but these lipids and others, such as plasmalogens, polyisoprenoids, and eicosanoids, are addressed in detail in later chapters.

ADVANCED CONCEPT BOX
THE INFORMATION CONTENT OF COMPLEX GLYCANS

Sugars are attached to each other in **glycosidic linkages** between a hemiacetal carbon of one sugar and a hydroxyl group of another sugar. Two glucose residues can be linked in many different linkages (i.e., α1,2; α1,3; α1,4; α1,6; β1,2; β1,3; β1,4; β1,6; α,α1,1; α,β1,1; β,β1,1) to give 11 different disaccharides, each with different chemical and biological properties. Two different sugars, such as glucose and galactose, can be linked either glucose → galactose or galactose → glucose, and these two disaccharides can have a total of 20 different isomers.

In contrast, two identical amino acids, such as two alanines, can only form one dipeptide, alanyl-alanine. And two different amino acids (e.g., alanine and glycine) can only form two dipeptides (e.g., alanyl-glycine and glycyl-alanine). As a result, sugars have the potential to provide a great deal of chemical information. As outlined in Chapters 17–19, carbohydrates bound to proteins and lipids in cell membranes can serve as recognition signals for both cell–cell and cell–pathogen interactions.

CLINICAL TEST BOX
REDUCING SUGAR ASSAY FOR BLOOD GLUCOSE

The original assays for blood glucose measured the reducing activity of blood. These assays work because glucose, at 5-mM concentration, is the major reducing substance in the blood. The Fehling and Benedict assays use alkaline cupric salt solutions. With heating, the glucose decomposes oxidatively, yielding a complex mixture of organic acids and aldehydes. Oxidation of the sugar reduces cupric ion (blue-green color) to cuprous ion (orange-red color) in solution. The color yield produced is directly proportional to the glucose content of the sample.

Reducing sugar assays do not distinguish glucose from other reducing sugars, such as fructose or galactose. In diseases of fructose and galactose metabolism, such as hereditary fructose intolerance or galactosemia (Chapter 17), these assays could yield positive results, creating the false impression of diabetes. Sucrose and gluconic acid are nonreducing sugars (see Figs 3.4 and 3.5), lacking a terminal aldehyde group, and yield a negative reaction in reducing sugar assays.

Fatty acids

Fatty acids exist in free form and as components of more complex lipids

As summarized in Table 3.2, most fatty acids are long, straight-chain alkanoic acids, commonly with 16 or 18 carbons. They may be saturated or unsaturated, the latter containing one to five double bonds, all in *cis* geometry. The double bonds are not conjugated but separated by methylene groups.

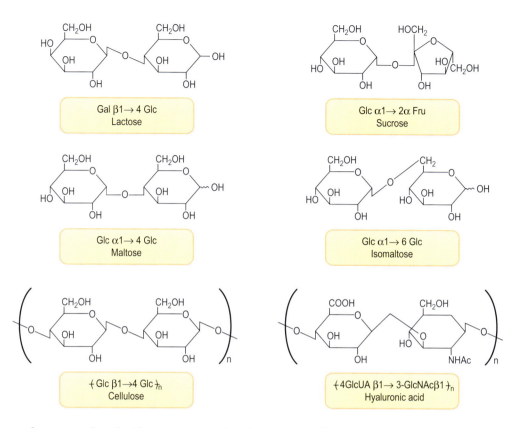

Fig. 3.5 **Structures of common disaccharides and polysaccharides.** Lactose (milk sugar); sucrose (table sugar); maltose and isomaltose, disaccharides formed on degradation of starch; and repeating disaccharide units of cellulose (from wood) and hyaluronic acid (from vertebral disks). Fru, fructose; Gal, galactose; Glc, glucose; GlcNAc, *N*-acetylglucosamine; GlcUA, glucuronic acid.

Table 3.2 Structure and melting point of naturally occurring fatty acids in the body					
Carbon atoms	**Chemical formula**		**Systematic name**	**Common name**	**Melting point (°C)**
Saturated fatty acids					
12 12:0	$CH_3(CH_2)_{10}COOH$		*n*-dodecanoic	Lauric	44
14 14:0	$CH_3(CH_2)_{12}COOH$		*n*-tetradecanoic	Myristic	54
16 16:0	$CH_3(CH_2)_{14}COOH$		*n*-hexadecanoic	Palmitic	63
18 18:0	$CH_3(CH_2)_{16}COOH$		*n*-octadecanoic	Stearic	70
20 20:0	$CH_3(CH_2)_{18}COOH$		*n*-eicosanoic	Arachidic	77
Unsaturated fatty acids					
16 16:1; ω-7, Δ^9	$CH3(CH2)5CH=CH(CH2)7COOH$			Palmitoleic	−0.5
18 18:1; ω-9, Δ^9	$CH_3(CH_2)_7CH=CH(CH_2)_7COOH$			Oleic	13
18 18:2; ω-6, $\Delta^{9,12}$	$CH_3(CH_2)_4CH=CHCH_2CH=CH(CH_2)_7COOH$			Linoleic	−5
18 18:3; ω-3, $\Delta^{9,12,15}$	$CH_3CH_2CH=CHCH_2CH=CHCH_2CH=CH(CH_2)_7COOH$			Linolenic	−11
20 20:4; ω-6, $\Delta^{5,8,11,14}$	$CH_3(CH_2)_4CH=CHCH_2CH=CHCH_2CH=CHCH_2CH=CH(CH_2)_3COOH$			Arachidonic	−50

For unsaturated fatty acids, the ω designation indicates the location of the first double bond from the methyl end of the molecule; the Δ superscripts indicate the location of the double bonds from the carboxyl end of the molecule. Unsaturated fatty acids account for about two-thirds of all fatty acids in the body; oleate and palmitate account for about one-half and one-quarter of total fatty acids, respectively.

Fatty acids with a single double bond are described as monounsaturated, and those with two or more double bonds are described as polyunsaturated fatty acids. The polyunsaturated fatty acids are commonly classified into two groups, **ω-3 and ω-6 fatty acids**, depending on whether the first double bond appears three or six carbons from the terminal methyl group. The melting point of fatty acids, as well as that of more complex lipids, increases with the chain length of the fatty acid but decreases with the number of double bonds. The **cis-double bonds** place a kink in the linear structure of the fatty acid chain, interfering with close packing, therefore requiring a lower temperature for freezing (i.e., they have a lower melting point).

Triacylglycerols (triglycerides)

Triglycerides are the storage form of lipids in adipose tissue

Fatty acids in plant and animal tissues are commonly esterified to glycerol, forming a triacylglycerol (triglyceride; Fig. 3.6), either oils (liquid) or fats (solid). In humans, triglycerides are stored in solid form in adipose tissue as fat. They are degraded to glycerol and fatty acids in response to hormonal signals, then released into plasma for metabolism in other tissues, primarily muscle and liver. The ester bond of triglycerides and other glycerolipids is also readily hydrolyzed in vitro by a strong base, such as NaOH, forming glycerol and free fatty acids. This process is known as **saponification;** one of the products, the sodium salt of the fatty acid, is soap.

Glycerol itself does not have a chiral carbon, but the numbering is standardized using the stereochemical numbering (*sn*) system, which places the hydroxyl group of C-2 on the left; thus all glycerolipids are derived from L-glycerol (see Fig. 3.6). Triglycerides isolated from natural sources are not pure compounds but mixtures of molecules with different fatty acid composition (e.g., 1-palmitoyl, 2-oleyl, 3-linoleoyl-L-glycerol), where the distribution and type of fatty acids vary from molecule to molecule. Thus fats are a mixture of many different triglycerides.

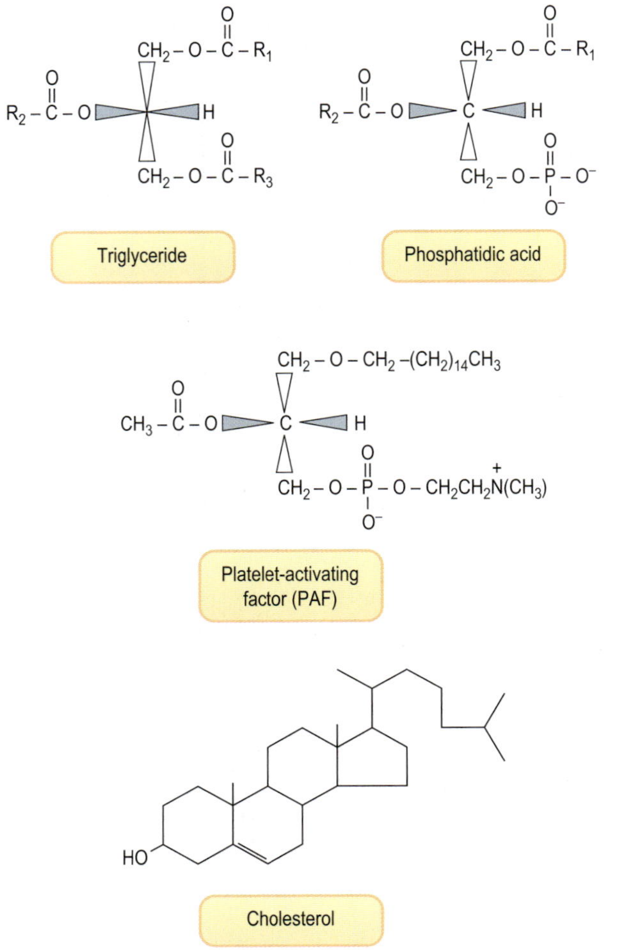

Fig. 3.6 **Structure of four lipids with significantly different biological functions.** Triglycerides are storage fats. Phosphatidic acid is a metabolic precursor of both triglycerides and phospholipids (see Fig. 3.7). Platelet-activating factor, a mediator of inflammation, is an unusual phospholipid, with a lipid alcohol rather than an esterified lipid at the *sn*-1 position, an acetyl group at *sn*-2, and phosphorylcholine esterified at the *sn*-3 position. Cholesterol is less polar than phospholipids; the hydroxyl group tends to be on the membrane surface, while the polycyclic system intercalates between the fatty acid chains of phospholipids.

⬥ ADVANCED CONCEPT BOX
BUTTER OR MARGARINE?

There is continuing debate among nutritionists about the health benefits of butter versus margarine in foods. Butter is rich in both cholesterol and triglycerides containing saturated fatty acids, both of which are dietary risk factors for atherosclerosis. Margarine contains no cholesterol and is richer in unsaturated fatty acids.

However, the unsaturated fatty acids in margarine are mostly the unnatural *trans*-fatty acids formed during the partial hydrogenation of vegetable oils. Like saturated fatty acids, *trans*-fatty acids are atherogenic, suggesting that there are comparable risks associated with the consumption of butter or margarine. The resolution of this issue is complicated by the fact that various forms of margarine - for example, soft-spread and hard-block types - vary significantly in their content of *trans*-fatty acids. Partially hydrogenated oils are more stable than the natural oils during heating; when used for deep-frying, they need to be changed less frequently. Despite the additional expense, the food and food-service industries have gradually shifted to the use of natural oils, rich in unsaturated fatty acids and without *trans*-fatty acids, for cooking and baking.

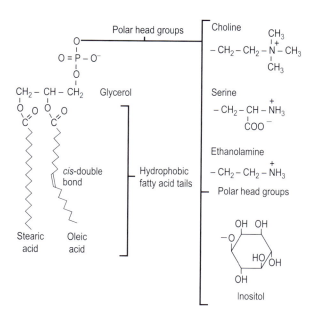

Fig. 3.7 **Structure of the major phospholipids of animal cell membranes.** Phosphatidylcholine, phosphatidylserine, phosphatidylethanolamine, and phosphatidylinositol.

Phospholipids

Phospholipids are the major lipids in biological membranes

Phospholipids are polar lipids derived from phosphatidic acid (1,2-diacyl-glycerol-3-phosphate; see Fig. 3.6). Like triglycerides, the glycerophospholipids contain a spectrum of fatty acids at the *sn*-1 and *sn*-2 positions, but the *sn*-3 position is occupied by phosphate esterified to an amino compound. The phosphate acts as a bridging diester, linking the diacylglyceride to a polar, nitrogenous compound, most frequently choline, ethanolamine, or serine (Fig. 3.7). Phosphatidylcholine (**lecithin**), for example, usually contains palmitic acid or stearic acid at its *sn*-1 position and an 18-carbon, unsaturated fatty acid (e.g., oleic, linoleic, or linolenic) at its *sn*-2 position. Phosphatidylethanolamine (cephalin) usually has a longer-chain polyunsaturated fatty acid at the *sn*-2 position, such as arachidonic acid. These complex lipids contribute charge to biological membranes (see Fig. 3.8): phosphatidylserine and phosphatidylinositol are anionic, whereas phosphatidylcholine and phosphatidylethanolamine are zwitterionic at physiologic pH and have no net charge. A number of other phospholipid structures with special functions are introduced in later chapters.

When phospholipids are dispersed in aqueous solution, they spontaneously form lamellar structures, and under suitable conditions, they organize into extended bilayer structures - not only lamellar structures but also closed vesicular structures termed **liposomes.** The liposome is a model for the structure of a biological membrane, a bilayer of polar lipids with the polar faces exposed to the aqueous environment and the fatty acid side chains buried in the oily, hydrophobic interior of the membrane. The liposomal surface membrane is a pliant, mobile, and flexible structure at body temperature.

Biological membranes also contain another important amphipathic lipid: cholesterol, a flat, rigid hydrophobic molecule with a polar hydroxyl group (see Fig. 3.6). Cholesterol is found in all biomembranes and acts as a modulator of membrane fluidity. At lower temperatures, it interferes with fatty acid chain associations and increases fluidity, but at higher temperatures, it tends to limit disorder and decrease fluidity. Cholesterol–phospholipid mixtures have properties intermediate between the gel and liquid crystalline states of the pure phospholipids; they form stable but supple membrane structures.

STRUCTURE OF BIOMEMBRANES

Eukaryotic cells have a plasma membrane and intracellular membranes that define compartments with specialized functions

Cellular and organelle membranes differ significantly in protein and lipid composition (Table 3.3). In addition to the major phospholipids described in Fig. 3.7, other important membrane lipids include cardiolipin, sphingolipids (sphingomyelin and glycolipids), and cholesterol, which are described in detail in later chapters. Cardiolipin (diphosphatidyl glycerol) is a significant component of the mitochondrial inner membrane, whereas sphingomyelin, phosphatidylserine, and cholesterol are enriched in the plasma membrane (see Table 3.3). Some lipids are distributed asymmetrically in the membrane; for example, phosphatidylserine (PS) and phosphatidylethanolamine (PE) are enriched on the inside, and phosphatidylcholine (PC) and sphingomyelin on the outside, of the red blood cell membrane. The protein-to-lipid ratio also differs among various biomembranes, ranging from about 80% (dry weight) lipid in the myelin sheath that insulates nerve cells to about 20% lipid

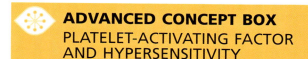

ADVANCED CONCEPT BOX
PLATELET-ACTIVATING FACTOR AND HYPERSENSITIVITY

Platelet-activating factor (PAF; see Fig. 3.6) contains an acetyl group at C-2 of glycerol and a saturated 18-carbon alkyl ether group linked to the hydroxyl group at C-1, rather than the usual long-chain fatty acids of phosphatidylcholine. It is a major mediator of hypersensitivity reactions, acute inflammatory reactions, and anaphylactic shock, and it affects the permeability properties of membranes, increasing platelet aggregation and causing cardiovascular and pulmonary changes, including edema and hypotension.

In allergic persons, cells involved in the immune response become coated with immunoglobulin E (IgE) molecules that are specific for a particular antigen or allergen, such as pollen or insect venom. When these individuals are reexposed to that antigen, antigen–IgE complexes form on the surface of the inflammatory cells and activate the synthesis and release of PAF.

Table 3.3 Phospholipid composition of organelle membranes from rat liver

	Mitochondria	Microsomes	Lysosomes	Plasma membrane	Nuclear membrane	Golgi membrane
Cardiolipin	18	1	1	1	4	1
Phosphatidylethanolamine	35	22	14	23	13	20
Phosphatidylcholine	40	58	40	39	55	50
Phosphatidylinositol	5	10	5	8	10	12
Phosphatidylserine	1	2	2	9	3	6
Phosphatidic acid	–	1	1	1	2	<1
Sphingomyelin	1	1	20	16	3	8
Phospholipids (mg/mg protein)	0.18	0.37	0.16	0.67	0.50	0.83
Cholesterol (mg/mg protein)	<0.01	0.01	0.04	0.13	0.04	0.08

This table shows the phospholipid composition (%) of various organelle membranes together with weight ratios of phospholipids and cholesterol to protein.

in the inner mitochondrial membrane. Lipids affect the structure of the membrane, the activity of membrane enzymes and transport systems, and membrane function in processes such as cellular recognition and signal transduction. Exposure of phosphatidylserine in the outer leaflet of the erythrocyte plasma membrane increases the cell's adherence to the vascular wall and is a signal for macrophage recognition and phagocytosis, mediating red cell turnover in the spleen.

The fluid mosaic model

The fluid mosaic model portrays cell membranes as flexible lipid bilayers with embedded proteins

The generally accepted model of biomembrane structure is the fluid mosaic model proposed by Singer and Nicolson in 1972. This model represents the membrane as a fluidlike phospholipid bilayer into which other lipids and proteins are embedded (Fig. 3.8). As in liposomes, the polar head groups of the phospholipids are exposed on the external surfaces of the membrane, with the fatty acyl chains oriented to the inside of the membrane. Whereas membrane lipids and proteins easily move on the membrane surface (lateral diffusion), "flip-flop" movement of lipids between the outer and inner bilayer leaflets rarely occurs without the aid of the membrane enzyme flippase.

Membrane proteins are classified as integral (intrinsic) or peripheral (extrinsic) membrane proteins. The former are embedded deeply in the lipid bilayer, and some of them traverse the membrane several times (**transmembrane proteins**) and have both internal and external polypeptide segments that participate in regulatory processes. In contrast, peripheral membrane proteins are bound to membrane lipids and/or integral membrane proteins (see Fig. 3.8); they can be removed from the membrane by mild denaturing agents, such as urea or mild detergent, without destroying the integrity of the membrane. In contrast, integral and transmembrane

proteins can be removed from the membrane only by treatments that dissolve membrane lipids and destroy the integrity of the membrane. Most of the transmembrane segments of integral membrane proteins form α-helices. They are composed primarily of amino acid residues with nonpolar side chains - about 20 amino acid residues forming six to seven α-helical turns are enough to traverse a membrane of 5 nm (50 Å) in thickness. The transmembrane domains interact with one another and with the hydrophobic tails of the lipid molecules, often forming complex structures, such as channels involved in ion-transport processes (see Fig. 3.8 and Chapter 4).

Membranes maintain the structural integrity, cellular recognition processes, and transport functions of the cell

There is growing evidence that many membrane proteins have limited mobility and are anchored in place by attachment to cytoskeletal proteins. Membrane substructures, described as lipid rafts, also demarcate regions of membranes with specialized composition and function. Specific phospholipids are also enriched in regions of the membrane involved in endocytosis and junctions with adjacent cells. However, fluidity is essential for membrane function and cell viability. For example, when bacteria are transferred to lower temperature, they respond by increasing the content of unsaturated fatty acids in membrane phospholipids, thereby decreasing the melting/freezing temperature and maintaining membrane fluidity at low temperature. The membrane also mediates the transfer of information and molecules between the outside and inside of the cell, including cellular recognition, signal transduction processes, and metabolite and ion transport; fluidity is essential for these functions. Overall, cell membranes, which are often viewed by microscopy as static, are well-organized, flexible, and responsive structures. In fact, the microscope picture is like a high-speed photo of a sporting event; it may look peaceful and still, but there's a lot of action going on.

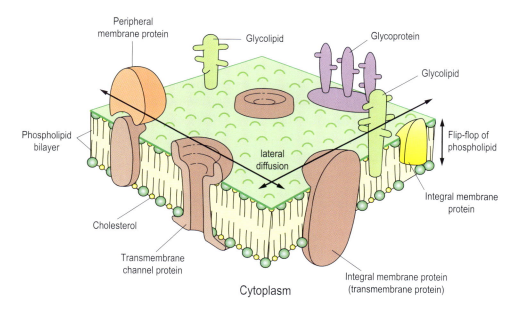

Peripheral membrane protein

Glycolipid

Glycoprotein

Glycolipid

Phospholipid bilayer

Flip-flop of phospholipid

lateral diffusion

Integral membrane protein

Cholesterol

Transmembrane channel protein

Cytoplasm

Integral membrane protein (transmembrane protein)

Fig. 3.8 **Fluid mosaic model of the plasma membrane.** In this model, proteins are embedded in a fluid phospholipid bilayer; some are on one surface (peripheral) and others span the membrane (transmembrane). Carbohydrates, covalently bound to some proteins and lipids, are not found on all subcellular membranes (e.g., mitochondrial membranes). On the plasma membrane, they are located almost exclusively on the outer surface of the cell.

 ADVANCED CONCEPT BOX
MEMBRANE PATCHES

Although the fluid mosaic model is basically correct, it is recognized that there are membrane regions with unique protein and lipid compositions. **Caveolae,** 50- to 100-nm plasma membrane invaginations, and lipid rafts are plasma membrane patches (microdomains) important for signal transduction and endocytosis. These patches are enriched in cholesterol and sphingolipids, and the interaction of the long saturated fatty acid tails of sphingolipids with cholesterol results in the stabilization of the fluid environment.

The patches are resistant to detergent solubilization and show high buoyant density on sucrose-density gradient centrifugation. Pathogens such as viruses, parasites, bacteria, and even bacterial toxins may enter into host cells through binding to specific components of caveolae. Classic examples of patches enriched in a particular protein are the purple membrane of *Halobacterium halobium* containing bacteriorhodopsin and gap junctions containing connexin. Bacteriorhodopsin is a light-driven proton pump that generates an H^+-concentration gradient across the bacterial membrane, providing energy for nutrient uptake for bacterial growth. **Gap junctions** between uterine muscle cells increase significantly during the late stages of pregnancy. They provide high-capacity channels between cells and permit coordinated contraction of the uterus during labor.

ADVANCED CONCEPT BOX
MEMBRANE-ANCHORING PROTEINS

Lateral movements of some membrane proteins are restricted by their tethering to macromolecular assemblies inside (cytoskeleton) and/or outside (extracellular matrix) the cell and, in some cases, to membrane proteins of adjacent cells (e.g., in tight junctions between epithelial cells).

Lateral diffusion of erythrocyte integral membrane proteins, band 3 (an anion transporter) and glycophorin, is limited by indirect interaction with spectrin, a cytoskeletal protein, through ankyrin and band 4.1 proteins, respectively. Such interactions are so strong that they limit lateral diffusion of band 3. Genetic defects in spectrin cause hereditary spherocytosis and elliptocytosis, diseases characterized by altered red cell morphology. Ankyrin mutation affects the localization of plasma-membrane proteins in cardiac muscle, causing cardiac arrhythmia, a risk factor for sudden cardiac death.

SUMMARY

Following the previous chapter on amino acids and proteins, this chapter provides a broader foundation for further studies in biochemistry by introducing the basic structural features and physical and chemical properties of two major dietary fuels and building blocks: carbohydrates and lipids.

- Carbohydrates are polyhydroxyaldehydes and ketones; they exist primarily in cyclic forms, which are linked to one another by glycosidic bonds.
- Glucose is the only monosaccharide that exists in the body in free form.
- Lactose and sucrose are important dietary disaccharides.
- Starch, cellulose, and glycogen are important homoglucan polymers of glucose.
- Carbohydrates may be linked to proteins and lipids to form glycoconjugates, known as glycoproteins and glycolipids.
- Lipids are hydrophobic compounds, commonly containing fatty acids esterified to glycerol.
- Fatty acids are long-chain alkanoic acids; unsaturated fatty acids contain one or more *cis*-double bonds, which decreases the melting (freezing) point of lipids.
- Triglycerides (triacylglycerols) are the storage form of lipids in adipose tissue.
- Phospholipids are amphipathic lipids found in biological membranes; they contain a phosphodiester at C-3 of glycerol, linking a diglyceride to an amino compound - most frequently choline, ethanolamine, or serine.

- The fluid mosaic model describes the essential roles of phospholipids, integral and membrane proteins, and other lipids in the structure and function of biological membranes.
- Biological membranes compartmentalize cellular functions and also mediate ion and metabolite transport, cellular recognition, signal transduction, and electrochemical processes involved in bioenergetics, nerve transmission, and muscle contraction.

FURTHER READING

Brand-Miller, J., & Buyken, A. E. (2012). The glycemic index issue. *Current Opinion in Lipidology, 23*, 62–67.

Goñi, F. M. (2014). The basic structure and dynamics of cell membranes: An update of the Singer-Nicolson model. *Biochimica et Biophysica Acta, 1838*, 1457–1476.

Jambhekar, S. S., & Breen, P. (2016). Cyclodextrins in pharmaceutical formulations ii: Solubilization, binding constant, and complexation efficiency. *Drug Discovery Today, 21*, 363–368.

Mensink, M. A., Frijlink, H. W., Van Der Voort, M. K., et al. (2015). Inulin, a flexible oligosaccharide i: Review of its physicochemical characteristics. *Carbohydrate Polymers, 130*, 405–419.

Taubes, G. (2008). *Good calories, bad calories: Fats, carbs, and the controversial science of diet and health*. New York, NY: Anchor Books.

RELEVANT WEBSITES

Carbohydrates:
- http://faculty.chemeketa.edu/lemme/CH%20123/Self-Tests/Carbohydrates.pdf
- http://home.earthlink.net/~dayvdanls/ReviewCarbos.htm
- http://mcat-review.org/carbohydrates.php
- http://www.biology-pages.info/C/Carbohydrates.html

Lipids:
- https://themedicalbiochemistrypage.org/lipids.php
- http://kitchendoctor.com/essays/soap.php

ACTIVE LEARNING

1. Compare the caloric value of starch and cellulose. Explain the difference.
2. Explain why disaccharides such as lactose, maltose, and isomaltose are reducing sugars, but sucrose is not.
3. What does the iodine number of a lipid indicate about its structure?
4. Review the industrial process for making soaps.
5. Review the history of models for biological membranes. What are the limitations of the original Singer–Nicolson model?

ABBREVIATIONS

Fru	Fructose
Gal	Galactose
GlcNAc	N-acetylglucosamine
GlcNH$_2$	Glucosamine
GlcUA	Glucuronic acid
Glc	Glucose
PC	Phosphatylcholine
PE	Phosphatidylethanolamine
PS	Phosphatidylserine

Membranes and Transport

John W. Baynes and Masatomo Maeda

INTRODUCTION

Biomembranes are not rigid or impermeable but highly mobile and dynamic structures

The plasma membrane is the gatekeeper of the cell; it is a fluid structure but also a strong hydrophobic barrier on the surface of the cell (Chapter 3). It controls not only the access and transport of inorganic ions, vitamins, and nutrients but also the entry of drugs and the exit of waste products. Integral transmembrane proteins have important roles in transporting molecules through the membrane and often maintain concentration gradients across the membranes; K$^+$, Na$^+$, and Ca^{2+} concentrations in the cytoplasm are maintained at ~140, 10, and 10^{-4} mmol/L, respectively, by transport proteins, whereas those outside (in the blood) are ~5, 145, and 1–2 mmol/L, respectively. The driving force for transport of ions and maintenance of ion gradients is directly or indirectly provided by ATP; and, in fact, most metabolic energy is used to drive transport processes that maintain ion and metabolite gradients across nerve and muscle membranes and in mitochondria in all tissues. The transport properties of membranes will be illustrated by several important examples.

TYPES OF TRANSPORT PROCESSES

Simple diffusion through the phospholipid bilayer

Some small, neutral molecules can traverse biomembranes by simple diffusion

Small, nonpolar molecules (e.g., O$_2$, CO$_2$, and N$_2$) and uncharged polar molecules (e.g., urea, ethanol, and small organic acids) move through membranes by simple diffusion without the aid of membrane proteins (Table 4.1 and Fig. 4.1A). The direction of net movement of these species is always "downhill," along the concentration gradient, from high to low concentration toward equilibrium.

The hydrophobicity of the molecules is an important requirement for simple diffusion across the membrane because the interior of the phospholipid bilayer is hydrophobic (Chapter 3). The rate of transport of small molecules is, in fact, closely related to their **partition coefficient** between oil and water.

Although water molecules can be transported by simple diffusion, channel proteins (see below) control the movement of water across most membranes, especially in the kidney for concentration of the urine. Mutation in a water-channel protein gene (aquaporin-2) causes diuresis in patients with **nephrogenic diabetes insipidus,** a disease characterized by excessive urination but without the hyperglycemia characteristic of diabetes mellitus (see Chapter 35).

Transport mediated by membrane proteins

Membrane proteins are required for transport of larger molecules across biomembranes

Transport of larger, polar molecules, such as amino acids or sugars, into a cell requires the involvement of membrane proteins known as **transporters,** also called porters, **permeases, translocases,** or carrier proteins. Transporters are as specific as enzymes for their substrates, and they work by one of two mechanisms: **facilitated diffusion** or **active transport.** Facilitated diffusion catalyzes the movement of a substrate through a membrane down a concentration gradient and does not require energy. In contrast, active transport is a process in which substrates are transported uphill, against

Table 4.1 Transport systems of biomembranes

Type		Example	Transport protein	Energy coupling	Specificity	Saturability	Rate (molecules / transport protein/s)
Passive transport or diffusion	Simple diffusion		−	−	−	−	
	Facilitated diffusion		+	−	+	+	
	Transporter	GLUT-1~5					~10^2
	Channel	H_2O, Na^+, K^+, Ca^{2+}, Cl^-					10^7–10^8
Active transport	Primary	Proton pumps	+	+	+	+	10^2–10^4
	Secondary	ABC transporters	+	+	+	+	10^0–10^2*
	Symporter	SGLT-1, 2, neutral amino acids					
	Antiporter	Cl^-/HCO_3^-, Na^+/Ca^{2+}, Na^+/H^+					
	Uniporter	Glutamate					

Transport systems are classified according to the role of transport proteins and energy coupling.
*The Cl^-/HCO_3^- antiporter is unusual among secondary active transport systems because its transport rate is high, at 10^5 molecules / transport protein/s.

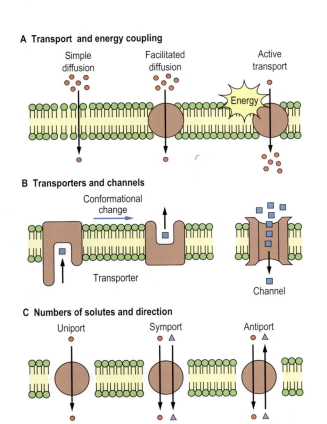

Fig. 4.1 **Various models of solute movement across membranes.**

ADVANCED CONCEPT BOX
ANTIBIOTICS AND MEMBRANE PERMEABILITY

Antibiotics act as **ionophores** and increase the permeability of membranes to specific ions; bactericidal effects of ionophores are attributed to a disturbance of the ion-transport systems of bacterial membranes. Ionophores facilitate the net movement of ions down their electrochemical gradients. There are two classes of ionophores: mobile ion carriers (or caged carriers) and channel formers (Fig. 4.2).

Valinomycin is a typical example of a mobile ion carrier. It is a cyclic peptide with a lipophilic exterior and an ionic interior. It dissolves in the membrane and diffuses between the inner and outer surfaces. K^+ binds in the central core of valinomycin, and the complex diffuses across the membrane, releasing the K^+, gradually dissipating the K^+ gradient. The carrier-type iono-phores, nigericin and monensin, exchange H^+ for Na^+ and K^+, respectively. Ionomycin and A23187 are Ca^{2+} ionophores.

The β-helical gramicidin A molecule, a linear peptide with 15 amino acid residues, forms a pore. The head-to-head dimer of gramicidin A makes a transmembrane channel that allows movement of monovalent cations (H^+, Na^+, and K^+).

Polyene antibiotics such as amphotericin B and nystatin exert their cytotoxic action by rendering the membrane of the target cell permeable to ions and small molecules. Formation of a sterol–polyene complex is essential for the cytotoxic function of these antibiotics because they display a selective action against organisms in which the membranes contain sterols. Thus they are active against yeasts, a wide variety of fungi, and other eukaryotic cells, but they have no effect on bacteria. Because their affinity toward ergosterol, a fungal membrane component, is higher than that for cholesterol, these antibiotics have been used for the treatment of topical infections of fungal origin.

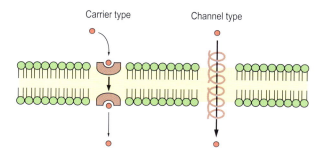

Fig. 4.2 **Mobile ion carriers and channel-forming ionophores.** Ionophores permit net movement of ions only down their electrochemical gradients.

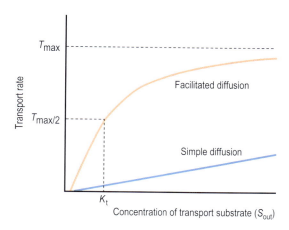

Fig. 4.3 **Comparison of the transport kinetics of facilitated diffusion and simple diffusion.** The rate of transport of substrate is plotted against the concentration of substrate in the extracellular medium. In common with enzyme catalysis, transporter-catalyzed uptake has a maximum transport rate, T_{max} (saturable). K_t is the concentration at which the rate of substrate uptake is half-maximal. For simple diffusion, the transport rate is slower and directly proportional to substrate concentration.

their concentration gradient. Active transport must be coupled with an energy-producing reaction (see Fig. 4.1A).

Saturability and specificity are important characteristics of membrane transport systems

The rate of facilitated diffusion is generally much greater than that of simple diffusion: transport proteins catalyze the transport process. In contrast to simple diffusion, in which the rate of transport is directly proportional to the substrate concentration, facilitated diffusion is a saturable process, having a maximum transport rate, T_{max} (Fig. 4.3). When the concentration of extracellular molecules (transport substrates) becomes very high, the T_{max} is achieved by saturation of the transport proteins with substrate. The kinetics of facilitated diffusion for substrates can be described by the same equations that are used for enzyme catalysis (e.g., Michaelis–Menten and Lineweaver–Burk types of equations; see Chapter 6):

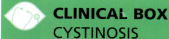

$$S_{out} + \text{transporter} \xrightleftharpoons{K_t} (S \cdot \text{transporter complex}) \longrightarrow S_{in}$$

where K_t is the dissociation constant of the substrate–transporter complex, and S_{out} is the concentration of transport substrate. Then the transport rate, t, can be calculated as

$$t = \frac{T_{max}}{1 + \dfrac{K_t}{S_{out}}}$$

where the K_t is the concentration that gives the half-maximal transport rate. The K_t for a transporter is conceptually the same as the K_m for an enzyme (Chapter 6).

The transport process is usually highly specific: each transporter transports only a single species of molecule or structurally related compounds. The red blood cell GLUT-1 transporter has a high affinity for D-glucose but a 10 to 20 times lower affinity for the related sugars, D-mannose and D-galactose. The enantiomer L-glucose is not transported; its K_t is more than 1000 times higher than that of the D-form.

CLINICAL BOX
CYSTINOSIS

An 18-month-old child presented with polyuria, failure to thrive, and an episode of severe dehydration. Urine dipstick testing demonstrated glucosuria and proteinuria, with other biochemical analyses showing generalized aminoaciduria and phosphaturia.

Comment
This is a classical presentation of infantile cystinosis, resulting from the accumulation of cystine in lysosomes because of a defect in the lysosomal transport protein, cystinosine. Cystine is poorly soluble, and crystalline precipitates form in cells throughout the body. In vitro experiments with cystine loading have shown that renal proximal tubular cells become ATP-depleted, resulting in impairment of ATP-dependent ion pumps with consequent electrolyte imbalances and metabolite losses.

Treatment with cysteamine increases the transport of cystine from lysosomes, delaying the decline in renal function. Cysteamine is a weak base; it forms a mixed disulfide with cysteine, which is then secreted through a cationic amino acid transporter. If untreated, renal failure occurs by 6–12 years of age. Unfortunately, there is a further accumulation of cystine in the central nervous system, despite therapy, with resulting long-term neurological damage.

Table 4.2 Classification of glucose transporters

Transporter	K_t for D-glucose transport (mmol)	Substrate	Major sites of expression
Facilitated diffusion (uniporter) (passive transport)			
GLUT-1	1–2	Glucose, galactose, mannose	Erythrocyte, blood–tissue barriers
GLUT-2	15–20	Glucose, fructose	Liver, intestine, kidney, pancreatic β-cells, brain
GLUT-3	1.8*	Glucose	Ubiquitous
GLUT-4	5	Glucose	Skeletal and cardiac muscles, adipose tissues
GLUT-5	6–11**	Fructose	Intestine
Na⁺-coupled symporter (active transport)			
SGLT-1	0.35	Glucose (2 Na⁺/1 glucose), galactose	Intestine, kidney
SGLT-2	1.6	Glucose (1 Na⁺/1 glucose)	Kidney

K_m values are determined from the uptake of 2-deoxy-D-glucose (*), a nonmetabolizable analogue of glucose, and fructose (**).

Characteristics of glucose transporters (uniporters)

Glucose transporters catalyze downhill transport of glucose into and out of cells

Glucose transporters are essential for facilitated diffusion of glucose into cells. The GLUT family of glucose transporters includes GLUT-1 to GLUT-5 (Table 4.2) and others. They are transmembrane proteins similar in size, all having about 500 amino acid residues and 12 transmembrane helices. GLUT-1,

in red blood cells, has a K_m of ~2 mmol/L; it operates at about 70% of T_{max} under fasting conditions (blood glucose concentration of 5 mmol/L; 90 mg/dL). This level of activity is sufficient to meet the needs of the red cell (Chapter 9). In contrast, pancreatic islet β-cells express GLUT-2, with a $K_m > 10$ mmol/L (180 mg/dL), so it operates at about 30% efficiency at 5-mM plasma glucose concentration. In response to the intake of food and the resulting increase in blood glucose concentration, GLUT-2 molecules respond by increasing the rate of glucose uptake into β-cells, stimulating insulin secretion (Chapter 31). Cells in insulin-sensitive tissues such as muscle and adipose have GLUT-4. Insulin stimulates translocation of GLUT-4 from intracellular vesicles to the plasma membrane, accelerating postprandial glucose uptake.

Transport by channels and pores

Membrane channels or pores are open, less selective conduits for transport of ions, metabolites, and even proteins across biomembranes

Channels are often pictured as tunnels across the membrane, in which binding sites for substrates (ions) are accessible from either side of the membrane at the same time (see Fig. 4.1B). Conformational changes do not participate in the translocation of substrates entering from one side of the membrane to exit on the other side. However, transmembrane voltage changes and ligand binding induce conformational changes in channel structure that have the effect of opening or closing the channels - processes known as **voltage or ligand "gating."** Movement of molecules through channels is fast in comparison with the rates achieved by transporters (see Table 4.1).

The terms *channel* and *pore* are sometimes used interchangeably. However, *pore* is used most frequently to describe more

CLINICAL BOX
DEFECTIVE GLUCOSE TRANSPORT ACROSS THE BLOOD–BRAIN BARRIER AS A CAUSE OF SEIZURES AND DEVELOPMENTAL DELAY

A male infant at the age of 3 months suffered from recurrent seizures. His cerebrospinal fluid (CSF) glucose concentrations were low (0.9–1.9 mmol/L; 16–34 mg/dL), and the ratio of CSF to blood glucose ranged from 0.19 to 0.33; the normal value is 0.65.

The potential causes of low CSF glucose concentrations, such as bacterial meningitis, subarachnoid hemorrhage, and hypoglycemia, were not present, and high CSF lactate values would be found in all these conditions except hypoglycemia. In contrast, the CSF lactate concentrations were consistently low (0.3–0.4 mmol/L; 3–4 mg/dL) compared with the normal value (~2 mmol/L; 20 mg/dL). These findings suggested a defect in transport of glucose from the blood to the brain.

Comment
Assuming that the activity of GLUT-1 glucose transporter in the erythrocyte reflects that of the brain microvessels, a transport assay using the patient's erythrocytes was carried out. The T_{max} for uptake of glucose by his erythrocytes was 60% of the mean normal value, suggesting a heterozygous defect. A ketogenic diet (a high-fat, low-protein, low-carbohydrate diet) was started because the brain can use ketone bodies as oxidizable fuel sources, and the entry of ketone bodies into the brain is not dependent on the glucose transporter system. The patient stopped having seizures within 4 days of beginning the diet.

open, somewhat nonselective structures that discriminate between substrates (e.g., peptides or proteins) on the basis of size. The term *channel* is usually applied to more specific ion channels.

Examples of pores important for cellular physiology

The **gap junction** between endothelial, muscle, and neuronal cells is a cluster of small pores, in which two cylinders of six **connexin** subunits in the plasma membranes join each other to form a pore about 1.2–2.0 nm (12–20 Å) in diameter. Molecules smaller than about 1 kDa can pass between cells through these gap junctions. Such cell–cell interchange is important for physiologic communication or coupling - for example, in the concerted contraction of uterine muscle during labor and delivery. Mutations of the genes encoding connexin 26 and connexin 32 cause deafness and Charcot–Marie–Tooth disease, respectively.

Mitochondrial proteins encoded by nuclear genes are transported to this organelle through pores in the outer mitochondrial membrane. Nascent polypeptide chains of secretory proteins and plasma-membrane proteins also pass through pores in the endoplasmic reticulum membrane during biosynthesis of the peptide chain. Nuclear pores have a radius of about 9.0 nm (90 Å), through which larger proteins and nucleic acids enter and leave the nucleus. Transport of macromolecules through channels and pores is commonly mediated by chaperone or escort proteins.

Active transport

Primary active transport systems use ATP directly to drive transport; secondary active transport uses an electrochemical gradient of Na⁺ or H⁺ ions, or a membrane potential produced by primary active transport processes

ATP is a high-energy product of metabolism and is often described as the "energy currency" of the cell (Chapter 8). The phosphoanhydride bond of ATP releases free energy when it is hydrolyzed to produce adenosine diphosphate (ADP) and inorganic phosphate. Such energy is used for biosynthesis, cell movement, and uphill transport of molecules against concentration gradients. Primary active transport systems use ATP directly to drive transport; secondary active transport uses an electrochemical gradient of Na⁺ or H⁺ ions or a membrane potential produced by primary active transport processes. Sugars and amino acids are generally transported into cells by passive transport - for example, GLUT transporters (Table 8.2) - or by secondary active transport systems.

Primary active transport systems use ATP to drive ion pumps (ion-transporting ATPases, or pump ATPases)

The pump ATPases are classified into four groups (Table 4.3). Coupling-factor ATPases (F-ATPases) in mitochondrial, chloroplast, and bacterial membranes hydrolyze ATP and transport hydrogen ions (H⁺). As discussed in detail in Chapter 8, the mitochondrial **F-ATPase** works in the backward direction, synthesizing ATP from ADP and phosphate as protons move down the electrochemical (concentration and charge) gradient generated across the inner mitochondrial membrane during oxidative metabolism. The product, ATP, is released into the mitochondrial matrix but is needed for biosynthetic reactions in the cytoplasm. ATP is transported to the cytoplasm through an **ATP–ADP translocase** in the mitochondrial inner membrane. This translocase is an example of an **antiport** system (see Fig. 4.1C); it allows one molecule of ADP to enter the mitochondrion only if one molecule of ATP exits simultaneously.

Cytoplasmic vesicles, such as lysosomes, endosomes, and secretory granules, are acidified by a **V-type (vacuolar) H⁺-ATPase** in their membranes. Acidification by this V-ATPase is important for the activity of lysosomal enzymes that have acidic pH optima and for the accumulation of neurotransmitters in secretory granules. The V-ATPase also acidifies the extracellular environments of osteoclasts in bone and renal epithelial cells. Defects in the osteoclast plasma membrane V-ATPase result in osteopetrosis (increased bone density), whereas mutation of the V-ATPase in collecting ducts of the kidney

Table 4.3 Primary active transporters in eukaryotic cells

Group	Member	Location	Substrate(s)	Functions
F-ATPase (coupling factor)	H^+-ATPase	Mitochondrial inner membrane	H^+	ATP synthesis driven by electrochemical gradient of H^+
V-ATPase (vacuolar)	H^+-ATPase	Cytoplasmic vesicles (lysosome, secretory granules), plasma membranes (ruffled border of osteoclast, kidney epithelial cell)	H^+	Activation of lysosomal enzymes, accumulation of neurotransmitters, turnover of bone, acidification of urine
P-ATPase (phosphorylation)	Na^+/K^+-ATPase	Plasma membranes (ubiquitous, but abundant in kidney and heart)	Na^+ and K^+	Generation of electrochemical gradient of Na^+ and K^+
	H^+/K^+-ATPase	Stomach (parietal cell in gastric gland)	H^+ and K^+	Acidification of stomach lumen
	Ca^{2+}-ATPase	Sarcoplasmic reticulum and endoplasmic reticulum	Ca^{2+}	Ca^{2+} sequestration into sarcoplasmic (endoplasmic) reticulum
	Ca^{2+}-ATPase	Plasma membrane	Ca^{2+}	Ca^{2+} excretion to outside of the cell
	Cu^{2+}-ATPase	Plasma membrane and cytoplasmic vesicles	Cu^{2+}	Cu^{2+} absorption from intestine and excretion from liver
ABC (ATP-binding cassette) transporter	P-glycoprotein	Plasma membrane	Various drugs	Excretion of harmful substances, multidrug resistance for anticancer drugs
	MRP	Plasma membrane	Glutathione conjugate	Detoxification, multidrug resistance
	CFTR*	Plasma membrane	Cl^-	c-AMP-dependent chloride channel, regulation of other channels
	TAP	Endoplasmic reticulum	Peptide	Presentation of peptides for immune response

Various examples of primary active transporters (ATP-powered pump ATPases) are listed, together with their locations.
*Some ABC transporters function as channels or channel regulators.
MRP, multidrug resistance–associated protein; CFTR, cystic fibrosis transmembrane conductance regulator; TAP, transporter associated with antigen processing.

causes renal tubular acidosis. F- and V-type ATPases are structurally similar, and they seem to be derived from a common ancestor. The ATP-binding catalytic subunit and the subunit forming the H^+ pathway are conserved between these ATPases.

P-ATPases form phosphorylated intermediates that drive ion translocation: the *P* refers to **p**hosphorylation. These transporters have an active-site aspartate residue that is reversibly phosphorylated by ATP during the transport process. The P-type Na^+/K^+-ATPase in various tissues and the Ca^{2+}-ATPase in the muscle sarcoplasmic reticulum have important roles in maintaining cellular ion gradients. Na^+/K^+-ATPases also create an **electrochemical gradient** of Na^+ that produces the driving force for uptake of nutrients from the intestine (see later discussion). The discharge of this electrochemical gradient is also fundamental to the process of nerve transmission. Mutations of P-ATPase genes cause Brody cardiomyopathy (Ca^{2+}-ATPase), familial hemiplegic migraine type 2 (Na^+/K^+-ATPase), and Menkes and Wilson's diseases (Cu^{2+}-ATPases).

ATP-binding cassette (ABC) transporters comprise the fourth active transporter family. *ABC* is the abbreviation for *ATP-binding cassette*, referring to an ATP-binding motif in the transporter (see Table 4.3). P-glycoprotein (P = permeability) and **multidrug resistance–associated protein (MRP)**, which have a physiologic role in excretion of toxic metabolites

and xenobiotics from cells, contribute to the resistance of cancer cells to chemotherapy. TAP transporters, a class of ABC transporters associated with antigen presentation, are required for initiating the immune response against foreign proteins; they mediate transport of peptides from the cytosol into the endoplasmic reticulum for induction of the immune response. Some ABC transporters are present in the peroxisomal membrane, where they appear to be involved in the transport of peroxisomal enzymes necessary for oxidation of very-long-chain fatty acids. Defects in ABC transporters are associated with a number of diseases, including cystic fibrosis (see Advanced Concept Box).

Uniport, symport, and antiport are examples of secondary active transport

Transport processes may be classified into three general types: **uniport** (monoport), **symport** (cotransport), and **antiport** (countertransport; see Fig. 4.1). Transport substrates move in the same direction during symport and in opposite directions during antiport. The proteins participating in these systems are termed uniporters, symporters, and antiporters, respectively (see Table 4.1). Active transport of ions across a membrane by a uniport system is facilitated by a transporter or channel and is driven by an **electrochemical gradient,** a combination

CLINICAL BOX
MENKES AND WILSON'S DISEASES

X-linked **Menkes disease** is a lethal disorder that occurs in 1 in 100,000 newborn infants and is characterized by abnormal and hypopigmented hair, a characteristic facies, cerebral degeneration, connective tissue and vascular defects, and death by the age of 3 years. A copper-transporting P-ATPase that is expressed in all tissues except liver is defective in this disease (Table 4.3). In patients with Menkes disease, copper enters intestinal cells but is not transported further, resulting in a severe copper deficiency. Subcutaneous administration of a copper histidine complex may be an effective treatment if started early.

The gene for **Wilson's disease** also encodes a copper-transporting P-ATPase and is 60% identical with that of the Menkes gene. It is expressed in liver, kidney, and placenta. Wilson's disease occurs in 1 in 35,000–100,000 newborns and is characterized by failure to incorporate copper into ceruloplasmin in the liver and to excrete copper from the liver into bile, resulting in toxic accumulation of copper in the liver and also in the kidney, brain, and cornea. Liver cirrhosis, progressive neurologic damage, or both occur during childhood to early adulthood. Chelating agents such as penicillamine and triethylamine tetramine are used for the treatment of patients with this disease. Oral zinc treatment may be useful to decrease the absorption of dietary copper. Copper is an essential trace metal and an integral component of many enzymes. However, it is toxic in excess because it binds to proteins and nucleic acids, enhances the generation of free radicals, and catalyzes the oxidation of lipids and proteins in membranes (Chapter 42).

ADVANCED CONCEPT BOX
ABC TRANSPORTER DISEASES

Human genome data suggests that there are about 50 genes for ABC transporters. An unusually wide range of diseases can result from defects in ABC transporters, including Tangier disease, Stargardt disease, progressive intrahepatic cholestasis, Dubin–Johnson syndrome, pseudoxanthoma elasticum, familial persistent hyperinsulinemic hypoglycemia of infancy (PHHI), adrenoleukodystrophy, Zellweger syndrome, sitosterolemia, and cystic fibrosis.

Cystic fibrosis (CF) is the most common potentially lethal autosomal recessive disease of Caucasian populations, affecting 1 in 2500 newborns. CF is usually manifested as exocrine pancreatic insufficiency, an increase in the concentration of chloride ions (Cl^-) in sweat, male infertility, and airway disease, which is the major cause of morbidity and mortality. The pancreatic and lung pathology results from the increased viscosity of secreted fluids (mucoviscidosis). CF is caused by mutations in the gene CFTR (cystic fibrosis transmembrane conductance regulator), which contains an ABC motif and encodes a Cl^- channel. ATP binding to CFTR is required for channel opening. The lack of this channel activity in epithelia of CF patients affects both ion and water secretion.

of the concentration gradient (chemical potential) and the voltage gradient (electrical potential) across the membrane. These forces may act in the same direction or in opposite directions. In symport systems, the movement of one substrate, such as a Na^+ ion, down its electrochemical gradient into the cell drags another substrate into the cell against its concentration gradient; in antiport systems, the movement of one substrate uphill, against its concentration gradient, is driven by counterport of second substrate (usually a cation such as Na^+ or H^+) down its electrochemical gradient.

In the case of Na^+ ions, the concentration difference between outside (145 mmol/L) and inside (12 mmol/L) the cell is about a factor of 10, being maintained by the Na^+/K^+-ATPase. The **Na^+/K^+-ATPase** is electrogenic, pumping out three Na^+ and pumping in two K^+ ions, generating an inside-negative membrane potential. K^+ leaks out through K^+ channels, down its concentration gradient (140 mmol/L to 5 mmol/L), further increasing the electrical potential. The concentration gradient of Na^+ ions and the electrical potential (inside-negative) power the import and export of other molecules with Na^+ against their concentration gradients by symporters and antiporters, respectively.

Examples of transport systems and their coupling

Ca^{2+} transport and mobilization in muscle

Membrane depolarization opens up voltage-dependent ion channels at the neuromuscular junction

Striated muscle (skeletal and cardiac) is composed of bundles of muscle cells (Chapter 37). Each cell is packed with bundles of actin and myosin filaments (myofibrils) that produce contraction. During muscle contraction, nerves at the neuromuscular junction stimulate local depolarization of the membrane by opening voltage-dependent Na^+ channels. The depolarization spreads rapidly into invaginations of the plasma membrane called transverse (T) tubules, which extend around the myofibrils (see Fig. 37.5).

Voltage-dependent Ca^{2+} channels (VDCC) located in the T tubules of skeletal muscle change their conformation in response to membrane depolarization, and they directly activate a Ca^{2+}-release channel in the sarcoplasmic reticulum membrane, a network of flattened tubules that surrounds each myofibril in the muscle cell cytoplasm (see Fig. 36.5). The escape of Ca^{2+} from the lumen (interior compartment) of the sarcoplasmic reticulum increases the cytoplasmic concentration of Ca^{2+} (depolarization-induced Ca^{2+} release) about 100-fold, from 10^{-4} mmol/L (0.0007 mg/L) to about 10^{-2} mmol/L (0.07 mg/dL), triggering ATP hydrolysis by myosin, which initiates muscle contraction. A Ca^{2+}-ATPase in the sarcoplasmic reticulum then hydrolyzes ATP to transport Ca^{2+} back out of the cytoplasm into the lumen of the sarcoplasmic reticulum, decreasing the cytoplasmic Ca^{2+} and allowing the muscle to relax (Fig. 4.4, left).

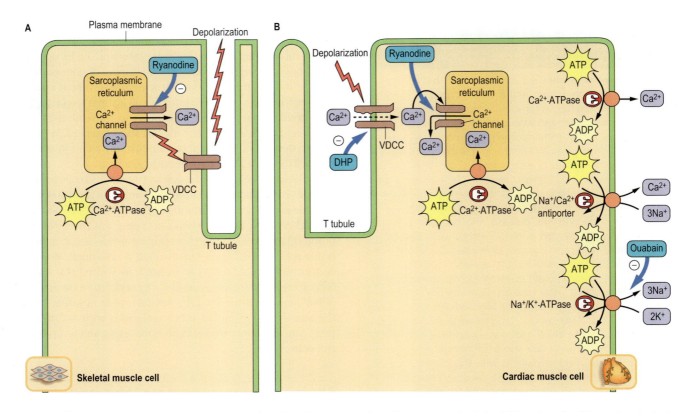

Fig. 4.4 Ca²⁺ movement in muscle contraction cycle. Roles of transporters in Ca²⁺ movements in skeletal (A) and cardiac (B) muscle cells during contraction. Thick arrows indicate the binding sites for inhibitors. In **skeletal muscle,** VDCCs directly activate the release of Ca²⁺ from the sarcoplasmic reticulum. The increased cytoplasmic Ca²⁺ concentration triggers muscle contraction. A Ca²⁺-ATPase in the sarcoplasmic reticulum pumps Ca²⁺ back into the lumen of the sarcoplasmic reticulum, decreasing the cytoplasmic Ca²⁺ concentration, and the muscle relaxes. In **heart muscle,** VDCCs allow entry of a small amount of Ca²⁺, which induces the release of Ca²⁺ from the lumen of sarcoplasmic reticulum. Two types of Ca²⁺-ATPases and an Na⁺/Ca²⁺-antiporter also pumps cytoplasmic Ca²⁺ out of the muscle cell. The Na⁺/Ca²⁺-antiporter uses the sodium (Na⁺) gradient produced by Na⁺/K⁺-ATPase to antiport Ca²⁺. Dihydropyridine (DHP; e.g., nifedipine) is a calcium-channel blocker used for the treatment of hypertension. Ryanodine is a potent inhibitor of the Ca⁺⁺ channel in the sarcoplasmic reticulum. Ouabain is a cardiac glycoside that inhibits the plasma membrane Na⁺/K⁺-ATPase. The resultant increase in intracellular Na⁺ limits the activity of the Na⁺/Ca⁺⁺ antiporter, leading to an increase in intracellular Ca⁺⁺ concentration.

In cardiac muscle, VDCCs permit the entry of a small amount of Ca²⁺, which then stimulates Ca²⁺ release through the Ca²⁺ channel from the lumen of the sarcoplasmic reticulum (Ca²⁺-induced Ca²⁺ release). Not only the sarcoplasmic reticulum Ca²⁺-ATPase but also an Na⁺/Ca²⁺-antiporter and a plasma membrane Ca²⁺-ATPase are responsible for pumping Ca²⁺ out of the cytoplasmic compartment of heart muscle (Fig. 4.4, right). The rapid restoration of ion gradients allows for rhythmic contraction of the heart.

Active transport of glucose into epithelial cells

A Na⁺/K⁺-ATPase drives uptake of glucose into intestinal and renal epithelial cells

The transport of blood glucose into cells is generally by facilitated diffusion because the intracellular concentration of glucose is typically less than that of blood (see Table 4.2). In contrast, the transport of glucose from the intestine into blood involves both facilitated diffusion and active transport processes

(Fig. 4.5). Active transport is especially important for maximal recovery of sugars from the intestine when the intestinal concentration of glucose falls below that in the blood. An Na⁺-coupled glucose symporter SGLT1, driven by a Na⁺ gradient formed by Na⁺/K⁺-ATPase, transports glucose uphill into the intestinal epithelial cell, whereas GLUT-2 facilitates the downhill movement of glucose from the epithelial cell into the portal circulation (see Fig. 4.5).

A similar pathway operates in the kidney. The renal glomerulus is an ultrafiltration system that filters small molecules from the blood. However, glucose, amino acids, many ions, and other nutrients in the ultrafiltrate are almost completely reabsorbed in the proximal tubules by symport processes. Glucose is reabsorbed primarily by sodium glucose transporter 2 (SGLT2; one-to-one Na⁺:Glc stoichiometry) into renal proximal tubular epithelial cells. Much smaller amounts of glucose are recovered by SGLT1 in a later segment of the tubule, which couples transport of one molecule of glucose to two sodium ions. The concentration of Na⁺ in the filtrate is 140 mmol/L (322 mg/dL), whereas that inside the epithelial cells is

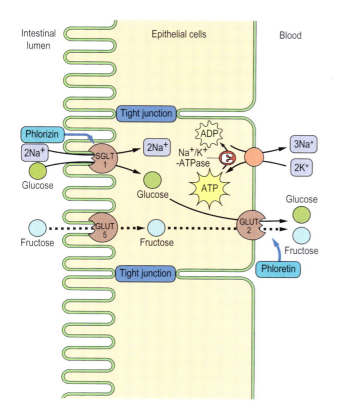

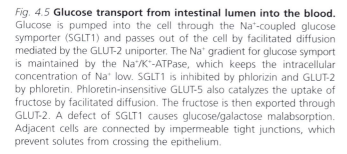

Fig. 4.5 **Glucose transport from intestinal lumen into the blood.** Glucose is pumped into the cell through the Na^+-coupled glucose symporter (SGLT1) and passes out of the cell by facilitated diffusion mediated by the GLUT-2 uniporter. The Na^+ gradient for glucose symport is maintained by the Na^+/K^+-ATPase, which keeps the intracellular concentration of Na^+ low. SGLT1 is inhibited by phlorizin and GLUT-2 by phloretin. Phloretin-insensitive GLUT-5 also catalyzes the uptake of fructose by facilitated diffusion. The fructose is then exported through GLUT-2. A defect of SGLT1 causes glucose/galactose malabsorption. Adjacent cells are connected by impermeable tight junctions, which prevent solutes from crossing the epithelium.

30 mmol/L (69 mg/dL), so that Na^+ flows "downhill" along its gradient, dragging glucose "uphill" against its concentration gradient. As in intestinal epithelial cells, the low intracellular concentration of Na^+ is maintained by an Na^+/K^+-ATPase on the opposite side of the tubular epithelial cell, which antiports three cytoplasmic sodium ions for two extracellular potassium ions, coupled with hydrolysis of a molecule of ATP.

Acidification of gastric juice by a proton pump in the stomach

P-ATPase in gastric parietal cells maintains the low pH of the stomach

The lumen of the stomach is highly acidic (pH ≈1) because of the presence of a proton pump (**H^+/K^+-ATPase**; P-ATPase in Table 4.3) that is specifically expressed in gastric parietal cells. The gastric proton pump is localized in intracellular

CLINICAL BOX
MODULATION OF TRANSPORTER ACTIVITY IN DIABETES

An ATP-sensitive K^+ channel (K_{ATP}) participates in the regulation of insulin secretion in pancreatic islet β-cells. When the blood concentration of glucose increases, glucose is transported into the β-cell through a glucose transporter (GLUT-2) and metabolized, resulting in an increase in cytoplasmic ATP concentration. The ATP binds to the ABC motif of the regulatory subunit of the K^+ channel, K_{ATP}-β, of the sulfonylurea receptor, SUR1, causing structural changes in the K_{ATP}-α subunit, which closes the K_{ATP} channel. This induces depolarization of the plasma membrane (decreased voltage gradient across the membrane) and activates voltage-dependent calcium (Ca^{2+}) channels (VDCC). The entry of Ca^{2+} stimulates exocytosis of vesicles that contain insulin.

Sulfonylureas such as tolbutamide and glibenclamide bind to K_{ATP}-β, stimulating insulin secretion, which decreases blood glucose concentration in diabetes. Defective K_{ATP} channels, which are unable to transport K^+, induce low blood glucose concentration - a condition called persistent hyperinsulinemic hypoglycemia of infancy (PHHI), which occurs in 1 per 50,000 persons - as a result of loss of K^+-channel function and continuous insulin secretion.

ADVANCED CONCEPT BOX
VARIOUS DRUGS INHIBIT TRANSPORTERS IN CARDIAC MUSCLE

Phenylalkylamine (verapamil), benzothiazepine (diltiazem), and dihydropyridine (DHP; nifedipine) are **Ca^{2+}-channel blockers** that inhibit VDCCs (Fig. 4.4). These drugs are used as **antihypertensive agents** to inhibit the increase in cytoplasmic Ca^{2+} concentration and thus the force of muscle contraction. In contrast, cardiac glycosides such as ouabain and digoxin increase heart muscle contraction and are used for the treatment of congestive heart failure. They act by inhibiting the Na^+/K^+-ATPase that generates the Na^+ concentration gradient used to drive export of Ca^{2+} by the Na^+/Ca^{2+} antiporter. Snake venoms, such as α-bungarotoxin, and tetrodotoxin from the puffer fish inhibit voltage-dependent Na^+ channels. Lidocaine, a Na^+-channel blocker, is used as a local anesthetic and antiarrhythmic drug. Inhibition of Na^+ channels represses transmission of the depolarization signal.

vesicles in the resting state. Stimuli such as histamine and gastrin induce fusion of the vesicles with the plasma membrane (Fig. 4.6A). The H^+/K^+-ATPase pump antiports two cytoplasmic protons and two extracellular potassium ions, coupled with hydrolysis of a molecule of ATP. The counter-ion Cl^- is secreted through a Cl^- channel, producing hydrochloric acid (HCl; gastric acid) in the lumen (Fig. 4.6B).

A

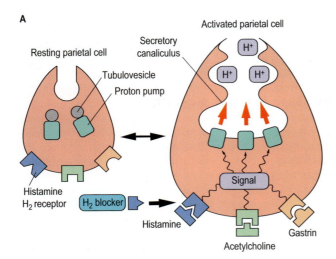

Resting parietal cell

Activated parietal cell

Secretory canaliculus

Tubulovesicle

Proton pump

Histamine H$_2$ receptor

H$_2$ blocker

Histamine

Signal

Acetylcholine

Gastrin

H$^+$

B

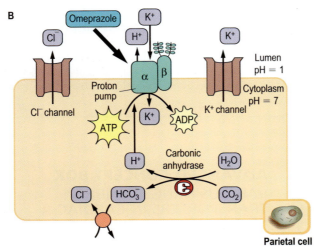

Omeprazole

K$^+$

Cl$^-$

H$^+$

K$^+$

α β

Cl$^-$ channel

Lumen pH = 1

Cytoplasm pH = 7

K$^+$ channel

Proton pump

ATP

K$^+$

ADP

H$^+$

Carbonic anhydrase

H$_2$O

Cl$^-$

HCO$_3^-$

CO$_2$

Parietal cell

Fig. 4.6 **Acid secretion from gastric parietal cells.** (A) Acid secretion is stimulated by extracellular signals and accompanied by morphologic changes in parietal cells, from resting (left) to activated (right). The proton pump (H$^+$/K$^+$-ATPase) moves to the secretory canaliculus (plasma membrane) from cytoplasmic tubulovesicles. H$_2$-blockers compete with histamine at the histamine H$_2$-receptor. (B) Ion balance in the parietal cell. The H$^+$ transported by the proton pump are supplied by carbonic anhydrase. Bicarbonate, the other product of this enzyme, is antiported with Cl$^-$, which is secreted through a Cl$^-$ channel. The potassium ions imported by the proton pump are again excreted by a K$^+$ channel. The proton pump has catalytic α- and glycosylated β-subunits. The drug omeprazole covalently modifies cysteine residues located in the extra-cytoplasmic domain of the α-subunit and inhibits the proton pump.

SUMMARY

■ Numerous substrates - such as ions; nutrients; small organic molecules, including drugs and peptides; and proteins - are transported across membranes by various transporters. These integral membrane proteins

CLINICAL BOX
INHIBITING THE GASTRIC PROTON PUMP AND ERADICATION OF *HELICOBACTER PYLORI*

Chronic strong-acid secretion by the gastric proton pump injures the stomach and the duodenum, leading to gastric and duodenal ulcers. Proton pump inhibitors such as omeprazole are delivered to parietal cells from the circulation after oral administration. Omeprazole is a prodrug: it accumulates in the acidic compartment because it is a weak base, and it is converted to the active compound under the acidic conditions in the gastric lumen. The active form covalently modifies cysteine residues located in the extracytoplasmic domain of the proton pump. H$_2$-blockers (receptor antagonists) such as cimetidine and ranitidine indirectly inhibit acid secretion by competing with histamine for its receptor (Fig. 4.6).

Comment

Infection of the stomach by *Helicobacter pylori* also causes ulcers and is associated with an increased risk of gastric adenocarcinoma. Recently, antibiotic treatment has been introduced to eradicate *H. pylori*. Interestingly, antibiotic treatment together with omeprazole is much more effective, possibly because of an increased stability of the antibiotic under the weakly acidic condition produced by proton pump inhibition.

ACTIVE LEARNING

1. Describe the similarities between the kinetics of enzyme action and transport processes. Compare the properties of various glucose transporters with those of hexokinase and glucokinase, both kinetically and in terms of physiologic function.
2. Identify a number of transport inhibitors used in clinical medicine (e.g., laxatives and inhibitors of gastric acid secretion).
3. Investigate the process of glucose transport across the blood–brain barrier, and explain the pathogenesis of hypoglycemic coma.
4. Study the role and specificity of ABC transporter in multidrug resistance to chemotherapeutic agents.

control the permeability properties of biological membranes.

■ Protein-mediated transport is a saturable process with high substrate specificity.

■ Facilitated diffusion is catalyzed by transporters that permit the movement of ions and molecules down concentration gradients, whereas uphill, or active, transport requires energy.

■ Primary active transport is catalyzed by pump ATPases that use energy produced by ATP hydrolysis.

■ Secondary active transport uses the electrochemical gradients of Na$^+$ and H$^+$ or the membrane potential produced by primary active transport processes. Uniport, symport, and antiport are examples of secondary active transport.

■ The expression of unique sets of transporters is important for specific cell functions, such as muscle contraction, nutrient and ion absorption by intestinal and renal epithelial cells, and secretion of acid from gastric parietal cells.

FURTHER READING

Chen, L. Q., Cheung, L. S., Feng, L., et al. (2015). Transport of sugars. *Annual Review of Biochemistry, 84*, 865–894.

Dlugosz, A., & Janecka, A. (2016). ABC transporters in the development of multidrug resistance in cancer therapy. *Current Pharmaceutical Design, 22*, 4705–4716.

Elborn, J. S. (2016). Cystic fibrosis. *Lancet, 388*, 2519–2531.

Kiela, P. R., & Ghishan, F. K. (2016). Physiology of intestinal absorption and secretion. *Best Practice and Research. Clinical Gastroenterology, 30*, 145–159.

Meinecke, M., Bartsch, P., & Wagner, R. (2016). Peroxisomal protein import pores. *Biochimica et Biophysica Acta, 1863*, 821–827.

Savarino, V., Dulbecco, P., de Bortoli, N., et al. (2017). The appropriate use of proton pump inhibitors (PPIs): Need for a reappraisal. *European Journal of Internal Medicine, 37*, 19–24.

Staudt, C., Puissant, E., & Boonen, M. (2016). Subcellular trafficking of mammalian lysosomal proteins: An extended view. *International Journal of Molecular Sciences, 18*, 1–25.

Watson, H. (2015). Biological membranes. *Essays in Biochemistry, 59*, 43–69.

Zhu, C., Chen, Z., & Jiang, Z. (2016). Expression, distribution and role of aquaporin water channels in human and animal stomach and intestines. *International Journal of Molecular Sciences, 17*, 1–18.

RELEVANT WEBSITES

General reviews:
  Human ABC transporters: https://www.youtube.com/watch?v=AYGnZHzXsLs
Animations:
  http://www.stolaf.edu/people/giannini/biological%20anamations.html
  https://www.youtube.com/watch?v=ovHYKlHYpyA

ABBREVIATIONS

ABC	ATP binding cassette
CF	Cystic fibrosis
GLUT	Glucose transporter
K_t	Concentration required for half-maximal rate of transport
MDR	Multidrug resistance-associated protein
SGLT	Na^+-coupled glucose transporter
T_{max}	Maximum rate of transport
VDCC	Voltage-dependent Ca^{2+}-channel

Oxygen Transport

John W. Baynes, Norma Frizzell, and George M. Helmkamp Jr.

INTRODUCTION

Vertebrates are aerobic organisms

Vertebrates have a closed circulatory system and a mechanism for extraction of O_2 from air (or water) and release of carbon dioxide (CO_2) in waste products. Inspired O_2 leads to an efficient utilization of metabolic fuels, such as glucose and fatty acids; expired CO_2 is a major product of cellular metabolism. This utilization of O_2 as a metabolic substrate is accompanied by the generation of reactive oxygen species (ROS) that are capable of damaging virtually all biological macromolecules (Chapter 42). Organisms protect themselves from radical damage in several ways: sequestering O_2, limiting production of ROS, and detoxifying them. **Heme proteins** participate in these protective mechanisms by sequestering and transporting oxygen. The major heme proteins in mammals are myoglobin (Mb) and hemoglobin (Hb). Mb is found primarily in skeletal and striated muscle, and it serves to store O_2 in the cytoplasm and deliver it on demand to the mitochondrion. Hb is restricted to erythrocytes, where it facilitates the transport of O_2 and CO_2 between the lungs and peripheral tissues. This chapter presents the molecular features of Mb and Hb, the biochemical and physiologic relationships between the structures of Mb and Hb and their interaction with O_2 and other small molecules, and the pathologic aspects of selected Hb mutations.

Properties of oxygen

Most oxygen in the body is bound to a carrier protein containing heme

Photosynthetic organisms release diatomic oxygen into the earth's atmosphere during energy production, contributing to the current level of 21% oxygen in air. In mixtures of gases, each component makes a specific contribution, known as its partial pressure (Dalton's law), that is directly proportional to its concentration. It is also customary to use the partial pressure of a gas as a measure of its concentration in physiologic fluids. For atmospheric O_2 at a barometric pressure (sea level) of 760 mmHg, or torr (101.3 kP, or kPa; 1 atmosphere absolute, or ATA), the partial pressure of oxygen, pO_2, is ~160 mmHg (21% of 760). The amount of O_2 in solution is, in turn, directly proportional to its partial pressure. Thus in the arterial blood (37°C, pH 7.4) the pO_2 is 100 mmHg, which produces a concentration of dissolved O_2 of 0.13 mmol/L. This level of dissolved O_2, however, is inadequate to support efficient aerobic metabolism.

Rather, the major fraction of O_2 transported in blood and stored in muscle is complexed with the iron (ferrous, Fe^{2+}) proteins Hb and Mb, respectively. Hb is a tetrameric protein with four O_2-binding sites (heme groups). In arterial blood with a Hb concentration of 150 g/L (2.3 mmol/L) and O_2 saturation of 97.4%, the contribution of protein-bound O_2 is about 8.7 mmol/L. This concentration represents a dramatic 67-fold increase over physically dissolved O_2. The total oxygen-carrying capacity of the arterial blood, in dissolved and protein-bound forms, is 8.8 mmol/L - almost 200 mL of dissolved oxygen per liter of blood, the equivalent of the oxygen content of a liter of air.

CHARACTERISTICS OF MAMMALIAN GLOBIN PROTEINS

Globins constitute an ancient family of soluble metalloproteins

Globins are a ubiquitous family of proteins, found in microorganisms, plants, invertebrates, and vertebrates. Present-day

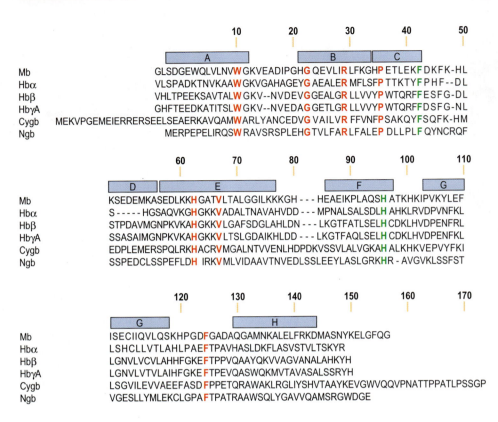

```
                10        20        30        40        50
                |         |         |         |         |
        ┌─────────────A─────────────┐┌──────B──────┐┌───C───┐
Mb      GLSDGEWQLVLNVW GKVEADIPGHG QEVLIR LFKGHP ETLEKF DKFK-HL
Hbα     VLSPADKTNVKAAW GKVGAHAGEYG AEALER MFLSFP TTKTYF PHF--DL
Hbβ     VHLTPEEKSAVTALW GKV--NVDEVG GEALGR LLVVYP WTQRFF ESFG-DL
HbγA    GHFTEEDKATITSLW GKV--NVEDAG GETLGR LLVVYP WTQRFF DSFG-NL
Cygb    MEKVPGEMEIERRERSEELSEAERKAVQAMW ARLYANCEDVG VAILVR FFVNFP SAKQYF SQFK-HM
Ngb     MERPEPELIRQSW RAVSRSPLEHG TVLFAR LFALEP DLLPLF QYNCRQF
```

```
                60        70        80        90       100       110
                |         |         |         |         |         |
        ┌──D──┐┌──────────E──────────┐      ┌─────F─────┐  ┌───G───┐
Mb      KSEDEMKASEDLKKH GATVLTALGGILKKKGH --- HEAEIKPLAQSH ATKHKIPVKYLEF
Hbα     S-----HGSAQVKGH GKKVADALTNAVAHVDD --- MPNALSALSDLH AHKLRVDPVNFKL
Hbβ     STPDAVMGNPKVKAH GKKVLGAFSDGLAHLDN --- LKGTFATLSELH CDKLHVDPENFRL
HbγA    SSASAIMGNPKVKAH GKKVLTSLGDAIKHLDD --- LKGTFAQLSELH CDKLHVDPENFKL
Cygb    EDPLEMERSPQLRKH ACRVMGALNTVVENLHDPDKVSSVLALVGKAH ALKHKVEPVYFKI
Ngb     SSPEDCLSSPEFLDH IRKVMLVIDAAVTNVEDLSSLEEYLASLGRKHR - AVGVKLSSFST
```

```
                120       130       140       150       160       170
                |         |         |         |         |         |
        ┌──G──┐      ┌─────────H──────────┐
Mb      ISECIIQVLQSKHPGDF GADAQGAMNKALELFRKDMASNYKELGFQG
Hbα     LSHCLLVTLAHLPAEF TPAVHASLDKFLASVSTVLTSKYR
Hbβ     LGNVLVCVLAHHFGKE FTPPVQAAYQKVVAGVANALAHKYH
HbγA    LGNVLVTVLAIHFGKE FTPEVQASWQKMVTAVASALSSRYH
Cygb    LSGVILEVVAEEFASD FPPETQRAWAKLRGLIYSHVTAAYKEVGWVQQVPNATTPPATLPSSGP
Ngb     VGESLLYMLEKCLGPA FTPATRAAWSQLYGAVVQAMSRGWDGE
```

Fig. 5.1 **Human globin amino acid sequences are highly conserved.** An alignment of human globins is depicted, with identical amino acid residues in orange. The two residues in green, PheCD1 (F) and HisF8 (H), are absolutely conserved in all metazoan globins. Helical segments in myoglobin are identified by the blue bars. Mb, myoglobin; Hbα, α-globin; Hbβ, β-globin; HbγA, γA-globin; Cygb, cytoglobin; Ngb, neuroglobin.

globins, with their spectacular diversity of function, are most likely derived from a single ancestral globin. Although the extent of amino acid identity among invertebrate and vertebrate globins varies widely and can often appear random, two features are noteworthy: the invariant residues PheCD1 and HisF8 and the characteristic patterns of hydrophobic residues in helical segments (Fig. 5.1). Human Mb consists of a single globin polypeptide (153 amino acid residues, 17,053 Da). Human Hb is a tetrameric assembly of two α-globin polypeptides (141 residues, 15,868 Da) and two β-globin polypeptides (146 residues, 15,126 Da). A single heme prosthetic group is noncovalently associated with each globin **apoprotein.**

The secondary structure of mammalian globins is dominated by a high proportion of α-helix, with more than 75% of the amino acids associated with eight helical segments. These α-helices are organized into a tightly packed, nearly spherical tertiary structure, designated the globin fold (Fig. 5.2). So universal is this overall tertiary structure among all globins that the conventional nomenclature for globin residues follows that defined initially for sperm whale Mb - namely, helices A, B, C, and so forth, starting at the N-terminus, separated by corners AB, BC, and so forth, with residues numbered within each helix and corner. For example, residue A14, an amino acid that participates in electrostatic stabilization between helix A and the GH corner, corresponds to Lys[15] in insect Hb, Lys[16] in Mb and α-globin, and Lys[17] in β-globin.

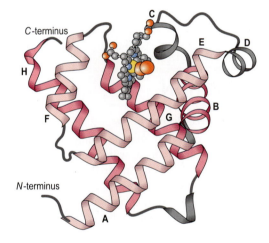

Fig. 5.2 **Myoglobin is a compact globular protein.** In this drawing of mammalian Mb, only the globin polypeptide backbone is shown, with emphasis on the high proportion of secondary structure (exclusively α-helix). The two-layer, three-over-three arrangement of α-helices is highlighted by the light and dark shades of red. The heme group is illustrated as a gray "ball-and-stick" structure, with iron (yellow) and a bound oxygen molecule (red).

Polar amino acids are located almost exclusively on the exterior surface of globin polypeptides and contribute to the remarkably high solubility of these proteins (e.g., 370 g/L [37% protein solution; 5.7 mmol/L] Hb in the erythrocyte). Amino acids that are both polar and hydrophobic, such as

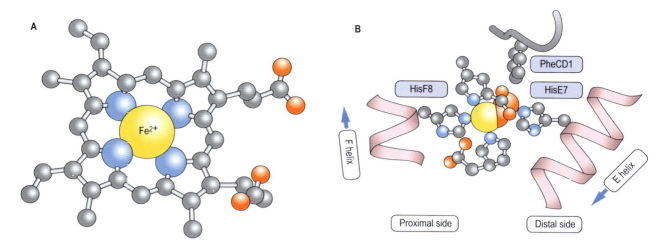

Fig. 5.3 **Heme is a complex of porphyrin and iron.** (A) In this view, the carbon framework of protoporphyrin IX, a conjugated tetrapyrrole ring, is shown in gray; O_2 molecules are red. Iron (yellow sphere) prefers six ligands in an octahedral coordination geometry; pyrrole nitrogen atoms (blue spheres) provide four of these. PheCD1 makes critical hydrophobic and electrostatic stacking interactions with the porphyrin ring. (B) In the oxygenated globin structure, the planar heme is positioned between the proximal and distal histidines (HisF8 and HisE7, respectively); only HisF8 has an imidazole nitrogen (blue sphere) close enough to bond with iron. The α-helices that contain these histidines are shown in pink. In deoxygenated globins, the sixth position remains vacant, leaving a pentacoordinated iron. In the oxygenated state, O_2 occupies the sixth position. Both porphyrin propionate moieties participate in hydrogen and electrostatic bonding interactions with globin side chains and solvent.

threonine, tyrosine, and tryptophan, are oriented with their polar functions toward the protein's exterior. Hydrophobic residues are buried within the interior, where they stabilize the folding of the polypeptide and form a pocket that accommodates the hydrophobic heme prosthetic group. Notable exceptions to this general distribution of amino acid residues in globins are the two histidines, in the E and F helices, that play indispensable roles deep within the heme pocket (Fig. 5.3). Their side chains are oriented perpendicular to and lay on either side of the heme prosthetic group. One of the side chain imidazole nitrogens of the invariant proximal histidine (HisF8) is close enough to bond directly to the pentacoordinate Fe^{2+} atom. On the opposite side of the heme plane, the distal histidine (HisE7), which is too far from the heme iron for direct bonding, functions to stabilize bound O_2 by hydrogen bonding.

Structure of the heme prosthetic group

Heme, the O_2-binding moiety common to Mb and Hb, is a porphyrin molecule to which an iron atom (Fe^{2+}) is coordinated

The Fe-porphyrin prosthetic group of heme is planar and hydrophobic, with the exception of two propionate groups that are exposed to solvent. Heme becomes an integral component of the **holoprotein** during polypeptide synthesis; it is heme that gives globins their characteristic purple-red color - purple in the deoxygenated state in venous blood, red in the oxygenated state in arterial blood.

Globins increase the aqueous solubility of the otherwise poorly soluble, hydrophobic heme prosthetic group. Once sequestered inside a hydrophobic pocket created by the folded globin polypeptide, heme is in a protective environment that minimizes the spontaneous oxidation of Fe^{2+} (ferrous) to Fe^{3+} (ferric: rusting) in the presence of O_2. Such an environment is also essential for globins to bind and release O_2. Should the iron atom become oxidized to the ferric state, heme can no longer interact reversibly with O_2, compromising its function in O_2 storage and transport.

Myoglobin: An oxygen storage protein

Mb binds O_2 that has been released from Hb in tissue capillaries and subsequently diffused into tissues

Located in the cytosol of skeletal, cardiac, and some smooth muscle cells, Mb stores a supply of O_2 that is readily available to cellular organelles, particularly the mitochondrion, that carry out oxidative metabolism. Mb is a monomeric heme protein; with its single ligand-binding site, the reversible reaction of Mb with O_2

$$Mb + O_2 \rightleftharpoons Mb{\cdot}O_2$$

may be described by the following equations:

$$K_a = [Mb{\cdot}O_2]/[Mb][O_2]$$

$$Y = [Mb{\cdot}O_2]/\{[Mb{\cdot}O_2] + [Mb]\}$$

where K_a is an affinity or equilibrium constant, and Y is the fractional O_2 saturation. Combining these two equations,

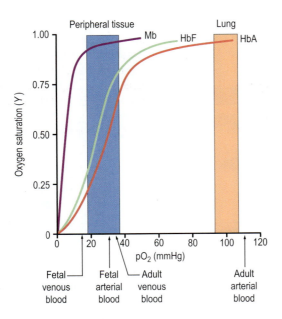

Fig. 5.4 Oxygen saturation curves of myoglobin and hemoglobin. Mb and Hb have different O_2 saturation curves. The fractional saturation (Y) of O_2-binding sites is plotted against the concentration of O_2 (pO_2 [mmHg]). Curves are shown for Mb, fetal Hb (HbF), and adult Hb (HbA). Also indicated, by arrows and shading, are the normal levels of O_2 measured in various adult and fetal blood samples.

expressing the concentration of O_2 in terms of its partial pressure (pO_2) and substituting the term P_{50} for $1/K_a$ yields the equation for the O_2 saturation curve of Mb:

$$Y = pO_2/\{pO_2 + P_{50}\}$$

By definition, the constant P_{50} is the value of pO_2 at which $Y = 0.5$, or half the ligand sites are occupied by O_2. In a plot of Y versus pO_2, the equation for ligand binding by Mb describes a hyperbola (Fig. 5.4) with a P_{50} of 4 mmHg. The low value of P_{50} reflects a high affinity for O_2. In the capillary beds of muscle tissues, pO_2 values are in the 20–40 mmHg range. Predictably, working muscles exhibit lower pO_2 values than muscles at rest. With its high affinity for O_2, myocyte Mb readily becomes saturated with O_2 that has entered from the blood. As O_2 is consumed during aerobic metabolism, it dissociates through mass action from Mb and diffuses into mitochondria, the power plants of the muscle cell. Whales and other diving mammals have unusually high concentrations of Mb in their muscle tissue; the Mb is thought to function as a large oxygen reservoir for prolonged periods under water.

Hemoglobin: An oxygen transport protein

Hb is the principal O_2-transporting protein in human blood; it is localized exclusively in erythrocytes

Adult Hb (HbA) is a tetrahedral array of two identical α-globin and two identical β-globin subunits, a geometry that predicts

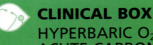

CLINICAL BOX
HYPERBARIC O_2 THERAPY FOR ACUTE CARBON MONOXIDE POISONING

A 22-year-old pregnant woman carrying a fetus of 31 weeks' gestational age was brought to the maternity clinic of a hospital for suspected CO poisoning.

The patient was experiencing headache, nausea, and visual abnormalities. She stated that her workplace had been undergoing repairs to the heating and ventilation systems during the past 2 weeks, and on the day of her hospital visit, the fire department had evacuated the building after detecting a high level of CO, 200 ppm, compared with a typical urban street level of 10 ppm. Her blood pressure was 116/68 mmHg with a pulse rate of 100 and respiratory rate of 24/min. Noteworthy in the patient's evaluation was a carboxy-Hb (COHb) component of 15% of total Hb at the time of admission (normal = 3%, but may exceed 10% in heavy smokers). Fetal monitoring indicated a fetal heart rate of 135, with occasional, moderate irregularities. Uterine contractions were occurring every 3–5 min.

The patient was treated in the hospital's hyperbaric O_2 chamber: 30 min at 2.5 ATA, then 60 min at 2.0 ATA. She also received magnesium sulfate intravenously to resolve the premature contractions. The patient was discharged 2 days later. She delivered a healthy female infant at 38 weeks of gestational age who, on examination at birth and at 6 weeks of age, exhibited no apparent sequelae to maternal exposure to CO or 100% O_2.

Comment
Carbon monoxide is a normal product of heme catabolism and has a range of physiologic activities in vascular, neuronal, and immunologic systems. Like O_2, CO also binds to heme prosthetic groups. Because the affinity of globin-bound heme for CO is about 250 times that for O_2, prolonged exposure of hemoglobin to exogenous CO would be virtually irreversible ($t_{1/2}$ for reversal in blood, 4–8 h) and lead to highly toxic levels of carboxy-Hb. Hyperbaric O_2 is the treatment of choice for severe or complicated CO poisoning.

The administration of 100% O_2 at 2–3 ATA creates arterial and tissue pO_2 values of 2000 mmHg and 400 mmHg, respectively (20 times normal). The immediate result is a reduction in the $t_{1/2}$ of carboxy-Hb in less than 30 min. Hyperbaric O_2 is also used in the treatment of decompression sickness, arterial gas embolism, radiation-induced or ischemic tissue injury, and severe hemorrhage.

several types of subunit–subunit interactions in the quaternary structure (Fig. 5.5). Importantly, within the Hb tetrahedron, each subunit is in contact with the other three. Experimental analysis of the quaternary structure indicates multiple non-covalent interactions (hydrogen bonds and electrostatic bonds) between each pair of dissimilar subunits - that is, at the α–β interfaces. In contrast, there are fewer and predominantly hydrophobic interactions between identical subunits at the α_1–α_2 or β_1–β_2 interfaces. The actual number and nature of

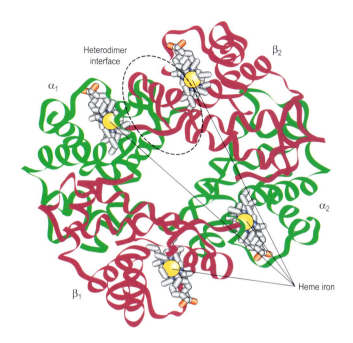

Fig. 5.5 **Hemoglobin is a tetramer of four globin subunits.** Hb is a tetrahedral complex of two identical α-globins (α₁ and α₂, green) and two identical β-globins (β₁ and β₂, maroon). With this geometry, each globin subunit contacts the other three subunits, creating the interfaces and interactions that define cooperativity. One of the heterodimer interfaces is outlined in a dashed oval.

contacts differ in the presence or absence of O₂. Strong associations within each αβ heterodimer and at the interface between the two heterodimers (see Fig. 5.5) are now recognized as major factors determining O₂ binding and release. Thus Hb is more appropriately considered a dimer of heterodimers (αβ)₂ rather than an α₂β₂ tetramer. Although a solution of HbA is theoretically a dynamic mixture of heterodimers and tetramers, under physiologic conditions (high Hb and neutral pH), the equilibria greatly favor the tetramer: 99.0% for oxygenated Hb and 99.9% for deoxygenated Hb.

Interactions of hemoglobin with oxygen

Hb binds oxygen cooperatively, with a Hill coefficient of ~2.7

As a gas-delivery vehicle, Hb must be able to bind O₂ efficiently as it enters the lung alveoli during respiration and to release O₂ to the extracellular environment with similar efficiency as erythrocytes circulate through tissue capillaries. This remarkable duality of function is achieved by cooperative interactions among globin subunits. When deoxygenated Hb becomes oxygenated, significant structural changes extend throughout the protein molecule. In the heme pocket, as a consequence of O₂ coordination to iron and a new orientation of atoms in the heme structure, the proximal histidine and helix F to which it belongs shift their positions (see Fig. 5.3).

This subtle conformational change triggers major structural realignments elsewhere within that globin subunit. In turn, these tertiary structural changes are transmitted, even amplified, in the overall quaternary structure, such that a 12–15° rotation and a 0.10-nm displacement of the α₁β₁ dimer relative to the α₂β₂ dimer take place. Because of the inherent asymmetry of the α₂β₂ tetramer, these combined motions result in quite dramatic changes within and, more importantly, between the αβ heterodimers. Because of structural changes in hemoglobin as a result of binding of oxygen and other effectors, the binding affinity for subsequent molecules of oxygen may be increased (positive **cooperativity**) or decreased (negative cooperativity).

Hb can bind up to four molecules of O₂ in a cooperative manner

With its multiple ligand-binding sites and structural changes in response to binding, the oxygen affinity and the fractional saturation of Hb are more complex functions than those of Mb. Consequently, the equation for the fractional O₂ saturation curve must be modified to the following:

$$Y = pO_2{}^n / \{pO_2{}^n + P_{50}{}^n\}$$

where the exponent n is the **Hill coefficient**. In a plot of Y versus pO_2 when $n > 1$, the equation for ligand binding describes a sigmoid (S-shaped) curve (see Fig. 5.4). The Hill coefficient, determined experimentally, is a measure of cooperativity among ligand-binding sites - that is, the extent to which the binding of O₂ to one subunit influences the affinity of O₂ to other subunits. For fully cooperative binding, n is equal to the number of sites (four in Hb), an indication that binding at one site maximally enhances binding at other sites in the same molecule. The normal Hill coefficient for adult Hb ($n = 2.7$) reflects strongly cooperative ligand binding. Hb has a considerably lower affinity for O₂, reflected in a P_{50} of 27 ± 2 mmHg compared with myoglobin ($P_{50} = 4$ mmHg). In the absence of cooperativity, even with multiple sites, the Hill coefficient would be 1 - that is, binding of one molecule of O₂ would not influence the binding of other molecules. Decreased or absent cooperativity is observed for Hb mutants that have lost functional subunit–subunit contacts (Table 5.1). The steepest slope of the saturation curve for Hb lies in a range of pO_2 that is found in most tissues (see Fig. 5.4). Thus relatively small changes in pO_2 will result in considerably larger changes in the interaction of Hb with O₂. Accordingly, slight shifts of the curve in either direction will also dramatically influence O₂ affinity.

Hemoglobin subunits may assume two different conformations that differ in O₂ affinity

The mechanism underlying the cooperativity in oxygen binding by hemoglobin involves a shift between two conformational states of the hemoglobin molecule that differ in oxygen affinity. These two quaternary conformations are known as the **T (tense) and R (relaxed) states**, respectively. In the T state, interactions between the heterodimers are stronger; in the R state, these noncovalent bonds are, in summation, weaker.

Table 5.1 Classification and examples of hemoglobinopathies

Classification	Common name	Mutation	Frequency	Biochemical changes	Clinical consequences
Abnormal solubility	HbC	$Glu^{6(\beta)} \rightarrow Lys$	Common	Intracellular crystallization of oxygenated protein; increased erythrocyte fragility	Mild hemolytic anemia; splenomegaly (enlarged spleen)
Decreased O_2 affinity	Hb Titusville	$Asp^{94(\alpha)} \rightarrow Asn$	Very rare	Heterodimer interface altered to stabilize T state; decreased cooperativity	Mild cyanosis (blue-purple skin coloration from deoxygenated blood)
Increased O_2 affinity	Hb Helsinki	$Lys^{82(\beta)} \rightarrow Met$	Very rare	Reduced binding of 2,3-BPG in T state	Mild polycythemia (increased erythrocyte count)
Ferric heme (methemoglobin)	HbM Boston	$His^{58(\alpha)} \rightarrow Tyr$	Occasional	Altered heme pocket (mutation of distal His)	Cyanosis of skin and mucous membranes; decreased Bohr effect
Unstable protein	Hb Gun Hill	$\Delta\beta 91–95$	Very rare	Misfolding caused by loss of Leu in heme pocket and shorter helix	Formation of Heinz bodies (inclusions of denatured Hb); jaundice (yellow coloration of integument and sclera); pigmented urine
Abnormal synthesis	Hb Constant Spring	$Tyr^{142(\alpha)} \rightarrow Gln$	Very rare	Loss of termination codon; decreased mRNA stability	α-Thalassemia (hemolytic anemia, splenomegaly and jaundice)

Hemoglobinopathies are usually classified according to the most prominent change to the protein's structure, function, or regulation. Initial identification of a mutation often involves electrophoretic or chromatographic analysis, as shown in Fig. 5.9 for HbSC, a double heterozygous genotype associated with a sickle cell disease–like phenotype. Δ, deletion mutant.

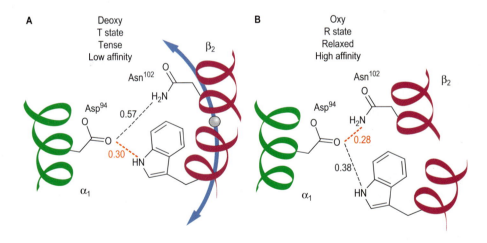

Fig. 5.6 **Noncovalent bonds differ in deoxygenated and oxygenated hemoglobin.** In the middle of the interface between the two $\alpha\beta$ heterodimers are the residues $Asp^{94(\alpha)}$ on the α_1-globin of one heterodimer and $Trp^{37(\beta)}$ and $Asn^{102(\beta)}$ on the β_2-globin of the other heterodimer (see dashed oval in Fig. 5.5). Each has side chain atoms capable of noncovalent interactions. (A) In the deoxygenated T state, the distance between the Asp and Trp residues favors a hydrogen bond, whereas the distance between Asp and Asn is too great. (B) As a result of the conformational changes that accompany the transition to the oxygenated R state, the distance between Asp and Trp is now too large, but the distance between Asp and Asn is compatible with the formation of a new hydrogen bond. Elsewhere along this interface, other bonds are created and broken. An identical alignment of residues and noncovalent interactions is found between the α_2- and β_1-globin monomers. Distances are shown in nanometers (nm). Hydrogen bonds are commonly 0.27–0.31 nm in length.

O_2 affinity is lower in the T state and higher in the R state. Transition between these states is accompanied by the breaking of existing noncovalent bonds and formation of new ones at the heterodimer interfaces (Fig. 5.6). Contact between the two $\alpha\beta$ heterodimers (see Fig. 5.5) is stabilized by a mixture of hydrogen and electrostatic bonds. Approximately 30 amino acids participate in the noncovalent interactions that characterize the deoxygenated and oxygenated Hb conformations.

Several models have been developed to describe the transition between the T and R states of Hb. At one extreme is a

Pulse oximetry (pulse-ox) is a noninvasive method of estimating the oxygen saturation of arterial Hb. Two physical principles are involved: first, the visible and infrared spectral characteristics of oxy- and deoxy-Hb are different; second, arterial blood flow has a pulsatile component that results from volume changes with each heartbeat. Transmission or reflectance measurements are made in a translucent tissue site with reasonable blood flow - commonly a finger, toe, or ear of adults and children or a foot or hand of infants. The photodetector and microprocessor of the pulse oximeter permit a calculation of oxygen saturation (**SpO₂** = peripheral capillary oxygen saturation) that typically correlates within 4%–6% of the value found by arterial blood gas analysis.

Pulse oximetry is used to monitor the cardiopulmonary status during local and general anesthesia, in intensive care and neonatal units, and during patient transport. Body movement, radiated ambient light, elevated bilirubin, and artificial or painted fingernails can interfere with pulse oximetry.

Conventional two-wavelength instruments "assume" that the optical measurements are associated with oxygenated and deoxygenated hemoglobins; they cannot discriminate among oxy-, carboxy-, and metHb. Newer technologies, however, utilize six or eight wavelengths and permit multiple Hb species discrimination with an accuracy of ±2% and precision of ±1%.

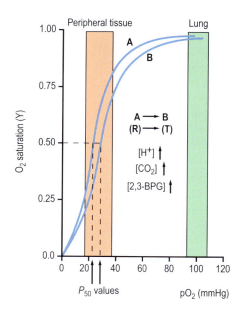

Fig. 5.7 **Allosteric effectors decrease the oxygen affinity of hemoglobin.** O_2 interaction with Hb is regulated by allosteric effectors. Under physiologic conditions, HbA exhibits a highly cooperative O_2 saturation curve. With an increase in the erythrocyte concentration of any of three allosteric effectors - H^+, CO_2, or 2,3-bisphosphoglycerate (2,3-BPG) - the curve shifts to the right (position B), indicating a decreased affinity for O_2 (increase in P_{50} value). Actions of the effectors that modulate O_2 affinity appear to be additive. Conversely, a decrease in any of the allosteric effectors shifts the curve to the left (position A). Increasing temperature will also shift the curve to the right. The sensitivity of O_2 saturation to H^+ is known as the Bohr effect. Normal ranges of O_2 measured in pulmonary and peripheral-tissue capillaries are indicated by shaded areas.

model in which each Hb subunit sequentially responds to O_2 binding with a conformational change, thereby permitting hybrid intermediates of the T and R states. At the opposite extreme is a model in which all four subunits switch concertedly; hybrid states are forbidden, and binding of O_2 to one subunit shifts the equilibrium of all subunits from the T to the R state simultaneously. The molecular structures of deoxygenated and partially and fully ligated Hb have been studied extensively by a broad range of thermodynamic and kinetic techniques, yet progress toward reconciling inconsistencies among classic and more recent models has been slow. These different viewpoints on conformational changes in multiple-subunit proteins are discussed further in the section on allosteric enzymes in Chapter 6.

ALLOSTERIC MODULATION OF THE OXYGEN AFFINITY OF HEMOGLOBIN

Allosteric proteins and effectors

Hb is an allosteric protein; its affinity for O_2 is regulated by small molecules

Hb is one of the best-studied examples of an allosteric protein. Allosteric effectors are small molecules that bind to proteins at sites that are spatially distinct from the ligand-binding sites,

thus their designation as **allosteric (other site) effectors.** Through long-range conformational effects, they alter the ligand- or substrate-binding affinity of the protein. Allosteric proteins are typically multiple-subunit proteins. The O_2-binding affinity of Hb is affected positively by O_2 as well as a number of chemically diverse allosteric effectors, including H^+, CO_2, and **2,3-bisphosphoglycerate** (2,3-BPG; Fig. 5.7). When an allosteric effector affects its own binding to the protein (at other sites), the process is termed **homotropic** (e.g., the effect of binding of O_2 at one site on Hb enhances the affinity for binding of O_2 to other sites on Hb). When the allosteric effector is different from the ligand whose binding is altered, the process is termed **heterotropic** (e.g., the effect of H^+ [pH] on the P_{50} for oxygen binding to Hb). These interactions lead to horizontal shifts in the O_2 binding curves (see Fig. 5.7).

Bohr effect

Acidic pH (protons) decreases the O_2 affinity of Hb

The O_2 affinity of Hb is exquisitely sensitive to pH, a phenomenon known as the Bohr effect. The **Bohr effect** is most readily described as a right shift in the O_2 saturation curve with decreasing pH. Thus an increased concentration of H^+ (decreased pH) favors an increased P_{50} (lower affinity) for O_2 binding to Hb, **equivalent to an H^+-dependent shift of Hb from the R to the T state**.

To understand the Bohr effect at the level of protein structure and to appreciate the role of H^+ as a heterotropic allosteric effector, it is important to recall that Hb is a highly charged molecule. The residues that participate in the Bohr effect include the N-terminal Val amino group of α-globin and the C-terminal His side chain of β-globin. The pK_a values of these weak acids differ sufficiently between the deoxygenated and oxygenated forms of Hb to cause the uptake of 1.2–2.4 protons by the deoxygenated, compared with the oxygenated, tetramer.

Identification of specific amino acid residues of the α- and β-globins that participate in the Bohr effect is complicated by differential interactions of other charged solutes with deoxy- and oxy-Hb. Thus a preferential binding of a given anion (i.e., Cl^- and/or organic phosphates) to deoxygenated Hb involves the alteration of the pKa of some cationic groups, thereby contributing to the overall observed Bohr effect. For example, there is compelling evidence showing that $Val^{1(\alpha)}$ is relevant to the Bohr effect only in the presence of Cl^-. The pK_a of this group shifts from 8.00 in deoxygenated Hb to 7.25 in oxygenated Hb in the presence of a physiologic concentration of Cl^- (≈ 100 mmol/L). Further, the participation of the $Val^{1(\alpha)}$ groups in the chloride-dependent Bohr effect is strongly modulated by CO_2 because of the formation of CO_2 (carbamino) adducts of Hb (described later in the chapter).

As Hb binds O_2, protons dissociate from selected weak-acid functions; conversely, in acidic media, protonation of the conjugate bases inhibits O_2 binding

During their circulation between pulmonary alveoli and peripheral tissue capillaries, erythrocytes encounter markedly different conditions of pO_2 and pH. The high pO_2 in the lungs promotes ligand saturation and forces protons from the Hb molecule to stabilize the R state. In the capillary bed, particularly in metabolically active tissues, the pH is slightly lower due to the production of acidic metabolites, such as lactate. Oxygenated Hb, upon entering this environment, will acquire some "excess" protons and shift toward the T state, promoting the release of O_2 for uptake by tissues for aerobic metabolism.

Effects of CO₂ and temperature

Like H^+, CO_2 is increased in venous capillaries and is a negative allosteric effector of the O_2 affinity of Hb

Closely related to the Bohr effect is the ability of CO_2 to alter the O_2 affinity of Hb. The increase in pCO_2 in venous capillaries decreases the affinity of Hb for O_2. Accordingly, a right shift in the ligand-saturation curve occurs as pCO_2 increases. It should be emphasized that the allosteric effector is, in fact, CO_2, not HCO_3^-: CO_2 forms a reversible covalent bond with the

unprotonated N-terminal amino groups of the globin polypeptides to form **carbamino adducts**:

$$Hb-NH_2 + CO_2 \rightleftharpoons Hb-NHCOO^- + H^+$$

This transient covalent chemical modification of Hb is not only a specialized example of allosteric control, resulting in a stabilization of deoxygenated Hb; it also represents one form of transport of CO_2 to the lungs for clearance from the body. Between 5% and 10% of the total CO_2 content of blood exists as carbamino adducts.

There is a strong physiologic correlation between pCO_2 and the O_2 affinity of Hb. CO_2 is a major product of mitochondrial oxidation and, like H^+, is particularly abundant in metabolically active tissues. Upon diffusing into blood, CO_2 can react with oxygenated Hb, shift the equilibrium toward the T state, and thereby promote the dissociation of bound O_2 (see Fig. 5.7). The vast majority of peripheral tissue CO_2, however, is hydrated by erythrocyte **carbonic anhydrase** to carbonic acid (H_2CO_3), a weak acid that dissociates partially to H^+ and HCO_3^-:

$$CO_2 + H_2O \rightleftharpoons H_2CO_3 \text{ enzyme-catalyzed reaction}$$

$$H_2CO_3 \rightleftharpoons H^+ + HCO_3^- \text{ spontaneous dissociation}$$

Interestingly, from both carbamino adduct formation and hydration/dissociation reactions involving CO_2, an additional pool of protons is generated. These are protons that become available to participate in the Bohr effect and facilitate O_2–CO_2 exchange. During its return to the lungs, blood transports two forms of CO_2: carbamino-Hb and the H_2CO_3/HCO_3^- acid–conjugate base pair. Blood and Hb are now exposed to a low pCO_2, and through mass action, the carbamino adduct formation is reversed, and binding of O_2 is again favored. Similarly, in the pulmonary capillaries, erythrocyte carbonic anhydrase converts H_2CO_3 to CO_2 and H_2O, which are expired into the atmosphere (see Chapter 36).

Working muscles not only produce the allosteric effectors H^+ and CO_2 as by-products of aerobic metabolism but also liberate heat. Because the binding of O_2 to heme is an exothermic process, **the O_2 affinity of Hb decreases with increasing temperature**. Thus the microenvironment of an exercising muscle profoundly favors a more efficient release of Hb-bound O_2 to the surrounding tissue.

Effect of 2,3-bisphosphoglycerate

2-3-Bisphoglycerate (2,3-BPG), an intermediate in carbohydrate metabolism, is an important allosteric effector of Hb

2,3-BPG is synthesized in human erythrocytes in a one-step shunt from the glycolytic pathway (Chapter 9). Like H^+ and CO_2, 2,3-BPG is an indispensable negative allosteric effector that, when bound to Hb, causes a marked increase in P_{50} (see Fig. 5.7). Were it not for the high erythrocyte concentration of 2,3-BPG (~4 mmol/L), the O_2 saturation curve of Hb would approach that of Mb!

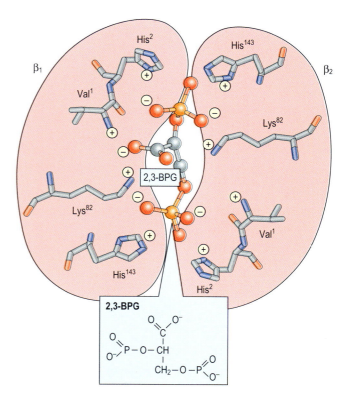

ADVANCED CONCEPT BOX
ARTIFICIAL HEMOGLOBINS

The supply-and-demand curves for whole blood and packed red cell availability and utilization point to an impending crisis and the need to develop alternatives. Red cell substitutes are transfusion alternatives that are potentially useful during major surgical procedures and hemorrhagic shock emergencies.

Three types of artificial O_2 carriers have been investigated: Hb-based oxygen carrier (HBOC), liposome- or nanoparticle-encapsulated Hb, and perfluorocarbon emulsions. HBOCs are hemoglobins derived from allogeneic, xenogeneic, or recombinant sources that have been modified by polymerization, crosslinkage, or conjugation. These modifications facilitate purification and sterilization, and they minimize toxicity and immunogenicity. They are also necessary to stabilize the extracellular Hb tetramers; otherwise, the hemoglobin dissociates into dimers and monomers in plasma and is excreted in urine. The artificial forms have O_2 affinity (P_{50}) in the range 16–38 mmHg, compared to ~27 mM for Hb, but they usually have diminished cooperativity (n = 1.3–2.1) and Bohr effects.

Several HBOCs have progressed through clinical evaluation, and some are used in medical procedures in some countries. Adverse effects are not uncommon with HBOCs. Increased vasoconstriction with subsequent hypertension occurs a result of increased binding of nitric oxide (NO), an endogenous regulator of vasodilation, by extracellular Hb. Other problems include increased heme oxidation to metHb, elevated iron deposition in tissues, gastrointestinal distress, neurotoxicity, and interference with diagnostic measurements. Molecular engineering of human Hb, now under way in a number of laboratories, seeks to improve the O_2 binding and allosteric properties of HBOCs and minimize the side effects. Packaging of hemoglobin in liposomes or nanocapsules, producing artificial red blood cells, is also a promising technology because this limits the escape of Hb into extravascular spaces.

Fig. 5.8 **2,3-Bisphosphoglycerate binds preferentially to deoxygenated hemoglobin.** On the surface of the deoxygenated Hb tetramer where the two β-globins (purple) interact, there is a cleft formed by the N-terminal amino acid residue (Val$^{1(β)}$) and the side chains of His$^{2(β)}$, Lys$^{82(β)}$, and His$^{143(β)}$ (stick models). This site consists of eight cationic groups, sufficient to bind with high affinity one molecule of 2,3-BPG (ball-and-stick model; phosphorus, orange), a molecule with five anionic groups at physiologic pH. This array of positive charges does not exist in oxygenated Hb. In fetal Hb (HbF), His$^{143(β)}$ is replaced by a Ser residue.

At one end of the twofold symmetry axis within the quaternary structure of Hb, there is a shallow cleft defined by cationic amino acids of the juxtaposed β-globin subunits (Fig. 5.8). A single molecule of 2,3-BPG binds to this site. **A critical consequence of the conformational differences between the T and R states is that deoxygenated Hb preferentially interacts with the negatively charged 2,3-BPG.** Multiple electrostatic interactions stabilize the complex between the polyanionic effector and deoxygenated Hb. The cleft is too narrow in fully oxygenated Hb to accommodate 2,3-BPG.

The importance of 2,3-BPG as a negative allosteric effector is underscored by observations that its concentration in the erythrocyte changes in response to various physiologic and pathologic conditions. During chronic hypoxia (decreased pO_2) secondary to pulmonary disease, anemia, or shock, the level of 2,3-BPG increases. Such compensatory increases have also been described in cigarette smokers and on adaptation to high altitudes. The net result is a greater stabilization of the deoxygenated, low-affinity T state and a further shift of the saturation curve to the right, thereby facilitating the release of more O_2 to tissues. Under most circumstances, the rightward shift has an insignificant effect on the O_2 saturation of Hb in the lungs.

SELECTED TOPICS

Interaction of hemoglobin with nitric oxide

Nitric oxide, a potent vasodilator, is stored on Hb as S-nitrosoHb (SNO-Hb)

Nitric oxide (NO) is a gaseous free radical capable of oxidative modification (nitration, nitrosation, nitrosylation) of biological macromolecules. Yet this highly reactive molecule, also known as **endothelium-derived relaxing factor (EDRF)**, is synthesized in endothelial cells and participates in normal vascular physiology, including vasodilation (smooth muscle), hemostasis (platelet), and adhesion molecule expression (endothelial cell).

Erythrocytes make up the largest intravascular reservoir of bioactive NO, and Hb is indispensable for its formation, storage, and release. SNO-Hb is the product of *S*-nitrosylation of the $Cys^{93\beta}$ side chains of Hb. These Cys thiol groups can accept NO by transfer from intracellular *S*-nitrosoglutathione or from heme-bound NO (nitrosyl-Hb). NO is released by exchange from SNO-Hb to Cys side chains of anion exchanger 1, an erythrocyte membrane protein that can then deliver NO to the plasma. The formation and breakdown of SNO-Hb are sensitive to pO_2; NO is released from Hb in response to hypoxia or on conversion to the T state, for example, in venous capillaries, where it induces vasodilation and increased blood flow.

Another remarkable process within the erythrocyte is the allosterically regulated conversion of nitrite (NO_2^-) to NO, a reaction performed by deoxygenated Hb. This intrinsic "nitrite reductase" activity takes advantage of the moderate NO_2^- concentration in the erythrocyte (up to 0.3 μmol/L). Although the chemistry is complex, the reaction is thought to yield a labile intermediate nitrosyl-metHb(ferric) that can readily transfer NO to $Cys^{93(\beta)}$ on oxygenated Hb.

ADVANCED CONCEPT BOX
ACUTE MOUNTAIN SICKNESS - TOO HIGH, TOO FAST

Acute mountain sickness (AMS) develops in individuals who ascend rapidly to ambient conditions of hypobaric oxygen. Symptoms of hypoxia include shortness of breath, rapid heart rate, headache, nausea, anorexia, and sleep disturbance. These can develop at altitudes of 2000 m (25% incidence) and higher to 4000 m or more (50% incidence). The most severe form is high-altitude cerebral edema (2% incidence), a potentially fatal condition characterized by ataxia and other neuromuscular and neurologic problems.

At 4000 m, the barometric pressure is 460 mmHg, leading to an ambient partial pressure of O_2 of 96 mmHg (sea level, 160). Physiologic calculations yield values of a tracheal pO_2 of 86 mmHg (sea level, 149), an alveolar pO_2 of 50 mmHg (sea level, 105), and an arterial pO_2 of 45 mmHg (sea level, 100). At this arterial partial pressure of O_2, Hb saturation is only 81% (see Fig. 5.4). Consequently, the O_2-carrying capacity of arterial blood decreases to 160 mL/L (sea level, 198). Hypoxia can also lead to overperfusion of vascular beds, endothelial leakage, and edema.

Humans adapt to high altitude (acclimatization) by several mechanisms. Hyperventilation is a critical short-term response that serves to decrease alveolar pCO_2 and, in turn, increase alveolar pO_2. Arterial pH is also increased during hyperventilation, leading to a higher affinity of Hb for O_2. A gradual increase in 2,3-BPG typically occurs in response to chronic hypoxia. Another important adaptive mechanism is polycythemia, an increase in erythrocyte concentration that results from erythropoietin stimulation of bone marrow cells. Within 1 week of acclimatization, the Hb concentration can increase by as much as 20% to provide near-normal arterial O_2 content.

Neuroglobin and cytoglobin: Minor mammalian hemoglobins

Two other globins have recently been identified in humans

Neuroglobin (Ngb) is expressed primarily in the central nervous system and some endocrine tissues; cytoglobin (Cygb) is ubiquitously expressed, primarily in cells of fibroblast origin. Tissue concentrations of both are < 1 mmol/L. The Ngb polypeptide has 151 amino acid residues (16,933 Da), whereas Cygb contains 190 residues (21,405 Da), with "extensions" of 20 amino acids at both the N- and C-termini (see Fig. 5.1). Both human proteins share only about 25% sequence identity with Mb and Hb. Yet all key elements of the globin fold are present: the three-over-three α-helix sandwich; the proximal and distal His residues; and a hydrophobic, heme-containing pocket.

In contrast to Mb and Hb, Ngb and Cygb contain hexacoordinate hemes for both the Fe^{2+} and the Fe^{3+} valency states. The distal HisE7, serving as the sixth ligand, must be displaced to permit binding of O_2. Yet the O_2 affinities of Ngb and Cygb are surprisingly high, with P_{50} values in the range of 1.0–7.5 mmHg and 0.7–1.8 mmHg, respectively, compared with a $P_{50} < 27$ mmHg for Hb. Binding of O_2 to the dimeric Cygb is cooperative (Hill coefficient = 1.2–1.7) but independent of pH. Conversely, monomeric Ngb exhibits a pH-dependent O_2 affinity. The functions of these minor globins remain elusive. Ngb appears to be comparable to Mb, mediating the delivery of O_2 to retinal mitochondria. Cygb is thought to function as an enzyme cofactor, supplying O_2 for the hydroxylation of Pro and Lys side chains in some proteins.

Hemoglobin variants

More than 95% of the Hb found in adult humans is **HbA**, with the $\alpha_2\beta_2$ globin subunit composition. HbA₂ accounts for 2%–3% of the total and has an $\alpha_2\delta_2$ polypeptide composition. **HbA₂** is elevated in β-thalassemia, a disease characterized by a deficiency in β-globin biosynthesis. Functionally, these two adult hemoglobins are indistinguishable. Not surprisingly, mutations of the gene encoding δ-globin are without clinical consequence.

Another minor Hb is **fetal Hb** (HbF); its subunits are α-globin and γ-globin. Although it accounts for no more than 1% of adult Hb, HbF predominates in the fetus during the second and third trimesters of gestation and in the neonate. Gene switching on chromosome 11 causes HbF to decrease shortly after birth. The most striking functional difference between HbF and HbA is its decreased sensitivity to 2,3-BPG. Comparison of the primary structures of the β- and γ- polypeptides reveals a replacement of $His^{143\beta}$ by Ser in γ-globin (see Fig. 5.1). Consequently, two of the cationic groups that participate in the binding of the anionic allosteric effector are no longer available (see Fig. 5.8). Predictably, the interaction of

CLINICAL BOX
A STUDENT WITH HYPERVENTILATION, NUMBNESS, AND DIZZINESS

A college student with severe muscle spasms in her arms, numbness in her extremities, some dizziness, and respiratory difficulty was brought to the student health center. The patient had been vigorously exercising in an attempt to relieve the stress of forthcoming examinations when she suddenly began to experience forced, rapid breathing. Suspecting hyperventilation, a health-care worker began to reassure the student and helped her recover by getting her to breathe into a paper bag. After 20 minutes, the spasms ceased, feeling returned to her fingers, and the lightheadedness resolved.

Comment
Alveolar hyperventilation is an abnormally rapid, deep, and prolonged breathing pattern that leads to respiratory alkalosis - that is, a profound decrease in pCO$_2$ and an increase in blood pH that can be attributed to an increased loss of CO$_2$ from the body. With decreased [CO$_2$] and [H$^+$], two allosteric effectors of O$_2$ binding and release, the affinity of Hb for O$_2$ increases sufficiently to reduce the efficiency of delivery of O$_2$ to peripheral tissues, including the central nervous system. Another characteristic of alkalosis is a decreased level of ionized calcium in plasma, a situation that contributes to muscle spasms and cramps. In general, hyperventilation may be triggered by hypoxemia, pulmonary and cardiac diseases, metabolic disorders, pharmacologic agents, and anxiety. See also Chapter 36.

2,3-BPG with HbF is weaker, resulting in an increased affinity for O$_2$ (P_{50} of 19 mmHg for HbF compared with 27 mmHg for HbA) and a greater stabilization of the oxygenated R state. **The direct benefit of this structural and functional change in the HbF isoform is a more efficient transfer of O$_2$ from maternal HbA to fetal Hb** (see Fig. 5.4). Separation of these and other Hb variants in the clinical laboratory is performed by electrophoretic and chromatographic analyses (Fig. 5.9).

CLINICAL TEST BOX
SEPARATION OF HEMOGLOBIN VARIANTS AND MUTANTS: DIAGNOSIS OF HEMOGLOBINOPATHIES

The mobility of a protein during electrophoresis or chromatography is determined by its charge and interaction with the matrix. Three commonly used techniques provide sufficient resolution to separate Hb variants differing in a single charge from HbA: electrophoresis, isoelectric focusing, and ion-exchange chromatography. Electrophoretic and chromatographic separations of Hb are illustrated in Fig. 5.9.

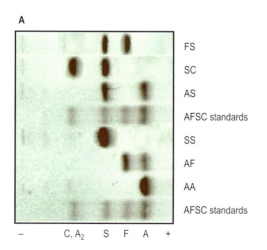
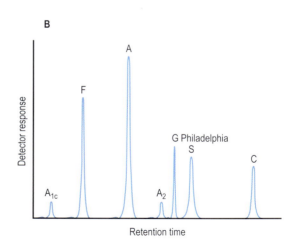

Fig. 5.9 **Normal and abnormal hemoglobins can be separated by electrophoretic and chromatographic methods.** (A) This panel shows cellulose acetate electrophoresis (pH 8.4) of blood samples obtained for neonatal screening. This rapid technique will tentatively identify HbS and HbC, two common mutant hemoglobins in the African American population. Additional tests are required for a definitive diagnosis. FS, Newborn with sickle cell disease; SC, Double heterozygote child with sickle cell–like disease; AS, Child with sickle cell trait; SS, Adult with sickle cell disease; AF, Normal neonate. (B) This trace illustrates high-pressure liquid chromatography (HPLC) with a cation-exchanger solid phase, a technique capable of separating and quantifying more than 40 hemoglobins. HPLC may also be used to measure HbA$_{1c}$, a glycated protein that is measured clinically as an index of mean blood glucose concentration in diabetes mellitus (Chapter 31). Also shown is the elution profile of Hb G Philadelphia (Asn$^{68(\alpha)}$→Lys), a common but benign variant that co-migrates with HbS on electrophoresis.

Sickle cell disease: A common hemoglobinopathy

In sickle cell disease (SCD), distortion of erythrocyte structure (sickling) limits capillary blood flow

Clinically, an individual with SCD presents with intermittent episodes of hemolytic anemia, resulting from chronic lysis of red cells, and painful vasoocclusive crises. Common features also include impaired growth, increased susceptibility to infections, and multiple-organ damage. In the African American population in the United States, SCD affects 90,000–100,000 individuals, a frequency of 0.2%; heterozygous, mostly asymptomatic carriers number 8% in this population.

SCD is caused by an inherited single-point mutation in the gene encoding β-globin, leading to the expression of the Hb **variant HbS**. Indeed, HbS has been studied biochemically, biophysically, and genetically for more than 50 years, making SCD the paradigm of a molecular disease. The mutation is $Glu^{6(\beta)} \rightarrow Val$: a surface-localized charged amino acid is replaced by a hydrophobic residue. Valine on the mutant β-globin subunit fits into a complementary pocket (sometimes called a sticky patch) formed on the β-globin subunit of a deoxygenated Hb molecule, a pocket that becomes exposed only upon the release of bound O_2 in tissue capillaries.

HbA remains a true solute at rather high concentrations, largely as a result of a polar exterior surface that is compatible and nonreactive with nearby Hb molecules. In contrast, HbS, when deoxygenated, is less soluble and has a more hydrophobic surface. It forms long filamentous polymers that readily precipitate, distorting erythrocyte morphology to the characteristic sickle shape. In the homozygous individual with SCD (HbS/HbS), the complex process of nucleation and polymerization occurs rapidly, producing about 10% of circulating erythrocytes that are sickled. In the heterozygous individual (HbA/HbS, sickle cell trait), the kinetics of sickling are decreased by at least a factor of 1000, thereby accounting for the asymptomatic nature of this genotype. In dilute solution, HbS has interactions with O_2 (P_{50} value, Hill coefficient) that are similar to those for HbA. However, the Bohr effect on concentrated HbS is more pronounced, leading to a greater release of O_2 in the capillaries and increased propensity for sickling.

Sickled erythrocytes exhibit less deformability. They no longer move freely through the microvasculature and often block blood flow, especially in the spleen and joints. Moreover, these cells lose water, become fragile, and have a considerably shorter life span, leading to **hemolysis** and **anemia (hemolytic anemia)**. Except during extreme physical exertion, the heterozygous individual appears normal. For reasons that remain to be elucidated, heterozygosity is associated with an increased resistance to malaria, which is caused by the infectious agent *Plasmodium falciparum* in the erythrocyte. This observation represents an example of a selective advantage that the HbA/HbS heterozygote exhibits over either the HbA/HbA normal or the HbS/HbS homozygote and probably

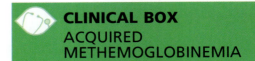

CLINICAL BOX
ACQUIRED METHEMOGLOBINEMIA

In a rural region of the state, a 4-month-old infant was seen at the local emergency room for episodes of seizures, breathing difficulty, and vomiting. The infant's skin and mucous membranes were bluish, indicating cyanosis. Analysis of arterial blood revealed a chocolate brown color, a normal pO_2, an O_2 saturation of 60%, and a metHb (ferric-heme) level of 35%.

The tentative cause of the acute toxic methemoglobinemia was found to be well water contaminated by a nitrate/nitrite concentration of 34 mg/L. The infant was treated successfully by intravenous administration of methylene blue (1–2 mg/kg) that serves to accelerate indirectly the enzymatic reduction of metHb to normal (ferrous) Hb by NADPH metHb reductase, which is normally a minor pathway for conversion of metHb to Hb.

Comment

MetHb is formed when the ferrous iron of heme is oxidized to ferric iron; it is produced spontaneously at a low rate and more rapidly in the presence of certain drugs, nitrites, and aniline dyes. In genetic forms of methemoglobinemia, mutation of either the proximal or the distal His to Tyr makes the heme iron more susceptible to oxidation (see Table 5.1). The extent of oxidation in Hb tetramers can range from one heme group to all four. Erythrocytes contain an NADH-cytochrome b_5 reductase, or NADH diaphorase, that is responsible for the majority of metHb reduction. Infants are particularly vulnerable to methemoglobinemia because their level of NADH-cytochrome b_5 reductase is half that of adults. Moreover, their higher level of HbF is more sensitive to oxidants compared with HbA.

offers an explanation for the persistence of HbS in the gene pool.

Other hemoglobinopathies

More than 1000 mutations in the genes encoding the α- and β-globin polypeptides have been documented

As with most mutational events, most lead to few, if any, clinical problems. There are, however, several hundred mutations that give rise to abnormal Hb with pathologic phenotypes. Hb mutants, or hemoglobinopathies, are usually named after the location (hospital, city, or geographical region) in which the abnormal protein was first identified. They are classified according to the type of structural change and altered function and the resulting clinical characteristics (see Tables 5.1 and 5.2). Although many of these mutants have predictable phenotypes, others are surprisingly pleiotropic in their impacts on multiple properties of the Hb molecule. With few exceptions, Hb variants are inherited as autosomal recessive traits. Occasionally, double heterozygotes are identified (e.g., HbSC; see Fig. 5.9).

CLINICAL BOX
ANALGESIC TREATMENT OF SICKLE CELL VASOOCCLUSIVE CRISES

Acute vasoocclusive crises are the most common problem reported by individuals with sickle cell disease (SCD); they are also the most frequent reason for emergency room treatment and hospital admission. Episodes of vasoocclusive pain are unpredictable and are often excruciating and incapacitating. The origin of this progressive pain involves altered rheologic and hematologic properties of erythrocytes attributable to HbS polymerization and aggregation. Microvascular dysfunction is precipitated by an inflammatory response, indicated by elevation of plasma acute-phase proteins. Ultimately, impaired vasomotor responses in arterioles and adhesive interactions between sickled erythrocytes and endothelial cells in postcapillary venules restrict blood flow to tissues throughout the body.

Epidemiologic data indicate that 5% of patients with SCD can expect to experience 3–10 episodes of severe pain annually. Typically, the pain crisis resolves within 5–7 days, but a severe crisis may cause pain that persists for weeks. To provide relief to the patient, nonnarcotic, narcotic, and adjuvant analgesics are used alone or in combination.

The severity and duration of the pain dictate the most appropriate analgesic regimen. Parenterally administered opioids are frequently used for the treatment of severe pain in vasoocclusive crises. Several recent studies suggest additional options for the patient and physician: continuous intravenous infusion of nonsteroidal anti-inflammatory drugs and continuous epidural administration of local anesthetics and opioid analgesics effectively decreased pain that was unresponsive to conventional measures. In addition to analgesia, oxygen therapy and fluid management are also initiated.

The volume of hemolysate required (<100 µL) makes these techniques suitable for neonatal and adult blood samples. Quantification is performed by scanning densitometry or absorption spectrometry. Indications of abnormalities in screening tests are followed by complete blood count (Table 5.2), additional protein analysis, and DNA analysis to identify specific mutations to the globin genes.

CLINICAL TEST BOX
COMPLETE BLOOD COUNT

A complete blood count (CBC) provides information on blood cell populations and their characteristics. Data are obtained from whole blood samples by automated hematology analysis. Some instruments also provide leukocyte differentials, reticulocyte count, and red cell morphology. A typical printout of the results for one individual and the reference range is shown in Table 5.2.

Table 5.2 Complete blood count (CBC)

Parameter	Patient (male)	Reference value (SI units)*
White blood cell count, WBC	6.82×10^9/L	$4.0–11.0 \times 10^9$/L
Red cell count, RBC	4.78×10^{12}/L	$4.0–5.2 \times 10^{12}$/L (F); $4.5–5.9 \times 10^{12}$/L (M)
Hemoglobin, Hb	6.1 mmol/L	7.4–9.9 mmol/L (F); 8.4–10.9 mmol/L (M)
Hematocrit, HCT	33.4%	41–46% (F); 37–49% (M)
Mean corpuscular volume, MCV	71.9 fL	80–96 fL
Mean corpuscular hemoglobin, MCH	21.3 pg/cell	26–34 pg/cell
Mean corpuscular hemoglobin concentration, MCHC	296 g/L	320–360 g/L
Red cell distribution width, RDW	17.7%	11.5–14.5%
Platelet count, PLT	274×10^9/L	$150–350 \times 10^9$/L
Mean platelet volume, MPV	8.6 fL	6.4–11.0 fL

*F, female; M, male; fL = 10^{-15} L; pg = 10^{-12} g. To convert mmol Hb/L to g Hb/dL, multiply by 0.01611. Automated laboratory evaluation of blood provides invaluable information for the monitoring and diagnosis of health and disease. The complete blood count, performed on a sample of whole blood, includes counts of red cells (erythrocytes), white cells (leukocytes), and platelets and quantitative indices of the red cells (MCV, MCH, MCHC, and RDW). The results describe the hematopoietic status of the bone marrow and the presence of anemia and its possible cause. Data presented are characteristic of an individual with iron deficiency anemia: low Hb, low MCV (microcytosis), and low MCH (hypochromia). See also reference values in Appendix 1.

SUMMARY

- This chapter describes two important proteins that reversibly interact with O_2: myoglobin (Mb), a tissue oxygen storage protein, and hemoglobin (Hb), a blood oxygen transport protein. Both use an ancient heme-containing polypeptide domain motif to sequester O_2 and increase its solubility.
- As a tetramer of globins, Hb is one of the best-characterized examples of cooperativity in ligand interactions. Conformational changes in both the tertiary and the quaternary structures characterize the transition between deoxygenated and oxygenated states. With its wide variety of effector molecules,

Hb is also a prototype of allosteric proteins and enzymes.

■ Protons, through the Bohr effect, and CO_2 promote the release of oxygen from hemoglobin in peripheral tissue. 2,3-Bisphosphoglycerate is also an important allosteric effector of Hb, decreasing the oxygen affinity of hemoglobin; this is an important adaptation to high altitude and in pulmonary disease.

■ Mutations in globin genes lead to a spectrum of structural and functional variants, some of which are pathogenic, such as HbS, which causes sickle cell disease.

FURTHER READING

Alayash, A. I. (2014). Blood substitutes: Why haven't we been more successful? *Trends in Biotechnology, 32,* 177–185.
Giardina, B., Mosca, D., & De Rosa, M. C. (2004). The Bohr effect of haemoglobin in vertebrates: An example of molecular adaptation to different physiological requirements. *Acta Physiologica Scandinavica, 182,* 229–244.
Goodman, M. A., & Malik, P. (2016). The potential of gene therapy approaches for the treatment of hemoglobinopathies: Achievements and challenges. *Therapeutic Advances in Hematology, 7,* 302–315.
Meier, E. R., & Rampersad, A. (2016). Pediatric sickle cell disease: Past successes and future challenges. *Pediatric Research, 81*(1–2), 249–258.
Roderique, J. D., Josef, C. S., Feldman, M. J., et al. (2015). A modern literature review of carbon monoxide poisoning theories, therapies, and potential targets for therapy advancement. *Toxicology, 334,* 45–58.
Thein, S. L. (2011). Milestones in the history of hemoglobin research. *Hemoglobin, 35,* 450–462.
Yuan, Y., Tam, M. F., Simplaceanu, V., et al. (2015). New look at hemoglobin allostery. *Chemical Reviews, 115,* 1702–1724.

RELEVANT WEBSITES

Anemia: Pathophysiologic consequences, classification, and clinical investigation: http://web2.airmail.net/uthman/anemia/anemia.html
Protein domain structures: http://themedicalbiochemistrypage.org/protein-structure.php
The red cell and anemia (detailed five-part presentation by pathologist E. Uthman): Blood cells and the CBC: http://web2.airmail.net/uthman/blood_cells.html
Sickle Cell Information Center (comprehensive site for both patients and professionals): http://www.scinfo.org/
Teaching cases, American Society of Hematology: http://teachingcases.hematology.org

ABBREVIATIONS

2,3-BPG	2,3-bisphosphoglycerate
COHb	Carboxyhemoglobin
Hb	Hemoglobin
HbA	Adult (normal) hemoglobin
HbA_{1c}	Glycated hemoglobin
HbF	Fetal hemoglobin
HbS	Sickle Cell hemoglobin
Mb	Myoglobin
metHb	Methemoglobin (Fe^{+3})
SCD	Sickle Cell disease
SNO-Hb	S-nitrosohemoglobin
SpO_2	Peripheral capillary oxygen saturation

Catalytic Proteins - Enzymes

Junichi Fujii

INTRODUCTION

Almost all biological functions are supported by chemical reactions catalyzed by biological catalysts called enzymes

Efficient metabolism is controlled by orderly, sequential, and branching metabolic pathways. Enzymes accelerate chemical reactions under physiologic conditions. However, an enzyme cannot alter the equilibrium for a reaction; it can only accelerate the reaction rate by decreasing the activation energy of the reaction (Fig. 6.1). Regulation of enzymatic activities allows metabolism to adapt to rapidly changing conditions. **Nearly all enzymes are proteins,** although some ribonucleic acid molecules, termed ribozymes, also have catalytic activity (Chapter 21). Based on analysis of the human genome, it is estimated that about a quarter of human genes encode for enzymes that catalyze metabolic reactions.

ENZYMATIC REACTIONS

Factors affecting enzymatic reactions

Effect of temperature

Enzymes have an optimum temperature at which they function most efficiently

In the case of an inorganic catalyst, the reaction rate increases with the temperature of the system, and high temperature may be used to accelerate a reaction. In contrast, enzymes normally function as catalysts at constant (ambient or body) temperature. In in vitro assays, however, enzyme activity increases with temperature but then declines at higher temperatures. This happens because enzymes, like all proteins, denature at high temperature and lose activity.

Effect of pH

Every enzyme has a pH optimum because ionizable amino acids, such as histidine, glutamate, and cysteine, participate in the catalytic reactions

Cytosolic enzymes have pH optima in the range of pH 7–8. Pepsin, which is secreted by gastric cells and functions in gastric juice, has a pH optimum of 1.5–2.0; trypsin and chymotrypsin have alkaline pH optima, consistent with their digestive activity in alkaline pancreatic juice; and lysosomal enzymes typically have acidic pH optima. The pH sensitivity of enzymes results from the effect of pH on the ionic charge of amino acid side chains of enzymes. Various solutes, including substrates, products, metal ions, and regulatory molecules, also affect the rate of enzymatic reactions.

Definition of enzyme activity

One international unit (IU) of enzyme catalyzes conversion of 1 μmol of substrate to product per minute

For the purposes of standardization, the activity of an enzyme is measured under defined conditions (temperature, pH, buffer, substrate and coenzyme concentration). The rate, or velocity (v), of an enzymatic reaction under these conditions is defined as the rate of conversion of substrate to product per unit of time. A unit of enzyme is a measure of the amount of enzyme. The **katal** is an international unit for the amount of enzyme that

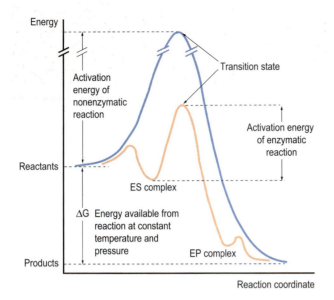

Fig. 6.1 **Reaction profile for enzymatic and nonenzymatic reactions.** The basic principles of an enzyme-catalyzed reaction are the same as those for any chemical reaction. When a chemical reaction proceeds, the substrate must gain activation energy to reach a point called the transition state of the reaction, at which the energy level is maximum. Because the **transition state** of the enzyme-catalyzed reaction has a lower energy than that of the uncatalyzed reaction, the reaction can proceed faster. ES complex, enzyme–substrate complex; EP complex, enzyme–product complex.

Table 6.1 Enzyme classification

Class	Reaction	Enzymes
1. Oxidoreductases	$A_{red} + B_{ox} \rightarrow A_{ox} + B_{red}$	Dehydrogenases, peroxidases
2. Transferases	$A\text{-}B + C \rightarrow A + B\text{-}C$	Hexokinase, transaminases
3. Hydrolases	$A\text{-}B + H_2O \rightarrow A\text{-}H + B\text{-}OH$	Alkaline phosphatase, trypsin
4. Lyases (synthases)	$X\text{-}A\text{-}B\text{-}Y \rightarrow A = B + XY$	Fumarase, dehydratases
5. Isomerases	$A \rightleftharpoons isoA$	Triose phosphate isomerase, phosphoglucomutase
6. Ligases (synthetases)	$A + B + ATP \rightarrow A\text{-}B + ADP + Pi$	Pyruvate carboxylase, DNA ligases

catalyzes the conversion of 1 mole of substrate into 1 mole of product per second (1 kat = 1 mol/s). Because the katal is generally a very small number, the much larger international unit (IU) is more commonly used as the standard unit of activity. The commonly used IU is the amount of enzyme that catalyzes the conversion of 1 micromole of substrate to product per min (1 IU = 1 µmol/min).

The specific activity of an enzyme is a measure of the number of IU/mg protein

The specific activity of an enzyme, a measure of activity per amount of protein, is expressed as µmol/min/mg of protein or IU/mg of protein. The specific activity of enzymes varies greatly among tissues, depending on the metabolic function of the tissue. The enzymes for cholesterol synthesis, for example, have a higher specific activity (IU/mg tissue) in liver than in muscle, consistent with the role of the liver in the biosynthesis of cholesterol. The specific activity of an enzyme is useful for estimating its purity - the higher the specific activity of an enzyme, the higher its purity, or homogeneity.

Reaction and substrate specificity

Most enzymes are highly specific for both the type of reaction catalyzed and the nature of the substrate(s)

The reaction that an enzyme catalyzes is determined chemically by the amino acid residues in the catalytic center of the enzyme. In general, the active site of the enzyme is composed of the substrate-binding site and the catalytic site. Substrate specificity is determined by the size, structure, charges, polarity, and hydrophobicity of the substrate-binding site. This is because the substrate must bind in the active site as the first step in the reaction, setting the stage for catalysis. Highly specific enzymes such as catalase and urease, which degrade H_2O_2 and urea, respectively, catalyze only one specific chemical reaction, but some enzymes have broader substrate specificity. The serine proteases are a typical example of such a group of enzymes. These are a family of closely related enzymes, such as the pancreatic enzymes chymotrypsin, trypsin, and elastase, that contain a reactive serine residue in the catalytic site. They catalyze the hydrolysis of peptide bonds on the carboxyl side of a limited range of amino acids in protein. Although they have similar structures and catalytic mechanisms, their substrate specificities are quite different because of structural features of the substrate binding site (Fig. 6.2).

All enzymes are assigned a four-digit enzyme classification (EC) number to organize the different enzymes that catalyze the many thousands of reactions. The first digit indicates membership of one of the six major classes of enzymes shown in Table 6.1. The next two digits indicate substrate subclasses and sub-subclasses; the fourth digit indicates the serial number of the specific enzyme. Isozymes are enzymes that catalyze the same reaction but differ in their primary structure and/or subunit composition. The activities of some tissue-specific enzymes and isozymes are measured in serum for diagnostic purposes (Fig. 6.3 and Table 6.2).

Roles of coenzymes

Helper molecules, referred to as coenzymes, play an essential part in many enzyme-catalyzed reactions

Enzymes with covalently or noncovalently bound coenzymes are referred to as **holoenzymes.** A holoenzyme without a

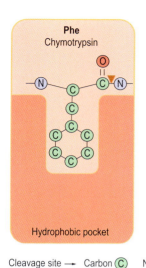

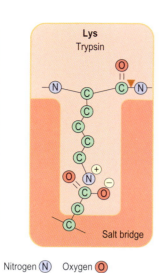

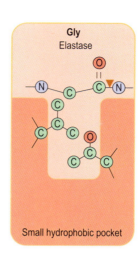

Fig. 6.2 Characteristics of the substrate-binding sites in the serine proteases chymotrypsin, trypsin, and elastase. In chymotrypsin, a hydrophobic pocket binds aromatic amino acid residues such as phenyl-alanine (Phe). In trypsin, the negative charge of the aspartate residue in the substrate-binding site promotes cleavage to the carboxyl side of positively charged lysine (Lys) and arginine (Arg) residues. In elastase, side chains of valine and threonine block the substrate-binding site and permit binding of amino acids with small or no side chains, such as glycine (Gly). ▼, site of hydrolysis by enzyme.

Cleavage site →   Carbon Ⓒ   Nitrogen Ⓝ   Oxygen Ⓞ

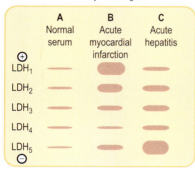

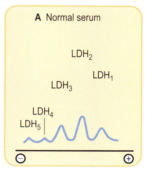

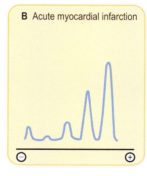

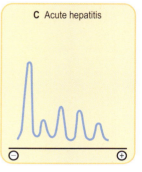

Fig. 6.3 Densitometric patterns of the lactate dehydrogenase (LDH) isozymes in the serum of patients diagnosed with myocardial infarction or acute hepatitis. Isozymes, differing slightly in charge, are separated by electrophoresis on cellulose acetate, visualized using a chromogenic substrate, and quantified by densitometry. Total serum LDH activity is also increased in these patients. Because hemolysis releases LDH from red blood cells and affects isozyme distribution and differential diagnosis, blood samples should be treated with care. The LDH measurements for the diagnosis of myocardial infarction have now been superseded by assay of plasma troponin and other biomarkers.

coenzyme is termed an **apoenzyme.** Coenzymes are divided into two categories. Soluble coenzymes bind reversibly to the protein moiety of the enzyme. They are often modified during the enzymatic reaction, then dissociate from the enzyme and are recycled by another enzyme; oxidoreductases, discussed in Chapter 8, have coenzymes that may be oxidized by one enzyme, then reduced and recycled by another. Coenzymes, such as coenzyme A, assist in the transport of intermediates from one enzyme to another during a sequence of reactions. Most coenzymes are vitamin derivatives. Derivatives of the B vitamins, niacin and riboflavin, act as coenzymes for oxidoreductase reactions. The structure and function of coenzymes are described in later chapters. **Prosthetic groups** are tightly bound, often covalently linked, to an enzyme and remain associated with the enzyme during the entire catalytic cycle. Some enzymes require inorganic (metal) ions, frequently termed **cofactors,** for their activity - for example, blood-clotting enzymes that

require Ca^{2+}, and oxidoreductases, which use iron, copper, and manganese.

ENZYME KINETICS

The Michaelis–Menten equation: A simple model of enzyme catalysis

Enzyme reactions are multistep in nature and comprise several partial reactions

In 1913, long before the structure of proteins was known, Leonor Michaelis and Maud Leonora Menten developed a simple model for the kinetics of enzyme-catalyzed reactions (Fig. 6.4). The Michaelis–Menten model assumes that the substrate S binds to the enzyme E, forming an essential intermediate, the

Table 6.2 Some enzymes used for clinical diagnosis

Enzyme	Tissue source(s)	Diagnostic use
AST	Heart, skeletal muscle, liver, brain	Liver disease
ALT	Liver	Liver disease (e.g., hepatitis)
Amylase	Pancreas, salivary gland	Acute pancreatitis, biliary obstruction
CK	Skeletal muscle, heart, brain	Muscular dystrophy, myocardial infarction
GGT	Liver	Hepatitis, cirrhosis
LDH	Heart, liver, erythrocytes	Lymphoma, hepatitis
Lipase	Pancreas	Acute pancreatitis, biliary obstruction
Alkaline phosphatase	Osteoblast	Bone disease, bone tumors
Acid phosphatase (PSA)	Prostate	Prostate cancer

AST, aspartate aminotransferase, formerly known as serum glutamate oxaloacetate transaminase (SGOT); ALT, alanine aminotransferase, formerly known as serum glutamate pyruvate transaminase (SGPT); CK, creatine phosphokinase; GGT, γ-glutamyl transpeptidase; LDH, lactate dehydrogenase; PSA, prostate-specific antigen (kallikrein 3).

 CLINICAL TEST BOX
TISSUE SPECIFICITY OF LACTATE DEHYDROGENASE ISOZYMES

A 56-year-old female was admitted to an intensive care unit. The patient had suffered from a slight fever for 1 week and reported some chest pain and difficulty breathing for the past 24 h. No abnormality was found on chest X-ray or by electrocardiography. However, a blood test showed white blood cells 12,100/mm³ (normal: 4000–9000/mm³), red blood cells 240 × 10⁴/mm³ (normal: 380–500 × 10⁴/mm³), hemoglobin 8.6 g/dL (normal: 11.8–16.0 g/dL), lactate dehydrogenase (LDH) 1400 IU/L (normal: 200–400 IU/L). Levels of other enzymes were normal. Based on the blood tests, the LDH isozyme profile, and other data, the patient was eventually diagnosed with malignant lymphoma.

Comment
LDH is a tetrameric oxidoreductase composed of two different 35-kDa subunits. The heart contains mainly the H-type subunit, and skeletal muscle and the liver mainly contain the M type, which are encoded by different genes. Five types of tetrameric isozymes can be formed from these subunits: H_4 (LDH_1), H_3M_1 (LDH_2), H_2M_2 (LDH_3), H_1M_3 (LDH_4), and M_4 (LDH_5). Because isozyme distributions differ among tissues, it is possible to diagnose tissue damage by assaying total LDH activity and then isozyme profiling (Fig. 6.3).

For hematological reference values, see Table 5.2 and Appendix 1.

 ADVANCED CONCEPT BOX
PROPORTION OF ENZYME GENES IN WHOLE HUMAN GENOME

About a quarter of genes encode enzymes. Names of enzyme groups with number and proportion (percentage in parentheses) in a total of 26,383 human genes were as follows: transferase, 610 (2.0); synthase and synthetase, 313 (1.0); oxidoreductase, 656 (2.1); lyase, 117 (0.4); ligase, 56 (0.2); isomerase, 163 (0.5); hydrolase, 1227 (4.0); kinase, 868 (2.8); nucleic acid enzyme, 2308 (7.5).

Original data (Venter et al., Science 291:1335, 2001) are quoted here, and so classification does not exactly match the nomenclature in Table 6.2.

 CLINICAL TEST BOX
ISOZYMES

Isozyme profiles are often performed in the clinical laboratory for diagnostic purposes (see Fig. 6.3). The definition of isozymes is often operational - that is, based on simple and reproducible substrate-specific assay methods that sometimes do not require precise knowledge of enzyme structure.

The term *isozyme* is commonly used to refer to (1) genetic variants of an enzyme; (2) genetically independent proteins with little homology; (3) heteropolymers of two or more noncovalently bound polypeptide chains; (4) unrelated enzymes that catalyze similar reactions, such as enzymes conjugated with different prosthetic groups or requiring different coenzymes or cofactors; and (5) different forms of a single polypeptide chain - for example, varying in carbohydrate composition, deamination of amino acids, or proteolytic modification.

enzyme-substrate (ES) complex, which then undergoes reaction on the enzyme surface and decomposes to E + P (product). The model assumes that E, S, and ES are all in rapid equilibrium with one another so that a steady-state concentration of ES is rapidly achieved and that decomposition of the ES complex to E + P is the **rate-limiting step** in catalysis. The overall reaction rate is directly dependent on the activation energy for decomposition of the ES complex (Fig. 6.1).

The catalytic constant, k_{cat}, also known as the turnover number, is a rate constant that describes how quickly an enzyme can catalyze a reaction. **The k_{cat} is defined as the number of substrate molecules converted to product per *enzyme molecule* per unit of time.** The proportion of ES, in relation to the total number of enzyme molecules $[E]_t$ - that is, the ratio $[ES]/[E]_t$ - limits the velocity of an enzyme (v) so that

$$v = k_{cat}[ES]$$

Because E, S, and ES are all in chemical equilibrium, the enzyme achieves maximal velocity, V_{max}, at very high (saturating) substrate concentrations [S], when [ES] ≈ [E]$_t$ (total enzyme). Thus for the dissociation of the ES complex, the law of mass action yields:

$$K_d = \frac{[E][S]}{[ES]}$$

Given that

$$[E]_t = [E] + [ES]$$

it can be shown that

$$\frac{[ES]}{[E]_t} = \frac{[S]}{K_m + [S]}$$

where $K_m = K_d$

Consequently, the velocity of the enzymatic reaction, v, is given by

$$v = \frac{k_{cat}[E]_t[S]}{k_m + [S]}$$

Because $k_{cat}[E]_t$ corresponds to the maximum velocity, V_{max}, that is attained at high (saturating) substrate concentrations, we obtain the Michaelis–Menten equation:

$$v = V_{max} \cdot \frac{[S]}{K_m + [S]}$$

Analysis of the previous equations indicates that the Michaelis constant, K$_m$, is expressed in units of concentration and corresponds to the substrate concentration at which v is 50% of the maximum velocity - that is, [ES] = ½[E]t and v = V$_{max}$/2 (Fig. 6.4)

K_m is a useful constant for estimating the affinity of an enzyme for its substrate. Enzymes with a high K_m require high substrate concentration for efficient activity, whereas those with low K_m

operate efficiently on trace levels of substrate. The Michaelis–Menten model is based on the following assumptions:

- E, S, and ES are in rapid equilibrium.
- There are no forms of the enzyme present other than E and ES.
- The conversion of ES into E + P is a rate-limiting, irreversible step. Although all enzyme-catalyzed reactions are theoretically reversible, initial velocities are normally measured when product concentration, and therefore the rate of the reverse reaction, is negligible.

Similar types of kinetic models have been developed for describing the kinetics of multisubstrate, multiproduct enzymes.

Use of the Lineweaver–Burk and Eadie–Hofstee plots

Alternative graphical analyses permit more accurate determination of the K$_m$ and V$_{max}$ of an enzyme

In a plot of reaction rate versus substrate concentration, the rate of the reaction approaches the maximum velocity (V_{max})

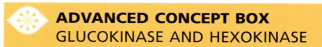

ADVANCED CONCEPT BOX
GLUCOKINASE AND HEXOKINASE

Hexokinase catalyzes the first step in glucose metabolism in all cells - namely, the phosphorylation reaction of glucose by adenosine triphosphate (ATP) to form glucose 6-phosphate (Glc-6-P):

glucose + ATP = glucose 6-phosphate + ADP

This enzyme has a low K_m for glucose (0.2 mmol/L) and is inhibited allosterically by its product, Glc-6-P. Because normal glucose levels in blood are about 5 mmol/L and intracellular levels are 0.2–2 mmol/L, hexokinase efficiently catalyzes this reaction (50%–90% of V_{max}) under normal conditions (e.g., in muscle).

Hepatocytes, which store glucose as glycogen, and pancreatic β-cells, which regulate glucose consumption in tissues and its storage in the liver by secreting insulin, contain an isozyme called glucokinase.

Glucokinase catalyzes the same reaction as hexokinase, but it has a higher K_m for glucose (10 mmol/L) and is not inhibited by the product, Glc-6-P. Because glucokinase has a much higher K_m than hexokinase, glucokinase phosphorylates glucose with increasing efficiency as blood glucose levels increase following a meal (see Fig. 6.4). One of the physiologic roles of glucokinase in the liver is to provide Glc-6-P for the synthesis of glycogen, a storage form of glucose, when blood glucose increases following a meal. In the pancreatic β-cell, glucokinase functions as the glucose sensor, activating glucose metabolism and energy production, leading to secretion of insulin. Mice lacking glucokinase in the pancreatic β-cell die within 3 days of birth of profound hyperglycemia because of failure to secrete insulin.

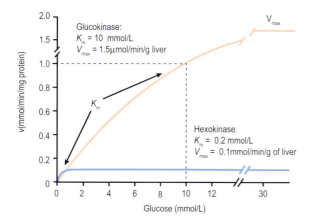

Fig. 6.4 **Properties of glucokinase and hexokinase.** Glucokinase and hexokinase catalyze the same reaction, phosphorylation of glucose to glucose 6-phosphate (Glc-6-P). They exhibit different kinetic properties and have different tissue distributions and physiologic functions.

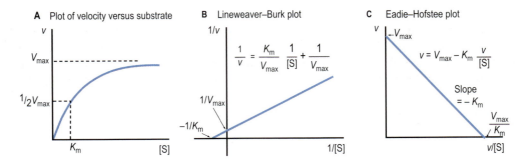

Fig. 6.5 **Enzyme kinetics plot.** Kinetic representations of the properties of enzymes. (A) Michaelis–Menten plot of velocity (v) versus substrate concentration ([S]). (B) Lineweaver–Burk plot. (C) Eadie–Hofstee plot.

asymptotically (Fig. 6.5A), so it is difficult to obtain accurate values for V_{max} and, as a result, K_m (substrate concentration required for half-maximal activity) by simple extrapolation. To solve this problem, several linear transformations of the Michaelis–Menten equation have been developed.

Lineweaver–Burk plot

The Lineweaver–Burk, or double-reciprocal, plot is obtained by taking the reciprocal of the Michaelis–Menten equation (Fig. 6.5B). By rearranging the equation, we obtain:

$$\frac{1}{v} = \frac{1}{V_{max}} + \frac{k_m}{V_{max}} \times \frac{1}{[S]}$$

This equation yields a straight line ($y = mx + b$), with $y = 1/v$, $x = 1/[S]$, m = slope, and b = y-intercept. Therefore a graph of $1/v$ versus $1/[S]$ (Fig. 6.5B) has a slope of K_m/V_{max}, a $1/v$-intercept of $1/V_{max}$, and a $1/[S]$-intercept of $-1/K_m$. Although the Lineweaver–Burk plot is widely used for kinetic analysis of enzyme reactions, because reciprocals of the data are calculated, a small experimental error - especially at low substrate concentration - can result in a large error in the graphically determined values of K_m and V_{max}. An additional disadvantage is that important data obtained at high substrate concentrations are concentrated into a narrow region near the $1/v$-axis.

Eadie–Hofstee plot

A second, widely used linear form of the Michaelis–Menten equation is the Eadie–Hofstee plot (Fig. 6.5C), described by the following equation:

$$v = V_{max} - K_m \times \frac{v}{[S]}$$

In this case, a plot of v versus $v/[S]$ has a y-axis (v-intercept) of V_{max}, an x-axis ($v/[S]$) intercept of V_{max}/K_m, and a slope of $-K_m$. The Eadie–Hofstee plot does not compress the data at high substrate concentrations.

MECHANISM OF ENZYME ACTION

Enzymatic reactions involve functional groups on amino acid side chains, coenzymes, substrates, and products

Enzymes vary significantly in their mechanism of action. In some cases, catalysis is carried out on a substrate noncovalently, reversibly bound to the enzyme. In other cases, a covalent intermediate is formed on and then released from the enzyme; in others, all the action takes place on a coenzyme that forms a covalent bond with substrate.

The serine proteases, introduced in Fig. 6.2, are representative of enzymes that form a covalent intermediate with their substrates. These enzymes cleave peptide bonds in proteins, and as in all enzymatic reactions, functional groups on amino acid side chains participate in the enzyme-catalyzed reaction. In the serine protease family, an active-site serine residue catalyzes cleavage of the peptide bond. The functional group on serine, a primary alcohol, is not among the more reactive functional groups in organic chemistry. To enhance its activity in serine proteases, this serine residue is part of a "catalytic triad," in the case of chymotrypsin: Asp^{102}, His^{57}, and Ser^{195} (Fig. 6.6). Concerted hydrogen bonding interactions between these amino acids increase the nucleophilicity of the serine residue so that it can attack the carbonyl carbon atom of the peptide bond in the substrate. Chymotrypsin is specific for

cleavage on the carboxyl side of peptide bonds containing aromatic amino acids, such as phenylalanine. The mechanism of the enzymatic reaction is outlined in Fig. 6.7, showing the formation and cleavage of an enzyme-bound intermediate.

Trypsin and elastase, two other digestive enzymes with different amino acid specificities (Fig. 6.2), are similar (homologous) to chymotrypsin in many respects. About 40% of the amino acid sequences of these three enzymes are identical, and their three-dimensional structures are very similar. All three enzymes contain the aspartate-histidine-serine catalytic triad, and all are inactivated by reaction of fluorophosphates with the active serine residue. The nerve gas **diisopropyl-fluorophosphate** forms a sterically hindered, very slowly hydrolyzed serine-diisopropylphospate ester and inhibits serine proteases.

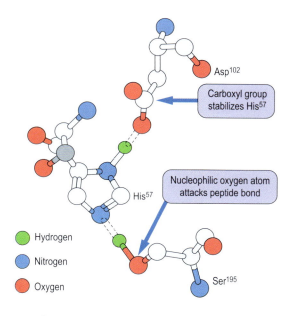

Fig. 6.6 **A schematic model of a catalytic triad of serine protease.**

Carboxyl group stabilizes His[57]

Nucleophilic oxygen atom attacks peptide bond

His[57]

Ser[195]

Asp[102]

● Hydrogen
● Nitrogen
● Oxygen

ENZYME INHIBITION

Among numerous substances affecting metabolic processes, enzyme inhibitors are particularly important. Many drugs, either naturally occurring or synthetic, act as enzyme inhibitors. Metabolites of these compounds may also inhibit enzyme activity. Most enzyme inhibitors act reversibly, but there are also irreversible inhibitors that permanently modify the target enzyme. Using Lineweaver–Burk plots, it is possible to distinguish three forms of reversible inhibition: competitive, uncompetitive, and noncompetitive inhibition.

Competitive inhibitors cause an apparent increase in K_m without changing V_{max}

An enzyme can be inhibited competitively by substances that are similar in chemical structure to the substrate. These compounds bind in the active site and compete with the substrate for the active site of the enzyme; they cause an apparent increase in K_m but no change in V_{max} (Fig. 6.8). The inhibition is the result of an effect not on enzyme activity but

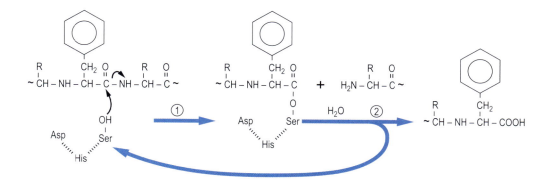

Fig. 6.7 **Mechanism of action of chymotrypsin.** The active-site serine residue attacks the carbonyl group of the peptide bond on the carboxyl side of a phenylalanine residue. The carboxy-terminal peptide is released, and the amino-terminal peptide remains an enzyme-bound intermediate - the amino-terminal peptide linked covalently through its carboxy-terminal phenylalanine esterified to the active-site serine residue. The ester bond is hydrolyzed in the second step of the reaction to release the amino-terminal peptide and regenerate active enzyme.

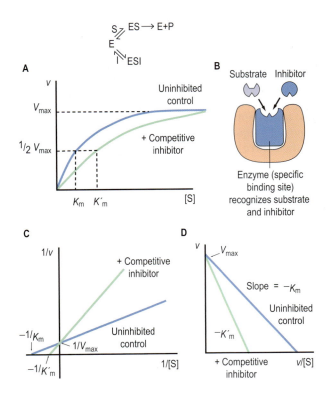

$$S \xrightarrow{\text{\hspace{1em}}} ES \rightarrow E+P$$
$$E$$
$$\xrightarrow{\text{\hspace{1em}}} ESI$$

A

B

Substrate   Inhibitor

Enzyme (specific binding site) recognizes substrate and inhibitor

C

D

Fig. 6.8 **Competitive enzyme inhibition.** (A) Plot of velocity versus substrate concentration. (B) Mechanism of competitive inhibition. (C) Lineweaver–Burk plot in the presence of a competitive inhibitor. (D) Eadie–Hofstee plot in the presence of a competitive inhibitor. K'_m is the apparent K_m in the presence of inhibitor.

on substrate access to the active site. The reaction scheme for competitive inhibition is

$$\begin{array}{c} E \overset{+S}{\underset{+I}{\rightleftharpoons}} ES \rightarrow E+P \\ \rightleftharpoons EI \end{array}$$

The inhibition constant (K_i) is the dissociation constant of the enzyme–inhibitor (EI) complex, and the lower the K_i (the tighter the binding), the more efficient the inhibition of enzyme activity. Regardless of the K_i, however, **the rate of the enzyme-catalyzed reaction in the presence of a competitive inhibitor can be increased by increasing the substrate concentration** because substrate, at higher concentration, competes more effectively with the inhibitor.

Uncompetitive inhibitors cause an apparent decrease in V$_{max}$

An uncompetitive inhibitor binds only to the enzyme–substrate complex and not to the free enzyme. The following equation shows the reaction scheme for uncompetitive inhibition. In this case, the K_i is the dissociation constant for the enzyme–substrate–inhibitor (ESI) complex.

$$E + S \rightleftharpoons ES \begin{array}{c} \overset{I}{\rightharpoonup} ESI \\ \searrow E+P \end{array}$$

CLINICAL BOX
TREATMENT WITH AN INHIBITOR OF ANGIOTENSIN-CONVERTING ENZYME (ACE)

A 50-year-old man was admitted to the hospital, suffering from general fatigue, a stiff shoulder, and headache. The patient was 1.8 m tall and weighed 84 kg. His blood pressure was 196/98 mmHg (normal below 140/90 mmHg; optimal below 120/80 mmHg) and his pulse was 74. He was diagnosed as hypertensive. The patient was given captopril, an angiotensin-converting enzyme (ACE) inhibitor. After 5 days' treatment, his blood pressure returned to near-normal levels.

Comment
Renin in the kidney converts angiotensinogen into angiotensin I, which is then proteolytically cleaved to angiotensin II by ACE. Angiotensin II increases renal fluid and electrolyte retention, contributing to hypertension. Inhibition of ACE activity is therefore an important target for hypertension treatment. Captopril inhibits ACE competitively, decreasing blood pressure. (See also Chapter 35.)

CLINICAL BOX
METHANOL POISONING CAN BE TREATED BY ETHANOL ADMINISTRATION

A 46-year-old male presented to the emergency room 7 h after consuming a large quantity of bootleg alcohol. He could not see clearly and complained of abdominal and back pain. Laboratory results indicated severe metabolic acidosis, a serum osmolality of 465 mmol/kg (reference range 285–295 mmol/kg), and serum methanol level of 4.93 g/L (156 mmol/L). With aggressive treatment, including an ethanol drip, bicarbonate, and hemodialysis, he survived and regained his eyesight.

Comment
Methanol poisoning is uncommon but extremely hazardous. Ethylene glycol (antifreeze) poisoning is more common and exhibits similar clinical characteristics. The most important initial symptom of methanol poisoning is visual disturbance. Laboratory evidence of methanol poisoning includes severe metabolic acidosis and increased plasma solute (methanol) concentration. Methanol is slowly metabolized to formaldehyde, which is then rapidly metabolized to formate by alcohol dehydrogenase. Formate accumulates during methanol intoxication and is responsible for the metabolic acidosis in the early stage of intoxication. In later stages, lactate may also accumulate as a result of formate inhibition of respiration. Ethanol is metabolized by alcohol dehydrogenase, which binds ethanol with much higher affinity than either methanol or ethylene glycol. Ethanol is therefore a useful agent to inhibit competitively the metabolism of methanol and ethylene glycol to toxic metabolites. The unmetabolized methanol and ethylene glycol are gradually excreted in urine. Early treatment with ethanol, together with bicarbonate to combat acidosis and hemodialysis to remove methanol and its toxic metabolites, yields a good prognosis.

The inhibitor causes a decrease in V_{max} because a fraction of the enzyme–substrate complex is diverted by the inhibitor to the inactive ESI complex. Binding of the inhibitor and an increase in stability of the ESI complex may also affect the dissociation of substrate, causing an apparent decrease in K_m (i.e., an apparent increase in substrate affinity).

Noncompetitive inhibitors may bind to sites outside the active site and alter both the K_m and the V_{max} of the enzyme

A noncompetitive (mixed) inhibitor can bind either to the free enzyme or to the enzyme–substrate complex typically at a site outside the active site. Noncompetitive inhibitors exhibit more complex effects and may alter both the K_m and the V_{max} of an enzymatic reaction. The following equation shows the reaction scheme observed for noncompetitive inhibition:

$$
\begin{array}{ccc}
\text{E} + \text{S} & \rightleftharpoons \text{ES} & \rightarrow \text{E} + \text{P} \\
+ & + & \\
\text{I} & \text{I} & \\
\updownarrow & \updownarrow & \\
\text{EI} & \text{ESI} &
\end{array}
$$

Many drugs and poisons irreversibly inhibit enzymes

Prostaglandins are key inflammatory mediators. Their synthesis is initiated by cyclooxygenase-mediated oxidation and cyclization of arachidonate under inflammatory conditions (Chapter 25). Compounds that suppress cyclooxygenase have anti-inflammatory activity. **Aspirin** (acetylsalicylic acid) inhibits cyclooxygenase activity by acetylating Ser[530], which blocks access of arachidonate to the active site of the enzyme. Other **nonsteroidal anti-inflammatory drugs (NSAID)**, such as indomethacin, inhibit cyclooxygenase activity by reversibly blocking the arachidonate binding site.

Disulfiram (**Antabuse**) is a drug used for the treatment of alcoholism. Alcohol is metabolized in two steps to acetic acid. The first enzyme, alcohol dehydrogenase, yields acetaldehyde, which is then converted into acetic acid by aldehyde dehydrogenase. The latter enzyme has an active-site cysteine residue that is irreversibly modified by disulfiram, resulting in accumulation of both alcohol and acetaldehyde in the blood. People who take disulfiram become sick because of the accumulation of acetaldehyde in blood and tissues, leading to alcohol avoidance.

Alkylating agents, such as iodoacetamide (ICH_2CONH_2), irreversibly inhibit the catalytic activity of some enzymes by modifying essential cysteine residues. **Heavy metals,** such as mercury and lead salts, also inhibit enzymes with active-site sulfhydryl residues. The mercury adducts are often reversible by thiol compounds. Eggs or egg whites are sometimes administered as an antidote for accidental ingestion of heavy metals. The egg-white protein ovalbumin is rich in sulfhydryl groups; it traps the free metal ions and prevents their absorption from the gastrointestinal tract.

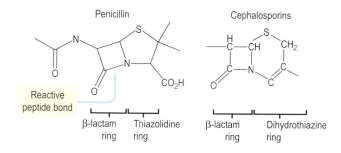

Fig. 6.9 **Structure of penicillin showing the reactive peptide bond in the β-lactam ring and core structure of cephalosporins.** Penicillins contain a β-lactam ring fused to a thiazolidine ring. Cephalosporins are another class of compounds containing the β-lactam ring fused to a six-membered dihydrothiazine ring. Because of their effectiveness and lack of toxicity, β-lactam compounds are widely used antibiotics. Bacteria with β-lactamase, which breaks the β-lactam ring, are resistant to these antibiotics.

ADVANCED CONCEPT BOX
ENZYME INHIBITION: TRANSITION-STATE INHIBITION AND SUICIDE SUBSTRATE

Enzymes catalyze reactions by inducing the transition state of the reaction. It should therefore be possible to construct molecules that bind very tightly to the enzyme by mimicking the transition state of the substrate. Transition states themselves cannot be isolated because they are not a stable arrangement of atoms, and some bonds are only partially formed or broken. But for some enzymes, analogs (*analogues* is the chiefly British spelling) can be synthesized that are stable but still have some of the structural features of the transition state.

Penicillin (Fig. 6.9) is a good example of a transition-state analog. It inhibits the transpeptidase that crosslinks bacterial cell-wall peptidoglycan strands, the last step in cell-wall synthesis in bacteria. It has a strained four-membered lactam ring that mimics the transition state of the normal substrate. When penicillin binds to the active site of the enzyme, its lactam ring opens, forming a covalent bond with a serine residue at the active site. Penicillin is a potent irreversible inhibitor of bacterial cell-wall synthesis, making the bacterium osmotically fragile and unable to survive in the body.

In many cases, irreversible inhibitors are used to identify active-site residues involved in enzyme catalysis and to gain insight into the mechanism of enzyme action. By sequencing or mass spectrometric analysis of the modified peptide, it is possible to identify the specific amino acid residue modified by the inhibitor and involved in catalysis.

REGULATION OF ENZYME ACTIVITY

There are multiple complementary mechanisms for regulation of enzyme activity

Generally, five independent mechanisms are involved in the regulation of enzyme activity:

- The expression of the enzyme protein from the corresponding gene changes in response to the cell's changing environment or metabolic demands.
- Enzymes may be irreversibly activated or inactivated by proteolytic enzymes.
- Enzymes may be reversibly activated or inactivated by covalent modification, such as phosphorylation.
- Allosteric regulation modulates the activity of key enzymes through reversible binding of small molecules at sites distinct from the active site in a process that is relatively rapid and, hence, the first response of cells to changing conditions.
- The rate of degradation of enzymes by intracellular proteases in the lysosome or by proteasomes in the cytosol also determines the half-life of enzymes and, consequently, enzyme activity over a much longer period of time (Chapter 22).

Proteolytic activation of digestive enzymes

Some enzymes are stored in subcellular organelles or compartments in an inactive precursor form

Several digestive enzymes are stored as inactive zymogens or proenzymes in secretory vesicles in the pancreas. The zymogens are secreted in pancreatic juice following a meal and are activated in the gastrointestinal tract. Trypsinogen is converted into trypsin by the action of intestinal enteropeptidase. Enteropeptidase, located on the inner surface of the duodenum, hydrolyzes an N-terminal peptide from the inactive trypsinogen. Rearrangement of the tertiary structure yields the proteolytically active form of trypsin. The active trypsin then digests other zymogens, such as procarboxypeptidase, proelastase, and chymotrypsinogen, as well as other trypsinogen molecules (Chapter 30). Through **cascade amplification**, an initial weak stimulus may be amplified in sequential parallel or serial steps. Similar proteolytic cascades are observed in blood clotting and fibrinolysis (dissolution of clots; Chapter 41), and cascade amplification is characteristic of intracellular signaling systems induced by hormones and cytokines (Chapters 25 and 27).

Allosteric regulation of rate-limiting enzymes in metabolic pathways

Allosteric enzymes display sigmoidal, rather than hyperbolic, plots of reaction rate versus substrate concentration

The substrate saturation curve for an isosteric (single-shape) enzyme is hyperbolic (see Fig. 6.5A). In contrast, allosteric

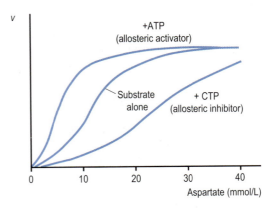

Fig. 6.10 **Allosteric regulation of aspartate transcarbamoylase (ATCase).** Plot of velocity (v) versus substrate concentration in the presence of an allosteric activator or allosteric inhibitor ATCase is an example of an allosteric enzyme. Aspartate (substrate) homotropically regulates ATCase activity, providing sigmoidal kinetics. CTP, an end product, heterotropically inhibits, but ATP, a precursor, heterotropically activates ATCase.

enzymes show sigmoidal plots of reaction velocity versus substrate concentration [S] (Fig. 6.10). An allosteric (other-site) effector molecule binds to the enzyme at a site that is distinct and physically separate from the substrate binding site and affects substrate binding (K_m) and/or k_{cat}. In some cases, the substrate may exert allosteric effects; this is referred to as a **homotropic** effect. If the allosteric effector is different from the substrate, it is referred to as a **heterotropic** effect. Homotropic effects are observed when the reaction of one substrate molecule with a multimeric enzyme affects the binding of a second substrate molecule at a different active site on the enzyme. The interaction between subunits makes the binding of substrate cooperative and results in a sigmoidal curve in the plot of v versus [S]. This effect is essentially identical to that described for the binding of O_2 to hemoglobin (Chapter 5), except that in the case of enzymes, substrate binding leads to an enzyme-catalyzed reaction.

Positive and negative cooperativity

Positive cooperativity (Fig. 6.11) indicates that the reaction of a substrate with one active site makes it easier for another substrate to bind or react at another active site. **Negative cooperativity** means that the reaction of a substrate with one active site makes it more difficult for a substrate to bind or react at the other active site. Because the affinity, or specific activity, of the enzyme changes with substrate concentration, it cannot be described by simple Michaelis–Menten kinetics. Instead, it is characterized by the substrate concentration giving a half-maximal rate, $[S]_{0.5}$, and the **Hill coefficient** (H; Chapter 5). The H-values are larger than 1 for enzymes with positive cooperativity and less than 1 for those with negative cooperativity. For most allosteric enzymes, intracellular substrate concentrations are poised near the $[S]_{0.5}$ so that the enzyme's activity responds to slight changes in substrate concentration.

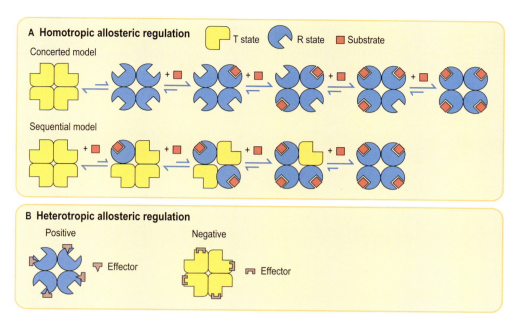

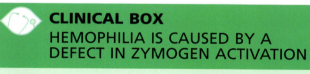

Fig. 6.11 **Schematic representation of allosteric regulation with positive cooperativity.** (A) In homotropic regulation, the substrate acts as an allosteric effector. Two models are presented. In the concerted model, all of the subunits convert from the T (tense; low affinity for substrate) into the R (relaxed; high affinity for substrate) state at the same time; in the sequential model, they change one by one, with each substrate-binding reaction. (B) In heterotropic regulation, the effector is distinct from the substrate, and it binds at a structurally different site on the enzyme. Positive and negative effectors stabilize the enzyme in R and T states, respectively.

CLINICAL BOX
HEMOPHILIA IS CAUSED BY A DEFECT IN ZYMOGEN ACTIVATION

A child was admitted to hospital with muscle bleeding affecting the femoral nerve. Laboratory findings indicated a blood-clotting disorder, hemophilia A, resulting from deficiency of factor VIII. Factor VIII was administered to the patient to restore blood-clotting activity.

Comment
Formation of a blood clot results from a cascade of zymogen-activation reactions. More than a dozen different proteins, known as blood-clotting factors, are involved. In the final step, the blood clot is formed by conversion of a soluble protein, fibrinogen (factor I), into an insoluble, fibrous product, fibrin, which forms the matrix of the clot. This last step is catalyzed by the serine protease, thrombin (factor IIa). Hemophilia is a disorder of blood clotting caused by a defect in one of the sequence of clotting factors. Hemophilia A, the major (85%) form of hemophilia, is caused by a defect of clotting factor VIII (see Chapter 41).

ADVANCED CONCEPT BOX
NUCLEOSIDE ANALOGS AS ANTIVIRAL AGENTS

Nucleoside analogs such as acyclovir and ganciclovir have been used for treatment of herpes simplex virus (HSV), varicella-zoster (VZV), and cytomegalovirus (CMV). They are pro-drugs that are activated by phosphorylation and terminate viral DNA synthesis by inhibiting the viral DNA polymerase reaction. The thymidine kinase (TK) of the viruses phosphorylate these compounds to their monophosphate form. Cellular kinases next add phosphates to form the active triphosphate compounds, which are competitive inhibitors of the viral DNA polymerase during DNA replication (Chapter 20).

Whereas viral TK has low substrate specificity and efficiently phosphorylates nucleoside analogs, cellular nucleoside kinases have high substrate specificity and barely phosphorylate the nucleoside analogs. Thus virus-infected cells are prone to be arrested at a specific cell-cycle stage, the G_2-M checkpoint (Chapter 28), but uninfected cells are resistant to the nucleoside analogs.

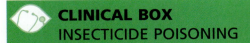

A 55-year-old man was spraying an insecticide containing organic fluorophosphates in a rice field. He suddenly developed a frontal headache, eye pain, and tightness in his chest, typical signs of overexposure to toxic organic fluorophosphates. He was taken to the hospital and treated with an intravenous injection of 2 mg of atropine sulfate, and he gradually recovered.

Comment
Organic fluorophosphates form covalent phosphoryl-enzyme complexes with both serine proteases and esterases, such as acetylcholinesterase, irreversibly inhibiting the enzymes. Acetylcholinesterase terminates the action of acetylcholine during neuromuscular activity (Chapter 26) by hydrolyzing the acetylcholine to acetate and choline. Inhibition of this enzyme prolongs the action of acetylcholine, leading to constant neuromuscular stimulation. Atropine competitively blocks acetylcholine binding and muscle stimulation at the neuromuscular junction.

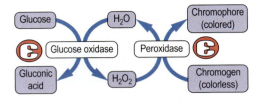

Fig. 6.12 **The glucose oxidase/peroxidase assay for blood glucose.** The color produced in this assay is directly proportional to blood glucose concentration.

ENZYMATIC MEASUREMENT OF BLOOD GLUCOSE

The glucose oxidase/peroxidase assay

In clinical laboratories, most compounds are measured by automated enzymatic methods

The most common assay for blood glucose concentration uses a mixture of glucose oxidase and peroxidase (Fig. 6.12). Glucose oxidase is highly specific for glucose but oxidizes only the β-anomer of the sugar, which represents ~64% of glucose in solution. The assay mixture is therefore supplemented with mutarotase, which rapidly catalyzes the interconversion of the anomers, enhancing assay sensitivity by ~50%. The H_2O_2 produced in the oxidase reaction is then used in a peroxidase reaction to oxidize a chromogen to yield a colored chromophore. The color yield is directly proportional to the glucose content of the sample. There are fluorometric versions of this assay for high sensitivity, and one commercial analyzer uses an oxygen electrode to measure the rate of decrease in oxygen concentration in the sample, which is also directly proportional to the glucose concentration.

Reagent strips and glucometers

People with diabetes normally monitor their blood glucose several times a day using reagent strips or glucose meters

The glucose reagent strips are impregnated with a glucose oxidase/peroxidase (GOP) reagent. In a manual version of this assay, the extent of color change on a dipstick is related to glucose concentration - typically on a scale of 1 to 4. Modern glucometers use a small drop of blood (~1 μL) and amperometric electrodes to measure the current produced by the redox reaction catalyzed by glucose dehydrogenase (GDH), which oxidizes glucose to gluconic acid but reduces a coenzyme rather than oxygen. These assays are commonly used where rapid or frequent measurements of blood glucose are required. When the GOP and GDH assays were compared at high altitude on a trek up Mount Kilimanjaro, the GOP assay, which depends on ambient oxygen, was found to have a greater error. Both methods were less accurate at the low temperatures at high altitude.

Kinetic assays

Kinetic assays are more rapid than endpoint assays

In the assay described in Fig. 6.12 and plotted for several glucose concentrations in Fig. 6.13A, the reaction is allowed to proceed to its endpoint - that is, until all the glucose has been oxidized - then the color change is measured. The color yield is then plotted against a standard to determine blood glucose concentration (Fig. 6.13B). High-throughput kinetic analyzers estimate the glucose concentration in a sample by measuring the initial rate of the reaction. Analysis of the kinetic plots in Fig. 6.13A, for example, indicates that both the endpoint and the initial rate of the glucose oxidase assay are dependent on glucose concentration. Thus the analyzer can measure the change in absorbance (or some other parameter) during the early stages of the reaction and compare this rate to that of a standard solution to estimate the glucose concentration (Fig. 6.13C). These assays are performed on flow-injection or centrifugal analyzers to ensure rapid mixing of reagents and sample.

Kinetic analyzers are inherently faster than endpoint assays because they estimate glucose concentration before the assay reaches its endpoint. These assays work because glucose oxidase and glucose dehydrogenase have a high K_m for glucose. At the concentrations of glucose found in blood, the rate of the oxidase reaction is proportional to glucose concentration - that is, in the first-order region of the Michaelis–Menten equation, where the substrate concentration is less than the K_m (see Fig. 6.4).

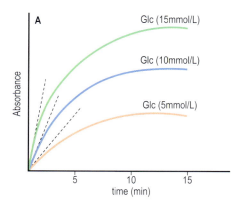

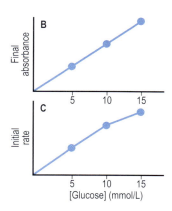

Fig. 6.13 **Glucose oxidase/peroxidase assays - endpoint versus kinetic assays.** (A) Graphical analysis of an endpoint assay. (B) The final (endpoint) absorbances are plotted as a function of glucose concentration, yielding a straight line. (C) Initial rates of reactions are estimated by multiple measurements early in the assay (dotted lines in frame A) and plotted versus glucose concentration. Nonlinear plots, when obtained, are analyzed by computer.

ACTIVE LEARNING

1. In a multistep sequence of enzymatic reactions, where is the most effective site for controlling the flux of substrate through the pathway? What effect will an inhibitor of a rate-limiting enzyme have on the concentration of substrates in a multistep pathway?
2. Most drugs are designed to inhibit specific enzymes in biological systems. The drug Prozac has had a profound effect on the medical treatment of depression. Review the history of the development of Prozac, illustrating the importance of specificity in the mechanism of drug action.
3. Discuss some examples of reversible and irreversible enzyme inhibitors used in medical practice.
4. Knockout (KO) mice are mice that lack a specific gene. Discuss the impact of KO mice on the direction of drug development in the pharmaceutical industry.

SUMMARY

▪ Most metabolism is catalyzed by highly specific biological catalysts called enzymes that have active sites designed for substrate recognition and catalysis. Their catalytic activity is dependent on coenzymes and cofactors, often derived from vitamins.

▪ The Michaelis–Menten equation is used to model enzyme kinetics and explains the relationship between substrate concentration and enzyme activity. The Michaelis constant is the substrate concentration at which an enzyme has half-maximal catalytic activity.

▪ Enzymes are strictly regulated by several mechanisms, including gene expression, zymogen activation, and

protein turnover. Both covalent and noncovalent modifications allow for sensitive, short-term changes in enzymatic activity.

▪ Enzyme activity can be inhibited (or activated) by synthetic compounds (drugs), exogenous compounds (toxins), and endogenous compounds (allosteric effectors).

▪ Assays of enzymes in blood and enzyme-based clinical assays are useful for diagnosis and monitoring of many clinical conditions.

FURTHER READING

Davies, G. J., & Williams, S. J. (2016). Carbohydrate-active enzymes: Sequences, shapes, contortions and cells. *Biochemical Society Transactions, 44,* 79–87.

Hetz, C., Chevet, E., & Oakes, S. A. (2015). Proteostasis control by the unfolded protein response. *Nature Cell Biology, 17,* 829–838.

Oakes, B. L., Nadler, D. C., & Savage, D. F. (2014). Protein engineering of Cas9 for enhanced function. *Methods in Enzymology, 546,* 491–511.

Pandya, C., Farelli, J. D., Dunaway-Mariano, D., et al. (2014). Enzyme promiscuity: Engine of evolutionary innovation. *Journal of Biological Chemistry, 289,* 30229–30236.

Pettinati, I., Brem, J., Lee, S. Y., et al. (2016). The chemical biology of human metallo-β-lactamase fold proteins. *Trends in Biochemical Sciences, 41,* 338–355.

Quirós, P. M., Langer, T., & López-Otín, C. (2015). New roles for mitochondrial proteases in health, ageing and disease. *Nature Reviews. Molecular Cell Biology, 16,* 345–359.

Roston, D., & Cui, Q. (2016). QM/MM analysis of transition states and transition state analogues in metalloenzymes. *Methods in Enzymology, 577,* 213–250.

RELEVANT WEBSITES

Clinical chemistry: http://www.labtestsonline.org/

MetaCyc metabolic pathways from all domains of life: http://metacyc.org/

The comprehensive enzyme information system: http://www.brenda-enzymes.org/

Enzyme nomenclature: http://www.chem.qmul.ac.uk/iubmb/enzyme/

IntEnz (integrated relational enzyme database): http://www.ebi.ac.uk/intenz/

ABBREVIATIONS

ALT	Alanine aminotransferase
AST	Aspartate aminotransferase
E	Enzyme
EP	Enzyme-product complex
ES	Enzyme-substrate complex
IU	International unit
K_i	Inhibition constant
K_m	Michaelis constant
LDH	lactate dehydrogenase
PSA	Prostate-specific antigen (kallikrein 3)
S	Substrate
SGOT	Serum glutamate oxaloacetate transaminase
SGPT	Serum glutamate pyruvate transaminase
V_{max}	Maximum velocity

Vitamins and Minerals
Marek H. Dominiczak

INTRODUCTION

Vitamins and trace elements are micronutrients essential for metabolism

Vitamins and trace elements form **prosthetic groups of enzymes** or serve as their **cofactors.** They participate in the metabolism of carbohydrates, fat, and proteins. A and D vitamins act as **hormones**. Vitamins and trace metals are important for cell growth, proliferation, and differentiation, and many of them affect immune phenomena.

Deficiency of a micronutrient may develop because of inadequate intake, poor absorption from the intestinal tract, inefficient utilization or increased loss, or increased demand. Such deficiencies of micronutrients lead to specific clinical syndromes. They may develop as a component of general malnutrition, may themselves be a cause of illness, or may develop during periods of increased demand such as pregnancy or the adolescent growth spurt. In old age, deficiencies may be associated with less efficient intestinal absorption (Chapter 30). They may also occur as complications of gastrointestinal surgery. Multiple micronutrient deficiencies are much more common than single ones. Finally, some vitamins and trace metals are toxic in excess.

Fat-soluble and water-soluble vitamins

The fat-soluble vitamins are A, D, E, and K, and the water-soluble vitamins are B_1, B_2, B_3, B_5, B_6, B_7 (biotin), B_9 (folic acid), B_{12}, and vitamin C.

FAT-SOLUBLE VITAMINS

Fat-soluble vitamins are stored in tissues

Fat-soluble vitamins are associated with body fat and are often stored in tissues, with circulating concentrations being kept relatively constant. For example, vitamin A is stored in the liver and is transported in plasma by specific binding proteins. Fat-soluble vitamins are not as readily absorbed from the diet as are water-soluble vitamins, but ample amounts are stored in tissues. With the exception of vitamin K, they do not act as coenzymes: vitamins A and D behave like hormones. Vitamins A and D, but not vitamin E or K, can be toxic in excess.

Fat malabsorption may lead to deficiencies of vitamins A, D, E, and K. It may occur as a consequence of diseases of liver or gallbladder, inflammatory bowel disease (Crohn's disease, celiac disease), and cystic fibrosis.

Vitamin A

Vitamin A is a generic term for **retinol, retinal**, and **retinoic acid**. Retinal and retinoic acid are active forms of vitamin A. The term *retinoids* has been used to define these substances as well as other synthetic compounds associated with vitamin A–like activity.

The provitamin of vitamin A is a plant pigment **β-carotene** and other carotenoids. All dietary forms of vitamin A are converted to retinol. Retinol, in turn, can be converted to retinal and retinoic acid. Retinol esters are transported from the intestine to the liver in the chylomicrons and chylomicron remnants (Fig. 7.1).

β-Carotene is water soluble and is found in plant food. Good sources of β-carotene are dark-green and yellow vegetables and tomatoes. Conversion of carotenoids to vitamin A is rarely 100% efficient, and the potency of foods is described in retinol activity equivalents (RAE); 1 μg of retinol is equivalent to 12 μg β-carotene, or 24 μg of other carotenes. Liver, fish oil, egg yolk, butter, and milk are good sources of preformed retinol and retinoic acid.

Vitamin A is stored in the liver and needs to be transported to its sites of action

Vitamin A is esterified in the liver by lecithin:retinol acyltransferase and stored in the form of retinyl esters (retinol palmitate), bound to the cytosolic retinol-binding proteins (CRBP). The stores in the liver can provide approximately 1 year's supply. Retinol is secreted from the liver bound to serum retinol-binding protein (RBP) and is taken up by cells via a membrane receptor.

Retinoic acid is thought to be transported to cells bound to either albumin or a specific retinoic acid–binding protein

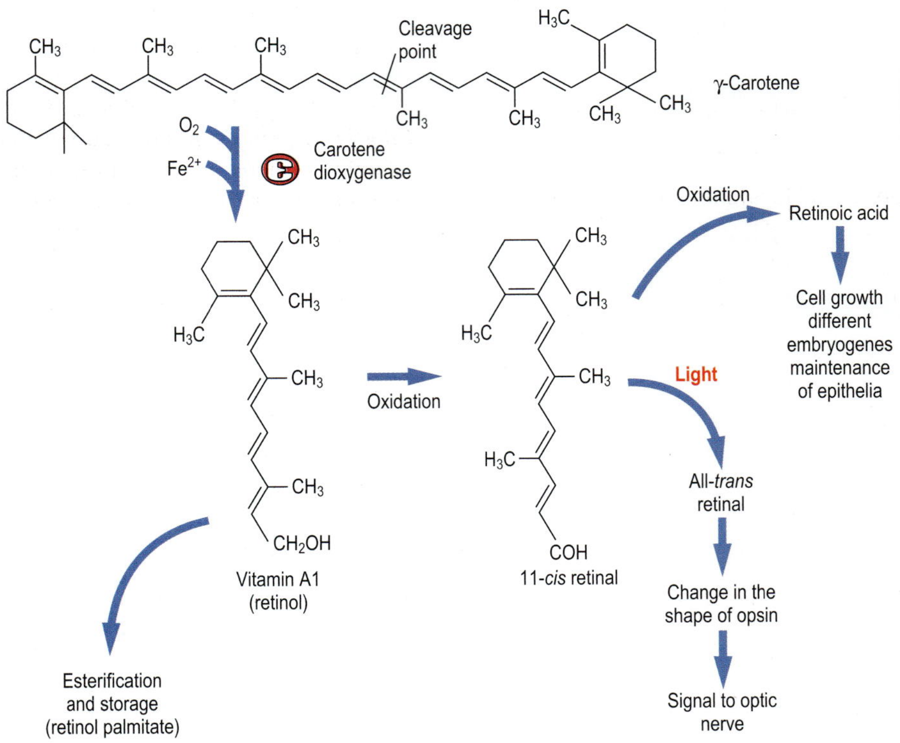

Fig. 7.1 **Structure, metabolism, and function of vitamin A.** Retinol is formed from the cleavage of beta carotene. Its ester is a storage form. Its oxidized derivative 11-*cis* retinal is light sensitive. In the eye rods, light striking 11-*cis* retinal associated with protein opsin in the cones of the retina transforms it into all-*trans* retinal. This transformation changes the shape of opsin, and this generates a signal to the optic nerve (see also Chapter 39 and Fig. 39.4). Retinoic acid, a product of 11-*cis* retinal oxidation, is a signaling molecule.

(RABP). **Retinoic acid is a signaling molecule.** It interacts with ligand-activated transcription factors, known as the nuclear retinoid receptors. The **retinoid acid receptors (RAR)** bind both all-*trans*- and 9-*cis*-retinoic acid, whereas the so-called **rexinoid receptors (RXR)** bind the 9-*cis* isomer only. These receptors can form **heterodimers**. RXR-type receptors can also interact with other nuclear receptors, such as those for vitamin D₃, thyroid hormones, or peroxisome proliferator-activated receptors (PPAR).

Retinoic acid is important in role in growth, differentiation, and proliferation of cells; in embryonic development and organogenesis; and also in the maintenance of epithelia.

Vitamin A deficiency presents as night blindness

The visual pigment rhodopsin, found in the rod cells of the retina, is formed by the binding of 11-*cis*-retinal to the apoprotein opsin. When rhodopsin is exposed to light, the retinal dissociates and is isomerized and reduced to all-*trans*-retinol (Fig. 7.1). This reaction is accompanied by a conformational change and elicits a nerve impulse perceived by the brain as light. The rod cells are responsible for vision in poor light. Therefore vitamin A deficiency presents as **defective night vision, or night blindness** (it is the most common symptom of vitamin A deficiency in children and pregnant women).

Because vitamin A affects the growth and differentiation of epithelial cells, its deficiency produces defective epithelialization and corneal softening and opacity (keratomalacia).

Severe vitamin A deficiency leads to permanent blindness

Vitamin A deficiency is the **commonest cause of blindness in the world.** Subclinical deficiency may also lead to increased susceptibility to infections. Severe vitamin A deficiency occurs mostly in the developing world, but it is also fairly common in patients with severe liver disease or fat malabsorption (e.g., cystic fibrosis).

Pregnant and lactating women are prone to vitamin A deficiency. The most vulnerable group are premature infants and, in the developing countries, breastfed children of mothers who themselves are vitamin A deficient.

Vitamin A is toxic in excess

Vitamin A is toxic in excess, with symptoms including increased intracranial pressure, headaches, double vision, dizziness, bone and joint pain, hair loss, dermatitis, hepatosplenomegaly, and diarrhea and vomiting. Increased intake of vitamin A is also associated with teratogenicity, and it **should be avoided during pregnancy.** It is virtually impossible to develop vitamin A toxicity by ingesting normal foods; however, toxicity may result from the use of vitamin A supplements.

Both vitamin A deficiency and excess can cause birth defects

Vitamin D

Vitamin D is a hormone, and in addition to its role in calcium homeostasis, it influences genes involved in cell proliferation, differentiation, and apoptosis.

It modulates growth, participates in immune function, and is antiinflammatory. Deficiency of vitamin D produces rickets in children and osteomalacia in adults.

Vitamin D is toxic in excess.

Vitamin D metabolism and actions are described in Chapter 38.

Vitamin E

Dietary vitamin E is a mixture of several compounds, known as tocopherols. Ninety percent of vitamin E present in human tissues is in the form of α-tocopherol (Fig. 7.2). It is absorbed from the diet in the small intestine with lipids. It is packed into the **chylomicrons,** and in the circulation, it is associated with lipoproteins.

Vitamin E is a membrane antioxidant

Vitamin E is the most abundant natural antioxidant, and because of its lipid solubility, it is associated with all lipid-containing structures: membranes, lipoproteins, and fat deposits. It protects lipids from oxidation by the reactive oxygen species (ROS). It is also involved in immune function, cellular signaling, and gene expression. α-Tocopherol inhibits the activity of protein kinase C (PKC) and affects cell adhesion as well as arachidonic acid metabolism.

The richest sources of naturally occurring vitamin E are vegetable oils, nuts, and green leafy vegetables.

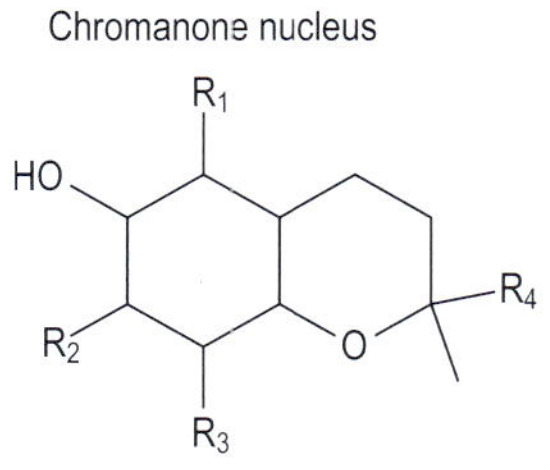

R_1–R_3			R_4
α-tocopherol	$R_1,R_2,R_3,$	Me	
β-tocopherol	$R_1,R_3,$	Me	$- CH_2(CH_2 - CH_2 - CH - CH_2)_3 -$ with CH_3
γ-tocopherol	$R_2,R_3,$	Me	
δ-tocopherol	$R_2,R_3,$	Me	

Fig. 7.2 **Structure of vitamin E family (tocopherols).** R_1–R_3 can be methylated in a variety of combinations. R_4 is a polyisoprenoid chain. Me, methyl.

Fat malabsorption reduces vitamin E absorption

Malabsorption of fat and abetalipoproteinemia may lead to vitamin E deficiency. Deficiency may also develop as a result of low vitamin E intake in pregnancy and newborn infants (mostly in preterm infants fed with formula milk with low vitamin E content). In premature infants, this causes **hemolytic anemia, thrombocytosis, and edema, as well as peripheral neuropathy, myopathy, and ataxia**.

Vitamin K

Vitamin K is a group of compounds that vary in the number of isoprenoid units in their side chain. Vitamin K circulates as phylloquinone (vitamin K_1), and its hepatic stores are in the form of menaquinones (vitamin K_2). The structure, nomenclature, and sources the vitamin K are outlined in Fig. 7.3. Absorption of vitamin K depends on the ability to absorb fat.

Vitamin K is necessary for blood clotting

Vitamin K is required for posttranslational modification of coagulation factors (factors II, VII, IX, and X; Chapter 41). All of these proteins are synthesized by the liver as inactive precursors and are activated by the carboxylation of specific glutamic acid residues by a vitamin K–dependent enzyme (Fig. 7.4). Prothrombin (factor II) contains 10 of these carboxylated residues, and all are required for this protein's specific chelation of Ca^{2+} ions during its function in the coagulation process.

Vitamin K is widely distributed in nature; its dietary sources are green leafy vegetables, fruits, dairy products, vegetable oils, and cereals. Vitamin K is also produced by the intestinal microflora.

Vitamin K deficiency causes bleeding disorders

Vitamin K supply by the intestinal microflora virtually ensures that dietary deficiency does not occur in humans, except for newborn infants. Rarely, deficiency may develop in those with liver disease or fat malabsorption. The deficiency is associated with bleeding disorders.

Premature infants are at particular risk of deficiency and may develop hemorrhagic disease of the newborn

Placental transfer of vitamin K to the fetus is inefficient. Immediately after birth, the circulating concentration decreases. The gut of the newborn is sterile; therefore for several days after birth, there is no source of vitamin K. Usually, the concentration normalizes when the absorption of food starts, but this might be delayed in preterm infants.

Inhibitors of vitamin K action are valuable antithrombotic drugs

Specific inhibitors of vitamin K–dependent carboxylation are used in the treatment of thrombosis-related diseases - for example, in patients with **deep vein thrombosis** and **pulmonary thromboembolism** or those with **atrial fibrillation**

Source	Structure	Group
Plants		Phylloquinone (vitamin K₁)
Animal tissue bacteria		Menaquinones (vitamin K₂)

Fig. 7.3 **Structures of the different forms of vitamin K.**

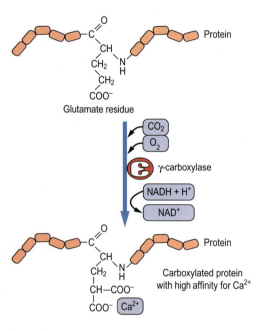

Glutamate residue

CO₂
O₂

γ-carboxylase

NADH + H⁺
NAD⁺

Protein

Carboxylated protein with high affinity for Ca²⁺

Fig. 7.4 **Vitamin K–mediated carboxylation of glutamate residues.** These carboxylated residues in a protein chain are required for Ca²⁺ chelation. AA, amino acid.

who are at risk of thrombosis. These are the drugs of the dicoumarin group (e.g., **warfarin**), which inhibit the action of vitamin K (Chapter 41). Warfarin is also used as rat poison, and vitamin K is the antidote for poisoning by this agent.

WATER-SOLUBLE VITAMINS

Vitamin B and vitamin C are water soluble

With the exception of vitamin B₁₂, the body has no storage capacity for water-soluble vitamins. As a consequence, they must be regularly supplied in the diet. Any excess is excreted in the urine.

B-complex vitamins

B-complex vitamins are essential for normal metabolism and serve as coenzymes in many reactions in carbohydrate, fat, and protein metabolism

The greater the caloric intake, the larger the requirement for B vitamins. Increased energy supply, in particular from simple carbohydrates, requires increased amounts of B vitamins. **High carbohydrate intake requires greater intake of thiamine and other B vitamins.** Therefore beriberi (see later discussion) might develop on a high-carbohydrate diet.

Vitamin B₁ (thiamine) is essential for carbohydrate metabolism

In its active form, **thiamine pyrophosphate (TPP),** vitamin B₁ is a coenzyme of pyruvate dehydrogenase (the E1 enzyme in the PDH complex; Chapter 10). It participates in oxidative decarboxylation of β-ketoglutarate and also in the metabolism of branched-chain amino acids. It is also a coenzyme for transketolase in the pentose phosphate pathway (Chapter 9), and it is important in the production of hydrochloric acid in the stomach.

Beriberi was the first-discovered deficiency disease

Severe thiamine deficiency results in **beriberi, either "dry"** (without fluid retention) **or "wet"** (associated with cardiac failure with edema). Beriberi is characterized primarily by neuromuscular symptoms and occurs in populations relying exclusively on polished rice for food. The signs and symptoms of deficiency may also be seen in the elderly or in low-income groups with poor diet.

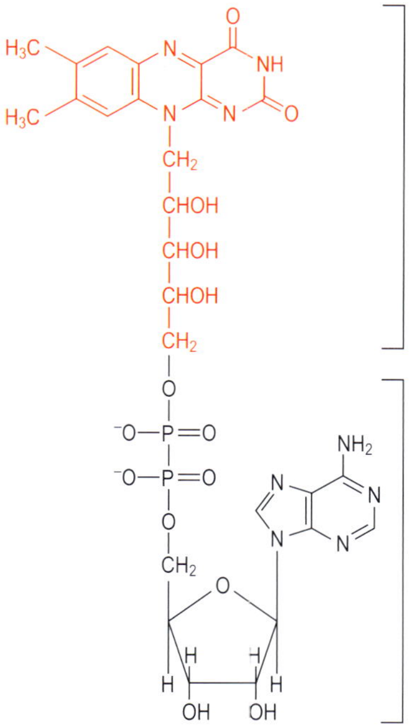

Fig. 7.5 **Vitamin B₂, riboflavin, forms part of flavin mononucleotide (FMN) and the flavin adenine dinucleotide (FAD, shown here).**

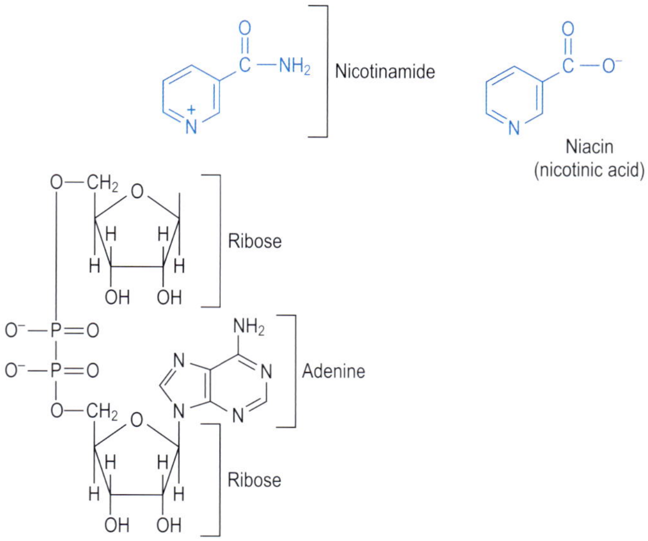

Fig. 7.6 **Vitamin B₃, niacin, forms part of nicotinamide adenine dinucleotide (NAD⁺, shown here) and nicotinamide adenine dinucleotide phosphate (NADP⁺).**

Thiamine deficiency is associated with alcoholism

Thiamine depletion can occur quickly (within approximately 14 days). Early symptoms are loss of appetite, constipation, and nausea. They may progress to depression, peripheral neuropathy, and unsteadiness. Further deterioration results in mental confusion (loss of short-term memory), ataxia, and loss of eye coordination. This combination, often seen in alcoholic patients, is known as **Wernicke–Korsakoff psychosis**. Wet beriberi is particularly associated with alcoholism.

Tests used to assess the thiamine status include its direct measurement by high-pressure liquid chromatography and the measurement of erythrocyte transketolase activity.

Vitamin B₂ (riboflavin) is required for FMN and FAD synthesis

Riboflavin is attached to the sugar alcohol ribitol. The molecule is colored, fluorescent, and decomposes in visible light but is heat stable. Flavin mononucleotide (FMN) and the flavin adenine dinucleotide (FAD) are formed by transfer of phosphate and adenosine monophosphate from ATP, respectively. They are coenzymes of the oxidoreductases, are tightly bound to the native enzyme, and participate in redox reactions (Fig. 7.5; Chapter 8).

Lack of riboflavin in the diet causes a deficiency syndrome that includes inflammation of the corners of the mouth (angular stomatitis), inflammation of the tongue (glossitis), and scaly dermatitis. Photophobia may also develop. Because of its light sensitivity, riboflavin deficiency may occur in newborn infants with jaundice who are treated with phototherapy. Hypothyroidism

is also known to affect the conversion of riboflavin to FMN and FAD.

To determine riboflavin status, **erythrocyte glutathione reductase** activity is measured.

Vitamin B₃ (niacin) is required for NAD⁺ and NADP⁺ synthesis

Niacin is a generic name for nicotinic acid or nicotinamide, both of which are essential nutrients. Niacin is active as part of the coenzyme nicotinamide adenine dinucleotide (NAD⁺) and nicotinamide adenine dinucleotide phosphate (NADP⁺), both of which participate in oxidoreductase-catalyzed reactions (Fig. 7.6). The active form of the vitamin required for the synthesis of NAD⁺ and NADP⁺ is nicotinate, and therefore nicotinamide must be deamidated before becoming available for synthesis of these coenzymes. **The requirement for niacin is related to energy expenditure.** Niacin can be synthesized from tryptophan and, hence, in the truest sense, is not a vitamin. The conversion is, however, very inefficient and cannot supply sufficient amounts of niacin. In addition, the conversion requires thiamine, pyridoxine, and riboflavin, and on marginal diets, such synthesis would be problematic.

Severe niacin deficiency results in dermatitis, diarrhea, and dementia

Niacin deficiency initially produces a superficial glossitis but may progress to **pellagra,** which is characterized by dermatitis, sunburn-like skin lesions in areas of the body exposed to sunlight and to pressure, and also by diarrhea and dementia. Untreated pellagra is fatal; however, in the modern world, pellagra is a medical curiosity. Certain drugs, such as the antituberculosis drug isoniazid, predispose to niacin deficiency. In contrast, very high doses of niacin can cause hepatotoxicity.

Vitamin B₆ (pyridoxine) participates in carbohydrate and lipid metabolism and is particularly important for amino acid metabolism

Vitamin B_6 is a mixture of pyridoxine, pyridoxal, pyridoxamine, and their 5′-phosphate esters. Pyridoxine is the major form of vitamin B_6 in the diet, and pyridoxal phosphate is its active form. It is absorbed in the jejunum.

Pyridoxine requirements increase with high protein intake

Pyridoxal phosphate and pyridoxamine are involved in more than 100 reactions in carbohydrate (including the glycogen phosphorylase reaction) and lipid metabolism; in the synthesis, catabolism, and interconversion of amino acids (Chapter 15); and in the metabolism of one-carbon units. Pyridoxine is required for the synthesis of the neurotransmitters serotonin and noradrenaline (Chapter 26); sphingosine, a component of sphingomyelin and sphingolipids (Chapter 18); and heme (Chapter 34). It influences immune function. Because of its role in amino acid metabolism, vitamin B_6 requirements increase with protein intake.

Vitamin B_6 is present in a wide variety of foods, such as fish, beef, liver, poultry, potatoes, and fruits (but not citrus fruits).

Pyridoxine deficiency causes neurologic symptoms and anemia

Vitamin B_6 deficiency in its mild form causes irritability, nervousness, and depression, progressing in severe deficiency to peripheral neuropathy, convulsions, and coma. Severe deficiency is also associated with a sideroblastic anemia (anemia characterized by the presence of nucleated red blood cells with iron granules). Dermatitis, cheilosis, and glossitis also occur. Decreased levels are observed in **alcoholism, obesity,** and **malabsorption states** (Crohn's disease, celiac disease, and ulcerative colitis), as well as in **end-stage renal disease** and in **autoimmune conditions**.

The drug **isoniazid**, by binding to pyridoxine, and the oral contraceptive pill, by increasing the synthesis of enzymes requiring the vitamin, may precipitate deficiency. The debate concerning the contraceptive pill continues, but it is generally accepted that there is an increased requirement for pyridoxine.

Assessment of pyridoxine status is based on the measurement of erythrocyte aspartate aminotransferase.

Vitamin B₇ (biotin) participates in carboxylation reactions in lipogenesis and gluconeogenesis and in the catabolism of the branched-chain amino acids

Biotin (formerly called vitamin H) serves as a coenzyme in multienzyme complexes involved in carboxylation reactions in lipogenesis and gluconeogenesis as well as in the catabolism of the branched-chain amino acids (Chapter 15). Biotin is normally synthesized by the intestinal flora, and this meets most of the body's requirements.

Symptoms of biotin deficiency include depression, hallucinations, muscle pain, and dermatitis. Children with multiple decarboxylase deficiency also develop immunodeficiency disease. Consumption of raw eggs can cause biotin deficiency because the egg-white protein avidin combines with biotin, preventing its absorption.

Vitamin B₉ (folic acid) derivatives are important in single-carbon-transfer reactions and are necessary for the synthesis of DNA

Folic acid (pteroyl-L-glutamic acid) exists in a number of derivatives collectively known as folates. It participates in **single-carbon-transfer reactions,** such as methylation (important in both metabolism and regulation of gene expression), and in the synthetic pathways of choline, serine, glycine, and methionine. Folic acid is also necessary for the synthesis of purines and pyrimidine thymine and, thus, for the **synthesis of nucleic acids**. Polymorphisms associated with variants of 5,10-methylenetetrahydrofolate reductase (MTHFR) gene, the key enzyme in folate metabolism, are associated with conditions such as colon cancer, spina bifida, and adult acute lymphocytic leukemia.

Folic acid is physiologically inactive until reduced to dihydrofolic acid. Its main forms are tetrahydrofolate, 5-methyl tetrahydrofolate (N^5MeTHF), and N^{10}-formyltetrahydrofolate-polyglutamate derived from N^5MeTHF predominant in fresh food. Before polyglutamates can be absorbed, they must be hydrolyzed by glutamyl hydrolase in the small intestine. The main circulating form of folate is the monoglutamate-N^5-THF.

Folic acid is present in liver, yeast, and green leafy vegetables (spinach) and fruits, including citrus fruits. Its sources also include folic acid–enriched cereals and grains. It can be measured by HPLC.

Structural analogues of folate are used as antibiotics and anticancer drugs

Not surprisingly, rapidly dividing cells have high requirements for folate because it is necessary for the synthesis of purines and pyrimidine thymine, all required for DNA synthesis (Chapter 16). Structural analogs of folate exhibit selective toxicity toward rapidly growing cells such as bacteria and cancer cells. This is the principle behind the development of drugs known as the **folic acid antagonists,** which are used as antibiotics (e.g., trimethoprim) and anticancer agents (methotrexate).

Folate deficiency is one of the commonest vitamin deficiencies

Causes of folate deficiency include inadequate intake, impaired absorption, impaired metabolism, and increased demand. The most common examples of increased demand are pregnancy and lactation. Folic acid requirements increase greatly as the blood volume and number of erythrocytes increase in pregnancy. By the third trimester of pregnancy, folic acid requirements double. Megaloblastic anemia in pregnancy (other than multiple pregnancy) is rare. However, folate deficiency increases the risk of **neural tube defects,** low **birth weight,** and **premature**

birth. In infants, it results in a decreased growth rate. Other causes of folate deficiency are **alcoholism, malabsorption, dialysis, and liver disease**. Folate deficiencies are seen in the elderly as a result of poor diet and poor absorption.

Folate deficiency in adults causes megaloblastic anemia

The failure to synthesize methionine and nucleic acids in folate-deficient states accounts for the signs and symptoms of **megaloblastic anemia** (i.e.. the presence of enlarged blast cells in the bone marrow). Macrocytic erythrocytes have fragile membranes and a tendency to hemolyze: a macrocytic anemia exists in association with a megaloblastic bone marrow. The hematologic abnormalities cannot be distinguished from vitamin B_{12} deficiency (see later discussion). The neurologic changes are also similar. Deficiency of folate also contributes to hyperhomocysteinemia. Many symptoms are nonspecific, such as loss of appetite, diarrhea, and weakness.

Adequate intake of folate around conception is essential

The common practice is to provide folate supplements during pregnancy. Supplementation during the periconception period (definitions of that period are variable; the one used in clinical studies is 4 weeks before and 8 weeks after conception) prevents spina bifida because the closure of the neural tube occurs between 22 and 28 days after conception.

Vitamin B_{12} forms part of the heme structure

Vitamin B_{12} (cobalamin) has a complex ring structure similar to the porphyrin of heme (Chapter 34) but is hydrogenated to a greater extent. The iron at the center of the heme ring is replaced by a cobalt ion (Co^{3+}). This is the only known function of cobalt in the body. In addition, a dimethylbenzimidazole ring is also part of the active molecule; it is essential for the chelation of the cobalt ion (Fig. 7.7) and in methionine synthesis.

Vitamin B_{12} participates in **nucleic acid synthesis**, in the **production of erythrocytes**, and also in the **recycling of folates**. Together with folate and vitamin B_6, it controls homocysteine metabolism, where it is a cofactor for methionine synthase, which converts homocysteine to methionine. It participates in the synthesis of the methyl donor molecule, the **S-adenosylmethionine**. Vitamin B_{12} is required in only one further reaction, that of L-methylmalonyl-CoA mutase, which converts methylmalonyl-CoA to succinyl-CoA. The coenzyme form of the vitamin in this case is 5′-deoxy-adenosyl cobalamin. Vitamin B_{12} is synthesized solely by bacteria. It is absent from all plants but is concentrated in the livers of animals in three forms: methylcobalamin, adenosylcobalamin, and hydroxycobalamin.

Vitamin B_{12} requires the intrinsic factor for its absorption

Cobalamin is released from foods by a gastric protease and HCl. It is bound to the intrinsic factor secreted by the parietal cells in the stomach, and it is absorbed in the distal ileum by receptor-mediated endocytosis. Vitamin B_{12} is excreted in the bile, and there is a marked enterohepatic circulation (Fig. 7.8).

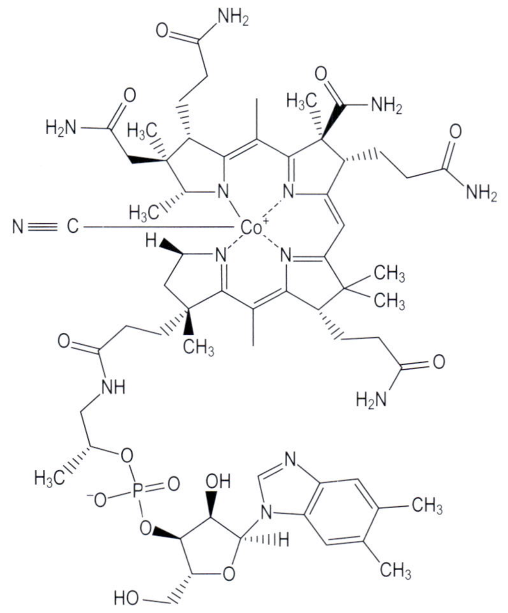

Fig. 7.7 **Vitamin B_{12}.** There is a cyano group (CN) attached to the cobalt; this is an artifact of extraction, but it is also the most stable form of the vitamin and, indeed, is the commercially available product. The cyano group does require removal for conversion to the active form of the vitamin.

Vitamin B_{12} is only present in animal products

Vitamin B_{12} is found only in animal products such as fish, dairy products, and meats, particularly organ meats such as liver and kidney. **Vegans are therefore at risk of developing a dietary deficiency of vitamin B_{12}.** Fortified breakfast cereals also contain the vitamin.

Vitamin B_{12} deficiency causes pernicious anemia

Vitamin B_{12} deficiency is characterized by anemia, fatigue, constipation, weight loss, diarrhea, and neurologic symptoms such as numbness and tingling, loss of balance, confusion, mood disturbances, and dementia. Deficiency can occur through several mechanisms. The most common one is pernicious anemia, an autoimmune condition that results in gastric atrophy and the lack of the intrinsic factor, which prevents vitamin absorption in the terminal ileum. Pernicious anemia affects 1%–3% of older adults. The intrinsic factor deficiency can also be caused by gastric surgery and by bariatric (weight-loss) surgery. A similar situation, albeit caused by a different mechanism, arises upon surgical removal of the ileum - for instance, in Crohn's disease. Deficiency may also be caused by hypochlorhydria associated with age.

The function of vitamin B_{12} needs to be considered together with folate

The functions of vitamin B_{12} and folate are interrelated, and a deficiency of either produces the same signs and symptoms.

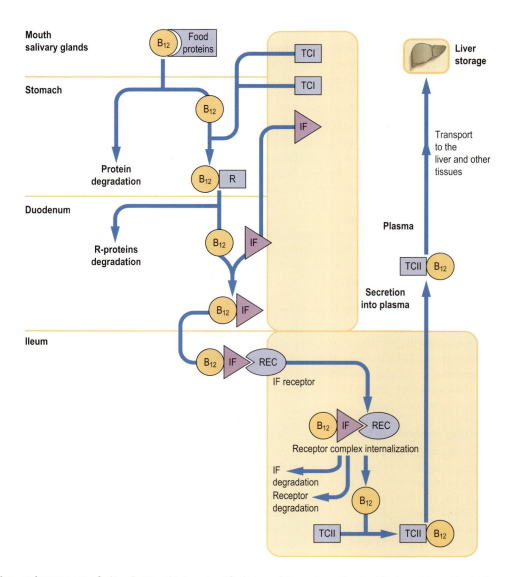

Fig. 7.8 **Absorption and transport of vitamin B₁₂.** This is a simplified view of the system. Simple diffusion of free vitamin B_{12} across the intestinal membrane accounts for 3% of transported vitamin, and complexing with intrinsic factor (IF) accounts for 97%. Vitamin B_{12} derivatives are released from food by peptic digestion and bind to several proteins known as R-proteins of which one is haptocorrin (transcobalamin I [TCI]) and other proteins (R proteins) produced by salivary glands. Only haptocorrin binding is shown here. In the duodenum, B_{12} is released from haptocorrin and binds to IF secreted by the parietal cells of the gastric mucosa. Lower down in the gastrointestinal tract, IF–B_{12} complex binds to specific receptor sites on the ileal mucosa. The rate-limiting factor for vitamin B_{12} absorption is the number of ileal receptor sites. Haptocorrin (TCI) and transcobalamin II (TCII) bind B_{12}, transporting it to the liver. Both TCII-B_{12} and TCI-B_{12} (not shown) complexes participate in the transport of vitamin B_{12} between tissues.

The reaction that involves both of these vitamins is the conversion of homocysteine to methionine (Fig. 7.9).

Megaloblastic anemia characteristic of vitamin B_{12} deficiency is probably due to a secondary deficiency of reduced folate and a consequence of the accumulation of N^5-methyltetrahydrofolate. A neurologic presentation can also develop in the absence of anemia. This is known as **subacute combined degeneration of the cord** and is probably secondary to a relative deficiency of methionine in the cord.

Deficiency of vitamin B_{12} results in the accumulation of methylmalonic acid and homocysteine, leading to **methylmalonic aciduria and homocystinuria**.

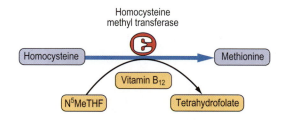

Fig. 7.9 **The "tetrahydrofolate trap."** Vitamin B_{12} and folate are involved in the conversion of homocysteine to methionine. An absence of vitamin B_{12} inhibits the reaction and leads to the buildup of N^5-methyltetrahydrofolate (N⁵MeTHF).

ADVANCED CONCEPT BOX
VITAMIN B₁₂ TRANSPORT PROTEINS

The intrinsic factor (IF) is a glycoprotein. Other cobalamin-binding proteins are the R-proteins including, the glycoprotein haptocorrin (TC I), and nonglycoprotein transcobalamin (TC II).

At an acid pH, the R proteins bind cobalamin more strongly than IF. In contrast to IF, they are normally degraded by pancreatic proteinases. Thus in pancreatic disease where they are not degraded, there is less cobalamin available to bind to IF, with loss of absorptive capacity for this vitamin.

In the final stages of the absorption process, the IF molecule binds to the ileal receptor in the presence of Ca^{2+} and at neutral pH. As the IF–B₁₂ complex crosses the ileal mucosa, in plasma, haptocorrin binds 70%–80% of B₁₂, and transcobalamin binds 20%–30%. Cobalamin bound to haptocorrin and transcobalamin is delivered to the tissues, where it binds to specific cell-surface receptors. It enters the cell by endocytosis, ultimately releasing the cobalamin as hydroxycobalamin. Subsequently, hydroxycobalamin is converted to methylcobalamin in the cytosol.

Vitamin B₁₂ must be supplemented during folate treatment

Folate supplementation without B₁₂ supplements can mask symptoms but lead to neurologic damage. Giving folate alone in a case of vitamin B₁₂ deficiency aggravates the neuropathy. Therefore if supplementation is required during the investigation of the cause of megaloblastic anemia, after blood and bone marrow specimens have been taken to confirm the diagnosis, folate needs to be given together with vitamin B₁₂.

The deficiency states of the B vitamins are summarized in Fig. 7.10. Finally, deficiency of a single B vitamin is rare; patients most often present with multiple deficiencies.

Pantothenic acid

Pantothenic acid is widely distributed in animals and plants

Pantothenic acid forms part of the molecule of coenzyme A (CoA; Fig. 7.11).

There is no evidence of deficiency in humans, except those on experimental diets.

Vitamin C

Vitamin C serves as a reducing agent. Its active form is ascorbic acid, which is oxidized during the transfer of reducing equivalents, yielding dehydroascorbic acid. The synthetic pathway and structure of vitamin C are shown in Fig. 7.12, and its antioxidant activity is illustrated in Chapter 42. It participates in the regeneration of another antioxidant vitamin,

α-tocopherol. Vitamin C takes part in the synthesis of collagen and epinephrine, in steroidogenesis, in the degradation of tyrosine, in the formation of bile acids, and also in the synthesis of L-carnitine and neurotransmitters. It improves absorption of nonheme iron and participates in bone mineral metabolism. Its prime function is to maintain metal cofactors in their lower valence states (e.g., Fe^{2+} and Cu^{2+}). In the synthesis of collagen, it is required specifically for the hydroxylation of proline (Chapter 19).

Vitamin C is absorbed in the intestine by a carrier-mediated, sodium-dependent transporter. It is reabsorbed in the renal proximal tubules. Progressively more vitamin C is excreted in urine as intake increases.

Humans cannot synthesize ascorbic acid; therefore it is an essential nutrient

Vitamin C is labile: it is easily destroyed by oxygen, metal ions, increased pH, heat, and light. Citrus, soft fruits, tomatoes, and peppers are rich sources of vitamin C.

Vitamin C deficiency causes scurvy and compromises immune function

Vitamin C deficiency causes defective collagen synthesis. **Scurvy** is characterized by capillary fragility, causing subcutaneous and other hemorrhages; muscle weakness; soft, swollen, bleeding gums; loosening of teeth; poor wound healing; and anemia. Fatigue, malaise, and depression also occur. The inability to maintain bone matrix in association with demineralization results in osteoporosis.

Vitamin C deficiency resulting in the full clinical picture of scurvy is now rare, except in older individuals. Milder forms of vitamin C deficiency are more common, and their manifestation includes easy bruising and the formation of petechiae (small, pinpoint hemorrhages under the skin). Immune function is also compromised. This reduction in immunocompetence has been the basis for providing megadoses of the vitamin to prevent the common cold and also for its role in cancer prevention. No clear evidence exists, however, to substantiate these claims first made by Linus Pauling in the 1970s. Vitamin C is certainly required for normal leukocyte function, and leukocyte vitamin C levels drop precipitously during the stress caused by either trauma or infection. Elderly individuals are at increased risk of deficiency, as are smokers and infants fed evaporated or boiled milk.

There is no evidence that vitamin C taken in excess is toxic. Theoretically, because it is metabolized to oxalate, there is a risk of the development of renal oxalate stones in susceptible individuals. However, this has not been substantiated in practice.

DIETARY SUPPLEMENTATION OF VITAMINS

Supplementation of some vitamins results in a clear health benefit. This includes supplementation of folic acid to women

Vitamin	Structure	Deficiency disease	Food source
Thiamine (vit B_1)	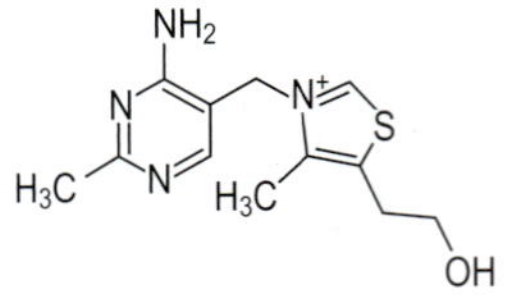	Beriberi	Seeds, nuts, wheatgerms, legumes, lean meat
Riboflavin (vit B_2)	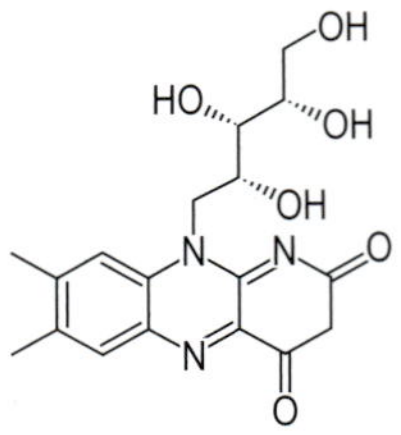	Pellagra	Meats, nuts, legumes
Niacin (vit B_3)	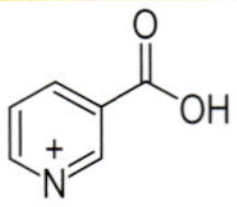	Pellagra	Meats, nuts, legumes
Panthothenic acid (vit B_5)	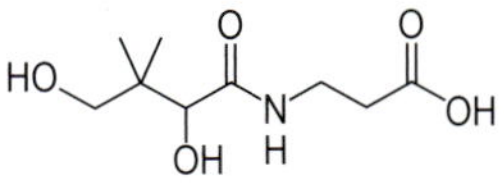		Yeast, grains, egg yolk, liver
Pyridoxine (vit B_6)	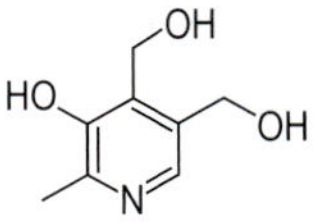	Neurologic symptoms	Yeast, liver, wheatgerm, nuts beans, bananas
Biotin (vit B_7)	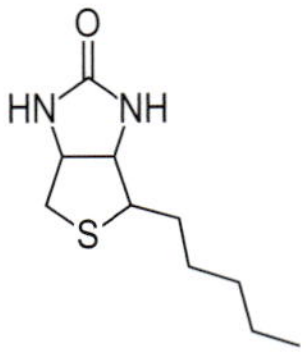	Neurologic symptoms, dermatitis conjunctivitis, brittle nails, hair loss	Corn, soy, egg yolk, liver, kidney, tomatoes
Folate (vit B_9)	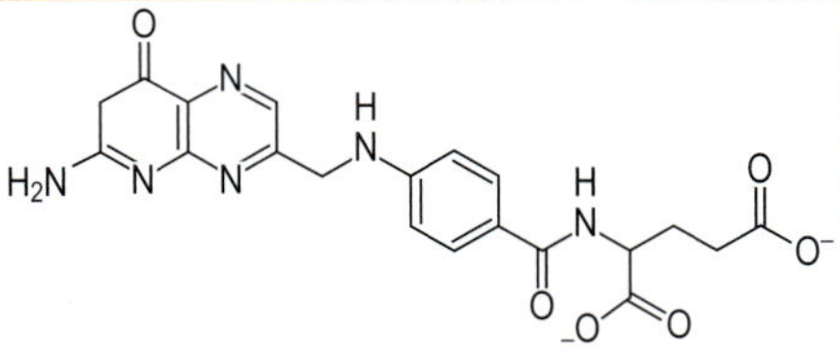	Anemia	Yeast, liver, leafy vegetables
Cobalamin (vit B_{12})	Complex	Pernicious anemia	Liver, kidney, egg, cheese

Fig. 7.10 **Structure, sources, and deficiency diseases of the B vitamins.**

who are pregnant or are planning pregnancy to prevent neural tube defects. Vitamin D provision to people living in areas of low sunlight has also been beneficial.

The benefits of vitamin supplementation in cancer and cardiovascular disease are uncertain

Because supplementation of folic acid and vitamin B_6 and B_{12} lowers the plasma homocysteine concentration, it has been suggested that it could be beneficial for the prevention of cardiovascular disease. There also were suggestions that supplementation of vitamins A, C, and E is protective against cancer. Some observational studies suggested that the supplementation of vitamins C and E could also be useful in the prevention of cardiovascular disease. However, prospective studies of this possibility yielded controversial results.

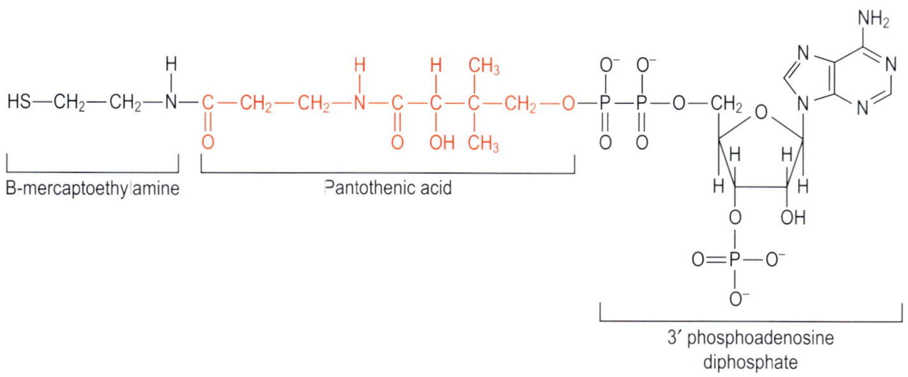

Fig. 7.11 **Pantothenic acid (vitamin B₅) forms part of the molecule of coenzyme A.**

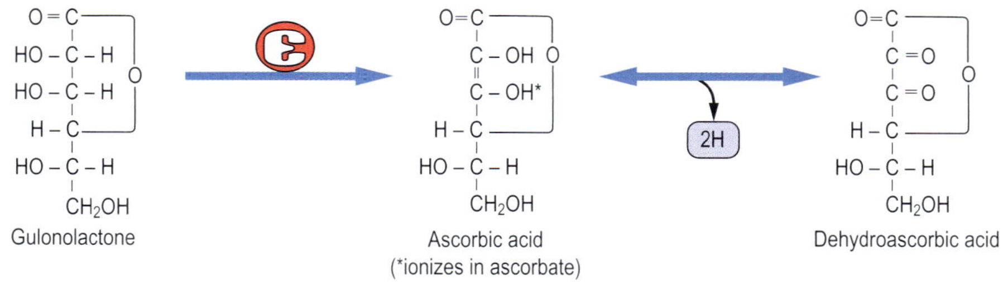

Fig. 7.12 **Structure and synthesis of vitamin C (ascorbic acid).** Note that the enzyme that converts gulonolactone to ascorbic acid is absent in humans and higher primates.

Vitamin supplementation can be harmful

As mentioned previously, high-dose vitamin supplementation may be harmful; an example is the reduction of bone mineral density, hepatotoxicity, and teratogenicity associated with high doses of vitamin A. Supplementation of β-carotene in smokers was also found to be harmful, resulting in an increase in lung cancer mortality.

Fruit and vegetables are the best sources of vitamins

In clinical studies, vitamins have been supplemented in a pure form, rather than as complete foodstuffs, and this might be why the benefit of supplementation was not evident. Clearly, there are benefits of eating diets rich in vegetables and fruits, which are the most important sources of vitamins. There is no reason to discourage people from taking vitamin supplements apart from proven instances of toxicity.

The role of vitamins in metabolism is summarized in Table 7.1.

MINERALS

Major minerals present in the human body are sodium, potassium, chloride, calcium, phosphate, and magnesium

The daily body requirements for minerals range from grams (sodium, calcium, chloride, phosphorus) to milligrams (iron, iodine, magnesium, manganese, molybdenum) to micrograms (zinc, copper, selenium, other trace elements). Many are essential for normal functioning of the body.

Sodium and chloride are important for the maintenance of the osmolality of the extracellular fluid and cell volume (Chapter 35). Sodium participates in electrophysiologic phenomena and, together with potassium, is essential for maintaining transmembrane potential and impulse transmission (Chapter 4). **Potassium** is the main intracellular cation. Potassium is contained in vegetables and fruit, particularly bananas, and in fruit juices. Dietary potassium intake needs to be limited in renal disease because of its impaired excretion and a consequent tendency to hyperkalemia (Chapter 35). Importantly, both hyperkalemia and hypokalemia may lead to life-threatening arrhythmias.

Magnesium functions as a cofactor for many enzymes and is also important in the maintenance of membrane electrical potential. Its role is linked to that of potassium and calcium. It is important for skeletal development and for the maintenance of electrical potential in nerve and muscle membranes. It is a cofactor for ATP-requiring enzymes and is important for DNA replication and for RNA synthesis. Magnesium deficiency develops during starvation, in individuals with malabsorption, and after the loss from the gastrointestinal tract in diarrhea and vomiting. It sometimes occurs as a result of diuretic treatment. It is also associated with acute pancreatitis and alcoholism. **Hypomagnesemia is often accompanied by hypocalcemia and hypokalemia.** Magnesium deficiency leads to muscle weakness and cardiac arrhythmias.

Table 7.1 Role of vitamins in metabolism

Vitamin		Metabolic role
Fat-soluble vitamins		
A	Retinol, retinal	Vision
A	Retinoic acid	Embryonic development; organogenesis; maintenance of epithelia; cell growth, proliferation, and differentiation
D	Cholecalciferol, ergocalciferol, and derivatives	Bone metabolism and calcium homeostasis
E	Tocopherols	ROS scavenging (membrane antioxidants)
K	2-Methyl-1,4-naphthoquinone (3-) derivatives	Blood clotting
Water-soluble vitamins		
B_1	Thiamine	Carbohydrate metabolism: pyruvate dehydrogenase, α-ketoglutarate dehydrogenase, amino acid metabolism
B_2	Riboflavin	Oxidoreductases, FMN, FAD
B_3	Niacin	Oxidoreductases, NAD^+, $NADP^+$
B_5	Pantothenic acid	Structure of coenzyme A
B_6	Pyridoxine	Carbohydrate, lipid, and amino acid metabolism; neurotransmitter synthesis; synthesis of sphingolipids; heme synthesis
B_7	Biotin	Carboxylation reactions, lipogenesis, gluconeogenesis, branched-chain amino acid metabolism
B_9	Folic acid	One-carbon-transfer reactions, choline synthesis of amino acids, synthesis of purines and pyrimidine (thymine)
B_{12}	Cobalamine	Heme structure, folate recycling, synthesis of methyl group donor S-adenosyl methionine
C	Ascorbic acid	Antioxidant function, collagen synthesis, bile acid synthesis, neurotransmitter synthesis

Calcium and phosphate are essential for bone metabolism, secretory processes, and cellular signaling. Plasma calcium concentration is regulated primarily by parathormone and vitamin D (Chapter 38). Calcium is present in milk and milk products and in some vegetables. Phosphates are abundant in plant and animal cells.

Iodine is essential for the synthesis of thyroid hormones (Chapter 27). The iodine content of food depends on the composition of the soil where it is grown. Marine fish and shellfish have the highest content. It is also present in freshwater fish, meat and dairy products, legumes, vegetables, and fruit.

Fluoride influences the structure of the bone and teeth enamel. In many areas, fluoride is added to municipal water supplies to prevent teeth decay. Excess leads to tooth discoloration and fragility of bones.

Iron metabolism

Iron is important in the transfer of molecular oxygen

Iron is a component of heme in hemoglobin and myoglobin (Chapter 5) and also cytochromes *a*, *b*, and *c* (Chapter 8). Altogether, there are 3–4 g of iron in the body, of which 75% is in hemoglobin and myoglobin and 25% is stored in tissues such as bone marrow, liver, and the reticuloendothelial system.

Dietary sources of iron include organ meats, poultry, fish and oysters, egg yolks, dried beans, dried figs and dates, and some green vegetables.

Iron is transported in plasma bound to transferrin

Iron is absorbed in the upper small intestine (Fig. 7.13). Meat and ascorbic acid increase its absorption, and vegetable fiber inhibits it. It is **transported in blood bound to transferrin** and is **stored as ferritin and hemosiderin**. Transferrin is normally about 30% saturated with iron. Iron is lost through the skin and through the gastrointestinal tract.

Dietary iron is in the ferric (Fe^{3+}) form. It is reduced in the gastrointestinal tract to divalent Fe^{2+} by ascorbate and a ferrireductase enzyme located in the intestinal brush border. Fe^{2+} is transported into the cells by a divalent metal transporter (which also transports most trace metals). The iron pool within the enterocyte is controlled by the iron regulatory proteins.

Erythrocyte content of iron affects its absorption from the intestine

When erythrocytes are iron rich, the iron is stored in the enterocytes incorporated into ferritin. Otherwise, it is transported through the basolateral membrane, where one of the transport-facilitating proteins, ferroxidase, also called

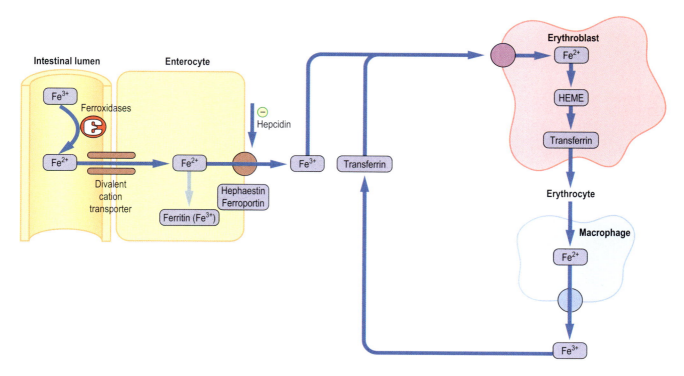

Fig. 7.13 **Iron metabolism.** Dietary iron is absorbed in the intestine and either stored in enterocytes as ferritin or transported out to plasma. Hephaestin and ferroportin are iron transporters located in the basolateral membrane of the enterocyte. In plasma, iron remains bound to transferrin. It is taken up by cells such as erythroblasts through the mediation of the membrane transferrin receptor. In erythroblasts, iron is incorporated into heme, then hemoglobin. Old erythrocytes are degraded by macrophages in the reticuloendothelial system. Liberated iron is released from cells and recycled bound to transferrin. Note that the dietary iron is in the ferric (Fe^{3+}) form. This is reduced to ferrous ion (Fe^{2+}) at the intestinal brush border. The transported form of iron is ferric again, but the form incorporated into heme is ferrous.

hephaestin, oxidizes Fe^{2+} to Fe^{3+}, which is then bound to transferrin in plasma. In the bone marrow, transferrin is taken up by erythrocyte precursors cells in a receptor-dependent manner. Within the cells, iron is released, again reduced to Fe^{2+}, and transported to the mitochondria for incorporation into heme. After destruction of the old erythrocytes by macrophages in the reticuloendothelial system, the iron is released as Fe^{2+}, reoxidized to Fe^{3+}, and loaded back onto transferrin. Fig. 7.13 shows the outline of iron metabolism.

Iron deficiency causes anemia

Iron requirements increase during growth and pregnancy. Iron deficiency results in **defective erythropoiesis** and in **normocytic or microcytic hypochromic anemia**. This is most likely to develop in infants and adolescents, in pregnant and menstruating women, and in the elderly. Iron deficiency most often develops as a result of abnormal blood loss, and therefore **a person presenting with iron-deficiency anemia always needs to be investigated for causes of bleeding**, particularly from the gastrointestinal tract. The assessment of iron status includes the measurements of transferrin and ferritin in plasma, hematologic variables, and the bone marrow smear. Humans do not have a mechanism to excrete iron, and free iron is toxic.

 CLINICAL BOX
HEMOCHROMATOSIS

Hemochromatosis is an autosomal recessive disorder resulting from the increased absorption of iron. It is the most common inherited disorder in persons of Northern European ancestry.

Iron accumulates in heart, liver, and pancreas and can cause liver cirrhosis, hepatocellular carcinoma, diabetes, arthritis, and heart failure. In the classic form of hemochromatosis, the mutated gene encodes the protein known as hereditary hemochromatosis protein (HFE), which is structurally similar to class I major histocompatibility antigens (Chapter 43). It is now known that mutations of other proteins can lead to a very similar clinical picture.

Zinc metabolism

Zinc is a trace element contained in approximately 100 enzymes associated with carbohydrate and energy metabolism, protein synthesis and degradation, and nucleic acid synthesis

Zinc plays a role in cellular transport and in immune function, cell division and growth, and protection from oxidative damage.

Spermatogenesis is also zinc-dependent. It plays a role in maintaining exocrine and endocrine pancreatic function. It is important in the maintenance of skin integrity and in wound healing.

Zinc shares transport mechanisms with copper and iron in the gut

On absorption, zinc is bound to metallothioneins, a family of cysteine-rich proteins, which also bind other divalent metal ions, such as copper. Synthesis of metallothioneins is dependent on the amount of trace metals present in the diet. Increased synthesis is part of the metabolic response to trauma and results in a reduction of serum zinc concentration.

Zinc deficiency is common

Increased losses of zinc occur in patients with major burns and in those with renal damage. Zinc loss in renal disease is due to its association with plasma albumin, and it accompanies urinary protein loss. Substantial amounts of zinc may also be lost during dialysis. A symptomatic deficiency may develop during intravenous feeding. Zinc is not stored in the body.

Sources of zinc include oysters (highest content), red meat, poultry, beans, and nuts. Note that phytates bind zinc. Zinc deficiency might be a result of malabsorption associated with gastrointestinal surgery, short bowel syndrome, Crohn's disease, and ulcerative colitis, and it may occur in liver and kidney disease. Chronic illnesses such as diabetes, malignancy, and chronic diarrhea also lead to deficiency. Pregnant women and alcoholics are prone to deficiency.

Zinc deficiency affects growth, skin integrity, and wound healing

In children, zinc deficiency is characterized by growth retardation, skin lesions, and impairment of immune function and sexual development. A specific inherited defect in the absorption of zinc from the gut was identified in the 1970s; it presented with severe skin lesions (**acrodermatitis enteropathica**), diarrhea, and loss of hair (alopecia). Zinc deficiency also leads to impairment in taste and smell and to **delayed wound healing.**

Zinc is probably the least toxic of the trace metals, but increased oral intake interferes with copper absorption and may lead to copper deficiency and anemia.

Zinc supplements are used in the treatment of diarrhea in children

Zinc supplementation was shown to reduce the severity and duration of diarrhea in children in developing countries and to prevent further episodes of diarrhea. Therefore zinc supplements are now recommended by WHO/UNICEF along with the oral rehydration treatment.

The usual method of assessing zinc status is the measurement of its plasma concentration. Many conditions and environmental factors affect its concentration in plasma, including inflammation, stress, cancer, smoking, steroid administration, and hemolysis.

CLINICAL BOX
A MAN TREATED WITH PARENTERAL NUTRITION WHO DEVELOPED A GENERALIZED RASH: ZINC DEFICIENCY

A 34-year-old man who required total intravenous feeding had been receiving the same prescription for 4 months, with no assessment of his trace-metal status. During this time, he continued to have major gastrointestinal losses and had intermittent pyrexia. He developed a rash across his face, head, and neck, with accompanying hair loss. He was clearly zinc deficient, with serum zinc concentration less than 1 µmol/L (6.5 µg/dL, reference range: 9–20 µmol/L; 60–130 µg/dL).

Comment

Patients with major catabolic illness and increased gastrointestinal losses have markedly increased zinc requirements. The zinc-depleted state this patient developed could aggravate his illness by preventing healing of his gastrointestinal lesions and by making him more susceptible to infection due to defects in his immune competence. Patients receiving intravenous feeding need to have their micronutrient status checked regularly.

Copper metabolism

Copper scavenges superoxide and other reactive oxygen species

One of the main roles of copper is the scavenging of superoxide and other reactive oxygen species. Copper is associated with **oxygenase enzymes**, including cytochrome oxidase and superoxide dismutase (the latter also requires zinc). Copper is also required for the crosslinking of collagen, being an essential component of lysyl oxidase.

Pathways of copper metabolism are shared with other metals

Absorption of copper from the gut is, similar to zinc, associated with metallothionein (Fig. 7.14). Copper availability in the diet is less affected by other dietary constituents than zinc, although high fiber intake reduces availability by complexing copper. In plasma, the absorbed copper is bound to albumin. The copper–albumin complex is quickly taken up by the liver. Within the hepatocyte, copper is associated with intracellular metallothioneins, which are also capable of binding zinc and cadmium. Copper is transported within the hepatocyte to sites of protein synthesis by a chaperone protein, and it is incorporated into apoceruloplasmin. The incorporation is catalyzed by an ATPase called ATP7B. Ceruloplasmin is then released into the circulation. The only mechanism of copper excretion is elimination in bile (Fig. 7.14). Refer also to the section.

Rare copper deficiency leads to anemia; skin and hair may also be affected

Rare copper deficiency is most likely to occur from reduced intake or excess loss (e.g., during renal dialysis). Deficiency

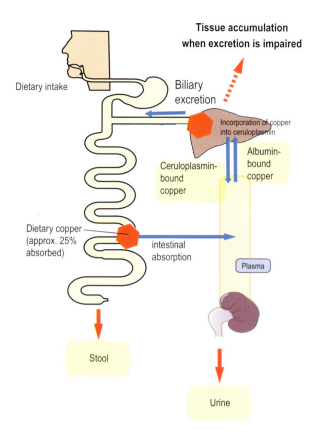

Fig. 7.14 **Copper metabolism.** Reproduced from Dominiczak MH. Medical Biochemistry Flash Cards. London: Elsevier, 2012, Card 42.

manifests itself as a **microcytic hypochromic anemia** resistant to iron therapy. There is also a reduction in the number of leukocytes in the blood (neutropenia) and degeneration of vascular tissue with bleeding, as a result of defects in the synthesis of elastin and collagen. In severe deficiency, skin depigmentation and alteration in hair structure also occur. The very rare Menkes' syndrome results from copper depletion caused by a deficiency of the intestinal ATP7B ATPase.

Copper excess causes liver cirrhosis

When taken orally, copper is generally nontoxic. However, in large doses, it accumulates in tissues. Chronic excessive intake results in liver cirrhosis. Acute toxicity is manifested by marked hemolysis and damage to both liver and brain cells. The latter is seen in the autosomal dominant inherited metabolic defect **Wilson's disease,** where the liver's capacity to synthesize ceruloplasmin is compromised. The cause is mutations in the gene coding for the ATP7B ATPase. This results in a reduced incorporation of copper into ceruloplasmin and in its cellular accumulation. The excess apoceruloplasmin is degraded. Copper accumulates in tissues such as the brain and cornea. Patients present with neurologic symptoms or liver cirrhosis and have typical **Kaiser–Fleischer rings** in the cornea. There is also a low plasma concentration of ceruloplasmin and high urinary copper excretion.

Selenium

Selenium is present in all cells as amino acids selenomethionine and selenocysteine

Selenium is a component of selenoproteins, which contain the amino acid selenocysteine. The antioxidant enzyme **glutathione peroxidase** is a selenoprotein, as are the **iodothyronine deiodinases**, enzymes that produce triiodothyronine (T_3) and reverse T_3 (rT_3). **Thioredoxin reductases** that participate in cell proliferation, apoptosis, and DNA synthesis also contain selenocysteine. Selenium affects functions of the immune system, including stimulation of differentiation of T cells and proliferation of activated T lymphocytes, as well as increase in the activity of natural killer cells. It also plays a role in spermatogenesis.

Selenium is absorbed in the small intestine. It remains protein bound in the circulation and is excreted in urine. Selenoprotein P possesses 10 selenocysteine residues, and it transports selenium in plasma from the liver to, primarily, the brain, testis, and kidney. Selenium is present in the diet as selenomethionine and selenocysteine. Brazil nuts are its richest source. Its dietary sources also include organ meats, fish (tuna) and shellfish, and cereals. Its content in plant-derived food depends on the content of the soil.

Selenium status may influence the risk of many chronic conditions

Low selenium is associated with a decline in immune function and with cognitive problems. Low concentration has been observed in individuals with epileptic seizures and also in pre-eclampsia. Deficiency of selenium can also develop during **total parenteral nutrition.** There is a rare selenium-responsive cardiomyopathy **(Keshan disease)**, which is endemic in China in areas of very low selenium intake. Selenium deficiency may result in chronic muscle pain, abnormal nail beds, and cardiomyopathy. Excess of selenium, on the other hand, leads to liver cirrhosis, splenomegaly, gastrointestinal bleeding, and depression.

Increased intake of selenium might be required during lactation. Several studies indicate a beneficial effect of selenium on the risk of lung, prostate, bladder, and other cancers. Single-nucleotide polymorphisms in selenoprotein genes were shown to be important in determining the risk of conditions such as various cancers, preeclampsia, and possibly cardiovascular disease.

Currently it seems that whereas people with a low selenium concentration may benefit from supplementation, supplementing it in those with normal or high values can actually be harmful.

Other metals

Numerous other trace metals are required for normal biological function - for example, manganese, molybdenum, vanadium, nickel, and cadmium. Some, similar to zinc and copper, form prosthetic groups of enzymes. These include **molybdenum** (xanthine oxidase) and **manganese** (superoxide dismutase and pyruvate carboxylase). **Chromium** has been associated with glucose tolerance.

Many of these metals were previously thought to be toxic; indeed, their environmental excess does result in toxicity, such as the renal toxicity observed in shipyard workers exposed to **cadmium** over long periods of time. As techniques for separation and analysis develop, other metals and other functions of known essential minerals will become known. This will lead to a better understanding of the epidemiology of certain diseases that may have, at least in part, an environmental etiology.

SUMMARY

◼ Vitamins function mostly as cofactors to enzymes.

◼ Fat-soluble vitamins can be stored in the adipose tissue, but there usually is only a short-term supply of the water-soluble vitamins.

◼ Dietary micronutrient deficiencies are most likely to occur in susceptible groups with increased demand or in people unable to maintain sufficient intake. Children, pregnant women, the elderly, alcoholics, and low-income groups are particularly vulnerable.

◼ High caloric intake increases the demand for B vitamins; high protein intake increases the demand for pyridoxine.

◼ Gastrointestinal disease and gastrointestinal surgery are potential causes of micronutrient deficiencies.

◼ Vitamin and trace metal supplements are particularly important in patients who remain on artificial diets and on parenteral nutrition.

◼ Although there are controversies regarding the supplementation some vitamins, the intake of fruit and vegetables as sources of micronutrients is unequivocally recommended.

ACTIVE LEARNING

1. Compare and contrast the deficiencies of vitamin B_{12} and folic acid.
2. When may an increased intake of a nutrient or energy precipitate vitamin deficiencies?
3. Is vitamin A supplementation safe?
4. Describe the clinical importance of copper.
5. Which vitamins play a role in the development of hyperhomocysteinemia?

FURTHER READING

Ala, A., Walker, A. P., Ashkan, K., et al. (2007). Wilson's disease. *Lancet, 369,* 397–408.

Asplund, K. (2002). Antioxidant vitamins in the prevention of cardiovascular disease: A systematic review. *J Int Med, 251,* 372–392.

Bhutta, Z. A., & Haider, B. A. (2008). Maternal micronutrient deficiencies in developing countries. *Lancet, 371,* 186–187.

Chan, Y. M., Bailey, R., & O'Connor, D. L. (2013). Folate. *Advances in Nutrition, 4,* 123–125.

Fisher Walker, C. L., & Black, R. E. (2012). Zinc treatment for serious infections in young infants. *Lancet, 379,* 2031–2033.

Hughes, C. F., Ward, M., Hoey, L., et al. (2013). Vitamin B12 and aging: Current issues and interaction with folate. *Annals of Clinical Biochemistry, 50,* 315–329.

Lonsdale, D. A. (2006). Review of the biochemistry, metabolism and clinical benefits of thiamin(e) and its derivatives. *eCAM, 3,* 49–59.

Rayman, M. (2012). Selenium and human health. *Lancet, 379,* 1256–1268.

Schneider, B. D., & Leibold, E. A. (2000). Regulation of mammalian iron homeostasis. *Current Opinion in Clinical Nutrition and Metabolic Care, 3,* 267–273.

RELEVANT WEBSITES

FAO Corporate Documents Repository - Human Vitamin and Mineral Requirements. Chapter 5: Vitamin B12: http://www.fao.org/docrep/004/Y2809E/y2809e0b.htm

Dietary reference values for energy: https://www.gov.uk/government/uploads/system/uploads/attachment_data/file/339317/SACN_Dietary_Reference_Values_for_Energy.pdf

FAO Corporate Document Repository. Human vitamin and mineral requirements: http://www.fao.org/docrep/004/Y2809E/y2809e01.htm#TopOfPage

MORE CLINICAL CASES

Please refer to Appendix 2 for more cases relevant to this chapter.

ABBREVIATIONS

CRBP	Cytosolic retinol-binding proteins
FMN	Flavin mononucleotide
FAD	Flavin adenine dinucleotide
HFE	Hereditary hemochromatosis protein
HPLC	High-performance liquid chromatography
IF	Intrinsic factor IF
MTHFR	5,10-methylenetetrahydrofolate reductase
NAD^+	Nicotinamide adenine dinucleotide
$NADP^+$	Nicotinamide adenine dinucleotide phosphate
N5MeTHF	5-methyl tetrahydrofolate
PDH	Pyruvate dehydrogenase
PKC	Protein kinase C
PPARs	Peroxisome proliferator–activated receptors

RABP	Retinoic acid–binding protein	rT3	Reverse T3
RAE	Retinol activity equivalent	T3	Triiodothyronine
RAR	Retinoid acid receptor	T4	Thyroxine
RBP	Serum retinol-binding protein	TCI	Transcobalamin I
ROS	Reactive oxygen species	TCII	Transcobalamin II
RXR	Rexinoid receptor	TPP	Thiamine pyrophosphate

8 Bioenergetics and Oxidative Metabolism

Norma Frizzell and L. William Stillway

INTRODUCTION

ATP is the central metabolic currency

Oxidation of metabolic fuels is essential to life. In higher organisms, fuels such as carbohydrates and lipids are metabolized oxidatively to carbon dioxide and water, generating a central metabolic currency, adenosine triphosphate (ATP). Most metabolic energy is produced by oxidation–reduction (redox) reactions in mitochondria. The regulation of energy metabolism is no small feat because warm-blooded animals have such variable demands for energy from such processes as thermogenesis at low temperatures and coupling of ATP synthesis with the rate of respiration during work and exercise. This chapter provides an introduction to the concept of free energy, the pathway of oxidative phosphorylation, and the transduction of energy from fuels into useful work. The pathways and specific molecules through which electrons are transported to oxygen and the mechanism of generation of ATP are described and related to the structure of the mitochondrion, the powerhouse of the cell and the major source of cellular ATP.

OXIDATION AS A SOURCE OF ENERGY

Energy content of foods

Nutrition and disorders such as obesity, diabetes, and cancer all require an understanding of thermodynamics. Obesity, for example, is a disorder in which there is an imbalance between energy intake and expenditure. It is therefore important that the energy content of foods be known. The commonly accepted energy values for the four major food categories are shown in Table 8.1; alcohol is included because it is a significant dietary component for some people. These values are obtained by completely burning (oxidizing) samples of each food in the laboratory in a bomb calorimeter. Biologically, about 40% of food energy is conserved as ATP, and the remaining 60% is liberated as heat.

The basal metabolic rate (BMR)

The BMR is a measure of the total daily energy expenditure by the body at rest

Virtually all of the chemical reactions in the body are exothermic, and the sum of all reactions at rest is called the basal metabolic rate (BMR), which can be measured by two basic methods: **direct calorimetry,** where the total heat liberated by an animal is measured over time, and **indirect calorimetry,** where the BMR is calculated from the quantity of oxygen consumed, which is directly related to the BMR. Heat production by mitochondria accounts for the largest portion of the BMR. Adult men (70 kg) have a BMR of about 7500 kJ (1800 kcal); women have about 5400 kJ (1300 kcal) per day. The BMR may vary by a factor of 2 between individuals, depending on age, sex, and body mass and composition. The BMR is measured under controlled conditions: after an 8-hour sleep, in the reclining position, in the postabsorptive state, typically after a 12-hour fast.

Another measure often used is the resting metabolic rate (RMR), which is virtually the same as the BMR but measured under less restrictive conditions. The RMR is a measure of minimum energy expenditure at rest; it is typically about 70% of total daily energy expenditure. Exercise scientists frequently use the term metabolic equivalent task (MET) as a measure of the rate of energy expenditure at rest. Slow to vigorous

Table 8.1 Energy content of the major classes of food

	Metabolic fuel (kJ/g)	Energy content (kcal/g)
Fats	38	9
Carbohydrates	17	4
Proteins	17	4
Alcohol	29	7

Note that the thermodynamic term kcal (energy required to increase the temperature of 1 kg [1 L] of water by 1°C) is equivalent to the common nutritional Calorie (capital C) - that is, 1 Cal = 1 kcal; 1 kcal = 4.2 kJ.

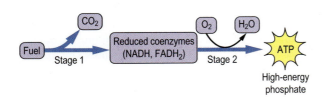

Fig. 8.1 **Stages of fuel oxidation.** NADH, reduced nicotinamide adenine dinucleotide; FADH$_2$, reduced flavin adenine dinucleotide.

walking is a 2- to 4-MET activity; vigorous running on a treadmill may consume energy at more than 15 MET (i.e., 15 times the resting metabolic rate).

Stages of fuel oxidation

The oxidation of fuels can be divided into two general stages: production of reduced nucleotide coenzymes during the oxidation of fuels and use of the free energy from the oxidation of the reduced coenzymes to produce ATP (Fig. 8.1).

FREE ENERGY

The direction of a reaction depends on the difference between the free energy of reactants and products

The Gibbs' free energy (ΔG) of a reaction is the maximum amount of energy that can be obtained from a reaction at constant temperature and pressure. The units of free energy are kcal/mol (kJ/mol). It is not possible to measure the absolute free energy content of a substance directly, but when reactant A reacts to form product B, the free-energy change in this reaction, ΔG, can be determined.

For the reaction A → B,

$$\Delta G = G_B - G_A$$

where G_A and G_B are the free energy of A (reactant) and B (product), respectively. All reactions in biological systems are considered to be reversible reactions, so the free energy of the reverse reaction, B → A, is numerically equivalent but opposite in sign to that of the forward reaction.

If there is a greater concentration of B than of A at equilibrium (i.e., $K_{eq} > 1$), the conversion A → B is favorable - that is, the reaction tends to move forward from a standard state in which A and B are present at equal concentrations. In this case, the reaction is said to be a spontaneous, or exergonic, reaction, and the free energy of this reaction is defined as negative - that is, $\Delta G < 0$, indicating that energy is liberated by the reaction. Conversely, if the concentration of A is greater than that of B at equilibrium, the forward reaction is termed unfavorable, nonspontaneous, or endergonic, and the reaction has a positive free energy - that is, when starting concentrations are equal, B tends to form A, rather than A to form B. In this case, energy input would be required to push the reaction A → B forward from its equilibrium position to the standard state in which A and B are present at equal concentrations. The total free energy available from a reaction depends on both its tendency to proceed forward from the standard state (ΔG) and the amount (moles) of reactant converted to product.

The free energy of metabolic reactions is related to their equilibrium constants by the Gibbs' equation

Thermodynamic measurements are based on standard-state conditions, where reactant and product are present at 1 molar concentrations, the pressure of all gases is 1 atmosphere, and the temperature is 25°C (298K). Most commonly, the concentrations of reactants and products are measured after equilibrium is attained. Standard free energies are represented by the symbol $\Delta G°$ and biological standard free-energy change by $\Delta G°'$, with the accent symbol designating pH 7. The free energy available from a reaction may be calculated from its equilibrium constant by the Gibbs' equation:

$$\Delta G°' = -RT \ln K'_{eq}$$

where T is absolute temperature (Kelvin), $\ln K'_{eq}$ is the natural logarithm of the equilibrium constant for the reaction at pH 7, and R is the ideal gas constant:

$$R = (8.3 \, \text{Jmol}^{-1}/\text{K or} : 2 \, \text{calmol}^{-1}/\text{K}).$$

Several common metabolic intermediates are listed in Table 8.2, along with the equilibrium constants and free energies for their hydrolysis reactions. Those intermediates with free-energy changes equal to or greater than that of ATP, the central energy transducer of the cell, are considered to be **high-energy compounds** and generally have either anhydride or thioester bonds. The lower-energy compounds listed are all phosphate esters and, in comparison, do not yield as much free energy on hydrolysis. The hydrolysis reaction of glucose-6-phosphate (Glc-6-P) is written as

$$\text{Glc-6-P} + H_2O \rightarrow \text{Glucose} + Pi$$

This reaction has a negative free energy and occurs spontaneously. The reverse reaction, synthesis of Glc-6-P from glucose and phosphate, would require the input of energy.

Table 8.2 Thermodynamics of hydrolysis reactions

Metabolite	K'_{eq}	$\Delta G^{\circ\prime}$ (kJ/mol)	(kcal/mol)
Phosphoenolpyruvate	1.2×10^{11}	−61.8	−14.8
Phosphocreatine	9.6×10^{8}	−50.2	−12.0
1,3-bisphosphoglycerate	6.8×10^{8}	−49.3	−11.8
Pyrophosphate	9.7×10^{5}	−33.4	−8.0
Acetyl coenzyme A	4.1×10^{5}	−31.3	−7.5
ATP	2.9×10^{5}	−30.5	−7.3
Glucose-1-phosphate	5.5×10^{3}	−20.9	−5.0
Fructose-6-phosphate	7.0×10^{2}	−15.9	−3.8
Glucose-6-phosphate	3.0×10^{2}	−13.8	−3.3

Equilibrium constants and free energy of hydrolysis of various metabolic intermediates at pH 7 (ΔG°).

CONSERVATION OF ENERGY BY COUPLING OF REACTIONS TO HYDROLYSIS OF ATP

ATP is a product of catabolic reactions and a driver of biosynthetic reactions

Living systems must transfer energy from one molecule to another without losing all of it as heat. Some of the energy must be conserved in a chemical form to drive nonspontaneous biosynthetic reactions. In fact, nearly half of the energy obtained from the oxidation of metabolic fuels is channeled into the synthesis of **ATP, a universal energy transducer in living systems**. ATP is often referred to as the common currency of metabolic energy because it is used to drive so many energy-requiring reactions. ATP consists of the purine base adenine, the five-carbon sugar ribose, and α, β, and γ phosphate groups (Fig. 8.2). The two phosphoanhydride linkages are said to be high-energy bonds because their hydrolysis

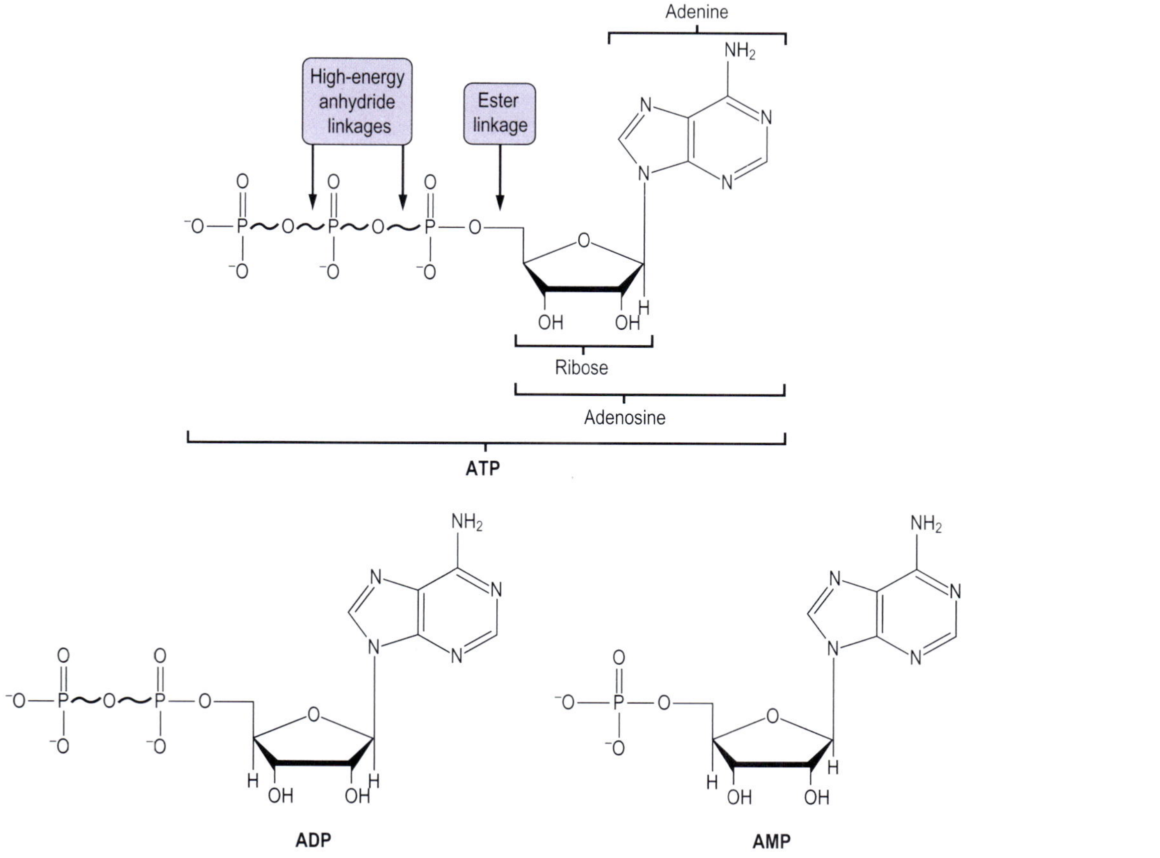

Fig. 8.2 **Structures of adenine nucleotides.** ATP is shown, together with its hydrolysis products, adenosine diphosphate (ADP) and adenosine monophosphate (AMP). ATP has two high-energy phosphoanhydride bonds, ADP has one, and AMP has only a low-energy phosphoester bond.

yields a large negative change in free energy. When ATP is used for metabolic work, these high-energy linkages are broken, and ATP is converted to ADP or AMP.

The free energy of a high-energy bond, such as the phosphate anhydride bonds in ATP, can be used to drive or push forward reactions that would otherwise be unfavorable. In fact, nearly all biosynthetic pathways are thermodynamically unfavorable, but they are made favorable by coupling various reactions with hydrolysis of high-energy compounds. For example, the first step in the metabolism of glucose is the synthesis of Glc-6-P (see Fig. 3.4). As shown in Table 8.2, this is not a favorable reaction: the hydrolysis of Glc-6-P ($\Delta G^{\circ\prime}$ = −13.8 kJ/mol, or −3.3 kcal/mol) is the favored reaction. However, as shown in the following series, the synthesis of Glc-6-P (reaction I) can be **energetically coupled** to the hydrolysis of ATP (reaction II), yielding a "net reaction" III that is favorable for the synthesis of Glc-6-P:

	$\Delta G^{\circ\prime}$
I: $Glc + Pi \rightarrow Glc\text{-}6\text{-}P + H_2O$	+3.3 kcal/mol
II: $ATP + H_2O \rightarrow ADP + Pi$	−7.3 kcal/mol
Net: $Glc + ATP \rightarrow Glc\text{-}6\text{-}P + ADP$	−4 kcal/mol

This is possible because of the high free energy, or "group transfer potential," of ATP. The physical transfer of the phosphate from ATP to glucose occurs in the active site of a kinase enzyme, such as glucokinase. This motif, in which ATP is used to drive biosynthetic reactions, transport processes, or muscle activity, occurs commonly in metabolic pathways.

MITOCHONDRIAL SYNTHESIS OF ADENOSINE TRIPHOSPHATE FROM REDUCED COENZYMES

Oxidative phosphorylation is the mechanism by which energy derived from fuel oxidation is conserved in the form of ATP

Metabolism of carbohydrates begins in the cytoplasm through the glycolytic pathway (see Chapter 9), whereas energy production from fatty acids occurs exclusively in the mitochondrion. Mitochondria are subcellular organelles about the size of bacteria. They are essential for aerobic metabolism in eukaryotes. Their main function is to oxidize metabolic fuels and conserve free energy by synthesizing ATP.

Mitochondria are bounded by a dual membrane system (Fig. 8.3). The outer membrane (OMM) contains enzyme and transport proteins, and via the pore-forming protein porin (P, also known as voltage-dependent anion channel), it is permeable to virtually all ions, small molecules (S), and proteins less than 10,000 Da. Large proteins must be transported via the **TOM** (translocase in the outer mitochondrial membrane) and **TIM** (translocase in the inner mitochondrial membrane) complexes. This is especially vital to the cell because almost all mitochondrial proteins are nuclear encoded and must be transported

into the mitochondrion. The **mitochondrial genome,** mtDNA, encodes 13 vital subunits of the proton pumps and ATP synthase. The **inner membrane (IMM)** is pleated with structures known as **cristae,** and it is impermeable to most ions and small molecules, such as nucleotides (including ATP), coenzymes, phosphate, and protons. Transporter proteins are required to selectively facilitate translocation of specific molecules across the inner membrane. The inner membrane also contains components of oxidative phosphorylation - the process by which the oxidation of reduced nucleotide coenzymes is coupled to the synthesis of ATP.

Transduction of energy from reduced coenzymes to high-energy phosphate

NAD⁺, FAD, and FMN are the major redox coenzymes

The major redox coenzymes involved in transduction of energy from fuels to ATP are nicotinamide adenine dinucleotide (NAD⁺), flavin adenine dinucleotide (FAD), and flavin mononucleotide (FMN; Fig. 8.4). During energy metabolism, electrons are transferred from carbohydrates and fats to these coenzymes, reducing them to NADH, FADH₂, and FMNH₂. In each case, two electrons are transferred, but the number of protons transferred differs. NAD⁺ accepts a hydride ion (H⁻) that consists of one proton and two electrons; the remaining proton is released into solution. FAD and FMN accept two electrons and two protons.

The oxidation of reduced nucleotides by the electron transport system produces a large amount of free energy. When the oxidation of 1.0 mole of NADH is coupled to the reduction of 0.5 mole of oxygen to form water, the energy produced is theoretically sufficient to synthesize 7.0 moles of ATP:

$$NADH + H^+ + \tfrac{1}{2}O_2 \rightarrow NAD^+ + H_2O$$

$$\Delta G^{\circ\prime} = -220 \text{ kJ/mol} \,(-52.4 \text{ kcal/mol})$$

$$ADP + Pi \rightarrow ATP + H_2O$$

$$\Delta G^{\circ\prime} = -30.5 \text{ kJ/mol} \,(-7.3 \text{ kcal/mol})$$

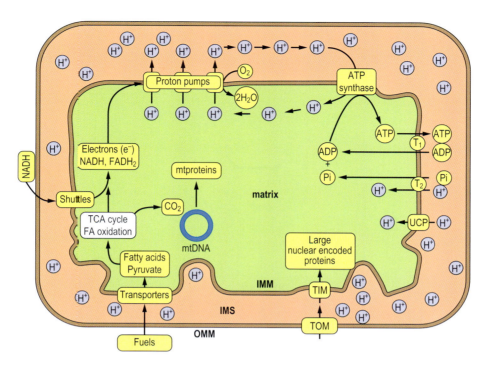

Fig. 8.3 **Mitochondrial structure and pathways of energy transduction: the mechanism of oxidative phosphorylation.** Major fuels, such as pyruvate from carbohydrates and fatty acids (FAs) from triglycerides, are transported into the matrix, where they are oxidized to generate CO_2 and the reduced nucleotide coenzymes NADH and $FADH_2$. Oxidation of these nucleotides via the electron transport system reduces oxygen to water and pumps protons by three proton pumps out of the matrix and into the intermembrane space (IMS), creating a pH gradient, which is the major contributor to the membrane potential. It should be noted that protons in the intermembrane space freely diffuse through the outer membrane via the protein porin, a proton channel, so the pH of the intermembrane space is approximately that of the cytosol. Although the membrane potential is mostly composed of the proton gradient, it actually consists of several electrochemical gradients and is expressed as a voltage. Controlled influx of protons through ATP synthase powers the synthesis of ATP by ATP synthase (F-ATPase; Table 4.3). Mitochondrial ATP is then exchanged for cytoplasmic ADP through the ADP–ATP translocase (T_1). Phosphate (Pi), which is also required for ATP synthesis, is transported by the phosphate translocase (T_2). The inner membrane also contains uncoupling proteins (UCP) that may be used to allow the controlled leakage of protons back into the matrix. OMM, outer mitochondrial membrane; IMM, inner mitochondrial membrane; mtproteins, mitochondrial proteins; mtDNA, mitochondrial DNA; TOM and TIM, protein translocase complexes in outer and inner mitochondrial membrane; TCA, tricarboxylic acid cycle.

Dividing 220.0 kJ/mol of $\Delta G°'$ available from the oxidation of NADH by $\Delta G°'$ 30.5 required for synthesis of ATP yields, theoretically, 7.0 mol ATP/mol NADH. As discussed in the next section, the actual yield is closer to 2.5 mol ATP / mol NADH oxidized.

The free energy of oxidation of NADH and $FADH_2$ is used by the electron transport system to pump protons into the intermembrane space. The energy produced when these protons reenter the mitochondrial matrix is used to synthesize ATP. This process is known as **oxidative phosphorylation** (see Fig. 8.3).

THE MITOCHONDRIAL ELECTRON TRANSPORT SYSTEM

The mitochondrial electron transport chain transfers electrons in a defined multistep sequence from reduced nucleotides to oxygen

The entire electron transport system, also known as the electron transport chain or respiratory chain, is located in the inner

---

ADVANCED CONCEPT BOX
METABOLIC FUNCTION OF ATP REQUIRES MAGNESIUM

ATP readily forms a complex with magnesium ion, and this complex is required in all reactions in which ATP participates, including its synthesis. A magnesium deficiency impairs virtually all of metabolism because ATP can neither be made nor utilized in adequate amounts.

mitochondrial membrane (Fig. 8.5). It consists of several large protein complexes and two small, independent components: ubiquinone and cytochrome *c*. The protein components are very complex; complex I, for example, which accepts electrons from NADH, contains at least 45 subunits. Each step in the electron transport chain involves a redox reaction where electrons are transferred from components with more negative reduction potentials to components with more positive reduction potentials. Electrons are conducted through this system

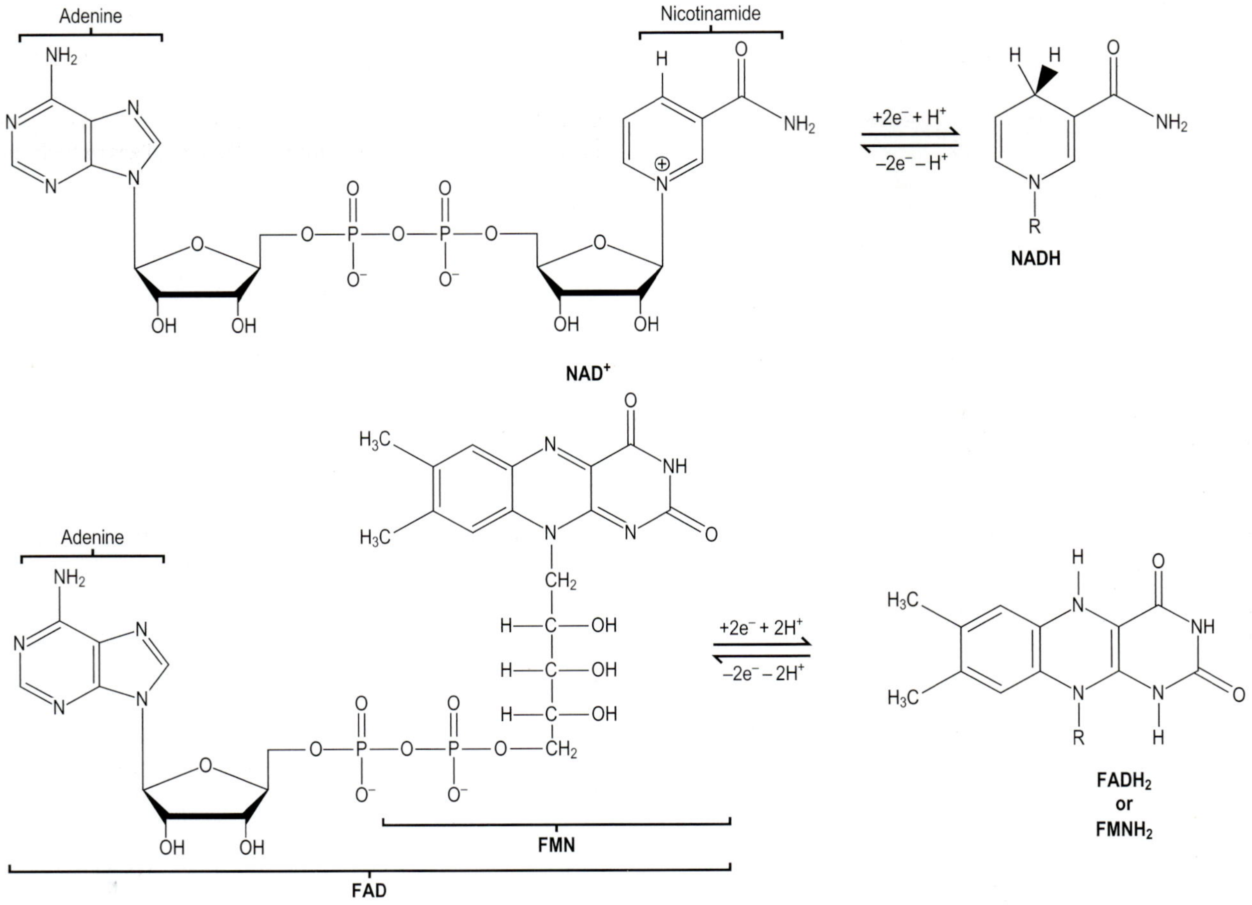

Fig. 8.4 **The structure of redox coenzymes.** NAD$^+$ and its reduced form, NADH (nicotinamide adenine dinucleotide), consists of adenine, two ribose units, two phosphates, and nicotinamide. FAD and its reduced form, FADH$_2$ (flavin adenine dinucleotide), consists of riboflavin, two phosphates, ribose, and adenine. FMN and FMNH$_2$ consist of riboflavin phosphate. The nicotinamide and riboflavin components of these coenzymes are reversibly oxidized and reduced during electron transfer (redox) reactions. NADH and FADH$_2$ are often called reduced nucleotides or reduced coenzymes.

in a defined sequence from reduced nucleotide coenzymes to oxygen, and the free-energy changes drive the transport of protons from the matrix into the intermembrane space via the three proton pumps. After each step, the electrons are at a lower energy state.

Electrons are funneled into the electron transport chain by several flavoproteins

There are four flavoproteins in the electron transport chain: complex I contains FMN, and the other three contain FAD. These flavoproteins all reduce the small, lipophilic molecule **ubiquinone (Q or coenzyme Q$_{10}$)** at the beginning of the common electron transport pathway, consisting of Q, complex III, cytochrome *c*, and complex IV.

$$\text{Flavoprotein}_{(reduced)} + Q \rightarrow \text{Flavoprotein}_{(oxidized)} + QH_2$$

Protons are pumped from the matrix into the intermembrane space by complexes I, III, and IV. Oxygen (O$_2$) is the final

electron acceptor at the end of the chain, and it is reduced to two water molecules by the transfer of four electrons from complex IV and four protons from the mitochondrial matrix compartment.

The efficiency of oxidative phosphorylation can be measured by dividing the amount of phosphate incorporated into ADP by the amount of atomic oxygen reduced. One atom of oxygen is reduced by two electrons (one electron pair):

$$ADP + Pi + \tfrac{1}{2}O_2 + 2H^+ + 2e^- \rightarrow ATP + H_2O$$

For each pair of electrons transported through complexes I, III, or IV, a sufficient number of protons is pumped by each complex for the synthesis of approximately 1.0 mole of ATP/ complex. If electron transport begins with an electron pair from NADH, about 2.5 moles of ATP are actually synthesized, whereas an electron pair from any of the other three FADH$_2$-containing flavoproteins yields about 1.5 moles of ATP because the proton-pumping capability of complex I is bypassed.

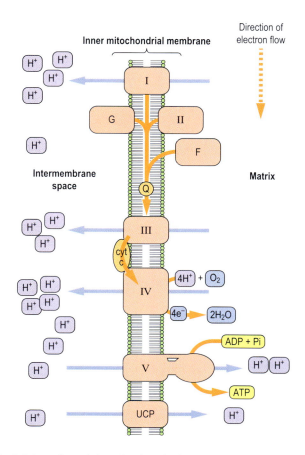

Fig. 8.5 **A section of the mitochondrial inner membrane with the electron transport system and ATP synthase.** I, complex I; II, complex II (succinate dehydrogenase); III, complex III; IV, complex IV; V, complex V, or ATP synthase; G, glycerol-3-phosphate dehydrogenase; F, fatty acyl CoA dehydrogenase; Q, ubiquinone; cyt c, cytochrome c; UCP, uncoupling protein.

Flavoproteins contain FAD or FMN prosthetic groups

Complex I, also called NADH–Q reductase or NADH dehydrogenase, is a flavoprotein containing FMN. It oxidizes mitochondrial NADH and transfers electrons through FMN and iron–sulfur (FeS) complexes to ubiquinone, providing enough energy to pump four protons from the matrix in the reaction:

$$NADH + Q + 5H^+_{matrix} \rightarrow NAD^+ + QH_2 + 4H^+_{intermembrane\ space}$$

Three other flavoproteins transfer electrons from oxidizable substrates via $FADH_2$ to ubiquinone (Q; see Fig. 8.5):

- Succinate–Q reductase (complex II, or succinate dehydrogenase of the TCA cycle; see Chapter 10) oxidizes succinate to fumarate and reduces FAD to $FADH_2$.
- Glycerol-3-phosphate–Q reductase, a part of the glycerol-3-P shuttle (see the following discussion), oxidizes cytoplasmic glycerol-3-P to dihydroxyacetone phosphate (DHAP) and reduces FAD to $FADH_2$.
- Fatty acyl-CoA dehydrogenase catalyzes the first step in the mitochondrial oxidation of fatty acids (Chapter 11) and also produces $FADH_2$.

Both FMN and FAD contain the water-soluble vitamin riboflavin. A dietary deficiency of riboflavin can severely impair the function of these and other flavoproteins.

TRANSFER OF ELECTRONS FROM NADH INTO MITOCHONDRIA

Electron shuttles

Electron shuttles are required for mitochondrial oxidation of NADH produced in the cytoplasmic compartment

NADH is produced in the cytosol during carbohydrate metabolism. NADH cannot cross the inner mitochondrial membrane,

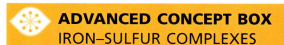

CLINICAL BOX
IRON DEFICIENCY LEADS TO ANEMIA

A 45-year-old woman complains of tiredness and appears pale. She is a vegetarian and is experiencing a monthly menstrual flow that is heavy and prolonged. Her hematocrit is 0.32 (reference range 0.36–0.46) and her hemoglobin concentration is 90 g/L (normal range 120–160 g/L; 12–16 g/dL).

Comment
Iron-deficiency anemia is a common nutritional problem and is especially common in menstruating and pregnant women because of their increased dietary requirement for iron. Men require about 1 mg iron/day, menstruating women about 2 mg/day, and pregnant women about 3 mg/day. Iron is required to maintain normal amounts of hemoglobin and the cytochromes and iron–sulfur complexes that are central to oxygen transport and energy metabolism. All of these processes are impaired in iron deficiency.

ADVANCED CONCEPT BOX
IRON–SULFUR COMPLEXES

Iron–sulfur complexes participate in redox reactions
Iron is an important constituent of heme proteins, such as hemoglobin, myoglobin, cytochromes, and catalase, but it is also associated with iron–sulfur (FeS) complexes or nonheme iron proteins that function as electron transporters in the mitochondrial electron transport system. The Fe_2S_2 and Fe_4S_4 types are shown in Fig. 8.6. In each case, the iron–sulfur center is bound to a peptide through cysteine residues. The FeS complexes undergo reversible distortion and relaxation during redox reactions. The redox energy is said to be conserved in the "conformational energy" of the protein.

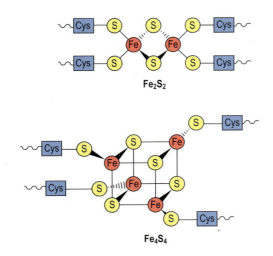

Fig. 8.6 **Iron–sulfur complexes.** Cys, cysteine.

and therefore it cannot be oxidized by the electron transport system. Two redox shuttles permit the oxidation of cytosolic NADH without its physical transfer into the mitochondrion. A characteristic feature of these shuttles is that they are powered by cytoplasmic and mitochondrial isoforms of the same enzyme, which catalyze opposing reactions on opposite sides of the membrane. The glycerol-3-P shuttle is the simpler of the two (Fig. 8.7, top). It transfers the electrons of NADH from the cytoplasm to the mitochondrion by reducing FAD to $FADH_2$. Cytoplasmic glycerol-3-P dehydrogenase catalyzes reduction of dihydroxyacetone-P (DHAP) with NADH to glycerol-3-P, regenerating NAD^+. The cytoplasmic glycerol-3-phosphate is oxidized back to DHAP by another glycerol-3-phosphate dehydrogenase isoform facing the outer surface of the inner mitochondrial membrane; this enzyme is a flavoprotein in which FAD is reduced to $FADH_2$. The electrons are then transferred to the common pathway via ubiquinone. Because the electrons are transferred to FAD, the yield of ATP from cytoplasmic NADH by this pathway is approximately 1.5 moles,

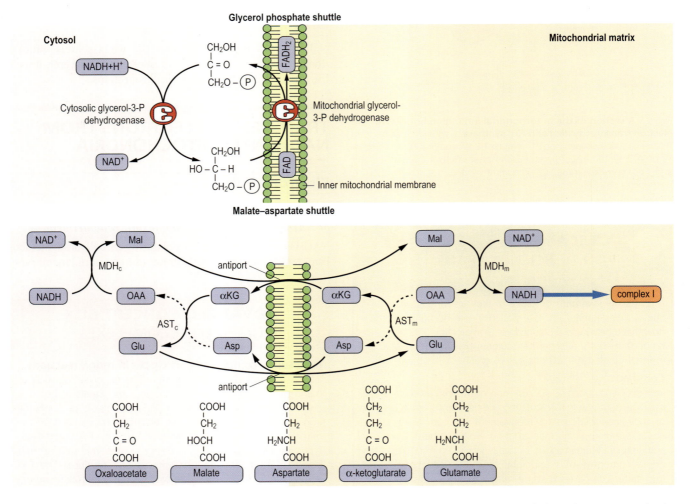

Fig. 8.7 **Redox shuttles in the inner mitochondrial membrane.** (Top) The glycerol phosphate shuttle. (Bottom) The malate–aspartate shuttle. MDH, malate dehydrogenase; AST, aspartate aminotransferase. Subscripts c and m refer to cytosolic and mitochondrial isozymes.

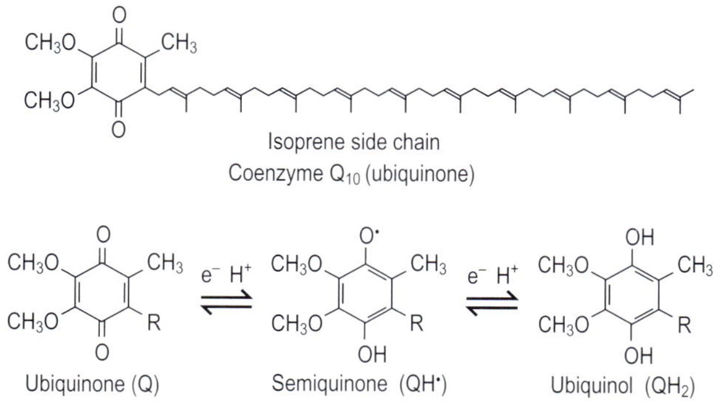

Isoprene side chain
Coenzyme Q_{10} (ubiquinone)

Ubiquinone (Q)   Semiquinone (QH·)   Ubiquinol (QH₂)

Fig. 8.8 **Coenzyme Q_{10}, or ubiquinone, accepts one or two electrons, transferring them from flavoproteins to complex III.** The semiquinone form is a free radical.

rather than the 2.5 moles available from mitochondrial NADH via the NADH-Q reductase complex (complex I).

Many cells (e.g., in skeletal muscle) use the glycerol-3-P shuttle, but the heart and liver rely on the malate–aspartate shuttle (Fig. 8.7, bottom), which yields 2.5 moles of ATP per mole of NADH. This shuttle is more complicated because the substrate, malate, can cross the inner mitochondrial membrane, but the membrane is impermeable to the product, oxaloacetate - there is no oxaloacetate transporter. The exchange is therefore accomplished by interconversion between α-keto-acids and α-amino acids, involving cytoplasmic and mitochondrial glutamate and α-ketoglutarate, and isozymes of glutamate-oxaloacetate transaminase (aspartate aminotransferase).

Ubiquinone (coenzyme Q_{10})

Ubiquinone transfers electrons from flavoproteins to complex III

Ubiquinone is so named because it is ubiquitous in virtually all living systems. It is a small lipid-soluble compound found in the inner membrane of animal and plant mitochondria and in the plasma membrane of bacteria. The primary form of mammalian ubiquinone contains a side chain of 10 isoprene units and is often called CoQ_{10}. It diffuses within the inner membrane, accepts electrons from the four major mitochondrial flavoproteins, and transfers them to complex III (QH_2–cytochrome c reductase). Ubiquinone can carry either one or two electrons (Fig. 8.8) and is also thought to be a major source of superoxide radicals in the cell (see Chapter 42).

Complex III: cytochrome c reductase

Complex III accepts electrons from ubiquinone and pumps four hydrogen ions across the inner mitochondrial membrane

This enzyme complex, also known as ubiquinone–cytochrome c reductase or QH_2–cytochrome c reductase, oxidizes ubiqui-

none and reduces cytochrome c. Reduced ubiquinone funnels electrons that it gathers from mitochondrial flavoproteins and transfers them to complex III. Electrons from ubiquinone are transferred through two species of cytochrome b to an FeS center, to cytochrome c_1, and finally to cytochrome c. Transport of two electrons to cytochrome c yields sufficient free-energy change and protons pumped to synthesize about 1 mole of ATP. The overall reaction is

$$QH_2 + 2cytc_{oxidized} + 2H^+_{matrix} \rightarrow$$
$$2Q + 2cytc_{reduced} + 4H^+_{intermembrane\ space}$$

Four protons are pumped during this reaction, two from fully reduced ubiquinone, and two from the matrix.

Cytochrome c

Cytochrome c is a peripheral membrane protein, shuttling electrons from complex III to complex IV

Cytochrome c, a small heme protein that is loosely bound to the outer surface of the inner membrane, shuttles electrons from complex III to complex IV. Each cytochrome c carries only one electron, so the reduction of O_2 to $2H_2O$ by complex IV requires four reduced cytochrome c molecules. The binding of cytochrome c to complexes III and IV is largely electrostatic, involving a number of lysine residues on the protein surface. Reduction of ferricytochrome c (Fe^{3+}) to ferricytochrome c (Fe^{2+}) by cytochrome c_1 leads to a change in the three-dimensional structure, charge distribution, and dipole moment of the protein, promoting the transfer of electrons to cytochrome a in complex IV (see Fig. 8.5). In response to oxidative stress and

ADVANCED CONCEPT BOX
CYTOCHROMES

Cytochromes, found in the mitochondrion and endoplasmic reticulum, are proteins that contain heme groups (Fig. 8.9), but which are not involved in oxygen binding or transport. The core structure of these heme groups is a tetrapyrrole ring similar to that of hemoglobin, sometimes differing only in the composition of the side chains. The heme group of cytochromes b and c_1 is known as iron protoporphyrin IX and is the same heme that is found in hemoglobin, myoglobin, and catalase. Cytochrome c contains heme C that is covalently bound to the protein through cysteine residues. Cytochromes a and a_3 contain heme A, which, like ubiquinone, contains a hydrophobic isoprene side chain. In hemoglobin and myoglobin, heme must remain in the ferrous (Fe^{2+}) state; in cytochromes, the heme iron is reversibly reduced and oxidized between the Fe^{2+} and Fe^{3+} states as electrons are shuttled from one protein molecule to another.

cell injury (Chapter 42), cytochrome c may be released from the inner mitochondrial membrane and leak into the cytosol, inducing apoptosis (cell death).

Complex IV

Complex IV, at the end of the electron transport chain, transfers electrons to oxygen, producing water

Complex IV, known as cytochrome c oxidase or cytochrome oxidase, exists as a dimer in the IMM. It oxidizes the mobile cytochrome c and conducts electrons through cytochromes a and a_3, finally reducing oxygen to water in a four-electron transfer reaction (Fig. 8.10). **Copper** is a common component of this and other oxidase enzymes. Small molecule poisons, such as **azide, cyanide,** and **carbon monoxide,** bind to the heme group of cytochrome a_3 in cytochrome c oxidase and inhibit complex IV. In common with complexes I and III, the cytochrome oxidase complex pumps protons out of mitochondria, providing for the synthesis of about 1 mole of ATP per pair of electrons transferred to oxygen. The actual number of protons pumped is four. In addition, four more are required in the reduction of O_2 to water. The overall reaction catalyzed by complex IV is

$$4cytc_{reduced} + 8H^+_{matrix} + O_2 \rightarrow$$
$$4cytc_{oxidized} + 2H_2O + 4H^+_{intermembrane\ space}$$

SYNTHESIS OF ADENOSINE TRIPHOSPHATE: THE CHEMIOSMOTIC HYPOTHESIS

According to the chemiosmotic hypothesis, mitochondria produce ATP using the free energy from the proton gradient

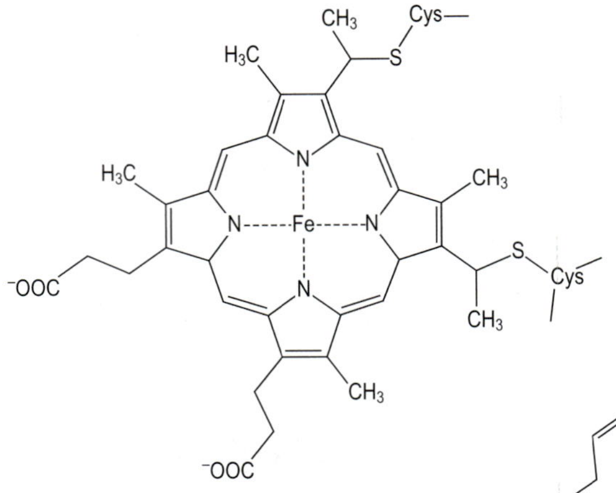

Heme group of cytochrome c (heme C)

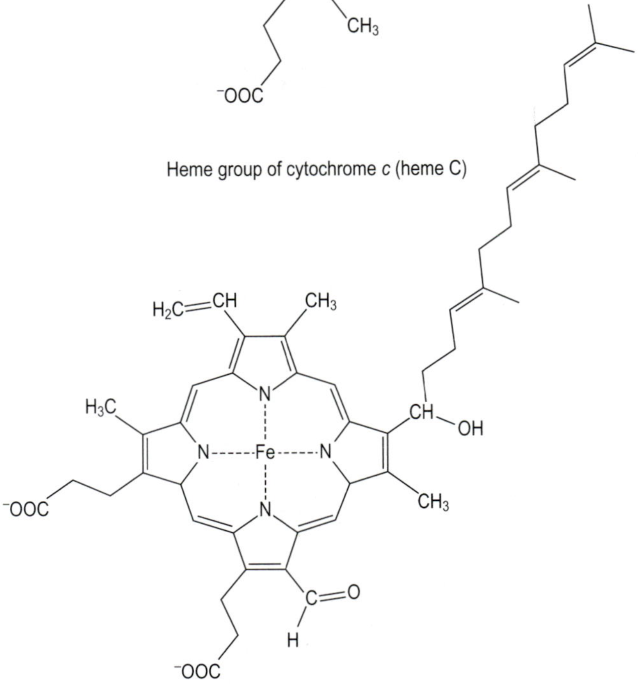

Heme group of cytochrome a (heme A)

Fig. 8.9 **Variations in heme structures among cytochromes.** The cytochromes are proteins that contain heme groups.

CLINICAL BOX
COPPER DEFICIENCY IN NEONATES

Copper is required in trace amounts for optimal human nutrition. Although copper deficiency is rare in adults, premature infants have low stores of copper and may suffer from its deficiency. This may lead to anemia and cardiomyopathy because of the failure to synthesize adequate amounts of cytochrome c oxidase and other enzymes, including several cuproenzymes involved in the synthesis of heme.

Comment

Copper deficiency can impair ATP production by inhibiting the terminal reaction of the electron transport chain, leading to pathology in the heart, where energy demand is high. Dietary formulas for premature infants must contain adequate copper; cow's milk alone is unsuitable because it is low in copper.

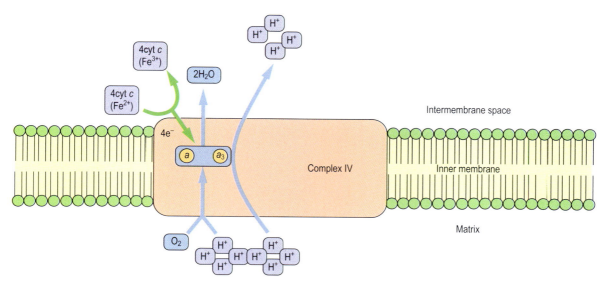

Fig. 8.10 **Complex IV.** Complex IV utilizes four electrons from cytochrome c and eight protons from the matrix. Four protons and electrons reduce oxygen to water. Four additional protons are pumped out of the matrix. Complex IV is regulated allosterically by ATP, by reversible phosphorylation/dephosphorylation, and by thyroid hormone (T_2, or diiodothyronine). *a*, cytochrome *a*; a_3, cytochrome a_3.

generated during oxidation of NADH and $FADH_2$. This energy is described as a **proton motive force,** an **electrochemical gradient** created by the proton concentration gradient and a proton charge differential (outside positive) across the inner mitochondrial membrane. To operate, it requires an inner membrane system that is impermeable to protons, except through ATP synthase or other complexes in a regulated fashion. When protons are pumped out of the matrix, the intermembrane space becomes more acidic and more positively charged than the matrix.

The ATP synthase complex (complex V) is an example of rotary catalysis

Lining the inner matrix face of the inner membrane of each mitochondrion are thousands of copies of the ATP synthase complex, also called complex V or F_0F_1-ATP synthase (F = coupling factor; see Chapter 4). ATP synthase is also called an ATPase because it can hydrolyze ATP, the thermodynamically preferred reaction. ATP synthase consists of two major complexes (Fig. 8.11). The inner membrane component, termed F_0, is the proton-driven motor with the stoichiometry of *a*, b_2, c_{10-14}. The *c*-subunits form the *c*-ring, which rotates in a clockwise direction in response to the flow of protons through the complex. Because the γ- and ε-subunits are bound to the *c*-ring, they rotate with it, inducing large conformational changes in the three-αβ dimers of the F_1 complex. The two β-proteins immobilize the second complex (F_1-ATP synthase).

F_1 has a stoichiometry of $α_3$, $β_3$, γ, δ, ε. The major part of F_1 consists of three αβ dimers arranged like slices of an orange, with the catalytic activity residing on the β-subunits. Each 120° rotation of the γ-subunit induces conformational changes in the αβ-dimeric subunits such that the nucleotide-binding sites alternate between three states: the first binds ADP and Pi, the second synthesizes ATP, and the third releases ATP, so each complete turn produces 3 ATP. This is known as the **binding-change mechanism** (Fig. 8.12). Surprisingly, the proton-motive free energy used by ATP synthase is not for ATP synthesis itself but for its release; when the proton gradient is too low to support ATP release, ATP remains stuck to ATP synthase, and further ATP production ceases. ADP and Pi are bound to the complex as soon as ATP leaves. The αβ-dimers are asymmetrical because each is in a different conformation at any given moment. This complex is a proton-driven motor, and it is an example of rotary catalysis. About three protons are required for the synthesis of each ATP. This complex acts independently of the electron transport chain; the addition of a weak acid, such as acetic acid, to a suspension of isolated mitochondria is sufficient to induce the biosynthesis of ATP in vitro.

P:O ratios

The P:O ratio is a measure of the number of high-energy phosphates (i.e., amount of ATP) synthesized per atom of oxygen consumed, or per mole of water produced. The P:O ratio can be calculated from the moles of ADP used to synthesize ATP and the atoms of oxygen taken up by mitochondria. For example, if 2.0 mmol of ADP is converted to ATP and 0.5 mmol of oxygen (1.0 milliatom of oxygen) is taken up, the P:O ratio is 2.0. As discussed earlier, the theoretical yield of ATP per mole of NADH is about 7.0 moles; however, by actual measurement with isolated mitochondria, **the P:O ratio for oxidation of metabolites that yield NADH is about 2.5, and the**

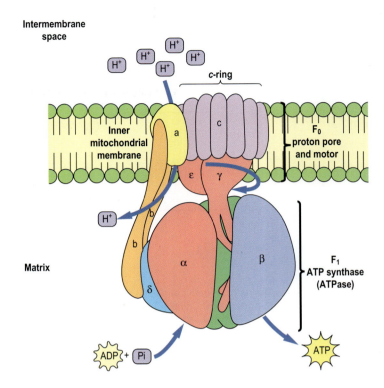

Fig. 8.11 **ATP synthase complex.** The ATP synthase complex consists of a motor (F_0) and generator (F_1). The proton pore involves the c-ring and the a-protein. The rotary component is the coiled-coil γ-subunit, which is bound to the ε-subunit and to the c-ring. The stationary component is the hexameric $α_3β_3$ unit, which is held in place by the δ-, b-, and a-proteins.

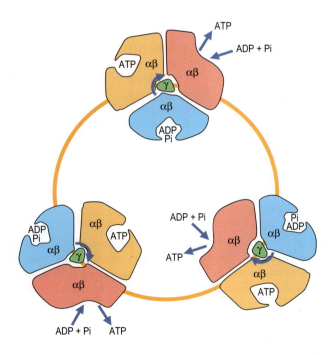

Fig. 8.12 **Binding-change mechanism of ATP synthase.** Powered by protons, the rotation of the γ-subunit of ATP synthase induces simultaneous conformational changes in all three αβ-dimers. Each 120° rotation results in ejection of an ATP, binding of ADP and Pi, and ATP synthesis.

ratio for those that yield $FADH_2$ is about 1.5. The remainder of the energy available from the oxidation of NADH and $FADH_2$ is released in the form of heat.

"Respiratory control" is the dependence of oxygen uptake by mitochondria on the availability of ADP

Normally, oxidation and phosphorylation are tightly coupled: substrates are oxidized, electrons are transported, and oxygen is consumed only when the synthesis of ATP is required (coupled respiration). Thus resting mitochondria consume oxygen at a slow rate, which can be greatly stimulated by addition of ADP (Fig. 8.13). ADP is taken up by the mitochondria and stimulates ATP synthase, which lowers the proton gradient. Respiration increases because the proton pumps are stimulated to reestablish the proton gradient. When the ADP is depleted, ATP synthesis terminates, and respiration returns to the original rate. Oxygen uptake also declines to the original rate when the concentration of ADP is depleted, and ATP synthesis terminates.

Mitochondria can become partially uncoupled if the inner membrane loses its structural integrity. They are said to be "leaky" because protons can diffuse through the inner membrane without involving ATP synthase. This occurs if isolated mitochondria are treated with mild detergents that disrupt the inner membrane or if they have been stored for a period of time. Such mitochondria are said to be "uncoupled";

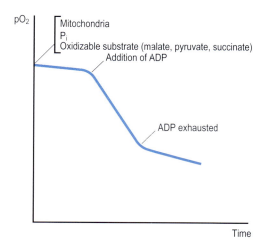

Fig. 8.13 **Effect of ADP on the uptake of oxygen by isolated mitochondria.** This may be studied in an isolated (sealed) system with an oxygen electrode and a recording device. The graph shows a typical recording of oxygen consumption (pO_2, partial pressure of oxygen) by normal mitochondria on introduction of ADP.

oxidation proceeds without production of ATP, and uncoupled mitochondria lose respiratory control because protons pumped by the electron chain bypass the ATPase and leak unproductively back into the matrix. The P:O ratio declines under these conditions.

The mechanism of respiratory control depends on the requirement for ADP and Pi binding to the ATP synthase complex: in the absence of ADP and Pi, protons cannot enter the mitochondrion through this complex, and oxygen consumption markedly decreases because the proton pumps cannot pump protons against a high proton back-pressure. This happens because the free energy of the electron transport reactions is sufficient to generate a pH gradient of only about two units across the membrane. If the pH gradient cannot be discharged for the production of ATP, the two-pH-unit gradient is established, and the pumps grind to a halt and stall. The electron transport chain becomes reduced, and substrate oxidation and oxygen consumption decrease. A little physical activity, with consumption of ATP and generation of ADP and Pi, opens up the ATPase channels, discharging the proton gradient and activating the electron transport chain and fuel and oxygen consumption. At a whole-body level, we breathe faster during exercise to provide the additional oxygen needed for increased oxidative phosphorylation.

Uncouplers

Uncouplers and uncoupling proteins are thermogenic

Uncouplers of oxidative phosphorylation dissipate the proton gradient by transporting protons back into mitochondria,

bypassing the ATP synthase. Uncouplers stimulate respiration and heat production because the system attempts to restore the proton gradient by oxidizing more fuel and pumping more protons out of mitochondria. **Uncouplers are typically hydrophobic compounds and either weak acids or bases, with pK_a near pH 7.** The classic uncoupler 2,4-dinitrophenol (DNP; Fig. 8.14) is protonated in solution on the outer, more acidic side of the inner mitochondrial membrane. Because of its hydrophobicity, it may then freely diffuse through the inner mitochondrial membrane. When it reaches the matrix side, it encounters a more basic pH, and the proton is released, effectively discharging the pH gradient. Other uncouplers include preservatives and antimicrobial agents, such as pentachlorophenol and p-cresol.

Uncoupling proteins (UCP)

According to the chemiosmotic hypothesis, the inner mitochondrial membrane is topologically closed. However, protons may also be transported into the matrix from the intermembrane space by routes other than the ATP synthase complex and inner membrane transporters. Much of the BMR is now thought to be mainly due to inner membrane components called uncoupling proteins (UCP). The first discovered was uncoupling protein-1 (UCP1), formerly known as **thermogenin,** which is found exclusively in **brown adipose tissue,** which is brown because of its high content of mitochondria. UCP1 provides body heat during cold stress in the young and in some adult animals (and can be induced upon mild cold exposure). It accomplishes this by uncoupling the proton gradient, allowing transport of protons but bypassing the ATPase, thereby generating heat (thermogenesis) instead of ATP. Uncoupling proteins are expressed at high levels in hibernating animals, permitting them to maintain body temperature without movement or exercise.

Four additional uncoupling proteins are expressed by the human genome: UCP2, UCP3, UCP4, and UCP5. Whereas UCP1 is exclusive to brown adipose tissue, UCP2 is expressed ubiquitously, UCP3 is mainly expressed in skeletal muscle, and UCP4 and UCP5 are expressed in the brain. Except for UCP1, the physiologic functions of these proteins are not well understood, but they could be of profound significance in our understanding of such health issues as diabetes, obesity, cancer, thyroid disease, and aging. As uncouplers, they have been linked to a number of fundamental functions. For example, there is strong evidence that obesity induces the synthesis of UCP2 in β-cells of the pancreas. This may play a role in the β-cell dysfunction found in type 2 diabetes because it lowers the intracellular concentration of ATP, which is required for secretion of insulin. The thyroid hormone (T_3) has been shown to stimulate thermogenesis in rats by promoting the synthesis of UCP3 in skeletal muscle. The common fever that is induced by infectious organisms is probably also due to uncoupling by UCPs.

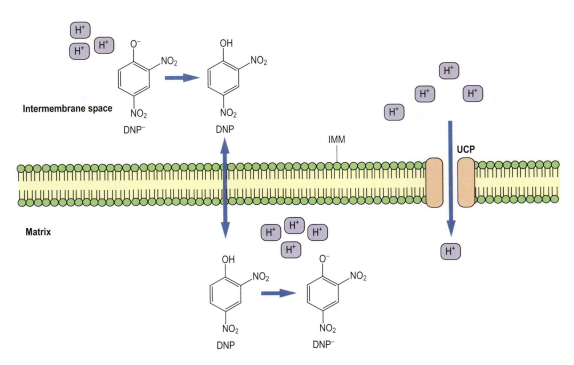

Fig. 8.14 **Proton transport by uncouplers.** Uncouplers transport protons into the mitochondrion, dissipating the proton gradient. DNP is an example of an exogenous uncoupler. The uncoupling proteins (UCP) are endogenous uncouplers in the IMM and are regulated by hormones. The gradient consisting of protons and other factors constitute the mitochondrial membrane potential (MMP), which is expressed in millivolts (mV). DNP, 2,4-dinitrophenol; IMM, inner mitochondrial membrane.

INHIBITORS OF OXIDATIVE METABOLISM

Electron transport system inhibitors

Inhibitors of electron transport selectively inhibit complexes I, III, or IV, interrupting the flow of electrons through the respiratory chain. This stops proton pumping, ATP synthesis, and oxygen uptake. Several inhibitors are readily available poisons that could be encountered in the practice of medicine - for example, the antidiabetic drug metformin, which at high concentrations inhibits complex I. Because metformin is not metabolized and is instead cleared via renal tubular secretion, clinicians must be mindful of metformin-associated lactic acidosis (MALA) in diabetic patients with impaired kidney function. It is noteworthy that genetic defects in respiratory-chain components often mimic the effects of these inhibitors, causing lactic acidosis because of increased reliance on glycolysis for ATP production (see Chapter 10).

Rotenone inhibits complex I (NADH–Q reductase)

Rotenone, a common insecticide, and some barbiturates (e.g., **amytal**) inhibit complex I. Because malate and lactate are oxidized by NAD^+, their oxidation will be decreased by rotenone.

However, substrates yielding $FADH_2$ can still be oxidized because complex I is bypassed, and electrons are donated to ubiquinone from $FADH_2$. Addition of ADP to a suspension of mitochondria supplemented with malate and phosphate (Fig. 8.15) markedly stimulates oxygen uptake as ATP synthesis occurs. Oxygen uptake is noticeably inhibited by rotenone, but when succinate is added, ATP synthesis and oxygen consumption resume until the supply of ADP is exhausted. Rotenone inhibition of complex I causes reduction of all components before the point of inhibition because they cannot be oxidized, whereas those after the point of inhibition become fully oxidized. This is known as a **crossover point**, and it can be determined spectrophotometrically because light absorption by respiratory-chain components changes according to redox state. Such analyses were used to define the sequence of components in the respiratory chain.

Antimycin A inhibits complex III (QH₂–cytochrome c reductase)

The inhibition of complex III by **antimycin A** prevents the transfer of electrons from either complex I or $FADH_2$-containing flavoproteins to cytochrome *c*. In this case, components preceding complex III become fully reduced, and those after it become oxidized. The oxygen uptake curve (Fig. 8.16) shows that the stimulation of respiration by ADP is inhibited by antimycin A, but the addition of succinate does not relieve the inhibition.

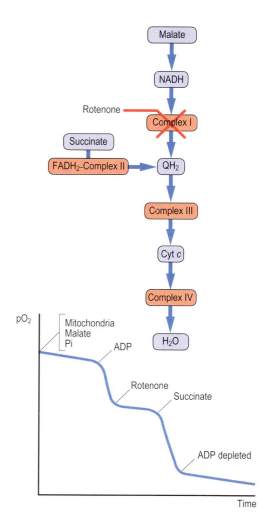

Fig. 8.15 **Inhibition of complex I.** Inhibitors such as rotenone inhibit oxygen uptake by mitochondria when NADH-producing substrates are being oxidized.

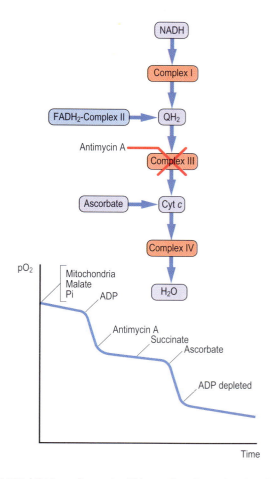

Fig. 8.16 **Inhibition of complex III by antimycin.** Antimycin A inhibits complex III, blocking transfer of electrons from both complex I and flavoproteins, such as complex II.

Ascorbic acid can reduce cytochrome c, and the addition of ascorbic acid restores respiration, illustrating that complex IV is unaffected by antimycin A.

Cyanide and carbon monoxide inhibit complex IV

Azide (N_3^-), cyanide (CN^-), and carbon monoxide (CO) inhibit complex IV (cytochrome c oxidase; Fig. 8.17). Because complex IV is the terminal electron transfer complex, its inhibition cannot be bypassed. All components preceding complex IV become reduced, oxygen cannot be reduced, none of the complexes can pump protons, and ATP is not synthesized. Uncouplers such as DNP have no effect because there is no proton gradient. Cyanide and carbon monoxide also bind to hemoglobin, blocking oxygen binding and transport (see Chapter 5). In these poisonings, both the ability to transport oxygen and the ability to synthesize ATP are impaired. The administration of oxygen is used for the treatment of such poisonings.

Oligomycin inhibits ATP synthase

Oligomycin inhibits respiration, but in contrast to electron transport inhibitors, it is not a direct inhibitor of the electron transport system. Instead, it inhibits the proton channel of ATP synthase. It causes an accumulation of protons outside the mitochondrion because the proton pumping system is still intact, but the proton channel is blocked. The addition of the uncoupler DNP after oxygen uptake has been inhibited by oligomycin illustrates this point: DNP dissipates the proton gradient and stimulates oxygen uptake as the electron transport system attempts to reestablish the proton gradient (Fig. 8.18).

Inhibitors of the ADP–ATP translocase

Most ATP is synthesized in the mitochondrion but used in the cytosol for biosynthetic reactions. Newly synthesized mitochondrial ATP and spent cytosolic ADP are exchanged

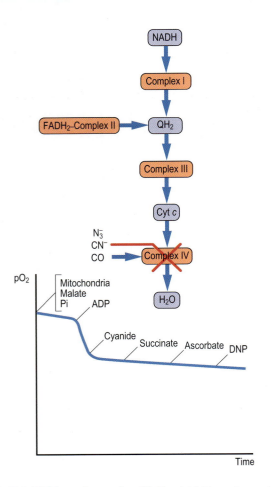

Fig. 8.17 **Inhibition of complex IV.** The inhibition of complex IV interrupts the transfer of electrons in the final step of electron transport. Electrons cannot be transferred to oxygen, and the synthesis of ATP is halted.

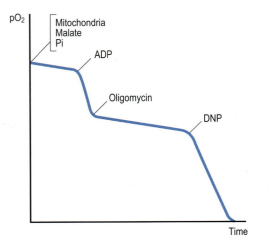

Fig. 8.18 **Oligomycin inhibition of oxygen uptake.** Oligomycin inhibits oxygen uptake in ATP-synthesizing mitochondria. Oligomycin inhibits ATP synthase and oxygen uptake in coupled mitochondria. However, DNP stimulates oxygen uptake after oligomycin inhibition by dissipating the proton gradient.

by a mitochondrial ADP–ATP translocase, representing about 10% of the protein in the inner mitochondrial membrane (see Fig. 8.3). This translocase can be inhibited by unusual plant and mold toxins, such as **bongkrekic acid** and **atractyloside**. Their effects are similar to those of oligomycin in vitro - a proton gradient builds up, and electron transport stops, but as with oligomycin, respiration can be reactivated by uncouplers.

REGULATION OF OXIDATIVE PHOSPHORYLATION

Respiratory control and feedback regulation

ADP is the key feedback regulator of oxidative phosphorylation

The oldest and simplest known mechanism of respiratory control depends on the supply of ADP. This is based on the fact that when added to isolated mitochondria, ADP stimulates respiration and ATP synthesis. When ADP is completely converted to ATP, respiration returns to the initial rate. Oxidative phosphorylation is also tightly coupled to fundamental pathways such as glycolysis, fatty acid oxidation, and the tricarboxylic acid cycle (see Chapters 9, 10, and 11) through feedback regulatory mechanisms, controlling the flux of fuel to mitochondria. Because oxidative phosphorylation depends on the supply of $FADH_2$, NADH, ADP, and Pi as well as the ATP/ADP ratio, the magnitude of the membrane potential, uncoupling, and hormonal factors, its modes of regulation are clearly complex.

Regulation by covalent modification and allosteric effectors (ATP–ADP)

The main target for regulating oxidative phosphorylation appears to be complex IV. It is phosphorylated in response to hormone action by cyclic-3′5′-adenosine monophosphate (cAMP)-dependent protein kinase (PKA) and dephosphorylated by a Ca^{2+}-stimulated protein phosphatase (see Chapter 12). Phosphorylation enables allosteric regulation by the ratio of ATP to ADP. A high ATP/ADP ratio inhibits and a low ratio stimulates oxidative phosphorylation. It is thought that the complex is normally phosphorylated and inhibited by ATP. With high Ca^{2+} levels, such as in muscle during exercise (see Chapter 37), the enzyme is dephosphorylated, the inhibition by ATP is abolished, and its activity is greatly stimulated, increasing ATP production. Based on the observation that in type 2 diabetes, ATP production is decreased when the β-subunit of ATP synthase is phosphorylated, it has been proposed that this complex is also regulated by phosphorylation/dephosphorylation.

Regulation by thyroid hormones

Thyroid hormones act at two levels in mitochondria. In rats, T_3 stimulates the synthesis of UCP2 and UCP3, which can uncouple the proton gradient, but this has not been documented in humans. Additionally, T_2 binds to complex IV on the matrix side, inducing slip in cytochrome c oxidase. The term *slip* means that complex IV pumps fewer protons per electron transported through the complex, resulting in increased thermogenesis. The action of T_3 could explain, in part, the long-term thermogenic effects of thyroid hormones, and T_2 could explain the short-term effects (see also Chapter 27).

Mitochondrial permeability transition pore (MPTP)

Located in the inner mitochondrial membrane, the MPTP is a nonselective pore that is a critical factor in cell death. It is normally closed but will open when cells are reperfused after a period of ischemia (**ischemic reperfusion injury [IRI]**; see Chapter 42), and small molecules will leave the mitochondrial matrix. The opening of the MPTP is now considered a key feature of IRI in which cellular damage is much greater than that produced by ischemia alone. Cascades of reactions occurring in response to IRI lead to apoptosis, necrosis, and cell death.

Ischemia, such as that found in heart attacks, is usually caused by a clot that blocks an artery. Clot busters such as streptokinase can be administered to dissolve clots and reperfuse ischemic cells. But if the ischemic state has been prolonged before administration of a clot buster, death may result from reperfusion injury and the opening of the MPTP. This occurs all too often in heart attack patients. Several drugs, such as cyclosporin A, inhibit the MPTP from opening and may protect cells from necrosis or apoptosis after the administration of a clot buster.

SUMMARY

- The electron transport system consists of electron carrier complexes that are located in the inner mitochondrial membrane.
- Oxidation of fuels leads to the production of reduced nucleotides, NADH and $FADH_2$, and four major flavoproteins feed electrons to ubiquinone, the first member of the common pathway of electron transport.
- Energy derived from the conductance of electrons through the electron transport system is used by three of the complexes to pump protons into the intermembrane space, creating an electrochemical gradient or proton motive force.
- The proton gradient is used to power ATP synthase for the synthesis of ATP by rotary catalysis as well as transport of intermediates across the inner membrane.

- Numerous toxins can severely impair the electron transport system, the ATP synthase, and the translocase that exchanges ATP and ADP across the inner mitochondrial membrane.
- The rate of ATP production by the electron transport system is regulated by modulation of the proton gradient, by allosteric modification and phosphorylation–dephosphorylation, and by thyroid hormones.
- At least five uncoupling proteins (UCP) with specific tissue distributions are found in the inner mitochondrial membrane, and they all regulate the membrane potential, energy expenditure, and thermogenesis.
- Chronic diseases or conditions such as diabetes, cancer, obesity, and aging all have metabolic links to dysregulation of oxidative phosphorylation through effects on the electron transport system and ATP synthase.
- The integrity of mitochondria and cells may be disrupted by ischemic reperfusion injury and the opening of the mitochondrial permeability transition pore, leading to death and tissue damage.

FURTHER READING

Acosta, M. J., Vazquez Fonseca, L., Desbats, M. A., et al. (2016). Coenzyme Q biosynthesis in health and disease. *Biochimica et Biophysica Acta, 1857,* 1079–1085.

Giachin, G., Bouverot, R., Acajjaoui, S., et al. (2016). Dynamics of human mitochondrial complex I assembly: Implications for neurodegenerative diseases. *Frontiers in Molecular Bioscience, 22*(3), 43.

Kwong, J. Q., & Molkentin, J. D. (2015). Physiological and pathological roles of the mitochondrial permeability transition pore in the heart. *Cell Metabolism, 21,* 206–214.

Lapuente-Brun, E., Moreno-Loshuertos, R., Acín-Pérez, R., et al. (2013). Supercomplex assembly determines electron flux in the mitochondrial electron transport chain. *Science, 340,* 1567–1570.

Picard, M., Taivassalo, T., Gouspillou, G., et al. (2011). Mitochondria: Isolation, structure and function. *Journal of Physiology, 589,* 4413–4421.

Pinadda, V., & Halestrap, A. P. (2012). The roles of phosphate and the phosphate carrier in the mitochondrial permeability transition pore. *Mitochondrion, 12,* 120–125.

Ruiz-Meana, M., Fernandez-Sanz, C., & Garcia-Dorado, D. (2010). The SR-mitochondria interaction: A new player in cardiac pathophysiology. *Cardiovascular Research, 88,* 30–39.

Shanbhag, R., Shi, G., Rujiviphat, J., et al. (2012). The emerging role of proteolysis in mitochondrial quality control and the etiology of Parkinson's disease. *Parkinson's Disease, 2012,* 382175. doi:10.1155/2012/382175.

Zhu, J., Vinothkumar, K. R., & Hirst, J. (2016). Structure of mammalian respiratory complex I. *Nature, 536,* 354–358.

RELEVANT WEBSITES

Movies:
ATP synthase: http://www.youtube.com/watch?v=PjdPTY1wHdQ
Animations:
ATP synthase: http://vcell.ndsu.nodak.edu/animations/atpgradient/index.htm
Virtual Cell Animation Center: http://vcell.ndsu.nodak.edu/animations/home.htm
Other resources:
Metformin monitoring: http://www.fda.gov/Safety/MedWatch/SafetyInformation/SafetyAlertsforHumanMedicalProducts/ucm494829.htm
Bioenergetics: http://www.bmb.leeds.ac.uk/illingworth/oxphos/
The Children's Mitochondrial Disease Network: http://www.cmdn.org.uk/
United Mitochondrial Disease Foundation: http://www.umdf.org/

ABBREVIATIONS

ATP	Adenosine triphosphate
BMR	Basal metabolic rate
DNP	Dinitrophenol
FAD	Flavin adenine dinucleotide
FMN	Flavin mononucleotide
IMM	Inner mitochondrial membrane
IMS	Intermembrane space
IRI	Ischemic reperfusion injury
MET	Metabolic equivalent task
mtDNA	Mitochondrial DNA
NAD(H)	Nicotinamide adenine dinucleotide
OMM	Outer mitochondrial membrane
R	Perfect gas constant
RMR	Resting metabolic rate
TIM	Transporter in inner membrane
TOM	Transporter in outer membrane
UCP	Uncoupling protein

Anaerobic Metabolism of Carbohydrates in the Red Blood Cell

John W. Baynes

LEARNING OBJECTIVES

After reading this chapter, you should be able to:

- Outline the sequence of reactions in anaerobic glycolysis, the central pathway of carbohydrate metabolism in all cells.
- Summarize the energetics of anaerobic glycolysis, including the reactions involved in the utilization and formation of ATP and the net yield of ATP during glycolysis.
- Identify the primary site of allosteric regulation of glycolysis and the mechanism of regulation of this enzyme.
- Identify steps in glycolysis that illustrate the use of coupled reactions to drive thermodynamically unfavored processes, including substrate-level phosphorylation.
- Explain the different roles of the pentose phosphate pathway in erythrocytes and nucleated cells.
- Describe the role of anaerobic glycolysis in the development of dental caries.
- Explain why glycolysis is essential for normal red cell functions, including consequences of deficiencies in glycolytic enzymes and the role of glycolysis in adaptation to high altitude.
- Explain the origin of drug-induced hemolytic anemia in persons with G6PD deficiency.

INTRODUCTION

Glycolysis is the central pathway of glucose metabolism in all cells

Glucose is the major carbohydrate on Earth, the backbone and monomer unit of cellulose and starch. It is also the only fuel that is used by all cells in our bodies. All of these cells, even the microbes in our intestines, begin the metabolism of glucose by a pathway termed *glycolysis* - that is, carbohydrate (glyco) splitting (lysis). Glycolysis is catalyzed by soluble cytosolic enzymes and is the ubiquitous, central metabolic pathway for glucose metabolism. The erythrocyte, commonly known as the red blood cell (RBC), is unique among all cells in the body: it uses glucose and glycolysis as its sole source of energy. Thus the RBC is a useful model for an introduction to glycolysis.

Pyruvate, a three-carbon carboxylic acid, is the end product of anaerobic glycolysis; 2 moles of pyruvate are formed per mole of glucose

In cells with mitochondria and oxidative metabolism, pyruvate is converted completely into CO_2 and H_2O; glycolysis in this setting is termed **aerobic glycolysis.** In RBCs, which lack mitochondria and oxidative metabolism, pyruvate is reduced to lactic acid, a three-carbon hydroxyacid, the product of **anaerobic glycolysis.** Each mole of glucose yields 2 moles of lactate, which are then excreted into the blood. Two molecules of lactic acid contain exactly the same number of carbons, hydrogens, and oxygens as one molecule of glucose (Fig. 9.1); however, there is sufficient free energy available from the cleavage and rearrangement of the glucose molecule to produce 2 moles of ATP per mole of glucose converted into lactate. The RBC uses most of this ATP to maintain electrochemical and ion gradients across its plasma membrane.

In the RBC, 10%–20% of the glycolytic intermediate 1,3-bisphosphoglycerate is diverted to the synthesis of 2,3-bisphosphoglycerate (2,3-BPG), an allosteric regulator of the O_2 affinity of Hb (Chapter 5). The **pentose phosphate pathway,** also a shunt from glycolysis, accounts for about 10% of glucose metabolism in the red cell. In the red cell, this pathway has a special role in protection against oxidative stress, whereas in nucleated cells, it also serves as a source of NADPH for biosynthetic reactions and pentoses for nucleic acid synthesis.

THE ERYTHROCYTE

The erythrocyte, or red blood cell, relies exclusively on blood glucose as a metabolic fuel

The erythrocyte, or red blood cell (RBC), represents 40%–45% of blood volume and more than 90% of the formed elements (erythrocytes, leukocytes, and platelets) in blood. The RBC is, both structurally and metabolically, the simplest cell in the body - the end product of the maturation of bone marrow reticulocytes. During its maturation, the RBC loses all its subcellular organelles. Without nuclei, it lacks the ability to synthesize DNA or RNA. Without ribosomes or an endoplasmic reticulum, it cannot synthesize or secrete protein. Because it cannot oxidize fats, a process requiring mitochondrial activity, the RBC relies exclusively on blood glucose as a fuel. Other dietary sugars, such as fructose from sucrose and high-fructose corn syrup and galactose from milk sugar (lactose), are

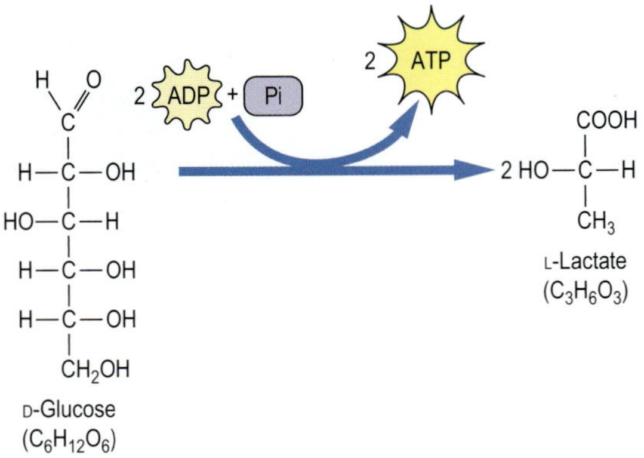

Fig. 9.1 Conversion of glucose to lactate during anaerobic glycolysis. One mole of glucose is converted to 2 moles of lactate during anaerobic glycolysis. No oxygen is consumed in this pathway, and no CO_2 is produced. There is a net yield of 2 moles of ATP per mole of glucose converted to lactate.

ADVANCED CONCEPT BOX
GLUCOSE UTILIZATION IN THE RED CELL

In a 70-kg person, there are about 5 L of blood and a little more than 2 kg (2 L) of RBCs. These cells constitute about 3% of total body mass and consume about 20 g (0.1 mole) of glucose per day, representing about 10% of total body glucose metabolism. The RBC has the highest specific rate of glucose utilization of any cell in the body, approximately 10 g of glucose/kg of tissue/day, compared with ~2.5 g of glucose/kg of tissue/day for the whole body.

In the RBC, about 90% of glucose is metabolized via glycolysis, yielding lactate, which is excreted into the blood. Despite its high rate of glucose consumption, the RBC has one of the lowest rates of ATP synthesis of any cell in the body, ~0.1 mole of ATP/kg tissue/day, reflecting the fact that anaerobic glycolysis recovers only a fraction of the energy available from complete combustion of glucose to CO_2 and H_2O.

converted to glucose, primarily in the liver. Metabolism of glucose in the RBC is entirely anaerobic, consistent with the primary role of the RBC in oxygen transport and delivery rather than its utilization.

GLYCOLYSIS

Overview

Pyruvate is the end product of anaerobic glycolysis

Glucose enters the RBC by facilitated diffusion via the insulin-independent glucose transporter GLUT-1. Glycolysis then proceeds through a series of phosphorylated intermediates,

starting with the synthesis of **glucose-6-phosphate** (Glc-6-P). During this process, which involves 10 enzymatically catalyzed steps, two molecules of ATP are expended (**investment** stage) to build up a nearly symmetric intermediate, fructose-1,6-bisphosphate (Fru-1,6-BP), which is then cleaved (**splitting** stage) to two three-carbon triose phosphates. These are eventually converted into lactate, with production of ATP, during the **yield** stage of glycolysis. The yield stage includes both redox and phosphorylation reactions, leading to formation of four molecules of ATP during the conversion of the two triose phosphates into lactate. The outcome is a net 2 moles of ATP per mole of glucose converted into lactate.

Glycolysis is a relatively inefficient pathway for extracting energy from glucose: the yield of 2 moles of ATP per mole of glucose is only about 5% of the 30–32 ATP that are available by complete oxidation of glucose to CO_2 and H_2O by mitochondria in other tissues (Chapter 10).

One might ask why a 10-step pathway is required to convert glucose to lactate; couldn't it have been done in fewer steps or by cleavage of one carbon at a time? The answer, from a metabolic point of view, is that glycolysis is not an isolated pathway; most glycolytic intermediates serve as branch points to other metabolic pathways. In this way, the metabolism of glucose intersects with the metabolism of fats, proteins, and nucleic acids, as well as other pathways of carbohydrate metabolism. Some of these metabolic interactions are shown in Fig. 9.2.

The investment stage of glycolysis

Two ATP are invested to prime the metabolism of glucose by glycolysis

Glucose-6-phosphate

Glucose is taken up into the red cell via the facilitated transporter GLUT-1 (Chapter 4); this protein accounts for about 5% of total red-cell membrane protein, so glucose transport is not rate limiting for glycolysis. Thus the steady-state concentration of glucose in the RBC is only ~20% lower than that in plasma. The first step in the commitment of glucose to glycolysis is the phosphorylation of glucose to Glc-6-P, catalyzed by the enzyme **hexokinase** (Fig. 9.3, top). The formation of Glc-6-P from free glucose and inorganic phosphate is energetically unfavorable, so a molecule of ATP must be expended, or *invested*, in the phosphorylation reaction; the hydrolysis of ATP is coupled to the synthesis of Glc-6-P. Glc-6-P is trapped in the RBC, along with other phosphorylated intermediates in glycolysis, because there are no transport systems for sugar phosphates in the plasma membranes of mammalian cells.

Fructose-6-phosphate

The second step in glycolysis is the conversion of Glc-6-P into Fru-6-P by **phosphoglucose isomerase** (Fig. 9.3, middle).

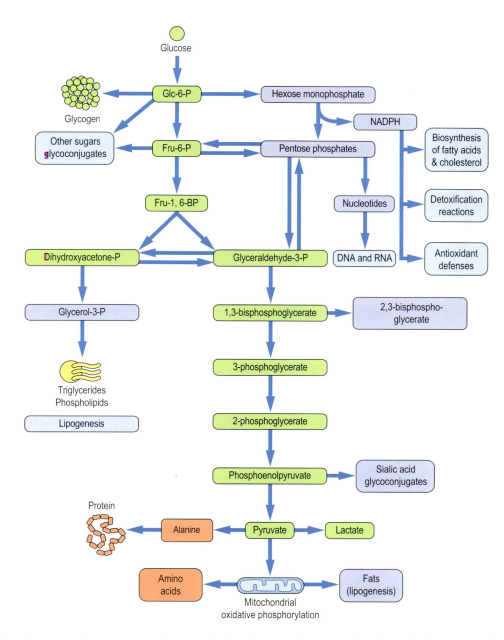

Fig. 9.2 **Interactions between glycolysis and other metabolic pathways.** The green-colored boxes indicate intermediates involved in the pathway of glycolysis. Other boxes illustrate some of the metabolic interactions between glycolysis and other metabolic pathways in the cell. Not all of these pathways are active in the red cell, which has limited biosynthetic capacity and lacks mitochondria. Glc-6-P, glucose-6-phosphate; Fru-6-P, fructose-6-phosphate; Fru-1,6-BP, fructose-1,6-bisphosphate.

Isomerases catalyze freely reversible equilibrium reactions - in this case, an aldose–ketose interconversion. A second molecule of ATP is invested to phosphorylate Fru-6-P at the C-1 position; the reaction is catalyzed by **phosphofructokinase-1** (PFK-1). The product, **fructose 1,6-bisphosphate** (Fru-1,6-BP), is a pseudosymmetric intermediate, with a phosphate ester on each end of the molecule. Like hexokinase, PFK-1 requires ATP as a substrate and catalyzes an essentially irreversible reaction. Both hexokinase and PFK-1 are important regulatory enzymes in glycolysis, but PFK-1 is the critical, commitment step. This

reaction directs glucose to glycolysis, the only pathway for the metabolism of Fru-1,6-BP.

The splitting stage of glycolysis

Fructose-1,6-BP is cleaved in the middle by a reverse aldol reaction

The **aldolase** reaction (Fig. 9.3, bottom) is a freely reversible equilibrium reaction, converting Fru-1,6-BP to two triose

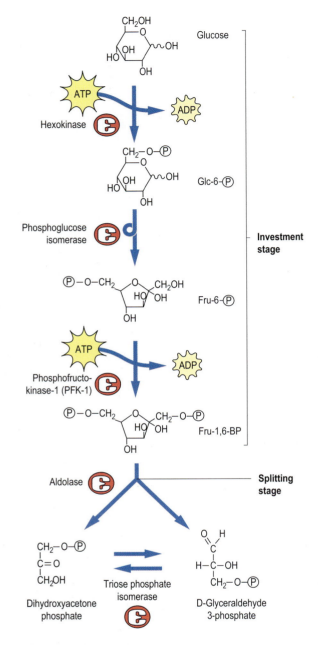

Fig. 9.3 **The investment and splitting stages of glycolysis.** Note the consumption of ATP at the hexokinase and phosphofructokinase-1 reactions. Glc-6-P, glucose-6-phosphate; Fru-6-P, fructose-6-phosphate; Fru-1,6-BP, fructose-1,6-bisphosphate.

phosphates, dihydroxyacetone phosphate and glyceraldehyde-3-phosphate, from the top and bottom halves of the Fru-1,6-BP molecule, respectively. Only the glyceraldehyde-3-phosphate continues through the yield stage of glycolysis, but **triose phosphate isomerase** catalyzes the interconversion of dihydroxyacetone phosphate and glyceraldehyde-3-phosphate so that both halves of the glucose molecule are eventually metabolized to lactate.

The yield stage of glycolysis: Synthesis of ATP by substrate-level phosphorylation

The yield stage of glycolysis produces 4 moles of ATP, yielding a net of 2 moles of ATP per mole of glucose converted into lactate

The synthesis of ATP during glycolysis is accomplished by kinases that catalyze **substrate-level phosphorylation,** a process in which a high-energy phosphate compound (X~P) transfers its phosphate to ADP, yielding ATP.

$$\text{Substrate-level phosphorylation:} \ X \sim P + ADP \rightarrow X + ATP$$

Glyceraldehyde-3-phosphate dehydrogenase (GAPDH)

GAPDH catalyzes a redox reaction, forming a high-energy acyl phosphate compound

To set the stage for substrate-level phosphorylation, the aldehyde group of glyceraldehyde-3-phosphate is oxidized to a carboxylic acid, and the energy available from the oxidation reaction is used, in part, to trap a phosphate from the cytoplasmic pool as an **acyl phosphate.** This reaction is catalyzed by glyceraldehyde-3-phosphate dehydrogenase (GAPDH), yielding the high-energy compound (X~P), 1,3-bisphosphoglycerate (1,3-BPG). The coenzyme NAD^+ is simultaneously reduced to NADH (Figs. 9.4 and 9.5).

The GAPDH reaction provides an interesting illustration of the role of enzyme-bound intermediates in the formation of high-energy phosphates. How does the oxidation of an aldehyde and the reduction of NAD^+ lead to the formation of an acyl phosphate bond in 1,3-BPG? How does the phosphate enter the picture and become activated to a high-energy state? The inhibition of GAPDH by thiol reagents such as iodoacetamide, p-chloromercuribenzoate, and N-ethylmaleimide points to involvement of an active-site sulfhydryl residue. The mechanism of action of this enzyme is described in Fig. 9.5.

Substrate-level phosphorylation

Substrate-level phosphorylation produces ATP from another high-energy phosphate compound

Phosphoglycerate kinase (PGK) catalyzes the transfer of the phosphate group from the high-energy acyl phosphate of 1,3-BPG to ADP, forming ATP. This substrate-level phosphorylation reaction yields the first ATP produced in glycolysis. The remaining phosphate group in 3-phosphoglycerate is an ester phosphate and does not have enough energy to phosphorylate ADP, so a series of isomerization and dehydration reactions is enlisted to convert the ester phosphate into a high-energy enol phosphate. The first step is to shift the phosphate to C-2 of glycerate, converting 3-phosphoglycerate into 2-phosphoglycerate, catalyzed by the enzyme **phosphoglycerate mutase** (Fig. 9.4). Mutases catalyze the transfer of functional groups within a molecule. Phosphoglycerate mutase

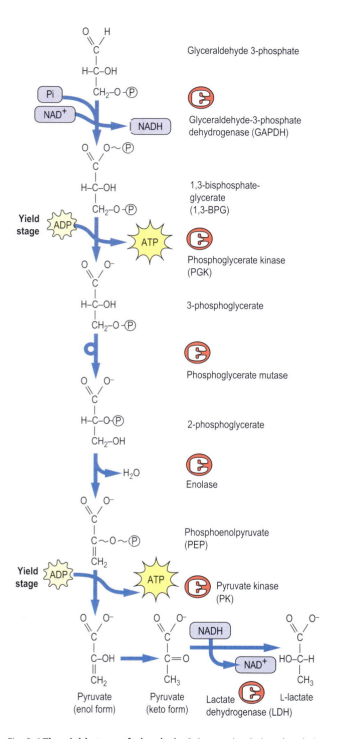

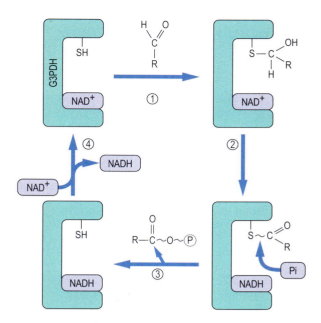

Fig. 9.4 **The yield stage of glycolysis.** Substrate-level phosphorylation reactions catalyzed by phosphoglycerate kinase and pyruvate kinase produce ATP, using the high-energy compounds 1,3-bisphosphoglycerate and phosphoenolpyruvate, respectively. Note that NADH produced during the glyceraldehyde-3-phosphate dehydrogenase reaction is recycled back to NAD+ during the lactate dehydrogenase reaction, permitting continued glycolysis in the presence of only catalytic amounts of NAD+.

Fig. 9.5 **Mechanism of the glyceraldehyde-3-phosphate dehydrogenase (GAPDH) reaction.** In Step 1, glyceraldehyde-3-P (RCHO) reacts with the active-site sulfhydryl group of GAPDH to form a thiohemiacetal adduct. In Step 2, the thiohemiacetal is oxidized to a thioester by NAD+, which is bound in the active site of the enzyme and is reduced to NADH. In Step 3, phosphate enters the active site and, in a phosphorylase reaction, cleaves the carbon–sulfur bond, displacing the 3-phosphoglycerate group, producing 1,3-bisphosphoglycerate and regenerating the sulfhydryl group. In Step 4, the enzyme exchanges NADH for NAD+, completing the catalytic cycle.

has an active-site histidine residue, and a phospho-histidine adduct is formed as an enzyme-bound intermediate during the phosphate transfer reaction.

2-Phosphoglycerate then undergoes a dehydration reaction, catalyzed by **enolase**, a (de)hydratase, to yield the high-energy phosphate compound phosphoenolpyruvate (PEP). PEP is used by **pyruvate kinase (PK)** to phosphorylate ADP, yielding pyruvate and the second ATP, again by substrate-level phosphorylation. It seems strange that the high-energy phosphate bond in PEP can be formed from the low-energy phosphate compound 2-phosphoglycerate by a simple sequence of isomerization and dehydration reactions. However, the thermodynamic driving force for these reactions is probably derived from charge–charge repulsion between the phosphate and carboxylate groups of 2-phosphoglycerate and the isomerization of enolpyruvate to pyruvate after the phosphorylation reaction.

Phosphoglycerate kinase and pyruvate kinase catalyze substrate-level phosphorylation reactions

The ATP-generating reactions of glycolysis produce 2 moles of ATP per mole of triose phosphate, or a total of 4 moles of ATP per mole of Fru-1,6-BP. After adjustment for the ATP invested in the hexokinase and PFK-1 reactions, the net energy yield is 2 moles of ATP per mole of glucose converted into pyruvate.

ADVANCED CONCEPT BOX
INHIBITION OF SUBSTRATE-LEVEL PHOSPHORYLATION BY ARSENATE

Arsenic is just below phosphorus in the periodic table of the elements, and it might be expected to share some of the properties and reactivity of phosphate. In fact, arsenate has pK_a values similar to those of phosphate and can actually be used by GAPDH, producing 1-arsenato-3-phosphoglycerate. However, the acyl–arsenate bond is unstable and hydrolyzes rapidly, and ATP is not generated by substrate-level phosphorylation. Although arsenate does not inhibit any of the enzymes of glycolysis, it dissipates the redox energy available from the GAPDH reaction and prevents the formation of ATP by substrate-level phosphorylation at the PGK reaction. In effect, arsenate *uncouples* the GAPDH and PGK reactions. Note that arsenic and arsenite are also toxic but have a different mechanism of action: they react with thiol groups in sulfhydryl enzymes, such as GAPDH (Fig. 9.5), irreversibly inhibiting their activity.

CLINICAL TEST BOX
INHIBITION OF ENOLASE BY FLUORIDE

Measurements of blood-glucose concentration are used for the diagnosis and management of diabetes. Frequently these measurements are made in the clinical laboratory more than 1 h after the collection of the blood sample. Because RBCs can metabolize glucose to lactate - even in a sealed, anoxic container - glucose in the blood will be consumed, and lactate will be produced, which will lead to acidification of the blood sample. These reactions proceed in RBCs, even at room temperature, so that both blood glucose concentration and pH will decrease during standing, possibly leading to a false diagnosis of hypoglycemia and/or acidemia.

Anaerobic metabolism of glucose can be prevented by adding an inhibitor of glycolysis to the blood collection tube. Sulfhydryl reagents would work - they are potent inhibitors of GAPDH - however, most blood samples are collected with a small amount of a much cheaper reagent, sodium fluoride, in the sample-collection vial. Fluoride is a strong competitive inhibitor of enolase, blocking glycolysis and lactate production in the RBC. It is an unusual competitive inhibitor because fluoride bears little resemblance to 2-phosphoglycerate. In this case, fluoride forms a complex with phosphate and Mg^{2+} in the active site of the enzyme, blocking access of the substrate.

Lactate dehydrogenase (LDH)

LDH regenerates NAD⁺ consumed in the GAPDH reaction, producing lactate, the end product of anaerobic glycolysis

Two molecules of pyruvate have exactly the same number of carbons and oxygens as one molecule of glucose; however,

CLINICAL BOX
PYRUVATE KINASE DEFICIENCY

A child presented with jaundice and abdominal tenderness, which developed after a severe cold. Laboratory tests revealed a low hematocrit and hemoglobin concentration, normochromatic erythrocytes with normal morphology, and mild reticulocytosis. Serum bilirubin was increased.

Comment

Pyruvate kinase deficiency is the most common of the hemolytic anemias that result from a deficiency of a glycolytic enzyme. It is an autosomal recessive disorder that occurs with a frequency of 1/10,000 (~1% gene frequency) in the world population. It is second only to G6PDH deficiency (see later discussion) as an enzymatic cause of hemolytic anemia. These diseases are diagnosed by measurement of erythrocyte levels of enzymes or metabolites, by demonstrating abnormalities in enzymatic activities, or by genetic analysis. Enzymatic defects in pyruvate kinase that have been characterized include thermal lability, increased K_m for PEP, and decreased activation by Fru-1,6-BP.

Pyruvate kinase deficiency varies significantly in severity, from a mild, compensated condition requiring little intervention, to a severe disease requiring transfusions. The anemia results from an inability to synthesize sufficient ATP for maintenance of RBC ion gradients and cell shape. Interestingly, patients may tolerate the anemia quite well. Even with mild anemia, the accumulation of 2,3-bisphosphoglycerate in their RBCs decreases the oxygen affinity of hemoglobin, promoting oxygen delivery to muscle during exercise and even to the fetus during pregnancy.

there is a deficit of four hydrogens - each pyruvate has four hydrogens, a total of eight hydrogens for two pyruvates, compared with 12 in a molecule of glucose. The "missing" four hydrogens remain in the form of the 2NADH and 2 H⁺ formed in the GAPDH reaction. Because NAD⁺ is present in only catalytic amounts in the cell and is an essential cofactor for glycolysis (and other reactions), there must be a mechanism for regeneration of NAD⁺ if glycolysis is to continue.

The oxidation of NADH is accomplished under anaerobic conditions by lactate dehydrogenase (LDH), which catalyzes the reduction of pyruvate to lactate by NADH + H⁺ and regenerates NAD⁺. In mammals, all cells have LDH, and lactate is the end product of glycolysis under anaerobic conditions. Under aerobic conditions, mitochondria oxidize NADH to NAD⁺ and convert pyruvate to CO_2 and H_2O so that lactate is not formed. Despite their capacity for oxidative metabolism, however, some cells may at times "go glycolytic," forming lactate (e.g., in muscle during oxygen debt and in phagocytes in pus or in poorly perfused tissues). Most of the lactate excreted into blood is retrieved by the liver for use as a substrate for gluconeogenesis (Chapter 12).

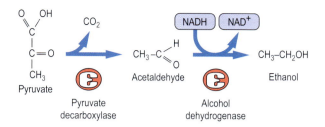

Fig. 9.6 **Anaerobic glycolysis in yeast.** Formation of ethanol by anaerobic glycolysis during fermentation. Pyruvate is decarboxylated by pyruvate decarboxylase, yielding acetaldehyde and CO_2. Alcohol dehydrogenase uses NADH to reduce acetaldehyde to ethanol, regenerating NAD^+ for glycolysis.

Fermentation

Fermentation is a general term for anaerobic metabolism of glucose, usually applied to unicellular organisms

Some anaerobic bacteria, such as lactobacilli, produce lactate, whereas others have alternative pathways for anaerobic oxidation of NADH formed during glycolysis. During fermentation in yeast, the pathway of glycolysis is identical to that in the RBC, except that pyruvate is converted into ethanol (Fig. 9.6). The pyruvate is first decarboxylated by pyruvate decarboxylase to acetaldehyde, releasing CO_2. The NADH produced in the GAPDH reaction is then reoxidized by alcohol dehydrogenase, regenerating NAD^+ and producing ethanol.

Ethanol is a toxic compound, and most yeast die when the ethanol concentration in their medium reaches about 12%–16%, which is the approximate concentration of alcohol in natural wines. Alcoholic beverages are a rich source of energy; alcohol yields ~7 kcal/g (29 kJ/g) by aerobic metabolism (see Table 8.1), intermediate between carbohydrates and lipids. As a food, alcoholic beverages are more stable during long-term storage compared with the fruits and vegetables from which they are produced. Beer, wine, cider, and mead also provide varying amounts of vitamins, minerals, phytochemicals, and xenobiotics.

Other fermented food products, which are estimated to account for a third of all foods eaten by humans worldwide, include pickles, sauerkraut, buttermilk, yogurt, sausage, some fish and meats, bread, cheese, and various sauces and condiments - even coffee and chocolate. Fermentation is an important source of the flavor and aroma of all of these foodstuffs. The acidic environment produced during fermentation limits spoilage and growth of pathogenic microorganisms.

There are as many as 1000 species of anaerobic bacteria in our intestines. These enterobacteria thrive in a symbiotic relationship with humans. They assist significantly in the digestion and extraction of energy from foodstuffs, are a source of biotin and vitamin K, provide protection against infection by pathogens, and promote gastrointestinal peristalsis. The species distribution also changes in response to the carbohydrate, fat, and protein content of our diet.

Regulation of glycolysis in erythrocytes

Glycolysis is regulated allosterically at three kinase reactions

Hexokinase

RBCs consume glucose at a fairly steady rate. They are not physically active like muscle, and they do not require energy for transport of O_2 or CO_2. Glycolysis in red cells appears to be regulated simply by the energy needs of the cell, primarily for maintenance of ion gradients. The balance between ATP consumption and production is controlled allosterically at three sites: the **hexokinase, phosphofructokinase-1,** and **pyruvate kinase** reactions (Fig. 9.2). Based on measurements of the V_{max} of the various enzymes in RBC lysates in vitro, hexokinase is present at the lowest activity of all glycolytic enzymes. Its maximal activity is about five times the rate of glucose consumption by the RBC, but it is subject to feedback (allosteric) inhibition by its product Glc-6-P. Hexokinase has 30% homology between its *N*- and *C*-terminal domains, the result of duplication and fusion of a primordial gene; binding of Glc-6-P to the *N*-terminal domain inhibits the activity of the enzyme and production of Glc-6-P at the active site in the *C*-terminal domain.

Phosphofructokinase-1 (PFK-1)

PFK-1 is the primary site of regulation of glycolysis

PFK-1 controls the flux of Fru-6-P to Fru-1,6-BP and, indirectly through the phosphoglucose isomerase reaction, the level of Glc-6-P and inhibition of hexokinase. PFK-1 is strongly inhibited by ambient ATP, so its activity varies with the energy status of the cell. Surprisingly, ATP is both a substrate (Fig. 9.3) and

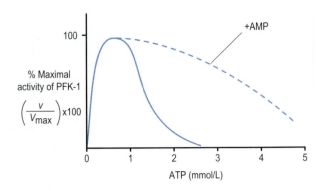

Fig. 9.7 **Allosteric regulation of phosphofructokinase-1 (PFK-1) by ATP.** AMP is a potent activator of PFK-1 in the presence of ATP.

Table 9.1 Regulation of glycolysis in the red cell	
Enzyme	**Regulator**
Hexokinase	Inhibited by glucose-6-P
Phosphofructokinase-1	Inhibited by ATP; activated by AMP
Pyruvate kinase	Activated by fructose-1,6-BP

an allosteric inhibitor (Fig. 9.7) of PFK-1, a dual function that permits fine control over the activity of the enzyme.

As shown in Fig. 9.7, the concentration of ATP in the RBC (~2 mmol/L) normally suppresses the activity of PFK-1. AMP, which is present at a much lower concentration (~0.05 mmol/L), relieves this inhibition. Because of their relative concentrations, a small fractional conversion of ATP to AMP in the RBC yields a large relative increase in AMP concentration, which activates PFK-1. ADP also relieves the inhibition of PFK-1 by ATP, but its concentration does not change as much with energy utilization. AMP not only relieves the inhibition of PFK-1 by ATP but also decreases the K_m for the substrate Fru-6-P, further increasing the catalytic efficiency of the enzyme.

Through allosteric mechanisms, the activity of PFK-1 in the red cell is exquisitely sensitive to changes in the energy status of the cell, as measured by the relative concentrations of ATP, ADP, and AMP. In effect, the overall activity of PFK-1, and thus the rate of glycolysis, depends on the cell's (AMP + ADP)/ATP concentration ratio. These products are interconvertible by the adenylate kinase reaction:

$$2\,ADP \rightleftharpoons ATP + AMP$$

When ATP is consumed and ADP increases, AMP is formed by the adenylate kinase reaction. The increase in AMP concentrations relieves the inhibition of PFK-1 by ATP, activating glycolysis. The phosphorylation of ADP during glycolysis, and then of AMP by the adenylate kinase reaction, gradually restores the ATP concentration, or **energy charge**, of the cell, and as the AMP concentration declines, the rate of glycolysis decreases to a steady-state level. Glycolysis operates at a fairly constant rate in the red cell, where ATP consumption is steady, but the activity of this pathway changes rapidly in response to ATP utilization in muscle during exercise.

Pyruvate kinase (PK)

In addition to regulation by hexokinase and PFK-1, pyruvate kinase in the liver is allosterically activated by Fru-1,6-BP,

CLINICAL BOX
GLYCOLYSIS IN TUMOR CELLS

Tumors are often said to "go glycolytic" - that is, to increase their reliance on glycolysis as a source of energy. The increase in glycolysis might result from inhibition of mitochondrial oxidative phosphorylation as a result of hypoxia, possibly because the metabolic requirements of rapidly dividing tumor cells exceed the supply of oxygen and nutrients from the blood. In these cases, the production and accumulation of lactate may become toxic to the tumor cell, contributing to necrosis and formation of a necrotic core in the tumor.

Some tumors secrete cytokines that promote angiogenesis (neovascularization), thereby increasing their fuel supply and enhancing tumor growth. Angiogenesis inhibitors, designed to inhibit the vascularization of the tumor, are being evaluated as a nonsurgical approach to tumor therapy. The ability to survive by relying on glycolysis in hypoxic environments may be an important factor in tumor survival and growth.

the product of the PFK-1 reaction. This process, known as feed-forward regulation, may be important in the RBC to limit the accumulation of chemically reactive triose phosphate intermediates in the cytosol.

Characteristics of regulatory enzymes

Regulatory enzymes are rate-limiting steps in metabolic pathways

Each of the three enzymes involved in regulation of glycolysis - hexokinase, PFK-1, and pyruvate kinase - has the characteristic features of a regulatory enzyme: (1) they are dimeric or tetrameric enzymes whose structure and activity are responsive to allosteric modulators, (2) they are present at low V_{max} in comparison with other enzymes in the pathway, and (3) they catalyze irreversible reactions.

The regulation of glycolysis in liver, muscle, and other tissues is more complicated than in the RBC (Table 9.1) because of greater variability in the rate of fuel consumption and the interplay between carbohydrate and lipid metabolism during aerobic metabolism. In these tissues, the amount and activity of the regulatory enzymes are controlled by other allosteric effectors, by covalent modification, and by induction or repression of enzyme activity.

SYNTHESIS OF 2,3-BISPHOSPHOGLYCERATE (2,3-BPG)

2,3-BPG is a negative allosteric effector of the oxygen affinity of hemoglobin

2,3-Bisphosphoglycerate (Fig. 9.8) is an important by-product of glycolysis in the RBC, sometimes reaching a concentration 5 mmol/L, which is ~25% of the molar concentration of hemoglobin (Hb) in the RBC. 2,3-BPG is the major phosphorylated intermediate in the erythrocyte, present at even higher concentrations than ATP (1–2 mmol/L) or inorganic phosphate (1 mmol/L). 2,3-BPG is a negative allosteric effector of the O_2 affinity of Hb. It decreases the O_2 affinity of hemoglobin, promoting the release of O_2 in peripheral tissue. The presence of 2,3-BPG in the RBC explains the observation that the O_2 affinity of purified adult Hb (HbA) is greater than that of whole RBCs. 2,3-BPG concentration increases in the RBC during adaptation to high altitude, in chronic obstructive pulmonary disease, and in anemia, promoting the release of O_2 to tissues when the O_2 tension and saturation of hemoglobin is decreased in the lung. **Fetal Hb (HbF) is less sensitive than HbA to the effects of 2,3-BPG;** the higher oxygen affinity of HbF, even in the presence of 2,3-BPG, promotes efficient transfer of O_2 across the placenta from HbA to HbF (see Chapter 5).

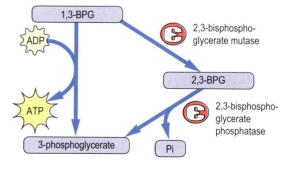

Fig. 9.8 **Pathway for biosynthesis and degradation of 2,3-bisphosphoglycerate (2,3-BPG).** BPG mutase catalyzes the conversion of 1,3-BPG to 2,3-BPG. This same enzyme has bisphosphoglycerate phosphatase activity, so it controls both the synthesis and the hydrolysis of 2,3-BPG. Note that this pathway bypasses the phosphoglycerate kinase reaction, so the net yield of ATP is decreased by 2 ATP/mol glucose.

THE PENTOSE PHOSPHATE PATHWAY

Overview

The pentose phosphate pathway is divided into an irreversible redox stage, which yields both NADPH and pentose phosphates, and a reversible interconversion stage, in which excess pentose phosphates are recycled into glycolytic intermediates

The pentose phosphate pathway is a cytosolic pathway present in all cells, so named because it is the primary pathway for formation of pentose phosphates for the synthesis of nucleotides for incorporation into DNA and RNA in nucleated cells. This pathway branches from glycolysis at the level of Glc-6-P - hence its alternative designation, the hexose monophosphate shunt. The pentose phosphate pathway is sometimes described as a shunt because when pentoses are not needed for biosynthetic reactions, the pentose phosphate intermediates are recycled back into the mainstream of glycolysis by conversion into Fru-6-P and glyceraldehyde-3-phosphate. This rerouting is especially important in the RBC and in nondividing, or quiescent, cells, where there is limited need for the synthesis of DNA and RNA.

NADPH is a major product of the pentose phosphate pathway in all cells

In tissues with active lipid biosynthesis (e.g., liver, adrenal cortex, or lactating mammary glands), the NADPH is used in redox reactions required for biosynthesis of cholesterol, bile salts, steroid hormones, and triglycerides. The liver also uses NADPH for hydroxylation reactions involved in the detoxification and excretion of drugs. The RBC has little biosynthetic activity but still shunts about 10% of glucose through the pentose phosphate pathway - in this case, almost exclusively for the production of NADPH. The NADPH is used primarily for the reduction of a cysteine-containing tripeptide, glutathione (GSH) (see Fig. 2.6), an essential cofactor for antioxidant protection (Chapter 42).

The redox stage of the pentose phosphate pathway: Synthesis of NADPH

NADPH is synthesized by two dehydrogenases in the first and third reactions of the pentose phosphate pathway

In the first step of the pentose phosphate pathway (Fig. 9.9), the **Glc-6-P dehydrogenase** (G6PDH) reaction produces NADPH by oxidation of Glc-6-P to 6-phosphogluconic acid lactone, a cyclic sugar ester. The lactone is hydrolyzed to 6-phosphogluconic acid by **lactonase**. Oxidative decarboxylation of 6-phosphogluconate, catalyzed by 6-phosphogluconate dehydrogenase, then yields the ketose sugar ribulose

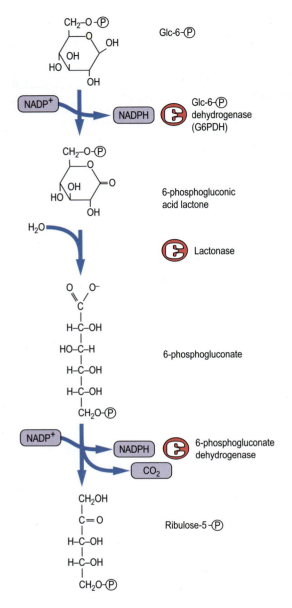

Fig. 9.9 **The redox stage of the pentose phosphate pathway.** A sequence of three enzymes forms 2 moles of NADPH per mole of Glc-6-P, which is converted into ribulose-5-phosphate, with evolution of CO_2 (Fig. 9.9).

5-phosphate, plus 1 mole of CO_2 and the second mole of NADPH.

G6PDH and 6-phosphogluconate dehydrogenase maintain a cytoplasmic ratio of $NADPH/NADP^+$ ~100. Interestingly, because NAD^+ is required for glycolysis, the ratio of $NADH/NAD^+$ in the cytoplasm is nearly the inverse, less than 0.01. Although the total concentrations (oxidized plus reduced forms) of NAD(H) and NADP(H) in the RBC are similar (~25 µmol/L), the cell maintains these two redox systems with similar redox potentials at such different set points in the same cell by isolating their metabolism through the specificity of cytoplasmic

dehydrogenases. **Glycolytic enzymes (GAPDH and LDH) use only NAD(H), whereas pentose phosphate pathway enzymes use only NADP(H).** There are no enzymes in the RBC that catalyze the reduction of NAD^+ by NADPH, so high levels of both NAD^+ and NADPH can exist simultaneously in the same compartment.

The interconversion stage of the pentose phosphate pathway

Excess pentose phosphates are converted to Fru-6-P and glyceraldehyde-3-P in the interconversion stage of the pentose phosphate pathway

In cells with active nucleic acid synthesis, ribulose-5-phosphate from the 6-phosphoglucose dehydrogenase reaction is isomerized to ribose-5-phosphate for the synthesis of ribo- and deoxyribonucleotides for RNA and DNA (Fig. 9.10, top). However, in red cells and nondividing (quiescent) nucleated cells, the pentose phosphates are routed back to glycolysis. This is accomplished by a series of equilibrium reactions in which 3 moles of ribulose-5-phosphate are converted into 2 moles of Fru-6-P and 1 mole of glyceraldehyde-3-phosphate. Certain restrictions are imposed on the interconversion reactions - they may be carried out only by transfer of two or three carbon units between sugar phosphates. Each reaction must also involve a ketose donor and an aldose receptor. **Isomerases** and **epimerases** convert ribulose-5-phosphate to the aldose- and ketose-phosphate substrates for the interconversion stage. **Transketolase, a thiamine-dependent enzyme,** catalyzes the two-carbon transfer reactions. **Transaldolase** acts similarly to the aldolase in glycolysis, except that the three-carbon unit is transferred to another sugar rather than released as a free triose phosphate for glycolysis.

As shown in Fig. 9.10 and Table 9.2, two molecules of ribulose 5-phosphate, the first pentose product of the redox stage, are converted into separate products: one molecule is isomerized to the aldose sugar ribose-5-phosphate, and the other is epimerized to xylulose-5-phosphate. Transketolase then catalyzes the transfer of two carbons from xylulose-5-phosphate to ribose-5-phosphate, yielding a seven-carbon ketose sugar, sedoheptulose-7-phosphate, and the three-carbon glyceraldehyde-3-phosphate. Transaldolase then catalyzes a three-carbon transfer between the two transketolase products, from sedoheptulose-7-phosphate to glyceraldehyde-3-phosphate, yielding the first glycolytic intermediate, Fru-6-P, and a residual erythrose-4-phosphate. A third molecule of xylulose-5-phosphate donates two carbons to erythrose-4-phosphate in a second transketolase reaction, yielding a second molecule of Fru-6-P and a molecule of glyceraldehyde-3-phosphate, both of which enter glycolysis.

Thus three five-carbon sugar phosphates (ribulose-5-phosphate) formed in the redox stage of the pentose phosphate pathway are converted into one three-carbon (glyceraldehyde-3-phosphate) and two six-carbon (fructose-6-phosphate)

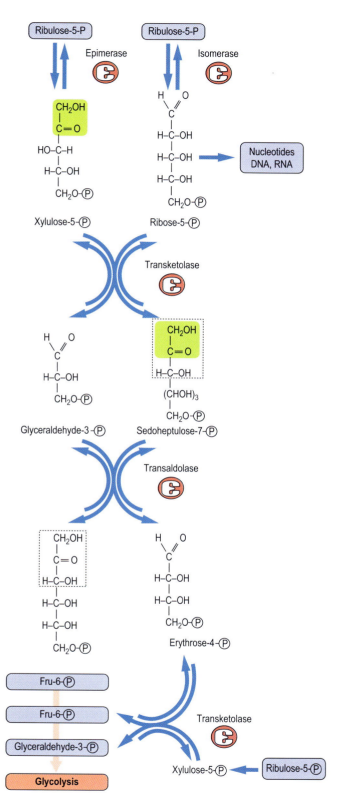

Fig. 9.10 **The interconversion stage of the pentose phosphate pathway.** The carbon skeletons of three molecules of ribulose-5-phosphate are shuffled to form two molecules of Fru-6-P and one molecule of glyceraldehyde 3-phosphate, which enter into glycolysis. All of these reactions are reversible.

Table 9.2 Summary of equilibrium reactions in the pentose phosphate pathway

Substrate(s)		Product(s)	Enzyme
Ribulose-5-P	⇌	Ribose-5-P	Isomerase
2 Ribulose-5-P	⇌	2 Xylulose-5-P	Epimerase
Xylulose-5-P + Ribose-5-P	⇌	Glyceraldehyde-3-P + Sedoheptulose-7-P	Transketolase
Sedoheptulose-7-P + Glyceraldehyde-3-P	⇌	Erythrose-4-P + Fructose-6-P	Transaldolase
Xylulose-5-P + Erythrose-4-P	⇌	Glyceraldehyde-3-P + Fructose-6-P	Transketolase
3 Ribulose-5-P	⇌	**Glyceraldehyde-3-P + 2 Fructose-6-P**	**Summary**

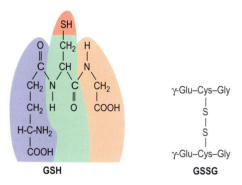

Fig. 9.11 **Glutathione.** Structure of reduced glutathione (GSH) and oxidized glutathione (GSSG). Note the isopeptide bond between the γ-carboxyl, rather than the α-carboxyl, of glutamic acid and the α-amino group of cysteine.

intermediates for glycolysis. In the RBC, these glycolytic intermediates continue through glycolysis to lactate, illustrating that glucose is only temporarily shunted away from the mainstream of glycolysis.

Antioxidant function of the pentose phosphate pathway

The pentose phosphate pathway protects against oxidative damage in the red cell

Glutathione (GSH) is a tripeptide γ-glutamyl-cysteinyl-glycine (Fig. 9.11). It is present in cells at 2–5 mmol/L, 99% in the reduced (thiol) form, and it is an essential coenzyme for the protection of the cell against a range of oxidative and chemical insults (Chapter 42). Most of the NADPH formed in the red cell is used by glutathione reductase to maintain GSH in the reduced state. During its function as a coenzyme for antioxidant activities, GSH is oxidized to the disulfide form, GSSG, which

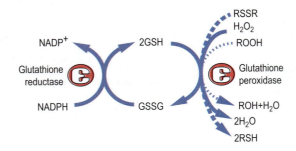

Fig. 9.12 **Antioxidant activities of glutathione.** GSH is the coenzyme for glutathione peroxidases, which detoxify hydrogen peroxide and organic (lipid) hydroperoxides. Hydrogen peroxide and lipid peroxides are formed spontaneously in the red cell, catalyzed by side reactions of heme iron during oxygen transport on hemoglobin (Chapter 41). GSH also reduces disulfide bonds in proteins (RSSR), formed during oxidative stress (Chapter 41), regenerating the native form of the protein (RSH).

is then regenerated by the action of glutathione reductase (Fig. 9.12).

GSH has a range of protective functions in the cell. Glutathione peroxidase (GPx) is found in all cells and uses GSH for detoxification of hydrogen peroxide and organic (lipid) peroxides in the cytosol and cell membranes (Fig. 9.12). Because GPx contains a selenocysteine residue in its active site, selenium, which is required in trace amounts in the diet, is often described as an antioxidant nutrient (see Chapter 7).

GSH also acts as an intracellular sulfhydryl buffer, maintaining exposed –SH groups on proteins and enzymes in the reduced state. Under normal circumstances, when proteins are exposed to O_2, their free sulfhydryl groups gradually oxidize to form disulfides, either intramolecularly or by intermolecular crosslinking with other proteins. In the red cell, GSH maintains the –SH groups of hemoglobin in the reduced state, inhibiting disulfide crosslinking and aggregation of the protein.

SUMMARY

This chapter describes two ancient metabolic pathways common to all cells in the body: glycolysis and the pentose phosphate pathway. The RBC, which lacks mitochondria and the capability for oxidative metabolism and obtains all of its ATP energy by glycolysis, is used as a model for introducing these pathways.

- Anaerobic glycolysis in the RBC provides a limited amount of ATP by conversion of the six-carbon sugar glucose to two molecules of pyruvate, a three-carbon ketoacid. Pyruvate is reduced to lactate and excreted from the cell.
- Through a series of sugar-phosphate intermediates, glycolysis provides metabolites for branch points to numerous other metabolic pathways

CLINICAL BOX
GLUCOSE-6-PHOSPHATE DEHYDROGENASE DEFICIENCY CAUSES HEMOLYTIC ANEMIA

Just before a planned departure to the tropics, a patient visited his physician, complaining of weakness and noting that his urine had recently become unexplainably dark. Physical examination revealed slightly jaundiced (yellow, icteric) sclera. Laboratory tests indicated a low hematocrit, a high reticulocyte count, and a significantly increased blood level of bilirubin. The patient had been quite healthy during a previous visit a month earlier when he received immunizations and prescriptions for antimalarial drugs.

Comment

A number of drugs, particularly primaquine and related antimalarials, undergo redox reactions in the cell, producing large quantities of reactive oxygen species (ROS; Chapter 42). The ROS cause oxidation of –SH groups in hemoglobin and peroxidation of membrane lipids. Some individuals have a genetic defect in Glc-6-P dehydrogenase (G6PDH), typically yielding an unstable enzyme that has a shorter half-life in the RBC or is unusually sensitive to inhibition by NADPH. In either case, because of the decreased activity of G6PDH and insufficient production of NADPH under stress, the cell's ability to recycle GSSG to GSH is impaired, and drug-induced oxidative stress leads to excessive damage and lysis of RBCs (hemolysis) and hemolytic anemia. Bilirubin, a brown pigment produced by heme metabolism, overloads hepatic detoxification pathways and also accumulates in plasma and tissues, causing jaundice. If the hemolysis is severe enough, Hb spills over into the urine, resulting in hematuria and dark-colored urine. Heinz bodies, disulfide crosslinked aggregates of hemoglobin, are also apparent in blood smears. G6PDH deficiency is typically asymptomatic, except in response to an oxidative challenge, which may be induced by drugs (antimalarials, sulfa drugs), diet (fava beans), or severe infection.

There are more than 200 known mutations of the *G6PDH* gene, yielding a wide variation in severity of disease. The RBC appears to be especially sensitive to oxidative stress because unlike other cells, it cannot synthesize and replace enzymes. Older cells, which have lower G6PDH activity, are therefore particularly affected. The activity of all enzymes in the RBC declines with the age of the cell, and cell death eventually results from the inability of to produce sufficient ATP for maintenance of cellular ion gradients. The gradual decline in activity of the pentose phosphate pathway in older cells is one mechanism leading to oxidative crosslinking of membrane proteins and loss of membrane elasticity, leading to entrapment and turnover of the RBC in the spleen.

- The rate of glycolysis is controlled by allosteric regulation of three kinases in the pathway: hexokinase, phosphofructose kinase-1, and pyruvate kinase.
- 2,3-bisphosphoglycerate, produced by isomerization of 1,3-bisphosphoglycerate, allosterically regulates the oxygen affinity of hemoglobin.

ACTIVE LEARNING

1. Why did evolution favor glucose as the blood sugar, rather than other sugars (e.g., galactose, fructose, or sucrose)?
2. Describe coupled enzymatic reactions, using only red-cell enzymes and a spectrometer for measuring NAD(P)(H) production or consumption, that could be used to measure blood glucose and lactate concentrations.
3. Explain the metabolic origin of acidosis in chronic obstructive pulmonary disease.

- Glc-6-P is oxidized to ribulose-5-P during the redox stage of the pentose phosphate pathway, producing 2 moles of NADPH. In all cells, NADPH provides antioxidant protection by maintaining the coenzyme glutathione in the reduced state; in nucleated cells, NADPH is required for many biosynthetic reactions.
- Ribulose-5-P is converted into glycolytic intermediates during the interconversion stage of the pentose phosphate pathway, catalyzed by isomerases and epimerases, including transaldolase and transketolase. One of the intermediates, ribose-5-P, may be used for the synthesis of nucleotides and ribonucleic and deoxyribonucleic acids (RNA, DNA) in nucleated cells.

FURTHER READING

Andoh, A. (2016). Physiological Role of Gut Microbiota for Maintaining Human Health. *Digestion, 93,* 176–181.
Bar-Even, A., Flamholz, A., Noor, E., et al. (2012). Rethinking glycolysis: On the biochemical logic of metabolic pathways. *Nature Chemical Biology, 8,* 509–517.
Katz, S. E. (2012). *The art of fermentation.* White River Junction, VT: Chelsea Green Publishing.
Koralkova, P., van Solinge, W. W., & van Wijk, R. (2014). Rare hereditary red blood cell enzymopathies associated with hemolytic anemia - Pathophysiology, clinical aspects, and laboratory diagnosis. *International Journal of Laboratory Hematology, 36,* 388–397.
Nicholson, J. K., Holmes, E., Kinross, J., et al. (2012). Host-gut microbiota metabolic interactions. *Science, 336,* 1262–1267.
Schwartz, L., Supuran, C. T., & Alfarouk, K. (2017). Anticancer agents, the Warburg effect and the hallmarks of cancer. *Anti-cancer Agents in Medicinal Chemistry, 17*(2), 164–170.

RELEVANT WEBSITES

Glycolysis – TED Ed: https://teded.herokuapp.com/on/akcpkhf0
Glycolysis: https://www.youtube.com/watch?v=EfGlznwfu9U
Pentose phosphate pathway: https://www.youtube.com/watch?v=EP_E-7jPnNs
Glycolytic enzyme deficiencies: https://www.youtube.com/watch?v=x41vJfWn9Y8

ABBREVIATIONS

1,3-BPG	1,3-bisphosphoglycerate
2,3-BPG	2,3-bisphosphoglycerate
Fru-1,6-BP	Fructose-1,6-bisphosphate
Fru-6-P	Fructose-6-phosphate
GAPDH	Glyceraldehyde-3-phosphate dehydrogenase
Glc-6-P	Glucose-6-phosphate
G6PDH	Glucose-6-phosphate dehydrogenase
GSH	Glutathione, reduced
GSSG	Glutathione, oxidized
LDH	Lactate dehydrogenase
PEP	Phosphoenolpyruvate
PFK-1	Phosphofructokinase-1
PK	Pyruvate kinase
RBC	Red blood cell

10
The Tricarboxylic Acid Cycle
Norma Frizzell and L. William Stillway

LEARNING OBJECTIVES

After reading this chapter, you should be able to:

- Outline the sequence of reactions in the tricarboxylic acid (TCA) cycle, and explain the purpose of the cycle.
- Identify the four oxidative enzymes in the TCA cycle and their products.
- Identify the two intermediates required in the first step of the TCA cycle and their metabolic sources.
- Identify four important metabolic intermediates synthesized from TCA-cycle intermediates.
- Describe how the TCA cycle is regulated by substrate supply, allosteric effectors, covalent modification, and protein synthesis.
- Explain why there is no net synthesis of glucose from acetyl-CoA.
- Explain the concept of "suicide substrate" as applied to the TCA cycle.
- Predict the metabolic consequences of TCA cycle defects in terms of metabolite accumulation and substrate diversion

INTRODUCTION

Located in the mitochondrion, the tricarboxylic acid (TCA) cycle, also known as the Krebs or citric acid cycle, is a shared pathway for the metabolism of all fuels. It oxidatively strips electrons from acetyl coenzyme A (acetyl-CoA), which is the common product of catabolism of fat, carbohydrate, and proteins, producing the majority of the reduced coenzymes that are used for the generation of adenosine triphosphate (ATP) in the electron transport chain. Although the TCA cycle does not use oxygen in any of its reactions, it requires oxidative metabolism in the mitochondrion for reoxidation of reduced coenzymes. The TCA cycle has two major functions: energy production and biosynthesis (Fig. 10.1).

FUNCTIONS OF THE TRICARBOXYLIC ACID CYCLE

Four oxidative steps provide free energy for ATP synthesis

A common end product of carbohydrate, fatty acid, and amino acid metabolism, acetyl-CoA (Fig. 10.2) is oxidized in the TCA cycle to produce reduced coenzymes by four redox reactions per turn of the cycle. Three produce reduced nicotinamide adenine dinucleotide (NADH), and the other produces reduced flavin adenine dinucleotide (FADH$_2$; Fig. 8.4). These reduced nucleotides provide energy for ATP synthesis by the electron transport system (Chapter 8). One high-energy phosphate, guanosine triphosphate (GTP), is also produced in the cycle by substrate-level phosphorylation. Nearly all metabolic carbon dioxide is produced by decarboxylation reactions catalyzed by pyruvate dehydrogenase and TCA cycle enzymes in the mitochondrion.

The TCA cycle provides a common ground for interconversion of fuels and metabolites

As discussed in subsequent chapters, in addition to its role in catabolism, the TCA cycle participates in the synthesis of glucose from amino acids and lactate during starvation and fasting (gluconeogenesis) and in the conversion of carbohydrates to fat following a carbohydrate-rich meal (lipogenesis). It is also a source of nonessential amino acids, such as aspartate and glutamate - which are synthesized directly from oxaloacetate and α-ketoglutarate, respectively - and of succinyl-CoA, which serves as a precursor to porphyrins for the synthesis of heme.

Acetyl-CoA is a common product of many catabolic pathways

The TCA cycle begins with acetyl-CoA (Fig. 10.2), which has three major metabolic precursors. Carbohydrates undergo glycolysis to yield pyruvate (Chapter 9), which can be taken up by mitochondria and oxidatively decarboxylated to acetyl-CoA by the pyruvate dehydrogenase complex. During lipolysis, triacylglycerols are converted to glycerol and free fatty acids, which are taken up by cells and transported into mitochondria, where they undergo oxidation to acetyl-CoA (Chapter 11). Lastly, proteolysis of tissue proteins releases constituent amino acids, many of which are metabolized to acetyl-CoA and TCA-cycle intermediates (Chapter 15).

The first version of the TCA cycle, proposed by Krebs in 1937, began with pyruvic acid, not acetyl-CoA. Pyruvic acid was decarboxylated and condensed with oxaloacetic acid through an unknown mechanism to form citric acid. The key intermediate, acetyl-CoA, was not identified until years later. It is tempting to begin the TCA cycle with pyruvic acid, unless it is recognized that fatty acids and many amino acids form acetyl-CoA by pathways that bypass pyruvate. In addition, the oxidation of ketone bodies and alcohol also generate acetyl-CoA for the TCA cycle (Chapters 11 and 34). It is for

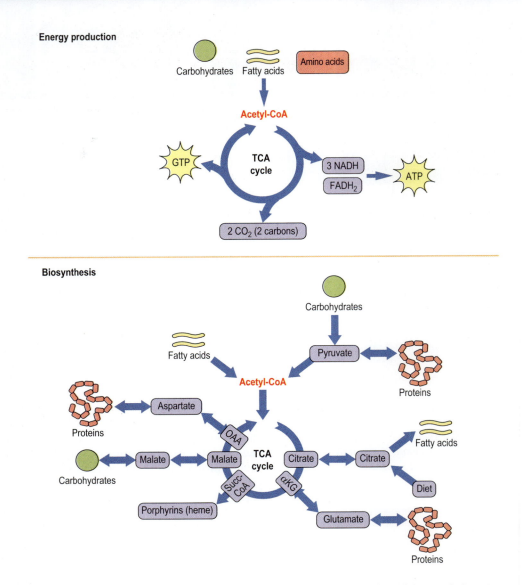

Energy production

Biosynthesis

Fig. 10.1 **Amphibolic nature of the TCA cycle.** The TCA cycle provides energy and metabolites for cellular metabolism. Because of the catabolic (top) and anabolic (bottom) nature of the TCA cycle, it is described as amphibolic. Acetyl-CoA is the common intermediate between metabolic fuels and the TCA cycle. αKG, α-ketoglutarate; FADH$_2$, reduced flavin adenine dinucleotide; GDP, guanosine diphosphate; NADH, reduced nicotinamide adenine dinucleotide; OAA, oxaloacetate; Succ-CoA, succinyl-CoA.

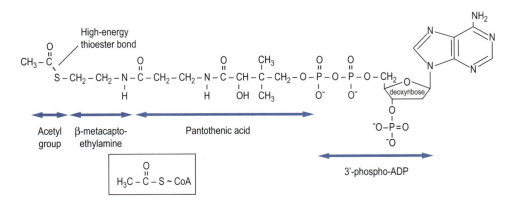

Fig. 10.2 **Structure of acetyl-CoA.** Coenzyme A is an adenine nucleotide, contains a pantothenic acid moiety, and terminates in a thiol group. The acetyl group is bound to the thiol group in a high-energy thioester linkage.

this reason that the TCA cycle is said to begin with acetyl-CoA, not pyruvic acid.

The TCA cycle is located in the mitochondrial matrix

Localization of the TCA cycle in the mitochondrial matrix is important metabolically; this allows identical intermediates to be used for different purposes inside and outside mitochondria. Acetyl-CoA, for example, cannot cross the inner mitochondrial membrane (IMM). The main fate of mitochondrial acetyl-CoA is oxidation in the TCA cycle, but in the cytoplasm, it is used for biosynthesis of fatty acids and cholesterol.

PYRUVATE CARBOXYLASE

Pyruvate may be directly converted to four different metabolites

Pyruvate is at a crossroads in metabolism. It may be converted in one step to lactate (lactate dehydrogenase), to alanine (alanine aminotransferase, ALT), to oxaloacetate (pyruvate carboxylase), and to acetyl-CoA (pyruvate dehydrogenase complex; Fig. 10.3). Depending on metabolic circumstances, pyruvate may be routed

toward gluconeogenesis (Chapter 12), fatty acid biosynthesis (Chapter 13), or the TCA cycle itself.

Pyruvate carboxylase, like most other carboxylases, uses CO_2; the coenzyme biotin (Fig. 10.4), a water-soluble vitamin; and ATP to drive the carboxylation reaction. The enzyme is a tetramer of identical subunits; each contains an allosteric site that binds acetyl-CoA, a positive heterotrophic modifier. Pyruvate carboxylase has an absolute requirement for acetyl-CoA; the enzyme does not work in its absence. An abundance of mitochondrial acetyl-CoA acts as a signal for the generation of additional oxaloacetate. For example, when lipolysis is stimulated, intramitochondrial acetyl-CoA levels rise, allosterically activating pyruvate carboxylase to produce additional oxaloacetate for gluconeogenesis (Chapter 12).

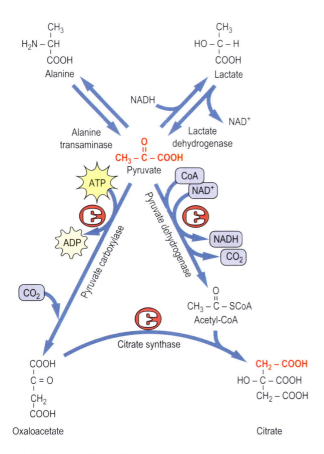

Fig. 10.3 **Pyruvate is at the crossroads of metabolism.** Pyruvate is readily formed from lactate or alanine. Acetyl-CoA and oxaloacetate are derived from pyruvate through the catalytic action of pyruvate dehydrogenase and pyruvate carboxylase, respectively. ADP, adenosine diphosphate.

CLINICAL TEST BOX
LACTIC ACIDOSIS

Lactic acid is measured in blood plasma in a clinical setting because its accumulation can result in rapid death. Lactic acid is produced metabolically by the reversible reduction of pyruvate with NADH by the enzyme lactate dehydrogenase (LDH). Both lactate and pyruvate coexist in metabolic systems, and the ratio of pyruvate:lactate is roughly proportional to the cytosolic ratio of NAD^+/NADH. Both lactate and pyruvate contribute to the acidity of biological fluid; however, lactate is usually present at higher concentrations and is more easily measured. Blood lactate may increase in chronic obstructive lung disease and during intense exercise, when the supply of oxygen is rate limiting for oxidative phosphorylation. Its measurement is usually indicated when there is metabolic acidosis, characterized by an elevated anion gap, $[Na^+] - ([Cl^-] + [HCO_3^-])$, indicating the presence of an unknown anion(s) in plasma. Although rare, lactic acidosis can be caused by metabolic defects in energy-producing pathways, such as some of the glycogen-storage diseases or in any enzyme in the pathways from pyruvate to the generation of ATP, including the pyruvate dehydrogenase complex, TCA cycle, electron transport system, or ATP synthase. Several pharmacological agents and environmental pesticides that interfere with components of the electron transport chain can also contribute to lactic acidosis.

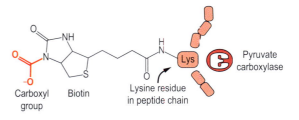

Fig. 10.4 **The carboxy-biotin intermediate.** Pyruvate carboxylase catalyzes carboxylation of pyruvate to oxaloacetate. The coenzyme biotin is covalently bound to pyruvate carboxylase and transfers the carbon originating from CO_2 to pyruvate (see Chapter 7).

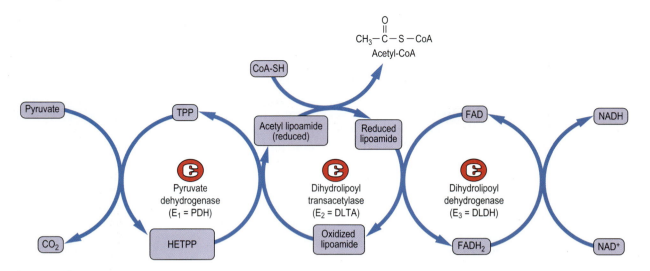

Fig. 10.5 **Mechanism of action of the pyruvate dehydrogenase complex.** The three enzyme components of the pyruvate dehydrogenase complex are pyruvate dehydrogenase (E_1 = PDH), dihydrolipoyl transacetylase (E_2 = DLTA), and dihydrolipoyl dehydrogenase (E_3 = DLDH). Pyruvate is first decarboxylated by the thiamine pyrophosphate-containing enzyme (E_1), forming CO_2 and hydroxyethyl-thiamine pyrophosphate (HETPP). Lipoamide, the prosthetic group on E_2, serves as a carrier in the transfer of the two-carbon unit from HETPP to coenzyme A (CoA). The oxidized, cyclic disulfide form of lipoamide accepts the hydroxyethyl group from HETPP. During this transfer reaction, the lipoamide is reduced, and the hydroxyethyl group is converted to an acetyl group, forming acetyldihydrolipoamide. Following transfer of the acetyl group to CoA, E_3 reoxidizes the lipoamide using FAD, and the $FADH_2$ is in turn oxidized by NAD^+, yielding NADH. The net reaction is: Pyr + NAD^+ + CoA-SH → acetyl-CoA + NADH + H^+ + CO_2.

THE PYRUVATE DEHYDROGENASE COMPLEX

The pyruvate dehydrogenase complex (PDC) serves as a bridge between carbohydrates and the TCA cycle (Fig. 10.5). PDC is one of several α-ketoacid dehydrogenases having analogous reaction mechanisms, including α-ketoglutarate dehydrogenase in the TCA cycle and α-ketoacid dehydrogenases associated with the catabolism of leucine, isoleucine, and valine. Its irreversibility explains in part why acetyl-CoA cannot yield a net synthesis of glucose (see later discussion). The complex functions as a unit consisting of the following three principal enzymes:

■ Pyruvate dehydrogenase (PDH)
■ Dihydrolipoyl transacetylase
■ Dihydrolipoyl dehydrogenase

Intermediates are tethered to the transacetylase component of the complex during the reaction sequence (Figs. 10.5 and 10.6). This optimizes the catalytic efficiency of the enzyme because the substrate does not equilibrate into solution.

Two additional enzymes of the complex, pyruvate dehydrogenase kinase and pyruvate dehydrogenase phosphatase, regulate its activity by covalent modification via reversible phosphorylation/dephosphorylation. There are four known isoforms of the kinase and two of the phosphatase; the relative amounts of each are cell specific.

Five coenzymes are required for PDC activity: thiamine pyrophosphate, lipoamide (lipoic acid bound in amide linkage to protein), CoA, FAD, and NAD^+. Four vitamins are required for their synthesis: thiamine, pantothenic acid, riboflavin, and nicotinamide. Deficiencies in any of these vitamins have obvious effects on energy metabolism. For example, increases in cellular concentrations of pyruvate and α-ketoglutarate are found in beriberi because of thiamine deficiency (Chapter 7). In this case, all the proteins are available but the relevant coenzyme is not, and the conversions of pyruvate to acetyl-CoA and α-ketoglutarate to succinyl-CoA are significantly decreased. Symptoms include cardiac and skeletal muscle weakness and neurologic disease. Thiamine deficiency is common in alcoholism and contributes to a condition known as Wernicke–Korsakoff syndrome (WKS) because distilled spirits are devoid of vitamins, and symptoms of beriberi are often observed.

ENZYMES AND REACTIONS OF THE TRICARBOXYLIC ACID CYCLE

The TCA cycle is a sequence of reactions for oxidation of acetyl-CoA to CO_2 and reduced nucleotides

The TCA cycle is a sequence of eight enzymatic reactions (Fig. 10.7), beginning with condensation of acetyl-CoA with

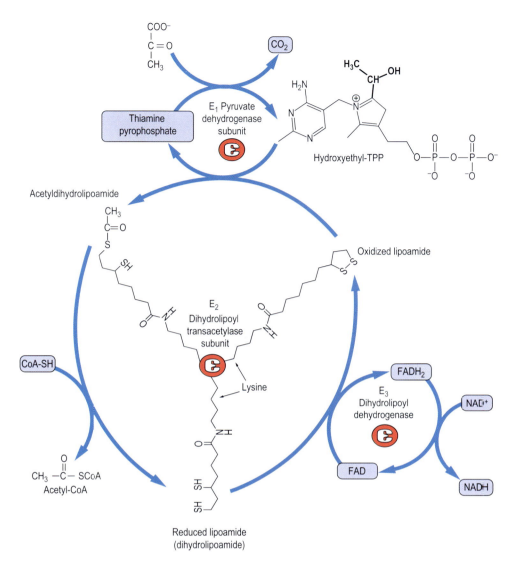

Fig. 10.6 **Lipoic acid in the pyruvate dehydrogenase complex.** The coenzyme lipoamide is attached to a lysine residue in the transacetylase subunit of pyruvate dehydrogenase. Lipoamide moves from one active site to another on the transacetylase subunit in a "swinging arm" mechanism. The structures of thiamine pyrophosphate (TPP) and lipoamide are shown.

oxaloacetate (OAA) to form citrate. The OAA is regenerated on completion of the cycle. Of the four oxidations in the cycle, two involve decarboxylations. Three dehydrogenases produce NADH, and one produces FADH$_2$. GTP, a high-energy phosphate, is produced at one step by substrate-level phosphorylation.

Citrate synthase

Citrate synthase begins the TCA cycle by catalyzing the condensation of acetyl-CoA and OAA to form citric acid. The reaction is driven by cleavage of the high-energy thioester bond of citryl-CoA, an intermediate in the reaction. The citrate

produced is an important precursor for de novo lipogenesis in the liver and adipose tissue in the fed state (Chapter 13).

Aconitase

Aconitase is an iron–sulfur protein that isomerizes citrate to isocitrate through the enzyme-bound intermediate *cis*-aconitate. The two-step reaction is reversible and involves dehydration followed by hydration. Although citrate is a symmetric molecule, aconitase works specifically on the OAA end of citrate, not the end derived from acetyl-CoA (Fig. 10.9). Such stereochemical specificity occurs because of the geometry of

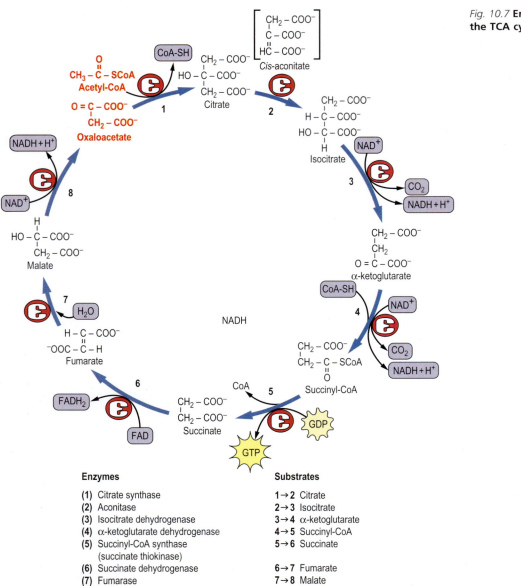

Fig. 10.7 **Enzymes and intermediates of the TCA cycle.**

Enzymes

(1) Citrate synthase
(2) Aconitase
(3) Isocitrate dehydrogenase
(4) α-ketoglutarate dehydrogenase
(5) Succinyl-CoA synthase
(succinate thiokinase)
(6) Succinate dehydrogenase
(7) Fumarase
(8) Malate dehydrogenase

Substrates

1→2 Citrate
2→3 Isocitrate
3→4 α-ketoglutarate
4→5 Succinyl-CoA
5→6 Succinate

6→7 Fumarate
7→8 Malate
8→1 Oxaloacetate

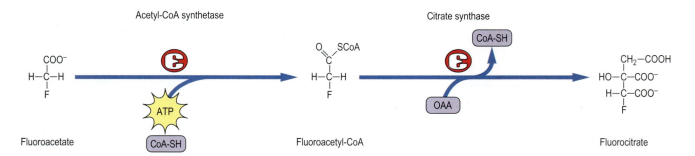

Fig. 10.8 **Toxicity of fluoroacetate: A suicide substrate.** Fluoroacetate is a competitive inhibitor of aconitase. OAA, oxaloacetate.

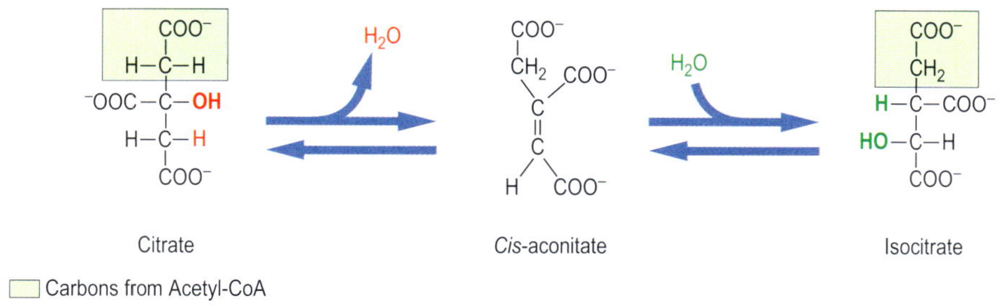

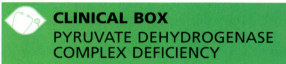

Citrate   *Cis*-aconitate   Isocitrate

Carbons from Acetyl-CoA

Fig. 10.9 **Specificity of isomerization during the aconitase reaction.**

CLINICAL BOX
PYRUVATE DEHYDROGENASE COMPLEX DEFICIENCY

Most children with PDH deficiency present in infancy with delayed development and reduced muscle tone, often associated with ataxia and seizures. Some infants have congenital malformations of the brain.

Comment

Without mitochondrial oxidation, pyruvate is reduced to lactate. The ATP yield from anaerobic glycolysis is less than a tenth of that produced from oxidation of glucose via the TCA cycle, so that both glucose utilization and lactate production are increased. The diagnosis is suggested by elevated lactate but with a normal lactate/pyruvate ratio (i.e., no evidence of hypoxia). A ketogenic diet and severe restriction of protein (<15%) and carbohydrate (<5%) improve mental development. Such treatment ensures that the cells use acetyl-CoA from fat metabolism. A few children show a reduction in plasma lactate on treatment with large doses of thiamine, but the outlook is generally poor.

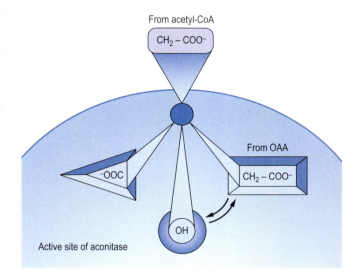

Fig. 10.10 **Stereochemistry of the aconitase reaction.** Aconitase converts achiral citrate to a specific chiral form of isocitrate. Binding of the adjacent C-3 hydroxyl (OH) and carboxylate (COO^-) groups of citrate on the enzyme surface places the carboxymethyl ($-CH_2-COO^-$) group, derived from the OAA end of the molecule, in touch with the third binding locus in the active site of aconitase. This assures the transfer of the OH group to the CH_2 group derived from OAA, indicated by arrows, rather than that derived from the acetyl group. OAA, oxaloacetate.

ADVANCED CONCEPT BOX
TOXICITY OF FLUOROACETATE: A SUICIDE SUBSTRATE

Fluoroacetate, originally isolated from plants, is a potent toxin. It is activated as fluoroacetyl-CoA and then condenses with OAA to form fluorocitrate (Fig. 10.8). Death results from inhibition of the TCA cycle by 2-fluorocitrate, a strong inhibitor of aconitase. Fluoroacetate is an example of a **suicide substrate**, a compound that is not toxic per se but is metabolically activated to a toxic product. Thus the cell is said to commit suicide by converting an apparently harmless substrate to a lethal toxin. Similar processes are involved in the activation of many environmental procarcinogens to carcinogens that induce mutations in DNA.

the active site of aconitase (Fig. 10.10). A cytosolic protein with aconitase activity, known as iron-response element binding protein (IRE-BP), functions in the regulation of iron storage.

Isocitrate dehydrogenase and α-ketoglutarate dehydrogenase

Isocitrate dehydrogenase and the α-ketoglutarate dehydrogenase complex catalyze two sequential oxidative decarboxylation reactions in which NAD^+ is reduced to NADH and CO_2 is

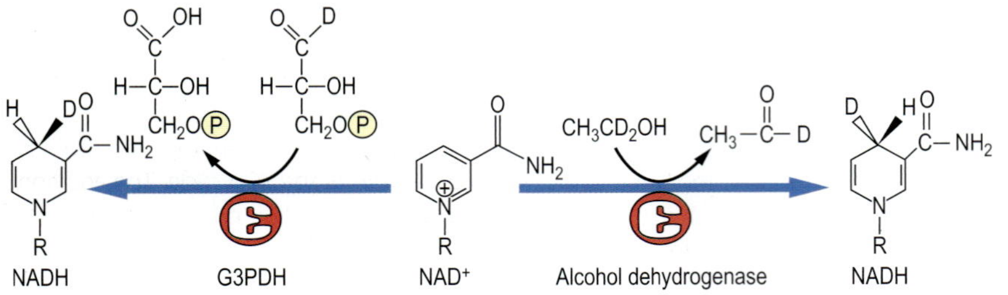

Fig. 10.11 **Stereochemistry of the reduction of NAD$^+$ by dehydrogenases.** Alcohol dehydrogenase places the hydrogen ion on the front face of the nicotinamide ring, while glyceraldehyde-3-phosphate dehydrogenase (G3PDH) places the hydrogen on the back face of the ring. The two positions can be discriminated using deuterated (D) substrates.

ADVANCED CONCEPT BOX
STEREOSPECIFICITY OF ENZYMES

Aconitase catalyzes isomerization at the OAA end of the citrate molecule. However, citrate has no asymmetric centers; it is achiral. How does aconitase know "which end is up"? The answer lies in the nature of citrate binding to the active site of aconitase, a process known as three-point attachment. As shown in Fig. 10.10, because of the geometry of the active site of aconitase, there is only one way for citrate to bind. This "three-point binding" places the OAA carbons in the proper orientation for the isomerization reaction, whereas the carbons derived from acetyl-CoA are excluded from the active site.

Although citrate is a symmetric or achiral molecule, it is termed *prochiral* because it is converted to a chiral molecule, isocitrate. Similar types of three-point binding processes are involved in transaminase reactions that produce exclusively L-amino acids from ketoacids. The reduction of the nicotinamide ring by NAD(H)-dependent dehydrogenases is also stereospecific. Some dehydrogenases place the added hydrogen exclusively on the front face of the nicotinamide ring (viewed with the amide group to the right), whereas others add hydrogen only to the back face (Fig. 10.11).

released. The first of these enzymes, isocitrate dehydrogenase, catalyzes the conversion of isocitrate to α-ketoglutarate. It is an important regulatory enzyme that is inhibited under energy-rich conditions by high levels of NADH and ATP, and it is activated when NAD$^+$ and ADP are produced by metabolism. Inhibition of this enzyme following a carbohydrate meal causes intramitochondrial accumulation of citrate, which is then exported to the cytosol, where it serves as a precursor for lipogenesis (Chapter 13) and an allosteric inhibitor of glycolysis at phosphofructokinase-1 (Chapter 9).

The second dehydrogenase, the α-ketoglutarate dehydrogenase complex, catalyzes the oxidative decarboxylation of α-ketoglutarate to NADH, CO_2, and succinyl-CoA, a high-energy thioester compound. Like the pyruvate dehydrogenase complex, this enzyme complex contains three subunits having the same designations as pyruvate dehydrogenase (E_1, E_2, and E_3). E_3 is identical in the two complexes and is encoded by the same gene. The reaction mechanisms and the cofactors thiamine pyrophosphate, lipoate, CoA, FAD, and NAD$^+$ are

the same. Both enzymes begin with an α-ketoacid, pyruvate or α-ketoglutarate, and both form a CoA ester, acetyl-CoA or succinyl-CoA, respectively.

At this point, the net carbon yield of the TCA cycle is zero; two carbons were introduced as acetyl-CoA, and two carbons were liberated as CO_2. Note, however, that because of the asymmetry of the aconitase reaction, neither of the CO_2 molecules produced in this first round trip through the TCA cycle originates from the carbons of the acetyl-CoA because they are derived from the OAA end of the citrate molecule. Both of the carbons that originated from acetyl-CoA remain in TCA-cycle intermediates, and they may appear in compounds produced in biosynthetic reactions branching from the TCA cycle, including glucose, aspartic acid, and heme. However, because of the loss of two CO_2 molecules at this point, there is no net synthesis of these metabolites from acetyl-CoA.

Animals cannot perform net synthesis of glucose from acetyl-CoA. This is an especially important concept in the understanding of starvation, diabetes, and ketogenesis because large amounts of acetyl-CoA are generated from fatty acids, but this process does not yield a net synthesis of glucose. "Net" synthesis is invoked because labeled carbons from acetyl-CoA eventually appear in glucose, making it appear that glucose is synthesized from acetyl-CoA. However, the investment of the two carbons of acetyl-CoA is dissipated by the two decarboxylation reactions in the TCA cycle.

Succinyl-CoA synthetase

Succinyl-CoA synthetase (succinate thiokinase) catalyzes the conversion of energy-rich succinyl-CoA to succinate and free CoA. The free energy of the thioester bond in succinyl-CoA is conserved by formation of GTP from GDP and inorganic phosphate (Pi). Because a high-energy thioester serves as the driving force for the synthesis of GTP, this is a substrate-level phosphorylation reaction, like the reactions catalyzed by phosphoglycerate kinase and pyruvate kinase in glycolysis (Chapter 9). GTP is used by enzymes such as phosphoenol-pyruvate carboxykinase (PEPCK) in gluconeogenesis (Chapter 12), in several steps in protein synthesis (Chapter 22), and in cell signaling (Chapter 25), but it is also readily equilibrated with ATP by the enzyme nucleoside diphosphate kinase:

$$GTP + ADP \rightleftharpoons GDP + ATP$$

CLINICAL BOX
DEFICIENCIES IN PYRUVATE METABOLISM IN THE TCA CYCLE

A 7-month-old-child showed progressive neurologic deterioration characterized by loss of coordination and muscle tone. He was unable to keep his head upright and had great difficulty moving his limbs, which were limp. He also suffered from unrelenting acidosis. Administration of thiamine had no effect. Measurements showed that he had elevated blood levels of lactate, α-ketoglutarate, and branched-chain amino acids. The child died a week later. Liver, brain, kidney, skeletal muscle, and heart were examined postmortem, and all gluconeogenic enzymes were shown to have normal activities, but both pyruvate dehydrogenase and α-ketoglutarate dehydrogenase were deficient. The defective component was shown to be dihydrolipoyl dehydrogenase (E_3), which is a single gene component required by all of the α-ketoacid dehydrogenases.

Comment
This is an example of one of the many variants of **Leigh's disease,** which is a group of disorders that are all characterized by lactic acidosis. Lactic acid accumulates under anaerobic conditions or because of any enzyme defect in the pathway from pyruvate to the synthesis of ATP. In this case, there are defects in both the pyruvate dehydrogenase and α-ketoglutarate complexes as well as other α-keto acid dehydrogenase complexes required for the catabolism of branched-chain amino acids. The failure of aerobic metabolism leads to increases in blood levels of lactate, α-ketoglutarate, and branched-chain amino acids. Tissues dependent on aerobic metabolism, such as brain and muscle, are most severely affected, so the clinical picture includes impaired motor function, neurologic disorders, and mental retardation. These diseases are rare, but deficiencies in pyruvate carboxylase and all the components of the pyruvate dehydrogenase complex (PDH) have been described, including the associated kinase and phosphatase enzymes (Fig. 10.12). In addition, several well-characterized mutations in the electron transport chain complexes also give rise to Leigh's disease.

ADVANCED CONCEPT BOX
THE MALONATE BLOCK

The malate dehydrogenase reaction played an important role in the elucidation of the cyclic nature of the TCA cycle. The addition of tricarboxylic acids (citrate, aconitate) and α-ketoglutarate was known to catalyze pyruvate metabolism - we now know that this is the result of the formation of catalytic amounts of OAA from these intermediates. In 1937, Krebs found that malonate, the three-carbon dicarboxylic acid homologue of succinate and competitive inhibitor of succinate dehydrogenase, blocked metabolism of pyruvate by minced muscle preparations. He also showed that malonate inhibition of pyruvate metabolism led to accumulation not only of succinate but also of citrate and α-ketoglutarate, suggesting that succinate was a product of pyruvate metabolism and that the tricarboxylic acids might be intermediates in this process. Interestingly, fumarate and OAA stimulated pyruvate oxidation and led to the accumulation of citrate and succinate during malonate block, suggesting that the three- and four-carbon acids might combine to form the tricarboxylic acids. The experiments with fumarate indicated that there were two paths between fumarate and succinate, one involving a reversal of the succinate dehydrogenase reaction, which was inhibited during malonate block, and the other involving conversion of fumarate to succinate through a series of organic acids. These observations, combined with Krebs's experience a few years earlier in the characterization of the urea cycle (Chapter 15), led to his description of the TCA cycle.

The next three reactions in the TCA cycle illustrate a common theme in metabolism for introducing a carbonyl group into a molecule:

- An FAD-dependent oxidation reaction to produce a double bond
- Addition of water across the double bond to form an alcohol
- Oxidation of the alcohol to a ketone

This same sequence occurs in the form of enzyme-bound intermediates during the oxidation of fatty acids (Chapter 11).

Succinate dehydrogenase

Succinate dehydrogenase is a flavoprotein containing the prosthetic group FAD. As described in Chapter 8, this enzyme is embedded in the IMM, where it is a part of complex II (succinate-Q reductase). The reaction involves oxidation of succinate to the *trans*-dicarboxylic acid fumarate, with reduction of FAD to $FADH_2$.

Fumarase

Fumarase stereospecifically adds water across the *trans* double bond of fumarate to form the α-hydroxy acid, L-malate.

Malate dehydrogenase

Malate dehydrogenase catalyzes the oxidation of L-malate to OAA, producing NADH, completing one round trip through the TCA cycle. The OAA may then react with acetyl-CoA, continuing the cycle of reactions.

ENERGY YIELD FROM THE TRICARBOXYLIC ACID CYCLE

During the course of the TCA cycle, each mole of acetyl-CoA generates sufficient reduced nucleotide coenzymes for the synthesis of ~9 moles ATP by oxidative phosphorylation.

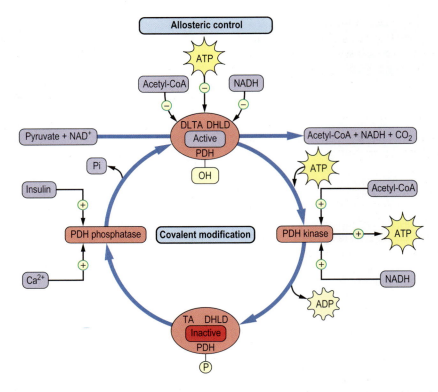

Fig. 10.12 **Regulation of the pyruvate dehydrogenase complex.** The pyruvate dehydrogenase complex regulates the flux of pyruvate into the TCA cycle. NAD(H), ATP, and acetyl-CoA exert both allosteric and covalent control of enzyme activity. PDH, pyruvate dehydrogenase; TA, dihydrolipoyl transacetylase; DHLD, dihydrolipoamide dehydrogenase subunit.

$$3\,NADH \rightarrow 7.5\,ATP$$

$$1\,FADH_2 \rightarrow 1.5\,ATP$$

Together with the GTP synthesized by substrate-level phosphorylation in the succinyl-CoA synthetase (succinate thiokinase) reaction, a total of ~10 ATP equivalents is available per mole of acetyl-CoA. Thus complete metabolism of a mole of glucose through glycolysis, the pyruvate dehydrogenase complex, and the TCA cycle yields ≈30–32 moles of ATP (Table 10.1). (The actual ATP yield depends on the route of transport of redox equivalents to the mitochondrion - that is, about 5 moles of ATP by the malate–aspartate shuttle and about 3 moles of ATP by the glycerol phosphate shuttle [Chapter 8].) In contrast, only 2 moles of ATP (net) are recovered by anaerobic glycolysis, in which glucose is converted to lactate (Chapter 9).

ANAPLEROTIC ("BUILDING UP") REACTIONS

As shown in Fig. 10.1, many TCA-cycle intermediates participate in biosynthetic processes, which deplete TCA-cycle intermediates. For example, the synthesis of 1 mole of heme requires 8 moles of succinyl-CoA. The TCA cycle would cease to function if the intermediates were not replenished because acetyl-CoA cannot yield a net synthesis of OAA. Anaplerotic (building up) reactions provide the TCA cycle with intermediates other than acetyl-CoA to maintain the activity of the cycle. Pyruvate carboxylase is a prime example of an enzyme that catalyzes an anaplerotic reaction. It converts pyruvate to OAA, which is required for initiation of the cycle. Malic enzyme in the cytoplasm also converts pyruvate to malate, which can enter the mitochondrion as a substrate for the TCA cycle. Aspartate is also a precursor of OAA by a transamination reaction, and α-ketoglutarate can be produced through an aminotransferase reaction from glutamate as well as by the glutamate dehydrogenase reaction. Several other "glucogenic" amino acids (Chapter 15) may also serve as sources of pyruvate or TCA-cycle intermediates, guaranteeing that the cycle never stalls because of a lack of intermediates.

REGULATION OF THE TRICARBOXYLIC ACID CYCLE

Pyruvate dehydrogenase and isocitrate dehydrogenase regulate TCA cycle activity

There are several levels of control of the TCA cycle. In general, the overall activity of the cycle depends on the availability of NAD+ for the dehydrogenase reactions. This, in turn, is linked to the rate of NADH consumption by the electron transport

Table 10.1 ATP yield from glucose during oxidative metabolism

Reaction	Mechanism	Moles ATP / Mole Glc
Hexokinase	Phosphorylation	−1
Phosphofructokinase	Phosphorylation	−1
G3PDH	NADH, oxidative phosphorylation	+5 (+3)*
Phosphoglycerate kinase	Substrate-level phosphorylation	+2
Pyruvate kinase	Substrate-level phosphorylation	+2
Pyruvate dehydrogenase	NADH, oxidative phosphorylation	+5
Isocitrate dehydrogenase	NADH, oxidative phosphorylation	+5
α-ketoglutarate dehydrogenase	NADH, oxidative phosphorylation	+5
Succinyl-CoA synthetase	Substrate-level phosphorylation (GTP)	+2
Succinate dehydrogenase	$FADH_2$, oxidative phosphorylation	+3
Malate dehydrogenase	NADH, oxidative phosphorylation	+5
TOTAL		32 (30)*

The yields of ATP shown are approximate because they are measured experimentally with live, isolated mitochondria, and there is some variability. Recent work suggests that the actual yields of ATP from NADH and FADH2 are about 2.5 and 1.5, respectively, yielding approximately 30–32 moles of ATP per mole of glucose. The oxidation of glucose in a bomb calorimeter yields 2870 kJ/mol (686 cal/mol), whereas the synthesis of ATP requires 31 kJ/mol (7.3 kcal/mol). Aerobic metabolism of glucose is therefore about 40% efficient (2870 kJ/mol glucose / 31 kJ/mole ATP = 93 theoretical moles of ATP/mol glucose; 36/93 = 39%).

*Electrons from cytosolic NADH can produce about 5 moles of ATP per mole of glucose via the malate–aspartate shuttle, but only about 3 via the glycerol-3-phosphate shuttle per mole of glucose (Chapter 8).

act as negative allosteric effectors of the enzyme complex. In addition, the pyruvate dehydrogenase complex has associated kinase and phosphatase enzymes that modulate the degree of phosphorylation of regulatory serine residues in the complex. NADH, acetyl-CoA, and ATP activate the kinase, which phosphorylates and inactivates the enzyme complex. In contrast, when these three compounds are low in concentration, the enzyme complex is activated both allosterically and by dephosphorylation by the phosphatase. This is an important regulatory process during fasting and starvation, when gluconeogenesis is essential to maintain blood glucose concentration. Active fat metabolism during fasting leads to increased NADH and acetyl-CoA in the mitochondrion, which leads to inhibition of pyruvate dehydrogenase and blocks the utilization of carbohydrate for energy metabolism in the liver. Under this condition, pyruvate, from such intermediates as lactate and alanine, is directed toward gluconeogenesis (Chapter 12). Conversely, insulin stimulates pyruvate dehydrogenase by activating the phosphatase in response to dietary carbohydrates. This directs carbohydrate-derived carbons into fatty acids (lipogenesis) via citrate synthase (Chapter 13). Ca^{2+} also affects PDC phosphatase activity in response to the increase in intracellular Ca^{2+} during muscle contraction (Chapter 37).

OAA is required for entry of acetyl-CoA into the TCA cycle, and at times, the availability of OAA appears to regulate the activity of the cycle. This occurs especially during fasting, when levels of ATP and NADH, derived from fat metabolism, are increased in the mitochondrion. The increase in NADH shifts the malate:OAA equilibrium toward malate, directing TCA-cycle intermediates toward malate, which is exported to the cytosol for gluconeogenesis. Meanwhile, acetyl-CoA derived from fat metabolism is directed toward the synthesis of ketone bodies because of the lack of OAA, regenerating CoA-SH and leading to the increase in ketone bodies in the plasma during fasting (Chapter 11).

Isocitrate dehydrogenase is a major regulatory enzyme within the TCA cycle. It is subject to allosteric inhibition by ATP and NADH and stimulation by ADP and NAD^+. During consumption of a high carbohydrate diet under resting conditions, the demand for ATP is diminished, and the level of carbohydrate-derived intermediates increases. Under these circumstances, increased insulin levels stimulate the pyruvate dehydrogenase complex, and the accumulation of ATP and NADH inhibits isocitrate dehydrogenase, causing mitochondrial accumulation of citrate. The citrate is then exported to the cytosol for the synthesis of fatty acids, which are exported from the liver for storage in adipose tissue as triglycerides. With an increase in energy demand (e.g., during muscle contraction), NAD^+ and ADP accumulate, and they stimulate isocitrate dehydrogenase.

Induction and repression, as well as proteolysis of enzyme proteins, such as pyruvate carboxylase and those in the pyruvate dehydrogenase complex and the TCA cycle, also play important regulatory roles. In fact, all of the TCA-cycle and associated enzymes are synthesized in the cytoplasm and transported

system, which ultimately depends on the rate of ATP utilization and production of ADP by metabolism. Thus as ATP is used for metabolic work, ADP is produced, then NADH is consumed by the electron transport system for ATP production, and NAD^+ is produced. The TCA cycle is activated, fuels are consumed, and more NADH is produced so that more ATP may be made.

There are several regulatory enzymes that affect the activity of the TCA cycle. The activity of the pyruvate dehydrogenase complex - and therefore the supply of acetyl-CoA from glucose, lactate, and alanine - is regulated by allosteric and covalent modifications (see Fig. 10.12). The products of the pyruvate dehydrogenase reaction, NADH and acetyl-CoA, as well as ATP, through a complex series of steps into the mitochondrion. Regulation can occur at the level of translation, transcription, and intracellular transport. Diet, for example, is known to control the expression of four pyruvate dehydrogenase kinases; one of them is induced in response to a high-fat diet and is repressed in response to a high-carbohydrate diet. Unfortunately, the regulation of the TCA cycle at the genetic and transport levels is not well understood.

Deficiencies in tricarboxylic acid–cycle enzymes

Germline mutations in several TCA-cycle enzymes are characteristic of some distinct cancer subtypes. Succinate dehydrogenase subunit mutations result in both pheochromocytomas and paragangliomas. Fumarate hydratase mutations are associated with increased fumarate production in renal, uterine, and cutaneous tumors in a syndrome known as hereditary leiomyoma and renal cell carcinoma (HLRCC). Mutations in the $NADP^+$-dependent isocitrate dehydrogenase 1 (IDH1) are the most frequent defect (~70%) in a range of glioma subtypes. IDH1 mutations lead to a gain of function to produce 2-hydroxyglutarate from α-ketoglutarate. These tumor cells appear to develop unique metabolic characteristics that promote their survival, even when TCA-cycle enzymes are defective. Cancer cells frequently use anaplerotic reactions to sustain their mitochondrial metabolism; for example, glutamine is converted to glutamate to replenish α-ketoglutarate. The α-ketoglutarate then undergoes reductive carboxylation (in contrast to oxidative decarboxylation during the forward operation of the TCA cycle) to isocitrate (via $NADP^+$-dependent IDH2), which is in turn converted to citrate to provide a precursor for the generation of fatty acids by the tumor cells. The role of TCA-cycle enzyme deficiencies in cancer is discussed in greater detail in the works cited in the Further Reading section.

SUMMARY

- The TCA cycle is the central, common pathway by which fuels are oxidized, and it also participates in major biosynthetic pathways.
- In its oxidative role, major products of the TCA cycle are GTP and the reduced coenzymes NADH and $FADH_2$, which furnish large amounts of free energy for the synthesis of ATP by oxidative phosphorylation.
- In its biosynthetic role, the TCA cycle provides essential intermediates for the synthesis of glucose, fatty acids, amino acids, and heme, as well as the ATP required for their biosynthesis.
- The activity of the TCA cycle is tightly regulated by substrate supply, allosteric effectors, and control of gene expression so that fuel consumption is tightly coupled to energy requirements.

ACTIVE LEARNING

1. In beriberi, the vitamin thiamine is deficient. Which intermediates would accumulate, and why?
2. Compare the regulation of the pyruvate dehydrogenase complex to the regulation of cytosolic enzymes by phosphorylation/dephosphorylation reactions.
3. Predict the consequences of deficiencies in TCA cycle enzymes such as succinate dehydrogenase, fumarase, or malate dehydrogenase.
4. Describe enzymatic assays for measurement of plasma or serum lactate in the clinical laboratory.

FURTHER READING

Akram, M. (2014). Citric acid cycle and role of its intermediates in metabolism. *Cell Biochemistry and Biophysics, 68*, 475–478.

Corbet, C., & Feron, O. (2017). Cancer cell metabolism and mitochondria: Nutrient plasticity for TCA cycle fueling. *Biochimica et Biophysica Acta, 1868*, 7–15.

Gerards, M., Sallevelt, S. C., & Smeets, H. J. (2016). Leigh syndrome: Resolving the clinical and genetic heterogeneity paves the way for treatment options. *Molecular Genetics and Metabolism, 117*, 300–312.

Marin-Valencia, I., Roe, C. R., & Pascual, J. M. (2010). Pyruvate carboxylase deficiency: Mechanisms, mimics and anaplerosis. *Molecular Genetics and Metabolism, 101*, 9–17.

Patel, K. P., O'Brien, T. W., Subramony, S. H., et al. (2012). The spectrum of pyruvate dehydrogenase complex deficiency: Clinical, biochemical and genetic features in 371 patients. *Molecular Genetics and Metabolism, 106*, 385–394.

Sciacovelli, M., & Frezza, C. (2016). Oncometabolites: Unconventional triggers of oncogenic signalling cascades. *Free Radical Biology and Medicine, 100*, 175–181.

Sudheesh, N. P., Ajith, T. A., Janardhanan, K. K., et al. (2009). Palladium alpha-lipoic acid complex formulation enhances activities of Krebs cycle dehydrogenases and respiratory complexes I–IV in the heart of aged rats. *Food and Chemical Toxicology, 47*, 2124–2128.

Vazquez, A., Jurre, J., Kamphorst, E. K., et al. (2016). Cancer metabolism at a glance. *Journal of Cell Science, 129*, 3367–3373.

Yang, M., Soga, T., Pollard, P. J., et al. (2012). The emerging role of fumarate as an oncometabolite. *Frontiers in Oncology, 2*, 85.

RELEVANT WEBSITES

TCA cycle animations:
https://www.youtube.com/watch?v=juM2ROSLWfw
https://www.youtube.com/watch?v=kp3bC5N5Jfo
https://www.youtube.com/watch?v=QQmlyMGeN9U&t=5s

ABBREVIATIONS

DLDH	Dihydrolipoyl dehydrogenase
DLTA	Dihydrolipoyl transacetylase
LDHq	Lactate dehydrogenase
OAA	Oxaloacetate
PDH	Pyruvate dehydrogenase
Succ-CoA	Succinyl-CoA
TCA cycle	Tricarboxylic acid cycle

Oxidative Metabolism of Lipids in Liver and Muscle

John W. Baynes

INTRODUCTION

Fats are normally the major source of energy in liver and muscle and in most other tissues, with two major exceptions: brain and red cells

Triglycerides are the storage and transport form of fats; fatty acids are the immediate source of energy. Fatty acids are released from triglyceride stores in adipose tissue, transported in plasma in association with albumin, and delivered to cells for metabolism. The catabolism of fatty acids is entirely oxidative; after they have been transported through the cytoplasm, their oxidation proceeds in both the peroxisome and the mitochondrion, primarily by a cycle of reactions known as **β-oxidation**. Carbons are released, two at a time, from the carboxyl end of the fatty acid; the major end products are acetyl coenzyme A (acetyl-CoA) and the reduced forms of the nucleotides $FADH_2$ and NADH. In muscle, the acetyl-CoA is metabolized via the tricarboxylic acid (TCA) cycle and oxidative phosphorylation to produce ATP. In liver, acetyl-CoA is converted largely to ketone bodies (**ketogenesis**), which are

water-soluble lipid derivatives that, like glucose, are exported for use in other tissues. Fat metabolism is controlled primarily by the rate of triglyceride hydrolysis (**lipolysis**) in adipose tissue, which is regulated by hormonal mechanisms involving **insulin, glucagon, epinephrine, and cortisol.** These hormones coordinate the metabolism of carbohydrates, lipids, and protein throughout the body (Chapter 31).

ACTIVATION OF FATTY ACIDS FOR TRANSPORT INTO THE MITOCHONDRION

Fatty acids are activated by formation of a high-energy thioester bond with coenzyme A

Fatty acids do not exist to a significant extent in free form in the body - salts of fatty acids are soaps; they would dissolve cell membranes. In blood, fatty acids are bound to albumin, which is present at ~0.5 mmol/L concentration (35 mg/mL) in plasma. Each molecule of albumin can bind six to eight fatty-acid molecules. In the cytosol, fatty acids are bound to a series of fatty acid–binding proteins that regulate their trafficking in the cytosol and between subcellular compartments. In the priming step for their catabolism, fatty acids are activated to their CoA derivative, using ATP as the energy source (Fig. 11.1). The carboxyl group is first activated to an enzyme-bound, high-energy acyl-adenylate intermediate formed by reaction of the carboxyl group of the fatty acid with ATP. The acyl group is then transferred to CoA by the same enzyme, **fatty acyl-CoA synthetase.** This enzyme is commonly known as fatty acid **thiokinase** because ATP is consumed in the formation of the thioester bond in acyl-CoA.

The length of the fatty acid dictates where it is activated to CoA

Short- and medium-chain fatty acids (Table 11.1) can cross the mitochondrial membrane by passive diffusion and are activated to their CoA derivative within the mitochondrion. Very long–chain fatty acids from the diet are shortened to long-chain fatty acids in peroxisomes. Long-chain fatty acids are the major components of storage triglycerides and dietary fats. They are activated to their CoA derivatives in the cytoplasm and are transported into the mitochondrion via the **carnitine shuttle.**

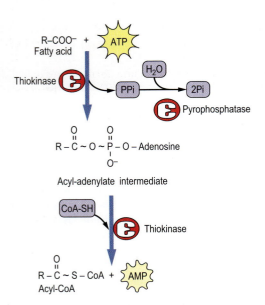

Fig. 11.1 **Activation of fatty acids by fatty acyl-CoA synthetase (thiokinase).** ATP forms an enzyme-bound acyl-adenylate intermediate, which is discharged by CoA-SH to form acyl-CoA. AMP, adenosine monophosphate; CoA-SH, coenzyme A; PPi, inorganic pyrophosphate.

Table 11.1 Metabolism of the four classes of fatty acids

Size class	Number of carbons	Site of catabolism	Membrane transport
Short chain	2–4	Mitochondrion	Diffusion
Medium chain	4–12	Mitochondrion	Diffusion
Long chain	12–20	Mitochondrion	Carnitine cycle
Very long chain	>20	Peroxisome	Unknown

The carnitine shuttle

The carnitine shuttle bypasses the impermeability of the mitochondrial membrane to coenzyme A

CoA is a large polar nucleotide derivative (Fig. 10.2) and cannot penetrate the mitochondrial inner membrane. Thus for the transport of long-chain fatty acids, the fatty acid is first transferred to the small molecule, carnitine, by **carnitine palmitoyl transferase-I** (**CPT-I**), located in the outer mitochondrial membrane. An **acyl-carnitine transporter**, or translocase, in the inner mitochondrial membrane mediates transfer of the acyl-carnitine into the mitochondrion, where **CPT-II** regenerates the acyl-CoA, releasing free carnitine. The carnitine shuttle (Fig. 11.2) operates by an antiport mechanism in which free carnitine and the acyl-carnitine derivative move

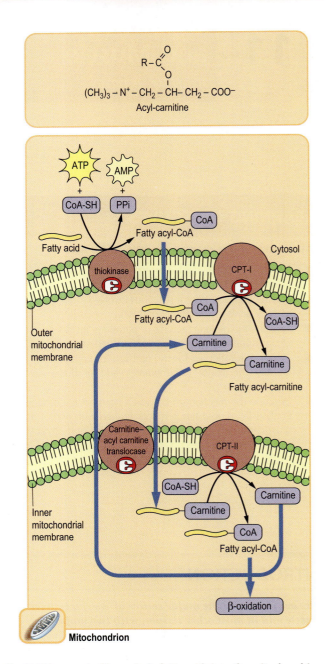

Fig. 11.2 **Transport of long-chain fatty acids into the mitochondrion.** The three components of the carnitine pathway include carnitine palmitoyl transferases (CPT) in the outer and inner mitochondrial membranes and the carnitine-acyl carnitine translocase.

in opposite directions across the inner mitochondrial membrane. The shuttle is an important site in the regulation of fatty acid oxidation. As discussed in the next chapter, the carnitine shuttle is inhibited by **malonyl-CoA** after the ingestion of carbohydrate-rich meals. Malonyl-CoA prevents the futile cycle in which newly synthesized fatty acids would be oxidized in the mitochondrion.

OXIDATION OF FATTY ACIDS

Mitochondrial β-oxidation

Oxidation of the β-carbon (C-3) facilitates sequential cleavage of acetyl units from the carboxyl end of fatty acids

Fatty acyl-CoAs are oxidized in a cycle of reactions involving oxidation of the β-carbon (C-3) to a ketone, hence the term *β-oxidation* (Figs. 11.3 and 11.4). The oxidation is followed by cleavage between the α- and β-carbons by a **thiolase**, rather than hydrolase, reaction; in this way, the high energy of the thioester bond is preserved to provide the thermodynamic driving force for subsequent reactions. One mole each of acetyl-CoA, $FADH_2$, and NADH is formed during each cycle, along with a fatty acyl-CoA with two fewer carbon atoms. For a 16-carbon fatty acid such as palmitate, the cycle is repeated seven times, yielding 8 moles of acetyl-CoA (Fig. 11.3), plus 7 moles of $FADH_2$ and 7 moles of NADH + H^+. This process occurs in the mitochondrion, and the reduced nucleotides are used directly for the synthesis of ATP by oxidative phosphorylation (Table 11.2).

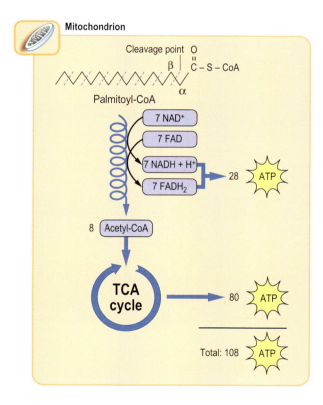

Fig. 11.3 **Overview of β-oxidation of palmitate.** In a cycle of reactions, the carbons of the fatty acyl-CoA are released in two-carbon acetyl-CoA units; the yield of 28 ATP from this β-oxidation is nearly equivalent to that from the complete oxidation of glucose. In liver, the acetyl-CoA units are then used for the synthesis of ketone bodies, and in other tissues, they are metabolized in the TCA cycle to form ATP. The complete oxidation of palmitate yields a net 106 moles of ATP, after correction for the 2-mole equivalents of ATP invested at the thiokinase reaction. The overall production of ATP per gram of palmitate is about twice that per gram of glucose because glucose is already partially oxidized in comparison with palmitate. For this reason, the caloric value of fats is about twice that of sugars (Table 11.2).

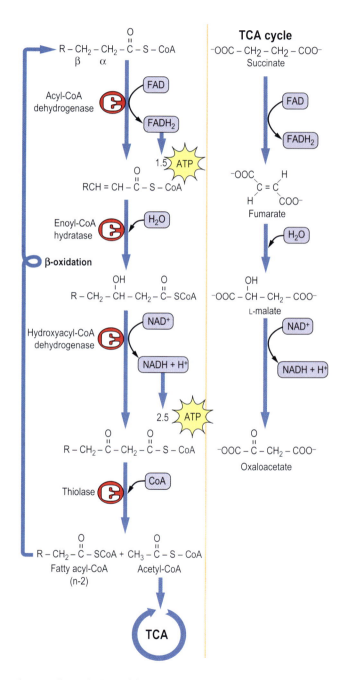

Fig. 11.4 **β-Oxidation of fatty acids.** Oxidation occurs in a series of steps at the carbon that is β to the keto group. Thiolase cleaves the resultant β-ketoacyl-CoA derivative to give acetyl-CoA and a fatty acid with two fewer carbon atoms, which then reenters the β-oxidation cascade. Note the similarity between these reactions and those of the TCA cycle, shown on the right.

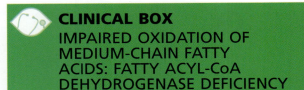

Substrate	Molecular weight	Net ATP yield (mol/mol)	ATP (mol/g)	Caloric value cal/g (kJ)
Glucose	180	36–38	0.2	4 (17)
Palmitate	256	129	0.5	9 (37)

Table 11.2 Comparative energy yield from glucose and palmitate

CLINICAL BOX

IMPAIRED OXIDATION OF MEDIUM-CHAIN FATTY ACIDS: FATTY ACYL-CoA DEHYDROGENASE DEFICIENCY

Fatty acyl-CoA dehydrogenase is not a single enzyme but a family of enzymes with chain-length specificity for oxidation of short-, medium-, and long-chain fatty acids; fatty acids are transferred from one enzyme to the other during chain-shortening β-oxidation reactions. Medium-chain fatty acyl-CoA dehydrogenase (MCAD) deficiency is an autosomal recessive disease characterized by hypoketotic hypoglycemia. It presents in infancy and is characterized by high concentrations of medium-chain carboxylic acids, acyl-carnitines, and acyl-glycines (intermediates in carnitine biosynthesis) in plasma and urine. Hyperammonemia may also be present as a result of liver damage. Concentrations of hepatic mitochondrial medium-chain acyl-CoA derivatives are also increased, limiting β-oxidation and recycling of CoA during ketogenesis. The inability to metabolize fats during fasting is life threatening because it limits gluconeogenesis and causes hypoglycemia. MCAD deficiency is treated by frequent feeding, avoidance of fasting, and carnitine supplementation. Deficiencies in short- and long-chain fatty acid dehydrogenases have similar clinical features.

The four steps in the cycle of β-oxidation are shown in detail in Fig. 11.4. Note the similarity between the sequence of these reactions and those from succinate to oxaloacetate in the TCA cycle. In common with succinate dehydrogenase, acyl-CoA dehydrogenase uses FAD as a coenzyme, and it is an integral protein in the inner mitochondrial membrane. Even the *trans* geometry of fumarate and the stereochemical configuration of L-malate in the TCA cycle are mirrored by *trans*-enoyl-CoA and L-hydroxyacyl-CoA intermediates in β-oxidation. The last step of the β-oxidation cycle is catalyzed by thiolase, which traps the energy obtained from the carbon–carbon bond cleavage as acyl-CoA, allowing the cycle to continue without the necessity of reactivating the fatty acid. The cycle continues until all of the fatty acid has been converted to acetyl-CoA, the common intermediate in the oxidation of carbohydrates and lipids.

Peroxisomal catabolism of fatty acids

Peroxisomes are essential for oxidation of very long–chain fatty acids; they release medium-chain fatty acids for oxidation in the mitochondrion.

Peroxisomes are subcellular organelles found in all nucleated cells. They are involved in the oxidation of a number of substrates, including urate, and very long–, long-, and branched-chain fatty acids. They are also the principal sites of production of hydrogen peroxide (H_2O_2) in the cell, accounting for nearly 20% of oxygen consumption in hepatocytes. Peroxisomes have a carnitine shuttle and conduct β-oxidation by a pathway similar to the mitochondrial pathway, except that their acyl-CoA dehydrogenase is an oxidase rather than a dehydrogenase. $FADH_2$ produced in this and other oxidation reactions, including α- and ω-oxidation (see the following discussion), is oxidized by molecular oxygen to produce H_2O_2. This pathway is energetically less efficient than β-oxidation in the mitochondrion, where ATP is produced by oxidative phosphorylation. Peroxisomal enzymes cannot oxidize short-chain fatty acids, so products such as butanoyl-, hexanoyl-, and octanoyl-carnitine are exported or diffuse from peroxisomes for further catabolism in the mitochondrion.

Peroxisomes also have anabolic functions. They are thought to have a role in the production of acetyl-CoA for biosynthesis of cholesterol and polyisoprenoids (Chapter 14), and they contain the dihydroxyacetone-phosphate acyltransferase required for synthesis of plasmalogens (Chapter 18).

Zellweger syndrome, resulting from defects in the import of enzymes into peroxisomes, is a severe multiorgan disorder that leads to death, usually at about 6 months of age; it is characterized by the accumulation of long-chain fatty acids in neuronal tissue, most likely because of the inability to turn over neuronal fatty acids. Fibrates are a class of hypolipidemic drugs that act by inducing peroxisomal proliferation in liver.

Alternative pathways of oxidation of fatty acids

Unsaturated fatty acids yield less FADH₂ when they are oxidized

Unsaturated fatty acids are already partially oxidized, so less $FADH_2$, and correspondingly less ATP, is produced by their oxidation. The double bonds in polyunsaturated fatty acids have *cis* geometry and occur at three-carbon intervals, whereas the intermediates in β-oxidation have *trans* geometry, and the reactions proceed in two-carbon steps. The metabolism of unsaturated fatty acids therefore requires additional isomerase and oxidoreductase enzymes, both to shift the position and to change the geometry of the double bonds.

Odd-chain fatty acids produce succinyl-CoA from propionyl-CoA

The oxidation of fatty acids with an odd number of carbons proceeds from the carboxyl end, like that of normal fatty acids,

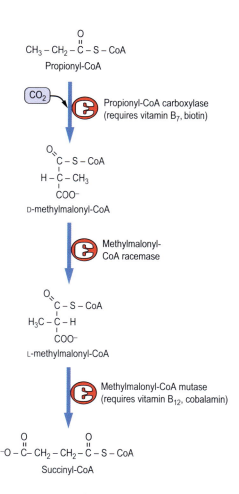

Fig. 11.5 Metabolism of propionyl-CoA to succinyl-CoA. Propionyl-CoA from odd-chain fatty acids is a minor source of carbons for gluconeogenesis. The intermediate, methylmalonyl-CoA, is also produced during catabolism of branched-chain amino acids. Defects in methylmalonyl-CoA mutase or deficiencies in vitamin B_{12} lead to methylmalonic aciduria.

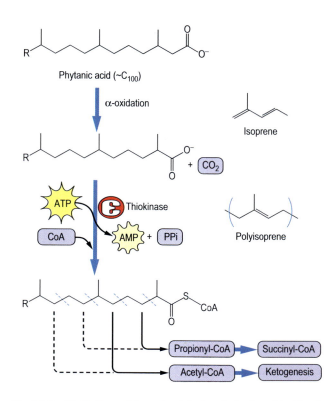

Fig. 11.6 α-Oxidation of branched-chain phytanic acids. The first carbon of phytanic acids is removed as carbon dioxide. In subsequent cycles of β-oxidation, acetyl-CoA and propionyl-CoA are released alternately.

except that propionyl-CoA is formed by the last thiolase cleavage reaction. The propionyl-CoA is converted to succinyl-CoA by a multistep process involving three enzymes and two vitamins **biotin** and **cobalamin** (Fig. 11.5). The succinyl-CoA enters directly into the TCA cycle.

α-Oxidation initiates oxidation of branched-chain fatty acids to acetyl-CoA and propionyl-CoA

Phytanic acids are branched-chain polyisoprenoid lipids found in plant chlorophylls. Because the β-carbon of phytanic acids is at a branch point, it is not possible to oxidize this carbon to a ketone. The first and essential step in the catabolism of phytanic acids is α-oxidation to a pristanic acid, releasing the α-carbon as carbon dioxide. Thereafter, as shown in Fig. 11.6, acetyl-CoA and propionyl-CoA are released alternately and in equal amounts. **Refsum's disease** is a rare neurologic disorder characterized by the accumulation of phytanic acid

deposits in nerve tissues as a result of a genetic defect in α-oxidation.

KETOGENESIS, A METABOLIC PATHWAY UNIQUE TO LIVER

Ketogenesis in fasting and starvation

Ketogenesis is a pathway for regenerating CoA from excess acetyl-CoA

The liver uses fatty acids as its source of energy for gluconeogenesis during fasting and starvation. Fats are a rich source of energy, and under conditions of fasting or starvation, liver mitochondrial concentrations of fat-derived ATP and NADH are high, inhibiting isocitrate dehydrogenase and shifting the oxaloacetate–malate equilibrium toward malate. TCA-cycle intermediates that are formed from amino acids released from muscle as part of the response to fasting and starvation (see Chapter 31) are also converted to malate in the TCA cycle. The malate exits the mitochondrion to take part in gluconeogenesis (Chapter 12). The resulting low level of oxaloacetate in hepatic mitochondria limits the activity of the TCA cycle,

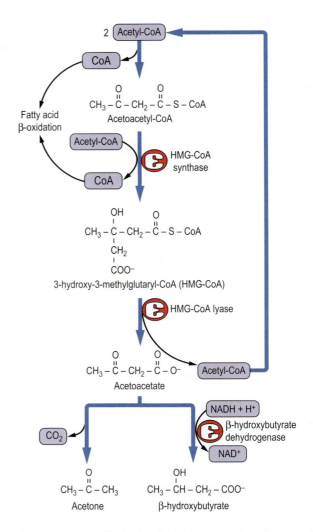

resulting in an inability to metabolize acetyl-CoA efficiently in the TCA cycle. Although the liver could obtain sufficient energy to support gluconeogenesis simply by the enzymes of β-oxidation, which generate both $FADH_2$ and NADH, the accumulation of acetyl-CoA, with concomitant depletion of CoA, eventually limits β-oxidation.

What does the liver do with the excess acetyl-CoA that accumulates in fasting or starvation?

The problem of dealing with excess acetyl-CoA is a critical one because CoA is present in only catalytic amounts in tissues, and free CoA is required to initiate and continue the cycle of β-oxidation, which is the primary source of ATP in the liver during gluconeogenesis. To recycle the acetyl-CoA, the liver uses a unique pathway known as ketogenesis, in which free CoA is regenerated, and the acetate group appears in blood in the form of three water-soluble lipid-derived products: **acetoacetate, β-hydroxybutyrate, and acetone**. The pathway of formation of these "**ketone bodies**" (Fig. 11.7) involves the synthesis and decomposition of **hydroxymethylglutaryl (HMG)-CoA** in the mitochondrion. The liver is unique in its content of HMG-CoA synthase and lyase, but it is deficient in the enzymes required for the metabolism of ketone bodies; the accumulating ketone bodies are exported into the blood.

Ketone bodies are taken up in extrahepatic tissues, including skeletal and cardiac muscle, where they are converted to CoA derivatives for metabolism (Fig. 11.8). Ketone bodies increase in plasma during fasting and starvation (Table 11.3) and are a rich source of energy. They are used in cardiac and skeletal muscle in proportion to their plasma concentration. During starvation, the brain also converts to the use of ketone bodies for more than 50% of its energy metabolism, sparing glucose and reducing the demand on the degradation of muscle protein for gluconeogenesis (see Chapters 12 and 31).

Fig. 11.7 **Pathway of ketogenesis from acetyl-CoA.** Ketogenesis generates ketone bodies from acetyl-CoA, releasing the CoA to participate in β-oxidation. The enzymes involved, HMG-CoA synthase and lyase, are unique to hepatocytes; mitochondrial HMG-CoA is an essential intermediate. The initial product is acetoacetic acid, which may be enzymatically reduced to β-hydroxybutyrate by β-hydroxybutyrate dehydrogenase or may spontaneously (nonenzymatically) decompose to acetone, which is excreted in urine or expired by the lungs.

Table 11.3 Plasma concentrations of fatty acids and ketone bodies in different nutritional states

Substrate	Plasma concentration (mmol/L)		
	Normal	**Fasting**	**Starvation**
Fatty acids	0.6	1.0	1.5
Acetoacetate	<0.1	0.2	1–2
β-Hydroxybutyrate	<0.1	1.0	5–10

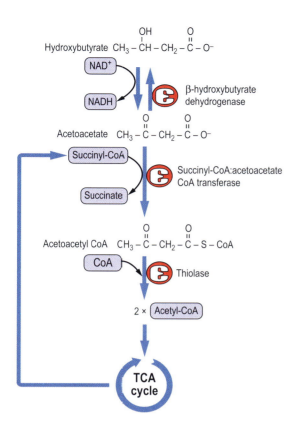

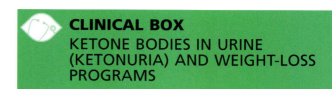

Fig. 11.8 **Catabolism of ketone bodies in peripheral tissues.** Succinyl-CoA:acetoacetate CoA transferase catalyzes the conversion of aceto-acetate to acetoacetyl-CoA. A thiokinase-type enzyme may also directly activate acetoacetate in some tissues.

Mobilization of lipids during gluconeogenesis

Carbohydrate and lipid metabolism are coordinately regulated by hormone action during the feed–fast cycle

Insulin, glucagon, epinephrine, and cortisol control the direction and rate of glycogen and glucose metabolism in the liver (Chapter 12). During fasting and starvation, hepatic gluco-neogenesis is activated by glucagon and requires the coordinated degradation of proteins and release of amino acids from muscle and the degradation of triglycerides and release of fatty acids from adipose tissue. The latter process, known as lipolysis, is controlled by the adipocyte enzyme **hormone-sensitive lipase,** which is activated by phosphorylation by cAMP-dependent protein kinase A in response to increasing plasma concentrations of glucagon (Chapters 12 and 31). Like gluconeogenesis, lipolysis is inhibited by insulin.

The activation of hormone-sensitive lipase has predictable effects - increasing the concentration of free fatty acids and glycerol in plasma during fasting and starvation (Fig. 11.9). Similar effects are observed in response to epinephrine during the stress response. Epinephrine activates glycogenolysis in the liver and lipolysis in adipose tissue so that both fuels, glucose and fatty acids, increase in the blood during stress. Cortisol exerts a more chronic effect on lipolysis and also causes insulin resistance. **Cushing's syndrome** (Chapter 27), in which there are high blood concentrations of cortisol, is characterized by hyperglycemia, muscle wastage, and redistribution of fat from glucagon-sensitive adipose depots to atypical sites, such as the cheeks, upper back, and trunk.

Regulation of ketogenesis

Ketogenesis is activated in concert with gluconeogenesis during fasting and starvation

Ketogenesis increases when hormone-sensitive lipase is activated by glucagon in adipose tissue during fasting and starvation and in diabetes. Under these conditions, plasma fatty acid concentration increases, and the liver uses these fatty acids to support gluconeogenesis. The energy is derived primarily from β-oxidation, and the product, acetyl-CoA, is metabolized by ketogenesis. Why isn't the acetyl-CoA used in the tricar-boxylic acid cycle?

During gluconeogenesis, glucagon activation of the cAMP cascade in liver inhibits glycolysis (Fig. 12.9), limiting pyru-vate flux from carbohydrates. Any pyruvate that is formed, mostly from lactate and alanine, is converted to oxaloacetate

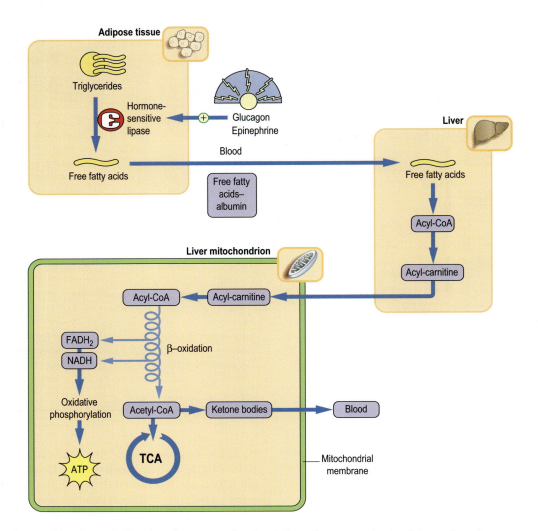

Fig. 11.9 **Regulation of lipid metabolism by glucagon and epinephrine.** Glucagon and epinephrine activate hormone-sensitive lipase in adipose tissue in coordination with activation of proteolysis in muscle and gluconeogenesis in liver. Metabolism of fatty acids through β-oxidation in liver yields ATP for gluconeogenesis. The acetyl-CoA is converted to and released to blood as ketone bodies. These effects are reversed by insulin after a meal.

CLINICAL BOX
DEFECTIVE KETOGENESIS: KETOGENESIS AS A RESULT OF A DEFICIENCY IN CARNITINE METABOLISM

The clinical presentation of deficiencies in carnitine metabolism occurs in infancy and is often life threatening. Characteristic features include hypoketotic hypoglycemia, hyperammonemia, and altered plasma free carnitine concentration. Hepatic damage, cardiomyopathy, and muscle weakness are common.

Comment

Carnitine is synthesized from lysine and α-ketoglutarate, primarily in the liver and kidney, and is normally present in plasma in a concentration of about 50 μmol/L (8 mg/dL). There are high-affinity uptake systems for carnitine in most tissues, including the kidney, which resorbs carnitine from the glomerular filtrate, limiting its excretion in urine. Homozygous deficiencies in carnitine transporters,

CPT-I and -II, and the translocase result in defects in long-chain fatty acid oxidation. Plasma and tissue carnitine concentrations decrease to < 1 μmol/L in carnitine transport deficiency because of both defective uptake into tissues and excessive loss in urine. On the other hand, plasma free carnitine may exceed 100 μmol/L (20 mg/dL) in CPT-I deficiency. In both translocase and CPT-II deficiency, total plasma carnitine may be normal, but it is mostly in the form of acyl-carnitine esters of long-chain fatty acids - in the former case because they cannot be transported into the mitochondrion; in the latter because of backflow from mitochondria. These diseases are treated by carnitine supplementation, by frequent high-carbohydrate feeding, and by avoidance of fasting.

CLINICAL BOX
HELLP AND AFLP SYNDROMES IN MOTHERS OF CHILDREN BORN WITH LCHAD (INCIDENCE 1 IN 200,000)

Long-chain L-3-hydroxyacyl-CoA dehydrogenase (LCHAD) deficiency can present in a wide variety of ways. Those affected are prone to episodes of nonketotic hypoglycemia but may develop fulminant hepatic failure, cardiomyopathy, rhabdomyolysis, and occasionally neuropathy and retinopathy. As with deficiencies in MCAD, treatment involves avoidance of fasting and diets enriched in medium-chain fatty acids.

Perhaps the most striking feature of this rare defect in fatty acid metabolism is the association with maternal HELLP (**h**emolysis, **e**levated **l**iver enzymes, and **l**ow **p**latelets) and AFLP (**a**cute **f**atty **l**iver of **p**regnancy). These potentially fatal obstetric emergencies may occur in mothers who are heterozygotes for LCHAD, especially if the child has LCHAD. These syndromes are also associated with another recessive fatty acid defect, carnitine palmitoyl-transferase-I deficiency.

ACTIVE LEARNING

1. Compare the metabolism of acetyl-CoA in the liver and muscle. Explain why the liver produces ketone bodies during gluconeogenesis. What prevents hepatic oxidation of acetyl-CoA?
2. Evaluate the evidence for the use of carnitine as a performance enhancer during exercise and as a supplement for geriatric patients.
3. Review the current use and mechanism of action of peroxisome proliferator drugs for the treatment of dyslipidemia and diabetes.
4. Compare the mechanisms underlying the development of ketoacidotic hyperglycemia and nonketotic hypoglycemia.

by pyruvate carboxylase, which is activated by acetyl-CoA (Fig. 12.9). The oxaloacetate is converted to malate for gluconeogenesis, and because of the low level of oxaloacetate, a substrate for citrate synthase, the acetyl-CoA is directed to ketogenesis rather than used for energy metabolism in the TCA cycle. The orientation toward ketogenesis is controlled by the energy charge of the liver. The high ATP concentration produced during fat metabolism inhibits the TCA cycle at the isocitrate dehydrogenase step (Chapter 10). Further, by respiratory control (Chapter 8), high ATP leads to an increase in the mitochondrial membrane potential, which inhibits the electron transport chain. The resulting increase in the NADH/NAD$^+$ ratio favors reduction of oxaloacetate to malate, which exits the mitochondrion for gluconeogenesis, rather than consumption in the tricarboxylic acid cycle.

In summary, during gluconeogenesis, acetyl-CoA produced by β-oxidation of fatty acids is converted to ketone bodies; it has nowhere else to go! The increase in ketone bodies in plasma (**ketonemia**) leads to their appearance in urine (**ketonuria**). In poorly controlled type 1 diabetes, the high rate of ketogenesis may lead to excessive ketonemia and possibly life-threatening diabetic **ketoacidosis** (Chapter 31).

SUMMARY

- Unlike carbohydrate fuels, which enter the body primarily as glucose or sugars that are converted to glucose, lipid fuels are heterogeneous with respect to chain length, branching, and unsaturation.

- The catabolism of fats is primarily a mitochondrial process but also occurs in peroxisomes.
- Using a variety of chain length–specific transport processes and catabolic enzymes, the primary pathways of catabolism of fatty acids involve their oxidative degradation in two-carbon units, a process known as β-oxidation, which produces acetyl-CoA.
- In most tissues, the acetyl-CoA units are used for ATP production in the mitochondrion.
- In liver, acetyl-CoA is catabolized to ketone bodies, primarily acetoacetate and β-hydroxybutyrate, by a mitochondrial pathway termed ketogenesis. The ketone bodies are exported from the liver for energy metabolism in peripheral tissue.
- Ketonemia and ketonuria develop gradually during fasting, whereas ketoacidosis may develop during poorly controlled diabetes, when fat metabolism is increased to high levels for support of gluconeogenesis.

FURTHER READING

Cahill, G. F., Jr. (2006). Fuel metabolism in starvation. *Annual Review of Nutrition*, *26*, 1–22.

Fukushima, A., & Lopaschuk, G. D. (2016). Acetylation control of cardiac fatty acid β-oxidation and energy metabolism in obesity, diabetes, and heart failure. *Biochimica et Biophysica Acta*, *1862*, 2211–2220.

Longo, N., Amat di San Filippo, C., & Pasquali, M. (2006). Disorders of carnitine transport and the carnitine cycle. *American Journal of Medical Genetics. Part C, Seminars in Medical Genetics*, *142*, 77–85.

Sass, J. O. (2012). Inborn errors of ketogenesis and ketone body utilization. *Journal of Inherited Metabolic Disease*, *35*, 23–28.

Tein, I. (2013). Disorders of fatty acid oxidation. *Handbook of Clinical Neurology*, *113*, 1675–1688.

Vishwanath, V. A. (2016). Fatty acid beta-oxidation disorders: A brief review. *Annals of Neurosciences*, *23*, 51–55.

Wanders, R. J. (2014). Metabolic functions of peroxisomes in health and disease. *Biochimie*, *98*, 36–44.

RELEVANT WEBSITES

Beta-oxidation: http://lipidlibrary.aocs.org/Biochemistry/
content.cfm?ItemNumber=39187
Carnitine: http://lpi.oregonstate.edu/mic/dietary-factors/L-carnitine
Overview of fatty acid oxidation: http://themedicalbiochemistrypage.org/
fatty-acid-oxidation.php
Peroxisomes: http://emedicine.medscape.com/article/1177387-overview
Peroxisomal disorders: http://emedicine.medscape.com/article/1177387
-overview

ABBREVIATIONS

CoA-SH	Acetyl-Coenzyme A
CPT-I, CPT-II	Carnitine palmitoyl transferase I and II
HMG-CoA	Hydroxymethylglutaryl-CoA
TCA cycle	Tricarboxylic acid cycle

Biosynthesis and Storage of Carbohydrate in Liver and Muscle
John W. Baynes

LEARNING OBJECTIVES

After reading this chapter, you should be able to:

■ Describe the structure of glycogen.

■ Identify the primary sites of glycogen storage in the body and the function of glycogen in these tissues.

■ Outline the metabolic pathways for synthesis and degradation of glycogen.

■ Describe the mechanism by which glycogen is mobilized in the liver in response to glucagon, in muscle during exercise, and in both tissues in response to epinephrine.

■ Explain the origin and consequences of glycogen storage diseases in liver and muscle.

■ Describe the mechanism for counterregulation of glycogenolysis and glycogenesis in the liver.

■ Outline the pathway of gluconeogenesis, including substrates, unique enzymes, and regulatory mechanisms.

■ Describe the complementary roles of glycogenolysis and gluconeogenesis in the maintenance of blood glucose concentration.

INTRODUCTION

The red cell and the brain have an absolute requirement for blood glucose for energy metabolism. Together, they consume about 80% of the 200 g of glucose consumed in the body per day. There are only about 10 g of glucose in the plasma and extracellular fluid volume, ~5% of the daily requirement, so that blood glucose must be replenished constantly. Otherwise, hypoglycemia develops and compromises brain function, leading to confusion and disorientation and possibly life-threatening coma at blood glucose concentrations below 2.5 mmol/L (45 mg/dL). We absorb glucose from our intestines for only 2–3 h after a carbohydrate-containing meal, so there must be a mechanism for maintenance of blood glucose between meals.

Glycogen, a polysaccharide storage form of glucose, is our first line of defense against declining blood glucose concentration. During and immediately after a meal, glucose is converted into glycogen, a process known as **glycogenesis,** in both the liver and muscle. The tissue concentration of glycogen is higher in the liver than in muscle, but because of the relative masses of muscle and liver, the majority of glycogen in the body is stored in muscle (Table 12.1).

Hepatic glycogenolysis and gluconeogenesis are required for maintenance of normal blood glucose concentration

Hepatic glycogen is gradually degraded between meals by the pathway of **glycogenolysis,** releasing glucose to maintain blood glucose concentration. However, total hepatic glycogen stores are barely sufficient for maintenance of blood glucose concentration during a 12-h fast.

During sleep, when we are not eating, there is a gradual shift from **glycogenolysis** to de novo synthesis of glucose, also a hepatic pathway, known as **gluconeogenesis** (Fig. 12.1). Gluconeogenesis is essential for survival during fasting or starvation, when glycogen stores are depleted. The liver uses amino acids from muscle protein as the primary precursor of glucose but also makes use of lactate from glycolysis and glycerol from fat catabolism. Fatty acids, mobilized from adipose tissue triglyceride stores, provide the energy for gluconeogenesis.

Glycogen is stored in muscle for use in energy metabolism

Muscle glycogen is not available for maintenance of blood glucose. Glucose obtained from blood and glycogen is used exclusively for energy metabolism in muscle, especially during bursts of physical activity. Although cardiac and skeletal muscles rely on fats as their primary source of energy, some glucose metabolism is essential for efficient fat metabolism in these tissues (see Chapter 37).

This chapter describes the pathways of glycogenesis and glycogenolysis in the liver and muscle and the pathway of gluconeogenesis in the liver.

STRUCTURE OF GLYCOGEN

Glycogen, a highly branched glucan, is the storage form of glucose in tissues

Glycogen is a branched polysaccharide of glucose. It contains only two types of glycosidic linkages, chains of $\alpha 1 \rightarrow 4$-linked glucose residues with $\alpha 1 \rightarrow 6$ branches spaced about every 4–6 residues along the $\alpha 1 \rightarrow 4$ chain (Fig. 12.2). Glycogen is closely related to **starch,** the storage polysaccharide of plants, but starch consists of a mixture of amylose and amylopectin. The amylose component contains only linear $\alpha 1 \rightarrow 4$ chains; the amylopectin component is more glycogen-like in structure but with fewer $\alpha 1 \rightarrow 6$ branches, about one per 12 $\alpha 1 \rightarrow 4$-linked

Table 12.1 Tissue distribution of carbohydrate energy reserves (70-kg adult)

Tissue	Type	Amount	% Of tissue mass	Calories
Liver	Glycogen	75 g	3%–5%	300
Muscle	Glycogen	250 g	0.5%–1.0%	1000
Blood and extracellular fluid	Glucose	10 g	—	40

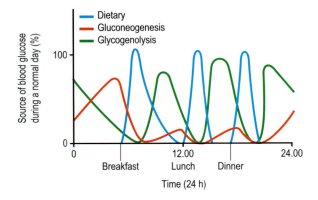

Fig. 12.1 **Sources of blood glucose during a normal day.** Between meals, blood glucose is derived primarily from hepatic glycogen. Depending on the frequency of snacking, glycogenolysis and gluconeogenesis may be more or less active during the day. Late in the night or in the early morning, after depletion of a major fraction of hepatic glycogen, gluconeogenesis becomes the primary source of blood glucose.

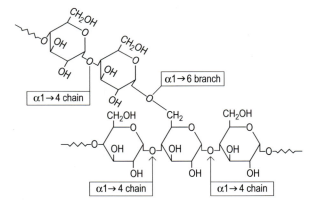

Fig. 12.2 **Close-up of the structure of glycogen.** The figure shows $\alpha1\rightarrow4$ chains and an $\alpha1\rightarrow6$ branch point. Glycogen is stored as granules in liver and muscle cytoplasm.

glucose residues. The gross structure of glycogen is dendritic in nature, expanding from a core sequence bound to a tyrosine residue in the protein **glycogenin** and developing into a final structure resembling a head of cauliflower. The enzymes of glycogen metabolism are bound to the surface of the glycogen particle; many terminal glucose molecules on the surface of

the molecule provide ready access for rapid release of glucose from the glycogen polymer.

PATHWAY OF GLYCOGENESIS FROM BLOOD GLUCOSE IN THE LIVER

Glycogenesis is activated in the liver and muscle after a meal

The liver is rich in the high-capacity, low-affinity (K_m >10 mmol/L) glucose transporter **GLUT-2**, making it freely permeable to glucose delivered at high concentration in portal blood during and after a meal (see Table 4.2). The liver is also rich in **glucokinase,** an enzyme that is specific for glucose and converts it to glucose 6-phosphate (Glc-6-P). Glucokinase (GK) is inducible by continued consumption of a high-carbohydrate diet. It has a high K_m, about 5–7 mmol/L, so that it is poised to increase in activity as portal glucose increases above the normal 5 mmol/L (100 mg/dL) blood glucose concentration. Unlike hexokinase, GK is not inhibited by Glc-6-P, so the concentration of Glc-6-P increases rapidly in the liver after a carbohydrate-rich meal, forcing glucose into all the major pathways of glucose metabolism: glycolysis, the pentose phosphate pathway, and glycogenesis (see Fig. 9.2). Glucose is channeled into glycogen, providing a carbohydrate reserve for maintenance of blood glucose during the postabsorptive state. Excess Glc-6-P in the liver, beyond that needed to replenish glycogen reserves, is then funneled into glycolysis, in part for energy production but primarily for conversion into fatty acids and triglycerides, which are exported from the liver for storage in adipose tissue. Glucose that passes through the liver causes an increase in peripheral blood glucose concentration after carbohydrate-rich meals. This glucose is used in muscle for synthesis and storage of glycogen and in adipose tissue as a source of glycerol for triglyceride biosynthesis.

The pathway of glycogenesis from glucose (Fig. 12.3A) involves four steps:

- Conversion of Glc-6-P into glucose-1-phosphate (Glc-1-P) by **phosphoglucomutase.**
- Activation of Glc-1-P to the sugar nucleotide uridine diphosphate (UDP)-glucose by the enzyme **UDP-glucose pyrophosphorylase.**
- Transfer of glucose from UDP-Glc to glycogen in $\alpha1\rightarrow4$ linkage by **glycogen synthase,** a member of the class of enzymes known as glycosyl transferases.
- When the $\alpha1\rightarrow4$ chain exceeds eight residues in length, **glycogen branching enzyme,** a transglycosylase, transfers some of the $\alpha1\rightarrow4$-linked sugars to an $\alpha1\rightarrow6$ branch, setting the stage for continued elongation of both $\alpha1\rightarrow4$ chains until they, in turn, become long enough for transfer by branching enzyme.

Glycogen synthase is the regulatory enzyme for glycogenesis, rather than UDP-glucose pyrophosphorylase, because UDP-glucose is also used for the synthesis of other sugars and as a glycosyl donor for the synthesis of glycoproteins, glycolipids,

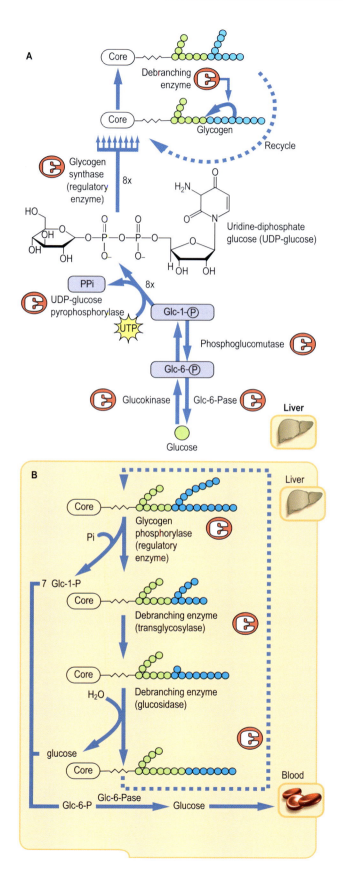

Fig. 12.3 **Pathways of glycogenesis (A) and glycogenolysis (B).**

and proteoglycans (Chapters 17–19). Pyrophosphate (PPi), the other product of the pyrophosphorylase reaction, is a high-energy phosphate anhydride. It is rapidly hydrolyzed to inorganic phosphate by pyrophosphatase. providing the thermodynamic driving force for biosynthesis of glycogen.

PATHWAY OF GLYCOGENOLYSIS IN THE LIVER

Hepatic glycogen phosphorylase provides for rapid release of glucose into the blood during the postabsorptive state

As with most metabolic pathways, separate enzymes, sometimes in separate subcellular compartments, are required for the forward and reverse pathways. The pathway of glycogenolysis (Fig. 12.3B) begins with removal of the abundant, external $\alpha 1 \rightarrow 4$-linked glucose residues in glycogen. This is accomplished not by a hydrolase but by **glycogen phosphorylase,** an enzyme that uses cytosolic phosphate and releases glucose from glycogen in the form of Glc-1-P. The Glc-1-P is isomerized by phosphoglucomutase to Glc-6-P, placing it at the top of the glycolytic pathway; the phosphorylase reaction, in effect, bypasses the requirement for ATP in the hexokinase or glucokinase reactions. In the liver, the glucose is released from Glc-6-P by **glucose-6-phosphatase** (Glc-6-Pase), and the glucose exits via the GLUT-2 transporter into the blood. The rate-limiting, regulatory step in glycogenolysis is catalyzed by phosphorylase, the first enzyme in the pathway.

Phosphorylase is specific for $\alpha 1 \rightarrow 4$ glycosidic linkages; it cannot cleave $\alpha 1 \rightarrow 6$ linkages. Further, this large enzyme cannot approach the branching glucose residues efficiently. Thus, as shown in Fig. 12.3B, phosphorylase cleaves the external glucose residues until the branches are three or four residues long, then **debranching enzyme,** which has both transglycosylase and glucosidase activity, moves a short segment of glucose residues bound to the $\alpha 1 \rightarrow 6$ branch to the end of an adjacent $\alpha 1 \rightarrow 4$ chain, leaving a single glucose residue at the branch point. This glucose is then removed by the exo-1,6-glucosidase activity of the debranching enzyme, allowing glycogen phosphorylase to proceed with degradation of the extended $\alpha 1 \rightarrow 4$ chain until another branch point is approached, setting the stage for a repeat of the transglycosylase and glucosidase reactions. About 90% of the glucose is released from glycogen as Glc-1-P, and the remainder, derived from the $\alpha 1 \rightarrow 6$ branching residues, is released as free glucose.

HORMONAL REGULATION OF HEPATIC GLYCOGENOLYSIS

Three hormones (insulin, glucagon, and cortisol) counterregulate glycogenolysis and glycogenesis

Glycogenolysis is activated in the liver in response to a demand for blood glucose, either because of its utilization during the postabsorptive state or in preparation for increased glucose

CLINICAL BOX
VON GIERKE'S DISEASE: GLYCOGEN STORAGE DISEASE CAUSED BY GLUCOSE-6-PHOSPHATASE DEFICIENCY

A baby girl was chronically cranky, irritable, sweaty, and lethargic, and she demanded food frequently. Physical evaluation indicated an extended abdomen resulting from an enlarged liver. Blood glucose, measured 1 h after feeding, was 3.5 mmol/L (70 mg/dL); normal value <5 mmol/L (100 mg/dL). After 4 h, when the child was exhibiting irritability and sweating, her heart rate was increased (pulse = 110), and blood glucose had declined to 2 mmol/L (40 mg/dL). These symptoms were corrected by feeding. A liver biopsy showed massive deposition of glycogen particles in the liver cytosol.

Comment
This child cannot mobilize glycogen. Because of the severity of hypoglycemia, the most likely mutation is in hepatic Glc-6-Pase, which is required for glucose production by both glycogenolysis and gluconeogenesis. Treatment involves frequent feeding with slowly digested carbohydrate (e.g., uncooked starch) and nasogastric drip-feeding during the night.

Table 12.2 Hormones involved in control of glycogenolysis

Hormone	Source	Initiator	Effect on glycogenolysis
Glucagon	Pancreatic α-cells	Hypoglycemia	Rapid activation
Epinephrine	Adrenal medulla	Acute stress, hypoglycemia	Rapid activation
Cortisol	Adrenal cortex	Chronic stress	Chronic activation
Insulin	Pancreatic β-cells	Hyperglycemia	Inhibition

utilization in response to stress. There are three major hormonal activators of glycogenolysis: glucagon, epinephrine (adrenaline), and cortisol (Table 12.2).

Glucagon is a peptide hormone (3500 Da) secreted from the **α-cells** of the endocrine pancreas. Its primary function is to activate hepatic glycogenolysis for maintenance of normal blood glucose concentration (normoglycemia). Glucagon has a short half-life in plasma, about 5 min, as a result of receptor binding, renal filtration, and proteolytic inactivation in the liver. Glucagon concentration in plasma therefore changes rapidly in response to the need for blood glucose. Blood glucagon increases between meals, decreases during a meal, and is chronically increased during fasting or on a low-carbohydrate diet (Chapter 31).

Hepatic glycogenolysis is also activated in response to both acute and chronic stress. The stress may be of the following types:

- Physiologic (e.g., in response to increased blood glucose utilization during exercise)
- Pathologic (e.g., as a result of blood loss [shock])
- Psychologic (e.g., in response to acute or chronic threats)

Acute stress, regardless of its source, causes an activation of glycogenolysis through the action of the **catecholamine hormone epinephrine,** released from the adrenal medulla. During prolonged or stressful exercise, both glucagon and epinephrine contribute to the stimulation of glycogenolysis and maintenance of blood glucose concentration.

Increased blood concentrations of the adrenocortical steroid hormone cortisol also induce glycogenolysis. Levels of the **glucocorticoid cortisol** vary diurnally in plasma but may be chronically elevated under continuously stressful conditions, including psychologic and environmental (e.g., cold) stress.

Glucagon serves as a general model for the mechanism of action of hormones that act by way of cell-surface receptors. Cortisol, which acts at the level of gene expression, is discussed in Chapters 23 and 25.

MECHANISM OF ACTION OF GLUCAGON

Glucagon activates glycogenolysis during the postabsorptive state

Glucagon binds to a hepatic plasma membrane receptor and initiates a cascade of reactions leading to mobilization of hepatic glycogen (Fig. 12.4) during the postabsorptive state. On the inside of the plasma membrane, there is a class of **signal transduction** proteins, known as **G-proteins,** that bind guanosine triphosphate (GTP) and guanosine diphosphate (GDP), nucleotide analogues of ATP and ADP. GDP is bound in the resting state. Binding of glucagon to the plasma membrane receptor stimulates the exchange of GDP for GTP on the G-protein, and the G-protein then undergoes a conformational change that leads to dissociation of its α-subunit, which then binds to and activates the plasma-membrane enzyme **adenylate cyclase.** This enzyme converts cytoplasmic ATP into **cyclic-3′,5′-AMP (cAMP),** a soluble mediator that is described as the "**second messenger**" for the action of glucagon (and other hormones). Cyclic AMP binds to the cytoplasmic enzyme **protein kinase A (PKA),** causing dissociation of inhibitory (regulatory) subunits from the catalytic subunits of the heterodimeric enzyme, relieving inhibition of PKA, which then phosphorylates serine and threonine residues on target proteins and enzymes.

The pathway for hormonal activation of glycogen phosphorylase (see Fig. 12.4) involves phosphorylation of many molecules of **phosphorylase kinase** by PKA, which then

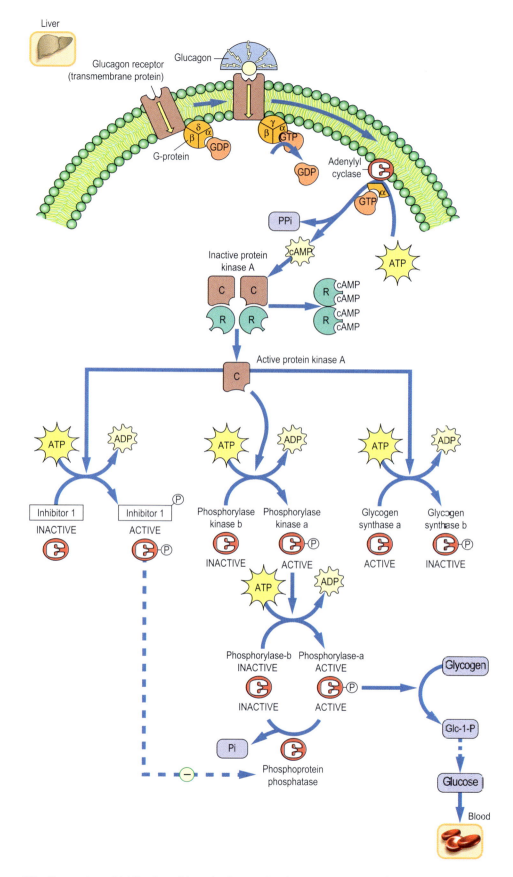

Fig. 12.4 **Cascade amplification system.** Mobilization of hepatic glycogen by glucagon. A cascade of reactions amplifies the hepatic response to glucagon binding to its plasma membrane receptor. cAMP is known as the second messenger of glucagon action. PKA indirectly activates phosphorylase via phosphorylase kinase and directly inactivates glycogen synthase. C, catalytic subunits; R, regulatory (inhibitory) subunits; PKA, protein kinase A.

A 30-year-old man consulted his physician because of chronic arm and leg muscle pains and cramps during exercise. He indicated that he had always had some muscle weakness and, for this reason, was never active in scholastic sports, but the problem did not become severe until he recently enrolled in an exercise program to improve his health. He also noted that the pain generally disappeared after about 15–30 min, and then he could continue his exercise without discomfort. His blood glucose concentration was normal during exercise, but serum creatine kinase (MM isoform from skeletal muscle) was elevated, suggesting muscle damage. Blood glucose declined slightly during 15 min of exercise, but unexpectedly, blood lactate also declined, rather than increased, even when he was experiencing muscle cramps. A biopsy indicated an unusually high level of glycogen in muscle, suggesting a **glycogen storage disease**.

Comment

This patient suffers from McArdle's disease, a rare deficiency of muscle phosphorylase activity. The actual enzyme deficiency must be confirmed by enzyme assay because a number of other mutations could also affect muscle glycogen metabolism. During the early periods of intense exercise, the muscle obtains most of its energy by metabolism of glucose, derived from glycogen. During cramps, which normally occur during oxygen debt, most of the pyruvate produced by glycolysis is excreted into the blood as lactate, leading to an increase in blood lactate concentration. In this case, however, the patient had cramps but did not excrete lactate, suggesting a failure to mobilize muscle glycogen to produce glucose. His recovery after 15–30 min results from epinephrine-mediated activation of hepatic glycogenolysis, which provides glucose to blood and relieves the deficit in muscle glycogenolysis. Treatment of McArdle's disease usually involves exercise avoidance or carbohydrate consumption before exercise. Otherwise, the course of the disease is uneventful.

ADVANCED CONCEPT BOX
G-PROTEINS

G-proteins are plasma-membrane, guanosine-nucleotide-binding proteins that are involved in signal transduction for a wide variety of hormones (Fig. 12.4; see also Chapter 25). In some cases, they stimulate (Gs); in other cases, they inhibit (Gi) protein kinases and protein phosphorylation. G-proteins are closely associated with hormone receptors in plasma membranes and consist of α, β, and γ subunits. The G_α-subunit binds GDP in the resting state. After hormone binding (ligation), the receptor recruits G-proteins, stimulating the exchange of GDP for GTP on the G_α-subunit. GTP binding leads to the release of the β- and γ-subunits, and the α-subunit is then free to bind to and activate adenylate cyclase. The hormonal response is amplified after receptor binding because a single receptor can activate many α-subunits. Hormonal responses are also turned off at the level of receptors and G-proteins by two mechanisms:
- The G_α-subunit has a sluggish guanosine triphosphate phosphatase (GTPase) activity that hydrolyzes GTP, with a half-time measured in minutes, so that it gradually dissociates from, and thereby ceases to activate, adenylate cyclase.
- Phosphorylation of the hormone receptor by protein kinase A decreases its affinity for the hormone, a process described as desensitization or hormone resistance.

ADVANCED CONCEPT BOX
PROTEIN KINASE A IS VERY SENSITIVE TO SMALL CHANGES IN cAMP CONCENTRATION

As illustrated in Fig. 12.4, cAMP-dependent PKA is a tetrameric enzyme with two different types of subunits (R_2C_2); the catalytic C-subunit has protein kinase activity, and the regulatory R-subunit inhibits the protein kinase activity. The R-subunit has a sequence of amino acids that would normally be recognized and phosphorylated by the C-subunit, except this sequence in R contains an alanine, rather than a serine or threonine, residue. Binding of two molecules of cAMP to each R-subunit induces conformational changes that lead to dissociation of a ($cAMP_2$-R_2) dimer from the C-subunits. The monomeric, active C-subunits then proceed to phosphorylate serine and threonine residues in target enzymes. PKA is not a typical allosteric enzyme in that the binding of the allosteric effector (cAMP) causes subunit dissociation; however, the complete activation of PKA involves cooperative binding of four molecules of cAMP to two R-subunits. PKA is fully activated at submicromolar concentrations of cAMP, so it is exquisitely sensitive to small changes in adenylate cyclase activity in response to glucagon.

phosphorylates and activates many molecules of glycogen phosphorylase. The net effect of these sequential steps, beginning with activation of many molecules of adenylate cyclase by G-proteins, is a **"cascade amplification"** system, not unlike that of a series of amplifiers in a radio or stereo set, resulting in a massive increase in signal strength within seconds after glucagon binding to the hepatocyte plasma membrane. Phosphorylase b - the inactive, unphosphorylated form of phosphorylase - is normally inhibited by ATP and glucose in the liver, but phosphorylation converts it to the active form, phosphorylase a (Fig. 12.4), activating glycogenolysis, forming Glc and Glc-1-P, which are converted to Glc-6-P and hydrolyzed to glucose for export into blood.

Table 12.3 Several mechanisms are involved in terminating the hormonal response to glucagon

1. Hydrolysis of GTP on G_α-subunit
2. Hydrolysis of cAMP by phosphodiesterase
3. Protein phosphatase activity

Glycogenolysis and glycogenesis are counterregulated by protein kinase A, which activates phosphorylase and inhibits glycogen synthase

Glycogenolysis and glycogenesis are opposing pathways. Theoretically, Glc-1-P produced by phosphorylase could be rapidly activated to UDP-glucose and reincorporated into glycogen. To prevent this wasteful, or **futile, cycle,** PKA also phosphorylates glycogen synthase - in this case, inactivating the enzyme. In this way, PKA coordinately activates phosphorylase (glycogenolysis) and inactivates glycogen synthase (glycogenesis). Other hepatic biosynthetic pathways - including protein, cholesterol, fatty acid, and triglyceride synthesis, as well as glycolysis - are also regulated by phosphorylation of key regulatory enzymes, generally limiting biosynthetic reactions and focusing liver metabolism in response to glucagon on the provision of glucose to blood for maintenance of vital body functions (see Chapter 31).

To balance the cascade of events amplifying the glycogenolytic response to glucagon, there are multiple redundant mechanisms to ensure rapid termination of the hormonal response (Table 12.3). In addition to the slow **GTPase** activity of the G_α-subunit, there is also a **phosphodiesterase** in the cell that hydrolyzes cAMP to AMP, permitting reassociation of the inhibitory and catalytic subunits of PKA, decreasing its protein kinase activity. There are also **phosphoprotein phosphatases** that remove the phosphate groups from the active, phosphorylated forms of phosphorylase kinase and phosphorylase. Another target of PKA is **inhibitor-1,** a phosphoprotein phosphatase inhibitor protein, which is activated by phosphorylation. Phosphorylated inhibitor-1 inhibits cytoplasmic phosphoprotein phosphatases, which would otherwise reverse the phosphorylation of enzymes and quench the response to glucagon (see Fig. 12.4). The decrease in cAMP concentration and PKA activity also leads to decreased phosphorylation of inhibitor-1, permitting increased activity of phosphoprotein phosphatases. Thus many mechanisms act in concert to ensure that hepatic glycogenolysis declines rapidly in response to increasing blood glucose and decreasing blood glucagon concentrations after a meal.

There are a number of autosomal recessive genetic diseases affecting glycogen metabolism (Table 12.4). These diseases, known as **glycogen storage diseases,** are characterized by the accumulation of glycogen granules in tissues, which eventually compromises tissue function. Predictably, glycogen storage diseases affecting hepatic glycogen metabolism are characterized by fasting hypoglycemia and may be life-threatening, whereas

Table 12.4 Major classes of glycogen storage diseases

Type	Name	Enzyme deficiency	Structural or clinical consequences
I	Von Gierke's	Glc-6-Pase	Severe postabsorptive hypoglycemia, lactic acidemia, hyperlipidemia
II	Pompe's	Lysosomal α-glucosidase	Glycogen granules in lysosomes
III	Cori's	Debranching enzyme	Altered glycogen structure, hypoglycemia
IV	Andersen's	Branching enzyme	Altered glycogen structure
V	McArdle's	Muscle phosphorylase	Excess muscle glycogen deposition, exercise-induced cramps and fatigue
VI	Hers'	Liver phosphorylase	Hypoglycemia, not as severe as type I

defects in muscle glycogen metabolism are characterized by rapid muscle fatigue during exercise.

MOBILIZATION OF HEPATIC GLYCOGEN BY EPINEPHRINE

Epinephrine activates glycogenolysis during stress, increasing blood glucose concentration

The catecholamine epinephrine (adrenaline) works through several distinct receptors on different cells. The best studied of these receptors are the α- and β-adrenergic receptors; they recognize different features of the epinephrine molecule, bind epinephrine with different affinities work by different mechanisms, and are inhibited by different classes of drugs. During severe hypoglycemia, glucagon and epinephrine work together to magnify the glycogenolytic response in the liver. However, even when blood glucose is normal, epinephrine is released in response to real or perceived threats, causing an increase in blood glucose to support a fight-or-flight response. **Caffeine** in coffee and **theophylline** in tea are inhibitors of phosphodiesterase and also cause an increase in hepatic cAMP and blood glucose. Like epinephrine, caffeine, administered in the form of a few strong cups of coffee, can also make us alert and responsive - and aggressive.

The epinephrine response augments the effects of glucagon on liver during severe hypoglycemia (metabolic stress) and also explains, in part, the rapid heartbeat, sweating, tremors, and anxiety associated with hypoglycemia. Epinephrine action on hepatic glycogenolysis proceeds by two pathways: through the epinephrine **β-adrenergic receptor**, which is similar to that for glucagon, involving a

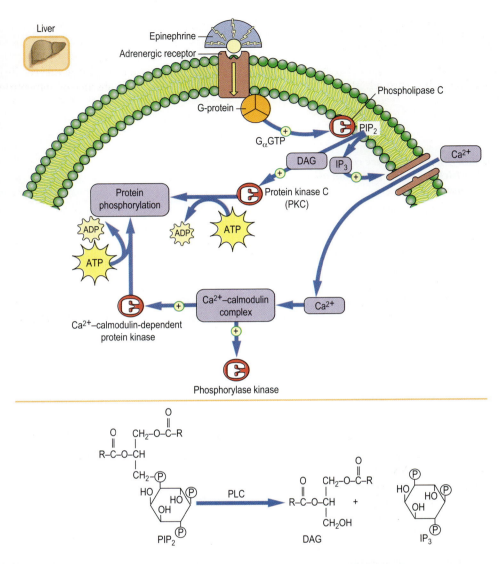

Fig. 12.5 **Mechanism of activation of protein phosphorylation (and thereby glycogenolysis) in the liver via the α-adrenergic receptor.** Diacylglycerol (DAG) and inositol trisphosphate (IP$_3$) are second messengers mediating the α-adrenergic response. PIP$_2$, phosphatidylinositol bisphosphate; PKC, protein kinase C. See also Chapter 24.

plasma membrane epinephrine-specific receptor, G-proteins, and cAMP; and through an α-adrenergic receptor, which works by a different mechanism. Binding to α-receptors also involves G-proteins - common elements in hormone signal transduction - but in this case, the G-protein is specific for activation of a membrane isozyme of **phospholipase C (PLC),** which is specific for cleavage of a membrane phospholipid, **phosphatidylinositol bisphosphate (PIP$_2$)** (Fig. 12.5). Both products of PLC action, **diacylglycerol (DAG)** and **inositol trisphosphate (IP$_3$),** act as second messengers of epinephrine action. DAG activates **protein kinase C (PKC),** which, like PKA, initiates phosphorylation of serine and threonine residues on target proteins. Simultaneously, IP$_3$ promotes the transport of Ca^{2+} into the cytosol. Ca^{2+} then binds to the cytoplasmic protein calmodulin, which binds to and activates phosphorylase kinase directly, leading to cAMP-independent

phosphorylation and activation of phosphorylase. A Ca^{2+}–calmodulin-dependent protein kinase and other enzymes are also activated, either by phosphorylation or by association with the **Ca^{2+}–calmodulin complex** (Fig. 12.5). Thus an intricate web of metabolic pathways is activated in response to stress, focusing on those involved in the mobilization of energy reserves.

GLYCOGENOLYSIS IN MUSCLE

Muscle lacks a glucagon receptor and glucose-6-phosphatase; it is not a source of blood sugar during hypoglycemia

The tissue localization of hormone receptors provides specificity to hormone action. Only those tissues with glucagon receptors respond to glucagon. Muscle may be rich in glycogen, even during hypoglycemia, but it lacks both the glucagon receptor and Glc-6-Pase. Therefore muscle glycogen cannot be mobilized to replenish blood glucose. Muscle glycogenolysis is activated in response to epinephrine through the cAMP-dependent **β-adrenergic receptor,** but the glucose is metabolized through glycolysis for energy production. This occurs not only during fight-or-flight situations but also in response to metabolic demands during prolonged exercise. In addition to this hormonal regulation during stress, there are also two important hormone-independent mechanisms for activation of glycogenolysis in muscle (Fig. 12.6). First, the influx of Ca^{2+} into the muscle cytoplasm in response to nerve stimulation

activates the basal, unphosphorylated form of phosphorylase kinase by the action of the Ca^{2+}–calmodulin complex. This hormone-independent activation of phosphorylase provides for rapid activation of glycogenolysis during short bursts of exercise, even in the absence of epinephrine action. A second mechanism for activation of muscle glycogenolysis involves direct allosteric activation of phosphorylase by AMP. Increased usage of ATP during a rapid burst of muscle activity leads to rapid accumulation of ADP, which is converted in part into AMP by the action of the enzyme **myokinase (adenylate kinase),** which catalyzes the reaction:

$$2\,ADP \rightleftharpoons ATP + AMP$$

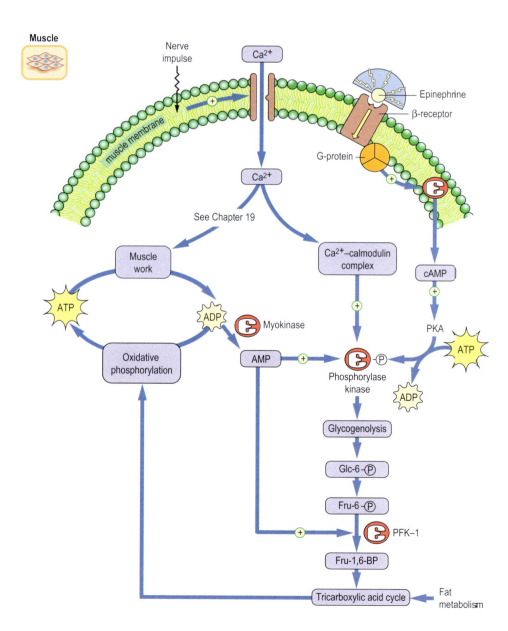

Fig. 12.6 **Regulation of protein kinase A (PKA) in muscle.** Activation of glycogenolysis and glycolysis in muscle during exercise. PFK-1, phosphofructokinase-1. Compare Fig. 8.4.

AMP activates both the basal and phosphorylated forms of phosphorylase, enhancing glycogenolysis in either the absence or the presence of hormonal stimulation. AMP also relieves inhibition of phosphofructokinase-1 (PFK-1) by ATP (see Chapter 9), stimulating the utilization of glucose through glycolysis for energy production. The stimulatory effects of Ca²⁺ and AMP ensure that the muscle can respond to its energy needs, even in the absence of hormonal input.

REGULATION OF GLYCOGENESIS

Insulin opposes the action of glucagon and stimulates gluconeogenesis

Glycogenesis, and energy storage in general, occurs during and immediately after meals. Glucose and other carbohydrates, rushing into the liver from the intestines via the portal circulation, are efficiently trapped to make glycogen. Excess glucose proceeds to the peripheral circulation, where it is taken up into muscle and adipose tissue for energy reserves or storage. We normally eat sitting down, rather than during exercise, so that the opposing pathways of uptake and storage versus mobilization and utilization of energy supplies are temporally compartmentalized functions in our lives.

Energy storage is under the control of the **polypeptide hormone insulin,** which is synthesized and stored in β-cells in the pancreatic islets of Langerhans (Chapter 30). Insulin is secreted in response to the rise in blood glucose after a meal, tracking blood glucose concentration. It has two primary functions in carbohydrate metabolism: first, insulin reverses the actions of glucagon in phosphorylation of proteins, turning off glycogen phosphorylase and activating glycogen synthase, promoting glucose storage; second, it stimulates the uptake of glucose into peripheral tissues (muscle and adipose tissue) through the GLUT-4 transporter, facilitating synthesis and storage of glycogen and triglycerides. Insulin also acts at the level of gene expression, stimulating the synthesis of enzymes involved in carbohydrate metabolism and storage and conversion of glucose into triglycerides. It also acts by more complex mechanisms as a growth hormone, stimulating protein synthesis and turnover during energy-rich conditions.

Protein tyrosine phosphorylation, rather than serine and threonine phosphorylation, is a characteristic feature of insulin and growth-factor signal transduction. Insulin binding to its transmembrane receptor (Fig. 12.7) stimulates dimerization of receptors, activating **tyrosine kinase** activity in the intracellular domain of the receptor. The insulin receptor **autophosphorylates** its tyrosine residues, enhancing its protein tyrosine kinase activity, and phosphorylates tyrosine residues in other intracellular effector proteins, which then activate secondary pathways. Among these are kinases that phosphorylate serine and threonine residues on proteins at sites and on proteins distinct from those phosphorylated by PKA and PKC. Insulin-dependent activation of GTPase, phosphodiesterase, and phosphoprotein phosphatases also checks the action of glucagon, which is typically present at high concentration in the blood at mealtimes - that is, several hours since the last meal.

The liver also appears to be directly responsive to ambient blood glucose concentration. The increase in hepatic glycogenesis begins more rapidly than the increase in insulin concentration in blood after a meal. Perfusion of the liver with glucose solutions in vitro, in the absence of insulin, also leads to inhibition of glycogenolysis and activation of glycogenesis. This appears to occur by direct allosteric inhibition of phosphorylase b by glucose and secondary stimulation of protein phosphatase activity.

Most, if not all, cells in the body are responsive to insulin in some way, but the major sites of insulin action, on a mass basis, are muscle and adipose tissue. These tissues normally have low levels of cell-surface glucose transporters, restricting the entry of glucose - they rely mostly on lipids for energy metabolism. In muscle and adipose tissue, insulin receptor tyrosine kinase activity induces movement of glucose transporter-4 (**GLUT-4**; see Table 4.2) from intracellular vacuoles to the cell surface, increasing glucose transport into the cell. The glucose is then used in muscle for the synthesis of glycogen and in adipose tissue to produce glyceraldehyde-3-phosphate, which is converted to glycerol-3-phosphate for the synthesis of triglycerides (Chapter 13). The insulin-stimulated, GLUT-4-mediated uptake of glucose into muscle and adipose tissue is the primary mechanism limiting the increase in blood glucose after a meal.

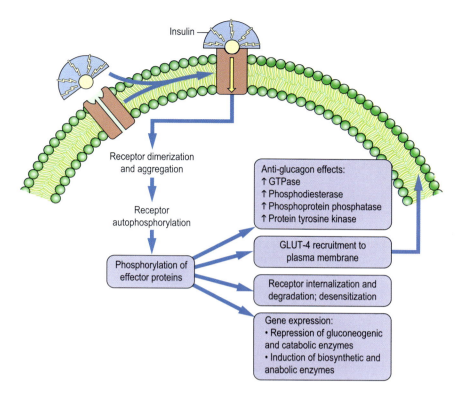

Fig. 12.7 **Mechanisms of insulin action.** Regulatory effects of insulin on hepatic and muscle carbohydrate metabolism. See also Chapter 30.

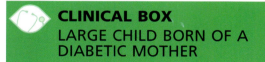

CLINICAL BOX
LARGE CHILD BORN OF A DIABETIC MOTHER

A baby boy, born of a poorly controlled, chronically hyperglycemic diabetic mother, was large and chubby (macrosomic) at birth (5 kg) but appeared otherwise normal. He declined rapidly, however, and within 1 h showed all the symptoms of hypoglycemia, similar to the case of a baby girl born of a malnourished mother (later in the chapter). The difference, in this case, was that the boy was obviously on the heavy side, rather than thin and malnourished.

Comment

This child has experienced a chronically hyperglycemic environment during uterine development. He adapted by increasing endogenous insulin production, which has a growth hormone–like activity, resulting in macrosomia. At birth, when placental delivery of glucose ceases, he has a normal blood glucose concentration and a substantial supply of hepatic glycogen. However, chronic hyperinsulinemia prior to birth probably represses gluconeogenic enzymes, and his high blood insulin concentration at birth promotes glucose uptake into muscle and adipose tissue. In the absence of a maternal source of glucose, insulin-induced hypoglycemia leads to a stress response, which was corrected by glucose infusion. After 1–2 days, his ample body mass will provide a good reservoir for the synthesis of blood glucose from muscle protein.

GLUCONEOGENESIS

Gluconeogenesis is required to maintain blood glucose during fasting and starvation

Unlike glycogenolysis, which can be turned on rapidly in response to hormonal stimulation, gluconeogenesis increases more slowly, depending on changes in gene expression, and reaches maximal activity over a period of hours (see Fig. 12.1); it becomes the primary source of our blood glucose concentration about 8 h into the postabsorptive state (Chapter 31). Gluconeogenesis requires both a source of energy for biosynthesis and a source of carbons for the formation of the backbone of the glucose molecule. The energy is provided by metabolism of fatty acids released from adipose tissue. The carbon skeletons are provided from three primary sources:

- Lactate produced in tissues such as the red cell and muscle
- Amino acids derived from muscle protein
- Glycerol released from triglycerides during lipolysis in adipose tissue

Among these, **muscle protein is the major precursor of blood glucose during fasting and starvation**; the rate of gluconeogenesis is often limited by the availability of substrate, including the rate of proteolysis in muscle or, in some cases, muscle mass. During prolonged fasting, malnutrition, or starvation, we lose both adipose and muscle mass. The fat is used for the general energy needs of the body and to support gluconeogenesis, whereas most of the amino acids in protein are converted into glucose. Urinary nitrogen (urea) excretion is also increased.

Gluconeogenesis from lactate

Gluconeogenesis uses lactate, amino acids, and glycerol as substrates for synthesis of glucose; fatty acids provide the energy

Gluconeogenesis from lactate is conceptually the opposite of anaerobic glycolysis but proceeds by a slightly different pathway, involving both mitochondrial and cytosolic enzymes (Fig. 12.8). During hepatic gluconeogenesis lactate is converted back into glucose, using, in part, the same glycolytic enzymes involved in the conversion of glucose into lactate. The lactate cycle involving the liver, red cells, and muscle, known as the **Cori cycle**, is discussed in detail in Chapter 31. At this point, we focus on the metabolic pathway for conversion of lactate to glucose.

A critical problem in the reversal of glycolysis is overcoming the irreversibility of three kinase reactions: **glucokinase (GK), phosphofructokinase-1 (PFK-1), and pyruvate kinase (PK)**. The fourth kinase in glycolysis, phosphoglycerate kinase (PGK), catalyzes a freely reversible equilibrium reaction: a substrate-level phosphorylation reaction, transferring a high-energy acyl phosphate in 1,3-bisphosphoglycerate to an energetically similar pyrophosphate bond in ATP. **To circumvent the three irreversible reactions in glycolysis, the liver uses four unique enzymes: pyruvate carboxylase (PC) in the mitochondrion and phosphoenolpyruvate carboxykinase (PEPCK) in the cytoplasm to bypass PK, fructose-1,6-bisphosphatase (Fru-1,6-BPase) to bypass PFK-1, and Glc-6-Pase to bypass GK** (see Fig. 12.8).

Gluconeogenesis from lactate involves its conversion into phosphoenolpyruvate (PEP), a process requiring investment of two ATP equivalents to form the high-energy enol–phosphate bond in PEP. Lactate is first converted into pyruvate by lactate dehydrogenase (LDH) and then enters the mitochondrion, where it is converted to oxaloacetate by PC, using **biotin** and ATP. Oxaloacetate is reduced to malate by the tricarboxylic acid (TCA)-cycle enzyme malate dehydrogenase, exits the mitochondrion, and is then reoxidized to oxaloacetate by cytosolic malate dehydrogenase. The cytosolic oxaloacetate is then decarboxylated by PEPCK, using GTP as a cosubstrate, yielding PEP. The energy for synthesis of PEP from oxaloacetate is derived from both the hydrolysis of GTP and the decarboxylation of oxaloacetate.

Glycolysis may now proceed backward from PEP until it reaches the next irreversible reaction, PFK-1. This enzyme is bypassed by a simple hydrolysis reaction, catalyzed by Fru-1,6-BPase without production of ATP, reversing the PFK-1 reaction and producing Fru-6-P. Similarly, the bypass of GK is accomplished by hydrolysis of Glc-6-P by Glc-6-Pase, without

production of ATP. The free glucose is then released from the liver into the blood.

Gluconeogenesis is fairly efficient - the liver can make a kilogram of glucose per day by gluconeogenesis and actually does so in poorly controlled, hyperglycemic diabetic patients. Normal glucose production, in the absence of dietary carbohydrate, is ~200 g/day, almost a half-pound of glucose. Gluconeogenesis from pyruvate is moderately expensive, requiring a net expenditure of the equivalent of 4 moles of ATP per mole of pyruvate converted into glucose (i.e., 2 mole ATP at the PC reaction and 2 moles of GTP at the PEPCK reaction). The ATP and GTP are provided by oxidation of fatty acids (Chapter 11).

Gluconeogenesis from amino acids and glycerol

Most amino acids are **glucogenic** (Chapter 15) - that is, after deamination, their carbon skeletons can be converted into glucose. **Alanine and glutamine are the major amino acids exported from muscle for gluconeogenesis.** Their relative concentrations in venous blood from muscle exceed their relative concentration in muscle protein, indicating considerable reshuffling of muscle amino acids to provide gluconeogenic substrates. As discussed in more detail in Chapter 15, alanine is converted directly into pyruvate by the enzyme alanine aminotransferase **(alanine transaminase [ALT])**, and then gluconeogenesis proceeds as described for lactate. Other amino acids are converted into TCA-cycle intermediates, then to malate for gluconeogenesis. Aspartate, for example, is converted into oxaloacetate by aspartate aminotransferase **(aspartate transaminase [AST])**, and glutamate into α-ketoglutarate by glutamate dehydrogenase. Some glucogenic amino acids are converted by less direct routes into alanine or intermediates in the TCA cycle for gluconeogenesis. The amino groups of these amino acids are converted into urea via the **urea cycle** in hepatocytes, and the urea is excreted in urine (Chapter 15).

Glycerol enters gluconeogenesis at the level of triose phosphates (see Fig. 12.8). After release of glycerol and fatty acids from adipose tissue into the plasma, the glycerol is taken up into the liver and phosphorylated by **glycerol kinase.** After the action of glycerol-3-phosphate dehydrogenase (see Fig. 8.7), glycerol enters the gluconeogenic pathway as dihydroxyacetone phosphate. Only the glycerol component of fats can be converted into glucose. Because PC and PEPCK are not required, incorporation of glycerol into glucose requires only 2 moles of ATP per mole of glucose produced.

Glucose cannot be synthesized from fatty acids!

As discussed in Chapter 11, metabolism of fatty acids involves their conversion in two carbon oxidation steps to form

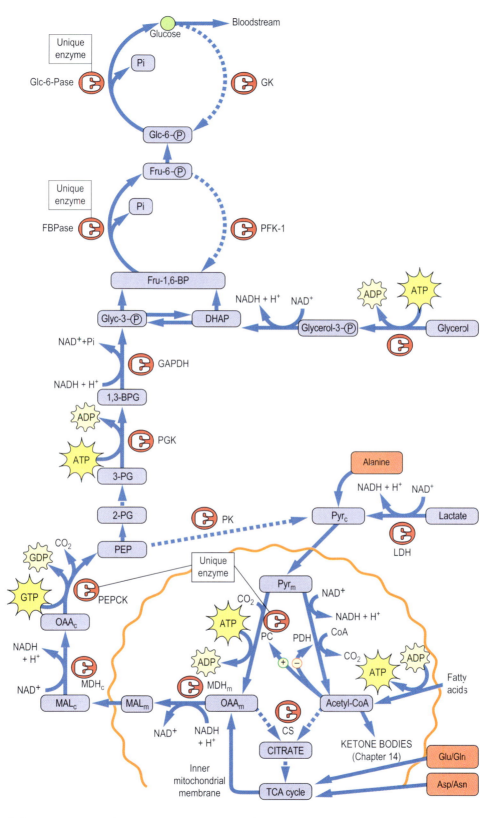

Fig. 12.8 **Pathway of gluconeogenesis.** Gluconeogenesis is the reverse of glycolysis. Unique enzymes overcome the irreversible kinase reactions of glycolysis. **Compartments:** c, cytoplasmic; imm, inner mitochondrial membrane; m, mitochondrial. **Enzymes:** CS, citrate synthase; Fru-1,6-BPase, fructose-1,6-bisphosphatase; GAPDH, glyceraldehyde-3-P dehydrogenase; Glc-6-Pase, glucose-6-phosphatase; GK, glucokinase; MDH, malate dehydrogenase; PC, pyruvate carboxylase; PDH, pyruvate dehydrogenase; PGK, phosphoglycerate kinase. **Substrates:** 2,3-BPG, bisphosphoglycerate; DHAP, dihydroxyacetone phosphate; Fru-1,6-BP, fructose-1,6-bisphosphate; Glyc-3-P, glyceraldehyde 3-phosphate; MAL, malate; OAA, oxaloacetate; PEP, phosphoenolpyruvate; PEPCK, PEP carboxykinase; Pyr, pyruvate; 3-PG, 3-phosphoglycerate. *Solid lines:* active during gluconeogenesis. *Dotted lines:* inactive during gluconeogenesis.

CLINICAL BOX
CHILD BORN OF MALNOURISHED MOTHER MAY HAVE HYPOGLYCEMIA

A baby girl was born at 39 weeks of gestation to a young, malnourished mother. The child was also thin and weak at birth and within 1 h after birth was showing signs of distress, including rapid heartbeat and respiration. Her blood glucose was 3.5 mmol/L (63 mg/dL) at birth and declined rapidly to 1.5 mmol/L (27 mg/dL) by 1 h, when she was becoming unresponsive and comatose. Her condition was markedly improved by the infusion of a glucose solution, followed by a carbohydrate-rich diet. She improved gradually over the next 2 weeks before discharge from the hospital.

Comment

During development in utero, the fetus obtains glucose exogenously from the placental circulation. However, after birth, the child relies at first on the mobilization of hepatic glycogen and then on gluconeogenesis for maintenance of blood glucose. Because of the malnourished state of the mother, this child was born with negligible hepatic glycogen reserves. Thus she was unable to maintain blood glucose homeostasis postpartum and rapidly declined into hypoglycemia, initiating a stress response. After surviving the transient hypoglycemia, she probably still lacked adequate muscle mass to provide a sufficient supply of amino acids for gluconeogenesis. Infusion of glucose, followed by a carbohydrate-rich diet, would address these deficits, but may not correct more serious damage from prolonged malnutrition during fetal development.

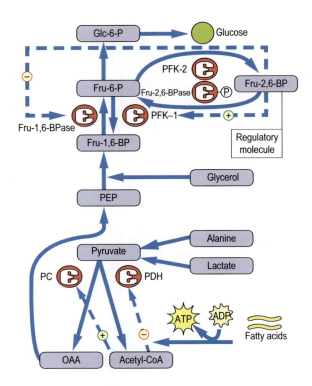

Fig. 12.9 **Regulation of gluconeogenesis.** Gluconeogenesis is regulated by hepatic levels of Fru-2,6-BP and acetyl-CoA. The upper part of the diagram focuses on the reciprocal regulation of Fru-1,6-BPase and PFK-1 by Fru-2,6-BP and the lower part on the reciprocal regulation of pyruvate dehydrogenase (PDH) and pyruvate carboxylase (PC) by acetyl-CoA.

acetyl-CoA, which is then metabolized in the TCA cycle after condensation with oxaloacetate to form citrate. Although the carbons of acetate are theoretically available for gluconeogenesis, during the pathway from citrate to malate, two molecules of CO_2 are eliminated at the isocitrate and α-ketoglutarate dehydrogenase reactions. Thus although energy is produced in the TCA cycle, the two carbons invested for gluconeogenesis from acetyl-CoA are lost as CO_2. For this reason, acetyl-CoA - and therefore even-chain fatty acids - cannot serve as substrates for *net* gluconeogenesis. However, odd-chain and branched-chain fatty acids, which form propionyl-CoA, can serve as minor precursors for gluconeogenesis. Propionyl-CoA is first carboxylated to methylmalonyl-CoA, which undergoes racemase and mutase reactions to form succinyl-CoA, a tricarboxylic acid cycle intermediate (see Chapter 11). Succinyl-CoA is converted into malate, which exits the mitochondrion and is oxidized to oxaloacetate. After decarboxylation by PEPCK, the three carbons of propionate are conserved in PEP and glucose.

Regulation of gluconeogenesis

Fructose-2,6-bisphosphate allosterically counterregulates glycolysis and gluconeogenesis

Like glycogen metabolism in liver, gluconeogenesis is regulated primarily by hormonal mechanisms. In this case, the regulatory process involves counterregulation of glycolysis and gluconeogenesis, largely by phosphorylation/dephosphorylation of enzymes, under the control of glucagon and insulin. The primary control points are the regulatory enzymes PFK-1 and Fru-1,6-BPase, which, in the liver, are exquisitely sensitive to the allosteric effector **fructose 2,6-bisphosphate (Fru-2,6-BP).** Fru-2,6-BP is an activator of PFK-1 and an inhibitor of Fru-1,6-BPase, counterregulating the two opposing pathways. As shown in Fig. 12.9, Fru-2,6-BP is synthesized by an unusual **bifunctional enzyme, phosphofructokinase-2/fructose-2,6-bisphosphatase (PFK-2/Fru-2,6-BPase),** which has both kinase and phosphatase activities. In the phosphorylated state, effected by glucagon through protein kinase A, this enzyme displays Fru-2,6-BPase activity, which reduces the level of Fru-2,6-BP. The decrease in Fru-2,6-BP simultaneously decreases the stimulation of glycolysis at PFK-1 and relieves inhibition of gluconeogenesis at Fru-1,6-BPase. In this way, glucagon-mediated phosphorylation of PFK-2/Fru-2,6-BP places the liver cell in a gluconeogenic mode. The coordinate, allosterically mediated increase in Fru-1,6-BPase and decrease in PFK-1 activities ensure that glucose made by gluconeogenesis is not consumed by glycolysis in a futile cycle but released into the blood by Glc-6-Pase. Similarly, any flux of glucose from glycogen through glycogenolysis, also induced by glucagon, is diverted to the blood, rather than to glycolysis, by inhibition of PFK-1. PK is also inhibited by phosphorylation by protein kinase A (PKA), providing an additional site for inhibition of glycolysis (Fig. 12.9).

When glucose enters the liver after a meal, **insulin** mediates the dephosphorylation of PFK-2/Fru-2,6-BPase, turning on its PFK-2 activity. The resultant increase in Fru-2,6-BP activates PFK-1 and inhibits Fru-1,6-BPase activity. Gluconeogenesis is inhibited, and glucose entering the liver is then incorporated into glycogen or routed into glycolysis for lipogenesis. Thus liver metabolism after a meal is focused on synthesis and storage of both carbohydrate and lipid energy reserves, which are used later - in the postabsorptive state - for maintenance of blood glucose and fatty acid homeostasis.

Gluconeogenesis is also regulated in the mitochondrion by acetyl-CoA. The increase in plasma fatty acids from adipose tissue, stimulated by glucagon to support gluconeogenesis (see Chapter 11), leads to an increase in hepatic acetyl-CoA, which is both an inhibitor of pyruvate dehydrogenase (PDH) and an essential allosteric activator of pyruvate carboxylase (PC; see Fig. 12.8). In this way, fat metabolism inhibits the oxidation of pyruvate and favors its use for gluconeogenesis in liver. In muscle during the fasting state, glucose utilization for energy metabolism is limited both by the low level of GLUT-4 in the plasma membranes (because of the low plasma insulin concentration) and by inhibition of PDH by acetyl-CoA. Active fat metabolism and high levels of acetyl-CoA in muscle promote the excretion of a significant fraction of pyruvate as lactate, even in the resting state. The carbon skeleton of glucose is returned to the liver via the Cori cycle (Chapter 31), and recycling of pyruvate into glucose, in effect, conserves muscle protein.

Conversion of fructose and galactose to glucose

As discussed in detail in Chapter 17, fructose is metabolized almost exclusively in the liver by the enzyme fructokinase. Fructose enters glycolysis at the level of triose phosphates, bypassing the regulatory enzyme, PFK-1. After consumption of fruit juices, Gatorade, or foods containing high-fructose corn syrup, large amounts of pyruvate may be forced on the mitochondrion for use in energy metabolism or fat biosynthesis. During a gluconeogenic state, this fructose may also proceed toward Glc-6-P, providing a convenient source of blood glucose. Gluconeogenesis from galactose is equally efficient because

Glc-1-P, derived from galactose 1-phosphate (Chapter 17), is readily isomerized to Glc-6-P by phosphoglucomutase. Fructose and galactose are good sources of glucose, independent of glycogenolysis and gluconeogenesis.

SUMMARY

- Glycogen is stored in two tissues in the body for different reasons: in the liver for short-term maintenance of blood glucose homeostasis and in muscle as a source of energy. Glycogen metabolism in these tissues responds rapidly to both allosteric and hormonal control.
- In the liver, the balance between glycogenolysis and glycogenesis is regulated by the balance between concentrations of glucagon and insulin in the circulation, which controls the state of phosphorylation of enzymes.
- Phosphorylation of enzymes under the influence of glucagon directs glycogen mobilization and is the most common condition in the liver (e.g., during sleep and between meals).
- Increases in blood insulin during and after meals promote dephosphorylation of the same enzymes, leading to glycogenesis. Insulin also promotes glucose uptake into muscle and adipose tissue for glycogen and triglyceride synthesis after a meal.
- Epinephrine increases phosphorylation of liver enzymes, enabling a burst in hepatic glycogenolysis and an increase in blood glucose for stress responses.
- Muscle is responsive to epinephrine but not to glucagon; in this case, the glucose produced by glycogenolysis is used for muscle energy metabolism - fight or flight. In addition, muscle glycogenolysis is responsive to intracellular Ca^{2+} and AMP concentrations, providing a hormone-independent mechanism for coupling glycogenolysis to normal energy consumption during exercise.
- Gluconeogenesis takes place primarily in the liver and is designed for maintenance of blood glucose during the fasting state. It is essential after 12 h of fasting, when the majority of hepatic glycogen has been consumed.
- The major substrates for gluconeogenesis are lactate, amino acids, and glycerol; fatty acid metabolism provides the energy. The major control point is at the level of phosphofructokinase-1 (PFK-1), which is activated by the allosteric effector Fru-2,6-BP.
- The synthesis of Fru-2,6-BP is under control of the bifunctional enzyme PFK-2/Fru-2,6-BPase, whose kinase and phosphatase activities are regulated by phosphorylation/dephosphorylation, under hormonal control by glucagon and insulin.

Table 12.5 General features of hormone action

1. Tissue specificity, determined by receptor distribution
2. Multistep, cascade amplification
3. Intracellular second messengers
4. Coordinate counterregulation of opposing pathways
5. Augmentation and/or opposition by other hormones
6. Multiple mechanisms of termination of response

Hormonal regulation of glucose metabolism illustrates fundamental principles of hormone action (see Chapter 27).

ACTIVE LEARNING

1. The inactivation of glycogenesis in response to epinephrine occurs in a single step by the action of PKA on glycogen synthase, whereas the activation of glycogenolysis involves an intermediate enzyme, phosphorylate kinase, which phosphorylates phosphorylase. Discuss the metabolic (dis) advantages of the two-step activation of glycogenolysis.
2. Investigate the use of inhibitors of gluconeogenesis for the treatment of type 2 diabetes.
3. Glucose-6-phosphatase is essential for the production of glucose in the liver but is not a cytosolic enzyme. Describe the activity and subcellular localization of this enzyme and the final stages of the pathway for production of glucose in the liver.
4. Discuss the rationale for both hormone-dependent and hormone-independent mechanisms of regulation of glycogen and glucose metabolism.

■ During fasting and active gluconeogenesis, glucagon mediates phosphorylation and activation of the phosphatase activity of PFK-2/Fru-2,6-BPase, leading to a decrease in the level of Fru-2,6-BP and a corresponding decrease in glycolysis; carbohydrate degradation is inhibited, and fats become the primary energy source during fasting and starvation. Oxidation of pyruvate is also inhibited in the mitochondrion by inhibition of PDH by acetyl-CoA, derived from fat metabolism.

■ After a meal, the decrease in phosphorylation of enzymes enhances PFK-2 activity; the increase in Fru-2,6-BP concentration activates PFK-1 and promotes glycolysis, providing pyruvate, which is converted to acetyl-CoA for lipogenesis. The actions of insulin, glucagon, and epinephrine illustrate many of the fundamental principles of hormone action (Table 12.5).

FURTHER READING

Adeva-Andany, M. M., González-Lucán, M., Donapetry-García, C., et al. (2016). Glycogen metabolism in humans. *BBA Clinical*, *5*, 85–100.

Bhattacharya, K. (2015). Investigation and management of the hepatic glycogen storage diseases. *Translational Pediatrics*, *4*, 240–248.

Chou, J. Y., Jun, H. S., & Mansfield, B. C. (2015). Type I glycogen storage diseases: Disorders of the glucose-6-phosphatase/glucose-6-phosphate transporter complexes. *Journal of Inherited Metabolic Disease*, *38*, 511–519.

Godfrey, R., & Quinlivan, R. (2016). Skeletal muscle disorders of glycogenolysis and glycolysis. *Nature Reviews. Neurology*, *12*, 393–402.

Kishnani, P. S., & Beckemeyer, A. A. (2014). New therapeutic approaches for Pompe disease: Enzyme replacement therapy and beyond. *Pediatric Endocrinology Reviews*, *12*(Suppl. 1), 114–124.

Ravnskjaer, K., Madiraju, A., & Montminy, M. (2016). Role of the cAMP Pathway in Glucose and Lipid Metabolism. *Handbook of Experimental Pharmacology*, *233*, 29–49.

RELEVANT WEBSITES

Glycogen: http://themedicalbiochemistrypage.org/glycogen.php
Glycogen storage diseases: http://emedicine.medscape.com/article/1116574-overview

ABBREVIATIONS

ALT	Alanine transaminase
AST	Aspartate transaminase
DAG	Diacylglycerol
Fru-1,6-BPase	Fructose-1,6-bisphosphatase
Fru-2,6-BPase	Fructose-2,6-bisphosphatase
GK	Glucokinase
Glc-6-Pase	Glucose-6-phosphatase
IP_3	Inositol trisphosphate
PC	Pyruvate carboxylase
PDH	Pyruvate dehydrogenase
PEP	Phosphoenolpyruvate
PEPCK	Phosphoenolpyruvate carboxykinase
PIP_2	Phosphatidylinositol bisphosphate
PFK	Phosphofructokinase
PFK-2/Fru-2,6-BPase	Phosphofructokinase-2/fructose-2, 6-bisphosphatase
PK	Pyruvate kinase
PKA	Protein kinase A
PKC	Protein kinase C
PPi	Pyrophosphate
UDP-Glc	Uridinediphosphate-glucose

13 Biosynthesis and Storage of Fatty Acids

Fredrik Karpe and Iain Broom

LEARNING OBJECTIVES

After reading this chapter, you should be able to:

- Describe the pathway of fatty acid synthesis, particularly the roles of acetyl-CoA carboxylase and the multifunctional enzyme fatty acid synthase.
- Outline short-term and long-term regulation of fatty acid synthesis.
- Explain the concepts of elongation and desaturation of the fatty acid chain.
- Describe the synthesis of triglycerides.
- Discuss the endocrine function of adipose tissue.

INTRODUCTION

Most fatty acids required by humans are supplied in the diet; however, the pathway for their de novo synthesis (**lipogenesis**) from two-carbon compounds is present in many tissues, such as liver, brain, kidney, mammary gland, and adipose tissue. It is also highly active in many cancers. In general, the pathway of de novo synthesis is **primarily active in situations of excess energy intake**, particularly in the form of excess carbohydrate. In this situation, carbohydrates and, to a lesser extent, amino acid precursors are converted to fatty acids, primarily in the liver but also in adipose tissue, and stored as **triacylglycerol** (TAG, also known as **triglyceride**) in cellular lipid droplets. The process is called de novo lipogenesis (DNL). Fatty acids generated through DNL in the liver will need to be transported to the tissue dedicated for long-term storage (i.e., adipose tissue). In the event this transport is not efficient enough, TAG will accumulate in the tissue not dedicated for fat storage; this is one process by which **"ectopic" lipid storage** can take place. The adipocyte in adipose tissue is dedicated to the storage of large quantities of TAG enabled by compartmentalization of TAG into a large intracellular unilocular lipid droplet with a machinery ensuring controlled uptake and release of fatty acids. This provides safe storage for large quantities of fatty acids.

The pathway for lipogenesis is not simply the reverse of oxidation of fatty acids (Chapter 11). Lipogenesis requires a completely different set of enzymes and is located in a different cellular compartment, the **cytosol**. Furthermore, it uses reduced nicotinamide adenine dinucleotide phosphate (NADPH) as a source of reductive power, as opposed to the nicotinamide adenine dinucleotide (NAD$^+$) required for β-oxidation.

The sterol regulatory element-binding proteins-1 (mainly SREBP1c but also SREBP1a) provide a master regulation of de novo lipogenesis through transcriptional control. The SREBP is an endoplasmic-reticulum-bound and membrane-sensing protein that undergoes proteolytic cleavage, enabling its transport to the nucleus. In the nucleus, SREBP binds to specific DNA sequences (the sterol regulatory elements or SRE) located in the control regions of the genes that encode enzymes needed for lipogenesis.

FATTY ACID SYNTHESIS

Fatty acids are synthesized from acetyl-CoA

The synthesis of fatty acids in mammalian systems can be considered as a two-stage process, with both stages requiring acetyl-CoA units and both employing multifunctional proteins in multienzyme complexes.

- Stage 1 is the formation of the key precursor malonyl-CoA from acetyl-CoA by acetyl-CoA carboxylase.
- Stage 2 is the elongation of the fatty acid chain in two-carbon increments by fatty acid synthase.

Note that the term lipogenesis is also used to cover both fatty acid synthesis and triacylglycerol (triglyceride) synthesis.

The preparatory stage: Acetyl-CoA carboxylase

Carboxylation of acetyl-CoA to malonyl-CoA is the committed step of fatty acid synthesis

In the first stage of fatty acid biosynthesis, acetyl-CoA, **mostly derived from carbohydrate metabolism**, is converted to malonyl-CoA by the action of the enzyme acetyl-CoA carboxylase (Fig. 13.1). There are two forms of acetyl-CoA carboxylase (ACC1 and ACC2). **ACC1 is located in the cytoplasm and committed to fatty acid synthesis**, whereas **ACC2 is in mitochondria, where it regulates fatty acid oxidation**. ACC2 inhibition results in reduced generation of malonyl-CoA, which in turn is an inhibitor of the carnitine-palmitoyl transferase 1 (CPT-1) allowing fatty acid uptake by the mitochondria. Through this inhibition, the fatty acid oxidation is reduced. ACC1 is a biotin-dependent enzyme with distinct enzymatic and carrier-protein function: its subunits

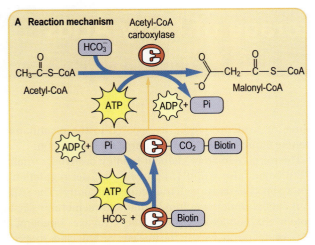

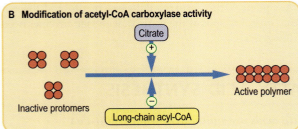

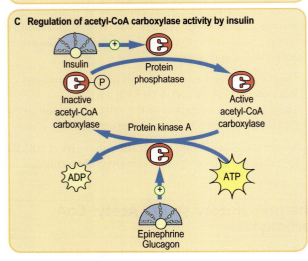

Fig. 13.1 **Conversion of acetyl-CoA to malonyl-CoA.** (A) Reaction catalyzed by the acetyl-CoA carboxylase. The enzyme has the covalently attached biotin, which is carboxylated using a molecule of ATP. (B) Acetyl-CoA carboxylase requires the presence of citrate for polymerization to its active form. (C) The activity of acetyl-CoA carboxylase is regulated by a phosphorylation–dephosphorylation mechanism. This in turn is controlled by hormones that regulate fuel metabolism: insulin, glucagon, and epinephrine.

serve as a biotin carboxylase, transcarboxylase, and biotin carboxyl carrier protein. The enzyme is synthesized in an inactive protomer form, with each protomer containing all of the previously described subunits, a molecule of biotin, and a regulatory allosteric site for the binding of citrate (a Krebs cycle metabolite) or palmitoyl-CoA (the end product of the

fatty acid biosynthetic pathway). The reaction itself takes place in stages: first, there is the carboxylation of biotin, involving adenosine triphosphate (ATP), followed by the transfer of this carboxyl group to acetyl-CoA to produce the malonyl-CoA. At this stage, the free enzyme–biotin complex is released.

As described previously, this process only allows the building up of fatty acid molecules with even numbers of carbon atoms, which is seen in eukaryote cells. However, propionyl-CoA is a substrate for the synthesis of fatty acids with an odd number of carbon atoms, but this is not seen in humans. Typically, the odd-chain fatty acids seen in humans originate from milk fat consumption because the bacterial/fermentation process in ruminants allows for the production of these fatty acids.

Acetyl-CoA carboxylase is subject to strict regulation

The protomers of acetyl-CoA carboxylase polymerize in the presence of **citrate** or **isocitrate**, producing the active form of the enzyme. The polymerization is inhibited by **palmitoyl-CoA** binding to the same allosteric site. The respective stimulatory and inhibitory effects of citrate and palmitoyl-CoA are entirely logical: under conditions of high citrate concentration, energy storage is desirable, but when palmitoyl-CoA, the product of the pathway, accumulates, a decrease in the synthesis of fatty acids is appropriate. There is an additional control mechanism, independent of the citrate or palmitoyl-CoA, involving phosphorylation and dephosphorylation of the enzyme molecule. This involves hormone-dependent protein phosphatase/kinase (Fig. 13.1). **Phosphorylation inhibits the enzyme, and dephosphorylation activates it.** Phosphorylation of the enzyme is promoted by glucagon or epinephrine, and dephosphorylation is promoted by the insulin, which is a lipogenic hormone. **Phosphorylation is also dependent on the activation of the AMP-activated protein kinase (AMPK).** Activated AMPK, as a sign of cellular depletion of ATP, will inhibit ACC2 and activate malonyl-CoA decarboxylase to alleviate the malonyl-CoA-dependent inhibition of CPT-1 and thereby allow mitochondrial fatty acid oxidation.

Dietary carbohydrate and fat intake also controls acetyl-CoA carboxylase

The carboxylation of acetyl-CoA to malonyl-CoA commits the pathway to fatty acid synthesis. This is why this enzyme is under such strict short-term control. Longer-term control is exerted by the induction or repression of enzyme synthesis affected by diet: synthesis of acetyl-CoA carboxylase is upregulated under conditions of high-carbohydrate/low-fat intake, whereas starvation or high-fat/low-carbohydrate intake leads to downregulation of synthesis of the enzyme.

Synthesizing a fatty acid chain: Fatty acid synthase

The second major step in fatty acid synthesis also involves a multienzyme complex, the fatty acid synthase. This enzyme

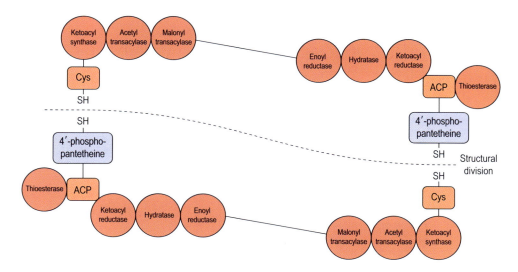

Fig. 13.2 **Structure of fatty acid synthase.** Fatty acid synthase is a dimer consisting of two large subunits arranged head to tail. It contains seven distinct enzyme activities and an acyl carrier protein (ACP). Cys, cysteine.

system is much more complex than acetyl-CoA carboxylase. The protein contains **seven distinct enzyme activities** and an **acyl carrier protein (ACP).** ACP, a highly conserved protein, replaces CoA as the entity that binds to the elongating fatty acid chain. The structure of this molecule is shown in Fig. 13.2 and consists of a dimer of large identical polypeptides arranged head to tail. Each monomer contains all seven enzyme activities and the ACP. It also contains a long **pantetheine group** that acts as a flexible "arm," making the molecule being synthesized available to different enzymes in the fatty acid synthetase complex. The function in fatty acid synthesis is shared between the two polypeptide chains.

Fatty acid synthase builds the fatty acid molecule up to 16-carbon length

The reaction proceeds after an initial priming of the cysteine (Cys-SH) group with acetyl-CoA, a reaction catalyzed by **acetyl transacylase** (Fig. 13.3). Then malonyl-CoA is transferred by **malonyl transacylase** to the -SH residue of the pantetheine group attached to the ACP in the other subunit. Next, **3-ketoacyl synthase** (the condensing enzyme) catalyzes the reaction between the previously attached acetyl group and the malonyl residue, liberating CO_2 and forming the 3-ketoacyl enzyme complex. This frees the cysteine residue on chain 1 that had been occupied by the acetyl-CoA. The 3-ketoacyl group subsequently undergoes sequential reduction, dehydration, and again reduction to form a saturated acyl–enzyme complex. The next molecule of malonyl-CoA displaces the acyl group from the pantetheine-SH group to the now free cysteine group, and the reaction sequence is repeated through six more cycles (seven cycles altogether). Once the 16-carbon chain (palmitate) is formed, the saturated acyl–enzyme complex activates the **thioesterase,** releasing the molecule

of palmitate from the enzyme complex. The two -SH sites are now free, allowing another cycle of palmitate synthesis to be initiated.

The synthesis of one palmitate molecule requires 8 molecules of acetyl-CoA, 7 ATP, 14 NADPH, and 14 H^+:

$$8Ac\text{-}CoA + 7ATP + 14NADPH + 14H^+$$
$$\rightarrow CH_3(CH_2)_{14}COO^- \text{ (palmitate)} + 14NADP^+ + 8CoA$$
$$+ 6H_2O + 7ADP + 7Pi + 7CO_2$$

In common with the acetyl-CoA carboxylase system, fatty acid synthase is also regulated by the presence of phosphorylated sugars via an allosteric effect as well as by induction and repression of the enzyme.

Alteration in the amount of enzyme protein is affected by the nutritional state

Rates of fatty acid synthesis are greatest when an individual follows a hypercaloric, high-carbohydrate/low-fat diet and are low during fasting/starvation or when eating a high-fat diet.

The malate shuttle

Malate shuttle allows recruitment of two-carbon units from the mitochondrion to the cytoplasm

The primary molecule required for the synthesis of fatty acids is acetyl-CoA. However, acetyl-CoA is generated in the mitochondria and cannot freely cross the inner mitochondrial membrane. As noted previously, fatty acid biosynthesis occurs in the cytosol. The malate shuttle is a mechanism allowing the transfer of two-carbon units from the mitochondria to the cytosol; it involves the **malate–citrate antiporter** (Fig. 13.4).

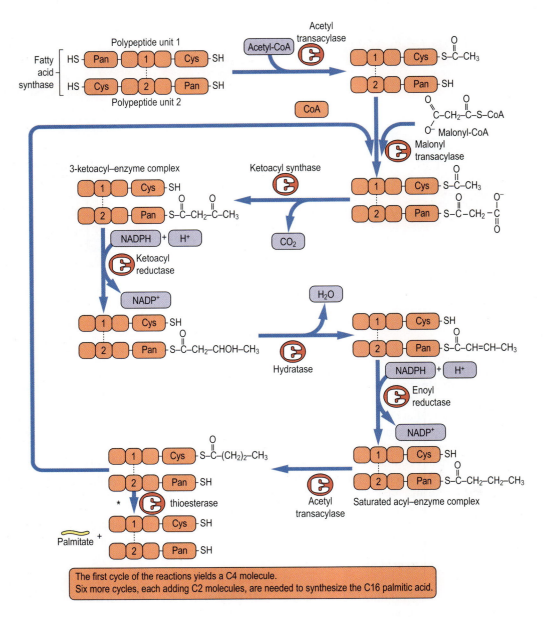

Fig. 13.3 **Reactions catalyzed by fatty acid synthase.** The synthesis of a fatty acid chain is initiated by a molecule of malonyl-CoA (C3), which reacts with the first molecule of acetyl-CoA (C2); this produces a C4 molecule (one carbon is lost as CO_2 during condensation of malonyl-CoA and acetyl-CoA). There are six more cycles, each adding 2C unit to the fatty acid chain (seven cycles altogether), and the result is a 16-carbon molecule of palmitate. NADPH, Reduced nicotinamide adenine dinucleotide phosphate; Pan, pantetheine. *This reaction occurs once the 16-carbon fatty acyl chain has been formed.

Pyruvate derived from glycolysis is decarboxylated to acetyl-CoA in the mitochondria; it subsequently reacts with oxaloacetate in the tricarboxylic acid (TCA) cycle (Chapter 10) to form citrate. Translocation of a molecule of citrate to the cytosol via the antiporter is accompanied by the transfer of a molecule of malate to the mitochondrion. In the cytosol, **citrate, in the presence of ATP and CoA, undergoes cleavage to acetyl-CoA and oxaloacetate by citrate lyase**. This makes acetyl-CoA available for carboxylation to malonyl-CoA and for the synthesis of fatty acids. The synthesis of fatty acids is also linked to glucose metabolism through the **pentose phosphate pathway,** which is the main provider of NADPH required for lipogenesis. Fructose is specifically channeled through this pathway and is very lipogenic. Some NADPH is also generated by the NADP+-linked decarboxylation of malate to pyruvate by the malic enzyme.

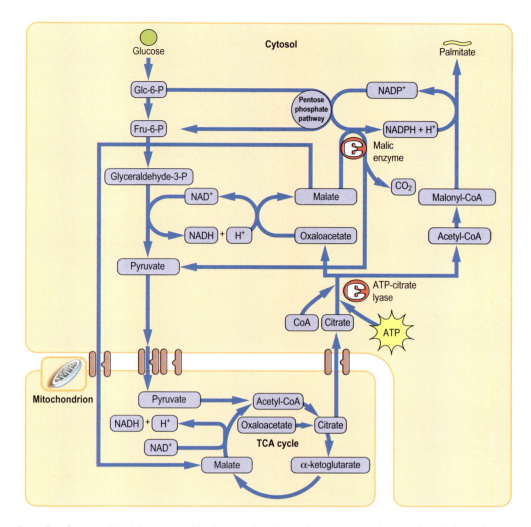

Fig. 13.4 **The malate shuttle.** Acetyl-CoA is generated in the mitochondria and cannot cross the mitochondrial membrane. The malate shuttle facilitates the transport of two-carbon units from the mitochondria to cytoplasm. Citrate, synthesized from acetyl-CoA and oxalate, is transported out of the mitochondria. In the cytosol, it is split back into acetyl-CoA and oxalate. Oxalate is then converted to malate, which returns to the mitochondrion - thus the "shuttle." Acetyl-CoA is resynthesized in the cytoplasm and enters lipogenesis. Note also the generation of NADPH in the pentose phosphate pathway and by the malic enzyme. Fru-6-P, fructose-6-phosphate; Glc-6-P, glucose-6-phosphate; NADH, reduced nicotinamide adenine dinucleotide.

 ADVANCED CONCEPT BOX

CHANGES IN ENZYME EXPRESSION IN RESPONSE TO FOOD INTAKE REGULATE STORAGE OF ENERGY SUBSTRATES

The fed state is associated with the induction of enzymes that increase fatty acid synthesis in the liver. Several enzymes are induced, including those involved in glycolysis (e.g., glucokinase [the hepatic form of hexokinase] and pyruvate kinase) as well as enzymes linked to increased production of NADPH (glucose-6-P dehydrogenase, 6-phosphogluconate dehydrogenase, and malic enzyme). Further, there is an increased expression of citrate lyase, acetyl-CoA carboxylase, fatty acid synthase, and Δ^9 desaturase.

Also, in the fed state, there is a concomitant repression of the key enzymes involved in gluconeogenesis. Phosphoenolpyruvate carboxykinase, glucose-6-phosphatase, and some aminotransferases are reduced in amount, either by a reduction in synthesis or by increased degradation (Chapter 31).

Fatty acid elongation

Elongation of a fatty acid chain beyond 16-carbon length requires another set of enzymes

Palmitate released from fatty acid synthase becomes a substrate for the synthesis of longer-chain fatty acids, with the exception of certain essential fatty acids (see following discussion). Chain elongation occurs by the addition of further two-carbon fragments derived from malonyl-CoA (Fig. 13.5). This process occurs on the endoplasmic reticulum by the action of yet another multienzyme complex: **fatty acid elongase**. The reactions occurring during chain elongation are similar to those involved in fatty acid synthesis, except that the fatty acid is attached to CoA rather than to the ACP. In fact, there are seven discrete fatty acid elongases with different tissue expressions and substrate specificities (ELOVL1-7; ELOVL stands for "elongation of very-long-chain fatty acids").

The substrates for the cytosolic fatty acid elongase include saturated fatty acids with a chain length of 10 carbons or more as well as unsaturated fatty acids. Very-long-chain (22- to 24-carbon) fatty acids are produced in the brain, and elongation of stearoyl-CoA (C_{18}) in the brain increases rapidly during myelination, producing the fatty acids required for the synthesis of sphingolipids.

Fatty acids can also be elongated in the mitochondria, where yet another system is used: it is NADH dependent and uses acetyl-CoA as a source of two-carbon fragments. It is simply the reverse of β-oxidation (Chapter 11), and the substrates for chain elongation are short- and medium-chain fatty acids containing fewer than 16 carbon atoms. During fasting and starvation, elongation of fatty acids is greatly reduced.

Desaturation of fatty acids

Desaturation reactions require molecular oxygen

The body has a requirement for mono- and polyunsaturated fatty acids, in addition to saturated fatty acids. Some of these need to be supplied in the diet; these two unsaturated fatty acids, linoleic and linolenic, are known as the essential fatty acids (EFAs). The desaturation system requires molecular oxygen, NADH, and cytochrome b_5. The process of desaturation, like that of chain elongation, occurs on the endoplasmic reticulum and results in the oxidation of both the fatty acid and NADH (Fig. 13.6).

In humans, the desaturase system is unable to introduce double bonds between carbon atoms beyond carbon-9 and the ω-(terminal methyl) carbon atom. Most desaturations occur between carbon atoms 9 and 10 (annotated as Δ^9 desaturations) - for example, those with palmitic acid producing palmitoleic acid (C-16:1, Δ^9) and those with stearic acid producing oleic acid (C-18:1, Δ^9). This step is catalyzed by stearoyl-CoA desaturase (SCD).

Essential fatty acids

The ω-3 and ω-6 fatty acids (or their precursors) must be supplied with diet

As discussed previously, the human desaturase is unable to introduce double bonds beyond C-9. On the other hand, two types of fatty acids - those having double bonds three carbons from the methyl end (**ω-3 fatty acids**) and six carbons from the methyl end (**ω-6 fatty acids**) - are required for phospholipid production and the synthesis of eicosanoids (C-20 fatty acids), precursors of important molecules such as prostaglandins, thromboxanes, and leukotrienes. Therefore, the ω-3 and ω-6 fatty acids (or their precursors) must be supplied in the diet. As it happens, they are obtained from **dietary vegetable oils** and **meats**, which contain the ω-6 fatty acid, linoleic acid (C-18:2, $\Delta^{9,12}$), and the ω-3 fatty acid, linolenic acid (C-18:3, $\Delta^{9,12,15}$). Linoleic acid is converted in a series of elongation and desaturation reactions to **arachidonic acid** (C-20:4, $\Delta^{5,8,11,14}$), the precursor for the synthesis of other **eicosanoids** in humans. Elongation and desaturation of linolenic acid produce eicosapentaenoic acid (EPA; C-20:5, $\Delta^{5,8,11,14,17}$), which

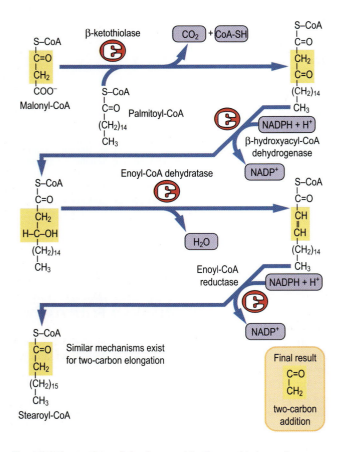

Fig. 13.5 **Elongation of the fatty acids.** Fatty acid elongation occurs on the endoplasmic reticulum and is carried out by a multienzyme complex, fatty acid elongase.

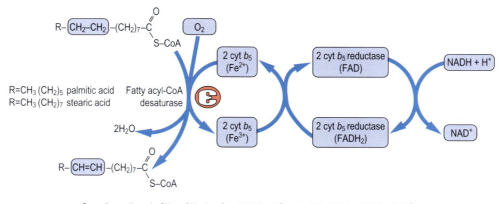

Overall reaction: $(-CH_2 - CH_2 -) + O_2 + NADH + H^+ \rightarrow (-CH = CH-) + 2H_2O + NAD^+$

Fig. 13.6 **Desaturation of fatty acids.** Desaturation of the fatty acids takes place in the endoplasmic reticulum. The reaction requires molecular oxygen, NADH$_2$, FADH$_2$, and cytochrome b_5. cyt b_5, cytochrome b_5; FAD, flavin adenine dinucleotide; FADH$_2$, reduced flavin adenine dinucleotide.

is a precursor of yet another series of eicosanoids. However, the elongation/desaturation of C-18:3, $\Delta^{9,12,15}$ to EPA occurs at a low rate; most of EPA in the human body derives from **fish consumption**.

STORAGE AND TRANSPORT OF FATTY ACIDS: SYNTHESIS OF TRIACYLGLYCEROLS (TRIGLYCERIDES)

Fatty acids derived from endogenous synthesis or from the diet are stored and transported as triacylglycerols known also as triglycerides

In both liver and adipose tissue, triacylglycerols (TAG) are produced by a pathway involving **phosphatidic acid** as an intermediate (Fig. 13.7). The source of glycerol-3-phosphate is, however, different in the two tissues. **Glycerol** is the source of phosphatidic acid in the liver. However, in the adipose tissue, due to the lack of glycerol kinase, **glucose** is the indirect source of glycerol, with the glycolytic metabolite dihydroxy-acetone phosphate being its immediate precursor. The first step from glycerol-3-phosphate is fatty acid acylation by glycerol-3-phosphate acyltransferase, for which the fatty acyl chain comes from a FA-acyl-CoA. The product is lysophosphatidic acid, which undergoes a second fatty acid acylation by **acyl-glycerol acyltransferase (AGPAT2)** to yield phosphatidic acid. This step is absolutely critical for adipocyte triacylglycerol synthesis: disruptive mutations in AGPAT2 leads to an inability to form triacylglycerol in adipose tissue, with congenital total lipodystrophy as a consequence. Phosphatidic acid is dephosphorylated by phosphatidic acid phosphatase to form **diacylglycerol** (DAG). Note that the DAG formed via this pathway resides in smooth endoplasmic reticulum and is thus compartmentalized from membrane or cytoplasmic formation of DAG

via the phospholipase C reaction of phosphatidylinositol. Typically, DAG formed via the TAG synthetic pathway have a mixture of saturated and monounsaturated fatty acids, whereas the cytoplasmic DAG has the typical fatty acid composition of phosphatidylinositol, which is 1-stearoyl-2-arachidonoyl-glycerol. Finally, TAG is formed from DAG by diacylglycerol acyltransferase (DGAT). These steps describe the so-called monoacylglycerol pathway, but TAG can also be formed via the Kennedy pathway, which would give an input at the phosphatidic acid step (see Further Reading).

Triacylglycerols produced in the liver on the smooth endoplasmic reticulum can only be transiently stored

The liver has the unique capacity to offload stored TAG by producing lipoprotein complexes also containing cholesterol, phospholipids, and apolipoproteins (the latter also synthesized on the endoplasmic reticulum) for export in the form of **very-low-density lipoprotein (VLDL)**. The VLDL is then assembled in the endoplasmic reticulum, transferred to the Golgi apparatus, and released into the bloodstream. To mobilize the transiently stored TAG, a lipolytic reaction occurs. It results in the formation of DAGs, which can then again enter the TAG synthetic pathway of VLDL assembly. The nature of this lipase is as yet not known but is of significant medical interest due to the complications of fatty liver disease. It is also possible that some TAGs enter the VLDL in the Golgi by the fusion of a primordial VLDL and an already-existing lipid droplet to produce the larger VLDL particles.

VLDL, once released into the bloodstream, is acted upon by **lipoprotein lipase (LPL).** This enzyme is found attached to the basement membrane glycoproteins of capillary endothelial cells and is active against both VLDL and chylomicrons (Chapter 33). The fatty acid of the TAG stored in adipose tissue will therefore reflect the mixture of fatty acids in the diet (delivered by chylomicrons) and the endogenous fatty acids delivered by VLDL. The latter will be composed of recirculated

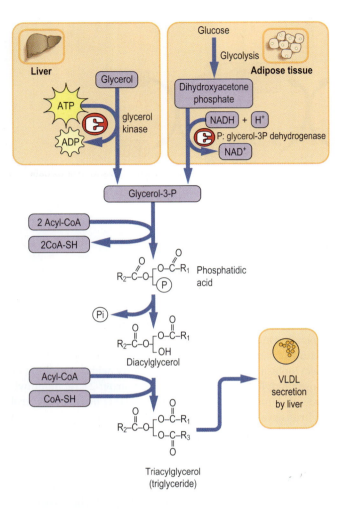

Fig. 13.7 **Triacylglycerol synthesis.** Triacylglycerols (triglycerides) are synthesized in the liver and in adipose tissue. The source of glycerol-3-P is different in the two tissues. In the liver, it is glycerol, but adipose tissue has no glycerol kinase activity. There, glycerol-3-P is generated from the glycolytic intermediate, dihydroxyacetone phosphate. The central "backbone" of the phosphatidic acid, the diacylglycerol and triacylglycerol molecule shown in the figure, consists of three carbon atoms saturated with hydrogens (compare Fig. 30.8). Note that triacylglycerols synthesized in the liver are subsequently packaged into the VLDL and exported to other tissues.

fatty acids (from adipose tissue) and DNL fatty acids from the liver. Beyond this, there might be a small component of DNL fatty acids generated within the tissue.

In the fed state, when adipose tissue is actively taking up fatty acids from the lipoproteins and storing them as TAG, the adipocytes synthesize LPL and secrete it into the capillaries of the adipose tissue. This increased synthesis and secretion of LPL is stimulated by insulin. Increased insulin levels also stimulate the uptake of glucose by adipose tissue and promote glycolysis. This has the net effect of producing increasing amounts of α-glycerophosphate, and it facilitates the synthesis of TAG within adipocytes. The skeletal muscle capillary bed also has LPL, but it is inhibited by insulin. Instead, **LPL is**

activated in skeletal muscle by its contractions or by adrenergic stimulation.

Insulin is an important hormone in relation to fatty acid synthesis and storage. It promotes glucose uptake in both the liver and adipose tissue. In the liver, by increasing fructose-2,6-bisphosphate levels, it stimulates glycolysis, thus increasing pyruvate production. By stimulating dephosphorylation of pyruvate dehydrogenase complex and thus activating this enzyme, insulin promotes production of acetyl-CoA, stimulating the TCA cycle and increasing citrate levels, which, in turn, through stimulation of the acetyl-CoA carboxylase, increase the rate of fatty acid synthesis (see also Chapter 31).

CLINICAL BOX
LIPID ABNORMALITIES IN ALCOHOLISM

A 36-year-old woman attending a well-woman clinic was found to have serum concentrations of triglyceride 73.0 mmol/L (6388 mg/dL) and cholesterol 13 mmol/L (503 mg/dL). After some initial prevarication, she admitted to drinking three bottles of vodka and six bottles of wine per week. When she discontinued alcohol, her triglyceride concentrations decreased to 2 mmol/L (175 mg/dL), and her cholesterol concentration decreased to 5.0 mmol/L (193 mg/dL). Three years later, the woman presented again with an enlarged liver and return of the lipid abnormality. Liver biopsy indicated alcoholic liver disease with steatosis (infiltration of the liver cells with fat).

Comment

In alcoholic individuals, the metabolism of alcohol produces increased amounts of reduced hepatic NADH. The increased $NADH^+/H^+/NAD^+$ ratio inhibits the oxidation of fatty acids. Fatty acids reaching the liver either from dietary sources or by mobilization from adipose tissue are therefore reesterified with glycerol to form triglycerides. In the initial stages of alcoholism, these are packaged with apolipoproteins and exported as very-low-density lipoproteins (VLDL). An increased concentration of VLDL, and hence of serum triglycerides, is often present in the early stages of alcoholic liver disease. As the liver disease progresses, there is a failure to produce the apolipoproteins and export the fat as VLDL; accumulation of triglycerides in the liver cells ensues. (See also Chapter 34)

REGULATION OF TOTAL BODY FAT STORES

Adipose tissue is an active endocrine organ

It has long been understood that increased energy intake without an appropriate increase in energy expenditure is associated with obesity, which is characterized by increased **adiposity,** meaning both the number of adipocytes and their fat content. In this sense, the quantity of stored TAG is merely a consequence of energy balance. However, it is now clear that adipose tissue, far from being an inert storage reservoir,

CLINICAL BOX
LIFESTYLE AND OBESITY

A 48-year-old ex-infantryman (height 1.91 m) presented with the problem of increasing weight over the previous 8 years since leaving the army. At the time of his retirement from active service, he had weighed 95 kg (209 lb), but at presentation, his weight was 193 kg (424.6 lb). His current occupation was that of truck driver. He denied any change in food intake since leaving the army but admitted to engaging in little or no exercise. Detailed inquiry indicated that his daily dietary intake provided between 12,600 and 16,800 kJ (3000 and 4000 kcal), with fat intake approaching 40%. The patient was initially placed on a healthy eating plan, with fat intake reduced to 35% of total calories. He was advised to exercise and preceded to swim three or four times per week. His weight immediately began to decrease, rapidly at first and then at 2–3 kg (4.4–6.6 lb) each month until it stabilized at 180 kg (396 lb). He was then placed on a high-protein/low-carbohydrate/low-fat diet, which induced a return of weight loss that continued for a further 4 months, resulting in a final weight of 173 kg (381 lb).

Comment

Obesity is increasingly prevalent in many parts of the world. Clinical obesity is now clearly defined in terms of height and weight through the body mass index (BMI), which is calculated as the weight in kilograms divided by the height in meters squared (see Chapter 32 for details).

A BMI of 25–30 kg/m² is classified as overweight or grade I obesity, BMI > 30 kg/m² is clinical or grade II obesity, and BMI > 40 kg/m² is classified as morbid or grade III obesity. Our patient had a BMI of 53 at presentation, falling to 48 after prolonged diet. If energy input exceeds output over time, then weight will increase. Obesity predisposes to several diseases. The most important is type 2 diabetes mellitus: 80% of this type of diabetes is associated with the obese state. Other associated illnesses include coronary heart disease, hypertension, stroke, arthritis, and gallbladder disease.

is hormonally active. Adipocytes produce **hormones** such as leptin, adiponectin, and resistin (collectively known as adipokines); **growth factors** such as vascular endothelial growth factor; and **proinflammatory cytokines** such as tumor necrosis factor α (TNF-α) and interleukin 6 (IL-6). Such hormonal signals, particularly leptin, may alter energy balance. This is further discussed in Chapter 32.

SUMMARY

- Fatty acid synthesis and storage are essential components of body energy homeostasis.
- Fatty acid synthesis takes place in the cytosol. Its committed step is the reaction catalyzed by acetyl-CoA carboxylase.

ACTIVE LEARNING

1. Describe how a growing fatty acid chain is transferred between the subunits of fatty acid synthase.
2. How are the eicosanoids synthesized?
3. Explain why the rate of lipolysis in the fed state is low.
4. Describe the committed step of fatty acid synthesis and its regulation.
5. What are the sources of acetyl-CoA for fatty acid synthesis?
6. Compare and contrast fatty acid synthesis and their oxidation.

- Elongation of the fatty acid chain (up to the length of 16 carbon atoms) is carried out by the dimeric fatty acid synthase, which possesses several enzyme activities. Both acetyl-CoA carboxylase and fatty acid synthase are subject to a complex regulation.
- The malate shuttle facilitates the transfer of two-carbon units from the mitochondria to cytoplasm for use in fatty acid synthesis.
- The reducing power for fatty acid synthesis in the form of NADPH is supplied by the pentose phosphate pathway and also by the malate shuttle.
- The essential unsaturated fatty acids are linoleic and linolenic acid. Linoleic acid is converted to arachidonic acid, which in turn serves as the precursor of prostaglandins.
- Adiposity signals are provided by adipokines, particularly leptin. Insulin is also important in the regulation of food intake.

FURTHER READING

Brown, M. S., Ye, J., Rawson, R. B., et al. (2000). Regulated intramembrane proteolysis: A control mechanism conserved from bacteria to humans. *Cell*, *100*, 391–398.

Gibellini, F., & Smith, T. K. (2010). The Kennedy pathway: De novo synthesis of phosphatidylethanolamine and pohosphatidylcholine. *IUMB Life*, *62*, 414–428.

Guillou, H., Zadravec, D., Martin, P. G., et al. (2010). The key roles of elongases and desaturases in mammalian fatty acid metabolism: Insights from transgenic mice. *Progress in Lipid Research*, *49*, 186–199.

Gurr, M. I., Harwood, J. L. K., & Frayn, K. N. (Eds.). (2008). *Lipid biochemistry: An introduction*. Oxford: Blackwell Science.

ABBREVIATIONS

ACC1, ACC2	Acetyl-CoA carboxylase
ACP	Acyl carrier protein
AGPAT2	Acylglycerol acyltransferase
AMPK	AMP-activated protein kinase
ATP	Adenosine triphosphate
BMI	Body mass index

CPT-1	Carnitine-palmitoyl transferase 1	Glc-6-P	Glucose-6-phosphate
DAG	Diacylglycerol	NAD^+	Nicotinamide adenine dinucleotide
DGAT	Diacylglycerol acyltransferase	NADH	Reduced nicotinamide adenine dinucleotide
DNL	De novo lipogenesis	SCD	Stearoyl-CoA desaturase
EFA	Essential fatty acid	SRE	Sterol regulatory element
ELOVL	Elongation of very-long-chain fatty acids	SREBP1c, SREBP1a	Sterol regulatory element-binding proteins-1
EPA	Eicosapentaenoic acid	TAG, TG	Triacylglycerol, also known as triglyceride
FAD	Flavin adenine dinucleotide	TCA	Tricarboxylic acid
FADH2	Reduced flavin adenine dinucleotide	TNF-α	Tumor necrosis factor α
Fru-6-P	Fructose-6-phosphate	VLDL	Very-low-density lipoprotein

Biosynthesis of Cholesterol and Steroids
Marek H. Dominiczak

INTRODUCTION

Cholesterol is essential for cell structure and function

Cholesterol is an essential component of mammalian cell membranes. It is also a precursor of the steroid hormones, vitamin D, and the bile acids. Moreover, the early stages of cholesterol synthesis provide substrates for the synthesis of compounds important for cell proliferation, for electron transport, and for combating oxidative stress (Fig. 14.1).

Excessive cholesterol intake and disorders in cholesterol transport and its handling by cells are linked to the development of atherosclerosis (Chapter 33).

Disorders of steroid hormone synthesis are responsible for a host of endocrine problems, and rare inherited enzyme deficiencies in the synthetic pathway of steroid hormones are seen in neonatal medicine. Cholesterol is excreted in bile and is also a major component of gallstones. The "Medical Map" of cholesterol is shown in Fig. 14.2.

Plasma cholesterol concentration depends on endogenous cholesterol synthesis and on its dietary intake

Humans synthesize approximately 1 g of cholesterol each day. A typical Western diet contains approximately 500 mg (1.2 mmol) of cholesterol daily, mainly in meat, eggs, and dairy products (Chapter 32). Under normal circumstances, 30%–60% of this is absorbed during passage through the gut. After intestinal absorption, cholesterol is transported to the liver and to peripheral tissues as a component of lipoprotein particles,

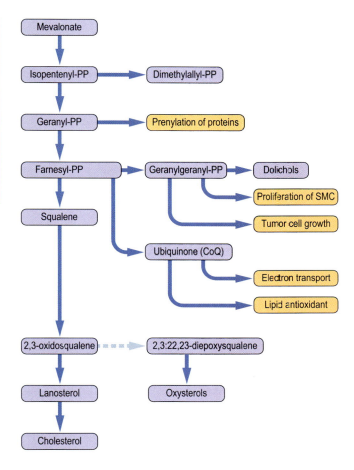

Fig. 14.1 **Cholesterol synthesis and related pathways.** The pathway of cholesterol synthesis is a source of compounds that participate in a variety of cell functions. These are shown in orange-colored boxes. (Modified from Charlton-Menys V, Durrington PN. Exp Physiol 2007; 93:27–42, with permission). SMC, smooth muscle cells; CoQ, coenzyme Q; PP, pyrophosphate.

the chylomicrons, and is then distributed to peripheral tissues by very-low-density lipoproteins (VLDL) and low-density lipoproteins (LDL). It is removed from cells by the high-density lipoproteins (HDL). We focus on lipoprotein metabolism in Chapter 33.

Humans cannot metabolize the sterol structure

Cholesterol is excreted by the liver in bile either in the form of bile acids or as free cholesterol. Most bile acids are reabsorbed in the terminal ileum and recycled back to the liver.

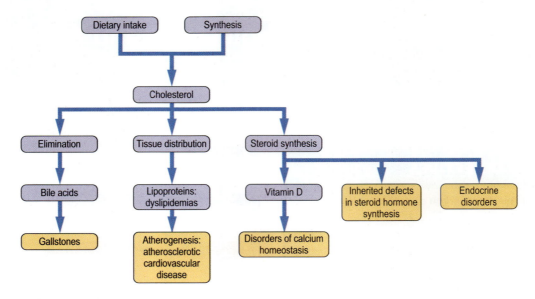

Fig. 14.2 **Clinical context of cholesterol synthesis and metabolism.**

THE CHOLESTEROL MOLECULE

The structure of cholesterol is shown in Fig. 14.3. It has a molecular weight of 386 Da and contains 27 carbon atoms, of which 17 are incorporated into the four fused rings A, B, C, and D of the cholestane structure. Two further carbons are in the methyl groups at the junctions of rings AB and CD, and eight are in the side chain. There is a solitary hydroxyl group on carbon 3 in ring A. It has just one double bond between carbon atoms 5 and 6 in ring B.

Cholesterol increases membrane fluidity

Cholesterol in membranes is held in the lipid bilayer by physical interactions between the planar steroid ring and the fatty acid chains. The absence of covalent bonding means that it may easily transfer in and out of the membrane. Membranes are fluid structures rich in phospholipids and sphingolipids, where both the lipid and protein molecules move and undergo conformational change (Chapter 4). At body temperature, the long hydrocarbon chains of the lipid bilayer are capable of considerable motion. Cholesterol is located between these hydrocarbon chains. **Cholesterol stabilizes the fluidity of membranes.** The more fluid the phospholipid bilayer becomes, the more permeable is the membrane.

Cholesterol is clustered in regions within the lipid bilayer. In such a cluster, there may be 1 mole of cholesterol per mole of phospholipid, whereas in adjacent areas, there may be no cholesterol. Therefore the membrane contains cholesterol-rich impermeable patches and more permeable cholesterol-free regions. Different cell organelles may vary substantially in cholesterol content. It is, for instance, virtually absent from the inner mitochondrial membrane.

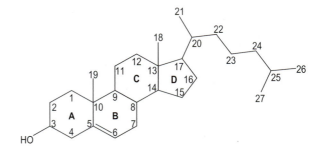

Fig. 14.3 **Structure of cholesterol.** A–D is the conventional notation used to describe the four rings in cholestane structure. Numbers 1–27 denote carbon atoms.

CHOLESTEROL IS ESTERIFIED WITHIN CELLS AND IN PLASMA

Cholesterol is poorly soluble in water. Only about 30% of circulating cholesterol occurs in the free form; the majority forms esters with long-chain fatty acids such as oleic and linoleic acids. Cholesteryl esters (CE) are even less soluble in water than free cholesterol. Cholesterol is esterified in the cells by the **acyl-CoA:cholesterol acyltransferase (ACAT)**, and CE are stored in lipid droplets in the endoplasmic reticulum. In the plasma, it is esterified by **cholesterol-lecithin acyltransferase** and is present mostly as CE in lipoproteins (Chapter 33).

Cholesterol is absorbed in the intestine by specific transporters

Dietary cholesterol is absorbed from the intestine via a membrane transporter known as the Nieman–Pick C1-like (NPC1L1) protein. Another transporter is the ATP-binding cassette G5/ G8, comprising two half-transporters: ABCG5 and ABCG8. These are involved in the secretion of other sterols into the bile. Mutations in these genes result in tissue accumulation of plant sterols **(sitosterolemia).** The drug **ezetimibe** suppresses the NPC1L1-mediated cholesterol transport and has been used in the treatment of hypercholesterolemia.

BIOSYNTHESIS OF CHOLESTEROL

Cholesterol is synthesized from acetyl-coenzyme A

The liver is the major site of cholesterol synthesis, and lesser amounts are synthesized in the intestine, adrenal cortex, and gonads. Virtually all human cells have the capacity to make cholesterol. Its synthesis requires a source of carbon atoms, a source of reducing power, and significant amounts of energy supplied by ATP. Acetyl-coenzyme A (acetyl-CoA) provides a high-energy starting point. Acetyl-CoA may be provided from the β-oxidation of long-chain fatty acids, from dehydrogenation of pyruvate, and also from the oxidation of ketogenic amino acids such as leucine and isoleucine. Reducing power is provided by reduced nicotinamide dinucleotide phosphate (NADPH) generated in the pentose phosphate pathway (Chapter 9).

Overall, the synthesis of 1 mole of cholesterol requires 18 moles of acetyl-CoA, 36 moles of ATP, and 16 moles of NADPH. All the biosynthetic reactions occur within the cytoplasm, although some of the required enzymes are bound to the ER membranes.

The first committed step in the pathway of cholesterol synthesis is the formation of mevalonic acid

Three molecules of acetyl-CoA are converted into the six-carbon mevalonic acid (Fig. 14.4). The first two steps occur in the cytoplasm and are condensation reactions leading to the formation of the 3-hydroxy-3-methylglutaryl-CoA (HMG-CoA). These reactions, catalyzed by acetoacetyl-CoA thiolase and HMG-CoA synthase, are the same as the ones in the synthesis of ketone bodies, although the latter occur within mitochondria.

The rate-limiting enzyme in the pathway is HMG-CoA reductase

The rate-limiting reaction is catalyzed by HMG-CoA reductase (HMGR) and leads to the formation of mevalonic acid. The reaction uses two molecules of NADPH.

HMGR is embedded in the ER. It is controlled on multiple levels: by feedback inhibition, by degradation rate, by phosphorylation (it is active in a nonphosphorylated state), and by changes in its gene expression. It is also affected by several hormones: insulin and triiodothyronine increase its activity, whereas glucagon and cortisol inhibit it. HMGR can be phosphorylated (and thus inhibited) by the "energy sensor" enzyme, the AMP-dependent kinase (AMPK; see Chapter 32).

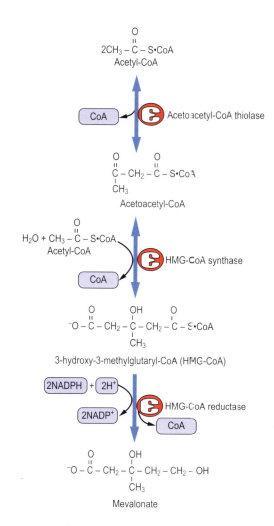

Fig. 14.4 **Pathway of cholesterol synthesis: Synthesis of mevalonic acid.** Mevalonic acid contains six carbon atoms derived from the three molecules of acetyl-CoA.

Farnesyl pyrophosphate is made up of three isoprene units

Three molecules of mevalonic acid are phosphorylated in two reactions requiring ATP. Subsequent decarboxylation yields the **isomeric 5-carbon isoprene units,** isopentenyl pyrophosphate and dimethylallyl pyrophosphate, which condense together to form 10-carbon geranyl pyrophosphate. Further condensation with isopentenyl pyrophosphate produces the 15-carbon atom molecule farnesyl pyrophosphate (Fig. 14.5). As well as being an intermediate in cholesterol biosynthesis, farnesyl pyrophosphate is the branching point for the synthesis of dolichol (a substrate for glycoprotein synthesis) and ubiquinone (Fig. 14.1).

Squalene is a linear molecule capable of a ring formation

Squalene synthase condenses two molecules of farnesyl pyrophosphate to form **squalene,** a 30-carbon hydrocarbon

ADVANCED CONCEPT BOX
MODULAR BUILDUP OF CHOLESTEROL MOLECULE

Isopentenyl diphosphate (IPP), also called the isoprene unit derivative, is precursor of large number of compounds, known as isoprenoids, in plants and animals.

It is also a 5-carbon building block of the steroid molecule. Two fused isoprene molecules are called terpene. In cholesterol synthesis, first, a condensation of two IPP isomers yields a 10-carbon terpene geranyl. Another added IPP forms la 15-carbon farnesyl. Two farnesol units fuse to form the 30-carbon squalene. The elimination of three methyl groups in the final stages of the pathway leads to the formation of cholesterol.

containing six double bonds (Fig. 14.6), which later enable it to fold into a ring similar to the steroid nucleus. Several intermediates are formed at this stage.

Squalene cyclizes to lanosterol

Before the ring is closed, squalene is converted to squalene 2,3-oxide by squalene monooxygenase. This NADPH-dependent enzyme inserts an oxygen molecule into the structure. Thereafter, cyclization is catalyzed by oxidosqualene cyclase, yielding lanosterol (Fig. 14.7).

In plants, there is a different product of squalene cyclization, termed cycloartenol, which is further metabolized to a range of phytosterols, including sitosterol.

Final stages of cholesterol biosynthesis occur on a carrier protein

Squalene, lanosterol, and all the subsequent intermediates in cholesterol synthesis are hydrophobic. In order for the final steps of the pathway to occur in an aqueous medium, these

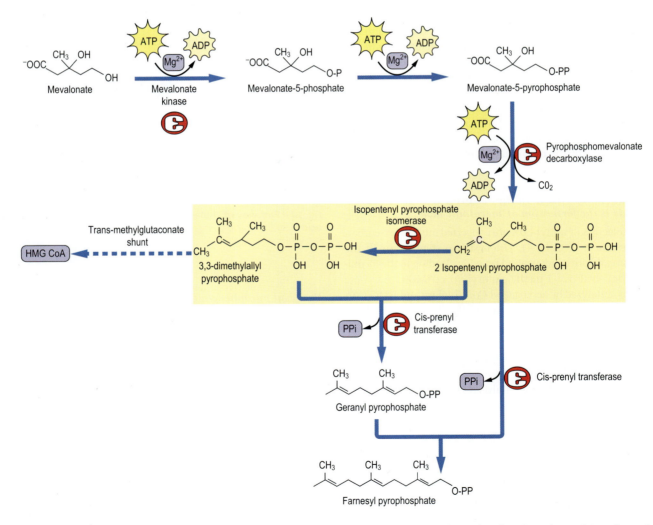

Fig. 14.5 **Pathway of cholesterol synthesis: Mevalonate to farnesyl pyrophosphate.** Farnesyl pyrophosphate is made up of three five-carbon isoprene units. ADP, adenosine diphosphate.

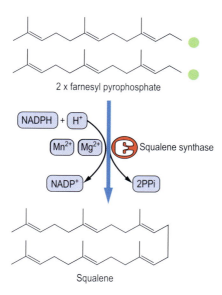

intermediates react while bound to a squalene- and sterol-binding protein. Conversion from the 30-carbon lanosterol to the 27-carbon cholesterol involves decarboxylations, isomerization, and reduction and results in the elimination of three methyl groups (Fig. 14.7).

Oxidation of the cholesterol side chain yields oxysterols

This is performed by a cytochrome P450 enzyme, cholesterol 24-hydroxylase (CYP46A1) present in the brain, and 25 hydroxylase (CYP25A1) and 27-hydroxylase (CYP27A1), present in other tissues. The 27-hydroxycholesterol can cross the blood–brain barrier without the need for an energy-requiring transporter. The 25-hydroxycholesterol regulates the liver X receptors (LXR). In the brain, through LXRs, it regulates expression of apolipoprotein E (an important transporter of cholesterol in the brain) and the transporters ABCA1, ABCG1, and ABCG4 present on astrocyte membranes.

Plant sterols and cholesterol precursors are markers of cholesterol absorption and metabolism

In the studies of cholesterol metabolism, the plant sterols campesterol, sitosterol, and biliary sterol 5α-cholestanol have

Fig. 14.6 **The pathway of cholesterol synthesis: Farnesyl pyrophosphate to squalene.** Squalene, still a linear molecule, results from the condensation of two molecules of 15-carbon farnesyl pyrophosphate. The six double bonds enable the squalene structure to fold into a ring later.

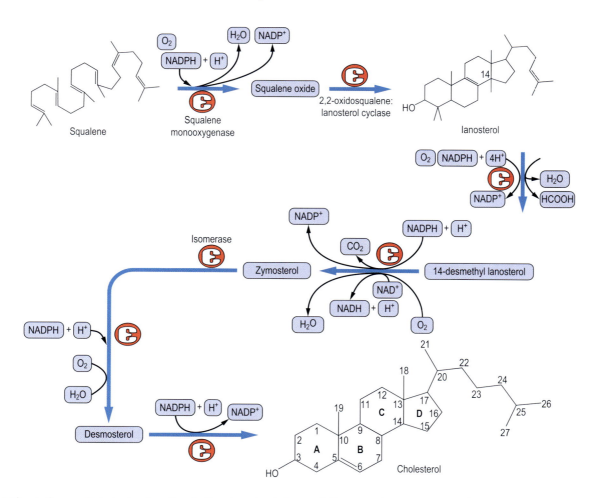

Fig. 14.7 **The pathway of cholesterol synthesis: Squalene to cholesterol.** These reactions occur on squalene- and sterol-binding proteins.

been used as markers of cholesterol absorption. Measurements of mevalonic acid, squalene, and lanosterol have been used as markers of cholesterol synthesis.

ADVANCED CONCEPT BOX
PCSK9 PROTEASE REGULATES DEGRADATION OF LDL RECEPTORS

Serine protease PCSK9 (proprotein convertase subtilisin / kexin type 9) regulates LDL receptors. PCSK9 is secreted from the liver, is present in plasma, and binds to the extracellular domain of the LDL receptor. After the LDL-receptor complex is internalized, PCSK9 prevents it from recycling to the membrane and channels it toward degradation. PCSK9 overexpression in transgenic mice lowers LDL receptor levels, decreasing the ability of the cell to take up cholesterol, thus elevating plasma cholesterol concentration. In **hypercholesterolemic individuals** with a gain-of-function mutation, PCSK9 has increased affinity for the LDL receptor. On the other hand, the loss-of-function mutation results in lower plasma cholesterol because it leads to more LDL receptors present in the membrane and thus increased cholesterol uptake from plasma. Monoclonal antibodies toward PCSK9 which suppress its activity, are now being used as cholesterol-lowering drugs.

Table 14.1 Regulation of intracellular cholesterol concentration

Processes that increase the free cholesterol concentration
De novo synthesis
Hydrolysis of intracellular cholesteryl esters by cholesterol ester hydrolase
Dietary intake of cholesterol
Receptor-mediated uptake of LDL: upregulation of LDL receptors
Processes that decrease intracellular free cholesterol concentration
Inhibition of de novo cholesterol synthesis
Downregulation of LDL receptors
Esterification of cholesterol by acyl-coenzyme A:cholesterol acyl transferase
Release of cholesterol from the cell to HDL
Conversion of cholesterol to bile acids or to steroid hormones
Factors that inhibit activity of HMG-CoA reductase
Decrease in concentration of HMG-CoA
High membrane concentration of cholesterol

Regulation of cellular cholesterol content

Cells acquire cholesterol from de novo synthesis and through external supply

Note that the "external supply" in the case of a cell does not necessarily equal diet. The exogenous cholesterol reaches cells predominantly as a component of lipoproteins, which bind to the apoB/E receptors present on the plasma membranes (Chapter 33). The lipoprotein/receptor complexes are taken up into the cell. In the cytoplasm, vesicles carrying the internalized complexes are acted upon by lysosomal enzymes, which separate the LDL from the receptor and hydrolyze cholesterol esters. Free cholesterol is released to the membrane. The LDL apoprotein B is degraded.

Synthesis of cholesterol de novo and delivery by lipoproteins are reciprocally related

Under normal circumstances, there is an inverse relationship between dietary cholesterol intake and the rate of cholesterol biosynthesis. This ensures a relatively constant supply of cholesterol to cells. It also explains why dietary restriction is only likely to achieve a moderate reduction in the plasma cholesterol concentration.

The synchronized regulation of intracellular cholesterol involves HMG-CoA reductase, the LDL receptor, 7α-hydroxylase, and a network of nuclear receptors. Intracellular (intramembrane) cholesterol concentration is a key factor regulating both cellular cholesterol synthesis and LDL receptors. Thus an increase in the free cholesterol concentration results in the following (Table 14.1 and Fig. 14.8):

- Reduction in the activity and expression of HMG-CoA reductase - this limits cholesterol synthesis.
- Downregulation of LDL receptors - this limits the cellular uptake of cholesterol.
- Increase in cholesterol and phospholipid efflux from cell to HDL - this decreases intracellular cholesterol.
- Increase in the rate of conversion of cholesterol to bile acids - this increases cholesterol elimination.

Sterol regulatory element-binding proteins (SREBP) are transcriptional regulators of cholesterol synthesis

SREBPs are synthesized as 120-kDa inactive precursors, which are integral part of the ER membrane. They bind to the ER protein known as the SREBP cleavage-activating protein (SCAP). The SCAP/SREBP complex transfers from the ER to the Golgi apparatus, where SREBPs are cleaved by a protease, releasing the active transcription factors, which in turn translocate to the nucleus and activate all the genes in the cholesterol synthetic pathway (Fig. 14.9).

This process is itself subject to an ingenious regulatory mechanism. Cholesterol molecules bind to sterol-sensing intermembrane domains (cholesterol "receptors") on the SCAP protein. This allows binding of the SCAP/SREBP complex to another ER protein, Insig-1 (Insig stands for "insulin-induced gene"). The stability of the SCAP/SREBP/Insig-1 complex is the key regulatory event. This is how it works: **When cholesterol is depleted,** the SCAP/SREBP complex dissociates from Insig-1 and travels to the Golgi apparatus. However, **when**

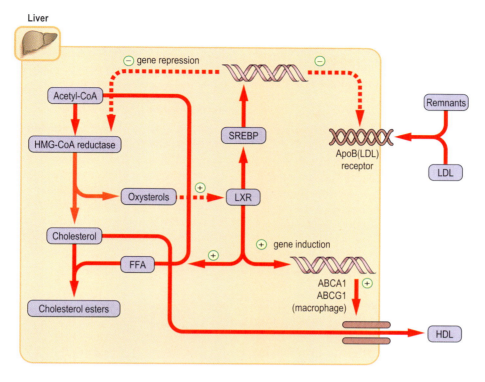

Fig. 14.8 **Regulation of intracellular cholesterol concentration.** Free membrane cholesterol and oxysterols regulate intracellular cholesterol concentration by inducing or suppressing gene expression. Note that an increase in the intracellular cholesterol concentration suppresses synthesis of HMG-CoA reductase and apoB/E receptor, at the same time increasing cholesterol esterification and its removal from cells. See text for details. FFA, free fatty acid; LXR, liver X receptor; SREBP, sterol regulatory element-binding protein.

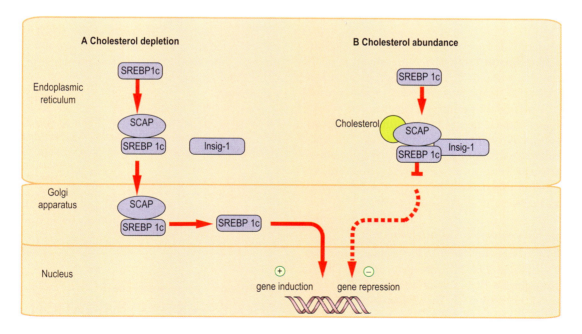

Fig. 14.9 **Control of transcription by sterol-regulated transcription factors (SREBP).** (A) When the membrane concentration of free cholesterol is low, the SCAP/SREBP complex transfers from the ER to Golgi apparatus. Proteolysis takes place, and the active transcription factor enters nucleus and initiates gene transcription. (B) When the membrane concentration of free cholesterol is high, conformational change in the SCAP protein, induced by binding of cholesterol, stabilizes its binding to the Insig-1. The complex remains in the ER with SREBP in inactive form, and transcription is repressed. See text for details. ER, endoplasmic reticulum; SREBP, sterol regulatory element-binding protein; SCAP, SREBP-cleavage-activating protein.

cholesterol concentration in the membrane is high, cholesterol binding to SCAP stabilizes the SCAP/SREBP/Insig-1 complex, blocking its movement to the Golgi. Consequently, there is a decrease in nuclear SREBP, and the transcription of relevant genes remains repressed. Cholesterol synthesis is inhibited (Fig. 14.9).

HMG-CoA reductase regulation by cholesterol involves enzyme degradation

HMGR possesses the sterol-sensing domain. When cholesterol level is high, HMGR, similarly to the SCAP/SREBP complex, binds to the Insig-1 protein. Here, however, the effect of the binding is different: it increases ubiquination of the enzyme and directs it toward degradation. The overall effect is inhibition of cholesterol synthesis.

SREBPs have wide-ranging effects on the synthesis of cholesterol and fatty acids

In addition to the effect on cholesterol synthesis, SREBPs **increase the expression of LDL receptor gene** and affect **fatty acid synthesis.** In mammals, there are two closely related SREBPs: SREBP1 and SREBP2. SREBP1 has two isoforms: SREBP1a and SREBP1c produced by the same gene by alternative splicing. SREBP2 regulates cholesterol synthesis and LDL-receptor gene expression, whereas SREBP1c controls fatty acid synthesis. SREBP1a induces all SREBP-responsive genes.

SREBP1c can be activated by liver X receptors in response to oxysterols

SREBP1c is upregulated by the LXRs. LXRs are **ligand-activated transcription factors** that are members of the nuclear receptor superfamily (Chapter 25). They form **heterodimers** with other similar molecules, such as the **retinoid X receptors** (RXR) and the **farnesyl X receptors** (FXRs; see Chapter 7). Resultant complexes bind to the LXR response elements on the DNA, regulating gene expression. LXRs also sense intracellular cholesterol concentration and contribute to regulating both its synthesis and its efflux from cells. However, it is not the cholesterol that binds to the LXR but oxysterols, such as 25-hydroxycholesterol or 27-hydroxycholesterol (Fig. 14.1).

SREBP1c regulates cholesterol efflux from cells

A high concentration of cholesterol in the hepatocyte induces, also through the LXR–SREBP1c mechanism, genes coding for cholesterol transporters that control its efflux from cells to HDL particles: the expression of ABCA1 (the transporter that controls efflux of cholesterol from cells to nascent HDL) and ABCG1 (the transporter that stimulates efflux of cholesterol to more mature HDL2 and HDL3). Another transcription factor, **peroxisome proliferator activated; receptor α** (PPARα), also regulates cholesterol efflux, acting through LXR (Chapter 33). PPARα is affected by a group of lipid-lowering drugs that are derivatives of the fibric acid (fibrates).

SREBP1c regulates fatty acid synthesis

A high intracellular cholesterol concentration also induces (through SREBP1c) genes coding for all the enzymes catalyzing fatty acid synthesis. Increased supply of fatty acids provides substrates for cholesterol esterification.

Statins inhibit HMG-CoA reductase

HMGR inhibitors, known as **statins,** lower cholesterol by binding to the HMG-CoA binding site on the enzyme and competitively inhibiting its activity. This results in a decrease in the intracellular cholesterol concentration. The decrease in free cholesterol stimulates expression of LDL receptors. LDL clearance increases, and the plasma LDL-cholesterol decreases. Hepatic HMGR exhibits a diurnal rhythm: its activity is at a peak about 6 h after dark and at a minimum about 6 h after exposure to light. Therefore statins are usually taken at night to ensure maximum effect.

CLINICAL BOX
A 50-YEAR-OLD MAN WITH HYPERCHOLESTEROLEMIA TREATED WITH A STATIN

Despite a strict low-cholesterol diet, a 50-year-old man with a family history of early cardiovascular disease had a serum cholesterol concentration of 8.0 mmol/L (309 mg/dL); desirable concentration is 4.0 mmol/L (<155 mg/dL). He also smoked 15 cigarettes per day. He was given smoking cessation advice and was prescribed a statin. He tolerated the therapy well, and 3 months later, his cholesterol was 5.5 mmol/L (212 mg/dL). The dose of the statin was increased, and after a further 3 months, his plasma cholesterol concentration was 4.1 mmol/L (158 mg/dL).

Comment

Partial inhibition of the HMGR brings about a lowering of total plasma cholesterol by 30%–50% and LDL-cholesterol by 30%–60%. A range of statins is now available; this follows the original discovery that compactin (later renamed mevastatin), a fungal metabolite isolated from *Penicillium citrinum,* had HMGR-inhibiting properties. Inhibition of HMGR leads to a decrease in the concentration of intracellular free cholesterol and to consequent increased expression of the cell membrane LDL receptors. The end result is the lowering of the plasma total cholesterol and LDL-cholesterol.

CHOLESTEROL ELIMINATION: THE BILE ACIDS

Liver removes cholesterol either in a free form or as bile acids

Bile acids are quantitatively the most abundant metabolic products of cholesterol. There are four main human bile acids

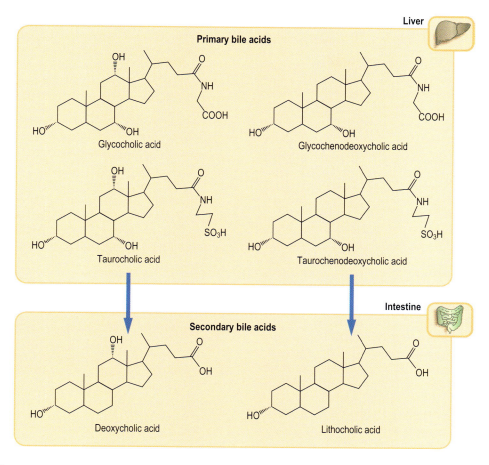

Fig. 14.10 **Bile acids.** Primary bile acids are synthesized in the liver. They are converted by the intestinal bacteria to secondary bile acids.

(Fig. 14.10). They all possess 24 carbon atoms; the terminal three carbons of the cholesterol side chain are removed. They have a saturated steroid nucleus and differ only in the number and position of hydroxyl groups.

Primary bile acids are synthesized in the liver

Cholic and **chenodeoxycholic acids,** the primary bile acids, are synthesized in the hepatic parenchymal cells. The rate-limiting step is the reaction catalyzed by the microsomal **7 α-hydroxylase** (a monooxygenase designated CYP7A1), which introduces a hydroxyl group at the 7α position.

Before their secretion, primary bile acids are **conjugated** through the carboxyl group, forming amide linkages with either **glycine** or **taurine.** In humans, there is a 3 : 1 ratio in favor of glycine conjugates. The secreted products are thus glyco-cholic, glycochenodeoxycholic, taurocholic, and taurocheno-deoxycholic acids. At physiologic pH, bile acids are present as sodium or potassium salts. The terms *bile acids* and *bile salts* are used interchangeably. These compounds are either directly secreted into the duodenum or stored in the gallbladder.

Together with water, phospholipids, cholesterol, and excretory products such as bilirubin, they form bile.

Liver X receptors participate in bile synthesis and secretion

LXRs coordinate expression of several genes relevant to cholesterol excretion, including cholesterol 7α-hydroxylase. Cholesterol is pumped into bile by **ABCG5 and ABCG8 transport proteins,** the expression of which is regulated by the LXRs. Cholesterol excretion into the bile is also regulated by other nuclear receptors: the farnesyl X receptor (FXR) heterodimerizes with RXR and binds to the bile acid response elements on the DNA. FXR acts as the cellular bile–acid sensor by binding bile acids and suppressing their synthesis.

Importantly, bile supersaturated with cholesterol facilitates formation of cholesterol gallstones.

Secondary bile acids are synthesized in the intestine

The secondary bile acids deoxycholic and lithocholic acid are formed within the intestine by the anaerobic bacteria (princi-pally *Bacteroides*) from the primary bile acids (Fig. 14.10). Only a proportion of primary bile acids is converted into secondary bile acids.

Bile acids assist the digestion of dietary fat

Secretion of bile and the emptying of the gallbladder are controlled by the gastrointestinal hormones hepatocrinin and cholecystokinin, respectively. They are released when partially digested food passes from the stomach to the duodenum. Once secreted into the intestine, the bile acids act as detergents (they possess polar carboxyl and hydroxyl groups), assisting the emulsification of ingested lipids; this aids the enzymatic digestion and absorption of dietary fat (Chapter 30).

Bile acids recirculate to the liver

Up to 30 g of bile acids pass from the bile duct into the intestine each day, but only 2% of this (approximately 0.5 g) is lost with the feces. Most are deconjugated and reabsorbed. Their passive reabsorption occurs in the jejunum and colon, but they are mostly taken up by active transport in the ileum. Reabsorbed bile acids are transported back to the liver via the portal vein, being noncovalently bound to albumin, and are re-secreted into the bile. The process is known as the **enterohepatic circulation.** Recirculation explains why bile contains both primary and secondary bile acids. The total bile acid pool amounts to only 3 g, and therefore they have to recirculate 5–10 times a day.

The 7α-hydroxylase is subject to feedback inhibition by the bile acids returning to the liver through the portal vein. Dietary bile acids also decrease the expression of 7α-hydroxylase. Bile acid metabolism is summarized in Fig. 14.11.

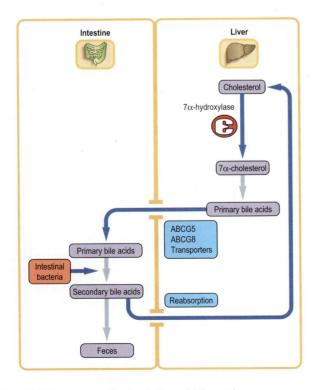

Fig. 14.11 **Enterohepatic circulation of bile acids.**

Cholesterol is excreted in the feces

Approximately 1 g of cholesterol is eliminated from the body each day through the feces: 50% of this is excreted as bile acids and the remainder as the isomeric saturated neutral sterols coprostanol (5β-) and cholestanol (5α-) produced by bacterial reduction of the cholesterol molecule.

Cholestyramine is a bile acid–binding resin that has been used to lower plasma cholesterol

Cholestyramine is a drug that binds bile acids and thus interrupts the enterohepatic circulation. This leads to an increase in 7α-hydroxylase activity and therefore to increased bile acid synthesis and increased bile acid excretion. As a result, cellular cholesterol synthesis and expression of LDL receptors increase. Cholestyramine was one of the first cholesterol-lowering drugs but now has been superseded by the statins.

> ### CLINICAL BOX
> ### A 45-YEAR-OLD WOMAN ADMITTED WITH ABDOMINAL PAIN AND VOMITING: GALLSTONES
>
> A 45-year-old woman complained of right upper quadrant abdominal pain and vomiting after eating fatty food. The only biochemical abnormality was a modestly raised alkaline phosphatase at 400 U/L (the upper reference limit is 260 U/L). An abdominal ultrasound was performed, and it showed that the gallbladder contained gallstones. She was referred to the surgeons.
>
> #### Comment
> Gallstones occur in up to 20% of the population of Western countries. Cholesterol-rich stones are formed within the gallbladder. Cholesterol is present in high concentrations in bile, being solubilized in micelles that also contain phospholipids and bile acids. When the liver secretes bile with a cholesterol-to-phospholipid ratio greater than 1:1, it is difficult to solubilize all the cholesterol in the micelles; thus there is a tendency for the excess to crystallize around any insoluble nuclei. This is compounded by further concentration of the bile in the gallbladder, resulting from reabsorption of water and electrolytes.
>
> The condition may be managed conservatively by reducing dietary cholesterol and by increasing the availability of bile acids that will assist with cholesterol solubilization in the bile and its excretion via the gut. Alternative treatment includes disintegration of stones by shock waves (lithotripsy) and surgery. Elevated alkaline phosphatase is a marker of cholestasis.

STEROID HORMONES

Cholesterol is the precursor of all steroid hormones

Mammals produce a wide range of steroid hormones, some of which differ only by a double bond or by the orientation of

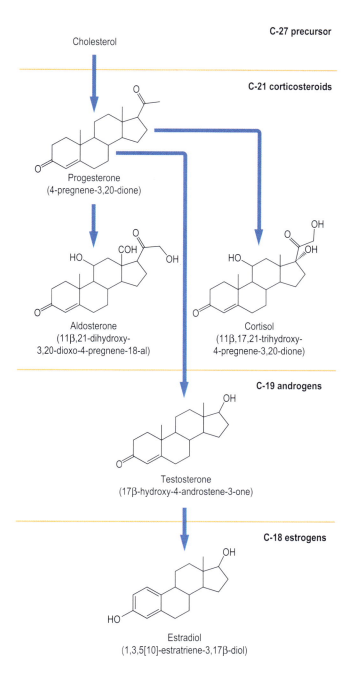

Fig. 14.12 **The most important human steroid hormones.** Their trivial and systematic names (in parentheses) are shown. For numbering of the atoms in a steroid molecule, see Fig. 14.1.

a hydroxyl group. Consequently, it has been necessary to develop a systematic nomenclature to detail their exact structures. There are three groups of steroid hormones (Fig. 14.12). The **corticosteroids** have 21 carbon atoms in the basic pregnane ring. The loss of the 2 carbon atoms from the cholesterol side chain produces the androstane ring and the hormones known as the **androgens.** Finally, the loss of the methyl group at carbon atom 19 as part of the aromatization of the A ring

results in the estrane structure found in the **estrogens.** The presence and position of double bonds, and the position and orientation of the functional groups on the basic nucleus, are characteristic for individual hormones.

Biosynthesis of the steroid hormones

Synthesis of steroid hormones occurs in three organs: adrenal cortex, testis, and ovary

A simplification used in practice is to consider the corticosteroids as the products of the adrenal cortex, the androgens as the products of the testis, and the estrogens as the products of the ovary. Such a simplified pathway of steroid synthesis is shown in Fig. 14.13 (see also Chapter 27 and Fig. 27.7). However, all three organs are capable of secreting small amounts of steroids belonging to other groups. In pathologic situations, such as a defect in steroidogenesis or a steroid-secreting tumor, a very abnormal pattern of steroid secretion may emerge.

Steroidogenesis is controlled by cytochrome P450 monooxygenases

Most of the enzymes involved in converting cholesterol into steroid hormones are cytochrome P450 proteins that require oxygen and NADPH. These enzymes catalyze the replacement of a carbon–hydrogen bond with a carbon–hydroxyl bond - hence the name *monooxygenase.* Hydroxylation of the adjacent carbon atoms precedes cleavage of the carbon–carbon bond. Comparison of the structure of cholesterol (Fig. 14.3)

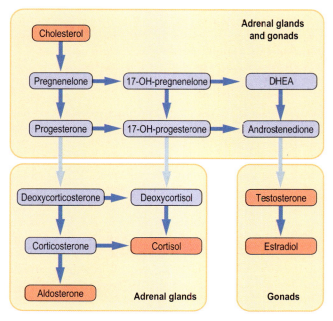

Fig. 14.13 **Overview of steroid hormone synthesis.** Note how the pathway branches from cholesterol, eventually leading to synthesis of mineralocorticoids (e.g., aldosterone), glucocorticoids (cortisol), androgens (testosterone), and estrogens (estradiol). DHEA, dehydroepiandrosterone.

with those of the steroid hormones (Fig. 14.12) demonstrates that the biosynthetic pathway largely consists of cleavage of carbon–carbon bonds and hydroxylation reactions. The enzymes involved have their own nomenclature in which the symbol CYP is followed by a specific suffix. Thus for instance, CYP21A2 refers to the enzyme that hydroxylates carbon atom 21.

CLINICAL BOX
SMITH–LEMLI–OPITZ SYNDROME: A DEFECT IN 7-DEHYDROCHOLESTEROL REDUCTASE

The syndrome presents at birth with microencephaly, short nasal root, small chin, high arched palate, and often midline cleft. There are often accompanying central nervous system (CNS) defects, polydactyly, and in males, ambiguous genitalia.

A defect in 7-dehydrocholesterol reductase was identified in 1993. The pathophysiology involves incomplete processing of embryonic signaling proteins (HH proteins), resulting in variable defects in different tissues.

Although some affected children die in infancy, the rest, if assisted in feeding, survive with severe mental retardation (IQ 20–40). Most also develop growth retardation. Treatment involves giving additional cholesterol to the child. This improves growth, but it appears to have no CNS benefits.

Corticosteroids

In the adrenal glands, the zona fasciculata and zona reticularis are places of synthesis of cortisol and adrenal androgens; the outer layer (zona glomerulosa) synthesizes aldosterone

Biosynthesis of cortisol, the main **glucocorticoid,** depends on the stimulation by pituitary adrenocorticotropic hormone (ACTH), which binds to its plasma membrane receptor. ACTH triggers intracellular events, including hydrolysis of CE stored in lipid droplets and activation of the cholesterol 20,22-desmolase, which converts C-27 cholesterol into pregnenolone, the first of the C-21 family of corticosteroids (Fig. 14.13). This is the rate-limiting step of steroidogenesis. Thereafter, conversion to cortisol requires a dehydrogenation–isomerization and three sequential hydroxylation reactions at C-17, C-21, and C-11, catalyzed by CYP enzymes (Fig. 14.13). The pathway is regulated by negative feedback control of ACTH secretion by cortisol (Chapter 27).

Aldosterone is the main **mineralocorticoid.** The main stimulus to its synthesis is not ACTH but angiotensin II (Chapter 35). Potassium is an important secondary stimulus. Angiotensin II and potassium work cooperatively to activate the first step

in the pathway: conversion of cholesterol into pregnenolone. *Zona glomerulosa* lacks the 17α-hydroxylase but has abundant amounts of 18-hydroxylase, which is the first step of a two-stage reaction forming the 18-aldehyde group of aldosterone (Fig. 14.13).

Androgens

Conversion of corticosteroids into androgens requires the C17–20 split and addition of 17α-hydroxyl group

The 17α-hydroxyl group is added before breaking the C17–C20 bond to yield the **androstane ring** structure (Fig. 14.13). The enzyme is abundant in the Leydig cells of the testis and in the granulosa cells of the ovary. However, in these two tissues, the same biosynthetic step is controlled by two different hormones. In the testis, the rate-limiting cholesterol side-chain cleavage step is stimulated by luteinizing hormone (LH), whereas in the ovary, it is stimulated by follicle-stimulating hormone (FSH).

Estrogens

Conversion of androgens into estrogens involves removal of the methyl group at C-19

The A ring undergoes two dehydrogenations, yielding the characteristic 1,3,5(10)-estratriene nucleus (Fig. 14.13). This aromatase is most abundant in the granulosa cells of the ovary. Many genetic defects have been identified in the CYP enzymes. These defects lead to abnormal steroid biosynthesis and to clinical disorders such as **congenital adrenal hyperplasia.**

ADVANCED CONCEPT BOX
ABNORMALITIES IN STEROID SYNTHESIS ARE REVEALED BY ALTERED PATTERNS OF URINARY STEROID METABOLITES

Steroid metabolites are excreted in urine mostly as water-soluble sulfate or glucuronic acid conjugates. The procedure used for their identification is gas chromatography–mass spectrometry (GC-MS); it is very similar to the methods adopted for the identification of anabolic steroids in sports. The first step in the analysis involves the enzymatic release of the steroids from these conjugates; this is followed by chemical derivatization to increase their stability and improve separation, which is carried out by gas chromatography on capillary columns at high temperatures. Final detection is by mass fragmentation: for each steroid metabolite, a unique ion fragmentation "fingerprint" is achieved, which allows positive identification and quantitation.

Mechanism of action of steroid hormones

Biological actions of the steroid hormones are diverse and are best considered as belonging to the trophic hormone system (Chapter 27).

Steroid hormones act via nuclear receptors

All steroid hormones act by binding to ligand-activated nuclear receptors. The superfamily of hormone receptors also includes receptors for the thyroid hormone triiodothyronine (T_3) and the active forms of vitamins A and D (Chapter 25). Adjacent to the hormone-binding domain of the receptor is a highly conserved DNA-binding domain characterized by the presence of two zinc fingers (Chapter 22). Binding of a steroid ligand facilitates translocation of the activated receptor to the nucleus and its binding to a specific steroid response element in the promoter regions of target genes (Chapter 22). Genetic variability in the structure of steroid receptors may be associated with a variable degree of hormone resistance and diverse clinical presentations. Refer also to the discussion of the steroid receptor in Chapter 23.

VITAMIN D

Vitamin D is derived from cholesterol and plays a key role in calcium metabolism. The actions and metabolism of vitamin D are described in Chapter 38.

Elimination of steroid hormones

Most steroid hormones are excreted in urine. There are two principal steps in this process. First, the removal of biological potency of a steroid is achieved by a series of reduction reactions. Second, the steroid structure is rendered water soluble by **conjugation to a glucuronide or sulfate,** usually through the C-3 hydroxyl group. Many different steroid hormone conjugates are present in urine. Urinary steroid profiling by gas chromatography–mass spectrometry (GC-MS) typically identifies more than 30 such steroids. Their relative concentrations may be used to pinpoint specific defects in the steroidogenic pathway (Fig. 14.14).

SUMMARY

- Cholesterol is an essential constituent of cell membranes and the precursor molecule for bile acids, steroid hormones, and vitamin D.
- Cholesterol is both supplied with the diet and synthesized de novo from acetyl-CoA.
- The rate-limiting enzyme in the cholesterol synthesis pathway is HMG-CoA reductase.
- The synthesis of bile acids and steroid hormones from cholesterol involves several hydroxylation reactions catalyzed by cytochrome P450 monooxygenases.

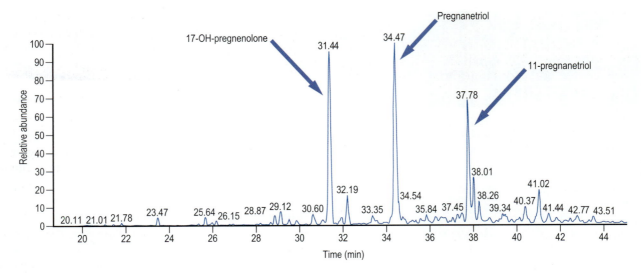

Fig. 14.14 Separation of urinary steroids by gas chromatography–mass spectrometry (GC-MS). In the clinical laboratory, measurement of urinary steroid metabolites helps diagnose inherited disorders of synthesis and metabolism of adrenal steroids and steroid-producing tumors. It is particularly valuable in identifying the site of the defect in congenital adrenal hyperplasia. These investigations are most often performed in neonates with ambiguous genitalia, children with precocious puberty, and patients with suspected Cushing's syndrome (Chapter 27). Shown here is a urinary steroid metabolite pattern from a **patient with 21-hydroxylase deficiency**. The most prominent steroid metabolites are 17-hydroxypregnenolone, pregnanetriol, and 11-oxo-pregnanetriol. X-axis: time at which the chromatographically separated steroid metabolites are detected by the mass spectrometer. Y-axis: relative abundance (quantity of ions).

FURTHER READING

Barnes, P. J., & Adcock, I. M. (2009). Glucocorticoid resistance in inflammatory diseases. *Lancet, 373*, 1905–1917.

Charlton-Menys, V., & Durrington, P. N. (2007). Human cholesterol metabolism and therapeutic molecules. *Experimental Physiology, 93*, 27–42.

Goldstein, J., DeBose Boyd, R. A., & Brown, M. S. (2006). Protein sensors for membrane sterols. *Cell, 124*, 35–46.

Griffiths, W. J., Abdel-Khalik, J., Hearn, T., et al. (2016). Current trends in oxysterol research. *Biochemical Society Transactions, 44*, 652–658.

Soyal, S. M., Nofziger, C., Dossena, S., et al. (2015). Targeting SREBPs for treatment of the metabolic syndrome. *Trends in Pharmacological Sciences, 36*, 406–416.

Vegiopoulos, A. A., & Herzig, S. (2007). Glucocorticoids, metabolism and metabolic diseases. *Molecular and Cellular Endocrinology, 275*, 43–61.

Young, S. G., & Fong, L. G. (2012). Lowering plasma cholesterol by raising LDL receptors – revisited. *The New England Journal of Medicine, 366*, 1154–1155.

RELEVANT WEBSITES

Cholesterol biosynthetic pathway - Rat Genome Database: http://rgd.mcw.edu/rgdweb/pathway/pathwayRecord.html?acc_id=PW:0000454

KEGG Pathway Database. Primary bile acid biosynthesis - Reference pathway: http://www.genome.jp/kegg/pathway/map/map00120.html

Bile acid biosynthesis - The Metabolomic Innovation Centre (TMIC). The Small Molecule Pathway Database (SMPDB): http://smpdb.ca/view/SMP00035

MORE CLINICAL CASES

Please refer to Appendix 2 for more cases relevant to this chapter.

ABBREVIATIONS

ABCG5, G8, A1, G1, and G4	ATP-binding cassette transporters
ACAT	Cholesterol acyltransferase
Acetyl-CoA	Acetyl-coenzyme A
ACTH	Adrenocorticotropic hormone
AMPK	AMP-dependent kinase
CE	Cholesterol ester
CNS	Central nervous system
FXR	Farnesyl X receptor
FSH	Follicle-stimulating hormone
GC-MS	Gas chromatography–mass spectrometry
HDL	High-density lipoproteins
HMG-CoA	3-hydroxy-3-methylglutaryl-CoA
HMGR	HMG-CoA reductase
IPP	Isopentenyl diphosphate
LDL	Low-density lipoproteins
LH	Luteinizing hormone
LXR	Liver X receptors
NADPH	Nicotinamide dinucleotide phosphate
NPC1L1	Niemann–Pick C1-like protein.
PCSK9	Proprotein convertase subtilisin/kexin type 9
PPARα	Peroxisome proliferator activated receptor-α
RXR	Retinoid X receptor
SCAP	SREBP-cleavage-activating protein
SREBP	Sterol regulatory element-binding protein
VLDL	Very-low-density lipoproteins

Biosynthesis and Degradation of Amino Acids

Allen B. Rawitch

LEARNING OBJECTIVES

After reading this chapter, you should be able to:

■ Describe the three mechanisms used by humans for removal of nitrogen from amino acids before the metabolism of their carbon skeletons.

■ Outline the sequence of reactions in the urea cycle, and trace the flow of nitrogen from amino acids into and out of the cycle.

■ Describe the role of vitamin B_6 in aminotransferase reactions.

■ Define the terms and give examples of glucogenic and ketogenic amino acids.

■ Summarize the factors that contribute to the input and the depletion of the pool of free amino acids in animals.

■ Summarize the sources and use of ammonia in animals, and explain the concept of nitrogen balance.

■ Identify the essential amino acids and the metabolic sources of the nonessential amino acids.

■ Explain the biochemical basis and the therapeutic rationale for treatment of phenylketonuria and maple syrup urine disease.

When amino acids are metabolized, the resulting excess nitrogen must be excreted. Because the primary form in which the nitrogen is removed from amino acids is ammonia, and because free ammonia is quite toxic, humans and most higher animals rapidly convert the ammonia derived from amino acid catabolism to urea, which is neutral, less toxic, and very soluble and is excreted in the urine. Thus **the primary nitrogenous excretion product in humans is urea, produced by the urea cycle in the liver.** Animals that excrete urea are termed ureotelic. In an average individual, more than 80% of the excreted nitrogen is in the form of urea (25–30 g/24 h). Smaller amounts of nitrogen are also excreted in the form of uric acid, creatinine, and ammonium ion.

The carbon skeletons of many amino acids may be derived from metabolites in central pathways, allowing the biosynthesis of some, but not all, the amino acids in humans. Amino acids that can be synthesized in this way are therefore not required in the diet (nonessential amino acids), whereas amino acids having carbon skeletons that cannot be derived from normal human metabolism must be supplied in the diet (essential amino acids). In the biosynthesis of nonessential amino acids, amino groups must be added to the appropriate carbon skeletons. This generally occurs through the transamination of an α-keto acid corresponding to the carbon skeleton of that specific amino acid.

INTRODUCTION

Amino acids are a source of energy from the diet and during fasting

In addition to their roles as building blocks for peptides and proteins and as precursors of neurotransmitters and hormones, the carbon skeletons of some amino acids can be used to produce glucose through gluconeogenesis, thereby providing a metabolic fuel for tissues that require or prefer glucose; such amino acids are designated as glucogenic or glycogenic amino acids. The carbon skeletons of some amino acids can also produce the equivalents of acetyl-CoA or acetoacetate and are termed ketogenic, indicating that they can be metabolized to give immediate precursors of lipids and ketone bodies. In an individual consuming adequate amounts of protein, a significant quantity of amino acids may also be converted to carbohydrate (glycogen) or fat (triacylglycerol) for storage. Unlike carbohydrates and lipids, amino acids do not have a dedicated storage form equivalent to glycogen or fat, but they may still provide a source of energy under some circumstances.

METABOLISM OF DIETARY AND ENDOGENOUS PROTEINS

Relationship to central metabolism

Muscle protein and adipose lipids are consumed to support gluconeogenesis during fasting and starvation

Although body proteins represent a significant proportion of potential energy reserves (Table 15.1), under normal circumstances, they are not used for energy production. In an extended fast, however, muscle protein is degraded to amino acids for the synthesis of essential proteins and to keto acids for gluconeogenesis to maintain blood glucose concentration as well as to provide metabolites for energy production. This accounts for the loss of muscle mass during fasting.

In addition to its role as an important source of carbon skeletons for oxidative metabolism and energy production, dietary protein must provide adequate amounts of those amino acids that we cannot make to support normal protein synthesis. The relationships of body protein and dietary protein to central amino acid pools and to central metabolism are illustrated in Fig. 15.1.

Digestion and absorption of dietary protein

For dietary protein to contribute to either energy metabolism or pools of essential amino acids, the protein must be digested to the level of free amino acids or small peptides and absorbed across the gut. Digestion of protein begins in the stomach with the action of pepsin, a carboxyl protease that is active in the very low pH found in the gastric environment. Digestion continues as the stomach contents are emptied into the small intestine and mixed with pancreatic secretions. These pancreatic secretions are alkaline and contain the inactive precursors of several serine proteases, including trypsin, chymotrypsin, and elastase, along with carboxypeptidases. The process is completed by enzymes in the small intestine (see Chapter 30). After any remaining di- and tripeptides are broken down in enterocytes,

the free amino acids are absorbed and transported to the portal vein, which carries them to the liver for energy metabolism, biosynthesis, or distribution to other tissues to meet similar needs.

Turnover of endogenous proteins

In addition to the ingestion, digestion, and absorption of amino acids from dietary protein, all the proteins in the body have a

Table 15.1 Storage forms of energy in the body

Stored fuel	Tissue	Amount (g)*	Energy (kJ)	(kcal)
Glycogen	Liver	70	1176	280
Glycogen	Muscle	120	2016	480
Free glucose	Body fluids	20	336	80
Triacylglycerol	Adipose	15,000	567,000	135,000
Protein	Muscle	6000	100,800	24,000

Proteins represent a substantial energy reserve in the body.
*In a 70-kg individual.
(Adapted with permission from Cahill, 1976.)

ADVANCED CONCEPT BOX
ALANINE AND INTERORGAN CARBON AND NITROGEN FLOW

Much of the carbon flow that occurs between peripheral tissues, such as skeletal muscle, and the liver is facilitated by the release of alanine into the blood by the peripheral tissues. The alanine is converted to pyruvate in the liver, and the nitrogen component is incorporated into urea. The pyruvate can be used for gluconeogenesis to produce glucose, which is released into the blood for transport back to peripheral tissues. This glucose–alanine cycle allows the net conversion of amino-acid carbons to glucose, the elimination of amino-acid nitrogen as urea, and the return of carbons to the peripheral tissues in the form of glucose.

The glucose–alanine cycle works in a fashion similar to the Cori cycle (Chapter 31), in which lactate, released from skeletal muscle, is used for hepatic gluconeogenesis, the key difference being that alanine also carries a nitrogen atom to the liver. Alanine and glutamine are released in approximately equal quantities from skeletal muscle and represent almost 50% of the amino acids released by skeletal muscle into the blood - an amount that far exceeds the proportion of these amino acids in muscle proteins. Thus there is substantial remodeling of protein-derived amino acids by transamination reactions before their release from muscle.

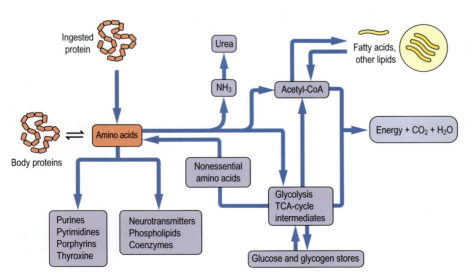

Fig. 15.1 **Metabolic relationships among amino acids.** The pool of free amino acids is derived from the degradation and turnover of body proteins and from the diet. The amino acids are precursors of important biomolecules, including hormones, neurotransmitters, and proteins, and also serve as a carbon source for central metabolism, including gluconeogenesis, lipogenesis, and energy production.

half-life or life span and are routinely degraded to amino acids and replaced with newly synthesized protein. This process of protein turnover is carried out in the lysosome or by proteasomes (Chapter 22). In the case of lysosomal digestion, protein turnover begins with engulfment of the protein or organelle in vesicles known as autophagosomes in a process called autophagy. The vesicles then fuse with lysosomes, and the protein, lipids, and glycans are degraded by lysosomal acid hydrolases. Cytosolic proteins are degraded primarily by proteasomes, which are high-molecular-weight complexes containing multiple proteolytic activities. This process is generally triggered by the attachment of a small protein (ubiquitin), although there are both ubiquitin-dependent and ubiquitin-independent pathways for degradation of cytosolic proteins.

AMINO ACID DEGRADATION

Amino acids destined for energy metabolism must be deaminated to yield the carbon skeleton

There are three mechanisms for removal of the amino group from amino acids.

- **Transamination** - the transfer of the amino group to a suitable keto acid acceptor (Fig. 15.2).
- **Oxidative deamination** - the oxidative removal of the amino group, resulting in keto acids, a reduced flavin coenzyme, and ammonia (see Fig. 15.3).
- **Removal of a molecule of water by a dehydratase** (e.g., serine or threonine dehydratase) - this reaction produces an

unstable imine intermediate that hydrolyzes spontaneously to yield an α-keto acid and ammonia (see Fig. 15.3).

The principal mechanism for removal of amino groups from the common amino acids is via transamination, or the transfer of amino groups from the amino acid to a suitable α-keto acid acceptor, most commonly to α-ketoglutarate or oxaloacetate, forming glutamate and aspartate, respectively. Several enzymes, called **aminotransferases (or transaminases)**, are capable of removing the amino group from most amino acids and producing the corresponding α-keto acid. Aminotransferase enzymes use pyridoxal phosphate, a cofactor derived from **vitamin B₆ (pyridoxine)**, as a key component in their catalytic

CLINICAL TEST BOX
MEASUREMENT OF BLOOD UREA NITROGEN

Serum urea (also reported by laboratories as BUN, or blood urea nitrogen) measurements are critical in monitoring patients with a variety of metabolic diseases in which the metabolism of amino acids may be affected and in tracking the condition of individuals with renal problems. The traditional methodology used for measuring blood urea has relied on the action of the enzyme urease, which converts urea to CO_2 and ammonia. The resulting ammonia can be detected spectrophotometrically by the formation of a colored compound on reaction with phenol or a related compound (the Berthelot reaction).

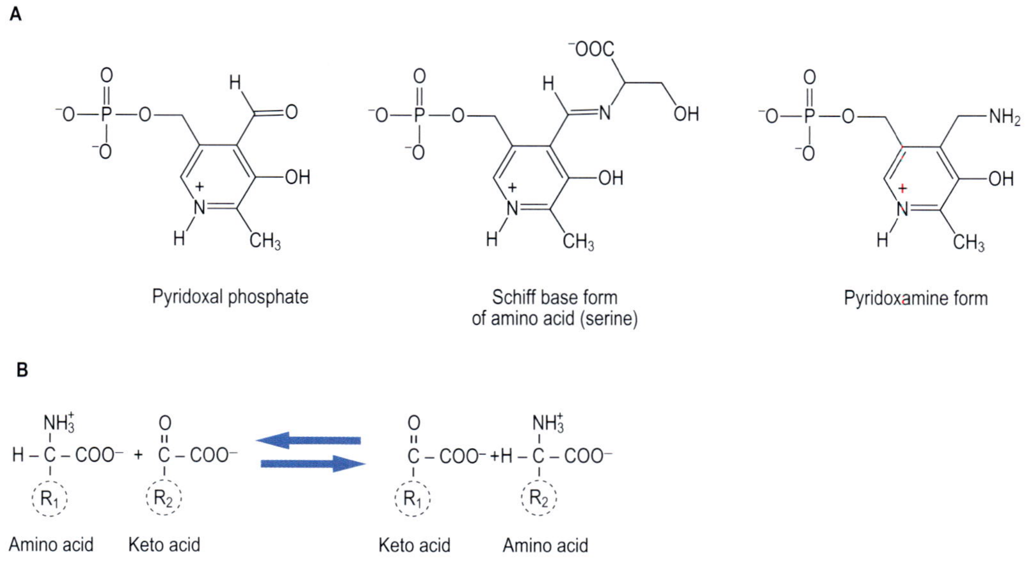

A

Pyridoxal phosphate

Schiff base form
of amino acid (serine)

Pyridoxamine form

B

Amino acid   Keto acid   Keto acid   Amino acid

Fig. 15.2 **The catalytic role of pyridoxal phosphate.** Aminotransferases, or transaminases, use pyridoxal phosphate as a cofactor. A pyridoxamine adduct acts as an intermediate in the transfer of an amino group between an α-amino acid and an α-keto acid. (A) Structures of the components involved. The cofactor, pyridoxal phosphate, is used in a variety of enzyme-catalyzed reactions involving both amino and keto compounds, including transamination and decarboxylation reactions. (B) Transamination involves both a donor α-amino acid (R₁) and an acceptor α-keto acid (R₂). The products are an α-keto acid derived from the carbon skeleton of R₁ and an α-amino acid from the carbon skeleton of R₂.

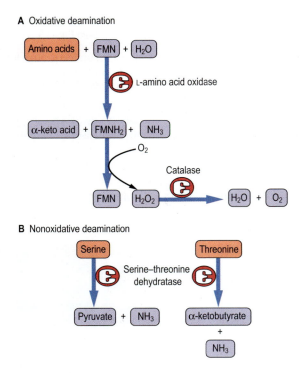

A Oxidative deamination

B Nonoxidative deamination

Fig. 15.3 **Deamination of amino acids.** The primary route for amino group removal is via transamination, but there are additional enzymes capable of removing the α-amino group. (A) L-amino acid oxidase produces ammonia and an α-keto acid directly, using flavin mononucleotide (FMN) as a cofactor. The oxidized form of the flavin must be regenerated using molecular oxygen; this reaction is one of several that produce H_2O_2. The peroxide is decomposed by catalase. (B) A second means of deamination is possible only for hydroxyamino acids (serine and threonine) through a dehydratase mechanism; the Schiff base imine intermediate hydrolyzes to form the keto acid and ammonia.

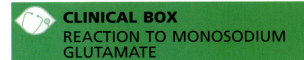

CLINICAL BOX
REACTION TO MONOSODIUM GLUTAMATE

A healthy 30-year-old woman experienced the sudden onset of headache, sweating, and nausea after eating at an Oriental restaurant. She felt weak and experienced some tingling and a sensation of warmth in her face and upper torso. The symptoms passed after about 30 min, and she experienced no further problems. Upon visiting her doctor the next day, she learned that some individuals react to foods containing high levels of the food additive monosodium glutamate, the sodium salt of glutamic acid. Monosodium glutamate is a common food additive used to enhance savory flavor in many foods. It is one of the principal substances responsible for the umami, or savory taste, sensation, which enhances the flavor effects of the other basic taste and taste-combination sensations.

Comment

The flu-like symptoms that develop, previously described as "Chinese-restaurant syndrome," have been attributed to central nervous system (CNS) effects of glutamate or its derivative, the inhibitory neurotransmitter γ-amino butyric acid (GABA). Interestingly, studies have shown that this phenomenon causes no permanent CNS damage and that although bronchospasm may be triggered in individuals with severe asthma, the symptoms are generally brief and completely reversible. Monosodium glutamate continues to be a widely used additive in many processed foods and is approved by the US Food and Drug Administration (FDA).

mechanism; pyridoxamine is an intermediate in the reaction. The structures of the various forms of vitamin B_6 and the net reaction catalyzed by aminotransferases are shown in Fig. 15.2.

Nitrogen atoms are incorporated into urea from two sources: glutamate and aspartate

The transfer of an amino group from one keto-acid carbon skeleton to another may seem to be unproductive and not useful in itself; however, when one considers the nature of the primary keto-acid acceptors that participate in these reactions (α-ketoglutarate and oxaloacetate) and their products (glutamate and aspartate), the logic of this metabolism becomes clear. The two nitrogen atoms in urea are derived exclusively from these two amino acids (Fig. 15.4). Ammonia, which is produced primarily from glutamate via the glutamate dehydrogenase (GDH) reaction (Fig. 11.5), enters the urea cycle as **carbamoyl phosphate.** The second nitrogen is contributed to urea by aspartic acid. Fumarate is formed in this process and may be recycled through the tricarboxylic acid (TCA) cycle to oxaloacetate, which can accept another amino group and

reenter the urea cycle, or the fumarate may be used for energy metabolism or gluconeogenesis. This process links the urea cycle in nitrogen metabolism to the TCA cycle and cellular energy metabolism. Thus the funneling of amino groups from other amino acids into glutamate and aspartate provides the nitrogen for urea synthesis in a form appropriate for the urea cycle (Fig. 15.4). The other pathways that lead to the release of amino groups from some amino acids through the action of amino acid oxidase or dehydratases (Fig. 15.3) make relatively minor contributions to the flow of amino groups from amino acids to urea.

The central role of glutamine

Ammonia is detoxified by incorporation into glutamine, then eventually into urea

In addition to the role of glutamate as a carrier of amino groups to GDH, glutamate serves as a precursor of glutamine, a process that consumes a molecule of ammonia. This is important because glutamine, along with alanine, is a key transporter of amino groups between various tissues and the

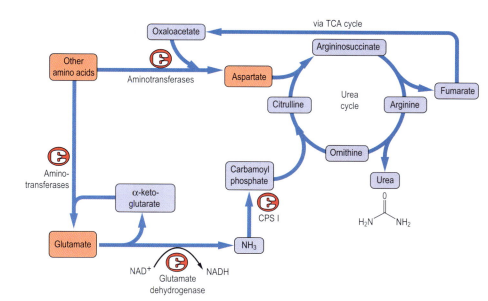

Fig. 15.4 **Sources of nitrogen atoms in the urea cycle.** Nitrogen enters the urea cycle from most amino acids via transfer of the α-amino group to either oxaloacetate or α-ketoglutarate to form aspartate or glutamate, respectively. Glutamate releases ammonia in the liver through the action of GDH (Fig. 15.5). The ammonia is incorporated into carbamoyl phosphate, and the aspartate combines with citrulline to provide the second nitrogen for urea synthesis. Oxaloacetate and α-ketoglutarate can be repeatedly recycled to channel nitrogen into this pathway. CPS I, carbamoyl phosphate synthetase-I.

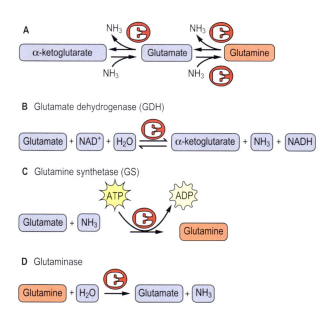

Fig. 15.5 **Relationships among glutamate, glutamine, and α-ketoglutarate.** The several forms of the carbon skeleton of glutamic acid have key roles in the metabolism of amino groups. (A) Three forms of the same carbon skeleton. (B) The glutamine dehydrogenase reaction is a reversible reaction that can produce glutamate from α-ketoglutarate or convert glutamate to α-ketoglutarate and ammonia. The latter reaction is important in the synthesis of urea because amino groups are fed to α-ketoglutarate via transamination from other amino acids. (C) Glutamine synthetase catalyzes an energy-requiring reaction with a key role in the transport of amino groups from one tissue to another; it also provides a buffer against high concentrations of free ammonia in tissues. (D) The second half of the glutamine transport system for nitrogen is the enzyme glutaminase, which hydrolyzes glutamine to glutamate and ammonia. This reaction is important in the kidney for the management of proton transport and pH control.

liver and is present in greater concentrations than most other amino acids in the blood. The three forms of the same carbon skeleton - α-ketoglutarate, glutamate, and glutamine - are interconverted via aminotransferases, glutamine synthetase, glutaminase, and GDH (see Fig. 15.5). Thus glutamine can serve as a buffer for ammonia utilization, as a source of ammonia, and as a carrier of amino groups. Because ammonia is quite toxic, a balance must be maintained between its production and utilization. A summary of the sources and pathways that use or produce ammonia is shown in Fig. 15.6. It should be noted that the GDH reaction is reversible under physiologic conditions, and if amino groups are required for amino acid and other biosynthetic processes, the reaction may run in the opposite direction.

The urea cycle and its relationship to central metabolism

The urea cycle is a hepatic pathway for disposal of excess nitrogen

Urea is the principal nitrogenous excretion product in humans (Table 15.2). The urea cycle (see Fig. 15.4) was the first metabolic cycle to be well defined; its description preceded that of the TCA cycle. The start of the urea cycle may be considered the synthesis of carbamoyl phosphate from an ammonium ion, derived primarily from glutamate via GDH (Fig. 15.5), and bicarbonate in liver mitochondria. This reaction requires two molecules of ATP and is catalyzed by the enzyme **carbamoyl phosphate synthetase I** (**CPS I**; Fig. 15.7), which is found at high concentration in the mitochondrial matrix.

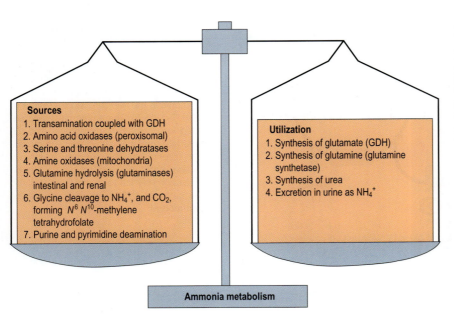

Fig. 15.6 **Balance in ammonia metabolism.** The balance between production and utilization of free ammonia is critical for maintenance of health. This figure summarizes the sources and pathways that use ammonia. Although most of these reactions occur in many tissues, *the synthesis of urea and the urea cycle are restricted to the liver.* Glutamine and alanine function as the primary transporters of nitrogen from peripheral tissues to the liver.

Sources
1. Transamination coupled with GDH
2. Amino acid oxidases (peroxisomal)
3. Serine and threonine dehydratases
4. Amine oxidases (mitochondria)
5. Glutamine hydrolysis (glutaminases) intestinal and renal
6. Glycine cleavage to NH_4^+, and CO_2, forming $N^6 N^{10}$-methylene tetrahydrofolate
7. Purine and pyrimidine deamination

Utilization
1. Synthesis of glutamate (GDH)
2. Synthesis of glutamine (glutamine synthetase)
3. Synthesis of urea
4. Excretion in urine as NH_4^+

Ammonia metabolism

Table 15.2 Urinary nitrogen excretion

Urinary metabolite	g excreted/24 h*	% of total
Urea	30	86
Ammonium ion	0.7	2.8
Creatinine	1.0–1.8	4–5
Uric acid	0.5–1.0	2–3

Approximate values in an average adult male.

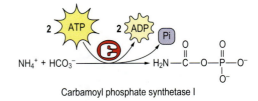

Carbamoyl phosphate synthetase I

Fig. 15.7 **Synthesis of carbamoyl phosphate.** The first nitrogen, derived from ammonia, enters the urea cycle as carbamoyl phosphate, synthesized by carbamoyl phosphate synthetase I in the liver.

The mitochondrial isozyme CPS I is unusual in that it requires *N*-acetylglutamate as a cofactor. It is one of two carbamoyl phosphate synthetase enzymes that have key roles in metabolism. The second, CPS II, is found in the cytosol, does not require *N*-acetylglutamate, and is involved in pyrimidine biosynthesis (Chapter 16).

Ornithine transcarbamoylase catalyzes the condensation of carbamoyl phosphate with the amino acid **ornithine** to form **citrulline**; see Fig. 15.4 for the pathway and Table 15.3 for the structures. In turn, the citrulline is condensed with aspartate to form argininosuccinate. This step is catalyzed by argininosuccinate synthetase and requires both ATP and aspartic acid; the reaction cleaves the ATP to adenosine monophosphate (AMP) and inorganic pyrophosphate (PPi; 2 ATP equivalents). The formation of argininosuccinate incorporates the second nitrogen atom destined for urea. Argininosuccinate is cleaved by argininosuccinase to arginine and fumarate, and the arginine is then cleaved by **arginase** to yield urea and ornithine, thus completing the cycle. The ornithine and fumarate can reenter the urea cycle and the TCA cycle, respectively, while the urea diffuses into the blood, is transported to the kidney, and is excreted in urine. The net process of ureagenesis is summarized in Table 15.4.

The urea cycle is split between the mitochondrial matrix and the cytosol

The first two steps in the urea cycle occur in the mitochondrion. The citrulline, which is formed in the mitochondrion, then moves into the cytosol by a specific passive transport system. The cycle is completed in the cytosol with the release of urea from arginine and the regeneration of ornithine. Ornithine is transported back across the mitochondrial membrane to continue the cycle. Carbons from fumarate, released in the argininosuccinase step, may also reenter the mitochondrion and be recycled by enzymes in the TCA cycle to oxaloacetate and ultimately to aspartate (Fig. 15.8), thus completing the second part of the urea cycle. *Urea synthesis occurs virtually exclusively in the liver,* and although the enzyme arginase is found in other tissues, its role is probably related more closely to ornithine requirements for polyamine synthesis than to the production of urea.

Table 15.3 Enzymes of the urea cycle

Enzyme	Reaction catalyzed	Remarks	Reaction product
Carbamoyl phosphate synthetase	Formation of carbamoyl phosphate from ammonia and CO_2	Fixes ammonia released from amino acids, uses 2 ATP, located in the **mitochondrion,** deficiency leads to high blood concentrations of ammonia and related toxicity	$$H_2N-\overset{\overset{\displaystyle O}{\|}}{C}-O-\overset{\overset{\displaystyle O}{\|}}{\underset{\underset{\displaystyle O^-}{\|}}{P}}-O^-$$ carbamoyl phosphate
Ornithine transcarbamoylase	Formation of citrulline from ornithine and carbamoyl phosphate	Releases Pi, an example of a transferase, located in the **mitochondrion,** deficiency leads to high blood concentrations of ammonia and orotic acid, as carbamoyl phosphate is shunted to pyrimidine biosynthesis	$$NH_2-\overset{\overset{\displaystyle O}{\|}}{C}-NH-(CH_2)_3-\overset{\overset{\displaystyle NH_3^+}{\|}}{CH}-COO^-$$ citrulline
Argininosuccinate synthetase	Formation of argininosuccinate from citrulline and aspartate	Requires ATP, which is cleaved to AMP + PPi – an example of a ligase, located in the **cytosol,** deficiency leads to high blood concentrations of ammonia and citrulline	$$\begin{array}{c}COO^-\\|\\NH-CH-CH_2-COO^-\\\|\|\\NH_2-C-NH-(CH_2)_3-\overset{\overset{\displaystyle NH_3^+}{\|}}{CH}-COO^-\end{array}$$ argininosuccinate
Argininosuccinase	Cleavage of argininosuccinate to arginine and fumarate	An example of a lyase, located in **cytosol,** deficiency leads to high blood concentrations of ammonia and citrulline	$$^-OOC-CH\!=\!CH-COO^-$$ $$NH_2 \qquad\qquad NH_2^+$$ $$NH_2-\overset{\overset{\displaystyle |}{}}{C}-NH-(CH_2)_3-\overset{\overset{\displaystyle |}{}}{CH}-COO^-$$ fumarate + arginine
Arginase	Cleavage of arginine to ornithine and urea	An example of a hydrolase, located in the **cytosol** and primarily in the liver, deficiency leads to moderately increased blood ammonia and high blood concentrations of arginine, urea is excreted and ornithine reenters the urea cycle	$$NH_2-\overset{\overset{\displaystyle O}{\|}}{C}-NH_2$$ $$NH_2-CH_2-CH_2-CH_2-\overset{\overset{\displaystyle NH_3^+}{\|}}{CH}-COO^-$$ urea + ornithine

Five enzymes catalyze the urea cycle in the liver. The first enzyme, CPS I, which fixes NH_4^+ as carbamoyl phosphate, is the regulatory enzyme and is sensitive to the allosteric effector, N-acetylglutamate.

Table 15.4 Urea synthesis

Component reactions in urea synthesis		
$CO_2 + NH_3 + 2$ ATP	→	Carbamoyl phosphate + 2 ADP + Pi
Carbamoyl phosphate + ornithine	→	Citrulline + Pi
Citrulline + aspartate + ATP	→	Argininosuccinate + AMP + PPi
Argininosuccinate	→	Arginine + fumarate
Arginine	→	Urea + ornithine
$CO_2 + NH_3 + 3$ ATP + aspartate	→	Urea + 2 ADP + AMP + 2 Pi + PPi + fumarate

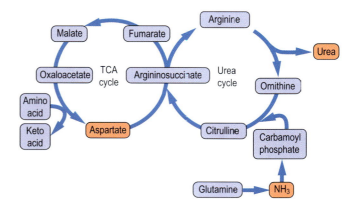

Fig. 15.8 **The tricarboxylic acid and urea cycles.** Analysis of the urea cycle reveals that it is really two cycles, with the carbon flow split between the primary urea synthetic process and the recycling of fumarate to aspartate; the latter cycle occurs in the mitochondrion and involves parts of the TCA cycle and an aminotransferase.

ADVANCED CONCEPT BOX
CARBAMOYL PHOSPHATE SYNTHESIS

The enzyme carbamoyl phosphate synthetase I (CPS I) is found in the mitochondrion and primarily in the liver; a second enzyme, CPS II, is found in the cytosol and in virtually all tissues. Although the product of both of these enzymes is the same - namely, carbamoyl phosphate - the enzymes are derived from different genes and function in ureagenesis (CPS I) or pyrimidine biosynthesis (CPS II), respectively. Additional differences between the two enzymes include their source of nitrogen (NH_3 for CPS I; glutamine for CPS II) and their requirement for N-acetylglutamate (required by CPS I but not by CPS II). Under normal circumstances, CPS I and II function independently and in different cellular compartments; however, when the urea cycle is blocked (e.g., as a result of a deficiency in ornithine transcarbamoylase), the accumulated mitochondrial carbamoyl phosphate spills over into the cytosolic compartment and may stimulate excess pyrimidine synthesis, resulting in a build-up of orotic acid in the blood and urine.

ADVANCED CONCEPT BOX
AMMONIA ENCEPHALOPATHY

The mechanisms involved in ammonia toxicity - the encephalopathy in particular - are not well defined. It is clear, however, that when its concentration builds up in the blood and other biological fluids, ammonia diffuses into cells and across the blood–brain barrier. The increase in ammonia causes an increased synthesis of glutamate from α-ketoglutarate and increased synthesis of glutamine. Although this is a normal detoxifying reaction in cells, when concentrations of ammonia are significantly increased, supplies of α-ketoglutarate in cells of the CNS may be depleted, resulting in inhibition of the TCA cycle and a decrease in ATP production. There may be additional mechanisms accounting for the bizarre behavior observed in individuals with high blood concentrations of ammonia. Changes in either glutamate, a major inhibitory neurotransmitter, or its derivative, γ-amino butyric acid (GABA), may also contribute to the CNS effects.

Regulation of the urea cycle

N-acetylglutamate (and indirectly, arginine) is an essential allosteric regulator of the urea cycle

The urea cycle is regulated in part by control of the concentration of **N-acetylglutamate,** the essential allosteric activator of CPS I. Arginine is an allosteric activator of *N*-acetylglutamate synthase and also a source of ornithine (via arginase) for the urea cycle. Concentrations of urea-cycle enzymes also increase or decrease in response to a high- or low-protein diets. Urea synthesis and excretion are decreased and NH_4^+ excretion is increased during acidosis as a mechanism to excrete protons into the urine. Although the details of this complex regulation are not completely defined, it is clear that both allosteric and genetic mechanisms are involved. Lastly, it should be noted that during

CLINICAL BOX
PARKINSON'S DISEASE

An otherwise healthy 60-year-old man noticed an occasional tremor in his left arm when relaxing and watching television. He also noticed occasional muscle cramping in his left leg, and his spouse noticed that he would occasionally develop a trance-like stare. A complete physical examination and consultation with a neurologist confirmed a diagnosis of Parkinson's disease. He was prescribed a medication that contained L-dihydroxyphenyl-alanine (L-DOPA) and a monoamine oxidase inhibitor (MAOI). L-DOPA is a precursor of the neurotransmitter dopamine, while monoamine oxidase is the enzyme responsible for the oxidative deamination and degradation of dopamine. His symptoms improved immediately, but he gradually experienced significant side effects from the medication, including involuntary movements and behavior or mood issues.

Comment

Parkinson's disease is caused by the death of dopamine-producing cells in the substantia nigra and the locus ceruleus. Although medication can markedly reduce the symptoms, the disease is progressive and may result in severe disability. Dopaminergic agonists often have side effects and also have limited effect on tremor, so other treatments, such as deep-brain stimulation or ablation, are used in selected cases. Monoamine oxidase is also involved in deamination of other amines in the brain, so monoamine oxidase inhibitors (MAOI) have many undesirable side effects. Transplantation of dopaminergic fetal tissue into the brain has been attempted but remains a controversial experimental treatment at present.

a fast, protein is broken down to free amino acids, which are used for gluconeogenesis. The increase in protein degradation during fasting results in increased urea synthesis and excretion as a mechanism to dispose of the released nitrogen.

Defects in any of the enzymes of the urea cycle have serious consequences. Infants born with defects in any of the first four enzymes in this pathway may appear normal at birth but rapidly become lethargic and hypothermic and frequently have difficulty breathing. Blood concentrations of ammonia increase quickly, followed by cerebral edema. The symptoms are most severe when early steps in the cycle are affected. However, a defect in any of the enzymes in this pathway is a serious issue and may cause hyperammonemia and lead rapidly to central nervous system (CNS) edema, coma, and death. Ornithine transcarbamoylase is the most common of these urea-cycle defects and shows an X-linked inheritance pattern. The remaining known defects associated with the urea cycle are autosomal recessive. A deficiency of arginase, the last enzyme in the cycle, produces less severe symptoms but is nevertheless characterized by increased concentrations of blood arginine and at least a moderate increase in blood ammonia. In individuals with high blood concentrations of ammonia, hemodialysis must be used, often followed by intravenous administration of sodium benzoate and phenylacetate.

CLINICAL TEST BOX
SCREENING FOR AMINO ACID METABOLIC DEFECTS IN THE NEWBORN

In most developed countries today, a spot of the blood of newborn infants is routinely collected on filter paper and tested for a series of compounds that are markers of inherited metabolic diseases. The number of markers tested for may vary from state to state in the United States but generally ranges from 10 to 30. Because of the need for rapid screening, small sample size, and reduced cost, older methodology is rapidly being replaced by technology that uses gas or liquid chromatography–mass spectrometry to measure the level of multiple markers simultaneously. The speed and high throughput capacity of this **metabolomics** technology allow rapid screening of 20 or more markers from dried blood spots and the identification of infants who are potential victims of these inborn errors of metabolism. This technology is also applied to the analysis of urine samples.

CLINICAL BOX
HEREDITARY HYPERAMMONEMIA

An apparently healthy 5-month-old female infant was brought to a pediatrician's office by her mother with a complaint of periodic bouts of vomiting and a failure to gain weight. The mother also reported that the child would oscillate between periods of irritability and lethargy. Subsequent examination and laboratory results revealed an abnormal electroencephalogram, a markedly increased concentration of plasma ammonia (323 mmol/L, 550 mg/dL; the normal range is 15–88 mmol/L, 25–150 mg/dL), and greater-than-normal concentrations of glutamine but low concentrations of citrulline. Orotate, a pyrimidine nucleotide precursor, was found in her urine.

Comment
The infant was admitted to the hospital and treated with intravenous benzoate and phenylacetate along with arginine. The benzoate and phenylacetate are metabolized to glycine and glutamate conjugates, which are excreted, with their nitrogen content, into the urine; arginine stimulates residual urea cycle activity. The infant improved rapidly and was discharged from the hospital on a low-protein diet with arginine supplementation. Subsequent biopsy of the patient's liver indicated that her hepatic ornithine transcarbamoylase activity was about 10% of normal.

The concept of nitrogen balance

A careful balance is maintained between nitrogen ingestion and secretion

Because there is no significant storage form of nitrogen or amino compounds in humans, nitrogen metabolism is quite dynamic. In an average, healthy diet, the protein content exceeds the amount required to supply essential and nonessential amino acids for protein synthesis, and the amount of nitrogen excreted is approximately equal to that taken in. Such a healthy adult would be said to be in "neutral nitrogen balance." When there is a need to increase protein synthesis, such as in recovering from trauma or in a rapidly growing child, amino acids are used for new protein synthesis, and the amount of nitrogen excreted is less than that consumed in the diet; the individual would be in "positive nitrogen balance." The converse is true in protein malnutrition: because of the need to synthesize essential body proteins, other proteins, particularly muscle proteins, are degraded, and more nitrogen is lost than is consumed in the diet. Such an individual would be said to be in "negative nitrogen balance." Fasting, starvation, and poorly controlled diabetes are also characterized by negative nitrogen balance as body protein is degraded to amino acids and their carbon skeletons are used for gluconeogenesis. The concept of nitrogen balance is clinically important because it reminds us of the continuous turnover of amino acids and proteins in the body (see Chapter 22).

METABOLISM OF THE CARBON SKELETONS OF AMINO ACIDS

Metabolism of amino acids interfaces with carbohydrate and lipid metabolism

When one examines the metabolism of the carbon skeletons of the 20 common amino acids, there is an obvious interface with carbohydrate and lipid metabolism. Virtually all the carbons can be converted into intermediates in the glycolytic pathway, the TCA cycle, or lipid metabolism. The first step in this process is the transfer of the α-amino group by transamination to α-ketoglutarate or oxaloacetate, providing glutamate and aspartate, the sources for the nitrogen atoms of the urea cycle (Fig. 15.9). The single exception to this is lysine, which does not undergo transamination. Although the details of pathways for the various amino acids vary, the general rule is that there is loss of the amino group, followed by either direct metabolism in a central pathway (glycolysis, the TCA cycle, or ketone-body metabolism) or one or more intermediate conversions to yield a metabolite in one of the central pathways. Examples of amino acids that follow the former scheme include alanine, glutamate, and aspartate, which yield pyruvate, α-ketoglutarate, and oxaloacetate, respectively. The branched-chain amino acids (leucine, valine, and isoleucine) and the aromatic amino acids (tyrosine, tryptophan, and phenylalanine) are examples of the latter, more complex pathways.

Amino acids may be either glucogenic or ketogenic

Depending on the point at which the carbons from an amino acid enter central metabolism, that amino acid may be considered to be either **glucogenic** or **ketogenic** - that is, possessing the ability to increase the concentrations of either

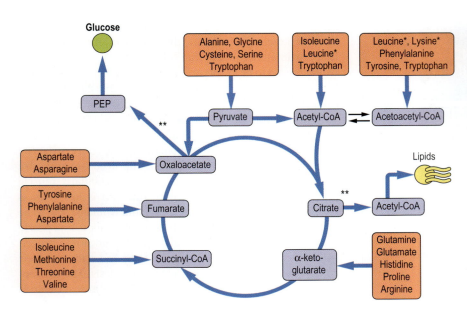

Fig. 15.9 **Amino acid metabolism and central metabolic pathways.** This figure summarizes the interactions between amino acid metabolism and central metabolic pathways. *The amino acids marked with an asterisk are ketogenic only. PEP, Phosphoenolpyruvate. ** Note that in addition to providing energy, carbons derived from amino acids can give rise to both glucose and fatty acids via oxaloacetate and citrate, respectively.

CLINICAL BOX
HOMOCYSTINURIA

A 21-year-old male was admitted to hospital after an episode of loss of speech and severe weakness on his right side. A diagnosis of ischemic stroke was made, and the patient was treated with anticoagulant therapy and improved. Laboratory results indicated substantially elevated levels of blood homocysteine. The patient made a significant recovery and was discharged on a modified diet along with supplements of vitamin B_6, folic acid, and vitamin B_{12}.

Comment

Homocystinuria is a relatively rare autosomal recessive condition (1 in 200,000 births) that results in a variety of symptoms, including mental retardation, vision problems, and thrombotic strokes and coronary artery disease at a young age. The condition is caused by lack of an enzyme that catalyzes the transfer of sulfur from homocysteine to serine, forming cysteine. Some of these patients respond to vitamin supplementation. Cross-sectional and retrospective studies suggest that even moderately elevated levels of homocysteine may be correlated with increased incidence of heart disease and stroke, but the jury is still out as to whether lowering homocysteine levels will reduce the development of these serious illnesses.

glucose or ketone bodies, respectively, when fed to an animal. Those amino acids that feed carbons into the TCA cycle at the level of α-ketoglutarate, succinyl-CoA, fumarate, or oxaloacetate and those that produce pyruvate can all give rise to the net synthesis of glucose via gluconeogenesis and are hence designated glucogenic. Those amino acids that feed carbons into central metabolism at the level of acetyl-CoA or acetoacetyl-CoA are considered ketogenic. Because of the nature of the TCA

cycle, no net flow of carbons can occur between acetate or its equivalent (e.g., butyrate or acetoacetate) from ketogenic amino acids to glucose via gluconeogenesis (Chapters 10 and 12).

Several amino acids, primarily those with more complex or aromatic structures, can yield both glucogenic and ketogenic fragments (see Fig. 15.9). Only the amino acids leucine and lysine are regarded as being exclusively ketogenic, and because of lysine's complex metabolism and lack of ability to undergo transamination, some authors do not consider it to be exclusively ketogenic. These classifications may be summarized as follows:

- **Glucogenic amino acids**: alanine, arginine, asparagine, aspartic acid, cysteine, cystine, glutamine, glutamic acid, glycine, histidine, methionine, proline, serine, valine
- **Ketogenic amino acids**: leucine, lysine
- **Both glucogenic and ketogenic amino acids**: isoleucine, phenylalanine, threonine, tryptophan, tyrosine

Metabolism of the carbon skeletons of selected amino acids

The 20 amino acids are metabolized by complex pathways to various intermediates in carbohydrate and lipid metabolism

Alanine, aspartate, and glutamate are examples of glucogenic amino acids. In each case, through either transamination or oxidative deamination, the resulting α-keto acid is a direct precursor of oxaloacetate via central metabolic pathways. Oxaloacetate can then be converted to PEP and subsequently to glucose via gluconeogenesis. Other glucogenic amino acids reach the TCA cycle or related metabolic intermediates through several steps after the removal of the amino group (Fig. 15.10).

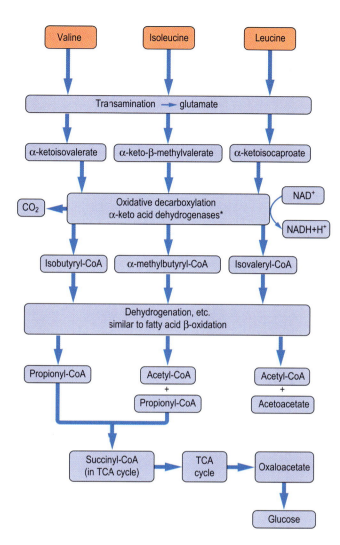

Fig. 15.10 **Degradation of branched-chain amino acids.** Metabolism of the branched-chain amino acids produces acetyl-CoA and acetoacetate. In the case of valine and isoleucine, propionyl-CoA is produced and metabolized, in two steps, to succinyl-CoA (Fig. 11.5). *The branched-chain amino acid dehydrogenases are structurally related to pyruvate dehydrogenase and α-ketoglutarate dehydrogenase and use the cofactors thiamine pyrophosphate, lipoic acid, flavin adenine dinucleotide, NAD⁺, and CoA.

Leucine is an example of a ketogenic amino acid. Its catabolism begins with transamination to produce 2-keto-isocaproate. The metabolism of 2-ketoisocaproate requires oxidative decarboxylation by a dehydrogenase complex to produce isovaleryl-CoA. Further metabolism of isovaleryl-CoA leads to the formation of 3-hydroxy-3-methylglutaryl-CoA, a precursor of both acetyl-CoA and the ketone bodies. The metabolism of leucine and the other branched-chain amino acids is summarized in Fig. 15.10. Note that propionyl-CoA derived from either amino acid degradation or odd-chain fatty acid metabolism is converted to succinyl-CoA (see Fig. 11.5) and may contribute to gluconeogenesis.

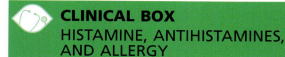

CLINICAL BOX
HISTAMINE, ANTIHISTAMINES, AND ALLERGY

An 8-year-old male child was referred to an allergy clinic due to repeated bouts of eczema with intense itching. He had no other known health issues. Previous treatment consisted of oral antihistamine medication, which provided some relief but did not prevent recurrence of the problem. After extensive testing, it was found that although he was marginally positive for an allergic reaction to dog and cat dander and to house dust mites, he was strongly positive for allergy to tomato. Examination of the boy's diet (he was quite fond of both pizza and spaghetti with tomato-based sauce) yielded a correlation of his bouts of eczema with his consumption of tomato-containing products. A dietary modification to avoid his allergic response to tomato products was initiated, and his symptoms became immediately less frequent and were well managed with oral antihistamine medication and the occasional use of topical steroid creams.

This is a good example of both the importance of appropriate allergy testing and the importance of antihistamines in the treatment of allergic reactions. This class of medication (there are many currently available) acts by interfering with the interaction of histamine with its receptor or inhibiting the production of histamine from its precursor, the amino acid histidine.

Tryptophan is a good example of an amino acid that yields both glucogenic and ketogenic precursors. After cleavage of its heterocyclic ring and a complex set of reactions, the core of the amino acid structure is released as alanine (a glucogenic precursor), whereas the balance of the carbons is ultimately converted to glutaryl-CoA (a ketogenic precursor). Fig. 15.11 summarizes key points in the catabolism of the aromatic amino acids.

BIOSYNTHESIS OF AMINO ACIDS

Evolution has left our species without the ability to synthesize almost half the amino acids required for the synthesis of proteins and other biomolecules

Humans use 20 amino acids to build peptides and proteins that are essential for the many functions of their cells. Biosynthesis of the amino acids involves the synthesis of the carbon skeletons for the corresponding α-keto acids, followed by addition of the amino group via transamination. However, humans are capable of carrying out the biosynthesis of the carbon skeletons of only about half of those α-keto acids in sufficient amounts. Amino acids that we cannot synthesize are termed **essential amino acids** and are required in the diet. Although almost all the amino acids can be classified as clearly essential or nonessential based on experimental studies of diet, a few require further qualification. For example, although cysteine is not generally considered an essential amino acid because

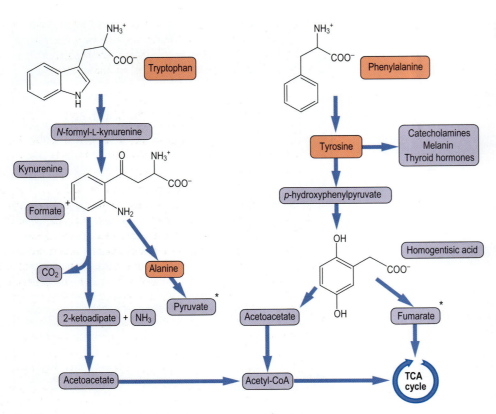

Fig. 15.11 **Catabolism of aromatic amino acids.** This figure summarizes the catabolism of the aromatic amino acids, illustrating the pathways that lead to ketogenic and glucogenic precursors derived from both tyrosine and tryptophan. *Both pyruvate and fumarate can lead to net glucose synthesis. They constitute the gluconeogenic portions of the metabolism of these amino acids.

it can be derived from the nonessential amino acid serine, its sulfur must come from the required, or essential, amino acid methionine. Similarly, the amino acid tyrosine is not required in the diet but must be derived from the essential amino acid phenylalanine. This relationship between phenylalanine and tyrosine will be discussed further in considering the inherited disease phenylketonuria (PKU). Although arginine can be synthesized as an intermediate of the urea cycle that meets the requirements of a normal, healthy adult, in growing children and in individuals recovering from trauma, it is considered an essential amino acid. Tables 15.5 and 15.6 list the nonessential and essential amino acids and the source of the carbon skeleton in the case of those not required in the diet.

Amino acids are precursors of many essential compounds

In addition to their role as the building blocks for peptides and proteins, amino acids are precursors of a number of neurotransmitters, hormones, inflammatory mediators, and carrier and effector molecules (Table 15.7). Examples of this include histidine, which serves as the precursor of histamine (the mediator of inflammation released by mast cells and lymphocytes), and glutamate, glycine, and aspartate, which are neurotransmitters. Additional examples include gamma aminobutyric acid (GABA), which is derived from glutamate, and tyrosine, which is derived from phenylalanine. Tyrosine is the precursor of the neurotransmitters 1,3-dihydroxyphenylalanine (DOPA), dopamine, and epinephrine; the thyroid hormones triiodothyronine and thyroxine; and melanin.

Table 15.5 Origins of nonessential amino acids

Amino acid	Source
Alanine	From pyruvate via transamination
Aspartic acid, asparagine, arginine, glutamic acid, glutamine, proline	From intermediates in the citric acid cycle
Serine	From 3-phosphoglycerate (glycolysis)
Glycine	From serine
Cysteine*	From serine; requires sulfur derived from methionine
Tyrosine*	Derived from phenylalanine via hydroxylation

*These are examples of nonessential amino acids that depend on adequate amounts of an essential amino acid.

INHERITED DISEASES OF AMINO ACID METABOLISM

In addition to deficiencies in the urea cycle, defects in the metabolism of the carbon skeletons of various amino acids were among the first disease states to be associated with simple

Table 15.6 Essential dietary amino acids

Mnemonic	Amino acid*	Notes or comments
P	Phenylalanine	Required in the diet also as a precursor of tyrosine
V	Valine	One of three branched-chain amino acids
T	Threonine	Metabolized like a branched-chain amino acid
T	Tryptophan	Its heterocyclic indole side chain cannot be synthesized in humans
I	Isoleucine	One of three branched-chain amino acids
M	Methionine	Provides the sulfur for cysteine and participates as a methyl donor in metabolism; the homocysteine is recycled
H	Histidine	Its heterocyclic imidazole side chain cannot be synthesized in humans
A	Arginine	Whereas arginine can be derived from ornithine in the urea cycle in amounts sufficient to support the needs of adults, growing animals require it in the diet
L	Leucine	A pure ketogenic amino acid
L	Lysine	Does not undergo direct transamination

*The mnemonic PVT TIM HALL is useful for recalling the names of the essential amino acids.

Table 15.7 Examples of amino acids as effector molecules or precursors

Amino acid	Effector molecule or prosthetic group
Arginine	Immediate precursor of urea, precursor of nitric oxide
Aspartate	Excitatory neurotransmitter
Glycine	Inhibitory neurotransmitter; precursor of heme
Glutamate	Excitatory neurotransmitter; precursor of γ-amino butyric (GABA), an inhibitory neurotransmitter
Histidine	Precursor of histamine, a mediator of inflammation and a neurotransmitter
Tryptophan	Precursor of serotonin, a potent smooth muscle contraction stimulator; precursor of melatonin, a regulator of circadian rhythm
Tyrosine	Precursor of the hormones and neurotransmitters catecholamines, dopamine, epinephrine, and norepinephrine, thyroxine

inheritance patterns. These observations gave rise to the concept of the genetic basis of inherited metabolic disease states, also known as **inborn errors of metabolism.** Garrod considered a number of disease states that appeared to be inherited in a Mendelian pattern, and he proposed a correlation between these abnormalities and specific genes, in which the disease state could be either dominant or recessive. Dozens of inborn errors of amino acid metabolism have now been described, and the molecular defect has been identified for many of them. Three classic inborn errors of metabolism that involve amino acids are discussed in some detail here.

Phenylketonuria (PKU)

The common form of PKU results from a deficiency of the enzyme phenylalanine hydroxylase. The hydroxylation of phenylalanine is a required step in both the normal degradation of the carbon skeleton of this amino acid and the synthesis of tyrosine (Fig. 15.12). When untreated, this metabolic defect

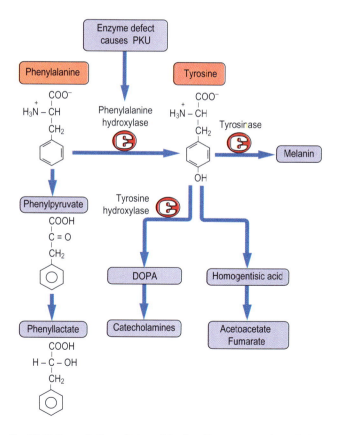

Fig. 15.12 **Degradation of phenylalanine.** To enter normal metabolism, phenylalanine must be hydroxylated by the enzyme phenylalanine hydroxylase. A defect in this enzyme leads to phenyl-ketonuria (PKU). Tyrosine is a precursor of acetyl-CoA and fumarate, catecholamine hormones, the neurotransmitter dopamine, and the pigment melanin. DOPA, dihydroxyphenylalanine.

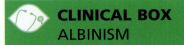

CLINICAL BOX
ALBINISM

A full-term infant, born to a normal and healthy mother and father, was observed to have a marked lack of pigmentation. The infant, who appeared to be otherwise normal, had blue eyes and very light blond, almost white, hair. This lack of pigmentation was confirmed as classic albinism on the basis of a family history and the establishment of a lack of the enzyme tyrosinase, which is responsible for a two-step hydroxylation of tyrosine to dihydroxyphenylalanine (DOPA) and a subsequent further oxidation to a quinone, a precursor of melanin in melanocytes.

Comment

The primary cause of albinism is a homozygous defect in either tyrosinase or an accessory P protein. A separate DOPA-producing enzyme, tyrosine hydroxylase, is involved in the biosynthesis of the catecholamine neurotransmitters, so albinos do not appear to have neurologic deficits. As a result of their lack of pigmentation, however, they are quite sensitive to damage from sunlight and must take added precautions against ultraviolet radiation from the sun. Albinos are generally very sensitive to bright light. They may have normal eyesight, in spite of the lack of pigmentation - retinal pigments are derived from carotene (vitamin A) rather than tyrosine - however, they are prone to eye problems.

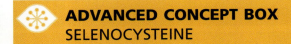

ADVANCED CONCEPT BOX
SELENOCYSTEINE

In addition to the 20 common amino acids found in proteins, a 21st amino acid has been discovered and shown to be an active-site amino acid in several enzymes, including the antioxidant enzyme glutathione peroxidase (Chapter 42) and 5'-deiodinases (important in the metabolism of thyroid hormones; Chapter 27). **Selenocysteine** is derived from serine and has unique chemical properties. It is because of the need for selenocysteine that trace amounts of selenium are required in the diet. It should be noted that although selenocysteine is incorporated per se into the enzymes in which it functions, a number of other unusual amino acids may be found in some proteins due to posttranslational modification. Examples of this can be seen in the collagens and connective tissue proteins that contain hydroxylated forms of proline and lysine, which are formed after the incorporation of proline and lysine into the protein polypeptide (see Chapter 19).

leads to excessive urinary excretion of phenylpyruvate and phenylacetate and severe mental retardation. In addition, individuals with PKU tend to have very light skin pigmentation; unusual gait, stance, and sitting posture; and a high frequency of epilepsy. In the United States, this autosomal recessive defect occurs in about 1 in 30,000 live births. Because of its frequency, and the ability to prevent the most serious consequences of the defect with a low-phenylalanine diet, newborns in most developed countries are routinely tested for blood concentrations of phenylalanine. Fortunately, with early detection and the use of a diet restricted in phenylalanine but supplemented with tyrosine, most of the mental retardation can be avoided. Mothers who are homozygous for this defect have a very high probability of bearing children with congenital defects and mental retardation unless their blood phenylalanine concentrations can be controlled by diet. The developing fetus is very sensitive to the toxic effects of high maternal concentrations of phenylalanine and related phenylketones. Not all hyperphenylalaninemias are caused by a defect in phenylalanine hydroxylase. In some cases, there is a defect in biosynthesis or reduction of a required tetrahydrobiopterin cofactor.

Alkaptonuria (black urine disease)

A second inherited defect in the phenylalanine–tyrosine pathway involves a deficiency in the enzyme that catalyzes the oxidation of homogentisic acid, an intermediate in the catabolism of tyrosine and phenylalanine. In this condition, which occurs in 1 in 1,000,000 live births, homogentisic acid accumulates and is excreted in urine. This compound oxidizes to alkaptone on standing or on treatment with alkali, giving the urine a dark color. Individuals with **alkaptonuria** ultimately suffer from the deposition of dark (ochre-colored) pigment in cartilage, with subsequent tissue damage, including severe arthritis. The onset of these symptoms is generally in the third or fourth decade of life. This autosomal recessive disease was the first of several that Garrod considered in proposing his initial hypothesis for inborn errors of metabolism. Although alkaptonuria is relatively benign compared with PKU, little is available in the way of treatment, other than symptomatic relief.

Maple syrup urine disease (MSUD)

The normal metabolism of the branched-chain amino acids leucine, isoleucine, and valine involves loss of the α-amino group, followed by oxidative decarboxylation of the resulting α-keto acid. This decarboxylation step is catalyzed by branched-chain keto acid decarboxylase, a multienzyme complex associated with the inner membrane of the mitochondrion. In approximately 1 in 300,000 live births, a defect in this enzyme leads to accumulation of the keto acids corresponding to these branched-chain amino acids in the blood and then to branched-chain ketoaciduria. When untreated or unmanaged, this condition may lead to both physical and mental retardation of the newborn and a distinct maple syrup odor of the urine. This defect can be partially managed with a low-protein or modified diet, but not in all cases. In some instances, supplementation with high doses of thiamine pyrophosphate, a cofactor for this enzyme complex, has been helpful.

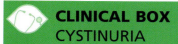

CLINICAL BOX
CYSTINURIA

A 21-year-old man came to the emergency room with severe pain in his right side and back. Subsequent investigation indicated a kidney stone as well as increased concentrations of cystine, arginine, and lysine in the urine. This patient exhibited the characteristic symptoms of cystinuria.

Comment

Cystinuria is an autosomal recessive disorder of intestinal absorption and proximal tubular reabsorption of dibasic amino acids; it does not result from a defect in cysteine metabolism per se. Because of the transport deficiency, cysteine, which is normally reabsorbed in the proximal renal tubule, remains in the urine. The cysteine spontaneously oxidizes to its disulfide form, cystine. Cystine is relatively insoluble and tends to precipitate in the urinary tract, forming kidney stones. The condition is generally treated by restricting the dietary intake of methionine (a biosynthetic precursor of cysteine), encouraging high fluid intake to keep the urine dilute, and more recently, using drugs that convert urinary cysteine to a more soluble compound that will not precipitate.

ACTIVE LEARNING

1. Tyrosine is included as a supplement in the diet plan for individuals with phenylketonuria. What is the rationale for this supplement? Compare the therapeutic approaches used for the treatment of the various forms of PKU in which phenylalanine hydroxylase is not affected.
2. Review the rationale for the use of levodopa, catechol-O-methyltransferase inhibitors, and monoamine oxidase inhibitors for the treatment of Parkinson's disease.
3. Review the pathways for biosynthesis of the neurotransmitters serotonin, melatonin, and dopamine and the catecholamines. What enzymes are involved in the inactivation of these compounds?

SUMMARY

- The catabolism of amino acids generally begins with the removal of the α-amino group, which is transferred to α-ketoglutarate and oxaloacetate and ultimately excreted in the form of urea.
- Because carbon skeletons corresponding to the various amino acids can be derived from or fed into the glycolytic pathway, the TCA cycle, fatty acid biosynthesis, and gluconeogenesis, amino acid metabolism should not be considered as an isolated pathway.
- Although amino acids are not stored like glucose (glycogen) or fatty acids (triglycerides), they have an important and dynamic role, not only in providing the building blocks for the synthesis and turnover of peptides and proteins, but also in normal energy metabolism, providing a carbon source for gluconeogenesis when needed and an energy source of last resort in starvation.
- Amino acids provide precursors for the biosynthesis of a variety of small signaling molecules, including hormones and neurotransmitters.
- The severe consequences of inherited diseases such as phenylketonuria and maple syrup urine disease illustrate the effects of abnormal amino acid metabolism.

FURTHER READING

Dietzen, D. J., Rinaldo, P., Whitley, R. J., et al. (2009). National academy of clinical biochemistry laboratory medicine practice guidelines: Follow-up testing for metabolic disease identified by expanded newborn screening using tandem mass spectrometry: Executive summary. *Clinical Chemistry, 55*, 1615–1626.

Kuhara, T. (2007). Noninvasive huma metabolome analysis for differential diagnosis of inborn errors of metabolism. *Journal of Chromatography B, 855*, 42–50.

MacLeod, E., Hall, K., & McGuire, P. (2016). Computational modeling to predict nitrogen balance during acute metabolic decompensation in patient with urea cycle disorders. *Journal of Inherited Metabolic Disease, 39*, 17–24.

Mitchell, J. J., Trakadis, Y. J., & Scriver, C. R. (2011). Phenylalanine hydroxylase deficiency. *Genetics in Medicine, 13*, 697–707.

Morris, S. M., Jr. (2006). Arginine: Beyond protein. *Am J Clin Nutr, 83*(Suppl.), 508S–512S.

Natesan, V., Mani, R., & Arumugam, R. (2016). Clinical aspects of urea cycle dysfunction and altered brain energy metabolism on modulation of glutamate receptors and transporters in acute and chronic hyperammonemia. *Biomed Pharmacother, 81*, 192–202.

Ogier de Baulny, H., & Saudubray, J. M. (2002). Branched-chain organic acidurias. *Seminars in Fetal and Neonatal Medicine, 7*, 65–74.

Saudubray, J. M., Nassogne, M. C., de Lonlay, P., et al. (2002). Clinical approach to inherited metabolic disorders in neonates: An overview. *Seminars in Fetal and Neonatal Medicine, 7*, 3–15.

Singh, R. H. (2007). Nutritional management of patients with urea cycle disorders. *Journal of Inherited Metabolic Disease, 30*, 880–887.

Summar, M. L., Dobbelaere, D., Brusilow, S., et al. (2008). Diagnosis, symptoms, frequency and mortality of 260 patients with urea cycle disorders from a 21-year, multicentre study of acute hyperammonaemic episodes. *Acta Paediatrica, 97*, 1420–1425.

Sun, R., Xi, Q., Sun, J., et al. (2016). In low protein diets, microRNA-19b regulates urea synthesis by targeting SIRT5. *Scientific Reports, 6*, 33291.

Wilcken, B. (2012). Screening for disease in the newborn: The evidence base for blood-spot screening. *Pathology, 44*, 73–79.

RELEVANT WEBSITES

Society for the Study of Inborn Errors of Metabolism (SSIEM): http://www.ssiem.org

Urea cycle disorders:
    http://www.ncbi.nlm.nih.gov/books/NBK1217/
    http://www.horizonpharma.com/urea-cycle-disorders/
Nitrogen metabolism: http://themedicalbiochemistrypage.org/
    nitrogen-metabolism.php
Parkinson's disease: http://www.mayoclinic.org/diseases-conditions/
    parkinsons-disease/basics/definition/con-20028488
Phenylketonuria: http://www.nlm.nih.gov/medlineplus/phenylketonuria.html

ABBREVIATIONS

BUN	Blood urea nitrogen
CPS	Carbamoyl phosphate synthetase
MAO	Monoamine oxidase
MAOI	Monoamine oxidase inhibitor
PKU	Phenylketonuria

16

Biosynthesis and Degradation of Nucleotides

Alejandro Gugliucci, Robert W. Thornburg, and Teresita Menini

LEARNING OBJECTIVES

After reading this chapter, you should be able to:

- Compare and contrast the structure and biosynthesis of purines and pyrimidines, highlighting differences between de novo and salvage pathways.
- Describe how cells meet their requirements for nucleotides at various stages in the cell cycle.
- Explain the biochemical rationale for using fluorouracil and methotrexate in chemotherapy.
- Describe the metabolic basis and therapy for classic disorders in nucleotide metabolism: gout, Lesch–Nyhan syndrome, and SCIDS.

- Salvage pathways that recycle preformed bases and nucleosides and provide an adequate supply of nucleotides for cells at rest
- Catabolic pathways for excretion of nucleotide degradation products, a process that is essential to limit the accumulation of toxic levels of nucleotides within cells (Impaired elimination or increased production of **uric acid,** the end product of purine metabolism, may cause gout and is associated with hypertension and metabolic syndrome.)
- Biosynthetic pathways for conversion of the ribonucleotides into the deoxyribonucleotides, providing precursors for DNA

Purines and pyrimidines

Nucleotides are formed from three components: a nitrogenous base, a five-carbon sugar, and phosphate

The nitrogenous bases found in nucleic acids belong to one of two heterocyclic groups, either purines or pyrimidines (Fig. 16.1). The major purines of both DNA and RNA are guanine and adenine. In DNA, the major pyrimidines are thymine and cytosine, while in RNA, they are uracil and cytosine; **thymine is unique to DNA and uracil is unique to RNA**.

When the nitrogenous bases are combined with a five-carbon sugar, they are known as nucleosides. When the nucleosides are phosphorylated, the resulting compounds are known as nucleotides. The phosphate can be attached at either the 5′ position or the 3′ position of the ribose, or both. Table 16.1 gives the names and structures of the most important purines and pyrimidines.

INTRODUCTION

Nucleotides, molecules composed of a pentose, a nitrogenous base, and phosphate, are key elements in cell physiology because they have the following roles:

- Precursors of DNA and RNA
- Components of coenzymes (e.g., NAD[H], NADP[H], FMN[H_2], and coenzyme A)
- Energy currency, driving anabolic processes (e.g., ATP and GTP)
- Carriers in biosynthesis (e.g., UDP for carbohydrates and CDP for lipids)
- Allosteric modulators of key enzymes in metabolism
- Second messengers in important signaling pathways (e.g., cAMP and cGMP)

We can synthesize purine and pyrimidine nucleotides from metabolic intermediates. In this way, although we ingest dietary nucleic acids and nucleotides, survival does not require their absorption and utilization. Because nucleotides are involved in so many levels of metabolism, they are important targets for chemotherapeutic agents used in the treatment of microbial and parasitic infections and cancer.

This chapter first describes the structure and then the metabolism of the two classes of nucleotides: **purines** and **pyrimidines.** The metabolic pathways are presented in four sections:

- De novo synthesis of nucleotides from basic metabolites, which is critical and sine qua non for growing cells

PURINE METABOLISM

De novo synthesis of the purine ring: Synthesis of inosine monophosphate (IMP)

Purines and pyrimidines are synthesized by both de novo and salvage pathways

The demand for nucleotide biosynthesis can vary greatly. It is high during the S-phase of the cell cycle, when cells are about to divide (Chapter 28). The process is therefore very active in growing tissues, embryonic and fetal tissue, and actively proliferating cells (e.g., hematopoietic [blood] cells and cancer cells) and during wound healing and tissue regeneration. Purine

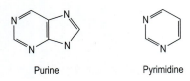

Fig. 16.1 **Classification of nucleotides.** Basic structure of purines and pyrimidines.

Table 16.1 Names and structures of important purines and pyrimidines

Structure	Free base	Nucleoside	Nucleotide
	Adenine	Adenosine	AMP ADP ATP cAMP
	Guanine	Guanosine	GMP GDP GTP cGMP
	Hypoxanthine	Inosine	IMP
	Uracil	Uridine	UMP UDP UTP
	Cytosine	Cytidine	CMP CDP CTP
	Thymine	Thymidine	TMP TDP TTP

The designation NTP refers to the ribonucleotide. The prefix d, as in dATP, is used to identify deoxyribonucleotides. dTTP is usually written as TTP, with the d-prefix implied.

and pyrimidine biosynthesis are energetically expensive processes subject to intracellular mechanisms that sense and effectively regulate the pool sizes of intermediates and products to avoid energy waste.

The raw materials for purine synthesis are CO₂, nonessential amino acids (Asp, Glu, Gly), and folic acid derivatives that act as single-carbon donors. Five molecules

of ATP are needed for the synthesis of IMP, the first purine product and common precursor of AMP and GMP. The starting material for synthesis of IMP is ribose 5-phosphate, a product of the pentose phosphate pathway (Chapter 9). The first step, catalyzed by **ribose-phosphate pyrophosphokinase (PRPP synthetase; phosphoribosylpyrophosphate synthetase),** generates the activated form of the pentose phosphate by transferring a pyrophosphate group from ATP to form 5-phosphoribosyl-pyrophosphate (PRPP; Fig. 16.2). In a series of 10 reactions, PRPP is converted to IMP. Most of the carbons and all of the nitrogens of the purine ring are derived from amino acids; one carbon is derived from CO_2 and two from **N¹⁰-formyltetrahydrofolate (THF),** a derivative of **folic acid** (see Fig. 16.9). Folic acid is a vitamin; therefore folate deficiency can impair purine synthesis, which can cause disease, notably anemia. On the other hand, an induced folate deficiency can be exploited clinically to kill rapidly dividing cells, which have a high demand for purine biosynthesis. The end product of this sequence of reactions is the ribonucleotide IMP; the purine base is called hypoxanthine, the nucleoside is inosine, and the nucleotide is inosine monophosphate.

Synthesis of ATP and GTP from IMP

IMP does not accumulate significantly within the cell; it is converted to both AMP and GMP. Two enzymatic reactions are required in each case (Fig. 16.3). Distinct enzymes, adenylate kinase and guanylate kinase, use ATP to synthesize the nucleotide mono- and diphosphates from the nucleotide monophosphates. Finally, a single enzyme, termed **nucleotide diphosphokinase,** converts diphosphonucleotides into nucleotide triphosphates. This is a wide-spectrum enzyme that has activity toward all nucleotide diphosphates, including pyrimidines and purines and both ribo- and deoxyribonucleotides for the synthesis of RNA and DNA, respectively.

Salvage pathways for purine nucleotide biosynthesis

In addition to de novo synthesis, cells can use preformed nucleotides obtained from the diet or from the breakdown of endogenous nucleic acids through salvage pathways. This is an important energy-saving mechanism. In mammals, there are two enzymes in the purine salvage pathway. **Adenine phosphoribosyl transferase (APRT)** converts free adenine into AMP (Fig. 16.4A). **Hypoxanthine-guanine phosphoribosyl transferase (HGPRT)** catalyzes a similar reaction for both hypoxanthine (the purine base in IMP) and guanine (Fig. 16.4B). Purine nucleotides are synthesized preferentially by salvage pathways, so long as the free nucleobases are available. This preference is mediated by inhibition of **amidophosphoribosyl transferase,** step 2 of the de novo pathway (Fig. 16.2) by AMP and GMP which act synergistically at distinct sites on

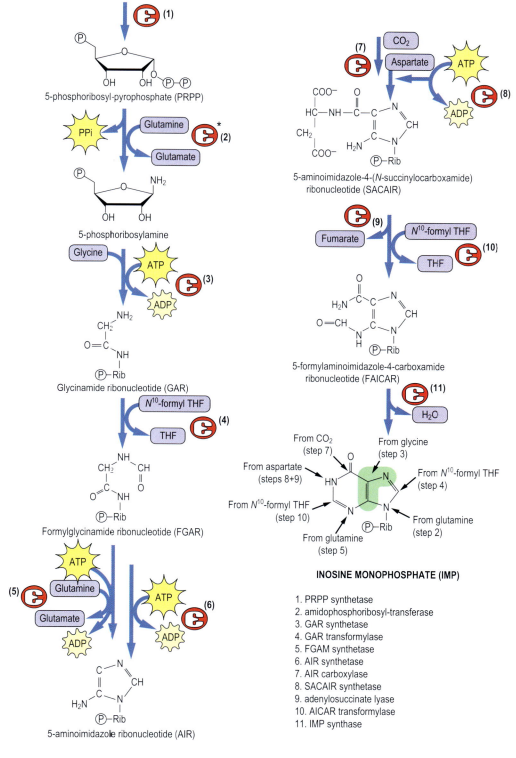

Fig. 16.2 **Synthesis of IMP.** *The asterisk identifies the regulatory enzyme amidophosphoribosyl transferase (2).

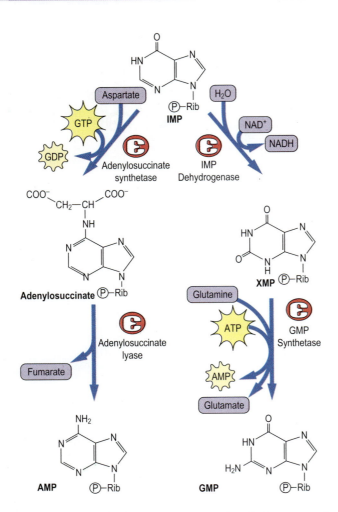

Fig. 16.3 **Conversion of IMP into AMP and GMP.** Two enzymatic reactions are needed in each branch of the pathway. XMP, xanthosine monophosphate.

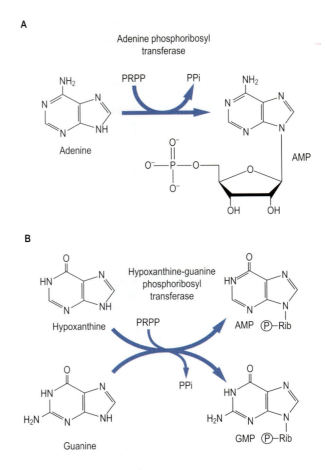

Fig. 16.4 **The purine salvage pathways.** (A) Adenine phosphoribosyl transferase. (B) Hypoxanthine-guanine phosphoribosyl transferase.

the enzyme. Note that step 2 is the site of inhibition of purine biosynthesis because PRPP is also used in other biosynthetic processes, including nucleotide salvage pathways.

Purine and uric acid metabolism in humans

Sources and disposal of uric acid

Uric acid is the end product of purine catabolism in humans

Uric acid, the end product of purine catabolism in humans, is not metabolized and must be excreted. However, the complex renal handling of urate, described later in the chapter, suggests an evolutionary advantage to having high circulating levels of urate. As noted in Chapter 42, uric acid is a circulating antioxidant. At pH 7.4, it is 98% ionized and therefore circulates as monosodium urate. This salt has poor solubility; the extracellular fluid becomes saturated at urate

concentrations a little above the upper limit of the reference range. Therefore there is a tendency for monosodium urate to crystallize in subjects with **hyperuricemia.** Crystallization is promoted by low temperature and pH in the extremities. The most obvious clinical manifestation of this process is gout, in which crystals form in cartilage, synovium, and synovial fluid. This can be accompanied by **renal calculi** (urate stones) and **tophi** (accumulation of sodium urate deposits in soft tissues). A sudden increase in urate production - for example, during chemotherapy when many cells die rapidly - can lead to widespread crystallization of urate in the joints but mainly in the urine, causing an acute **urate nephropathy.**

There are three sources of purines in humans: de novo synthesis, salvage pathways, and diet. The body urate pool (and thus plasma uric acid concentration) is governed by the relative rates of urate formation and excretion. More than half of urate is excreted by the kidney; the rest is excreted by the intestines, where bacteria dispose of it. In the kidney, urate is filtered and almost totally reabsorbed in the proximal tubule. Distally, both secretion and absorption occur, so overall urate clearance amounts to about 10% of the filtered load (i.e., 90%

ADVANCED CONCEPT BOX
SALVAGE PATHWAYS ARE THE PRINCIPAL SOURCE OF NUCLEOTIDES IN LYMPHOCYTES

In humans, resting T lymphocytes, immune system cells produced in the thymus (Chapter 43), meet their routine metabolic requirements for nucleotides through the salvage pathway, but de novo synthesis is required to support the growth of rapidly dividing cells. The salvage of nucleotides is especially important in HIV-infected T lymphocytes. In asymptomatic patients, resting lymphocytes show a block in de novo pyrimidine biosynthesis and correspondingly reduced pyrimidine pool sizes. After activation of the T-lymphocyte population, these cells cannot synthesize sufficient new DNA. The activation process leads to cell death, contributing to the decline in the T-lymphocyte population during the late stages of HIV infection.

The salvage pathways are especially important for many parasites as well. Some parasites, such as *Mycoplasma*, *Borrelia*, and *Chlamydia*, have lost the genes required for the de novo synthesis of nucleotides. These organisms prey metabolically on their host using preformed metabolites, including nucleotides.

CLINICAL BOX
GOUT RESULTS FROM AN EXCESS OF URIC ACID

Diagnosis
The diagnosis of **gout** is primarily clinical and supported by the demonstration of hyperuricemia. About 90% of gout patients appear to excrete urate at an inappropriately low rate for the plasma concentration, whereas about 10% have excessive production. Gouty arthritis has a typically hyperacute onset (less than 24 h), with severe pain, swelling, redness, and warmth in the joint(s), characteristically in first metatarsophalangeal joint (the big toe) but also at the elbow, knees, and other joints. It is confirmed by the presence of tophi, or sodium urate crystals, in the synovial fluid. The crystals are needle-shaped, are seen inside neutrophils, and have negative birefringence when viewed with polarized light.

Pathogenesis
Urate crystals in joints are phagocytized by neutrophils (leukocytes in blood and tissues). The crystals damage cellular membranes, and release of lysosomal enzymes in the joint precipitates an acute inflammatory reaction. Several cytokines enhance and perpetuate the inflammation, and phagocytic cells, monocytes, and macrophages aggravate the inflammation.

Management
The acute attack is managed with antiinflammatory agents, including steroidal (e.g. prednisone) and nonsteroidal antiinflammatory drugs (NSAID). Dietary changes (less meat and alcohol, increased water intake, weight reduction) and changes in concurrent drug therapies, such as diuretics, may be helpful. Probenecid, a uricosuric drug, is commonly employed to reduce uricemia. Colchicine, a microtubule disruptor, may also be used during an acute attack to inhibit phagocytosis and inflammation. If the patient is already a hyperexcretor, or tophi or renal disease is present, then allopurinol is used. Allopurinol is an inhibitor of xanthine oxidase (Fig. 16.5). Allopurinol undergoes the first oxidation to yield alloxanthine, but it cannot undergo the second oxidation. Alloxanthine remains bound to the enzyme, acting as a potent competitive inhibitor. The recently marketed febuxostat is a new-generation xanthine oxidase inhibitor that works with a similar mechanism. It produces a noncompetitive blockade of the molybdenum pterin center of the enzyme. Action of xanthine oxidase inhibitors leads to reduced formation of uric acid and accumulation of xanthine and hypoxanthine, which are 10 times more soluble and are easily excreted in urine. Another recently approved drug, lesinurad, works by inhibition of urate reabsorption (therefore increasing elimination) at the level of URAT1, an organic anion transporter.

is retained in the body. Normally, urate excretion increases if the filtered load is increased. Because of the role of the kidney in urate metabolism, kidney diseases can lead to urate retention and urate precipitation in the kidney (stones) and urine. Dietary purines account for about 20% of excreted urate. Therefore restricting purines in the diet (less meat) can reduce urate levels by only 10%–20%.

Endogenous formation of uric acid

Each of the purine nucleotide monophosphates (IMP, GMP, and AMP) can be converted into its corresponding nucleosides by 5'-nucleotidase. The enzyme purine nucleoside phosphorylase then converts the nucleosides inosine or guanosine into the free purine bases hypoxanthine and guanine as well as ribose-1-P. Hypoxanthine is oxidized, and guanine is deaminated to yield xanthine (Fig. 16.5). Two other enzymes, **AMP deaminase** and **adenosine deaminase,** convert the amino group of AMP and adenosine into IMP and inosine, respectively, which are then converted to hypoxanthine. In effect, guanine is directly converted to xanthine, whereas inosine and adenine are converted to hypoxanthine, then to xanthine.

Xanthine oxidase (XO), the final enzyme in this pathway, catalyzes a two-step oxidation reaction, converting hypoxanthine to xanthine, then xanthine to uric acid. Uric acid is the final metabolic product of purine catabolism in primates, birds, reptiles, and many insects. Other organisms, including most mammals, fish, amphibians, and invertebrates, metabolize uric acid to more soluble products, such as allantoin (see Fig. 16.5).

Hyperuricemia and gout

Most persons with hyperuricemia remain asymptomatic throughout life, but there is no gout without hyperuricemia

Plasma urate concentration is, on average, higher in men than in women; tends to rise with age; and is usually elevated

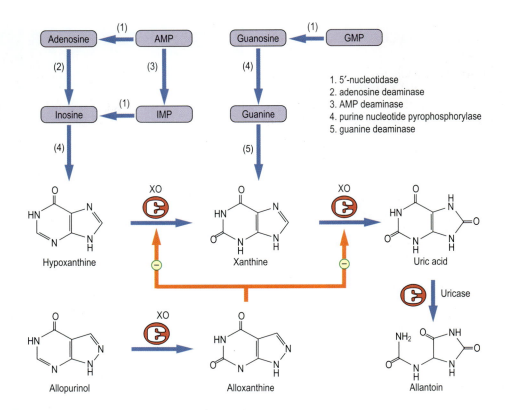

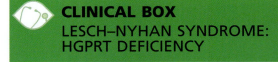

Fig. 16.5 **Degradation of purines and biochemical basis of allopurinol treatment of gout.** Inhibition of xanthine oxidase (XO) by alloxanthine is the mechanism involved in allopurinol treatment of gout. The enzyme uricase is missing in primates (including humans) but is commonly used for measurement of serum uric acid levels in humans. (1) 5′-nucleotidase; (2) adenosine deaminase; (3) AMP deaminase; (4) purine nucleotide pyrophosphorylase; (5) guanine deaminase.

in obese subjects and subjects in the higher socioeconomic groups; gout has been known for millennia as a "rich man's disease." Higher levels of uric acid correlate with high sugar, meat, and alcohol consumption. The risk of gout, a painful disease resulting from precipitation of sodium urate crystals in joints and dermis, increases with higher plasma urate concentrations. Hyperuricemia can occur due to increased formation, decreased excretion of uric acid, or both. Decreased renal excretion of urate can result from a decrease in filtration and/or secretion. Many factors (including drugs and alcohol) also affect the tubular handling of urates and can cause or increase hyperuricemia.

PYRIMIDINE METABOLISM

As with the purines, the pyrimidines (uracil, cytosine, and thymine) are also synthesized through a complex series of reactions using raw materials readily available in cells. One important difference is that the pyrimidine base is made first and the sugar added later (Fig. 16.6), whereas purines are assembled on a ribose-5-P scaffold (Fig. 16.2). Uridine monophosphate (UMP) is the precursor of all pyrimidine nucleotides. The de novo pathway produces UMP, which is then converted to cytidine

CLINICAL BOX
LESCH–NYHAN SYNDROME: HGPRT DEFICIENCY

The gene encoding HGPRT is located on the X chromosome. Its deficiency results in a rare X-linked recessive disorder, Lesch–Nyhan syndrome. The lack of HGPRT causes accumulation of PRPP, which is also the substrate for the enzyme amidophosphoribosyl transferase. This stimulates purine biosynthesis by up to 200-fold. Because of increased purine synthesis, the degradation product, uric acid, also accumulates to high levels. Elevated uric acid leads to a crippling gouty arthritis and severe neuropathology, resulting in mental retardation, spasticity, aggressive behavior, and a compulsion toward self-mutilation by biting and scratching.

triphosphate (CTP) and thymidine triphosphate (TTP). Salvage pathways also recover preformed pyrimidines.

De novo pathway

Pyrimidine and purine nucleoside biosynthesis share several common precursors: CO_2, amino acids (Asp, Gln), and for thymine, N^5,N^{10}-methylenetetrahydrofolate (**N^5,N^{10}-methylene-THF**; see Fig. 16.9). The pathway for biosynthesis of UMP is outlined in Fig. 16.6. The first step, catalyzed by the enzyme **carbamoyl phosphate synthetase II (CPS II)**, uses bicarbonate, glutamine, and 2 moles of ATP to form carbamoyl phosphate (CPS I is used in the synthesis of arginine in the urea cycle; Chapter 15). Most of the atoms required for formation of the pyrimidine ring are derived from aspartate, added in a single step by **aspartate transcarbamoylase** (ATCase). Carbamoyl aspartate is then cyclized to dihydroorotic acid by the action of the enzyme dihydroorotase. Dihydroorotic acid is oxidized to **orotic acid** by a mitochondrial enzyme, dihydroorotate dehydrogenase. Leflunomide, a specific inhibitor of this enzyme, is used for the treatment of rheumatoid arthritis because blockage of this step inhibits lymphocyte activation and thereby limits inflammation. The ribosyl-5′-phosphate group from PRPP is then transferred onto orotic acid to form orotidine monophosphate (OMP). Finally, OMP is decarboxylated to form UMP. UTP is synthesized in two enzymatic phosphorylation steps by the actions of UMP kinase and nucleotide diphosphokinase. CTP synthetase converts UTP into CTP by amination of UTP (Fig. 16.7, left). This step completes the synthesis of the ribonucleotides for the synthesis of RNA.

Metabolic channeling by multienzymes improves efficiency

In bacteria, the six enzymes of pyrimidine (UMP) biosynthesis exist as distinct proteins. However, during the evolution of mammals, the first three enzymatic activities became fused together into **CAD**, a single multifunctional polypeptide encoded by a single gene. The name of the enzyme derives from its three activities: **carbamoyl phosphate synthetase**, **aspartate transcarbamoylase, and dihydroorotase**. The final two enzymatic activities of pyrimidine biosynthesis, orotate phosphoribosyl transferase and orotidylate decarboxylase, are also fused into a single enzyme, UMP synthase. As with the fatty acid synthase complex (Chapter 13), this fusion of sequential enzyme activities avoids the diffusion of the metabolic intermediates into the intracellular milieu, thereby improving the metabolic efficiency of the individual steps.

Pyrimidine salvage pathways

As with the purines, free pyrimidine bases, available from the diet or from the breakdown of nucleic acids, can be recovered by several salvage enzymes. Uracil phosphoribosyl transferase (UPRTase) is similar to the enzymes of the purine salvage pathways. This enzyme also activates some chemotherapeutic agents, such as 5-fluorouracil (FU) or 5-fluorocytosine (FC). A uridine-cytidine kinase and a more specific thymidine kinase catalyze the phosphorylation of these nucleosides; nucleotide kinases and diphosphokinase complete the salvage process.

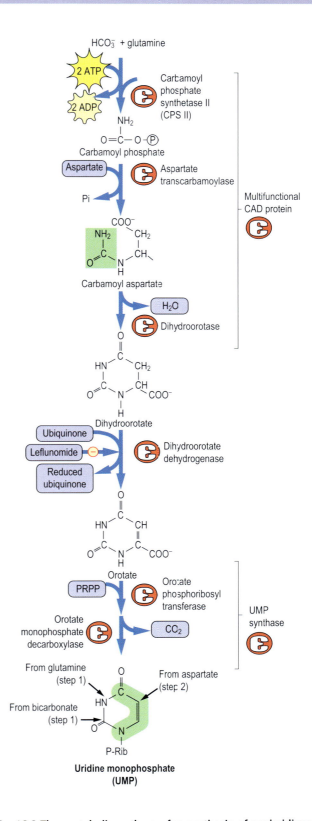

Fig. 16.6 **The metabolic pathway for synthesis of pyrimidines.** Formation of orotic acid and UMP, the first pyrimidine nucleotide.

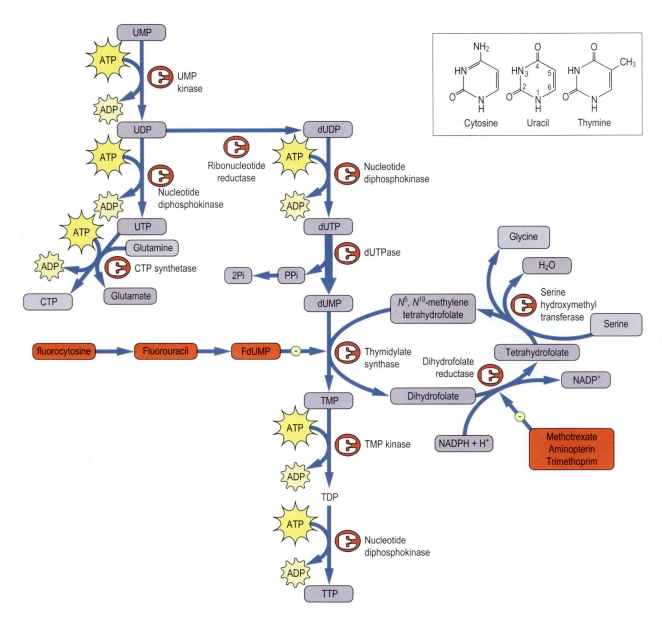

Fig. 16.7 **Synthesis of pyrimidine triphosphates.** Synthesis of thymidine is inhibited by fluorodeoxyuridylate (FdUMP), methotrexate, aminopterin, and trimethoprim at the indicated sites.

FORMATION OF DEOXYNUCLEOTIDES

Ribonucleotide reductase

Ribonucleotide reductase catalyzes reduction of ribose to deoxyribose in nucleotides for the synthesis of DNA

Because DNA uses deoxyribonucleotides instead of the ribonucleotides found in RNA, cells require pathways to convert ribonucleotides into the deoxy forms. The adenine, guanine, and uracil deoxyribonucleotides are synthesized from their corresponding ribonucleotide diphosphates by direct reduction of the 2'-hydroxyl by the enzyme **ribonucleotide reductase**, as shown for dUDP in Fig. 16.8. The reduction of the 2'-hydroxyl of ribose uses a pair of protein-bound sulfhydryl groups (cysteine residues). The hydroxyl group is released as water, and the cysteines are oxidized to cystine during the reaction. To regenerate an active enzyme, the disulfide must be reduced back to the original sulfhydryl pair by disulfide exchange; this is accomplished by reaction with a small protein, **thioredoxin.** Thioredoxin, a highly conserved Fe-S protein, is in turn reduced by the flavoprotein thioredoxin reductase.

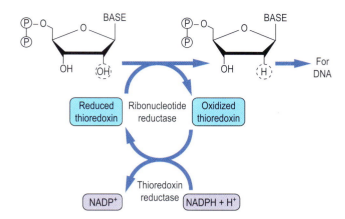

Fig. 16.8 **Formation of deoxyribonucleotides, except TTP, by ribonucleotide reductase.** Thioredoxin and NADPH (from the pentose phosphate pathway) are required for recycling of the enzyme.

A unique pathway to thymidine triphosphate

Thymine is synthesized by a complex reaction pathway, providing many opportunities for chemotherapy

The nucleotide deoxy-TMP, abbreviated as TMP rather than dTMP because thymine is unique to DNA, is synthesized by a special pathway involving methylation of the deoxyribose form of uridylate, dUMP (Fig. 16.7). The TMP biosynthetic pathway leads from UMP to UDP, then, through ribonucleotide reductase, to dUDP. The dUDP is then phosphorylated to dUTP, which creates an unexpected biochemical problem. DNA polymerase does not effectively discriminate between the two deoxyribonucleotides dUTP and TTP; the only difference is a methyl group at C-5. DNA polymerase incorporates dUTP into DNA in vitro, but this reaction would lead to high rates of mutagenesis in vivo. Therefore cells limit the concentration of dUTP by rapid hydrolysis of dUTP to dUMP, catalyzed by a highly specific low K_m (~1 μM) and kinetically rapid enzyme dUTPase. This enzyme cleaves a high-energy bond and releases pyrophosphate, which is rapidly hydrolyzed to phosphate, shifting the equilibrium ever further toward the formation of dUMP. The dUMP is converted to TMP by **thymidylate synthase (TS)**, using N^5,N^{10}-methylene-THF as the methyl donor; the dihydrofolate product is recycled by the action of the enzymes **dihydrofolate reductase** and serine hydroxymethyl transferase. Two rounds of phosphorylation of TMP yield TTP for the synthesis of DNA.

The synthesis of TTP is a roundabout pathway but provides opportunities for chemotherapy through inhibition of TMP biosynthesis (Fig. 16.7). There is only one reaction in pyrimidine synthesis that requires a THF derivative: conversion of dUMP to TMP, catalyzed by thymidylate synthase. This reaction is often rate limiting for cell division. Indeed, folate deficiency impairs cell replication, especially the replication of rapidly

ADVANCED CONCEPT BOX
CHEMOTHERAPEUTIC TARGETS: FOLATE RECYCLING AND THYMIDYLATE SYNTHASE

Fluorodeoxyuridylate (FdUMP) is a specific **suicide inhibitor** of thymidylate synthase. In FdUMP, a highly electronegative fluorine replaces the carbon-5 proton of uridine. This compound can begin the enzymatic conversion into dTMP by forming the enzyme–FdUMP covalent complex; however, the covalent intermediate cannot accept the donated methyl group from methylene THF, nor can it be broken down to release the active enzyme. The result is a suicide complex in which the substrate is covalently locked at the active site of thymidylate synthase. The drug is frequently administered as **fluorouracil,** and the body's normal metabolism converts the fluorouridine into FdUMP. Fluorouracil is used in the treatment of breast, colorectal, gastric, and uterine cancers.

Fluorocytosine is a potent antimicrobial agent. Its mechanism of action is similar to that of FdUMP; however, it must first be converted into fluorouracil by the action of cytosine deaminase. The fluorouracil is subsequently converted into FdUMP, which blocks thymidylate synthase, as previously explained. Although cytosine deaminase is present in most fungi and bacteria, it is absent in animals and plants. Therefore, in humans, fluorocytosine is not converted into fluorouracil and is nontoxic, whereas in the microbes, metabolism of fluorocytosine results in cell death.

Aminopterin and **methotrexate** are folic acid analogs (Fig. 16.9) that bind about 1000-fold more tightly to dihydrofolate reductase (DHFR) than does dihydrofolate. In this manner, they competitively, almost irreversibly, block the synthesis of dTMP. These compounds are also competitive inhibitors of other THF-dependent enzyme reactions used in the biosynthesis of purines, histidine, and methionine. Trimethoprim binds to DHFR, and it binds more tightly to bacterial DHFRs than it does to mammalian enzymes, making it an effective antibacterial agent. Folate analogs are relatively nonspecific chemotherapeutic agents. They poison rapidly dividing cells - not just cancer cells but also hair follicles, hematopoietic cells, and gut epithelial cells, causing the loss of hair, anemia, and the gastrointestinal side effects of chemotherapy. Beyond these roles, methotrexate in low doses is used to treat rheumatoid arthritis, inhibiting lymphocyte proliferation. Moreover, given the role of inflammation in atherosclerosis, major multicenter studies are currently evaluating low-dose methotrexate to reduce the risk for cardiovascular disease.

dividing cells. Thus folate deficiency is a frequent cause of anemia; bone marrow cells involved in erythropoiesis and hematopoiesis are among the most rapidly dividing cells in the body. As outlined in the Advanced Concept Box (above), inhibition of thymidylate synthase, either directly or by inhibition of THF recycling, provides a special opportunity for chemotherapy, targeting synthesis of DNA precursors in rapidly dividing cancer cells.

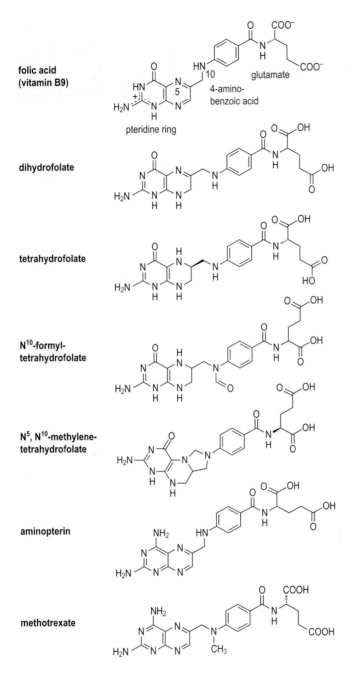

Fig. 16.9 **Structure of folic acid and related coenzymes and chemotherapeutic agents.**

both purines and pyrimidines are induced during the S-phase of cell division. Covalent and allosteric regulation also play an important role in the control of nucleotide synthesis. The multimeric protein CAD is activated by phosphorylation by protein kinases in response to growth factors, increasing its affinity for PRPP and decreasing inhibition by UTP. Both of these changes favor biosynthesis of pyrimidines for cell division.

Mole per mole, pyrimidine biosynthesis parallels purine biosynthesis, suggesting the presence of a coordinated control. Among them, one of the key points is the PRPP synthase reaction. PRPP is a precursor for all the ribo- and deoxyribonucleotides. PRPP synthase is inhibited by both pyrimidine and purine nucleotides.

Ribonucleotide reductase coordinates the biosynthesis of all four deoxynucleotides

Because a single enzyme is responsible for the conversion of all ribonucleotides into deoxyribonucleotides, this enzyme is subject to a complex network of feedback regulation. Ribonucleotide reductase contains several allosteric sites for metabolic regulation. Levels of each of the dNTPs modulate the activity of the enzyme toward the other NDPs. By regulating the enzymatic activity of deoxyribonucleotide synthesis as a function of the concentration of the different dNTPs, often described as "cross-talk" between the pathways, the cell ensures that the proper ratios of the different deoxyribonucleotides are produced for normal growth and cell division.

Catabolism of pyrimidine nucleotides

In contrast to the degradation of purines to uric acid, pyrimidines are degraded to soluble compounds, which are readily eliminated in urine and are not a frequent source of pathology. Orotic acidurias may occur in the rare cases when enzymes in the pyrimidine catabolic pathways are defective. Otherwise, the pyrimidine nucleotides and nucleosides are converted to the free bases, and the heterocyclic ring is cleaved, yielding **β-aminoisobutyrate** as the main excretion product, plus some ammonia and CO_2.

De novo nucleotide metabolism is highly regulated

Ribonucleotide reductase is the allosteric enzyme that coordinates a balanced supply of deoxynucleotides for synthesis of DNA

Because nucleotides are required for mammalian cells to proliferate, the enzymes involved in the de novo synthesis of

SUMMARY

■ Nucleotides are synthesized primarily from amino acid precursors and phosphoribosyl pyrophosphate by complex, metabolically expensive, multistep pathways.

■ De novo nucleotide metabolism is required for cell proliferation, but salvage pathways also play a prominent role in nucleotide metabolism.

CLINICAL BOX
SEVERE COMBINED IMMUNODEFICIENCY SYNDROMES (SCIDS) ARE CAUSED BY IMPAIRED PURINE SALVAGE PATHWAYS

SCIDS are fatal disorders resulting from defects in both cellular and humoral immune function. SCIDS patients cannot efficiently produce antibodies in response to an antigenic challenge. Approximately 50% of patients with the autosomal recessive form of SCIDS have a genetic deficiency in the purine salvage enzyme **adenosine deaminase.** The pathophysiology involves lymphocytes of both thymic and bone marrow origin (T and B lymphocytes) as well as "self-destruction" of differentiated cells after antigen stimulation. The precise cause of cell death is not yet known, but it may involve the accumulation of adenosine, deoxyadenosine, and dATP in lymphoid tissues, accompanied by ATP depletion. dATP inhibits ribonucleotide reductase and therefore DNA nucleotide synthesis. The finding that deficiency of the next enzyme in the purine salvage pathway, nucleoside phosphorylase, is also associated with an immune deficiency disorder suggests that integrity of the purine salvage pathway is critical for normal differentiation and function of immuno-competent cells in humans.

CLINICAL BOX
REVERSE EVOLUTION: URICASE AS A NEW TREATMENT FOR REFRACTORY GOUT

Most of the drugs employed to treat patients with gout have been used for more than 40 years. More recently, as our physiologic understanding of gout has improved, new innovative treatments have been developed and introduced in the market, such as enzyme therapy by administration of uricase. Pegloticase, a recombinant uricase, is a novel treatment option for patients suffering from chronic and refractory gout. The porcine uricase enzyme has been combined with polyethylene glycol (PEG), which increases its plasma half-life to 2 weeks, making its intravenous injection an alternative approach for the treatment of patients with symptomatic gout for whom existing hypouricemic agents are unsuccessful or contraindicated.

Human trials show that pegloticase maintains uric acid concentrations below 7 mg/dL in patients with chronic gout. These recombinant uricases may have a place in the treatment of severe gout, particularly in patients with severe and tophaceous gout to promote tophi dissolution.

ADVANCED CONCEPT BOX
THE YIN AND YANG OF XANTHINE OXIDASE: BEYOND URIC ACID PRODUCTION

Xanthine oxidase (XO) is a ubiquitous cytosolic flavoprotein that controls the rate-limiting step in purine catabolism. The oxidation of xanthine to uric acid produces $FADH_2$, and the reoxidation of $FADH_2$ produces reactive oxygen species (ROS; superoxide and hydrogen peroxide), which are toxic at high concentrations in the cell. An excess of ROS production is associated with many acute and chronic diseases, including ischemia-reperfusion injury (IRI), cardiovascular disease, microvascular syndromes, metabolic syndrome, and cancer (Chapter 42). XO, among other enzymes, contributes to the generation of excess ROS in these conditions. In IRI, the ROS are produced during reperfusion of the tissue (i.e., during the recovery phase). Allopurinol, an XO inhibitor, is being evaluated as adjuvant therapy to limit ROS production during recovery from myocardial infarction and stroke. In contrast, XO is also being conjugated to antitumor antibodies in experimental studies to direct ROS production to the tumor environment to kill cancer cells. Thus, although XO is a lead actor in purine catabolism, it also plays other roles in pathology and therapy.

ADVANCED CONCEPT BOX
FRUCTOSE CAN INCREASE PLASMA URIC ACID LEVELS, WHICH CAN BE IMPLICATED IN METABOLIC SYNDROME - HOW?

In the past few years, strong epidemiologic evidence has shown a connection between fructose consumption (especially in the form of sugar-sweetened beverages, including fruit juices) and increases in plasma uric acid. This is associated in many cases with hypertension and metabolic syndrome. Two straightforward, integrative biochemical connections can mechanistically explain these associations. As shown in Chapter 12, fructose reaches the liver and is metabolized essentially only there. It bypasses the two key regulatory steps in glycolysis; therefore surges of fructose (think of two big glasses of soda or apple juice, containing 40 g or more than 200 mM fructose) lead to unrestricted phosphorylation of fructose, which consumes ATP. The resultant ADP is recycled to ATP by nucleoside diphosphokinase, leading to accumulation of AMP. AMP is converted to uric acid, which can inhibit AMP kinase, a master regulator enzyme. Its inhibition favors stimulates hepatic lipogenesis, glucose secretion, and cholesterol biosynthesis, all associated with metabolic syndrome. Uric acid is also a quencher of NO, leading to increased blood pressure.

ACTIVE LEARNING

1. Compare the roles of de novo synthesis and the salvage pathways of nucleotide synthesis in various cell types (e.g., erythrocytes, lymphocytes, and muscle and liver cells).
2. In addition to its activity as a xanthine oxidase inhibitor, what other activities of allopurinol might contribute to its efficacy for the treatment of gout?
3. Discuss the use of thymidylate synthetase inhibitors and folate analogs for treatment of diseases other than cancer (e.g., arthritis, psoriasis).
4. Review the role of folates in metabolism, and explain the effects of folate deficiency and the rationale for folate supplementation during pregnancy.
5. Why is reduction in alcohol intake recommended for persons susceptible to gout.

■ Both classes of nucleotides (purines and pyrimidines) are synthesized as precursors (IMP, UMP), which are then converted into the DNA precursors (dATP, dGTP, dCTP, TTP).

■ With the exception of TTP, ribonucleotides are converted to deoxyribonucleotides by ribonucleotide reductase. TTP is synthesized from dUMP by a special pathway involving folates.

■ Salvage pathways have proven useful for the activation of pharmaceutical agents, whereas the uniqueness of the pathway for synthesis of TTP has provided a special target for chemotherapeutic inhibition of DNA synthesis and cell division in cancer cells.

■ High plasma concentrations of uric acid, the final product of purine catabolism in humans, can lead to gout and kidney stones and is associated with metabolic syndrome.

FURTHER READING

Agarwal, A., Banerjee, A., & Banerjee, U. C. (2011). Xanthine oxidoreductase: A journey from purine metabolism to cardiovascular excitation-contraction coupling. *Critical Reviews in Biotechnology, 31*, 264–280.

Doghramji, P. P. (2015). Hot topics in primary care: Update on the recognition and management of gout: More than the great toe. *The Journal of Family Practice, 64*(Suppl. 12), S31–S36.

Gangjee, A., Jain, H. D., & Kurup, S. (2008). Recent advances in classical and non-classical antifolates as antitumor and antiopportunistic infection agents. *Anti-cancer Agents in Medicinal Chemistry, 8*, 205–231.

Garay, R. P., El-Gewely, M. R., Labaune, J. P., et al. (2012). Therapeutic perspectives on uricases for gout. *Joint, Bone, Spine: Revue Du Rhumatisme, 79*, 237–242.

Johnson, R. J. (2015). Why focus on uric acid? *Current Medical Research and Opinion, 31*(Suppl. 2), 3–7.

Jordan, K. M. (2012). Up-to-date management of gout. *Current Opinion in Rheumatology, 24*, 145–151.

Jurecka, A. (2009). Inborn errors of purine and pyrimidine metabolism. *Journal of Inherited Metabolic Disease, 32*, 247–263.

Lee, B. E., Toledo, A. H., Anaya-Prado, R., et al. (2009). Allopurinol, xanthine oxidase, and cardiac ischemia. *Journal of Investigative Medicine, 57*, 902–909.

Maiuolo, J., Oppedisano, F., Gratteri, S., et al. (2016). Regulation of uric acid metabolism and excretion. *International Journal of Cardiology, 213*, 8–14.

Nyhan, W. L. (1997). The recognition of Lesch–Nyhan syndrome as an inborn error of purine metabolism. *Journal of Inherited Metabolic Disease, 20*, 171–178.

Shannon, J. A., & Cole, S. W. (2012). Pegloticase: A novel agent for treatment-refractory gout. *The Annals of Pharmacotherapy, 46*, 368–376.

Wu, A. H., Gladden, J. D., Ahmed, M., et al. (2016). Relation of serum uric acid to cardiovascular disease. *International Journal of Cardiology, 213*, 4–7.

RELEVANT WEBSITES

Gout: http://www.niams.nih.gov/Health_Info/Gout/default.asp
Lesch–Nyhan Syndrome: http://emedicine.medscape.com/article/1181356-overview
SCIDS:
http://www.scid.net
http://themedicalbiochemistrypage.org/nucleotide-metabolism.php

ABBREVIATIONS

APRT	Adenosine phosphoribosyl transferase
ATCase	Aspartate transcarbamoylase
CAD	Carbamoyl phosphate synthetase-Aspartate transcarbamoylase-Dihydroorotase
CPS-II	Carbamoyl phosphate synthetase II
HGPRT	Hypoxanthine-guanine phosphoribosyl transferase
IMP	Inosine monophosphate
N^5-N^{10}-THF	N^5-N^{10}-tetrahydrofolate
PRPP	Phosphoribosyl pyrophosphate
SCIDS	Severe Combined Immunodeficiency Syndrome
THF	Tetrahydrofolate

Complex Carbohydrates: Glycoproteins

Alan D. Elbein (deceased) and Koichi Honke

smaller amounts of carbohydrate than of protein, typically from just a few percent carbohydrate to 10%–15% sugar by weight.

Proteoglycans (see Fig. 17.1B and Chapter 19) contain as much as 50%–60% carbohydrate. In these molecules, the sugar chains are long, unbranched polymers that may contain hundreds of monosaccharides. These saccharide chains have a repeating disaccharide unit, generally made up of a uronic acid and an amino sugar.

Most proteins in cell-surface membranes that function as receptors for hormones or participate in other important membrane-associated processes such as cell–cell interactions are glycoproteins. Many of the membrane proteins of the endoplasmic reticulum or Golgi apparatus, as well as those proteins that are secreted from cells, including serum and mucous proteins, are also glycoproteins. In fact, glycosylation is the major enzymatic modification of proteins in the body. The addition of sugars to a protein can occur either at the same time and location as protein synthesis is occurring in the endoplasmic reticulum (i.e., cotranslationally) or after the completion of protein synthesis and after the protein has been transported to the Golgi apparatus (i.e., posttranslationally). The functions of the carbohydrate chains of the resulting glycoproteins are diverse (Table 17.1).

INTRODUCTION

Glycoconjugates include glycoproteins, proteoglycans, and glycolipids

Many mammalian proteins are glycoproteins - that is, they contain sugars covalently linked to specific amino acids in their structures. There are two major types of sugar-containing proteins that occur in animal cells, generally referred to as glycoproteins and proteoglycans. Along with glycolipids, which are presented in the next chapter, all of these compounds are part of the group of sugar-containing macromolecules called **glycoconjugates**.

Glycoproteins (Fig. 17.1A) have short glycan chains; they can have up to 20 sugars but usually contain between 3 and 15 sugars. These oligosaccharides are highly branched, they do not have a repeating unit, and they usually contain amino sugars (*N*-acetylglucosamine or *N*-acetylgalactosamine), neutral sugars (D-galactose, D-mannose, L-fucose), and the acidic sugar sialic acid (*N*-acetylneuraminic acid). Glycoproteins generally do not contain uronic acids, acidic sugars that are a major part of the proteoglycans. Glycoproteins usually contain much

STRUCTURES AND LINKAGES

Sugars are attached to specific amino acids in proteins

Sugars can be attached to protein in either **N-glycosidic** linkages or **O-glycosidic** linkages. N-linked oligosaccharides (*N*-glycans) are widespread in nature and are characteristic of membrane and secretory proteins. The attachment of these oligosaccharides to protein involves a **glycosylamine** linkage between an *N*-acetylglucosamine (GlcNAc) residue and the amide nitrogen of an asparagine residue (Fig. 17.2A). The asparagine that serves as an acceptor of this oligosaccharide must be in the **consensus sequence** Asn-X-Ser (Thr) to be recognized as the acceptor by the oligosaccharide transferring enzyme (see below). However, not all asparagine residues, even those in this consensus sequence become glycosylated, indicating that other factors such as protein conformation or other properties of the protein may be involved.

O-linked oligosaccharides (*O*-glycans) are most commonly found in proteins of mucous fluids but also occur frequently on the same membrane and secretory proteins that contain the *N*-glycans. The *O*-glycans typically contain three or more

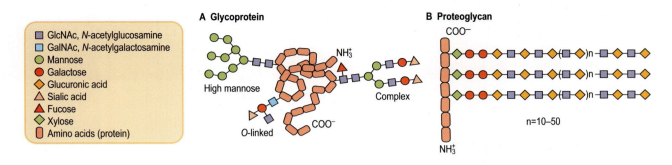

Fig. 17.1 **Generalized model of the structure of glycoproteins and proteoglycans.**

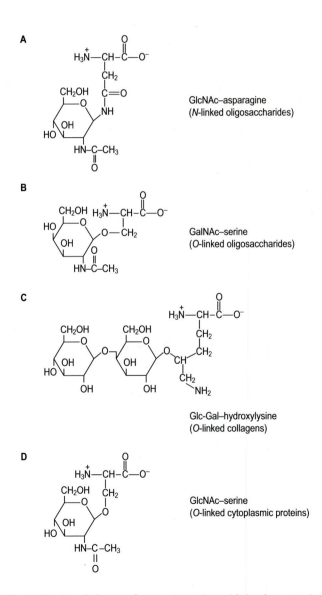

Fig. 17.2 **Various linkages of sugars to amino acids in glycoproteins.** GlcNAc, N-acetylglucosamine.

Table 17.1 Function of carbohydrates on glycoproteins

- Assist in protein folding to correct conformation
- Enhance protein solubility
- Stabilize the protein against denaturation
- Protect the protein from proteolytic degradation
- Target the protein to specific subcellular locations
- Serve as recognition signals for carbohydrate-binding proteins (lectins)

---

sugars in linear or branched chains, attached to the protein by a glycosidic linkage between an N-acetylgalactosamine (GalNAc) residue and the hydroxyl group of either a serine or a threonine residue on the protein (Fig. 17.2B; see Fig. 17.4). There does not appear to be a consensus sequence of amino acids for O-linked glycosylation, although there is an increased frequency of proline residues at the −1 and +3 positions, a preference for neighboring acidic amino acids, and a decreased frequency of aromatic and bulky amino acids near sites of O-glycosylation. These correlations suggest that O-glycosylated serine or threonine residues are near turns in the peptide chain on the hydrophilic surface of the protein.

A glucosyl-galactose disaccharide is frequently linked to the hydroxyl group of hydroxylysine residues in the fibrous protein, collagen (Fig. 17.2C). **Hydroxylysine** is an uncommon amino acid, found only in collagens and proteins with collagenous domains. Hydroxylysine is not directly incorporated into protein as such but is produced by posttranslational hydroxylation of lysine residues. Lysyl hydroxylase requires vitamin C as a cofactor; vitamin C is frequently used to expedite wound healing. Collagen is first synthesized in the cell as a precursor form called procollagen. Procollagens are usually synthesized as N-linked glycoproteins, but the N-glycan is removed as part of that peptide that is cleaved from procollagen during its maturation to collagen. Only the O-linked disaccharides remain on the mature collagen molecule. The less-glycosylated collagens tend to form ordered, fibrous structures, such as occur

—

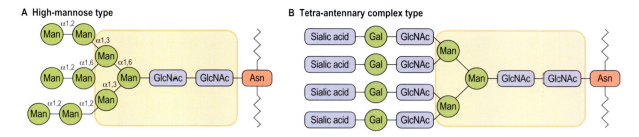

Fig. 17.3 **Typical structures of high-mannose and complex *N*-linked oligosaccharides.** The core structure (shaded area) is common to both structures. Asn, asparagine; Gal, galactose; GlcNAc, N-acetylglucosamine; Man, mannose.

in tendons, while the more heavily glycosylated collagens are found in meshwork structures, such as basement membranes in the vascular wall and renal glomerulus (see Chapter 19).

A single GlcNAc is attached to the hydroxyl group of serine or threonine residues on a number of cytoplasmic and nuclear proteins (Fig. 17.2D). This *O*-linked GlcNAc (*O*-GlcNAc) is linked to specific serine and threonine residues that become phosphorylated by protein kinases during hormonal stimulation or other signaling events. The enzyme that adds the GlcNAc is widespread, but how it is controlled is still not clear. There is a second enzyme that removes the GlcNAc from the serine and threonine residues, similar to the contrasting regulatory roles of protein kinases and phosphatases. The GlcNAc modification (***O*-GlcNAcylation**) may represent a mechanism that allows the cells to block phosphorylation of specific serine and threonine residues on selected proteins while allowing others to still be phosphorylated. Then the GlcNAc can be removed under appropriate conditions to allow phosphorylation. The donor substrate of *O*-GlcNAcylation is UDP-GlcNAc (see below), which is derived from glucose. *O*-GlcNAcylation is dependent on the intracellular UDP-GlcNAc level, which is correlated with extra-cellular glucose concentration. *O*-GlcNAcylation of proteins involved in the insulin signaling pathway brings about insulin resistance in skeletal muscle, adipose tissue, and pancreatic β-cells, which causes type 2 diabetes. *O*-GlcNAcylation also regulates transcription factors as well as the proteasome, which is involved in protein turnover (Chapter 22).

A novel class of *O*-linked glycans in which mannose is linked to serine or threonine residues is found on the muscle and nerve-specific protein dystroglycan. A typical *O*-mannose glycan consists of GlcNAc, galactose, and sialic acid, which are attached to the core mannose in this order. *O*-mannose glycans serve as linkers between the intracellular cytoskeleton and the extracellular matrix to maintain myocyte function. Deficiency in the biosynthesis of *O*-mannose glycans causes muscular dystrophy.

One other amino acid that can serve as a site for glycosylation is tyrosine. The only example of this linkage is in the protein glycogenin, found at the core of glycogen (see Chapter 12). **Glycogenin** is a self-glucosylating protein that initially attaches

a glucose to the hydroxyl group of one of its tyrosine residues. The protein then adds a number of other glucoses to the protein-linked glucose to make an oligosaccharide, which serves as the acceptor for glycogen synthase.

N-glycans have either "high-mannose' or "complex" structures built on a common core

Although there are a large number of different carbohydrate structures produced by living cells, most of the oligosaccharides on glycoconjugates have many sugars and glycosidic linkages in common. All *N*-glycans have oligosaccharide chains that are branched structures, having a common core of three mannose residues and two GlcNAc residues (Fig. 17.3A,B) but differing considerably beyond the core region to give high-mannose and complex types of chains. The reason for this similarity in structure is that the high-mannose type of *N*-linked oligosaccharide is the biosynthetic precursor for all other *N*-glycans. As indicated in the following discussion (see Fig. 17.11), the oligosaccharide is initially assembled on a carrier lipid in the endoplasmic reticulum as a high-mannose structure, then transferred to protein. It may remain as a high-mannose structure, especially in lower organisms but in animals, the oligosaccharide undergoes a number of processing steps in the endoplasmic reticulum and Golgi apparatus that involve removal of some mannoses and addition of other sugars. As a result, beyond the core region, the oligosaccharides give rise to a vast array of structures that are referred to as high-mannose structures (Fig. 17.3A) and complex chains (Fig. 17.3B).

Complex oligosaccharides are so named because of their more complex sugar compositions, including galactose, sialic acid, and L-fucose. Complex chains have terminal trisaccharide sequences composed of sialic acid→galactose→GlcNAc attached to each of the branched core mannoses (Fig. 17.3B). L-Fucose may also be found attached to a core GlcNAc (Fig. 17.1A), a terminal galactose (Fig. 18.12), or a penultimate GlcNAc (Fig. 17.9). In common with sialic acid, fucose is usually a terminal sugar on oligosaccharides - that is, no other sugars are attached to it. Some of the complex oligosaccharides have two trisaccharide sequences, one attached to each of the branched core mannoses, and are therefore called biantennary complex chains, whereas others have three (triantennary) or four (tetra-antennary) of the trisaccharide structures (Fig. 17.3B). More than 100 different complex oligosaccharide structures have now been identified on various cell-surface proteins, providing great diversity (**microheterogeneity**) as mediators of cellular recognition and chemical signaling events.

General structures of glycoproteins

A glycoprotein may have a single N-glycan chain, or it may have several of these types of oligosaccharides. Furthermore, the N-glycans may all have identical structures, or they may be quite different in structure. For example, the influenza virus coat glycoproteins, hemagglutinin and neuraminidase, are both glycoproteins, which usually have seven N-glycan chains, of which five are biantennary complex chains and two are high-mannose structures. Thus a range of related structures is commonly found in a single glycoprotein, and in fact, multiple different structures may also be found at a single site on different glycoprotein molecules. **Microheterogeneity** of oligosaccharide structures results from incomplete processing on some chains during their biosynthesis (see Fig. 17.12). As a result, some of the oligosaccharides on a glycoprotein may be complete complex chains while others may be only partially processed. Such diversity in the processing of N-glycans is controlled by many factors, e.g. structure near the N-glycosylation site. In general, N-glycans exposed on the surface of a folded protein are modified by the processing enzymes, whereas those shielded within the structure of the protein are inaccessible to the enzymes.

Many N-linked glycoproteins also contain O-glycans of the type shown in Fig. 17.4. The number of O-glycans varies considerably depending on the protein and its function. For example, the low-density lipoprotein (LDL) receptor is present in plasma membranes of smooth muscle cells and fibroblasts and functions to bind and endocytose circulating LDL, delivering cholesterol to the cell. The LDL receptor has two N-glycans that are located near the LDL-binding domain and a cluster of O-glycans near the membrane-spanning region. As shown in Fig. 17.5, this receptor has a membrane-spanning region of hydrophobic amino acids, an extended region of amino acids on the external side of the plasma membrane that contains the cluster of O-glycans and a functional domain that is involved in binding LDL (see Chapter 33). Although the two N-glycans are near the functional domain, they do not play a role in binding LDL. Instead, their function appears to be in helping the protein fold into the proper conformation in the endoplasmic reticulum so that it can be translocated to the Golgi apparatus. The negatively charged O-glycans, each having a sialic acid, are believed to function to keep the protein in an extended state and to prevent it from folding back on itself.

Structure–function relationships in mucin glycoproteins

Mucins are glycoproteins that are secreted by epithelial cells lining the respiratory, gastrointestinal, and genitourinary tracts. These proteins are very large in size, with subunits having molecular weights of more than 1 million daltons and having as much as 80% of their weight as carbohydrate. **Mucins are uniquely designed for their function,** with about one-third of the amino acids being serines or threonines and most of these being substituted with an O-glycan. Because most of these oligosaccharides carry a negatively charged sialic acid,

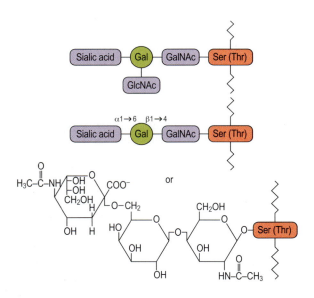

Fig. 17.4 **Typical structures of O-linked oligosaccharides.**

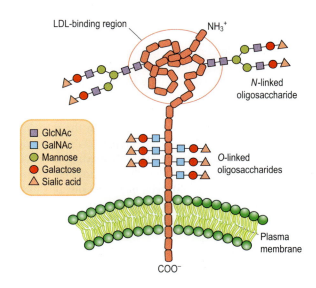

Fig. 17.5 **Model of the low-density lipoprotein (LDL) receptor.** (See also Chapter 32 and compare Fig. 32.2.)

ADVANCED CONCEPT BOX
THE STRUCTURE OF *N*-GLYCANS DEPENDS ON THE ENZYME COMPLEMENT OF THE CELL

The final structure of the *N*-glycan chain of a given glycoprotein is not coded in the genes for the protein but depends on the enzyme complement of the cell making that oligosaccharide. All cells appear to have the necessary enzymes to produce the lipid-linked saccharide precursor of the *N*-linked high-mannose chains, and they can therefore glycosylate any membrane protein that has the appropriate asparagine in the right sequence and protein conformation. However, the glycosyltransferases and glycosidases involved in processing the oligosaccharide to its final complex structure are not so widely distributed, and a given glycosyltransferase may be present in one type of cell but not in another. For example, one cell type may have the GlcNAc transferase (GlcNAc T-IV or V) necessary to attach a second GlcNAc on the 2-linked α-mannoses to make a triantennary or tetra-antennary chain, whereas another cell may not have these GlcNAc transferases. Such a cell will only make biantennary chains. Enveloped viruses, such as the influenza virus or HIV, are examples of this phenomenon because their *N*-glycan structures reflect that of the cell in which they are grown; viruses use the cellular machinery to make all of their structures, and therefore their glycoproteins will have carbohydrate structures characteristic of the infected cell. For the virus, this is beneficial because its proteins will not be recognized as foreign proteins and will escape immune surveillance. In addition, it allows the virus to attach to host cell receptors and fuse with host cell membranes by interacting with host lectins. In the biotechnology industry, this means that although a given protein will have the identical amino acid sequence regardless of cell type, it will have different oligosaccharide structures depending on the cell in which it is expressed. These differences in carbohydrate structure may affect the conformation and functional properties of the protein and limit its use in protein- or enzyme-replacement therapy. In fact, many cells used to express "human" proteins are bioengineered to contain the complement of enzymes needed to properly glycosylate the target protein.

and these negative charges are in close proximity, they repel each other and prevent the protein from folding, causing it to remain in an extended state. Thus the protein solution is highly viscous, forming a protective barrier on the epithelial surface, providing lubrication between surfaces, and facilitating transport processes, such as the movement of food through the gastrointestinal system. There is a wide range of complex linear and branching oligosaccharide structures on mucins, including blood-group antigens (see Chapter 18). Some oligosaccharides participate in interaction and binding to various bacterial cell surfaces. This property may play a significant role in bacterial sequestration and elimination, limiting colonization and infection.

INTERCONVERSIONS OF DIETARY SUGARS

Cells can use glucose to make all the other sugars they need

Humans have a dietary requirement for some essential fatty acids, amino acids, and vitamins, but all the sugars that they need to make glycoconjugates can be synthesized from blood sugar (i.e., D-glucose). Fig. 17.6 presents an overview of the sequence of reactions involved in interconversion of sugars in mammalian cells. All of these sugar interconversion reactions involve sugar phosphates or sugar nucleotides.

Formation of galactose, mannose, and fucose from glucose

Glucose is phosphorylated by hexokinase (or glucokinase in the liver) as it enters the cell. Glucose-6-phosphate (Glc-6-P) can then be converted by a mutase (phosphoglucomutase) to form Glc-1-P, which reacts with uridine triphosphate (UTP) to form UDP-Glc, catalyzed by the enzyme UDP-Glc pyrophosphorylase (Fig. 17.6). This enzyme is named for the reverse reaction in which the phosphate of Glc-1-P acts to cleave the pyrophosphate bond of UTP to form UDP-Glc and pyrophosphate (PPi); cleavage of the high-energy bond of PPi by pyrophosphatase provides the driving force for the reaction. This is the same pathway used in the liver and muscle for incorporation of glucose into glycogen (Chapter 12). UDP-Glc is epimerized to UDP-galactose (UDP-Gal) by UDP-Gal 4-epimerase, providing UDP-Gal for the synthesis of glycoconjugates.

Glc-6-P may also be converted to fructose-6-phosphate (Fru-6-P) by the glycolytic enzyme phosphoglucose isomerase, and Fru-6-P may be isomerized to mannose-6-phosphate (Man-6-P) by phosphomannose isomerase. The Man-6-P is then converted by a mutase (phosphomannomutase) to Man-1-P, which reacts with GTP to form GDP-Man. GDP-Man is the form of mannose that is used in the formation of *N*-linked oligosaccharides and is also the precursor for the formation of activated fucose, GDP-L-fucose. Mannose is present in our diet in small amounts, but it is not an essential dietary component because it can be readily produced from glucose. However, dietary mannose can also be phosphorylated by hexokinase to Man-6-P, and it then enters metabolism through phosphomannose isomerase.

Metabolism of galactose

Although animal cells can make all the galactose they need from glucose via UDP-Gal 4-epimerase, galactose is still a significant component of our diet because it is one of the sugars that make up the milk disaccharide lactose. The pathway of

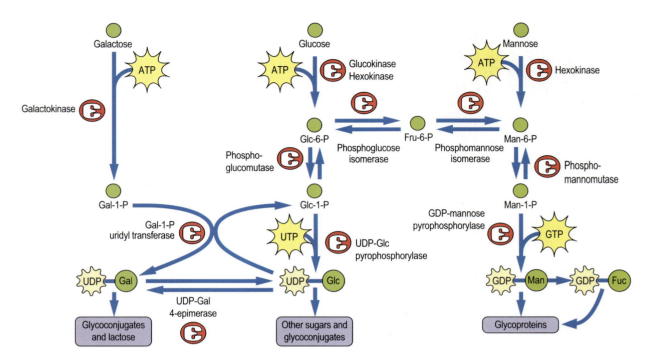

Fig. 17.6 **Interconversions of glucose, mannose, galactose, and their nucleotide sugars.** Fuc, fucose; Gal-1-P, galactose-1-phosphate; Glc-1-P, glucose-1-phosphate; Man-1-P, mannose-1-phosphate.

galactose metabolism requires three enzymes (Fig. 17.6). Dietary galactose is transported to the liver, where it is phosphorylated by a specific kinase (galactokinase) that attaches phosphate to the hydroxyl group on carbon-1 (rather than carbon-6) to form galactose-1-phosphate (Gal-1-P). Humans lack a UDP-Gal pyrophosphorylase, so the conversion of Gal-1-P to Glc-1-P involves the participation of UDP-Glc. The enzyme Gal-1-P uridyltransferase catalyzes an exchange between UDP-Glc and Gal-1-P to form UDP-Gal and Glc-1-P (Fig. 17.6). The UDP-Gal is used for the synthesis of glycoconjugates, and the Glc-1-P can be converted to Glc-6-P by phosphoglucomutase; thus the original galactose molecule enters glycolysis.

UDP-Glc is present in only micromolar concentrations in cells so that its availability for galactose metabolism would be quickly exhausted were it not for the presence of the third enzyme, UDP-Gal-4-epimerase. This enzyme catalyzes the equilibrium between UDP-Glc and UDP-Gal, providing a constant source of UDP-Glc during galactose metabolism. The reactions catalyzed by (1) **galactokinase**, (2) **Gal-1-P uridyltransferase**, and (3) **UDP-Gal 4-epimerase** are summarized as follows, illustrating the roundabout way by which galactose enters mainstream metabolic pathways:

$$(1)\ \text{Gal} + \text{ATP} \rightarrow \text{Gal-1-P} + \text{ADP}$$
$$(2)\ \text{Gal-1-P} + \text{UDP-Glc} \rightarrow \text{Glc-1-P} + \text{UDP-Gal}$$
$$(3)\ \text{UDP-Gal} \rightleftharpoons \text{UDP-Glc}$$
$$\overline{\text{Net}: \text{Gal} + \text{ATP} \rightarrow \text{Glc-1-P} + \text{ADP}}$$

Metabolism of fructose

Fructose accounts for about half the sugar in both sucrose (table sugar) and high-fructose corn syrup

Fructose can be metabolized by two pathways in cells, as shown in Fig. 17.7. It can be phosphorylated by hexokinase, an enzyme that is present in all cells; however, hexokinase has a strong preference for glucose as a substrate, and glucose, which is present at a concentration of about 5 mmol/L in blood, is a strong competitive inhibitor of the phosphorylation of fructose. The primary pathway of fructose metabolism, which is especially important after a meal, involves the hepatic enzyme fructokinase. This enzyme is a very specific kinase that phosphorylates fructose at carbon-1 (like galactokinase, rather than glucokinase or hexokinase) to give fructose-1-phosphate (Fru-1-P). The liver aldolase is called **aldolase B,** and it is different in substrate specificity from the muscle aldolase A because aldolase B can cleave both Fru-1-P and Fru-1,6-P, whereas aldolase A will only cleave Fru-1,6-P_2. Thus, in the liver, the products of fructose cleavage by aldolase B are dihydroxyacetone phosphate and glyceraldehyde (not glyceraldehyde-3-P). The glyceraldehyde must then be phosphorylated by triose kinase to be metabolized in glycolysis.

It should be noted that in the liver, fructose enters glycolysis at the level of the triose phosphate intermediates, rather than as Fru-6-P in muscle. Thus glycolytic metabolism of ingested

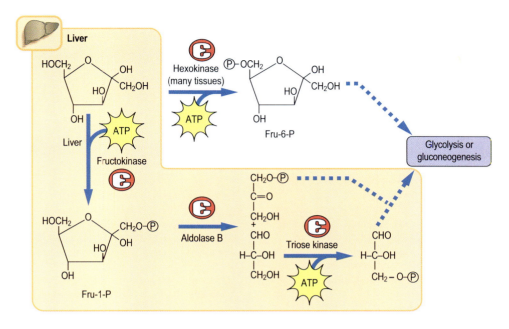

Fig. 17.7 **Metabolism of fructose by fructokinase or hexokinase.**

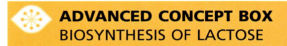

ADVANCED CONCEPT BOX
BIOSYNTHESIS OF LACTOSE

Lactose Synthase and α-Lactalbumin

Lactose (galactosyl-β1,4-glucose) is synthesized from UDP-Gal and glucose in the mammary glands during lactation. Lactose synthase is formed by the binding of **α-lactalbumin** to the galactosyltransferase that normally participates in the biosynthesis of *N*-glycans. α-Lactalbumin, which is expressed only in mammary glands and only during lactation, converts the galactosyltransferase to lactose synthase by lowering the enzyme's K_m for glucose by about three orders of magnitude, from 1 mol/L to 1 mmol/L, leading to the preferential synthesis of lactose, rather than galactosylation of glycoproteins. α-Lactalbumin is the only known example of a **"specifier" protein** that alters the substrate specificity of an enzyme.

fructose is not subject to regulation at the usual control points, hexokinase and phosphofructokinase. By circumventing these two rate-limiting steps, fructose provides a rapid source of energy in both aerobic and anaerobic cells. This was part of the rationale behind the development of high-fructose drinks such as Gatorade. The significance of the fructokinase, as opposed to the hexokinase, pathway of fructose metabolism is indicated by the pathology of hereditary fructose intolerance (see Clinical Box).

OTHER PATHWAYS OF SUGAR NUCLEOTIDE METABOLISM

UDP-GlcUA

UDP-Glc is the precursor of a number of other sugars, such as glucuronic acid, xylose, and galactose, which are required for proteoglycan and/or glycoprotein synthesis. The reactions that lead to the formation of these other sugars are outlined in Figs. 17.6 and 17.8. A two-step oxidation of UDP-Glc by the enzyme UDP-Glc dehydrogenase leads to the formation of the activated form of glucuronic acid, UDP-GlcUA (Fig. 17.8). This sugar nucleotide is the donor of glucuronic acid, both for the formation of proteoglycans (see Chapter 19), and for the detoxification and conjugation reactions that occur in the liver to remove bilirubin, drugs, and xenobiotics (see Chapter 34). UDP-GlcUA is also the precursor of UDP-xylose, a pentose sugar nucleotide (Fig. 17.8). UDP-GlcUA undergoes a decarboxylation reaction that removes carbon-6 to form UDP-xylose, the activated form of xylose. Xylose is the linkage sugar between protein and glycan in proteoglycans (Fig. 17.1B and Chapter 19). Xylose is also present on many plant glycoproteins, as part of their *N*-linked oligosaccharides, and is partly responsible for allergic reactions to peanut and nut proteins.

GDP-Man and GDP-Fuc

Guanosine diphosphate-mannose (GDP-Man) is the donor substrate for most mannosyltransferases. As shown in Fig. 17.6,

CLINICAL BOX
GALACTOSEMIA: A BABY WHO DEVELOPED JAUNDICE AFTER BREASTFEEDING

An apparently normal newborn baby began to vomit and develop diarrhea after breastfeeding. These problems, together with dehydration, continued for several days, when the child began to refuse food and developed jaundice indicative of liver damage, followed by hepatomegaly and then lens opacifications (cataracts). Measurement of glucose in the blood by a glucose oxidase assay (Chapter 6) indicated that the concentration of glucose was low, consistent with a failure to absorb foods. However, glucose measured by a colorimetric method that measures total reducing sugar (i.e., any sugar that is capable of reducing copper under alkaline conditions) indicated that the concentration of sugar was quite high in both the blood and the urine. The reducing sugar that accumulated was eventually identified as galactose, indicating an abnormality in galactose metabolism known as **galactosemia**. This finding was consistent with the observation that when milk was removed from the diet and replaced with an infant formula containing sucrose rather than lactose, the vomiting and diarrhea stopped, and hepatic function gradually improved.

Comment
The accumulation of galactose in the blood most often is the result of a deficiency in the enzyme Gal-1-P uridyl transferase (classic form of galactosemia), which prevents the conversion of galactose to glucose and leads to the accumulation of Gal and Gal-1-P in tissues. The accumulated Gal-1-P interferes with phosphate and glucose metabolism, leading to widespread tissue damage, organ failure, and mental retardation. In addition, accumulation of galactose in tissues results in galactose conversion, through the **polyol pathway,** to galactitol, which in the lens results in osmotic stress and development of cataracts (compare diabetic cataracts; Chapter 31). Another form of galactosemia is caused by galactokinase deficiency, but in this case, Gal-1-P does not accumulate, and complications are milder.

CLINICAL BOX
HEREDITARY FRUCTOSE INTOLERANCE: A CHILD WHO DEVELOPED HYPOGLYCEMIA AFTER EATING FRUIT

A child was brought into the emergency room suffering from nausea, vomiting, and symptoms of hypoglycemia along with sweating, dizziness, and trembling. The parents indicated that these attacks occurred shortly after eating fruit (which contains fruit sugar, fructose) or candy (sucrose). As a result of these symptoms, the child was developing a strong aversion to fruit, so the mother was providing a large supplementation of multivitamin preparations. The child was below normal weight, but he had not exhibited any of the described unusual symptoms during the period of time when he was breastfeeding. A series of clinical tests demonstrated some cirrhosis of the liver and a normal glucose tolerance test. However, reducing substances were detected in the urine, and these reducing substances did not react in the glucose oxidase test (i.e., they were not due to glucose). A **fructose tolerance test** was ordered using 3 g fructose/m^2 of body surface area, given intravenously in a single and rapid push. Within 30 min, the child displayed symptoms of hypoglycemia. Blood glucose analysis confirmed this and revealed that the hypoglycemia was greatest after 60–90 min. Fructose concentrations reached a maximum (3.3 mmol/L) after 15 min and gradually decreased to zero by 3 h. Plasma phosphate concentration fell by 50%, and tests for the enzymes alanine aminotransferase and aspartate aminotransferase indicated that they were elevated after about 90 min. The urine was also positive for fructose.

Comment
Hereditary fructose intolerance is caused by a deficiency of aldolase B in the liver (Fig. 17.7). The results of a fructose tolerance test demonstrate the accumulation of fructose and its derivatives in blood and urine. The elevation of liver enzymes, alanine, and aspartate aminotransferase, as well as jaundice and other symptoms, indicates liver damage and suggests that Fru-1-P affects the intermediary metabolism of carbohydrates in a manner similar to that of Gal-1-P in galactosemia.

it is produced from Man-6-P and is also the precursor to GDP-L-fucose (GDP-Fuc), which is the donor substrate for all fucosyltranferases. Fucose is a 6-deoxyhexose - that is, an important sugar participating in many recognition reactions in biological events, such as inflammatory response (Fig. 17.9). Conversion of GDP-Man to GDP-Fuc involves a complex series of oxidative and reductive steps as well as epimerizations. Deficiency in the GDP-Fuc transporter that translocates GDP-Fuc from the cytosol into the Golgi lumen is associated with a defective inflammatory response and increased susceptibility to infection (leukocyte adhesion deficiency II [LADII]). In this disease, depletion of GDP-Fuc in the Golgi lumen blocks the biosynthesis of the **leukocyte recognition signal, sialyl-Lewis-X** structure (see Fig. 17.9).

Amino sugars

Fru-6-P is the precursor of amino sugars

Fig. 17.10 shows the pathway of formation of GlcNAc, GalNAc, and sialic acid. The initial reaction involves the transfer of an amino group from the amide nitrogen of glutamine to Fru-6-P to produce glucosamine-6-P (GlcN-6-P). An acetyl group is then transferred from acetyl-CoA to the amino group of the GlcN-6-P to form GlcNAc-6-P, which is converted to its activated form, UDP-GlcNAc, by sequential mutase and pyrophosphorylase reactions. In addition to its role as a GlcNAc donor, UDP-GlcNAc can also be epimerized to UDP-GalNAc. With few exceptions, all amino sugars in glycoconjugates are acetylated;

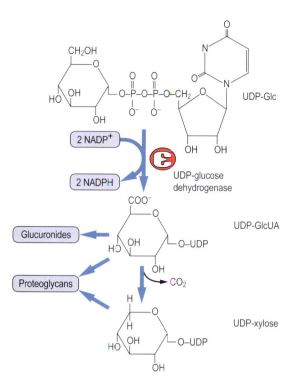

Fig. 17.8 Conversion of UDP-Glc to UDP-glucuronic acid (UDP-GlcUA) and UDP-xylose. Note that oxidation of UDP-Glc is a two-step reaction, from alcohol to aldehyde, then to an acid. Both reactions are catalyzed by UDP-Glc dehydrogenase.

thus they are neutral and do not contribute any ionic charge to the glycoconjugates.

Sialic acid

UDP-GlcNAc is the precursor of N-acetylneuraminic acid (NeuAc), also referred to as sialic acid. Sialic acid, a nine-carbon N-acetylamino-ketodeoxyglyconic acid, is produced by the condensation of an amino sugar with **phosphoenolpyruvate** (Fig. 17.10). Cytidine monophosphate neuraminic acid (CMP-NeuAc) is the activated form of sialic acid and is the sialic acid donor in biosynthetic reactions. CMP-sialic acid is the only nucleoside monophosphate sugar donor in glycoconjugate metabolism.

BIOSYNTHESIS OF OLIGOSACCHARIDES

N-glycan assembly begins in the endoplasmic reticulum

The synthesis of N-glycans begins with the transfer of two GlcNAc residues to a membrane-bound lipid, called dolichyl phosphate. Mannose and glucose residues are added to build a lipid-linked oligosaccharide intermediate, which is transferred "en bloc" to protein in the lumen of the endoplasmic reticulum (Fig. 17.11). **Dolichols** are long-chain polyisoprenol derivatives usually having about 120 carbon atoms (about 22–26 isoprene

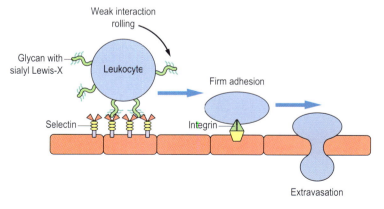

Fig. 17.9 Carbohydrate-dependent cell–cell interactions in inflammation. Sialyl Lewis-X, a tetrasaccharide antigen that forms part of the membrane structure of leukocytes, is recognized by a carbohydrate-binding protein, selectin, on the surface of endothelial cells. The sialyl Lewis-X-selectin interaction mediates the initial weak binding that results in rolling of the leukocytes along the endothelial monolayer. It facilitates the firm adhesion mediated by the protein–protein interactions leading to extravasation.

ADVANCED CONCEPT BOX
CARBOHYDRATE-DEPENDENT CELL–CELL INTERACTIONS

An important example of carbohydrate-dependent cell–cell interactions occurs during inflammation. An injury to, or infection of, the vascular endothelial cells elicits an inflammatory response that causes the release of cytokines, such as tumor necrosis factor-α (TNF-α) and interleukin-1 (IL-1), from the damaged tissue. These cytokines attract leukocytes to the site of injury or infection to remove the damaged tissue or the invading organisms. Leukocytes must be able to stop or exit from the blood flow and attach to the injured tissue. They are able to do this because they have a carbohydrate ligand on their surface that is recognized by a **lectin** (carbohydrate-binding protein) that becomes exposed on the surface of the damaged endothelial cells. The carbohydrate ligand is a tetrasaccharide called the sialyl Lewis-X antigen (Fig. 17.9), which is a component of a glycoprotein or glycolipid on the surface of the leukocyte. The sialyl Lewis-X antigen is recognized by lectins, **E-selectin and P-selectin,** that are expressed on the surface of the endothelial cells in response to cytokine stimulation. Fig. 17.9 illustrates the sequence of events occurring during vascular adhesion and extravasation of leukocytes to inflamed tissue. The sialyl Lewis-X–selectin interaction mediates the initial step of the leukocytes–endothelium interaction, which is described as tethering, followed by rolling of leukocytes along the endothelial cell surface. Although this carbohydrate–protein binding is weak and transient, multiple interactions slow down the leukocytes circulating under a strong shear force in blood and permit firm protein–protein interactions between leukocyte cell-surface integrins and their receptors. Eventually, the leukocytes migrate through the endothelium into the underlying tissue.

A similar interaction of L-selectin expressed on the lymphocytes with a sialyl Lewis-X–like oligosaccharide expressed on the endothelial cells of the high endothelial venules (HEV) enables lymphocytes circulating in the bloodstream to enter a lymph node by a similar mechanism. This process is called **lymphocyte homing.** While these carbohydrate–protein interactions play a critical role in the immune system, they can be dangerous and life threatening under other circumstances. Some cancer cells use these carbohydrate–protein interactions to facilitate their metastasis through the bloodstream. There is active research on developing drugs whose structure is similar to carbohydrates (glycomimetic) that will block the vascular adhesion of tumor cells and prevent metastasis.

Comment

Lectin–carbohydrate interactions in vivo involve many different lectins with carbohydrate-specific recognition sites. Once the carbohydrate structure is known and the protein-binding site has been mapped, it may be possible to design compounds that mimic the carbohydrate structure. These synthetic compounds should bind at the carbohydrate-binding site of the lectin and block the natural interaction. One of the difficulties with this approach is that the individual binding interactions are weak, and multiple cell–cell contacts are required; these multiple interactions may be difficult to block by small-molecule drugs. A second problem is that synthesis of specific oligosaccharides is difficult and expensive, and because of their short half-lives in the circulation, large quantities may have to be injected frequently for effective therapy.

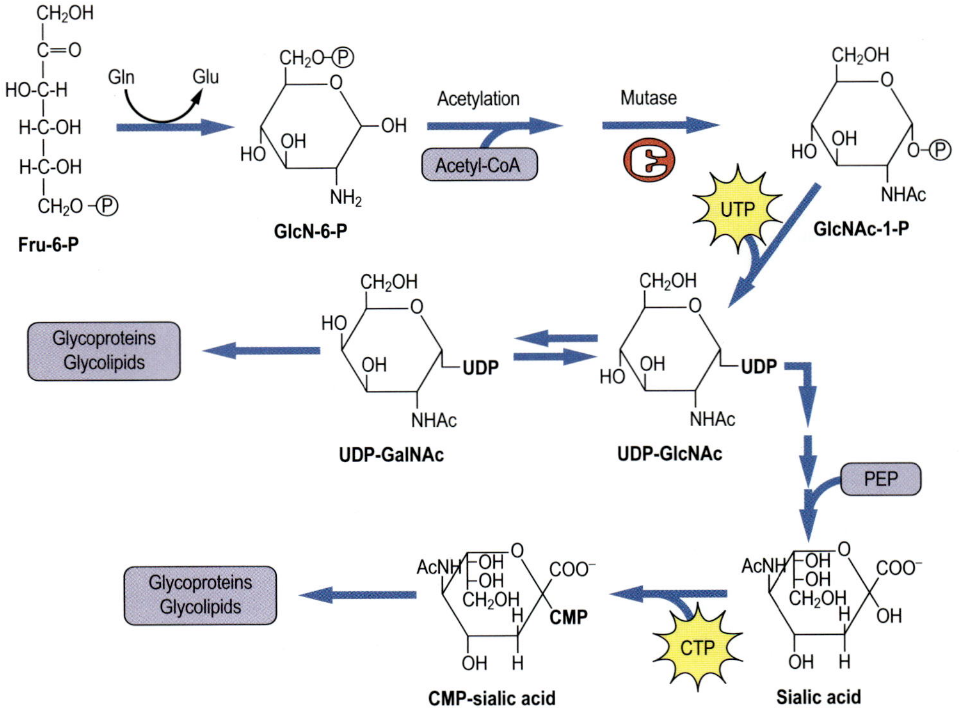

Fig. 17.10 **Synthesis of amino sugars and sialic acid.** Acetyl-CoA, acetyl coenzyme A; GlcN-6-P, glucosamine-6-phosphate; GlcNAc-6P, N-acetylglucosamine-6-phosphate; GalNAc, N-acetylgalactosamine; HNAc, AcHN, acetamide group; PEP, phosphoenolpyruvate.

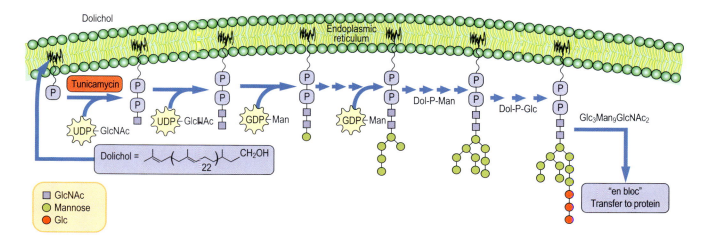

Fig. 17.11 **Synthesis of *N*-linked oligosaccharides in the endoplasmic reticulum.** Tunicamycin is an inhibitor of the GlcNAc phosphotransferase that the catalyzes the first step in glycan synthesis. GlcNAc, *N*-acetylglucosamine; Dol, dolichol; Man, mannose.

units) with a phosphate group at one end. They are synthesized in membranes using the same machinery that is used to make cholesterol, but in contrast to cholesterol, the dolichols remain as long straight chains. The length of the chain requires it to snake through the phospholipid bilayer, providing a strong anchor for the growing oligosaccharide chain.

The first sugar to be added to dolichyl-P from UDP-GlcNAc is GlcNAc-1-P by a GlcNAc-1-P transferase to produce dolichyl-P-P-GlcNAc. A second GlcNAc is added to the first GlcNAc from UDP-GlcNAc, followed by addition of four to five mannose residues from GDP-Man. Dolichyl-P-Man and dolichyl-P-Glc serve as glycosyl donors for the remaining mannoses and the three glucoses residues. Each of the sugars is transferred by a specific glycosyltransferase located in or on the endoplasmic reticulum membrane. The glucoses are not found on any of the N-linked oligosaccharides on glycoproteins but are removed by glucosidases in the endoplasmic reticulum. Why are they added in the first place? They serve two very important functions. First of all, the presence of glucoses on the lipid-linked oligosaccharide has been shown to expedite the transfer of oligosaccharide from lipid to protein - the transferring enzyme (oligosaccharide transferase) has a preference for oligosaccharides that contain three glucoses and transfers those oligosaccharides to protein much faster. Second, the glucoses are important in directing protein folding in the endoplasmic reticulum (see the following discussion).

Intermediate processing continues in the endoplasmic reticulum (ER) and Golgi apparatus

In a series of trimming or pruning reactions (Fig. 17.12), all three glucoses are removed in the ER. The oligosaccharide may then remain as a high-mannose oligosaccharide, or it may be further processed to a complex oligosaccharide structure. One or more mannoses may be removed in the ER, and the folded protein is then translocated to the Golgi apparatus, where three or four additional mannoses may be removed to leave the core structure of three mannose and two GlcNAc residues.

In the *cis*-Golgi, GlcNAc residues are added to each of the mannoses in the core. Then the protein enters the *trans*-Golgi fraction, where the remaining sugars of the trisaccharide sequences (i.e., galactose, sialic acid, and fucose) can be added to make a variety of different complex chains. The final structure of the oligosaccharide chains depends on the glycosyltransferase complement of the cell.

O-glycans

O-glycans are synthesized in the Golgi apparatus

In contrast to the biosynthesis of N-glycans, the synthesis of the O-glycans occurs only in the Golgi apparatus by the stepwise addition of sugars from their sugar nucleotide donors to the protein. No lipid intermediates are involved in O-glycan formation. Fig. 17.13 outlines the stepwise sequence of reactions that are involved in the assembly of an oligosaccharide chain on salivary mucin. In this sequence, GalNAc is first transferred from UDP-GalNAc to serine or threonine residues on the protein by a GalNAc transferase in the Golgi apparatus. The resulting GalNAc-serine protein serves as the acceptor for galactose and then sialic acid, transferred from their sugar nucleotides (UDP-Gal and CMP-sialic acid) by Golgi galactosyltransferases and sialyltransferases. Other Golgi glycosyltransferases are involved in the stepwise biosynthesis of more complex mucin oligosaccharides and in the synthesis of O-glycans in proteoglycans and collagens (see Chapter 19). There are more than 100 glycosyltransferases involved in glycoconjugate synthesis in a typical cell.

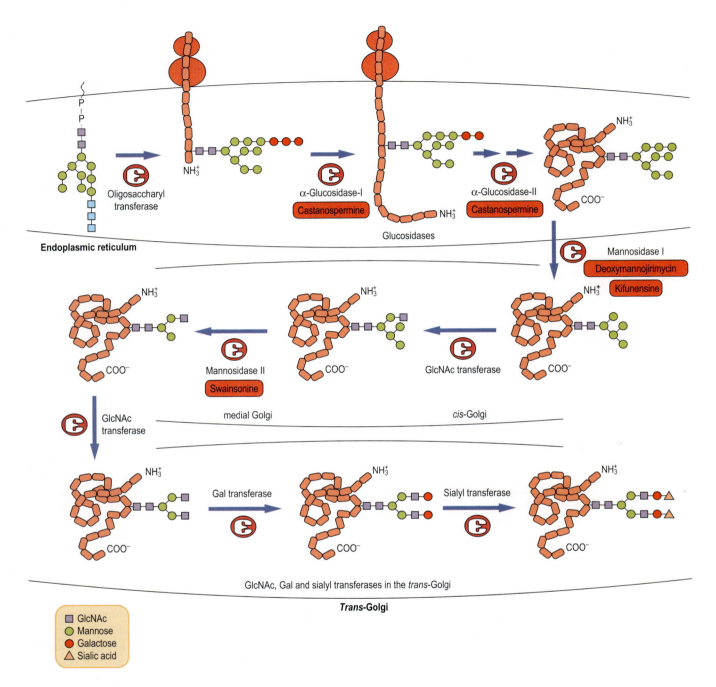

Fig. 17.12 **Processing of *N*-linked oligosaccharides from high-mannose to complex forms.** Glycoproteins are transported between the endoplasmic reticulum and Golgi compartments in vesicles. Inhibitors of glycan processing enzymes are shown in red. GlcNAc, *N*-acetylglucosamine.

FUNCTIONS OF THE OLIGOSACCHARIDE CHAINS OF GLYCOPROTEINS

N-*glycans have an important role in protein folding*

Resident proteins in the endoplasmic reticulum, known as **chaperones,** assist newly synthesized proteins to fold into their proper conformations. Two of these chaperones, calnexin and calreticulin, bind to unfolded glycoproteins by recognition of high-mannose oligosaccharides that still contain a single glucose remaining on their structures after the glucosidases have removed two of the three glucoses. Not all of the glycoproteins synthesized in the cell require assistance in folding, but for those that do, the rate of folding is greatly accelerated by the chaperones. Incorrectly folded or unfolded proteins do

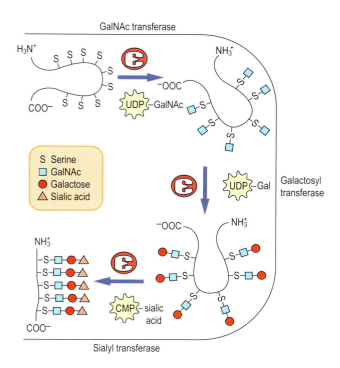

Fig. 17.13 Biosynthesis of O-linked oligosaccharides of mucins in the Golgi apparatus. GalNAc, N-acetylgalactosamine.

ADVANCED CONCEPT BOX
INHIBITORS OF GLYCOPROTEIN BIOSYNTHESIS

Inhibitors of the biosynthesis of N-glycans have been identified, and these compounds have proven to be valuable reagents for studies on the role of specific carbohydrate structures in glycoprotein function. **Tunicamycin** is a glycoside antibiotic that inhibits the first step in the synthesis of N-glycans - that is, the formation of dolichyl-PP-GlcNAc (see Fig. 17.11). Tunicamycin has varied effects on glycoprotein synthesis and on cells, from benign to profound. In some cases, the protein portion of the glycoprotein is synthesized, but without its carbohydrate, it is misfolded, is aggregated, and is degraded in the cell. Thus treatment of cells with tunicamycin frequently induces endoplasmic reticulum (ER) stress (see Chapter 22).

Other inhibitors prevent specific steps in the processing pathway. Many are plant alkaloids that structurally resemble the sugars glucose and mannose and inhibit the pruning glycosidases (see Fig. 17.12). Castanospermine inhibits the ER glucosidases, whereas kifunensine, deoxymannojirimycin, and swainsonine each inhibit a different processing mannosidase. These drugs prevent the formation of complex chains and are therefore useful to evaluate structure–function relationships. Some compounds have been tested against HIV and against some cancers and have shown positive inhibitory effects. However, they also have adverse effects on enzymes in normal cells and are therefore not useful for drug therapy. With more specific compounds, it may be possible to manipulate glycan structures for therapeutic purposes.

not undergo normal transport to the Golgi apparatus, and if they do not fold properly, they either precipitate in the endoplasmic reticulum or, in most cases, are exported to the cytoplasm for degradation by the ubiquitin–proteasome system (see Chapter 22).

Oligosaccharides containing Man-6-P target lysosomal enzymes to the lysosome

Lysosomes are subcellular organelles involved in the hydrolysis and turnover of many cellular organelles and proteins. They contain a variety of hydrolytic enzymes with acidic pH optima. Most of these lysosomal enzymes are N-linked glycoproteins that are synthesized and glycosylated in the endoplasmic reticulum and Golgi apparatus. The sorting of lysosomal enzymes occurs in the cis-Golgi. Proteins destined to be transported to the lysosomes contain a cluster of lysine residues that come together as a result of the protein folding into its proper conformation. As shown in Fig. 17.14, this cluster of lysine residues serves as a docking site for an enzyme, GlcNAc-1-P transferase, that transfers a GlcNAc-1-P from UDP-GlcNAc to terminal mannose residues on the high-mannose chains of the lysosomal enzymes. A second enzyme, called an uncovering enzyme, then removes the GlcNAc, leaving the phosphate residues still attached to the mannoses on the high-mannose chains. The resulting Man-6-P residues on the high-mannose structure are now recognized by a Golgi protein called the Man-6-P receptor, which directs the enzyme to the lysosomes. Thus the **Man-6-P residues are a targeting signal** used by the cell to sort out those proteins that are destined to go to lysosomes and separate them from other proteins being synthesized in the Golgi apparatus. The Man-6-P receptor is also present on the cell surface, so even extracellular enzymes that have this signal are endocytosed and transported to the lysosomes.

The oligosaccharide chains of glycoproteins generally increase the solubility and stability of proteins

Because oligosaccharides are hydrophilic, they increase the solubility of proteins in the aqueous environment. Thus most of the proteins that are secreted from cells are glycoproteins, including plasma proteins, excepting plasma albumin. These glycoproteins and enzymes generally have high stability to heat, chemical denaturants, detergents, acids, and bases. Enzymatic removal of the carbohydrate from many of these proteins greatly reduces their stability to stress. Indeed, when glycoproteins are synthesized in cells in the presence of glycosylation inhibitors - such as tunicamycin, which prevents the production and therefore the attachment of the N-glycan chain - many of these proteins become insoluble and form inclusion bodies in the cells as a result of incorrect folding and/or decreased hydrophilicity.

Sugars are involved in chemical recognition interactions with lectins

N-glycans on the mammalian cell surface play critical roles in cell–cell interactions and other recognition processes. One

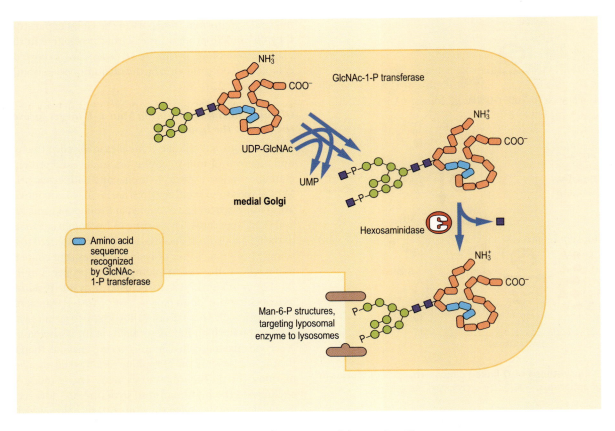
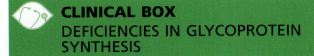
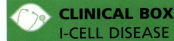

Fig. 17.14 **Targeting of lysosomal enzymes to lysosomes.** GlcNAc, *N*-acetylglucosamine; Man, mannose.

CLINICAL BOX
DEFICIENCIES IN GLYCOPROTEIN SYNTHESIS

The **congenital disorders of glycosylation (CDG)** are a recently described group of rare genetic diseases that affect the biosynthesis of glycoproteins. All patients show multisystem pathology, with severe involvement of the nervous system. Three distinct classes have been identified thus far and are characterized by a deficiency in the structure of the carbohydrate moiety of serum glycoproteins, lysosomal enzymes, or membrane glycoproteins. The diagnosis of the disease is routinely made by electrophoresis of serum transferrin. In CDG, the transferrin contains less sialic acid, and therefore the protein migrates more slowly. The decrease in sialic acid results from a defect in the biosynthesis of the underlying oligosaccharide structure. Although a change in the migration of serum transferrin indicates that the patient is suffering from one of the CDG, it does not identify the specific lesion. That can only be done by either characterizing the structure of the altered oligosaccharide chain(s) to determine what sugars or structures are missing or doing a profile of key enzymes in the biosynthetic pathways, since the absence of any of these enzymes will affect the final oligosaccharide structure.

Comment
The basic defects in this group of diseases appear to be in the synthesis or processing of *N*-glycans. However, defects in phosphomannose isomerase and phosphomannomutase (Fig. 17.6) have also been identified as causes of CDG.

CLINICAL BOX
I-CELL DISEASE

I-cell disease (mucolipidosis II) and pseudo-Hurler polydystrophy (mucolipidosis III) are rare inherited diseases that are caused by deficiencies in the machinery that targets lysosomal enzymes to lysosomes. Clinical presentation includes severe psychomotor retardation, coarse facial features, and skeletal abnormalities; death usually occurs in the first decade. In cultured fibroblasts taken from patients with mucolipidosis II, newly synthesized lysosomal enzymes are secreted into the extracellular medium rather than being targeted correctly to the lysosomes. Mesenchymal cells, especially fibroblasts, contain numerous membrane-bound vacuoles in the cytoplasm containing fibrillogranular material. These deposits are called inclusion bodies, and this is the origin of the name I-cell disease.

Comment
I-cell disease results from a deficiency in the synthesis of the targeting signal, Man-6-P residues, on high-mannose oligosaccharides. The mutation is most commonly an absence of GlcNAc-1-P transferase, but defects in the uncovering enzyme also occur. It is likely that absence of the Man-6-P receptor protein would yield the same phenotype. In I-cell disease, the lysosomes, lacking the full spectrum of hydrolase enzymes, become engorged with indigestible substances.

cell may contain on its cell surface a carbohydrate-recognizing protein, known as a **lectin,** that binds to a specific oligosaccharide structure on the surface of the complementary cell. The interaction between these two chemical interfaces mediates a specific chemical recognition between the cells, and such a process is a key factor in fertilization, inflammation, infection, development, and differentiation.

Carbohydrate–protein interactions are also important in non-self interactions. Many pathogens use this mechanism to recognize their target cells. *Escherichia coli*, for example, and some other Gram-negative enteric bacteria have short, hair-like projections called pili on their surfaces. These pili have mannose-binding lectins at their tips that can recognize and bind to high-mannose oligosaccharides on the brush border membranes of intestinal epithelial cells. This interaction allows the bacteria to be retained in the intestine. The influenza virus uses a hemagglutinin protein on its surface to bind to sialic acid residues on glycoproteins and glycolipids on the surfaces of target cells.

Variations in mucin structure appear to have a role in the specificity of fertilization, cell differentiation, development of the immune response, and virus infectivity. Glycoprotein ZP3, which is present on the zona pellucida of the mouse egg, functions as a receptor for sperm during fertilization. Enzymatic removal of *O*-glycans from ZP3 results in loss of sperm receptor activity, whereas removal of the *N*-glycans has no effect on sperm binding. The isolated *O*-glycans obtained from ZP3 also have sperm-binding activity and inhibit sperm–egg interaction and fertilization in vitro. Differences between the *O*-glycan structures of cytotoxic lymphocytes and helper cells involved in the immune response are also believed to be important in mediating cellular interactions during the immune response.

ADVANCED CONCEPT BOX
TOXICITY OF RICIN AND OTHER LECTINS

Lectins are found in a variety of foods, including beans, peanuts, and dry cereals. Many plant lectins are toxic to animal cells. In edible plants, these may be less of a problem if the foods are cooked because the lectins are denatured, then digested by gastrointestinal proteases. On the other hand, lectins in uncooked plants are very resistant to proteases and can therefore cause serious problems. They bind to cells in the gastrointestinal tract, inhibiting enzyme activities, food digestion, and nutrient absorption and causing gastrointestinal distress and allergic reactions.

Ricin, produced by the castor bean plant, is among the most poisonous proteins known. These types of toxic lectins are usually composed of several subunits, one of which is the carbohydrate-recognizing or carbohydrate-binding site, whereas the other subunit is an enzyme that, for example, can catalytically inactivate ribosomes. Thus a single molecule of this catalytic subunit entering a cell can completely block protein synthesis in that cell. Other toxic lectins include modeccin, abrin, and mistletoe lectin I.

SUMMARY

- Glycosylation is the major posttranslational modification of tissue proteins.
- Glycosylation is a multicompartment activity, involving sugar interconversions and activation in the cytosolic compartment, building of complex structures on lipid intermediates in the ER, and glycosylation and pruning reactions in the ER and Golgi apparatus. The outcome is an amazingly diverse range of oligosaccharide structures on proteins.
- Sugars on glycoconjugates can serve a number of different functions, including:
  - Modifying the physical properties of the protein (solubility, stability, and/or viscosity)

CLINICAL BOX
CHANGES IN SUGAR COMPOSITION AND/OR STRUCTURE CAN BE DIAGNOSTIC MARKERS OF SOME TYPES OF CANCER

Changes in glycosylation of both proteins and lipids have been consistently reported on cell-surface glycoconjugates of various types of cancer cells, including melanomas, ovarian cancer, and hepatocellular carcinoma. Although these changes are not the cause of the disease, they are being evaluated as diagnostic tools for early detection of disease. The enzyme GlcNAc transferase V (the transferase involved in adding a second [branching] GlcNAc residue to a mannose residue to make a triantennary complex chain) is over-expressed in some transformed cells, resulting in increased branching and production of larger *N*-linked oligosaccharides. Changes in *O*-linked oligosaccharides have also been reported - for example, increased levels of sialyl Lewis-X antigen, which are thought to contribute to metastasis. Changes in the amount and sialylation of mucins are also associated with metastasis of lung and colon carcinoma cells and are being studied for their usefulness as diagnostic or prognostic biomarkers. There is also evidence that changes in the level of fucose on some glycoproteins regulate the biological phenotype of cancer cells, and in fact, fucosylation of the protein α-fetoprotein (AFP-L3) has been used clinically as a marker for hepatocellular carcinoma.

Comment
The structure and composition of glycoproteins and glycolipids are altered in tumor cells, compared with normal cells. Although these changes may not cause the cancer, they may have a significant effect on clinical outcome (e.g., if they limit leukocyte infiltration, assist in evading immune surveillance, or facilitate metastasis). Analysis of oligosaccharide structures may be useful for early detection and diagnostic purposes, and manipulation of oligosaccharide structure may prove useful in the treatment of some cancers.

Singh, R. S., Walia, A. K., & Kanwar, J. R. (2016). Protozoa lectins and their role in host-pathogen interactions. *Biotechnology Advances, 34*, 1018–1029.

van Putten, J. P., & Strijbis, K. (2017). Transmembrane mucins: Signaling receptors at the intersection of inflammation and cancer. *Journal of Innate Immunity, 9*(3), 281–299.

Vliegenthart, J. F. (2017). The complexity of glycoprotein-derived glycans. *Proceedings of the Japan Academy, Ser. B, Physical and Biological Sciences, 93*, 64–86.

Zacchi, L. F., & Schulz, B. L. (2016). N-glycoprotein macroheterogeneity: Biological implications and proteomic characterization. *Glycoconjugate Journal, 33*, 359–376.

ACTIVE LEARNING

1. Why do eukaryotic cells use lipid-linked oligosaccharides as intermediates in the synthesis of *N*-glycans but not *O*-glycans?
2. Do animal cells need amino sugars and uronic acids in the diet to synthesize complex carbohydrates? If not, why not? Review the use of glucosamine-chondroitin supplements for the treatment of arthritis.
3. Describe the role of carbohydrate-dependent cell–cell interactions during the development of the nervous or immune system.

- Aiding in the folding of the protein
- Participating in the targeting of the protein to its proper location in the cell
- Mediating cell–protein and cell–cell recognition during fertilization, development, inflammation, and other processes
- Numerous human diseases involve defects in sugar metabolism, including galactosemia and hereditary fructose intolerance, leukocyte adhesion deficiency, congenital disorders of glycosylation (CDG), and lysosomal storage diseases.

FURTHER READING

Behera, S. K., Praharaj, A. B., Dehury, B., et al. (2015). Exploring the role and diversity of mucins in health and disease with special insight into non-communicable diseases. *Glycoconjugate Journal, 32*, 575–613.

Bode, L. (2015). The functional biology of human milk oligosaccharides. *Early Human Development, 91*, 619–622.

Brooks, S. A. (2017). Lectin histochemistry: Historical perspectives, state of the art, and the future. *Methods in Molecular Biology, 1560*, 93–107.

Etulain, J., & Schattner, M. (2014). Glycobiology of platelet-endothelial cell interactions. *Glycobiology, 24*, 1252–1259.

Frenkel, E. S., & Ribbeck, K. (2015). Salivary mucins in host defense and disease prevention. *Journal of Oral Microbiology, 7*, 29759.

Hennet, T., & Cabalzar, J. (2015). Congenital disorders of glycosylation: A concise chart of glycocalyx dysfunction. *Trends in Biochemical Sciences, 40*, 377–384.

Jegatheesan, P., & De Bandt, J. P. (2017). Fructose and NAFLD: The multifaceted aspects of fructose metabolism. *Nutrients, 9*(3).

Manning, J. C., Romero, A., Habermann, F. A., et al. (2017). Lectins: A primer for histochemists and cell biologists. *Histochemistry and Cell Biology, 147*, 199–222.

Mason, C. P., & Tarr, A. W. (2015). Human lectins and their roles in viral infections. *Molecules : A Journal of Synthetic Chemistry and Natural Product Chemistry, 20*, 2229–2271.

RELEVANT WEBSITES

Congenital disorders of glycosylation: https://rarediseases.org/rare-diseases/congenital-disorders-of-glycosylation/

Galactosemia: http://www.galactosemia.org/understanding-galactosemia/

O-GlcNAc modification of proteins: https://www.ncbi.nlm.nih.gov/books/NBK1954/

Glycoprotein biosynthesis: http://www.ccrc.uga.edu/~lwang/bcmb8020/N-glycans-A.pdf

Glycoprotein topics: http://www.glycoforum.gr.jp/science/word/glycoprotein/GP_E.html

Hereditary fructose intolerance: http://www.bu.edu/aldolase/HFI/

I-cell disease: http://emedicine.medscape.com/article/945460-overview

Plant lectins: http://poisonousplants.ansci.cornell.edu/toxicagents/lectins.html

ABBREVIATIONS

CDG	Congenital disease of glycosylation
CMP-NeuAc	CDP-neuraminic (sialic) acid
Dol	Dolichol
ER	Endoplasmic reticulum
AFP-L3	α-fetoprotein
Fru-1-P	Fructose-1-phosphate
Fru-1,6-P	Fructose-1,6-bisphosphate
Gal-1-P	Galactose-1-phosphate
GalNAc	N-acetylgalactosamine
GDP-Fuc	Guanosine diphosphate fucose
GDP-Man	Guanosine diphosphate mannose
GlcNAc	N-acetylglucosamine
LDL	Low density lipoprotein
Man-6-P	Mannose-6-phosphate
NeuAc	Neuraminic (sialic) acid
UDP-Gal	Uridine diphosphate galactose
UDP-GalNAc	Uridine diphosphate N-acetylgalactosamine
UDP-Glc	Uridine diphosphate glucose
UDP-GlcNAc	Uridine diphosphate N-acetylglucosamine
UDP-Xyl	Uridine diphosphate xylose

LEARNING OBJECTIVES

After reading this chapter, you should be able to:

- Describe how the various glycerol-based phospholipids are synthesized and how they are interconverted.
- Describe the multiple roles of cytidine nucleotides in the activation of intermediates in phospholipid synthesis.
- Describe the various types of sphingolipids and glycolipids that occur in mammalian cells and their functions.
- Explain the etiology of lysosomal storage diseases, their pathology, and the rationale for enzyme-replacement therapy for treatment of these diseases.

INTRODUCTION

Complex lipids encompass the glycerophospholipids, introduced in Chapter 3, and the sphingolipids. These molecules are found mostly in two locations, either embedded in biological membranes or in circulating lipoproteins. The sphingolipids are almost exclusively found in cell membranes, primarily the plasma membrane. They carry a wide range of carbohydrate structures that face toward the exterior environment and, like glycoproteins, have a range of recognition functions. A major difference between these two classes of lipids is that glycerophospholipids are saponifiable (except plasmalogens), whereas **sphingolipids** contain no alkali-labile ester bonds. Thus it was convenient to isolate sphingolipids from tissues by saponification, then extract the remaining lipids into an organic solvent. Once isolated, the characterization of the glycan structure of the sphingolipids was technically challenging to ascertain. Therefore the structures were, for a long time, unknown and mysterious, leading to their name: sphinx-like, or sphingolipids.

This chapter discusses the structure, biosynthesis, and function of the two major classes of polar lipids: glycerophospholipids and sphingolipids. In preparation for this chapter, it might help to review the structure of phospholipids in Chapter 3.

SYNTHESIS AND TURNOVER OF GLYCEROPHOSPHOLIPIDS

Synthesis of glycerophospholipids

There are many species of glycerophospholipids with a distinct composition of polar head groups and hydrophobic acyl groups (see Chapter 3). With regard to the acyl groups, saturated fatty acids are usually esterified at the sn-1 position, whereas unsaturated fatty acids are esterified at the sn-2 position. Biosynthesis of glycerophospholipids first proceeds by the de novo pathway, and subsequently the originally attached fatty acids in the de novo pathway are replaced with new ones in the remodeling pathway. Through this remodeling pathway, the diversity and asymmetry of the acyl groups are generated.

De novo pathway

Phospholipids are in a constant state of synthesis, turnover, and remodeling

The de novo pathway begins with sequential reactions, in which glycerol-3-P is acylated by transfer of two fatty acids from acyl-CoA to produce **phosphatidic acid** (PA) via the intermediate, lysophosphatidic acid (Fig. 18.1). Then PA is dephosphorylated to **diacylglycerol** (DAG) by a specific cytosolic phosphatase. Alternatively, PA reacts with cytidine triphosphate (CTP) to yield the activated phosphatidic acid **cytidine diphosphate (CDP)-DAG**. Phosphatidic acid and DAG are common intermediates in the synthesis of both triglycerides (triacylglycerols) and phospholipids. All animal cells, except for erythrocytes, are able to synthesize phospholipids de novo, whereas triglyceride synthesis occurs mainly in the liver, adipose tissue, and intestinal cells. The starting material, **glycerol-3-phosphate,** is formed in most tissues by reduction of the glycolytic intermediate dihydroxyacetone phosphate (DHAP). In the liver, kidney, and intestine, glycerol-3-P can also be formed directly via phosphorylation of glycerol by glycerol kinase. DHAP may also be acylated by the addition of a fatty acid to the 1-hydroxyl group; this intermediate is then reduced and acylated to PA.

The biosynthesis of the major phospholipid **phosphatidylcholine** (PC; also known as **lecithin**) from DAG requires

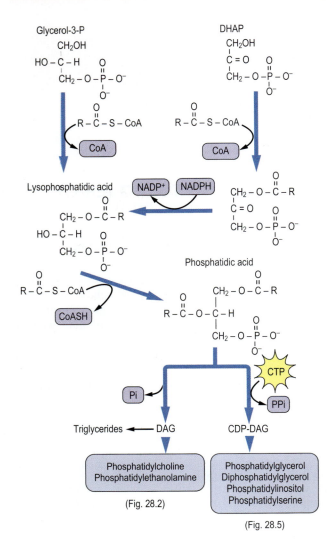

(Fig. 28.2)

(Fig. 28.5)

Fig. 18.1 **De novo pathway to synthesis of glycerophospholipids.** CDP, cytidine diphosphate; CDP-DAG, CDP-diacylglycerol; CTP, cytidine triphosphate; CoAS, coenzyme A; DHAP, dihydroxyacetone phosphate; Pi, inorganic phosphate; PPi, inorganic pyrophosphate.

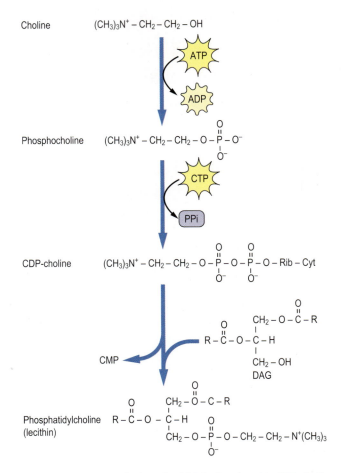

Fig. 18.2 **Formation of phosphatidylcholine by the CDP-choline pathway.** This pathway is an extension of the bottom left side of Fig. 18.1. Cyt, cytosine; CDP, cytidine diphosphate; CMP, cytidine monophosphate; DAG, diacylglycerol; Rib, ribose; CTP, cytidine triphosphate.

activation of choline to CDP-choline. In this series of reactions, shown in Fig. 18.2, the choline "head group" is converted to phosphocholine and then activated to **CDP-choline** by a pyrophosphorylase reaction. The pyrophosphate bond is cleaved, and phosphocholine (choline phosphate) is transferred to DAG to form PC. This reaction is analogous to the transfer of GlcNAc-6-P to dolichol or the high-mannose core of lysosomal enzymes, in which both the sugar and a phosphate are transferred from the nucleotide derivative. **Phosphatidylethanolamine** (PE) is formed by a similar pathway using CTP and phosphoethanolamine to form CDP-ethanolamine. Both PC and PE can react with free serine by an exchange reaction to form phosphatidylserine (PS) and the free base, choline or ethanolamine (Fig. 18.3).

Large amounts of PC are needed in the liver for the biosynthesis of lipoproteins and bile. In a secondary hepatic pathway, which is a necessary supplement to the CDP-choline pathway in times of starvation, PC can also be formed by methylation of PE with the methyl donor **S-adenosylmethionine (SAM;** Figs. 18.3 and 18.4). This methylation pathway involves the sequential transfer of three activated methyl groups from three molecules of SAM. PE used in this pathway is supplied from PS by a specific mitochondrial decarboxylase (Fig. 18.3).

PS and other phospholipids with an alcohol head group (e.g., phosphatidylglycerol [PG] and phosphatidylinositol [PI]) are synthesized by an alternative pathway. In this case, PA is activated by CTP, yielding CDP-DAG (see Fig. 18.5); the PA group is then transferred to free serine, glycerol, or inositol to form PS, PG, or PI, respectively. A second PA may also be added to phosphatidylglycerol to form 1,3-diphosphatidylglycerol (DPG). This lipid, known commonly as **cardiolipin,** is found almost exclusively in the inner mitochondrial membrane; it represents about 20% of phospholipids in heart mitochondria

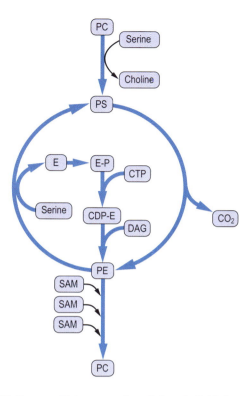

Fig. 18.3 **Pathways of interconversion of phospholipids by exchange of head groups, by methylation, or by decarboxylation.** CDP, cytidine diphosphate; CTP, cytidine triphosphate; DAG, diacylglycerol; E, ethanolamine; PC, phosphatidylcholine; PE, phosphatidylethanolamine; PC, phosphatidylserine; SAM, *S*-adenosylmethionine.

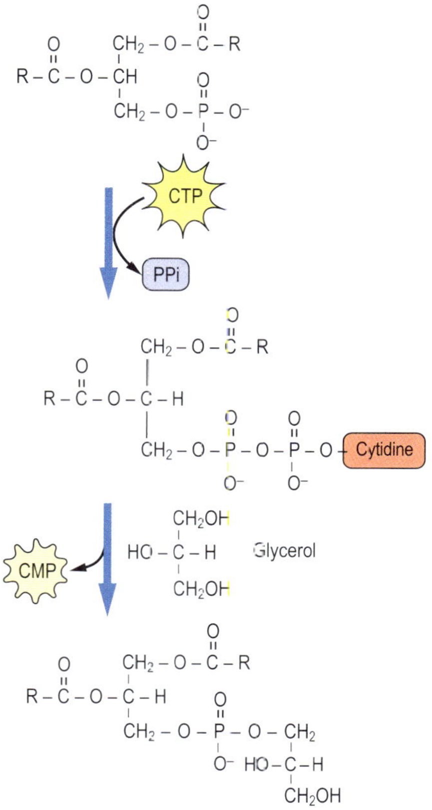

Fig. 18.5 **Formation of phosphatidylglycerol by activation of phosphatidic acid to form CDP-DAG, and transfer of DAG to glycerol.** This pathway is an extension of the lower right side of Fig. 18.1. CMP, cytidine monophosphate; CTP, cytidine triphosphate.

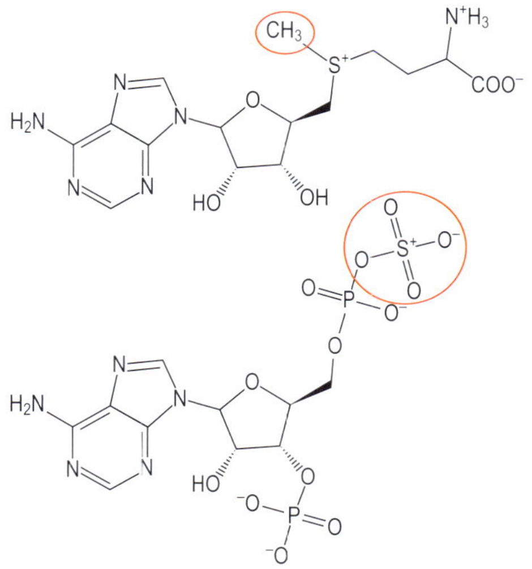

Fig. 18.4 **Structures of the methyl and sulfate donors involved in the synthesis of membrane lipids.** SAM, *S*-adenosylmethionine; PAPS, 3'-phosphoadenosine-5'-phosphosulfate (active sulfate).

and is required for efficient activity of electron transport complexes III and IV and the ATP:ADP translocase.

Plasmalogens are a second major class of mitochondrial lipids and are enriched in nerve and muscle tissue; in the heart, they account for nearly 50% of total phospholipids. The

biosynthesis of plasmalogens proceeds from DHAP: it is first acylated at C-1, then the acyl group exchanges with a lipid alcohol to form an ether lipid. The ether lipid is desaturated, leading eventually to a 1-alkenylether-2-acyl-phospholipid. The function of plasmalogens versus diacylphospholipids is not clear, but there is some evidence that they are more resistant to oxidative damage, which may provide protection against oxidative stress in tissues with active aerobic metabolism (see Chapter 42).

Remodeling pathway

The acyl groups of glycerophospholipids are highly diverse and distributed in an asymmetric manner between the *sn*-1 and *sn*-2 position of glycerol; polyunsaturated fatty acids, such as arachidonate, are found predominately at the *sn*-2 position. The composition of fatty acyl groups in phospholipids also varies among tissues and membranes and with the nature of the head group: choline, ethanolamine, serine, inositol, or glycerol. The diversity and asymmetry of phospholipids are not explained by the de novo pathway because phosphatidic

CLINICAL BOX
SURFACTANT FUNCTION OF PHOSPHOLIPIDS: ACUTE RESPIRATORY DISTRESS SYNDROME

Acute respiratory distress syndrome (ARDS) accounts for 15%–20% of neonatal mortality in Western countries. The disease affects premature infants, and its incidence is directly related to the degree of prematurity.

Comment

Immature lungs do not have enough type II epithelial cells to synthesize sufficient amounts of the phospholipid **dipalmitoyl phosphatidylcholine (DPPC).** This phospholipid makes up more than 80% of the total phospholipids of the extracellular lipid layer that lines the alveoli of normal lungs. DPPC decreases the surface tension of the aqueous surface layer of the lungs, facilitating opening of the alveoli during inspiration. Lack of surfactant causes the lungs to collapse during the expiration phase of breathing, leading to ARDS. The maturity of the fetal lung can be assessed by measuring the lecithin:sphingomyelin ratio in amniotic fluid. If there is a potential problem, a mother can be treated with a glucocorticoid to accelerate maturation of the fetal lung. ARDS is also seen in adults in whom the type II epithelial cells have been destroyed as a result of the use of immunosuppressive drugs or certain chemotherapeutic agents.

ADVANCED CONCEPT BOX
GLYCOSYLPHOSPHATIDYLINOSITOL MEMBRANE ANCHORS

Phosphatidylinositol is an integral component of the glycosylphosphatidylinositol (GPI) structure that anchors various proteins to the plasma membrane (Fig. 18.7). In contrast to other membrane phospholipids, including most of the membrane phosphatidylinositol, GPI has a glycan chain containing glucosamine and mannose attached to the inositol. Ethanolamine connects the GPI-glycan to the carboxyl terminus of the protein. Many membrane proteins in eukaryotic cells are anchored by a GPI structure, including alkaline phosphatase and acetylcholinesterase, which have roles in bone mineralization and nerve transmission, respectively. In contrast to integral or peripheral membrane proteins, GPI-anchored proteins may be released from the cell surface by phospholipase C in response to regulatory processes.

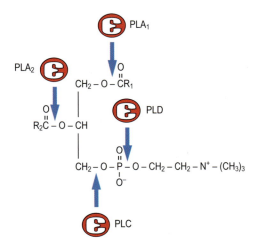

Fig. 18.6 **Sites of action of phospholipases on phosphatidylcholine.** PLA_1, PLA_2, PLC, and PLD are phospholipases A_1, A_2, C, and D, respectively.

acid and DAG are common precursors of both triglycerides and phospholipids. Instead, the redistribution of fatty acids in phospholipids is accomplished by remodeling pathways through the concerted action of **phospholipase A_2** (PLA_2) and **lysophospholipid acyltransferases** (LPLAT), which remove, replace and, in the process, redistribute fatty acids in phospholipids. Not until the last decade have the LPLAT enzymes been identified; they play an essential role in (re)incorporation of polyunsaturated fatty acids into phospholipids.

Turnover of phospholipids

Phospholipids are in a continuous state of turnover in most membranes. This occurs as a result of oxidative damage, during inflammation, and through activation of phospholipases, particularly in response to hormonal stimuli. As shown in Fig. 18.6, there are a number of phospholipases that act on specific bonds in the phospholipid structure. Phospholipase A_2 (PLA_2) and **phospholipase C** (PLC) are particularly active during the inflammatory response and in signal transduction. Phospholipase B (not shown) is a lysophospholipase that removes the second acyl group after the action of PLA_1 or PLA_2. The lysophospholipids may be degraded or recycled (reacylated).

SPHINGOLIPIDS

Structure and biosynthesis of sphingosine

Sphingolipids are a complex group of amphipathic, polar lipids. They are built on a core structure of the long-chain amino alcohol sphingosine, which is formed by oxidative decarboxylation and condensation of palmitate with serine. In all sphingolipids, the long-chain fatty acid is attached to the amino group of the sphingosine in an amide linkage (Fig. 18.8). Because of the alkaline stability of amides, compared with esters, sphingolipids are nonsaponifiable, which facilitates their separation from alkali-labile glycerolipids.

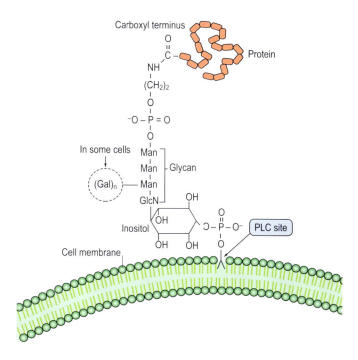

Fig. 18.7 **Structure of the glycosylphosphatidylinositol (GPI) anchor and its attachment to proteins.** Gal, galactose; GlcN, glucosamine; Man, mannose; PLC, phospholipase C.

Fig. 18.8 **Structures of sphingosine and sphingomyelin.**

The synthesis of the **sphingosine** base of sphingolipids involves condensation of palmitoyl-CoA with serine, in which the carbon-1 of serine is lost as carbon dioxide. The product of this reaction is converted in several steps to sphingosine, which is then N-acylated to form **ceramide** (N-acylsphingosine). Ceramide (see Fig. 18.9) is the precursor and backbone structure of both sphingomyelin and glycosphingolipids.

Sphingomyelin

Sphingomyelin is the only sphingolipid that contains phosphate and is the major phospholipid in the myelin sheath of nerves

Sphingomyelin (see Fig. 18.8) is found in plasma membranes, subcellular organelles, the endoplasmic reticulum, and

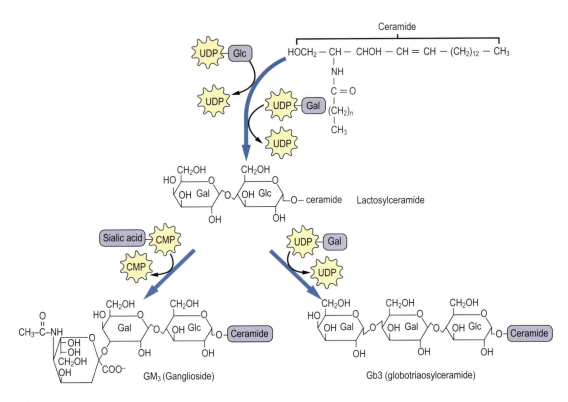

Fig. 18.9 **An outline of transferase reactions for elongation of glycolipids and formation of gangliosides.**

mitochondria. It comprises 5%–20% of the total phospholipids in most cell types and is mostly localized in the plasma membrane. The phosphocholine group in sphingomyelin is transferred to the terminal hydroxyl group of the sphingosine by a transesterification reaction with phosphatidylcholine. The fatty acid composition varies, but long-chain fatty acids are common, including lignoceric (24:0), cerebronic (2-hydroxylignoceric), and nervonic (24:1) acids. Although they are not essential fatty acids, these fatty acids are important for the developing brain and are present in breast milk.

Glycolipids

Sphingolipids containing covalently bound sugars are known as glycosphingolipids, or glycolipids. As with glycoconjugates in general, the structure of the oligosaccharide chains is highly variable. In addition, the glycosyltransferase distribution and glycosphingolipid content of cells vary during development and in response to regulatory processes.

Glycolipids can be classified into three main groups: neutral glycolipids, **sulfatides,** and gangliosides. In all of these compounds, the polar head group, comprising the sugars, is attached to ceramide by a glycosidic bond at the terminal hydroxyl group of the sphingosine. Fig. 18.9 illustrates the structure and biosynthesis of some of the simpler glycolipids. Neutral glycolipids contain only neutral and amino sugars.

Glucosylceramide (GlcCer) and galactosylceramide (GalCer) are the smallest members of this class of compounds and serve as the nucleus for the elaboration of more complex structures. Sulfatides are formed by the addition of sulfate from the sulfate donor, **3'-phosphoadenosine-5'-phosphosulfate (PAPS)** (Fig. 18.4), yielding, for example, GalCer 3-sulfate. Finally, glycolipids containing sialic acids (N-acetylneuraminic acid [NeuAc]) are termed gangliosides.

Structure and nomenclature of gangliosides

Gangliosides are glycosphingolipids containing sialic (N-acetylneuraminic) acid

The term *ganglioside* refers to glycolipids that were originally identified in high concentrations in ganglia in the central nervous system. In general, more than 50% of the sialic acid in these cells is present in gangliosides. Gangliosides are also found in the surface membranes of cells of most extraneural tissues, but in these tissues, they account for less than 10% of the total sialic acid.

The nomenclature used to identify the various gangliosides is based on the number of sialic acid residues contained in the molecule and on the sequence of the carbohydrates (Fig. 18.10). GM refers to a ganglioside with a single (mono) sialic acid, whereas GD, GT, and GQ would indicate two, three, and four

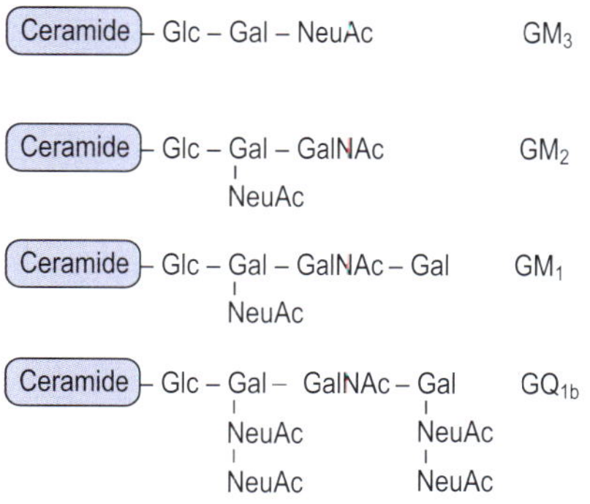

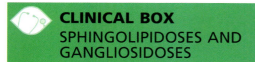

| Ceramide – Glc – Gal – NeuAc | GM₃ |

Ceramide – Glc – Gal – NeuAc GM₃

Ceramide – Glc – Gal – GalNAc GM₂
                         |
                       NeuAc

Ceramide – Glc – Gal – GalNAc – Gal GM₁
                         |
                       NeuAc

Ceramide – Glc – Gal – GalNAc – Gal GQ₁b
                         | |
                       NeuAc   NeuAc
                         | |
                       NeuAc   NeuAc

Fig. 18.10 **Generalized structures of gangliosides.** Glc, glucose; Gal, galactose; NeuAc, *N*-acetylneuraminic acid; GalNAc, *N*-acetylgalactosamine.

CLINICAL BOX
SPHINGOLIPIDOSES AND GANGLIOSIDOSES

Tay–Sachs disease is a gangliosidosis in which ganglioside GM₂ accumulates as a result of an absence of lysosomal hexosaminidase A (see Fig. 18.11). Individuals with this disease usually have mental retardation and blindness and die between 2 and 3 years of age. **Fabry's disease** is a sphingolipidosis resulting from a deficiency of lysosomal α-galactosidase and accumulation of globotriaosylceramide (Gb3; see Table 18.1). The symptoms of Fabry's disease are skin rash, kidney failure, and pain in the lower extremities. Patients with this condition benefit from kidney transplants and usually live into early to mid-adulthood. Most of these lysosomal storage diseases appear in several forms (variants) resulting from different mutations in the genome. Some lysosomal storage diseases and some variants are more severe and debilitating than others. Although lysosomal storage diseases are relatively rare, they have had a major impact on our understanding of the function and importance of lysosomes.

Comment
When cells die, biomolecules, including glycosphingolipids and glycoproteins, are degraded to their individual components. Fig. 18.11 presents the pathway for the degradation of ganglioside GM₁ in the lysosomes. A number of lysosomal diseases result from the absence of an essential glycosidase in this chain of hydrolase reactions (see Table 18.1). The sphingolipidoses are characterized by lysosomal accumulation of the substrate of the missing enzyme, which interferes with normal lysosomal function in turnover of biomolecules.

CLINICAL BOX
GAUCHER'S DISEASE: A MODEL FOR ENZYME-REPLACEMENT THERAPY

Gaucher's disease is a lysosomal storage disease in which afflicted individuals are missing the enzyme β-glucosidase (also known as glucocerebrosidase). This enzyme removes the final sugar from the ceramide, allowing the lipid portion to be further degraded in the lysosomes. This disease is characterized by hepatomegaly and neurodegeneration, but there are milder variants that are amenable to treatment by enzyme replacement therapy.

For treatment of Gaucher's disease, exogenous β-glucosidase was successfully targeted to the lysosomes of macrophages. To do this, it was necessary to produce the recombinant replacement enzyme with *N*-glycan chains containing terminal mannose residues. This was done by cleaving the glycans of the enzyme produced in mammalian cells with a combination of sialidase (neuraminidase), β-galactosidase, and β-hexosaminidase to trim the complex chains down to the mannose core. An alternative recombinant glucosidase has been produced in a baculovirus-infected insect cell system. Both enzymes have a high-mannose oligosaccharide; although they do not contain Man-6-P residues, they are recognized by a macrophage cell-surface receptor for high-mannose oligosaccharides; the enzymes are endocytosed and end up in the lysosomal compartment, where they hydrolyze glucosyl-ceramide. The recombinant enzymes are administered intravenously. The success in using recombinant glucocerebrosidase for the treatment of Gaucher's disease has stimulated the development of other lysosomal hydrolases for the treatment of lysosomal storage diseases.

LYSOSOMAL STORAGE DISEASES RESULTING FROM DEFECTS IN GLYCOLIPID DEGRADATION

The complex oligosaccharides on glycolipids are built up, one sugar residue at a time, in the Golgi apparatus and are degraded in a similar stepwise fashion but in the opposite direction by a series of exoglycosidases in lysosomes (Fig. 18.11). Defects in sequential degradation of glycolipids lead to a number of **lysosomal storage diseases,** known as sphingolipidoses and gangliosidoses (Table 18.1). These diseases are autosomal recessive in inheritance. Heterozygotes are asymptomatic, indicating that a single copy of the gene for a functional enzyme is sufficient for apparently normal turnover of glycolipids. Like I-cell disease (Chapter 17), the sphingolipidoses are characterized by the accumulation of undigested lipids in inclusion bodies in the cells.

sialic acid residues in the molecule, respectively. The number after the GM (e.g., GM₁) refers to the structure of the oligosaccharide. These numbers were derived from the relative mobility of the glycolipids on thin-layer chromatograms; the larger (e.g., GM₁) gangliosides migrate the slowest.

Table 18.1 Some lipid storage diseases

Disease	Symptoms	Major storage product	Deficient enzymes
Tay–Sachs	Blindness, mental retardation, death between 2nd and 3rd year	GM_2 ganglioside	Hexosaminidase A
Gaucher's	Liver and spleen enlargement, mental retardation in infantile form	Glucocerebroside	β-Glucosidase
Fabry's	Skin rash, kidney failure, pain in lower extremities	Ceramide trihexoside	α-Galactosidase
Krabbe's	Liver and spleen enlargement, mental retardation	Galactocerebroside	β-Galactosidase

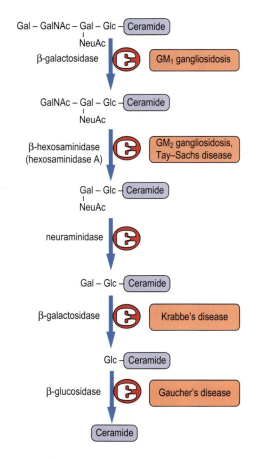

Fig. 18.11 **Lysosomal pathway for turnover (degradation) of ganglioside GM_1 in human cells.** Various enzymes may be missing in specific lipid storage diseases, as indicated in Table 18.1. Gal, galactose; GalNAc, *N*-acetylgalactosamine; Glc, glucose; NeuAc, *N*-acetylneuraminic acid.

 CLINICAL BOX
FABRY'S DISEASE (INCIDENCE 1 IN 100,000)

A 30-year-old man was found to have proteinuria at an insurance medical examination. He had been seen over a number of years from around age 10 with headaches, vertigo, and shooting pains in his arms and legs. No diagnosis was made, and he had grown accustomed to these problems. The physician carefully examined his perineum and scrotum, identifying small, raised, red angiokeratoma.

Comment

This man was diagnosed with Fabry's disease, which often takes years before a diagnosis is confirmed by measuring α-galactosidase A activity. The principal endothelial depositions of a ceramide trihexoside (Gal-α1-4-Gal-β1-4-Glc-β-ceramide; Gb3) occur in the kidney (leading to proteinuria and renal failure), the heart and brain (leading to myocardial infarction and stroke), and around blood vessels supplying nerves (leading to painful paresthesiae). Historically, most patients experienced end-stage renal disease, requiring transplantation. However, recombinant enzyme-replacement therapy appears to clear the deposited Gb3, and initial studies suggest that renal function is maintained.

ABO BLOOD GROUP ANTIGENS

Blood transfusion replenishes the oxygen-carrying capacity of blood in persons who suffer from blood loss or anemia (see Chapter 5). The term ***blood transfusion*** is something of a misnomer because it involves only the infusion of washed and preserved red cells. The membranes of red blood cells contain a number of blood group antigens, of which the ABO blood group system is the best understood and most widely studied.

The ABO blood group antigens are complex carbohydrates present as components of glycoproteins or glycosphingolipids of red cell membranes (Fig. 18.12). The H locus codes for a fucosyltransferase, which adds fucose to a galactose residue in a glycan chain. Individuals with type A blood have, in addition to the H substance, an A gene that codes for a specific GalNAc transferase that adds GalNAc α1,3 to the galactose residue of **H substance** to form the A antigen. Individuals with type B blood have a B gene that codes for a galactosyl transferase that adds galactose α1,3 to the galactose residue of H substance to form the B antigen. Individuals with type AB blood have both the GalNAc and the Gal transferases, and their red blood cells contain a mixture of A and B substances. Those with type O blood have only H substance on their red cell membranes; they do not make either enzyme. Enzymes such as coffee bean α-galactosidase can remove the galactose from type B red cells, an approach that is being tested for increasing the supply of type O (universal donor) red cells.

An individual may have type A, type B, type AB, or type O blood. Individuals with type A cells develop natural antibodies

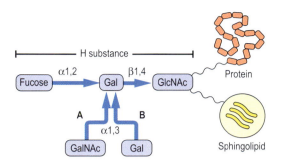

Fig. 18.12 **Relationship between the H, A, and B blood group substances.** The terminal oligosaccharide is linked through other sugars to proteins and lipids of the red cell membrane. GlcNAc, *N*-acetylglucosamine; GalNAc, *N*-acetylgalactosamine; Gal, galactose.

in their plasma that are directed against and will agglutinate type B and type AB red blood cells; those with type B red cells develop antibodies against A substance and will agglutinate type A and type AB blood. Persons with type AB blood have neither A nor B antibodies and are called **universal recipients** because they can be transfused with cells of either blood type. Individuals with type O blood have only H substance, not A or B substance, on their red blood cells and are **universal donors** because their red blood cells are not agglutinated by either A or B antibodies; however, they may accept blood only from a type O donor.

The ABO antigens are present on most cells in the body, but they are referred to as blood group antigens because of their association with transfusion reactions. The transfusion reaction is the result of the reaction of host antibodies with transfused red cells, resulting in complement-mediated hemolysis (see Chapter 41). Although the transfusion reaction demonstrates the role of carbohydrates in recognition of the foreign red cells, the physiologic function of blood group substances is unclear. Persons with an O genotype are generally as healthy as those with A or B genotype. However, there is some evidence that specific phenotypes may confer differential resistance to disease; for example, people with type A and type O blood appear to be more susceptible to smallpox and cholera, respectively.

The **Lewis blood group** antigens correspond to a set of fucosylated glycan structures. The Lewis-A antigen (Lewis[a]) is synthesized by a fucosyltransferase that transfers a fucose residue to a GlcNAc residue in a glycan chain (Fig. 18.13), and the Lewis[b] antigen is synthesized by the action of a second fucosyltransferase, which transfers fucose to the terminal galactose residue in the same glycan chain. Note the similarity of these structures to the sialyl Lewis-X antigen in Fig. 17.9 and the ABO antigens in Fig. 18.12. There are 13 fucosyltransferase genes in the human genome. Changes in fucosylation of glycans are associated with differentiation, development, carcinogenesis, and metastasis.

The **P blood group** antigens expressed on the globo-series of glycosphingolipids are distributed in red cells and other tissues. Again, the glycans in this blood group are synthesized

by the sequential action of distinct glycosyltransferases. The physiologic function of these blood groups is unknown, but P antigens are associated with urinary tract infections and parvovirus infections. Uropathogenic strains of *Escherichia coli* express lectins that bind to the Galα1,4Gal moiety of the P[k] and P$_1$ antigens. More work is needed to understand the genetics and biochemistry of these and other blood group antigens as well as their roles in physiology and disease.

ACTIVE LEARNING

1. Compare the role of plasmalogens versus diacylglycerol-phospholipids in cell membranes.
2. Discuss the challenges in the development of a vaccine to protect against trypanosomiasis.
3. Review current therapeutic approaches for the diagnosis and treatment of acute respiratory distress syndrome (ARDS).
4. Review the current status of enzyme-replacement therapy for the treatment of lysosomal storage diseases. What other genetic diseases are treated by this therapy?

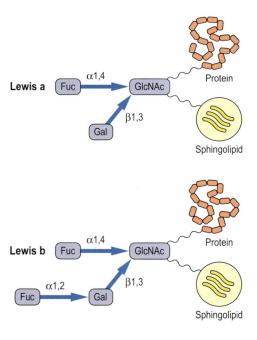

Fig. 18.13 **Structure of Lewis blood group antigens.**

properties as surfactants, as cofactors for membrane enzymes, and as components of signal transduction systems.

■ The primary route for de novo biosynthesis of phospholipids involves the activation of one of the components (either DAG or the head group) with CTP to form a high-energy intermediate, such as CDP-diacylglycerol or CDP-choline.

■ Phospholipids undergo maturation in the remodeling pathway, in which acyl groups at the *sn*-2 position are replaced with new ones, yielding diversity and asymmetry of the hydrophobic moiety of phospholipids.

■ Glycosphingolipids function as receptors for cell–cell recognition and interactions and as binding sites for symbiotic and pathogenic bacteria and for viruses. Carbohydrate structures on the glycosphingolipids of red cell membranes are also antigenic determinants responsible for the ABO and other blood types.

■ Glycosphingolipids are degraded in lysosomes by a sequence of reactions that involve a stepwise removal of sugars from the nonreducing end of the molecule, with each step involving a specific lysosomal exoglycosidase. Inherited lysosomal storage diseases result from defects in degradation of sphingolipids.

SUMMARY

■ Complex polar lipids are essential components of all cell membranes.
■ Phospholipids are the major structural lipids of all membranes, but they also have important functional

FURTHER READING

Belický, Š., Katrlík, J., & Tkáč, J. (2016). Glycan and lectin biosensors. *Essays in Biochemistry, 60,* 37–47.

Cooling, L. (2015). Blood groups in infection and host susceptibility. *Clinical Microbiology Reviews, 28,* 801–870.

Desnick, R. J., & Schuchman, E. H. (2012). Enzyme replacement therapy for lysosomal diseases: Lessons from 20 years of experience and remaining challenges. *Annual Review of Genomics and Human Genetics, 13,* 307–335.

Ezgu, F. (2016). Inborn errors of metabolism. *Advances in Clinical Chemistry, 73,* 195–250.

Franchini, M., & Liumbruno, G. M. (2013). ABO blood group: Old dogma, new perspectives. *Clinical Chemistry and Laboratory Medicine, 51*, 1545–1553.

Han, S., & Mallampalli, R. K. (2015). The role of surfactant in lung disease and host defense against pulmonary infections. *Annals of the American Thoracic Society, 12*, 765–774.

Heider, S., Dangerfield, J. A., & Metzner, C. (2016). Biomedical applications of glycosylphosphatidylinositol-anchored proteins. *Journal of Lipid Research, 57*, 1778–1788.

Johannes, L., Wunder, C., & Shafaq-Zadah, M. J. (2016). Glycolipids and lectins in endocytic uptake processes. *Molecular Biology, 428*, 4792–4818.

Oder, D., Nordbeck, P., & Wanner, C. (2016). Long-term treatment with enzyme replacement therapy in patients with Fabry disease. *Nephron, 134*, 30–36.

Pralhada Rao, R., Vaidyanathan, N., Rengasamy, M., et al. (2013). Sphingolipid metabolic pathway: An overview of major roles played in human diseases. *Journal of Lipid Research, 2013*, 178910.

Stirnemann, J., Belmatoug, N., & Camou, F. (2017). A review of Gaucher disease pathophysiology, clinical presentation and treatments. *International Journal of Molecular Sciences, 18*, 441.

Unione, L., Gimeno, A., & Valverde, P. (2017). Glycans in infectious diseases: A molecular recognition perspective. *Current Medicinal Chemistry, 2017*. Advance online publication.

RELEVANT WEBSITES

Blood groups: http://www.bloodbook.com/type-sys.html

Essential fatty acids: http://lpi.oregonstate.edu/mic/other-nutrients/essential-fatty-acids

Gaucher's disease: https://www.ninds.nih.gov/Disorders/All-Disorders/Gaucher-Disease-Information-Page

Glycosylphosphatidylinositol anchors: https://www.ncbi.nlm.nih.gov/books/NBK1966/

Paroxysmal nocturnal hemoglobinuria: http://emedicine.medscape.com/article/207468-overview

Sphingolipids: http://themedicalbiochemistrypage.org/sphingolipids.php

Tay–Sachs disease: https://www.ninds.nih.gov/Disorders/All-Disorders/Tay-Sachs-Disease-Information-Page

ABBREVIATIONS

ARDS	Acute respiratory distress syndrome
CDP	Cytidine diphosphate
CDP-DAG	CDP-diacylglycerol
DAG	Diacylglycerol
DPPC	Dipalmitoylphosphatidylcholine
GPI	Glycosylphosphatidylinositol anchor
LPLAT	Lysophospholipid acyltransferase
PAPS	Phosphoadenosine-5'-phosphosulfate
PNH	Paroxysmal nocturnal hemoglobinuria
PS	Phosphatidic acid
PC	Phosphatidylcholine
PE	Phosphatidylethanolamine
PI	Phosphatidylinositol
PLA2	Phospholipase A2
PLC	Phospholipase C
PS	Phosphatidylserine
SAM	S-adenosylmethionine

19 The Extracellular Matrix

Gur P. Kaushal, Alan D. Elbein (deceased), and Wayne E. Carver

LEARNING OBJECTIVES

After reading this chapter, you should be able to:

■ Describe the composition, structure, and function of the extracellular matrix (ECM) and its components, including collagens, noncollagenous proteins, hyaluronic acid, and glycosaminoglycans/proteoglycans.

■ Outline the sequence of steps in the biosynthesis and posttranslational modification of collagens and elastin, including the structure and synthesis of crosslinks.

■ Describe the pathways of biosynthesis and the turnover of proteoglycans.

■ Describe the role of link proteins in the formation of the extracellular matrix and the structure and function of integrins as receptors for ECM components.

■ Describe the pathology of several diseases associated with defects in ECM components.

INTRODUCTION

The extracellular matrix (ECM) is a complex network of secreted macromolecules located in the extracellular space. Historically, the ECM has been described as simply providing a three-dimensional framework for the organization of tissues and organs; however, it has become increasingly clear that it plays a central role in regulating basic processes, including proliferation, differentiation, migration, and even survival of cells. The macromolecular network of the ECM is made up of collagens, elastin, noncollagenous glycoproteins, and proteoglycans that are secreted by a variety of cell types. The components of the ECM are in intimate contact with their cells of origin and form a three-dimensional gelatinous bed in which the cells thrive (Fig. 19.1). Proteins in the ECM are also bound to the cell surface, so they transmit mechanical signals resulting from stretching and compression of tissues. The relative abundance, distribution, and molecular organization of ECM components vary enormously, depending on tissue type, developmental stage, and pathologic status. Variations in the composition, accumulation, and organization of the ECM dramatically impact the biomechanical, structural, and functional properties of the tissue. Changes in these ECM characteristics are associated with chronic diseases, such as arthritis, atherosclerosis, cancer, and fibrosis.

COLLAGENS

Collagens are the major proteins in the ECM

The collagens are a family of proteins that comprise about 30% of total protein mass in the body and are found to varying degrees in all tissues and organs. To date, more than 25 types of collagens have been identified that are broadly subclassified by their function, domain structure, and supramolecular organization. The collagen family can be generally divided into fibril-forming collagens (fibrillar) and nonfibrillar collagens. Collagen fibers are the most abundant structural components of the ECM. Their flexibility and high tensile strength play important roles in tissue architecture and integrity. Table 19.1 lists the types of collagens and their general distribution.

Triple-helical structure of collagens

The left-handed triple-helical structure of collagen is unique among proteins

All collagens share a common structural motif: the **collagen triple helix.** Collagen molecules are composed of three individual polypeptides known as α chains. The collagen triple helix is formed by folding of the three component α polypeptide chains. X-ray diffraction analysis indicates that the three left-handed helical polypeptide chains are wrapped around one another in a rope-like fashion to form a superhelix, or supercoiled, structure (Fig. 19.2). The left-handed helix is more extended than the α-helix of globular proteins, having nearly twice the rise per turn and only 3.0, rather than 3.6, amino acids per turn of the helix. Every third amino acid is glycine because only this amino acid, with the smallest side chain, fits into the crowded central core. The characteristic repeating sequence of collagen is **Gly-X-Y**, where X and Y can be any amino acid, but most often, X is proline and Y is hydroxyproline. Because of their restricted rotation and bulk, proline and hydroxyproline confer rigidity to the helix. The intra- and interchain helices are stabilized by hydrogen bonds, largely between peptide NH and C=O groups. The side chains of the X and Y amino acids point outward from the helix and thus are on the surface of the protein, where they form lateral interactions with other triple helices or proteins.

A

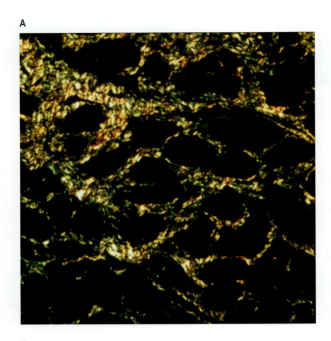

B

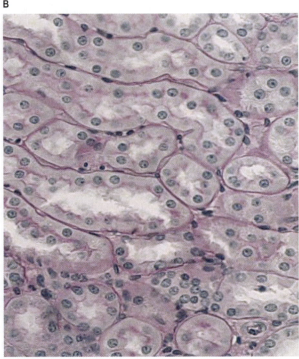

Fig. 19.1 (A) Light micrograph of picrosirius red-stained extracellular matrix in heart tissue, showing the insoluble collagen and elastin proteins. These proteins form a sheath around the cells and are embedded in a soluble, gelatinous matrix of polysaccharides and glycoconjugates, hyaluronic acid, and proteoglycans. The cells interact with ECM components, responding to mechanical signals through cell-surface proteins, including integrins, laminin, and fibronectin. (B) Periodic acid–Schiff (PAS) stain of renal tubular basement membranes. The PAS stain is specific for the proteoglycan component of the ECM (see Chapter 35).

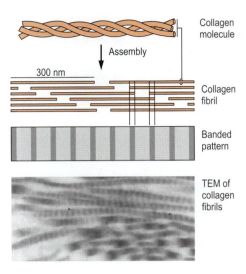

Fig. 19.2 **Three-dimensional structure of collagen.** Individual collagen polypeptide strands assume a left-handed, α-helical tertiary structure. They then associate to form a triple-stranded, right-handed superhelical quaternary structure characteristic of the collagen molecule. Collagen molecules associate in a staggered manner to form collagen fibrils that form a characteristic banding pattern. TEM, transmission electron microscopy.

Each collagen has one or more triple-helical domains, whose length can vary among collagen types. The mature forms of fibrillar collagens consist essentially of very long triple-helical regions, some more than 1000 amino acids, or about 300 nm, in length. Nonfibrillar collagens may contain less than 10% of their amino acids in the triple-helical structure.

Fibril-forming collagens

Fibrillar collagens provide tensile strength to tendons, ligaments, and skin

Type I is the most abundant fibrillar collagen and occurs in a wide variety of tissues, whereas other collagen types have a more limited tissue distribution (see Table 19.1). Type I and related fibrillar collagens form well-organized, banded fibrils and provide high tensile strength to the skin, tendons, and ligaments due to covalent bonding between collagen molecules. As indicated previously, collagens are trimers composed of three α-helical polypeptide chains (see Fig. 19.2). The type I collagen molecule is a heterotrimer being composed of two α1(I) polypeptide chains and one α2(I) polypeptide chain. Each of these polypeptide chains contains about 1000 amino acids and has a triple-helical domain structure along almost the entire length of the collagen molecule. The collagen fibrils are formed by the lateral association of triple helices in a "quarter-staggered" alignment, in which each collagen molecule is displaced by about one-quarter of its length relative to its nearest neighbor (Fig. 19.2). The **quarter-staggered array** is responsible for the banded appearance of collagen fibrils in connective tissues. The fibrils are stabilized by both noncovalent forces and interchain crosslinks derived from lysine residues.

Table 19.1 Members of the collagen family: Classification and distribution of different collagen types

Type	Class	Distribution
I	Fibrillar	Widely distributed, including skin, tendon, bone, heart, and ligaments (accounts for approximately 90% of all collagens)
II	Fibrillar	Cartilage, developing cornea, and vitreous humor
III	Fibrillar	Prominent in loose connective tissues and extensible tissues (e.g., skin, lung, uterus, and vascular system)
IV	Basement membrane forming	Basement membranes of epithelia, muscle, etc.
V	Fibrillar	Widely expressed in connective tissue of multiple organs, including liver, cornea, spleen, and others
VI	Basement membrane forming	Most connective tissues; particularly abundant immediately surrounding chondrocytes of cartilage
VII	Basement membrane forming	Present in anchoring fibrils of skin, uterus, esophagus, and other organs
VIII	Network forming	Blood vessels
IX	FACIT	Associated with collagen type II fibrils in cartilage
X	Network forming	Cartilage
XI	Fibril forming	Associated with type I and type II collagens in cartilage, bone, and placenta
XII	FACIT	Embryonic tendon and skin
XIII	Transmembrane	Widely distributed, including bone, cartilage, skin, intestine, striated muscle and others
XIV	FACIT	Fetal skin, placenta, and tendons
XV	Multiplexin (multiple triple helix domains and interruptions)	Heart and skeletal muscle
XVI	FACIT	Widely distributed; associated with fibroblasts and vascular smooth muscle cells
XVII	Transmembrane	Epithelia
XVIII	Multiplexin	Associated with epithelial and vascular basement membranes
XIX	FACIT	Blood vessels
XX	FACIT	Cornea, tendons, and cartilage
XXI	FACIT	Heart, skeletal muscle, and dense connective tissues
XXII	FACIT	Heart, skeletal muscle, articular cartilage, and skin
XXIII	Transmembrane	Heart, retina, and metastatic tumor cells
XXIV	Fibrillar	Embryonic eye and bone; associated with type I collagen fibrils
XXV	Transmembrane	Brain

FACIT, fibril-associated collagen with interrupted triple helices.

Nonfibrillar collagens

Nonfibrillar, lattice-forming collagens are major structural components of basement membranes

Nonfibrillar collagens are a heterogeneous group containing triple-helical segments of variable length, interrupted by one or more intervening nonhelical segments. This group includes basement membrane collagens (the type IV family), fibril-associated collagens with interrupted triple helices (FACIT), transmembrane collagens, and collagens with multiple triple-helical domains with interruptions, known as multiplexins.

Many of the nonfibrillar collagens associate with the fibrillar collagens, forming microfibrils and network, or mesh-like, structures. Type IV collagen assembles into a flexible mesh-like network in **basement membranes.** Basement membranes are relatively thin layers of ECM found on the basal aspect of epithelial cells and surrounding some other cell types, including myocytes, Schwann cells, and adipocytes. The basement membrane has a number of functions, including anchorage of cells to surrounding connective tissue and filtration. Collagen type IV contains a long triple-helical domain interrupted by short noncollagenous sequences. These interruptions in the

CLINICAL BOX
OSTEOGENESIS IMPERFECTA

A 6-year-old boy was seen in the emergency department with a broken tibia and fibula occurring during a soccer game. His 6-foot-tall father explained that he had broken his legs four times while at school. The father's teeth were slightly transparent and discolored.

Comment

Osteogenesis imperfecta (OI), also called brittle bone disease, is a congenital disease caused by multiple genetic defects in the synthesis of type I collagen. It is characterized by fragile bones, thin skin, abnormal teeth, and weak tendons. The majority of individuals with this disease have mutations in genes encoding α1(I) or α2(I) collagen polypeptides. Many of these mutations are single-base substitutions that convert glycine in the Gly-X-Y repeat to bulky amino acids, preventing the correct folding of the collagen polypeptide chains into a triple helix and their assembly into collagen fibrils. The dominance of type I collagen in bone explains why the bones are predominantly affected. However, there is remarkable clinical variability characterized by bone fragility, osteopenia, variable degrees of short stature, and progressive skeletal deformities. The most common form of OI - with a presentation that is sometimes mistaken for child abuse - has a good prognosis, with fractures decreasing after puberty, although the general reduction in bone mass means that lifetime risk remains high. Patients frequently develop deafness due to osteosclerosis, partly from recurrent fractures of the stapes. Bisphosphonate drugs, which inhibit osteoclast activity and thereby inhibit normal bone turnover, have reduced the incidence of fractures. Long-term follow-up studies are under way.

helical domain block continued association of two triple helices, oblige them to find another partner, and thus contribute to the formation of a lattice-type structure within the basement membrane. Anomalies in type IV collagen in the kidney basement membrane result in glomerular diseases, including **Goodpasture's syndrome**. This is a rare autoimmune disease caused by the production of antibodies that specifically bind to type IV collagen of basement membranes. The symptoms of this syndrome progress from blood in the urine (hematuria) to urine containing excessive protein (proteinuria) and eventually to kidney failure.

Synthesis and posttranslational modification of collagens

Collagen synthesis begins in the rough endoplasmic reticulum (RER)

The steps in the synthesis of most fibrillary collagens are similar and involve the constitutive secretory pathway used by cells. Collagen α chains are synthesized in the RER as long precursors, pro-α chains, or preprocollagen molecules, which then undergo extensive modifications in the Golgi apparatus and

extracellular space (Fig. 19.3). Preprocollagen is synthesized initially with a hydrophobic signal sequence that facilitates binding of ribosomes to the endoplasmic reticulum. Post-translational modification of the protein begins with removal of the signal peptide in the ER, yielding **procollagen.** Three different hydroxylases then add hydroxyl groups to proline and lysine residues, forming 3- and 4-**hydroxyprolines** and δ-**hydroxylysine.** These hydroxylases require ascorbate (vitamin C) as a cofactor (Fig. 19.3). Vitamin C deficiency leads to **scurvy** as a result of alterations in collagen synthesis and crosslinking.

O-linked glycosylation occurs by the addition of galactosyl residues to hydroxylysine by galactosyl transferase; a disaccharide is formed by the addition of glucose to galactosyl hydroxylysine by a glucosyl transferase (Fig. 19.3). These enzymes have strict substrate specificity for hydroxylysine or galactosyl hydroxylysine, and they glycosylate only those peptide sequences that are in noncollagenous domains. *N*-linked glycosylation also occurs on specific asparagine residues in nonfibrillar domains. The nonfibrillar collagens, with a greater extent of nonhelical domains, are more highly glycosylated than fibrillar collagens. Thus the extent of glycosylation may influence fibril structure, interrupting fibril formation and promoting the interchain interactions required for a meshwork structure. Intra- and interchain disulfide bonds are formed in the *C*-terminal domains by a protein disulfide isomerase, facilitating the association and folding of peptide chains into a triple helix (Fig. 19.3). At this stage, the **procollagen** is still soluble and contains additional nonhelical extensions at its *N*- and *C*-terminals.

Procollagen is finally modified to collagen in the Golgi apparatus

After assembly into a triple helix, procollagen is transported from the RER to the Golgi compartment, where it is packaged into secretory vesicles, then exported to the extracellular space by exocytosis. The nonhelical extensions of the procollagen are removed in the extracellular space by specific *N*- and *C*-terminal **procollagen proteinases** (Fig. 19.3). The collagen molecules (formerly called tropocollagen) then self-assemble into insoluble collagen fibrils, which are further stabilized by the formation of aldehyde-derived intermolecular crosslinks. **Lysyl oxidase** (not to be confused with the lysyl hydroxylase involved in the formation of hydroxylysine) oxidatively removes (deaminates) the ε-amino group of some lysine and hydroxylysine residues, producing reactive aldehyde derivatives known as **allysine and hydroxyallysine.** The aldehyde groups now form aldol condensation products with neighboring aldehyde groups, generating crosslinks both within and between triple-helical molecules. They may also react with the amino groups of unoxidized lysine and hydroxylysine residues to form Schiff base (imine) crosslinks (Fig. 19.4). The initial products may rearrange or be dehydrated or reduced to form stable crosslinks, such as **lysinonorleucine.** Studies with β-aminopropionitrile, which inhibits the enzyme lysyl oxidase, establish that collagen

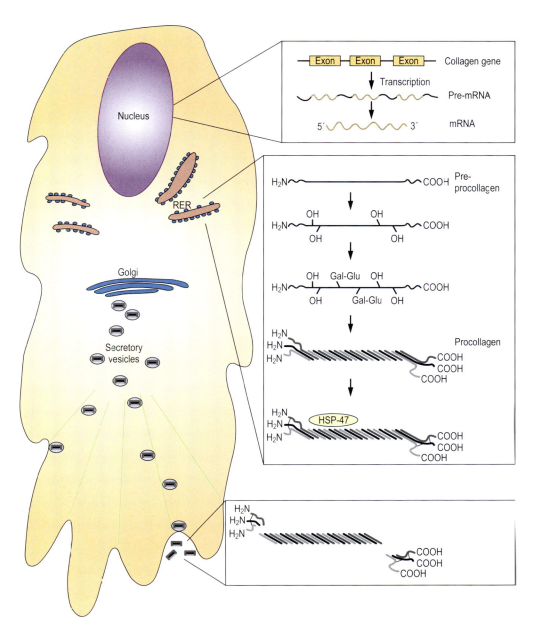

Fig. 19.3 **Biosynthesis and posttranslational processing of collagen.** The formation of collagen fibrils is a complex multistep process that begins with transcription of collagen α-chain mRNA in the nucleus. The collagen mRNA is transported to the cytoplasm, where it associates with the rough endoplasmic reticulum (RER). In the RER, translation of the polypeptides (termed pre-procollagens at this stage) occurs, which includes propeptides at the amino and carboxy termini. While in the RER, the polypeptides are modified by hydroxylation of specific proline and lysine amino acids (vitamin C–dependent), glycosylation by the addition of O- and N-linked oligosaccharides, and formation of intrachain and disulfide bonds in the N- and C-terminal regions. The α-chain polypeptides associate to form triple-stranded procollagen molecules, which are stabilized by interchain hydrogen bonds and association with chaperone proteins, such as heat shock protein 47 (HSP-47). The soluble procollagen molecules are transported to the Golgi complex, where they are packaged into secretory vesicles. The procollagen-containing secretory vesicles are transported to the cell surface, a process that is dependent on microtubules and associated motor proteins. This is followed by exocytosis of the procollagen molecules and subsequent cleavage of the N- and C-terminal, nonhelical propeptides by N- and C-terminal proteinases. The collagen molecules then self-assemble to form collagen fibrils, typically in "coves" on the cell surface. The fibrils are stabilized by the formation of covalent crosslinks, a process mediated by lysyl oxidase (not shown).

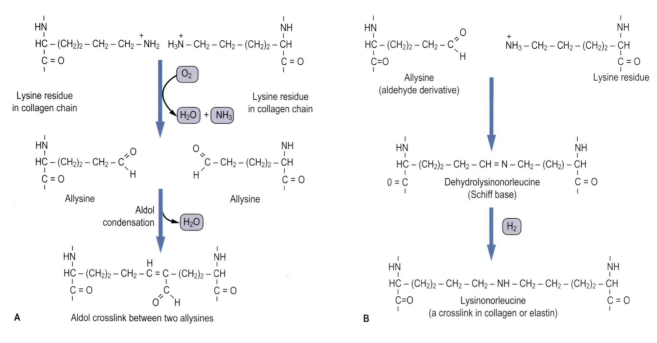

Fig. 19.4 **Collagen crosslink formation.** Allysine (and hydroxyallysine) are precursors of collagen crosslink formation by (A) aldol condensation and (B) Schiff base (imine) intermediates.

crosslink formation is a major determinant of tissue mechanical properties and strength. Inhibition of lysyl oxidase can result in **lathyrism,** a diet-induced disease characterized by deformation of the spine, dislocation of joints, demineralization of bones, aortic aneurysms, and joint hemorrhages. Lathyrism can be caused by chronic ingestion of the sweet pea *Lathyrus odoratus,* the seeds of which contain β-aminopropionitrile, an irreversible inhibitor of lysyl oxidase.

NONCOLLAGENOUS PROTEINS IN THE EXTRACELLULAR MATRIX

Elastin

Weak hydrophobic interactions between valine residues permit the flexibility and extensibility of elastin

The flexibility required for the function of blood vessels, lungs, ligaments, and skin is imparted by a network of elastic fibers in the ECM of these tissues. The predominant protein of elastic fibers is elastin. Unlike the multigene collagen family, there is only one gene for elastin, coding for a polypeptide about 750 amino acids long. In common with collagens, it is rich in glycine and proline residues, but elastin is more hydrophobic: one in seven of its amino acids is a valine. Unlike collagens, elastin contains little hydroxyproline and no hydroxylysine or carbohydrate chains, and it does not have a regular secondary

structure. Its primary structure consists of alternating hydrophilic and hydrophobic lysine and valine-rich domains. The lysines are involved in intermolecular crosslinking, whereas the weak interactions between valine residues in the hydrophobic domains impart elasticity to the molecule.

The soluble monomeric form of elastin initially synthesized on the RER is called tropoelastin. Except for some hydroxylation of proline, tropoelastin does not undergo posttranslational modification. During the assembly process in the extracellular space, lysyl oxidase generates allysine in specific sequences: -Lys-Ala-Ala-Lys- and -Lys-Ala-Ala-Ala-Lys- (Fig. 19.5). As with collagen, the reactive aldehyde of allysine condenses with other allysines or with unmodified lysines. Allysine and dehydrolysinonorleucine on different tropoelastin chains also condense to form pyridinium crosslinks - heterocyclic structures known as **desmosine** or **isodesmosine** (Fig. 19.5). Because of the way in which elastin monomers are crosslinked in polymers, elastin can stretch in two dimensions.

Other major ECM glycoproteins

Fibronectin and laminin have multiple binding sites for ECM proteins and proteoglycans

Fibronectin is a glycoprotein present as a structural component of the ECM and also in plasma as a soluble protein. Fibronectin is a dimer of two identical polypeptide subunits, each of 230 kDa, joined by a pair of disulfide bonds at their C-terminals.

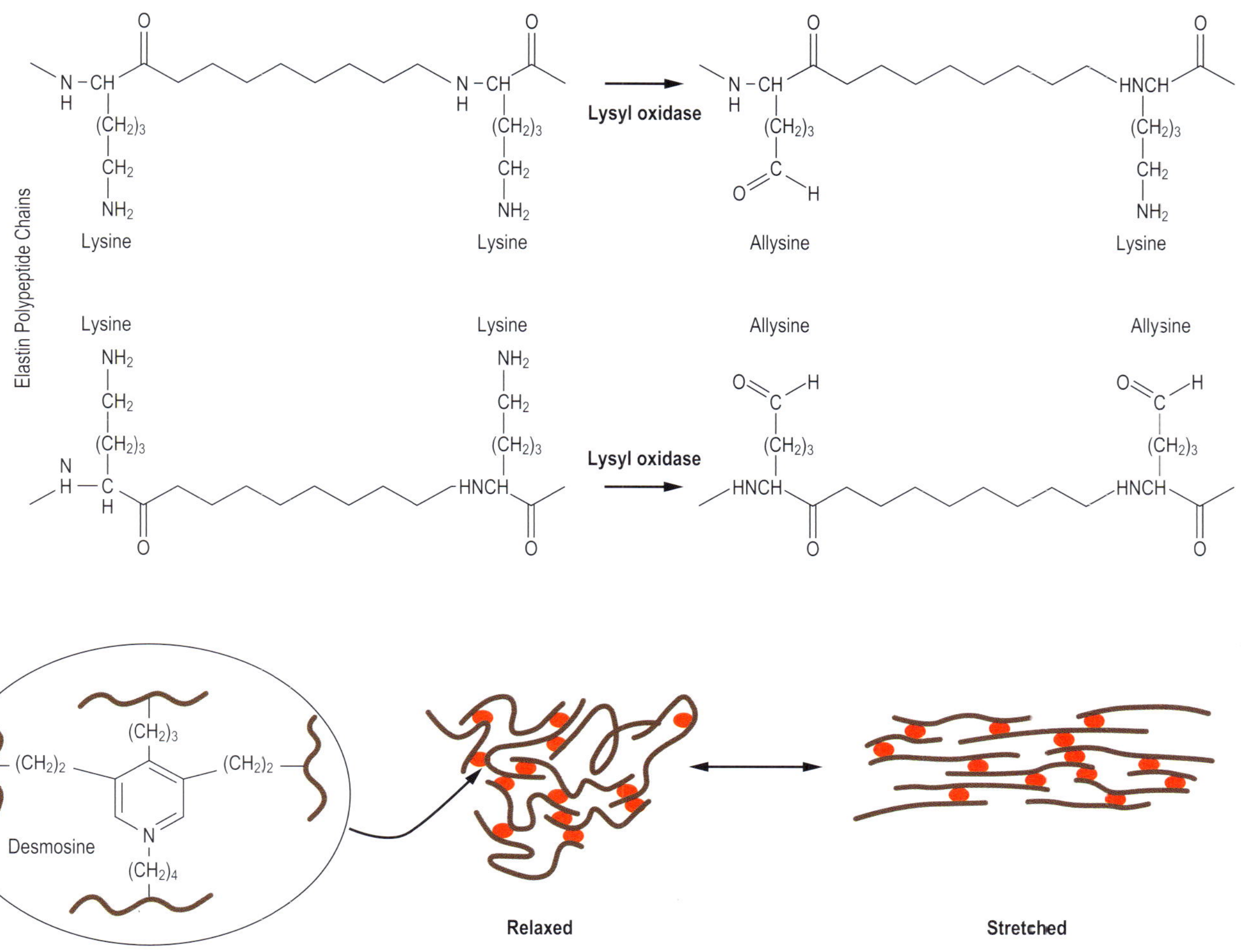

Fig. 19.5 **Desmosine - a multichain crosslink in elastin.** Allysine residue formation is mediated by lysyl oxidase. Allysine and dehydrolysinonorleucine residues in adjacent elastin chains react to form the three-dimensional elastic polymer, crosslinked by desmosine. These crosslinks between elastic fibers allow them to stretch and return to their original conformation when relaxed.

CLINICAL BOX
MARFAN'S SYNDROME: CAUSED BY MUTATIONS IN FIBRILLIN GENE

The ultrastructure of elastic fibers reveals elastin as an insoluble, polymeric, amorphous core covered with a sheath of microfibrils that contribute to the stability of the elastic fiber. The predominant constituent of microfibrils is the glycoprotein fibrillin. Marfan's syndrome is a relatively rare genetic disease of connective tissues caused by mutations in the fibrillin gene (frequency: 1 in 10,000 births). People with this disease have typically tall stature, long arms and legs, and arachnodactyly (long, "spidery" fingers). The disease in a mild form causes loose joints, deformed spine, floppy mitral valves (leading to cardiac regurgitation), and eye problems such as lens dislocation. In severely affected individuals, the aortic wall is prone to rupture because of defects in elastic fiber formation.

Each subunit is organized into multiple domains, known as type I, II, and III domains. Typically, 12 type I domains, two type II domains, and 15–17 type III domains organize to form a fibronectin polypeptide. The functionality of the fibronectin protein is determined by the binding affinity of specific domain sequences for other ECM components and the cell surface. The type I domains interact with fibrin, heparin (see below), and collagen; type II domains bind collagen; and type III domains are involved in binding to heparin and the cell surface. The specific interactions have been further mapped to short stretches of amino acids. For instance, a short peptide containing **Arg-Gly-Asp (RGD)**, present in the type III domain of fibronectin, binds to the integrin family of proteins present on cell surfaces. This sequence is not unique to fibronectin but is also found in other proteins in the ECM. At least 20 different tissue-specific isoforms of fibronectin have been identified, all produced by alternative splicing of a single precursor messenger ribonucleic acid (mRNA). The alternative splicing is regulated not only in

CLINICAL BOX
MUSCULAR DYSTROPHIES

Muscular dystrophies are a heterogeneous group of genetic disorders that result in a progressive decline in muscle strength and structure. To date, mutations have been identified in more than 30 genes that result in muscular dystrophies. Many of the identified gene products are components of the ECM–cell surface–cytoskeletal complex of muscle cells. In particular, one class of muscular dystrophy is caused by mutations in the α2 chain of laminin-2. These mutations prevent normal polymer formation of laminin-2 and result in abnormal basement membrane organization surrounding skeletal muscle fibers of patients with this muscular dystrophy.

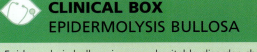

CLINICAL BOX
EPIDERMOLYSIS BULLOSA

Epidermolysis bullosa is a rare heritable disorder characterized by severe blistering of the skin and epithelial tissue. Three kinds are known:
- **Simplex:** blistering in the epidermis, caused by defects in keratin filaments
- **Junctional:** blistering in the dermal–epidermal junction, caused by defects in laminin
- **Dystrophic:** blistering in the dermis, caused by mutations in the gene encoding type VII collagen

Epidermolysis bullosa illustrates the multifactorial nature of connective tissue diseases that have similar clinical features.

a tissue-specific manner but also during embryogenesis, wound healing, and oncogenesis.

Laminins are a family of noncollagenous glycoproteins found in basement membranes and expressed in variant forms in different tissues. They are large (850 kDa) heterotrimeric molecules composed of α, β, and γ chains. To date, five α, four β, and three γ chains have been identified, which can associate to produce at least 15 different laminin variants. The three interacting chains in a heterotrimer are arranged in an asymmetric cruciform, or cross-shaped, molecule, held together by disulfide linkages. Laminins undergo reversible self-assembly in the presence of calcium to form polymers, contributing to the elaborate mesh-like network in the basement membrane. Like fibronectin, laminins interact with cells through multiple binding sites in several domains of the molecule. Laminin polymers are also connected to type IV collagen by a single-chain protein, **nidogen/entactin,** which has a binding site for collagen and, in common with fibronectin, also has an RGD sequence for integrin binding. Nidogen plays a central role in the formation of crosslinks between laminin and type IV collagen, generating a scaffold for anchoring of cells and ECM molecules in the basement membrane.

PROTEOGLYCANS

Proteoglycans are the gel-forming components of the ECM and comprise what has classically been called the "ground substance." They are composed of core proteins containing covalently bound sugars (glycosaminoglycans [GAGs]). The peptide chains of proteoglycans are usually more rigid and extended than the protein portion of glycoproteins, and the proteoglycans contain much larger amounts of carbohydrate - typically more than 95% carbohydrate. Proteoglycans have incredible diversity in the number of GAGs attached to their cores, ranging from 1 (decorin) to more than 200 (aggrecan).

Table 19.2 Structure and distribution of glycosaminoglycans

Glycosaminoglycan	Characteristic disaccharide	Sulfation	Tissue location
Hyaluronic acid	[4GlcUAβ1–3GlcNAcβ1]	None	Joint and ocular fluids
Chondroitin sulfates	[4GlcUAβ1–3GalNAcβ1]	GalNAc	Cartilage, tendons, bone, and heart valves
Dermatan sulfate	[4IdUAα1–3GalNAcβ1]	IdUA, GalNAc	Skin, heart valves, and blood vessels
Heparan sulfate	[4IdUAα1–4GlcNAcβ1]	GlcNAc	Cell surfaces and basement membranes
Heparin	[4IdUAα1–4GlcNAcβ1]	GlcNH₂, IdUA	Mast cells and basophils
Keratan sulfates	[3Galβ1–4GlcNAcβ1]	GlcNAc	Cartilage, cornea, and bone

GalNAc, N-acetylgalactosamine; GlcNH₂, glucosamine; GlcUA, D-glucuronic acid; IdUA, L-iduronic acid.

Structure of proteoglycans

Glycosaminoglycans are the polysaccharide components of proteoglycans

GAGs are linear, unbranched oligosaccharides that are much longer than those of glycoproteins and may contain more than 100 sugar residues in a linear chain. GAGs have a repeating disaccharide unit, usually composed of a uronic acid and an amino sugar (Table 19.2), and are polyanionic because of the many negative charges of the carboxyl groups of the uronic acids and from sulfate groups attached to some of the hydroxyl or amino groups of the sugars. The **disaccharide repeat** is different for each type of GAG but is usually composed of a hexosamine and a uronic acid residue, except in the case of keratan sulfate, in which the uronic acid is replaced by galactose. The amino sugar in GAGs is either glucosamine ($GlcNH_2$) or galactosamine ($GalNH_2$), both of which are present mostly in their N-acetylated forms (GlcNAc and GalNAc); however, in some of the GAGs (e.g., heparin, heparan sulfate), the amino group is sulfated rather than acetylated. The uronic acid is usually D-glucuronic acid (GlcUA), but in some cases (e.g., dermatan sulfate, heparin), it may be **L-iduronic acid (IdUA)**. With the exception of hyaluronic acid and keratan sulfate, all the GAGs are attached to protein by a core trisaccharide, Gal-Gal-Xyl; the xylose is linked to a serine or threonine residue of the core protein. Keratan sulfate is also attached to protein, but in that case, the linkage is through either an N-linked oligosaccharide (keratan sulfate I) or an O-linked oligosaccharide (keratan sulfate II). Hyaluronic acid, which has the longest polysaccharide chains, is the only GAG that is not attached to a core protein.

Synthesis and degradation of proteoglycans

The structure of glycosaminoglycans is determined by the cell's complement of glycosyl and sulfotransferases

Proteoglycans are synthesized by a series of glycosyl transferases, epimerases, and sulfotransferases, beginning with the synthesis of the **core trisaccharide (Xyl→Gal→Gal)** while the protein is still in the RER. Synthesis of the repeating oligosaccharide and other modifications take place in the Golgi apparatus. As with the synthesis of glycoproteins and glycolipids, separate enzymes are involved at each step. For example, there are separate galactosyl transferases for the two galactose units in the core, separate GlcUA transferases for the core and repeating disaccharides, and separate sulfotransferases for the C-4 and C-6 positions of the GalNAc residues of chondroitin sulfates. Phosphoadenosine phosphosulfate (PAPS) is the sulfate donor for the sulfotransferases. These pathways are illustrated in Fig. 19.6 for chondroitin-6-sulfate.

Defects of proteoglycan degradation lead to mucopolysaccharidoses

The degradation of proteoglycans occurs in lysosomes. The protein portion is degraded by lysosomal proteases, and the GAG chains are degraded by the sequential action of a number of different lysosomal acid hydrolases. The stepwise degradation of GAGs involves exoglycosidases and sulfatases, beginning from the external end of the glycan chain. This may involve the removal of sulfate by a sulfatase, then removal of the terminal sugar by a specific glycosidase, and so on. Fig. 19.7 shows the steps in the degradation of heparan sulfate. As with degradation of glycosphingolipids, if one of the enzymes involved in the stepwise pathway is missing, the entire

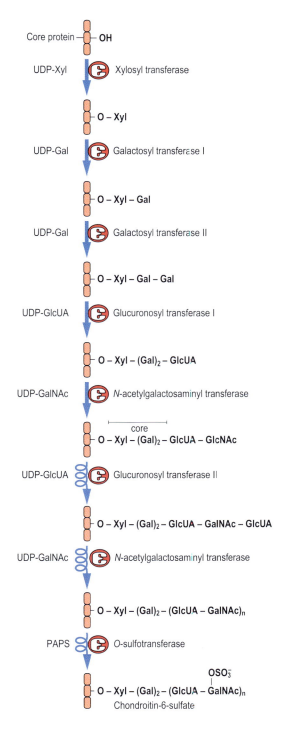

Fig. 19.6 **Synthesis of the proteoglycan chondroitin-6-sulfate.** Several enzymes participate in this pathway. Xyl, xylose.

degradation process is halted at that point, and the undegraded molecules accumulate in the lysosome. The lysosomal storage diseases resulting from the accumulation of GAGs are known as **mucopolysaccharidoses** (Table 19.3) because of the original designation of GAGs as mucopolysaccharides. There are more

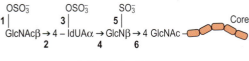

1. GlcNAc-6-sulfatase
2. Hexosaminidase
3. Iduronate sulfatase
4. Iduronidase
5. N-sulfatase
6. Glucosaminidase

Fig. 19.7 **Degradation of heparan sulfate.** This proceeds by a defined sequence of lysosomal hydrolase activities.

Table 19.3 Enzymatic defects characteristic of various mucopolysaccharidoses

Syndrome	Deficient enzyme	Product accumulated in lysosomes and secreted in urine
Hunter's	Iduronate sulfatase	Heparan and dermatan sulfate
Hurler's	α-Iduronidase	Heparan and dermatan sulfate
Morquio's A	Galactose-6-sulfatase	Keratan sulfate
Morquio's B	β-Galactosidase	Keratan sulfate
Sanfilippo's A	Heparan sulfamidase	Heparan sulfate
Sanfilippo's B	N-Acetylglucosaminidase	
Sanfilippo's C	N-Acetylglucosamine-6-sulfatase	

ADVANCED CONCEPT BOX
MECHANISMS OF THE ANTICOAGULANT EFFECT OF HEPARIN

Heparin is a heterogeneous (3000–30,000 kDa), polyanionic oligosaccharide activator of antithrombin III (AT). AT is a slow but quantitatively important inhibitor of thrombin (factor X) and other factors (IX, XI, XII) in the blood-clotting cascade (Chapter 41). When heparin binds to AT, it converts AT from a slow inhibitor to a rapid inhibitor of coagulating enzymes. Heparin interacts with a lysine residue in AT and induces a conformational change that promotes covalent binding of AT to the active serine centers of coagulating enzymes, forming a ternary complex and inhibiting procoagulant activity. Heparin then dissociates from the complex and can be recycled for anticoagulation.

The smallest, most active component of heparin is a pentasaccharide (GlcN-[N-sulfate-6-O-sulfate]-α1,4-GlcUA-β1,4-GlcN-[N-sulfate-3,6-di-O-sulfate]-α1,4-IdUA-[2-O-sulfate]-α-1,4-GlcN-[N-sulfate-6-O-sulfate]), which has a K_d of ~10 μM for binding to ATIII. Heparin has an average half-life of 30 min in the circulation, so it is commonly administered by infusion. Heparin does not have fibrinolytic activity; therefore it will not lyse existing clots. In addition to its anticoagulant activity, heparin also releases several enzymes from proteoglycan binding sites on the vascular wall, including lipoprotein lipase, which is often assayed as heparin-releasable plasma lipoprotein lipase activity or post-heparin lipase. Lipoprotein lipase is inducible by insulin, and decreased activity of this enzyme delays plasma clearance of chylomicrons and very low-density lipoprotein (VLDL), contributing to hypertriglyceridemia in diabetes.

than a dozen such mucopolysaccharidoses resulting from defects in degradation of GAGs. In general, these diseases can be diagnosed by the identification of specific GAG chains in the urine followed by assay of the specific hydrolases in leukocytes or fibroblasts.

Functions of the proteoglycans

One of the major roles of proteoglycans is to provide structural support to tissues, especially cartilage and connective tissue. In cartilage, large aggregates, composed of chondroitin sulfate and keratan sulfate chains linked to their core proteins, are noncovalently associated with hyaluronic acid via **link proteins,** forming a jelly-like matrix in which the collagen fibers are embedded. This macromolecule, a **"bottlebrush" structure** known as **aggrecan** (Fig. 19.8), provides both rigidity and stability to connective tissue. Because of their negative charge, the GAGs bind large amounts of monovalent and divalent cations: a cartilage proteoglycan molecule of 2 × 10^6 Da would have an aggregate negative charge of about 10,000. The maintenance of electrical neutrality consequently requires a high concentration of counter-ions. These ions draw water into the ECM, causing swelling and stiffening of the matrix, the result of tension between osmotic forces and binding interactions between proteoglycans and collagen. The structure and hydration of the ECM allow for a degree of rigidity, combined with flexibility and compressibility, enabling the tissue to withstand torsion and shock. The hyaluronic acid–proteoglycan–collagen aggregates in vertebral and articular disks have some of the viscoelastic properties of "silly putty" - bounce plus resilience - cushioning the impact between bones. These disks compress during the course of the day, expand elastically during the night, and deform gradually with age.

COMMUNICATION OF CELLS WITH THE EXTRACELLULAR MATRIX

Integrins are plasma membrane proteins that bind to and transmit mechanical signals between the ECM and intracellular proteins

Several cell surface receptors have been identified that mediate the interactions of cells with the ECM, including integrins, discoidin domain receptors, dystroglycan, and others. Of

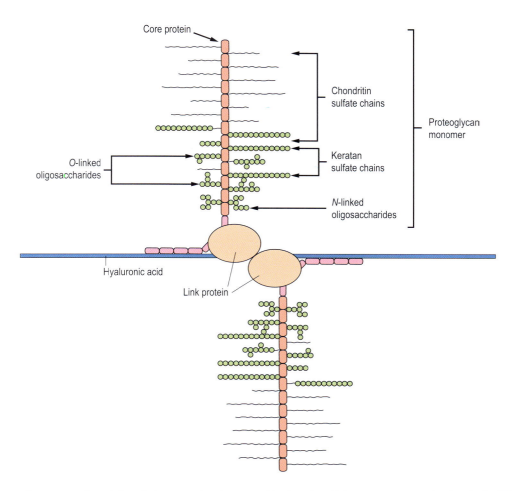

Fig. 19.8 **Structure of aggrecan.** Associations between proteoglycans and hyaluronic acid form an aggrecan structure in the ECM. The extension of this structure yields a three-dimensional array of proteoglycans bound to hyaluronic acid, which creates a stiff matrix, or "bottlebrush," structure in which collagen and other ECM components are embedded.

these, the **integrins** appear to be the most ubiquitous form of ECM receptors. Integrins are heterodimers of α and β chains that have been loosely grouped into subfamilies based on the component β chain. To date, 18 α and 8 β chains have been identified in mammals. Through various combinations of α and β chains, more than 20 different functional integrin heterodimers have been described. The specific combination of α and β chains dictates the specific ECM ligand for a particular integrin heterodimer. However, multiple integrin heterodimers can bind to some ECM components. For instance, $\alpha_4\beta_1$, $\alpha_5\beta_1$, and $\alpha_v\beta_3$ all interact with fibronectin through the RGD sequence. Adding to this complexity, several integrin heterodimers bind to multiple ECM components. For instance, $\alpha_v\beta_3$, which was originally described as a vitronectin receptor, can interact with not only vitronectin but also fibronectin, fibrinogen, and osteopontin.

In a functional integrin, both the α and β chains span the cell membrane (Fig. 19.9). Typically, each chain has a large extracellular domain, a single transmembrane domain, and a short cytoplasmic tail. The extracellular region of the integrin heterodimer interacts with ECM components in a divalent cation–dependent manner. The integrins are in an optimal position to transmit physical or mechanical signals from the ECM to the interior of the cell. These physical signals can be further distributed through the cell via the actin-containing cytoskeleton and ultimately modulate gene expression in the nucleus. Physical signals from the ECM can also be transduced into biochemical events in the cytoplasm of the cell via integrins. Unlike some other types of receptors, integrins do not themselves possess enzymatic activity. However, integrins associate with a number of cytoplasmic protein kinases, including focal adhesion kinase and Src. Activation of integrins initiates enzymatic cascades via these associated kinases, initiating changes in cell behavior and gene expression.

SUMMARY

■ The ECM contains a complex array of fibrillar and network-forming collagens, elastin fibers, a stiff

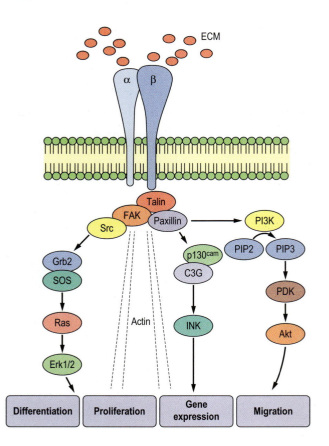

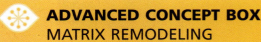

Fig. 19.9 **Organization of integrins.** The α and β chains span the cell membrane, interacting with the ECM outside the cell and the cytoskeleton and signaling molecules inside. In this manner, integrins can transduce signals from the ECM into biochemical and mechanical events in the cytoplasm that ultimately lead to alterations in cell morphology and function. The ovals contain abbreviations for components of the complex signaling cascade that conveys information from the integrin molecule to the nucleus of the cell.

ADVANCED CONCEPT BOX
MATRIX REMODELING

The ECM is in a constant state of synthesis and degradation, repair and remodeling - for example, during cell migration, morphogenesis and angiogenesis, and in response to inflammation and injury. ECM turnover is mediated primarily by a family of **matrix metalloproteinases (MMP)**, about 30 zinc endoproteinases with specificity for different components of the ECM. The MMP family includes collagenases, stromelysins, matrilysins, and elastases. These enzymes, with broad substrate specificities, catalyze the degradation of collagen, aggrecan, and accessory ECM proteins, such as fibronectin and laminin.

MMPs may be integral plasma membrane proteins, bound to the plasma membrane by a glycosylphosphatidylinositol (GPI) glycan anchor (see Fig. 18.7), or secreted into the extracellular space. They exist as zymogens until activated locally by proteolytic cleavage in response to cellular signals or extracellular enzymes, such as thrombin and plasmin, activated during blood clotting and fibrinolysis. As with the cascade of protease reactions involved in blood coagulation, there are also tissue inhibitors of MMPs, known as TIMPs, a family of four proteins that inactivate MMPs and limit the spread of damage. The balance between the activation and inhibition of MMPs is critical to the integrity and function of the ECM; alterations in MMP activity are associated with skeletal dysplasias, coronary artery disease, arthritis, and metastasis.

ADVANCED CONCEPT BOX
EXTRACELLULAR MATRIX AND TISSUE ENGINEERING

Over the past decade, the interest in producing replacement tissues through tissue engineering has grown considerably. The ultimate goal of tissue engineering is to combine appropriate cells and biomaterials to produce tissue equivalents that mimic normal tissues and organs and can replace damaged or diseased tissues. Because the biological and mechanical properties of tissues are determined in part by the heterogeneous composition and organization of the ECM, the successful generation of tissue equivalents will require the development of appropriate three-dimensional ECM scaffolds.

An attractive therapeutic approach is to combine undifferentiated stem cells with appropriate scaffolds and biochemical factors to promote differentiation of the cells along particular lines, depending on the specific replacement tissue desired. Properties of the ECM scaffold - including ECM composition, porosity, and mechanical properties - have important effects on stem cell differentiation. Culture of mesenchymal stem cells in scaffolds of relatively high stiffness tends to promote the formation of bone-like tissue and the formation of osteoblasts, whereas culture of the same stem cells in less stiff scaffolds results in the formation of cartilage cells or chondroblasts. These and other studies illustrate that physical and mechanical cues from the ECM are important in regulating the differentiation of stem cells. Advances in tissue engineering and production of replacement tissues will require a thorough understanding of the normal and pathologic ECM.

ACTIVE LEARNING

1. Discuss the characteristics and roles of the major families of collagen proteins.
2. Compare the structure of heparin, its mechanism of action, and its route and frequency of administration to that of other common anticoagulants, such as aspirin and coumarin derivatives.
3. Review the consequences of genetic defects in the sulfation of proteoglycans.
4. Discuss biomimetic ECM materials as investigational tools and as therapeutic devices.

gelatinous matrix of proteoglycans, and a number of glycoproteins that mediate the interaction of these molecules with one another and with the cell surface.

▪ The heterogeneity of both the protein and the carbohydrate components of the ECM provides for great diversity in the structure and function of the ECM in various tissues.

▪ Interactions between ECM components afford structure, stability, and elasticity to the ECM and provide a route for communication between the intra- and extracellular environments in tissues.

FURTHER READING

Couchman, J. R., & Pataki, C. A. (2012). An introduction to proteoglycans and their localization. *Journal of Histochemistry and Cytochemistry*, 60, 885–897.

Curry, A. S., Pensa, N. W., Barlow, A. M., et al. (2016). Takings cues from the extracellular matrix to design bone-mimetic regenerative scaffolds. *Matrix Biology*, 52–54, 397–412.

Gaggar, A., & Weathington, N. (2016). Bioactive extracellular matrix fragments in lung health and disease. *Journal of Clinical Investigation*, 126, 3176–3184.

Ghatak, S., Maytin, E. V., Mack, J. A., et al. (2015). Roles of proteoglycans and glycosaminoglycans in wound healing and fibrosis. *International Journal of Cell Biology*, 2015, 834893.

Ingber, D. E. (2008). Tensegrity-based mechanosensing from macro to micro. *Progress in Biophysics and Molecular Biology*, 97, 163–179.

Mittal, R., Patel, A. P., Debs, L. H., et al. (2016). Intricate functions of matrix metalloproteinases in physiological and pathological conditions. *Journal of Cell Physiology*, 231, 2599–2621.

Prydz, K. (2015). Determinants of glycosaminoglycan (GAG) structure. *Biomolecules*, 5, 2003–2022.

Theocharis, A. D., Skandalis, S. S., Gialeli, C., et al. (2016). Extracellular matrix structure. *Advanced Drug Delivery Reviews*, 97, 4–27.

Triggs-Raine, B., & Natowicz, M. R. (2015). Biology of hyaluronan: Insights from genetic disorders of hyaluronan metabolism. *Word Journal of Biological Chemistry*, 26, 110–120.

Wraith, J. E. (2013). Mucopolysaccharidoses and mucolipidosis. *Handbook of Clinical Neurology*, 113, 1723–1729.

Yamauchi, M., & Sricholpech, M. (2012). Lysine post-translational modifications of collagen. *Essays in Biochemistry*, 52, 113–133.

Yigit, S., Dinjaski, N., & Kaplan, D. L. (2016). Fibrous proteins: At the crossroads of genetic engineering and biotechnological applications. *Biotechnology and Bioengineering*, 113, 913–929.

RELEVANT WEBSITES

The extracellular matrix: http://themedicalbiochemistrypage.org/extracellularmatrix.php

Ehlers–Danlos syndrome: https://rarediseases.org/rare-diseases/ehlers-danlos-syndrome/

Marfan's syndrome: https://rarediseases.org/rare-diseases/marfan-syndrome/

Mucopolysaccharidoses:
 https://rarediseases.org/rare-diseases/mucopolysaccharidoses/
 https://www.orpha.net/data/patho/Pub/en/Mucopolysaccharidoses_En_2013.pdf

Scurvy: http://www.bbc.co.uk/history/british/empire_seapower/captaincook_scurvy_01.shtml

ABBREVIATIONS

ECM	Extracellular matrix
GAG	Glycosaminoglycan
IdUA	Iduronic acid
MMP	Matrix metalloproteinase
OI	Osteogenesis imperfecta
RER	Rough endoplasmic reticulum
RGD	Arg-gly-asp recognition sequence
TIMP	Tissue inhibitor of MMPs

Deoxyribonucleic Acid

Alejandro Gugliucci, Robert W. Thornburg, and Teresita Menini

LEARNING OBJECTIVES

After reading this chapter, you should be able to:

- Describe the composition and structure of DNA based on the Watson–Crick model, including the concepts of directionality and complementarity in DNA structure.
- Describe the packaging of DNA in the nucleus.
- Explain how replication of DNA is achieved with high fidelity.
- Discuss the enzymes involved, the activities at replication forks, and the structures and intermediates participating in the replication process.
- Outline the mechanism by which replication is controlled in the eukaryotic cell.
- Describe the types of damage to DNA and the mechanisms involved in DNA repair.
- Describe the mechanism of action of antiretroviral therapy for treatment of AIDS.
- Describe the principles of hybridization and Southern and Northern blotting.
- Describe several applications of DNA cloning and recombinant DNA technology.
- Define RFLP and SNPs, and explain their use.

INTRODUCTION

Cellular nucleic acids exist in two forms, deoxyribonucleic acid (DNA) and ribonucleic acid (RNA). Approximately 90% of the nucleic acid within cells is RNA, and the remainder is DNA, which is the repository of genetic information. This chapter will first examine the structure of DNA, the manner in which it is stored in chromosomes in the nucleus, and the mechanisms involved in its biosynthesis and repair. We will then explore DNA recombinant technology, which allowed for the current flurry of applications in research, clinical medicine, and forensics.

STRUCTURE OF DEOXYRIBONUCLEIC ACID

DNA is an antiparallel dimer of nucleic acid strands

DNA is composed of nucleotides containing the sugar deoxyribose. Deoxyribose is missing the hydroxyl group at the 2'-position of ribose. The chains of DNA are polymerized through a phosphodiester linkage from the 3'-hydroxyl of one ribose to the 5'-hydroxyl of the next ribose (Fig. 20.1A). Thus DNA is a duplex linear polymer of deoxyribose 3',5'-phosphate, with purine and pyrimidine bases attached to carbon-1' of the deoxyribose subunit.

Using base composition determined by Chargaff as well as X-ray diffraction photographs of DNA taken by Rosalind Franklin, James Watson and Francis Crick proposed a structure for DNA in 1953. This model proposed that DNA was composed of **two intertwined complementary strands**, with hydrogen bonds holding the strands together (Fig. 20.1B). The basic simplicity of this structure was consistent with the observation by Chargaff that in all DNA, the molar content of A is equal to that of T, and the molar content of G is equal to that of C. Although some of the details of the model have been modified, the Watson–Crick hypothesis was rapidly accepted, and its essential elements have remained unchanged since originally proposed.

Watson and Crick model of DNA

As originally presented by Watson and Crick, DNA is composed of two strands, wound around each other in a right-handed, helical structure, with the base pairs in the middle and the deoxyribosyl phosphate chains on the outside. The orientation of the DNA strands is **antiparallel** - that is, the strands run in opposite directions. The nucleotide bases on each strand interact with the nucleotide bases on the other strand to form base pairs (Fig. 20.2). The base pairs are planar and are oriented nearly perpendicular to the axis of the helix. Each base pair is held together by hydrogen bonding between a purine and a pyrimidine. Consistent with this pairing and the predominant tautomeric forms of the nitrogen bases, guanine forms three hydrogen bonds with cytosine, and adenine forms two with thymine. Because of the specificity of this interaction between purines and pyrimidines on the opposite strands, the opposing strands of DNA are said to have complementary structures. The composite strength of the numerous hydrogen bonds formed between the bases of the opposite strands and the hydrophobic interactions and Van der Waals forces acting among the stacking bases is responsible for the extreme stability of the DNA double helix. The hydrogen bonds between strands are affected by temperature and ionic strength, and stable complementary structures can be formed at room temperature with as few as six to eight nucleotides.

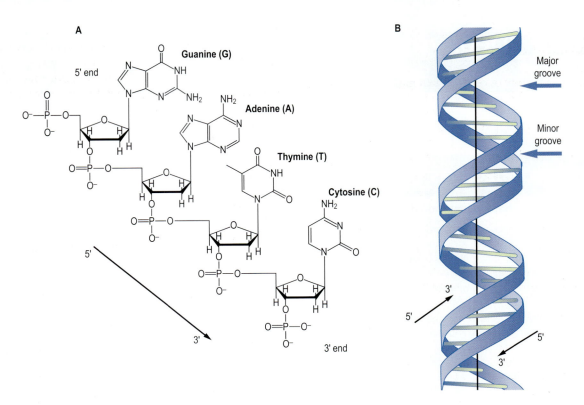

Fig. 20.1 **Structure of DNA.** (A) A tetranucleotide sequence of DNA showing each of the nucleotides normally found in DNA. The deoxyribose sugars are missing the 2′-hydroxyl that is present in the ribose sugars found in RNA. By convention, DNA is read from the 5′ to 3′ end, so the sequence of this tetranucleotide is 5′-GATC-3′. (B) A graphic representation of the structure of B-DNA, the major form of DNA in the cell. The base pairs in the middle are aligned nearly perpendicular to the helical axis. The major groove and the minor groove are shown. Note that the strands are antiparallel.

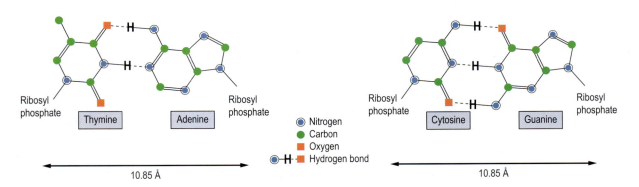

Fig. 20.2 **Watson–Crick base pairing of nucleotides in DNA.** The AT base pairs form two hydrogen bonds, and the GC base pairs form three hydrogen bonds. Thus GC-rich regions are more stable than AT-rich regions.

Three-dimensional DNA

The three-dimensional structure of the DNA **double helix** is such that the deoxyribosyl phosphate backbones of the two strands are slightly offset from the center of the helix. Because of this, the grooves between the two strands are of different sizes. These grooves are termed the major groove and the minor groove (see Fig. 20.1B). The major groove is more open and exposes the nucleotide base pairs. The minor groove is more constricted, being partially blocked by the deoxyribosyl moieties linking the base pairs. Binding of proteins to DNA occurs mostly in the major groove and is specific for the nucleotide sequence of DNA. This binding is very specific and is the key interaction that regulates DNA function; it determines which genes will be expressed, as the proteins involved are transcription factors.

Alternative forms of DNA may help to regulate gene expression

Although the majority of cellular DNA molecules exist in the B-form described, alternative forms of DNA (at least six) also exist. When the relative humidity of B-form DNA falls to less than 75%, the B-form undergoes a reversible transition into the A-form of DNA. In the A-form, the nucleotide base pairs are tilted 20° relative to the helical axis, and the helix diameter is increased compared with the B-form (Fig. 20.3). The A-form is observed in vivo when the DNA strands contain tracks of polypurine (and complementary polypyrimidine) residues. These regions do not efficiently bind histones and are therefore unable to form nucleosomes (see below), resulting in nucleosome-free (exposed) regions of DNA.

In Z-DNA, which forms when the sequence of DNA consists of alternating purine/pyrimidine stretches, the base pairs flip 180° relative to the sugar nucleotide bond. This results in a novel conformation of the base pairs relative to sugar phosphate backbones, yielding a form of DNA with a zigzag configuration (hence the name Z-DNA) along the sugar–phosphate backbone. Surprisingly, this change in conformation leads to the formation of a left-handed DNA helix. The Z-DNA form is favored at high ionic concentrations in vitro, but it is also induced at normal ionic concentrations by methylation of cytosine residues, a form of **epigenetic modification** of DNA (Chapter 23). Protein-binding interactions with these alternative forms of DNA, which are widely distributed in the genome, are involved in the regulation of gene expression.

The digital linear code (base pairing) in the DNA double helix has a significant component that acts by altering, along its length, the shape and stiffness of the molecule. In this way, one region of DNA is structurally differentiated from another, which provides another level of encoded information in three-dimensional space. These local shape and stiffness variations permit superhelical structures and three-dimensional spatial interactions in DNA. The superhelical density behaves as an analog regulatory mode as opposed to the more frequently accepted purely digital information content.

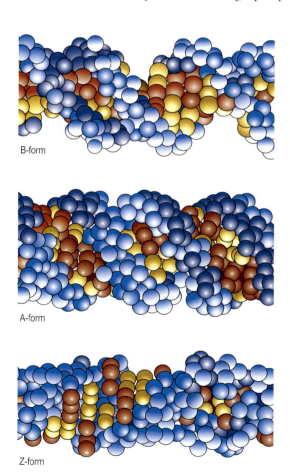

Fig. 20.3 **The structures of different forms of DNA include the B-, A-, and Z-forms.** The sugar–phosphate backbone of the DNA strands is colored blue. The nucleotide bases forming the internal base pairs are yellow for pyrimidines (thymine and cytosine) and red for purines (adenine and guanine).

Separated DNA strands can reassociate to form duplex DNA

Complementary strands of DNA spontaneously hybridize to form helical structures

Because the DNA strands are complementary and are held together only by noncovalent forces, they can be separated into individual strands. This strand separation, denaturation, or melting of DNA is commonly induced by heating the solution. The dissociation is reversible, and on cooling, the complementary nucleotide sequences reanneal to reform their original base pairs. Because adenine and thymine interact through two hydrogen bonds and guanine and cytosine through three (see Fig. 20.2), AT-rich regions melt at lower temperatures than GC-rich regions in DNA. The denaturation of DNA can also be induced locally by enzymes or DNA-binding proteins. The promoter region of DNA contains a TATA sequence (the TATA box), an easily melted region of DNA that facilitates the unwinding of DNA during the early stages of gene expression (Chapter 23).

The human genome

The human genome contains 20,000–25,000 different protein coding genes spread over 23 chromosome pairs.

Genes are unique DNA sequences that code for proteins and are present in single copies or at most only a few copies per genome. There are also several types of repeated DNA sequences within the genome. These are divided into two major classes: middle repetitive (<10 copies per genome) and highly repetitive (>10 copies per genome).

Some middle-repetitive DNA consists of genes that specify transfer and ribosomal ribonucleic acids, which are involved in protein synthesis (Chapter 22), and histone proteins that are part of the nucleosome (see the following discussion). Other middle-repetitive DNA sequences have no known useful function but may participate in DNA strand association and chromosomal rearrangements during meiosis. The best-characterized highly repetitive sequence in humans is known as the Alu sequence. Between 300,000 and 500,000 Alu I repeats of about 300 base pairs are scattered throughout the human genome, comprising 3%–6% of the total DNA. Individual repeats of the Alu sequence may vary by 10%–20% in identity. Similar sequences are found in other mammals and in lower eukaryotes.

Satellite DNA

Satellite DNA was originally identified as a subfraction of DNA with a buoyant density slightly lower than that of genomic DNA because of its higher content of AT base pairs. It consists of clusters of short, species-specific, nearly identical sequences that are repeated in tandem hundreds of thousands of times. These clusters lack protein-coding genes and are mainly found near the centromeres of chromosomes, suggesting that they may function to align the chromosomes during cell division to facilitate recombination. Because these repetitive sequences cover long stretches of chromosomes (hundreds to thousands of kilobase pairs; kbp), determining the sequence of satellite DNA and sequencing the centromere region of DNA are major challenges to completing the noncoding sequence of eukaryotic genomes.

Mitochondrial DNA

The nucleus of eukaryotic cells contains the majority of the DNA in the cell - genomic DNA. However, DNA is also found in mitochondria and in plant chloroplasts, which is consistent with **endosymbiont theories** for the origins of these cellular organelles - namely, that they are parasites that adapted to intracellular life by symbiosis.

The mitochondrial genome is small in size, is circular, and encodes relatively few proteins

In humans, the mitochondrial genome encodes 22 tRNAs, 2 rRNAs, and 13 mitochondrial proteins that are involved in the respiratory apparatus, including subunits of NADH dehydrogenase, cytochrome *b*, cytochrome oxidase, and ATPase.

The remaining proteins that are found in mitochondria (about 1000) are produced from nuclear genes, synthesized in the cytoplasm on "free" ribosomes (Chapter 22), then imported into the mitochondrion. This import process requires a special *N*-terminal **mitochondrial-import sequence** of about 25 amino acids in length that forms an amphipathic helix that interacts with transporter and chaperone proteins in the inner and outer mitochondrial membrane and matrix. Those few proteins that are encoded by the mitochondrial genome are synthesized in the mitochondrion, using machinery similar that used in the cytoplasm for the synthesis of non-mitochondrial proteins.

DNA is compacted into chromosomes

Chromosomes are compact, highly organized forms of DNA

In eukaryotes, nuclear DNA is arranged in superstructures termed chromosomes. Each chromosome contains between 48 million and 240 million base pairs. The B-form of DNA has a length of 3.4 Å per base pair. Therefore chromosomes have lengths of 1.6–8.2 cm, which is much longer than a cell. To fit into the nucleus, DNA is condensed almost 10,000-fold into an organized structure. Interactions between DNA and cations - such as Na^+, Mg^{2+}, and the polyamines such as **spermine** and **spermidine** - play an important role in the physical properties and biological function of DNA. Even in dilute solutions, approximately three out of four DNA charges are neutralized by a cation that is in some sense "bound." This neutralization facilitates compaction of DNA into densely packaged chromatin and deformation of DNA by proteins.

Chromatin contains DNA, RNA, and protein, plus inorganic and organic counterions

In the native chromosome, DNA is complexed with RNA and an approximately equal mass of protein. These DNA–RNA–protein complexes are termed chromatin. The majority of the proteins in chromatin are histones. Histones are a highly conserved family of proteins that are involved in the packing and folding of DNA within the nucleus. There are five classes of histones, termed H1, H2A, H2B, H3, and H4. They are all rich (>20%) in positively charged, basic amino acids (lysine and arginine). These positive charges interact with the negatively charged, acidic phosphate groups of the DNA strands to reduce electrostatic repulsion and permit tighter DNA packing.

Nucleosomes are the building blocks of chromatin

The histone proteins associate into a complex termed a nucleosome (Fig. 20.4). Each of these complexes contains two molecules each of H2A, H2B, H3, and H4 and one molecule of H1. The nucleosome protein complex is encircled with about 200 base pairs of DNA that form two coils around the nucleosome core. The H1 protein associates with the outside of the nucleosome core to stabilize the complex. By forming nucleosomes, the packing density of DNA is increased about sevenfold.

The **nucleosomes** are also organized into other, more tightly packed structures, termed 300-Å chromatin filaments. These filaments are constructed by winding the nucleosome particles into a spring-shaped solenoid structure with about six nucleosomes per turn (see Fig. 20.4). The solenoid is stabilized by head-to-tail associations of the H1 histones. Finally, the chromatin filaments are compacted into the mature chromosome using a nuclear scaffold. The scaffold is about 400 nm in diameter and forms the core of the chromosome. The filaments are dispersed around the scaffold to form radial loops

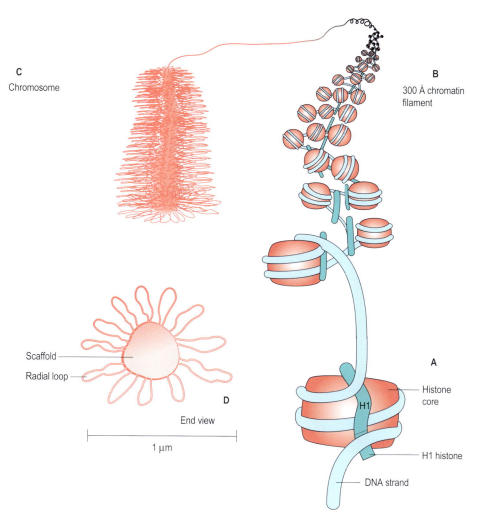

C
Chromosome

B
300 Å chromatin filament

Scaffold
Radial loop

D
End view
1 µm

A
H1
Histone core
H1 histone
DNA strand

Fig. 20.4 **Structures involved in chromosome packaging.** (A) The nucleosome core is composed of two subunits each of H2A, H2B, H3, and H4. The core is twice wrapped with DNA, and the H1 histone binds to the completed complex. (B) The 300-Å chromatin filament is formed by wrapping the nucleosomes into a spring-shaped solenoid. (C) The chromosome is composed of the 300-Å filaments, which bind to a nuclear scaffold, forming large loops of chromatin material. (D) The end view of a chromosome shows the central nuclear scaffold surrounded by the radial loops of chromatin. The diameter of a chromosome is about 1 µm.

about 300 nm in length. The final diameter of a chromosome is about 1 µm, compared to the 1.6–8.4 cm length of the DNA.

Telomeres

Telomeres are nucleoprotein complexes that cap the 3' ends of the eukaryotic chromosomes. They are essential for cell viability. These structures consist of tandem repeats of short, G-rich, species-specific oligonucleotides. In humans, the repeated sequence is TTAGGG. Telomeres can contain as many as 1000 copies of this sequence. During the synthesis of telomeres, the enzyme **telomerase,** a ribonucleoprotein complex, adds preformed hexanucleotide repeats to the 3' end of the chromosome, using the telomere RNA as a template; there is no requirement for a DNA template. In human somatic cells, telomeric DNA shortens in each cell division until it cannot exercise its end-protective functions (e.g., avoiding recognition of chromosome tips as double-stranded breaks). The shortening of telomeres after many cell replications has been linked to the development of cellular senescence. If telomeres turn out to be dysfunctional as a result of disproportionate shortening or defects in their intrinsic proteins, they trigger pathways that restrict cell proliferation. Telomere-based chromosome instability has been proposed as one driving force in oncogenesis.

THE CELL CYCLE IN EUKARYOTES

Fig. 20.5 shows the various phases of the growth and division of eukaryotic cells, known as the cell cycle. The G_1 (growth) phase is a period of cell growth that occurs before DNA replication. The phase during which DNA is synthesized or replicated is termed the S (synthesis) phase. A second growth phase, termed G_2 (gap), occurs after DNA replication but before cell division. The mitosis, or M, phase is the period of cell division. After mitosis, the daughter cells either reenter the G_1 phase or enter a quiescent phase termed G_0, when growth and replication cease. The passage of cells through the cell cycle is tightly

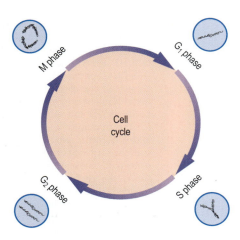

Fig. 20.5 **Stages of the cell cycle.** G_1 and G_2 are growth phases that occur before and after DNA synthesis, respectively. DNA replication occurs during the S phase. Mitosis occurs during the M phase, producing new daughter cells that can reenter the G_1 phase (compare Fig. 29.1).

ADVANCED CONCEPT BOX
DIFFERENCES BETWEEN VIRAL, BACTERIAL, AND EUKARYOTIC DNA

Although the essential constituents of DNA are the same along the tree of life, there are significant differences in the way it is organized, stored, and located between viruses, bacteria, and eukaryotes. Viral DNA (there are RNA and DNA viruses) is usually double stranded but may also be single stranded. It is usually protected and surrounded by lipid and protein, with no known regulatory role except the essential purpose of transferring to a bacterial or eukaryotic host. Bacterial DNA is not separated from the rest of the cells as it is in eukaryotes. Histone-like binding proteins are present in many bacteria, where they play an architectural role but do not form nucleosomes. Bacteria also have circular DNAs called plasmids that can replicate outside the host genome. Transfer of plasmids is one mechanism that bacteria use to develop antibiotic resistance; plasmids are also key tools of molecular biology (discussed later in the chapter). Eukaryotic DNA is for the most part secluded in the nucleus of cells, where it constitutes 10% of the nuclear mass in the form of nucleosomes and chromosomes.

controlled by a variety of proteins termed cyclin-dependent kinases (see Chapter 28).

DNA REPLICATION

DNA is replicated by separating and copying the strands

For cells to divide, their DNA must be duplicated during the S phase of the cell cycle. The structure of the DNA double helix and its complementarity suggested the mechanism for DNA replication - strand separation followed by strand copying. The separated parent strands serve as templates for the synthesis of the new daughter strands. This method of DNA replication is described as **semiconservative**; each replicated duplex daughter DNA molecule contains one parental strand and one newly synthesized strand.

DNA replication

The site at which DNA replication is initiated is termed the **origin of replication**.

In prokaryotes, a DNA-binding protein termed DnaA binds to repeated nucleotide sequences located within the origin. Binding of 20–30 DnaA molecules to the origin of replication induces unwinding, which separates the strands in an AT-rich region adjacent to the DnaA-binding sites. Next, the hexameric protein DnaB binds to the separated DNA strands. DnaB has **helicase** activity that catalyzes ATP-mediated unwinding of the DNA helix. DNA **gyrase** also participates in separation of the strands. As this complex continues unwinding the DNA strands in both directions from the origin of replication, single-stranded DNA-binding proteins coat the separated strands to inhibit their reassociation.

Once the strands are sufficiently separated, another protein, termed DNA **primase,** is added, resulting in the formation of

a **primosome complex** at the **replication fork.** The primosome synthesizes short ($n \leq 10$) RNA oligonucleotides complementary to each parental DNA strand. These oligonucleotides serve as primers for DNA synthesis. Once each RNA primer has been laid down, two **DNA polymerase III** complexes are assembled, one at each of the primed sites. In addition to its polymerase activity, one of the subunits of DNA polymerase III has a **proofreading** exonuclease activity, which corrects mismatches and assures fidelity in replication of DNA.

DNA synthesis proceeds in opposite directions along the leading and lagging strands of the template DNA

Because of the unidirectional 5′-to-3′ synthetic activity of the polymerase and the antiparallel nature of the two strands, the synthesis of DNA along the two strands is different (Fig. 20.6). The two daughter strands being synthesized are termed the leading strand and the lagging strand. DNA synthesis proceeds along the leading strand in a 5′-to-3′ direction, producing a single, long, continuous strand. However, because DNA synthesis adds new nucleotides only at the 3′ end of the elongating DNA strand, DNA polymerase III cannot synthesize the lagging strand in one long continuous piece as it does for the leading strand. Instead, the lagging strand is synthesized in small fragments, 1000–5000 base pairs in length, termed **Okazaki fragments** (see Fig. 20.6). The primosome remains associated with the lagging strand and continues periodically to synthesize RNA primers complementary to the separated strand. As DNA polymerase III moves along the parental DNA strand, it initiates the synthesis of Okazaki fragments at the RNA primers, elongating different fragments from each primer.

proceeds along a DNA template. During DNA replication, DNA polymerase I removes the RNA primer and replaces it with DNA. Finally, DNA **ligase** joins the lagging-strand DNA fragments to form a continuous strand.

Eukaryotes stringently regulate DNA replication

Eukaryotic DNA synthesis is remarkably similar to prokaryotic DNA synthesis. However, eukaryotes have many more origins of replication. These are activated simultaneously during the S phase of the cell cycle, permitting rapid replication of the entire chromosome. To ensure that excess amounts of unfinished, replicating DNA do not accumulate, cells use a protein termed **licensing factor** that is present in the nucleus before replication. After each round of replication, this factor is inactivated or destroyed, preventing further replication until more licensing factor is synthesized later in the cell cycle.

DNA REPAIR

There are typically more than 10,000 modifications of DNA per cell per day

Because DNA is the reservoir of genetic information within the cell, it is extremely important to maintain the integrity of DNA. Therefore the cell has developed multiple highly efficient mechanisms for the repair of modified or damaged DNA.

DNA can be damaged by numerous types of endogenous and exogenous agents that cause nucleotide modifications, deletions, insertions, sequence inversions, and transpositions. Some of this damage is secondary to chemical modification of DNA by alkylating agents (including many carcinogens), reactive oxygen species (Chapter 42), and ionizing radiation (ultraviolet or radioactive). Both the sugar and bases of DNA are subject to modification, yielding an estimated 10,000 to 100,000 modifications of DNA per cell per day. The nature of this damage is quite variable, including modification of single bases, single- or double-strand breaks, and crosslinking between bases or bases and proteins. Oxidative damage is probably the most common form of DNA damage; it is increased in inflammation, by smoking, and in aging and age-related diseases, including atherosclerosis, diabetes, and neurodegenerative diseases (Chapter 29). If not repaired, the accumulated damage will lead to permanent changes in the structure of DNA, setting the stage for the loss of cellular function, cell death, or cancer.

Multiple enzymatic pathways repair a wide range of chemical modifications of DNA

Chemical modification of the nucleotides in the DNA strand leads to mismatches during DNA synthesis. After chromosomal replication, the resulting daughter strand contains a different DNA sequence (mutation) from the parent strand. Cells use excision repair to remove alkylated nucleotides and other unusual base analogs, thereby protecting the DNA sequence from mutations. The unmodified strand serves as the template for the repair process.

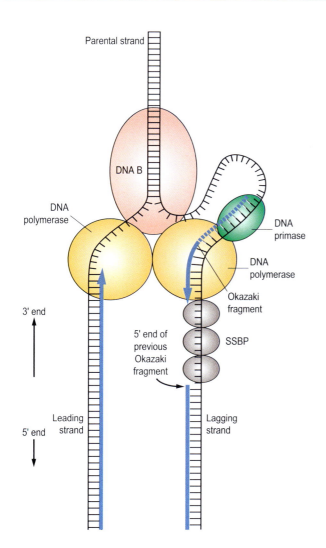

Fig. 20.6 **DNA synthesis.** DNA synthesis occurs at a replication fork, producing new strands termed the leading strand and the lagging strand. The "railroad tracks" represent double-stranded DNA. Some of the enzymes involved in DNA synthesis are shown: DNA B (helicase), DNA primase, DNA polymerase, and single-strand DNA binding protein (SSBP). The leading strand is replicated in a continuous fashion. However, for the lagging strand, RNA primers are periodically added by the DNA primase along the strand. DNA polymerase III elongates these RNA primers to form Okazaki fragments. When the Okazaki fragment is complete, the DNA polymerase III on the lagging strand will shift to the next RNA primer to initiate another Okazaki fragment. The exonuclease activity of DNA polymerase I removes the RNA primers and replaces them with DNA. DNA ligase seals the gaps in the DNA strands to complete synthesis of the lagging strand.

When the 3′ end of the elongating Okazaki fragment reaches the 5′ end of the previously synthesized fragment, DNA polymerase III releases the template and finds another RNA primer farther back along the lagging strand, synthesizing another Okazaki fragment. Eventually, the Okazaki fragments are joined by **DNA polymerase I.** This enzyme, which also has a role in DNA repair, has an exonuclease activity that permits it to remove and replace a stretch of nucleotides as it

CLINICAL BOX
ANTIRETROVIRAL THERAPY FOR HIV INFECTION

HIV infection results in a profound weakening of the immune system that makes the patient susceptible to a range of bacterial, fungal, protozoal, and viral superinfections. **Kaposi's sarcoma** may also develop; it is a cancer-like disease of the blood vessels caused by infection with human herpesvirus-8 (HHV-8). Effective treatments of the HIV viral infection rely on detailed knowledge of the viral life cycle. For the AIDS virus, the viral genome is RNA. In the infected cell, it is copied into a DNA form by a viral enzyme termed **reverse transcriptase**. Reverse transcriptase is an error-prone enzyme that does not have the proofreading capabilities of DNA polymerase III. Six drug classes have been developed for the treatment of HIV, and more than 25 individual drugs are on the market. They are used in combination to attack several phases of the viral cycle; the protocol is known as highly active antiretroviral therapy (HAART) and combines at least two nucleoside reverse-transcriptase inhibitors (NRTI) with one non-nucleoside reverse-transcriptase inhibitor or a protease inhibitor or drug from the other classes. A key therapeutic approach for the treatment of AIDS takes advantage of the enzyme's lack of specificity in the choice of complementary substrates. Several important antiviral drugs are therefore nucleotide analogs that inhibit reverse transcriptase (NRTI), including AZT (azido-2',3'-dideoxythymidine; Fig. 20.7). AZT, for example, is metabolized to the thymine triphosphate (TTP) analog azido-TTP. The HIV reverse transcriptase misincorporates azido-TTP into the reverse-transcribed viral genome, which blocks further chain elongation because the 3'-azido group cannot form a phosphodiester bond with subsequent nucleoside triphosphates. The inability to synthesize DNA from the viral RNA template results in inhibition of viral replication. The life cycle of HIV spans about 1.5 days from entry into a cell, replication, assembly, and release of new viral particles to infection of other cells. HIV lacks *proofreading* enzymes to correct errors occurring during conversion of its RNA into DNA via reverse transcription. Its short life cycle and high error rate cause the virus to mutate very rapidly, causing large genetic variability of HIV. Most of the mutations are not pathogenic, but some have a natural selection advantage over their parent, allowing them to evade the human immune system and antiretroviral drugs. The more actively the virus replicates, the greater the possibility that a strain resistant to antiretroviral drugs will appear. If antiretroviral therapy is incorrectly employed, these multidrug-resistant strains can turn out to be the dominant genotypes very promptly. Improper serial use of reverse-transcriptase inhibitors such as zidovudine, didanosine, zalcitabine, stavudine, and lamivudine may result in multi-drug-resistant (for greater readability) mutations.

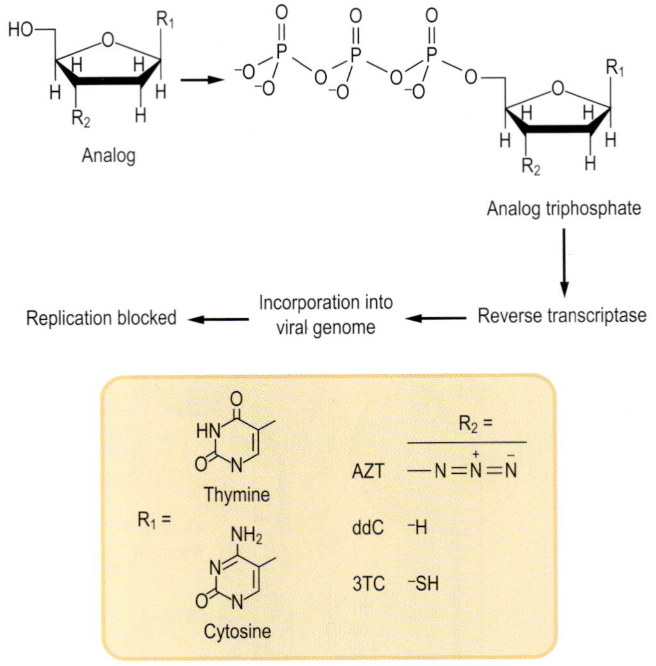

Fig. 20.7 **Mechanism of action of antiretroviral chemotherapeutic agents.** This class of inhibitors includes several compounds with slightly different chemical structures in the nucleobase structure and in substitution at the 3'-carbon of the sugar ring. Structures of some of the most widely used drugs are shown. These compounds are metabolized to the triphosphate form via normal cellular metabolism. The triphosphate analogs are then incorporated into the viral genome by reverse transcriptase. This blocks viral DNA synthesis because the modified 3' end R_2 of the viral DNA molecule is not a substrate for additional rounds of DNA synthesis. AZT, azido-2',3'-dideoxythymidine; ddC, 2',3'-dideoxycytidine; 3TC, 2',3'-dideoxy-3'-thiacytidine.

(Fig. 20.8). The primary mechanism for repair of these intra-strand thymine dimers is an excision repair mechanism. An endonuclease, specific for this type of modification, cleaves the dimer-containing strand near the thymine dimer, and a small portion of that strand is removed. DNA polymerase I, the same enzyme that is involved in DNA biosynthesis, then recognizes and fills in the resulting gap. DNA ligase completes the repair by rejoining the DNA strands.

Deamination: Excision repair

Those nucleotides that contain amines, cytosine and adenosine, may spontaneously deaminate to form uracil or hypoxanthine, respectively. When these bases are found in DNA, specific **N-glycosylases** remove them. This produces base-pair gaps that are recognized by specific apurinic or apyrimidinic endonucleases that cleave the DNA near the site of the defect. An exonuclease then removes the stretch of the DNA strand containing the defect. A repair DNA polymerase replaces the DNA, and finally, DNA ligase rejoins the DNA strand. This repair mechanism is also referred to as excision repair.

UV light produces thymine dimers: nucleotide excision repair

When short-wavelength ultraviolet (UV) light interacts with DNA, adjacent thymine bases undergo an unusual dimerization, producing a cyclobutylthymine dimer in the DNA strand

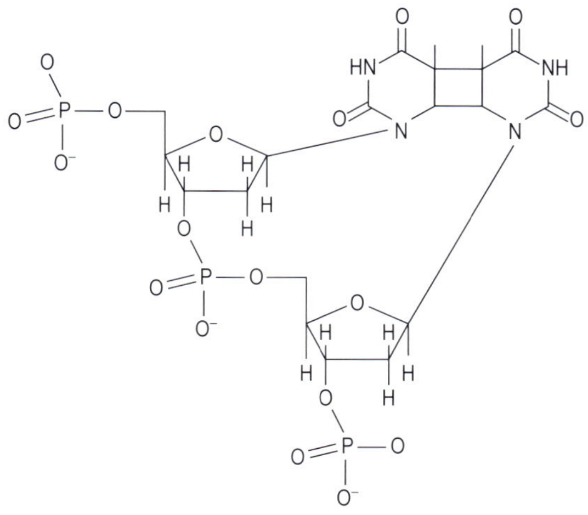

Fig. 20.8 **Thymine dimer.** A thymine dimer consists of a cyclobutane ring joining a pair of adjacent thymine nucleotides.

CLINICAL BOX
XERODERMA PIGMENTOSUM

Xeroderma pigmentosum (XP) is a group of rare, life-threatening, autosomal recessive disorders (incidence = 1/250,000) that are marked by extreme sensitivity to sunlight. Upon exposure to sunlight or ultraviolet (UV) radiation, the skin of XP patients erupts into pigmented spots resembling freckles. Multiple carcinomas and melanomas appear early in life, exacerbated by sun exposure, and the majority of patients succumb to cancer before reaching adulthood.

XP is the result of a defect in repair of UV-induced thymine dimers in DNA. There are at least eight polypeptides (genes) involved in recognition, unwinding, and excision repair of UV-induced thymine dimers. Patients with XP must avoid direct sunlight, fluorescent light, halogen light, or any other source of UV light. An experimental form of protein therapy, currently undergoing clinical evaluation, involves the application of a skin lotion containing the missing protein or enzyme. Ideally, this protein will enter the skin cells and stimulate the repair of UV-damaged DNA. However, protection occurs only where the lotion can be applied. For example, this treatment does not address the neurologic problems that affect about 20% of XP patients.

Depurination

Single-base-pair alterations also include depurination. The purine-N-glycosidic bonds are especially labile, so an estimated three to seven purines are removed from DNA per minute per cell. Specific enzymes recognize these depurinated sites, and the base is replaced without interruption of the phosphodiester backbone.

Strand breaks

Single-stranded breaks are frequently induced by ionizing radiation. These are repaired by direct ligation or by excision repair mechanisms. Double-stranded breaks are produced by ionizing radiation and some chemotherapeutic agents. Otherwise, double-stranded ends of DNA are rare in vivo; they are found at the end of chromosomes and in some specialized complexes involved in gene rearrangement. A specialized enzyme system is designed to recognize and rejoin these ends, but if the ends drift away from one another, the damage is not readily repaired.

Mismatch repair

Errors that escape the proofreading activity of DNA polymerase III appear in newly synthesized DNA in the form of nucleotide mismatches. Although they are readily repairable, the critical issue is the identification of the strand to be repaired: Which nucleotide strand is the daughter strand containing the error? In bacterial systems, mismatch repair is accomplished by postreplicative methylation of DNA at adenine residues in specific sequences spaced along the genome; methylation does not affect base pairing. Newly synthesized strands lack methylated adenine residues, so the mismatch repair system enzymes scan the DNA, identify the mismatch, and then repair the unmethylated strand by excision repair. A similar approach is used to correct mismatches occurring during synthesis of

mammalian DNA. Defects in mismatch repair are associated with hereditary nonpolyposis colon cancer, an autosomal dominant condition in humans.

8-Oxo-2'-deoxyguanosine

More than 20 different oxidative modifications of DNA have been characterized; the most studied is 8-oxo-2'-deoxyguanosine (8-oxoG; Fig. 20.9). During the process of DNA replication, mismatches between the modified 8-oxoG nucleoside in the template strand and incoming nucleotide triphosphates result in G-to-T transversions, thereby introducing mutations into the DNA strand. Although excision repair mechanisms are effective, 8-oxoG, like other modified bases, may be reincorporated into DNA after excision.

Recently, a mammalian protein, MTH1, was characterized that specifically degrades 8-oxo-dGTP, thereby preventing misincorporation of this altered nucleotide into DNA. Gene targeting was used to develop an MTH1 knockout mouse. Compared with the wild-type animal, the knockout showed a greater number of tumors in lung, liver, and stomach, illustrating the importance of this (and other) postrepair protection mechanisms.

In lung cells, inhalation of some particulate materials results in an increase in 8-oxoG levels. The inflammatory process may play a role in asbestos-induced formation of lung tumors. Smoking also induces oxidative damage and increases levels of DNA oxidation products in lungs, blood, and urine. 8-Oxo-2'-deoxyguanosine is eliminated via renal filtration. Therefore its urinary concentration is used as a sensitive biomarker for oxidative stress in many clinical studies (Chapter 42).

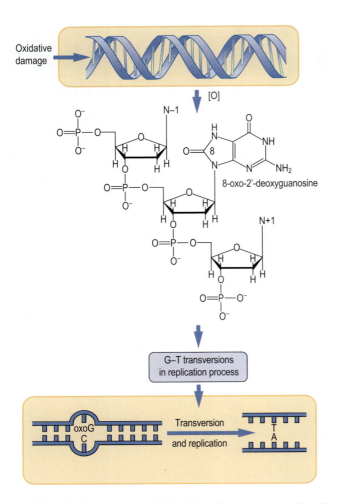

Fig. 20.9 **Oxidative damage to DNA.** 8-Oxo-2'-deoxyguanosine (oxoG) is an oxidative modification of DNA that causes mutations during replication of DNA. Replication of the strand containing oxoG frequently yields a pyrimidine A in the complementary strand, which, on further replication, yields an AT base pair instead of the original GC base pair.

RECOMBINANT DNA TECHNOLOGY

DNA sequencing, hybridization, and cloning are fundamental techniques of genetic engineering

Our current ability to analyze and manipulate genomes began with reports in the 1970s of methods to cleave DNA at specific sites, to insert new DNA fragments into bacterial plasmids, and to sequence regions of DNA more than just a few nucleotides long. This has led to an explosion in knowledge, technical achievements, and biological and medical applications of recombinant DNA technology. This technology is now widely used for the following applications: (a) production of human proteins in scales large enough to use in treatment of disease, (b) diagnosis of disease or prediction of predisposition to a disease, (c) prediction of individual response to drugs (pharmacogenomics), (d) production of proteins for vaccines, (e) forensic medicine, (f) studies in anthropology and human

CLINICAL TEST BOX
AMES TEST FOR MUTAGENS

Mutagens are chemical compounds that induce changes in the DNA sequence. A large number of natural and man-made chemicals are mutagenic. To evaluate the potential to mutate DNA, the biochemist Bruce Ames developed a simple test using special *Salmonella typhimurium* strains that cannot grow in the absence of histidine (His⁻ phenotype). These histidine auxotrophic strains contain nucleotide substitutions or deletions that prevent the production of histidine biosynthetic enzymes.

To test for mutagenesis, mutant bacteria are seeded on a culture medium lacking histidine; the suspected mutagen is added to the medium. The action of the mutagen occasionally results in the reversal of the histidine mutation, yielding a revertant strain that can now synthesize histidine and will grow in its absence. The mutagenicity of a compound is scored by counting the number of colonies that have grown (i.e., reverted to the His⁺ phenotype). There is a good correlation between results of the Ames mutagenicity test and direct tests of carcinogenic activity in animals.

Some chemicals (**procarcinogens**) are not mutagenic per se but are activated to mutagenic compounds during metabolic processes (e.g., during drug detoxification in the liver or kidney). Benzopyrene, for example, is not mutagenic, but during its detoxification in the liver, it is converted to diol epoxides, which are potent mutagens and carcinogens. To provide sensitivity for detecting procarcinogens, the culture medium for the Ames test is supplemented with an extract of liver microsomes, a subfraction of tissue rich in smooth endoplasmic reticulum containing drug-metabolizing enzymes.

CLINICAL BOX
CANCER TREATMENT NEWS: TWO NEW PROTEIN TARGETS TO COUNTERACT "RELAPSE" AND "DRUG RESISTANCE"

Current cancer treatments such as ionizing radiation and chemotherapy target DNA. Their rationale is clear: these treatments disrupt the genome, and a balance is struck between preventing cancer cells from dividing and proliferating while not irreversibly damaging healthy, less rapidly dividing cells. Nonetheless, cancer cells have a broad array of DNA repair mechanisms to limit injury. For this reason, DNA repair systems are targets of adjuvant therapy used to enhance the sensitivity of cancer cells to DNA-targeted agents. Base excision repair and nucleotide excision repair are key mechanisms of DNA repair. There are two protein targets associated with the hallmark relapse and drug-resistance phenomena seen during chemotherapy: excision repair cross-complementation group 1 (ERCC1) and DNA polymerase beta. The former is a key player in nucleotide excision repair; the latter is the error-prone polymerase of base excision repair. Only a few ERCC1 inhibitors have been discovered, but more than 60 have been found for DNA polymerase beta. The discovery of potent and tumor-specific inhibitors of these enzymes should improve current therapies where resistance develops, including bleomycin, alkylating agents, and cisplatin.

evolution, (g) understanding of molecular mechanisms of disease, and (h) gene therapy. Before these developments, genes in humans were known almost exclusively by their effects - that is, from phenotypes and disease; genes were concepts rather than structures. Gradually, it became possible to see exactly what a gene was and to determine if genes were normal or mutated. A major step in the process was recognition that single strands of nucleic acids will form double-stranded (ds) pairs with each other only if the sequences are highly complementary. Just as antibodies can detect single proteins in the midst of thousands of others, nucleic acid sequences will bind only to their complement in the presence of millions of nonmatching sequences. A second major advance was the discovery of restriction enzymes, which convert chromosomal DNA into discrete fragments of useful length. After separation by size, these smaller fragments could be detected by nucleic acid probes, then also sequenced. Although many of the procedures used for analysis of DNA in the 20th century are mostly of historical interest today, some knowledge of them is necessary both for reading the older literature and for understanding modern recombinant DNA technology. The ability to splice and recombine fragments of DNA into viruses, bacterial plasmids, and even chromosomes has revolutionized the production of many clinically important human proteins and vaccines.

Here we provide an overview of some of the general techniques for forming so-called recombinant DNA and for cloning of this DNA.

PRINCIPLES OF MOLECULAR HYBRIDIZATION

Hybridization is based on the annealing properties of DNA

Hybridization is a process by which a piece of DNA or RNA of known nucleotide sequence, which can range in size from as little as 15 base pairs (bp) to several hundred kilobases, is used to identify a region or fragment of DNA containing complementary sequences. The first piece of DNA or RNA is called a probe. Probe DNA will form a complementary base pair with another strand of DNA, often termed the target, if the two strands are complementary and a sufficient number of hydrogen bonds is formed.

For molecular hybridization, it is essential that the probe and target are initially single stranded

Probes can vary in both their size and their nature (DNA, RNA, or oligonucleotide). However, one essential feature of any hybridization reaction is that both the probe and the target must be free to base pair with one another. For DNA hybridization, the two strands of DNA must first be separated by thermal or chemical treatment, a process called DNA **denaturation,** or **melting.** Once both probe and target DNA are single stranded, mixing of the two under conditions that favor the formation of a double-stranded helix will allow complementary

bases to recombine. This process is called DNA **annealing** or **reassociation,** and when a probe strand reacts with a target strand, the complex is termed a **heteroduplex.**

Formation of probe–target heteroduplexes is key to the usefulness of molecular hybridization

The conditions under which DNA hybridization occurs and the reliability and specificity, or stringency, of hybridization are affected by several factors:

- **Base composition:** GC pairs have three hydrogen bonds compared with the two in an AT pair. Double-stranded DNA with a high GC content is therefore more stable and has a higher melting temperature (T_m).
- **Strand length:** The longer a strand of DNA, the greater the number of hydrogen bonds between the two strands. Longer strands require higher temperatures or stronger alkali treatment to denature them; stability varies dramatically with length for very short probes, but above a few hundred base pairs, stability is relatively insensitive to length and is determined primarily by base composition.
- **Reaction conditions:** High cation concentration (typically Na^+) favors double-stranded DNA because the negative charges on the sugar–phosphate backbone are shielded from each other. High concentrations of urea or formamide favor single-stranded DNA because these reagents reduce base-stacking and can compete for hydrogen bond formation. Hybridizations are said to be carried out at **low stringency** when conditions strongly favor duplex formation, permitting some mismatch in the DNA duplex, and at **high stringency** when only matched, complementary duplexes are formed.

Thus by appropriate selection of conditions (high stringency), a small 30- to 50-bp probe can require a perfect match to form a stable hybrid with its target. Conversely, under low stringency, a longer probe (e.g., 500 bp) might react with targets that contain multiple nucleotide mismatches or mutations (Fig. 20.10).

The stability of a nucleic acid duplex can be assessed by determining its melting temperature (T_m)

The melting temperature (T_m) is the temperature at which 50% of a double-stranded duplex has dissociated into single-strand form. For relatively long DNA probes, T_m is determined primarily by base composition, with AT-rich DNA melting at a lower temperature than GC-rich DNA. For humans and other mammals, the average GC content is about 40%, and the melting temperature in moderate salt is about 87°C. For short oligonucleotides, such as the primers used in polymerase chain reactions (PCR), effects of length, composition, and even the various dinucleotide sequences must be taken into consideration. This is because double-stranded DNA is stabilized by the degree of overlap by the stacked bases in successive nucleotides, and this varies depending on the specific nucleotide neighbors of a particular base. Computer programs are widely available to predict T_m values.

A Hybridization characteristics using a large conventional probe (>200 bases)

Match	Perfect	Single base mismatch	Multiple mismatch
Stringency	High	Intermediate	Low
Example	Human target + human probe 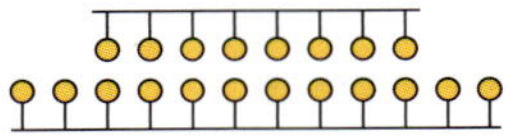	Human target + human probe with mutation 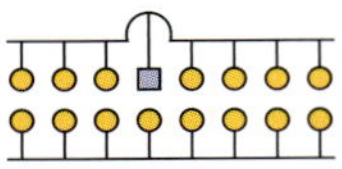	Human target + mouse probe 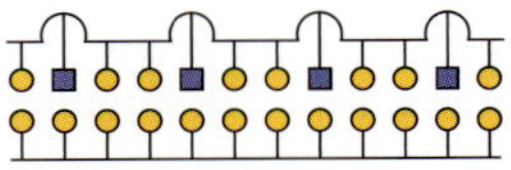
Stability	Stable	Stable	Stable

B Hybridization characteristics using a small oligonucleotide probe

Match	Perfect	Single base mismatch	
Stringency	High	High	
Example	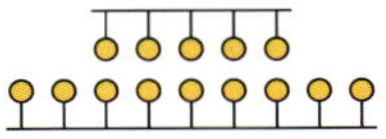	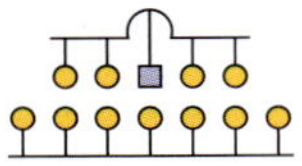	
Stability	Stable	Unstable	

Fig. 20.10 **Probe–template hybridization.** (A) Large probes (e.g., 200 bases or more) can form stable heteroduplexes with the target DNA even if there are a significant number of noncomplementary bases in conditions of low stringency. (B) Oligonucleotide probes, in contrast, may discriminate between targets that differ by a single base under stringent conditions.

Probes must have a label to be identified

Implicit in the use of probes to identify pieces of complementary DNA is the notion that if hybridization occurs, the heteroduplex can be specifically detected. Thus the probe is labeled so that the probe–target duplex can be identified. The labels generally fall into two categories, either isotopic (i.e., involving radioactive atoms) or nonisotopic (e.g., end-labeling probes with fluorescent tags or small ligand molecules). Use of fluorescent tags and laser detection has become far more widespread in the past few years. Still, some techniques involving probe hybridization and also studies of protein binding to DNA use radioisotopes such as ^{32}P, ^{35}S, or ^{3}H and, as such, require a method for detecting and localizing the radioactivity. The most common method involves the process of **autoradiography**. Autoradiography allows information from a solid phase (e.g., a gel or fixed-tissue sample) to be detected and saved in two-dimensional form as an exposed photographic image.

Southern blots are the prototype for methods that use specific hybridization probes to identify sequences in DNA or RNA

One of the fundamental steps in the evolution of molecular biology was the discovery that DNA could be transferred (blotted) from a semisolid gel (e.g., agarose or polyacrylamide) onto a nitrocellulose membrane in such a way that the membrane could act as a record of the DNA information in the gel

and could be used for multiple-probe experiments. The process whereby the DNA is transferred to the membrane was first described by Edward Southern. Subsequent blotting techniques used laboratory jargon for the transfer of RNA (Northern) and proteins (Western), and the jargon has become the standard nomenclature.

Restriction enzymes: Use of restriction enzymes to analyze genomic DNA

Restriction enzymes cleave DNA at specific nucleotide sequences

Restriction endonucleases cleave double-stranded DNA. These enzymes are sequence specific, and each enzyme acts at a limited number of sites in DNA called recognition, or cutting, sites. Restriction endonucleases are part of the bacterial "immune system." Bacteria methylate their own DNA at specific sites for which they produce a restriction enzyme, protecting it from their own restriction enzymes, but cleave unmethylated infecting viral or bacteriophage DNAs at specific sites, thereby inactivating the virus and restricting viral infection.

If DNA is digested by a restriction enzyme, the DNA will be reduced to fragments of varying sizes depending on how many cutting sites for that restriction enzyme are present in the DNA. The cutting sites are frequently **palindromic sequences,** sites

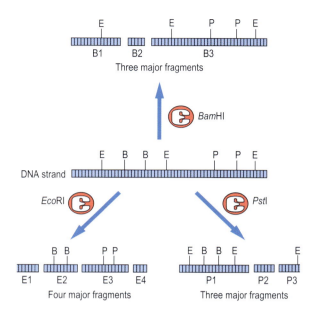

Fig. 20.11 **Restriction enzyme digestion of DNA.** Digestion of a DNA molecule by several different restriction enzymes may result in many different fragments, even though the apparent size of the fragments is similar. For example, fragments E1 and P3 are of similar size but are clearly different pieces of DNA. E, *Eco*RI site; B, *Bam*HI site; P, *Pst*I site.

at which the base sequence reading 5' to 3' on one strand is the same as the sequence reading 3' to 5' on the complementary strand of a double helix. It is important to note that each enzyme will cut DNA into a unique set of fragments (Fig. 20.11). Many restriction enzymes recognize sites that are typically four (e.g., HaeIII), six (e.g., *Eco*RI), or eight nucleotides (e.g., NotI) in length (Table 20.1). Variation in just one nucleotide within the recognition sequence makes a sequence completely resistant to a particular enzyme.

The frequency of the cutting sites for various enzymes varies with the length of the recognition site. Cut sites for an enzyme with a four-base recognition site, such as HaeIII, would occur by chance once per 256-bp sequence. Cut sites for an enzyme with an eight-base recognition site, such as NotI, would occur only once in about 656,000 base pairs. Thus frequent cutters typically generate many small fragments, whereas rare cutters generate fewer and larger fragments. These differences can be exploited in the analysis of gene structure and chromosomal location.

DNA fragments, blotted onto a solid gel phase, are used as a template for exposure to a range of molecular probes

If DNA is digested by a restriction enzyme, the resulting digest can be separated on the basis of size by gel electrophoresis. Agarose gel electrophoresis is commonly used to separate fragments ranging in size from 100 bases to approximately 20 kb in length (above 40 kb, resolution is minimal). After electrophoresis, the gels are soaked in a strong alkali solution

to denature the DNA. The single-stranded fragments can then be transferred to a nitrocellulose or nylon membrane to which they bind readily and, if preserved properly, permanently. The process of transfer involves the passage of solute through the gel, passively carrying the DNA and producing an image of the gel on the membrane (Fig. 20.12). The membrane may then be probed with an oligonucleotide or DNA fragment (Southern blot), for use in genotyping, paternity testing, or identification of cells incorporating a gene during a cloning experiment, for example, as described later in the chapter.

Restriction-fragment-length polymorphisms (RFLP) and single-nucleotide polymorphisms (SNP)

Analysis of restriction fragment length may be used to detect a mutation or polymorphism in a gene

If a change in DNA sequence creates or destroys a recognition site that yields a fragment detected by a probe, then the altered length of that fragment can be detected by Southern blotting. **When the change involves just one nucleotide, it is called a single-nucleotide polymorphism (SNP).** If a cleavage site is created, the fragment becomes smaller; if the cleavage site is eliminated, the fragment becomes larger. The different patterns generated as a result of a mutation or gene variant are known as restriction-fragment-length polymorphisms (RFLPs; Fig. 20.13). Such RFLPs can be used either to identify disease-causing mutations, resulting from a single point mutation creating or abolishing a restriction site, or to study variation in noncoding DNA for use in the study of genetic linkage. As an example, James Watson's DNA sequence was revealed a few years ago. He was found to have more than 3 million SNPs as compared with the "standard"

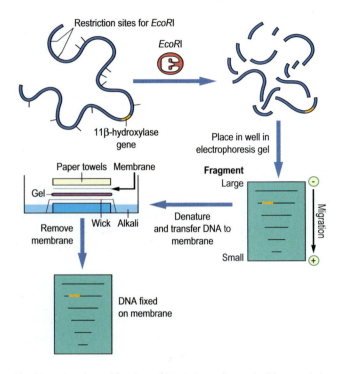

Fig. 20.12 **Southern blotting of DNA.** DNA digested with a restriction enzyme is size-fractionated by agarose electrophoresis. The agarose gel is then placed in alkali to denature the DNA. The now single-stranded DNA can pass from the gel to the membrane (typically nylon or nitrocellulose) as buffer solution flows upward by capillary action, forming a permanent record of the digested DNA.

human genome published in 2003. RFLP and SNP maps of the human genome have been constructed that serve as anchors to better study single-gene and polygenic diseases.

RFLP analysis can also detect larger pathologic changes in the DNA sequence, either deletions or duplications. Large deletions of a gene may abolish restriction sites; this leads to the disappearance of a fragment on a Southern blot in homozygous individuals. Alternatively, if a DNA duplication event occurs, a new gene may be formed, which has a different pattern of restriction sites that allow detection of the new gene. This type of hybridization is performed using large probes (0.5–5.0 kb) and is performed under moderate stringency - that is, it is sufficiently rigid to allow hybridization of probe and target but also to tolerate minor differences, for example, in noncoding DNA.

Low-stringency hybridization of a probe to a Southern blot of digested DNA may allow genes related to, but not identical to, the starting gene to be identified. Many genes exist in families or have nonfunctional, nearly identical copies elsewhere in the genome (pseudogenes), and thus hybridization of a probe may identify one or more restriction fragments corresponding to related genes. Similarly, related genes in different species may be identified by using a single probe that can hybridize at low stringency to complementary sequences in blots of DNA from mice, rats, or other species.

CLONING OF DNA

Cell-based cloning

Bacterial plasmids are bioengineered to optimize their use as vectors

Cell-based cloning relies on the ability of replicating cells (e.g., bacteria) to permit replication of so-called recombinant DNA

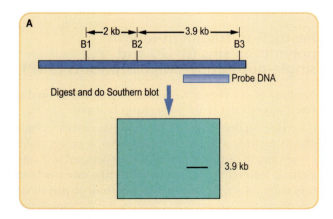

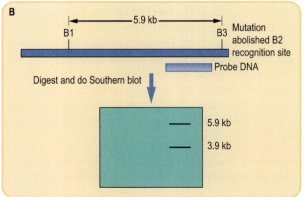

Fig. 20.13 **Restriction-fragment-length polymorphisms (RFLP).** Variations in the nucleotide sequence of DNA, either due to natural variation in individuals or as a result of a DNA mutation, can abolish the recognition sites for restriction enzymes. This means that when DNA is digested with the enzyme whose site is abolished, the size of the resulting fragments is altered. Southern blotting and probe hybridization can be used to detect this change. Results are shown for a representative gene from (A) homozygous normal and (B) heterozygous mutant individuals. B, *Bam*HI restriction site. The probe DNA is visualized by radioactivity or fluorescence.

CLINICAL BOX
USE OF RFLPS FOR DETECTION OF THE SICKLE CELL GENE

A 24-year-old Afro-Caribbean pregnant woman was referred for prenatal counseling. Her younger brother had sickle cell anemia, her partner was known to be a carrier of the sickle cell mutation (sickle cell trait), and she wanted to know if her child would develop sickle cell anemia.

Because the patient is at risk of being a carrier, she opted to have chorionic villus sampling (CVS) performed to detect the presence or absence of the sickle cell mutation in her child. Analysis of her own DNA revealed that she was a carrier, and the CVS showed that the child was also a carrier and would not develop sickle cell anemia.

Comment

Occasionally, a mutation will directly abolish or create a restriction site and thus allow the use of a restriction-based method to demonstrate the presence or absence of the mutant allele. One widely examined mutation is the A > T substitution at codon 6 in the sequence for the β-globin gene responsible for sickle-cell disease (see Chapter 5). This results in a glutamine-valine (Glu-Val) mutation in the amino-acid sequence β-globin and also abolishes a recognition site for MstII (CCTN[A > T]GG) in the β-globin gene. Digestion of normal human DNA with MstII and probing the Southern blot with a probe specific for the promoter of the β-globin gene yields a single band of 1.2 kb because the nearest MstII site is 1.2 kb upstream in the 5' region of the gene. The abolition of the codon 6 restriction site means that the fragment size seen when probing MstII digested DNA is now 1.4 kb because the next MstII site is located 200 bases downstream in the intron after exon 1. Thus patients with sickle cell anemia will show only one band, 1.4 kb; carriers will have two bands, one 1.4 kb and the other 1.2 kb; and unaffected individuals will have a single 1.2-kb band.

within them. Recombinant DNA refers to any DNA molecule that is artificially constructed from two pieces of DNA not normally found together. One piece of DNA will be the target DNA that is to be amplified, and the other will be the replicating **vector** or replicon, a molecule capable of initiating DNA replication in a suitable host cell.

Today, the majority of cell-based cloning is performed using bacterial cells. In addition to the bacterial chromosome, bacteria may contain extrachromosomal double-stranded DNA that can undergo replication. One such example is the bacterial plasmid. **Plasmids** are circular, double-stranded DNA molecules that undergo intracellular replication and are passed vertically from the parent cell to each daughter cell. However, unlike the bacterial chromosome, plasmids used in these techniques are copied many times during each cell division. Thus plasmids are ideal carriers for the amplification of target DNA and thus the encoded protein; they are also engineered to contain antibiotic resistance genes, which permits the selection of infected host cells. Target DNA is introduced into a plasmid

by using restriction enzymes to cut target and plasmid DNA so that the target DNA and the linearized vector DNA will have complementary sticky ends (Fig. 20.14). DNA ligase then covalently joins the target to the ends of the vector to form a closed circular recombinant plasmid. Once the target DNA is incorporated into the plasmid vector, the next step is to introduce the plasmid into a host cell to allow replication to occur. The cell membrane of bacteria is selectively permeable and prevents the free passage of large molecules such as DNA in and out of the cell. However, the permeability of cells can be altered temporarily by factors such as electric currents (electroporation) or high-solute concentration (osmotic stress) so that the membrane becomes temporarily permeable, and DNA can enter the cell. Such a process renders the cells competent: they can take up foreign DNA from the extracellular fluid, a process known as **transformation.** However, this process is generally inefficient, so only a small fraction of cells may take up plasmid DNA, and often only a single plasmid per bacterium is introduced during transformation. Yet it is this process of cellular uptake of plasmid DNA that forms a critical step in cell-based cloning. Individual recombinant DNAs are easily resolved from one another because they are taken up by separate cells that can be isolated simply by spreading them on an agar surface.

After transformation, the cells are allowed to replicate, usually on a standard agar plate containing a suitable antibiotic (see Fig. 20.14B) to kill cells that do not harbor the plasmid containing the antibiotic resistance gene. This selection or screening process, based on antibiotic resistance, is an important step because of the low efficiency of the uptake of plasmid DNA into bacteria. Colonies (clones of single surviving cells) are then "picked" and transferred to tubes for growth in liquid culture and a second phase of exponential increase in cell number. This work is done automatically in microplate systems so that, from a single cell and a single molecule of DNA, an extremely large number of cells containing multiple, identical recombinant plasmids can be generated in a relatively short time (Fig. 20.15). Recovery of the plasmid DNA is easy because it is a small, covalently intact circle, readily separated from the bacterial chromosomal DNA by a variety of techniques, such as gel electrophoresis or ultracentrifugation.

The bacterial cell is then grown in culture, and the target protein is recovered after lysis of the cells. Alternatively, the plasmid might encode a protein with a signal sequence so that it is secreted into the medium; the signal sequence would be removed afterward.

The technology for producing protein pharmaceuticals is a complex, multistep process, often protected by trade secrets. For the bacterial synthesis of recombinant insulin (see the accompanying box), for example, there is no gene or mRNA for the sequence of insulin - insulin is synthesized as preproinsulin, which is processed in pancreatic β-cells to yield the secreted hormone (Chapter 31). The synthesis of human insulin in a bacterial system might involve the incorporation of the proinsulin gene into a plasmid, transformation into a bacterial host, synthesis of proinsulin, spontaneous disulfide

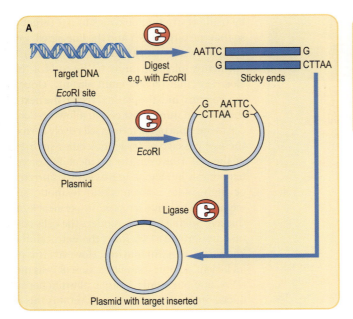
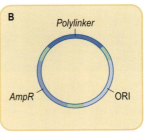

Fig. 20.14 **Formation of a plasmid containing a target gene for cloning.** (A) DNA containing the target gene is digested with a restriction enzyme that will produce "sticky ends" - for example, *Eco*RI. The plasmid also has a restriction site for *Eco*RI, so when digested with *Eco*RI, it becomes a linear DNA strand with "sticky ends" complementary to the target. Upon ligation, the target and vector form a recombinant molecule. (B) Structure of a typical plasmid. The plasmid contains a gene conferring resistance to the antibiotic ampicillin (AmpR) and a polylinker region containing approximately 10 different restriction-enzyme recognition sites, which serve as sites for insertion of target DNA. The plasmid also contains ORI, the site for origin of DNA replication.

crosslinking, processing by endopeptidases to remove the C-peptide, then folding to produce the active insulin molecule. The proteolytic processing might happen in the cell or after isolation of the proinsulin; intracellular processing would require encoding the protease in the bacterial plasmid. Other strategies might be imagined, such as synthesis of the A and B chains in separate bacterial hosts, then extracellular association into the active hormone. It might also be possible to design a protein product that would be secreted from the bacterial cell, then processed ex vivo to remove the secretory sequence and C-peptide.

Future directions

Cloning of DNA is a rapidly evolving field in biomedical research and modern medicine. It is the basic methodology for the production of genetically modified organisms (GMO), including agricultural products and transgenic and knockout animals. More sophisticated eukaryotic expression systems, including human tumor cells, hen's eggs, and plant cells, are now commonly used for the production of protein pharmaceuticals. In some cases, these cells are engineered to contain specific processing enzymes (e.g., glycosyltransferases) for posttranslational modification of the protein. The β-glucosidase used for enzyme-replacement therapy in Gaucher's disease (Chapter 18) is produced in bioengineered Chinese hamster ovary (CHO) cells. The enzyme secreted from these cells contains a mannose-6-phosphate signal,

so it is taken up into lysosomes after intravenous injection. *Humanized* proteins may also be synthesized in murine cells, then processed by glycosidases and/or glycosyl transferases to yield a protein with the proper posttranslational modifications for use in human plasma or cells. In the not-too-distant future, it may be possible to bypass all of these steps by gene therapy - that is, by incorporating the gene of interest directly into the relevant human cells using viral vectors.

It must be said that some of the excessive optimism harbored by the Human Genome Project and the trumpeting that this major achievement, completed in 2003, would quickly illuminate the pathogenicity (and therefore targets for treatment) of disease has been slow to come after almost 15 years. Too much emphasis was put into molecular biology without realizing that expression of proteins, interactions, fluxes, and metabolism go far beyond a linear coding sequence. This is why we now are tackling the proteome, the lipidome, the metabolome, and so forth and using systems biology to interpret the stream of data coming from these experiments.

SUMMARY

■ The human genome is composed of DNA, an antiparallel, double-stranded helical polymer of deoxyribonucleotides, stabilized by hydrogen binding between complementary bases.

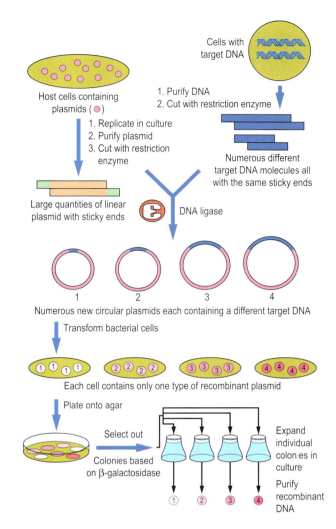

Fig. 20.15 **Cell-based DNA cloning.** An example of cloning genomic DNA using bacterial cells. In general, each transformed bacterium will take up only a single plasmid molecule. Therefore individual bacterial colonies will contain many identical copies of just one particular recombinant DNA.

- DNA is packaged in the chromosome in a highly organized, condensed structure known as chromatin.
- The replication of DNA is a complex, tightly regulated process. Genetic information is replicated by a semiconservative mechanism in which the parental strands are separated, and both act as templates for daughter DNA.
- DNA is essentially the only polymer in the body that is repaired, rather than degraded, after chemical or biological modification. Repair mechanisms generally involve excision of modified bases and replacement, using the unmodified strand as a template.
- Recombinant DNA technology employs DNA cleavage, hybridization, and cloning techniques that are useful for diagnosis of genetic diseases and production of human proteins for treatment of disease.

CLINICAL BOX
PRODUCTION OF RECOMBINANT PROTEINS: INSULIN

A 13-year-old girl was admitted with dehydration, vomiting, and weight loss. Her blood glucose level was 19.1 mmol/L (344 mg/dL), and she had ketonuria. A diagnosis of type 1 diabetes mellitus was made. She was started on recombinant human insulin, was rehydrated, and made a prompt recovery.

Comment
Prior to the advent of recombinant DNA technology, insulin therapy involved the use of animal insulins, most commonly pork or beef, which were chemically similar but not identical to human insulin. As a result of these differences, animal insulins often led to the development of antibodies, which reduced the efficacy of the insulin and could lead to treatment failures.

Insulin was the first clinically important human molecule to be produced by means of recombinant DNA technology. Following the cloning of the human insulin gene, large-scale production of pure human insulin was possible by inserting the cloned gene into a cell-based amplification system. Large amounts of insulin gene copies were produced and were then expressed in either bacteria or yeast, and the resulting purified insulin was made available for use in the treatment of diabetic patients. By this means, human recombinant insulin has largely replaced animal insulin in the treatment of diabetes. Other important recombinant human peptides used clinically include growth hormone, erythropoietin, and parathyroid hormone.

ADVANCED CONCEPT BOX
VECTOR SYSTEMS FOR CLONING LARGE DNA FRAGMENTS

One critical consideration in recombinant DNA technology is the size of the target DNA. Conventional bacterial plasmids, although convenient to work with, are limited in the size of insert they can accept; 1–2 kb (about 600 amino acids, representing a 75,000-kDa protein) is the common size of the insert, with an upper limit of 5–10 kb. Some modified plasmid vectors called **cosmids** can accept larger fragments up to 20 kb. Another commonly used vector that has the ability to accept larger DNA fragments is the **bacteriophage lambda** (λ). This viral particle contains a double-stranded DNA genome packaged within a protein coat. The λ-phage can infect *Escherichia coli* cells with high efficiency and introduce its DNA into the bacterium. Infection leads to the replication of viral DNA and the synthesis of new viral particles, which can then lyse the host cell and infect neighboring cells to repeat the process. The viral DNA is then re-isolated to obtain the recombinant DNA.

Larger inserts can also be cloned by using modified chromosomes from either bacteria **(bacterial artificial chromosomes [BACs])** or yeast **(yeast artificial chromosomes [YACs])**. Such vectors can accommodate DNA fragments up to 1–2 Mb. BACs have been particularly important in putting together the sequence of the human genome.

ACTIVE LEARNING

1. Several organizations offer DNA analysis for genealogical research. What types of analyses are performed? How does the analysis of male DNA differ from that of female DNA? Why?
2. Discuss the uses of RFLPs and SNPs in genetic counseling and forensic medicine.
3. Review the range of drug and multidrug therapies currently in use for treatment of HIV/AIDS.

FURTHER READING

Baeshen, N. A., Baeshen, M. N., Sheikh, A., et al. (2014). Cell factories for insulin production. *Microbial Cell Factories, 13*, 141.

Brázda, V., & Coufal, J. (2017). Recognition of local DNA structures by p53 protein. *International Journal of Molecular Sciences, 18*, 375.

Mukherjee, S. (2016). *The gene: An intimate history*. New York, NY: Simon & Schuster.

Nieto Moreno, N., Giono, L. E., Cambindo Botto, A. E., et al. (2015). Chromatin, DNA structure and alternative splicing. *FEBS Letters, 589*, 3370–3378.

Sanchez-Garcia, L., Martín, L., Mangues, R., et al. (2016). Recombinant pharmaceuticals from microbial cells: A 2015 update. *Microbial Cell Factories, 15*, 33.

Stryjewska, A., Kiepura, K., Librowski, T., et al. (2013). Biotechnology and genetic engineering in new drug development. Part I. DNA technology and recombinant proteins. *Pharmacological Reports, 65*, 1075–1085.

Travers, A., & Muskhelishvili, G. (2015). DNA structure and function. *The FEBS Journal, 282*, 2279–2295.

Travers, A. A., Muskhelishvili, G., & Thompson, J. M. (2012). DNA information: From digital code to analogue structure. *Philosophical Transactions. Series A, Mathematical, Physical, and Engineering Sciences, 370*, 2960–2986.

Venter, J. C. (2011). Genome sequencing anniversary: The human genome at 10 – successes and challenges. *Science, 331*, 546–547.

Watson, J. D. (1980). *The double helix: A personal account of the discovery of the structure of DNA*. New York, NY: W. W. Norton.

RELEVANT WEBSITES

DNA structure: http://www.chemguide.co.uk/organicprops/aminoacids/dna1.html

Watson and Crick discovery - *Nature*: http://www.nature.com/scitable/topicpage/discovery-of-dna-structure-and-function-watson-397

Encoding of biological information - *Nature*: http://www.nature.com/scitable/topicpage/dna-is-a-structure-that-encodes-biological-6493050

National Human Genome Research Institute: https://www.genome.gov/11006943/human-genome-project-completion-frequently-asked-questions/

Hybridization probes: http://www.biogene.com/ApplicationNotes/Analysis/Application/Hybridisation_Probes.htm

DNA cloning: https://www.khanacademy.org/science/biology/biotech-dna-technology/dna-cloning-tutorial/a/overview-dna-cloning

DNA Learning Center: https://www.dnalc.org/resources/animations/cloning101.html

ABBREVIATIONS

8-oxoG	8-oxo-2'-deoxyguanosine
PCR	Polymerase chain reaction
RFLP	Restriction fragment length polymorphism
SNP	Single nucleotide polymorphism
XP	Xeroderma pigmentosum

21 Ribonucleic Acid

Robert W. Thornburg

LEARNING OBJECTIVES

After reading this chapter, you should be able to:

- Identify the major types of cellular RNA and the function of each.
- Describe the major steps in the transcription of an RNA molecule.
- Explain the function of the different RNA polymerase enzymes.
- Describe the major differences between prokaryotic and eukaryotic mRNAs.
- Describe the different processing and splicing events that occur during the synthesis of eukaryotic mRNAs.
- Explain how small RNAs regulate mRNA expression.

INTRODUCTION

Transcription is defined as the synthesis of a ribonucleic acid (RNA) molecule using deoxyribonucleic acid (DNA) as a template

Transcription is the series of enzymatic processes that result in the transfer of genetic information stored in double-stranded DNA into a single-stranded RNA molecule. Three major classes of RNAs are involved in the conversion of the nucleotide sequence of the genome into the amino acid sequence of proteins: ribosomal RNA (rRNA), transfer RNA (tRNA), and messenger RNA (mRNA). In addition, there is a recently described class of small RNAs that function in protein/RNA complexes that join, cleave, or edit other mRNAs to alter gene expression inside cells. Each of the primary classes of RNA has a distinctive size and function (Table 21.1), described by its sedimentation rate in an ultracentrifuge (S, Svedberg units) or its number of bases (nt, nucleotides, or kb, kilobases). Prokaryotes have the same primary classes of RNA as eukaryotes, but sizes and structural features differ:

- Ribosomal RNA (rRNA) from prokaryotes consists of three different sizes of RNA, whereas rRNA from eukaryotes consists of four different sizes of RNA. These RNAs interact with each other and with proteins to form a **ribosome**, which is the basic machinery on which protein synthesis takes place.

- Transfer RNAs (tRNA) are 65–110 nt in length; they function as amino acid carriers and recognition molecules that identify the nucleotide sequence of an mRNA and translate that sequence into the amino acid sequence of proteins.

- Messenger RNAs (mRNA) represent the most heterologous class of RNAs found in cells. mRNAs generally range in size from ~500 nt to ~6 kb (some rare but important mRNAs are >100 kb). mRNAs are carriers of genetic information, defining the sequence of all proteins in the cell. They represent the "working copy" of the genome.

To explain the complex series of events that leads to the production of these three primary classes of RNA, this chapter is divided into five sections. The first section deals with the structure of the major classes of RNA and the steps involved in their formation. The second section describes the main enzymes involved in transcription. The third describes the three steps (initiation, elongation, and termination) required to produce an active mRNA. The fourth describes modifications that are made to the primary products of transcription (post-transcriptional processing). The final section describes the newly emerging area of micro-RNAs, which function to regulate gene expression at the RNA level.

MOLECULAR ANATOMY OF RIBONUCLEIC ACID MOLECULES

In contrast to DNA, RNAs are single stranded and contain uracil instead of thymine

The RNAs produced by both prokaryotes and eukaryotes are single-stranded nucleic acid molecules that consist of adenine, guanine, cytosine, and uracil nucleotides joined to one another by phosphodiester linkages. The start of an RNA molecule is known as its 5′ end, and the termination of the RNA is the 3′ end. Even though RNAs are single stranded, they fold back on themselves to form double-helical secondary structures that are important for their function. These secondary structures, known as **hairpin loops** (Fig. 21.1), are the result of intramolecular base pairing that occurs between complementary nucleotides within a single RNA molecule.

rRNAs: the ribosomal RNAs

Eukaryotic rRNAs are synthesized as a single RNA transcript that is ~13-kb (45-S) long. This large primary transcript is

Table 21.1 General classes of RNA

RNA	Size and length	Percent of total cellular RNA	Function
rRNA	28 S, 18 S, 5.8 S, 5 S (23 S, 16 S, 5 S)*	80	Interact to form ribosomes
tRNA	65–110 nt	15	Adapter
mRNA	0.5–6+ kb	5	Directs synthesis of cellular proteins

*Size of rRNA in prokaryotic cells.
nt, nucleotides; kb, kilobases; S, svedberg units.

Table 21.2 rRNAs and ribosomes

Cell type	rRNA	Subunit	Size	Intact ribosome
Prokaryotic	23 S, 5 S*	Large	50 S	70 S
	16 S	Small	30 S	
Eukaryotic	28 S, 5.8 S, 5 S	Large	60 S	80 S
	18 S	Small	40 S	

*Size of rRNA in cells.
S, svedberg units.

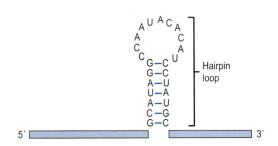

Fig. 21.1 **RNA hairpin loop.** RNA (and DNA) can form secondary structures called hairpin loops. These structures form when complementary bases within an individual RNA share hydrogen bonds and form base pairs. Hairpin loops are important in the regulation of transcription in both prokaryotic and eukaryotic cells.

processed into 28-S, 18-S, 5.8-S, and 5-S (~3-kb, 1.5-kb, 160-nt, and 120-nt, respectively) rRNAs (Table 21.1). The 28-S, 5.8-S, and 5-S rRNAs associate with ribosomal proteins to form the large ribosomal subunit. The 18-S rRNA associates with a different set of proteins to form the small ribosomal subunit (Table 21.2). The large ribosomal subunit with its RNA and proteins has a characteristic size of 60 S; the small ribosomal subunit has a size of 40 S. These two subunits interact to form a functional 80-S ribosome (see Chapter 22). Prokaryotic rRNAs interact in a similar manner to form ribosomal subunits that have a slightly smaller size, reflecting the difference in prokaryotic and eukaryotic rRNA transcript size (Table 21.2).

tRNA: the molecular cloverleaf

Prokaryotic and eukaryotic tRNAs are similar in both size and structure. They exhibit extensive secondary structure and contain several **modified ribonucleotides** that are derived from the normal four ribonucleotides. All tRNAs have a similar fold, with four distinct loops that have been described conventionally as a **cloverleaf** structure (Fig. 21.2A); however, X-ray crystal structures of tRNAs show that the true structure of the folded cloverleaf is an L-shaped molecule (Fig. 21.2B). The D loop contains several modified bases, including methylated cytosine and dihydrouridine (D), for which the loop is named. The **anticodon loop** is the structure responsible for recognition of the complementary codon of an mRNA molecule: specific interaction of an anticodon of the tRNA with the appropriate codon in the mRNA is due to base pairing between these two complementary trinucleotide sequences. A variable loop, 3–21 nt in length, exists in most tRNAs, but its function is unknown. Finally there is a TψC loop, which contains a modified base, pseudouridine (ψ). Another prominent structure found in all tRNA molecules is the **acceptor stem.** This structure is formed by base pairing between the nucleotides at each end of the tRNA. The last three bases found at the extreme 3′ end remain unpaired and always have the same sequence: 5′-...CCA-3′. The amino acid to be incorporated into protein is attached to the 3′ end of the acceptor stem via an ester bond between the 3′ hydroxyl group of the terminal adenosine of the tRNA and the carboxyl group of the amino acid (see Chapter 22).

mRNA: prokaryotic and eukaryotic mRNAs differ significantly in structure and processing

Prokaryotes and eukaryotes have dramatically different life cycles. Therefore it is not surprising that there are differences in the structures of their genes, in their mechanisms of transcription, and in the structures of their mRNAs. In fact, we can exploit these differences with novel antibiotic inhibitors that target unique portions of the prokaryotic life cycle. Because there are a number of major differences between prokaryotic and eukaryotic mRNAs, these will be discussed in the following sections. Briefly, these differences are as follows:

- Transcriptional units that differ in structure: prokaryotic mRNAs are polycistronic; eukaryotic mRNAs are monocystronic (Fig. 21.3).
- Compartmentalization of transcription and translation: prokaryotes synthesize RNA and protein in a single compartment, the cytoplasm; eukaryotes separate these events in the nucleus and cytoplasm.
- Protection at their 5′ and 3′ ends: the ends of prokaryotic mRNAs are naked; eukaryotic mRNAs are protected by a 5′ cap and a 3′ poly(A) tail.
- Processing of mRNAs: prokaryotic mRNAs are not processed; eukaryotic mRNAs contain introns that are spliced out.

A major difference between prokaryotic and eukaryotic mRNAs relates to the transcriptional unit structure. In prokaryotes, transcriptional units are generally polycistronic,

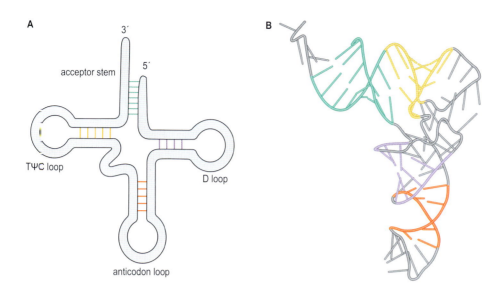

Fig. 21.2 **The structure of a tRNA molecule.** (A) The prototypical tRNA molecule consists of three hairpin-turn structures labeled the TψC loop, anticodon loop, and D loop. The three-dimensional structure of the molecule is generated by complementary base pairing between nucleotides within a single RNA. All tRNAs have this basic structure. (B) X-ray crystallographic analysis of a tRNA shows the L-shaped folded structure of the molecule, including the base pairing that holds the structure together. The colors of the loops in frame A are retained in the folded structure in frame B.

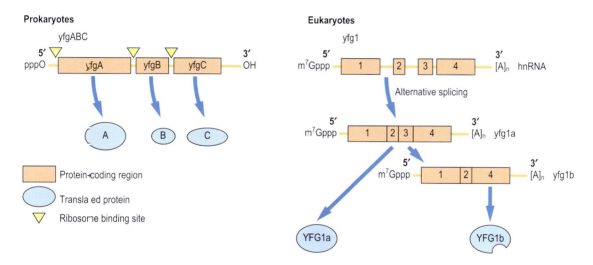

Fig. 21.3 **Prototypical structures of prokaryotic (polycistronic) and eukaryotic mRNAs.** Prokaryotic mRNAs have naked ends (triphosphate at the 5′ end and hydroxyl at the 3′ end). The boxes indicate those portions of the mRNA that encode a protein. Inverted triangles indicate location of ribosome-binding sites. The three genes in the prokaryotic cistron are translated into three different proteins. Other prokaryotic cistrons may encode up to 10 different proteins in a single mRNA. Nascent eukaryotic mRNA transcripts **(heterogeneous nuclear RNA [hnRNA])** contain both exons (boxes) and introns (lines). Eukaryotic mRNAs are protected by a 7-methylguanine nucleotide cap (m⁷Gppp) at the 5′ end and a poly(A) tail ([A]n) at the 3′ end of the mRNA. After splicing, the mature mRNAs consist only of exons plus the 5′ and 3′ UTRs. Alternatively, spliced mRNAs are translated into different protein isoforms. *yfg*, your favorite gene; UTR, untranslated region.

containing multiple protein-coding regions (Fig. 21.3), whereas in eukaryotes, each transcriptional unit generally codes for only a single protein. The **polycistronic mRNAs** of prokaryotes have individual start and stop codons at the beginning and end of each **open reading frame**, the sequence of mRNA that specifies the sequence of the polypeptide chain. Each stop codon is closely followed by another ribosome-binding site and

a translational start site that functions for the next open reading frame. In some cases, multiple proteins may be synthesized from a single eukaryotic gene transcript by **frameshifting**, in which alternative start sites produce different open reading frames and different proteins.

A second major difference between prokaryotic and eukaryotic mRNAs is the compartmentalization of transcription and translation. Because prokaryotes lack a nucleus, transcription and translation are intimately coupled in the cytoplasm; in fact, prokaryotic translation at the 5′ mRNA end is usually initiated before transcription at the 3′ end is finished. By coupling these processes. prokaryotes increase the rate at which proteins are expressed. This is consistent with the relatively short life cycles of prokaryotes. In contrast, eukaryotic cells separate transcription in the nucleus from translation in the cytoplasm. Although this arrangement slows response time for protein production, it allows for a more subtle control of protein expression.

The posttranscriptional processing of mRNAs is also significantly different in prokaryotes and eukaryotes. Because of their importance, these differences are detailed in a separate section dealing with posttranscriptional processing of RNAs. Briefly, eukaryotes protect the 5′ and 3′ ends of mRNAs by adding specific molecular structures (**5′ cap** and **poly[A] tail**) that function to reduce mRNA turnover. Eukaryotic genes also contain introns, sequences that interrupt the nascent transcripts and must be removed to produce mature mRNAs.

RIBONUCLEIC ACID POLYMERASES

RNA polymerases transcribe defined segments of DNA into RNA with a high degree of selectivity and specificity

The enzymes responsible for the synthesis of RNA are called RNA polymerases (RNAPol). In contrast to DNA polymerases (Chapter 20), RNA polymerases do not require a primer to initiate RNA synthesis. The RNA polymerases consist of two high-molecular-weight subunits and many smaller subunits, all of which are necessary for accurate transcription. Prokaryotes contain a single RNA polymerase that synthesizes all RNAs; however, eukaryotes contain three different RNA polymerases, termed RNA polymerase I, II, and III.

Each eukaryotic polymerase specializes in transcription of one class of RNA

■ RNAPol I transcribes ribosomal RNAs. All rRNAs are produced from a single transcriptional unit that is sub-

sequently processed to produce the 28-S, 18-S, 5.8-S, and 5-S rRNAs.
■ RNAPol II transcribes most genes within a eukaryotic cell, including all protein-coding genes that yield mRNA. RNAPol II is exquisitely sensitive to α-amanitin, a potent and toxic transcription inhibitor found in some poisonous mushrooms. RNAPol II also transcribes noncoding RNAs that produce micro-RNAs (discussed later in the chapter).
■ RNAPol III transcribes most of the small cellular RNAs, including the tRNAs.

MESSENGER RIBONUCLEIC ACID: TRANSCRIPTION

Transcription is a dynamic process involving interaction of enzymes with DNA to produce RNA molecules

It is convenient to divide transcription into three stages: initiation, elongation, and termination. Much can be learned about initiation from the structure of yeast RNAPol II. This enzyme consists of a 12-subunit core, and its structure is an excellent model for the human enzyme. It cycles between two alternative conformations. The first is an open form shaped like a cupped hand, with a cleft for binding the DNA molecule and associated transcription factors near the transcription start point. After melting and dissociation of the bound duplex DNA, the complex undergoes a large conformational change that closes the cleft, forming a clamp around the **antisense** or **template strand** of the DNA. The sense (nontemplate) strand is not bound. Then a specific protein *(rbp4/7)* binds to the base of the clamp, locking the clamp in the closed state, which is then competent for transcript elongation. During elongation, the RNAPol II enzyme proceeds along the antisense or template strand, producing a **complementary RNA** that is identical to the sense strand of the DNA (Fig. 21.4), except that the thymine residues in DNA are substituted by uracil residues in RNA. The yeast RNAPol II also appears to be a good model for the function of the RNAPol I and III enzymes because the core subunits are shared among the various enzymes.

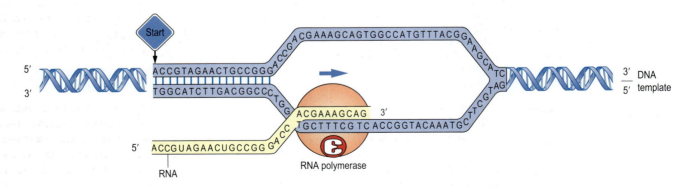

Fig. 21.4 **Transcription.** Transcription involves the synthesis of an RNA by RNA polymerase using DNA as a template. The RNA polymerase holoenzyme uses the antisense strand of DNA to direct the synthesis of an RNA molecule that is complementary to this strand.

The bacterial RNAPol is similar to the eukaryotic enzyme complexes, except the bacterial enzyme contains fewer subunits and, unlike the eukaryotic enzyme, requires only a single general transcription factor (α-factor) to recognize the promoter and recruit the RNA polymerase to initiate transcription.

CLINICAL BOX
α-AMANITIN POISONING: PICKING THE WRONG MUSHROOM

An otherwise healthy young woman arrives at the emergency room in the early morning with severe nausea, abdominal cramping, and copious diarrhea. The patient's vital signs show tachycardia, and the skin has poor turgor, indicating dehydration. While giving her medical history, the patient explains that her symptoms began suddenly, about 6 h after she had eaten dinner. Suspecting food poisoning, the patient is asked to recall everything eaten over the past 24 h. The patient reports that she had eaten mushrooms for dinner and added that the mushrooms were picked on a recent hike through the woods. The patient is started aggressively on saline and electrolytes to replenish lost fluids and given activated charcoal to absorb any residual or recirculating toxins in the gastrointestinal tract. The patient appears to stabilize over the next 24 h and is alert; however, she remains lethargic, and the skin begins to take on a yellowish tinge. Blood work shows reduced blood glucose, elevated serum aminotransferases, and increased prothrombin time, all indicative of hepatic stress. Amylase and lipase levels are normal, indicating no pancreatic involvement, and urinalysis indicates no renal involvement. The doctor consults a gastroenterologist, who advises increased monitoring of hepatorenal function and continued aggressive intravenous fluid and electrolyte treatment. After approximately 5 days, the patient recovers. What is the biochemical basis of this woman's illness?

Comment
About 95% of all mushroom fatalities in North America are associated with ingestion of mushrooms from the genus *Amanita*. These species produce a toxin, α-amanitin, that binds to RNAPol II and inhibits its function. The first cells to encounter the toxin are those lining the digestive tract. Cells incapable of synthesizing new mRNAs die, causing acute gastrointestinal distress. Liver failure is a serious complication of α-amanitin ingestion due to the induction of apoptosis in liver cells. Jaundice and liver function tests (transaminase, alkaline phosphate, bilirubin, aminotransferase levels, and prothrombin time) indicate the level of hepatic involvement (see Chapter 34). Most accidental mushroom exposures occur in children younger than 6 years old, who absorb a larger toxin dose per kilogram of body weight because of their size. However, even in adults, ingestion of a single *A. phalloides* mushroom can be fatal. Mortality ranges from 10% to 20% of all patients. No specific amatoxin antidote is available, although administration of high doses of penicillin G displaces amanitin from circulating plasma proteins, thereby promoting its excretion.

Initiation

Initiation begins with site-specific interaction of the RNA polymerase with DNA

Because most genomic DNA does not encode proteins, identification of transcription start sites is crucial to obtain desired mRNAs. Special sequences termed promoters recruit the RNA polymerase to the transcription start site (Fig. 21.5). Promoters are usually located in front (upstream) of the gene that is to be transcribed (see Chapter 23). However, RNA polymerase III promoters are located within the gene.

Prokaryotic genes generally contain simple promoters, which are rich in adenine (A) and thymine (T). The presence of these nucleotides facilitates separation of the two DNA strands because hydrogen bonding between A-T base pairs is weaker than that between G-C base pairs. Comparisons of large numbers of prokaryotic promoters have identified two common conserved regions. These are located about 10 nt and 35 nt upstream from the transcriptional start site (Fig. 21.5). The -10 sequence is known as the **TATA box.** This sequence binds the prokaryotic general transcription factor (σ-factor) that interacts and recruits the RNA polymerase to the promoter. Strong promoters tend to match a consensus sequence, whereas the sequences of weaker promoters differ from the consensus sequence and bind the σ-factor and the RNA polymerase less tightly and thus show reduced levels of transcription.

In eukaryotic RNAPol II promoters, **regulatory elements** (specific short DNA sequences) termed **upstream activation sequences (UASes),** enhancers, repressors, CAATT, and TATA box sequences are spread over several hundred to several thousand nucleotides. Individual transcription factors (activators or repressors) recognize and bind to these UASes. The control of initiation and the regulation of gene expression are outlined in detail in Chapter 22.

Elongation

Elongation is the process by which single nucleotides are added to the growing RNA chain

In prokaryotes, elongation is a relatively simple process. Ribonucleotides bind to an entry site on the RNA polymerase. If the incoming ribonucleotide matches the next base on the DNA template (i.e., forms compatible Watson–Crick base-pairing), the incoming ribonucleotide is transferred into the polymerase active site, and a new phosphodiester bond is formed. If it does not match, the ribonucleotide is released, and the process is repeated until the correct ribonucleotide is found. After the formation of the phosphodiester bond, the RNA polymerase moves along the template DNA strand. It is thought that the RNA polymerase accomplishes this by oscillating a small helical region of the RNA polymerase molecule between straight and bent conformations, permitting the polymerase to ratchet about 3 Å (~ 1 nucleotide step) along

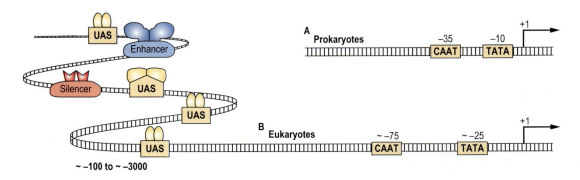

Fig. 21.5 **Prokaryotic and eukaryotic promoters.** (A) Prokaryotic promoters contain a TATA box at about 10 nt from the transcriptional start site (+1) and a CAAT box about 35-nt upstream from the +1 site. (B) Eukaryotic promoters also have TATA and CAAT boxes (slightly different from the prokaryotic boxes); however, these boxes are shifted upstream from the positions of prokaryotic boxes. Further upstream from the core promoter is a series of regulatory elements. These elements vary from promoter to promoter and can contain upstream activation sequences (UASes) that are recognized by one or several transcription factors. In addition, transcriptional enhancers and transcriptional silencers recognize specific elements that can exist in eukaryotic promoters (see Chapter 23).

the antisense strand. After translocation, another new nucleotide is added.

In eukaryotes, after RNA polymerase II initiates transcription, a pair of negative elongation regulatory factors (NELF and DSIF) traps the RNA polymerase in the starting position. An RNA protein complex, termed P-TEFb, is a kinase that phosphorylates these two inhibitory molecules, thereby releasing the RNA polymerase to continue RNA synthesis.

Vesicular stomatitis virus (VSV) and HIV produce viral proteins that stabilize the RNA polymerase complex, either directly or by recruiting host factors. The HIV protein TAT (a transactivating regulatory protein) is one of the better understood of these stabilization proteins. Upon interaction with RNA polymerase, the TAT protein rapidly recruits the P-TEFb complex, resulting in increased transcription of the full-length viral RNA at the expense of cellular RNAs.

Elongation can be a rapid process, occurring at the rate of ~40 nt per second. For elongation to occur, the double-stranded DNA must be continually unwound so that the template strand is accessible to the RNA polymerase. DNA **topoisomerases** I and II, enzymes associated with the transcription complex, move along the template with the RNA polymerase, separating DNA strands so that they are accessible for RNA synthesis.

Termination

Termination of transcription is catalyzed by multiple mechanisms in both prokaryotes and eukaryotes.

At the 3′-end of a transcriptional unit, the RNA polymerases terminate RNA synthesis at defined sites. Transcriptional termination mechanisms are much better understood in prokaryotes than in eukaryotes. In prokaryotes, termination occurs via one of two well-characterized mechanisms that require the formation of hairpin loops in the RNA secondary structure. In *rho*-dependent termination, the RNA transcript encodes a binding site for an ATP-dependent helicase, termed

rho, that unwinds the RNA transcript from DNA. It "chases" the RNA polymerase but is slower than RNA polymerase. A *rho*-termination site near the end of the transcriptional unit causes the RNA polymerase to pause, allowing the *rho* protein to catch up and unwind the RNA:DNA duplex displacing the RNA polymerase from the template, thereby stopping transcription. In *rho*-**in**dependent termination, a hairpin loop is formed just upstream of a sequence of six to eight uridine (U) residues located near the 3′ end of the transcript. The formation of this hairpin structure dislodges the RNA polymerase from the DNA template, resulting in termination of RNA synthesis.

In eukaryotes, the three RNA polymerases employ different mechanisms to terminate transcription. RNAPol I uses a specific protein, termination factor 1 (TTF1), that binds to an 18-nt terminator site located about 1000 nt downstream of the rRNA sequence. When RNAPol I encounters the TTF1 bound to DNA, a releasing factor releases the polymerase from the rRNA gene. RNAPol III uses a mechanism that is similar to bacterial *rho*-independent termination; however, the length of the uridine (U) stretch is shorter, and there is no requirement for an RNA secondary structure to dislodge RNAPol III. The mechanism of termination by RNAPol II, which transcribes most eukaryotic genes, is not well understood, in part because the RNAPol II products are immediately processed by removal of the nascent 3′ end and, immediately thereafter, the addition of a polyadenosine (poly[A]) tail.

POSTTRANSCRIPTIONAL PROCESSING OF RIBONUCLEIC ACIDS

The prokaryotic life strategy is to replicate as rapidly as possible when conditions support growth. Eukaryotes have a more controlled life strategy that invests more fully in increased regulation to achieve stable growth but limits rapid reproduction. Both

CLINICAL BOX
A STUBBORN MICROBE

A young charity worker reports to your clinic. He has just returned from a prolonged period of work overseas. He complains of fever, weight loss, fatigue, and night sweats. He has a productive cough. When telling his medical history, he relates that a local physician treated him with rifampicin, a powerful inhibitor of bacterial RNA polymerase, but his condition was not improved. In fact, he complains that his condition has worsened. On physical exam, you note that he has abnormal breath sounds in the upper lobes of the lungs. You suspect tuberculosis, so you order a tuberculin skin test, and because the culture of mycobacteria can take weeks, you also order a polymerase chain reaction (PCR) test (Chapter 24) specific for the assay of *Mycobacterium tuberculosis* DNA. You admit the young man to an isolation room. The next day, the PCR-based test returns positive for *M. tuberculosis,* and after 72 h, the tuberculin skin test shows an induration 10 mm in diameter, indicating a rather strong response. The patient asks you why the antibiotics have not worked.

Comment

Antibiotics work by targeting specific functions in the cell. Rifampicin is a potent inhibitor of prokaryotic RNA polymerases, but not eukaryotic RNA polymerases. Although rifampicin is one of the indicated antibiotics for tuberculosis, the patient's condition has worsened, causing you to suspect that this young man may have an antibiotic-resistant or multidrug-resistant (MDR) form of tuberculosis. Antibiotic-resistant forms are increasingly common in tuberculosis, as they are in many bacterial diseases. You order growth tests on the mycobacterium isolate to determine if the strain is indeed multidrug-resistant tuberculosis (MDR-TB), and you immediately start the patient on a multidrug regimen designed to combat MDR-TB. After 2 weeks of daily dosing, the patient can be switched to dosing of two to three times per week. Vital staining of sputum with fluorescein diacetate (FDA), which indicates living bacilli after initial antibiotic treatment, is recommended to confirm MDR-TB. Continued treatment of MDR-TB can last for 18 to 24 months, and consultations should be made with an expert on MDR-TB. Because many patients do not complete the full antibiotic regimen, relapse is high for MDR-TB, from 20% to 65%.

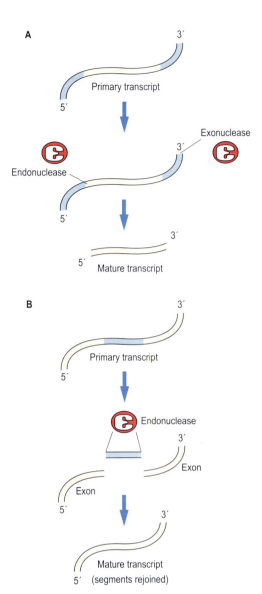

Fig. 21.6 **RNA processing.** There are two general types of RNA processing events. Processing of an RNA transcript can involve (A) the removal of excess sequences by the action of endonucleases and exonucleases as in the processing of rRNA and tRNA genes, or (B) the removal of excess sequences and the rejoining of segments of the newly transcribed RNA as in splicing of mRNAs.

strategies work well for each type of organism, as evidenced by the rich diversity of life on Earth; consequently, mechanisms of RNA synthesis and processing have evolved to optimize each life strategy.

Pre-rRNA and pre-tRNA

rRNAs and tRNAs are synthesized as larger precursors (pre-RNAs) that are processed to yield mature transcripts (Fig. 21.6)

In prokaryotes, a single 30-S (~6.5-kb) rRNA transcript contains specific leader and trailer regions located at the 5' and 3' ends

of the transcript as well as one copy each of the 23-S, 16-S, and 5-S rRNAs. This arrangement is clearly advantageous to maintain the ratio of large to small ribosomal subunits. The rRNA genes also contain a number of tRNAs that are embedded in the pre-rRNA transcript. The rRNA transcript must be processed to liberate the various functional RNAs.

In prokaryotes, processing of the pre-rRNA requires several RNases. Ribonuclease III (RNase III) cleaves the pre-rRNA in double-stranded regions that occur at each end of the 16-S and 23-S rRNAs. Their cleavage liberates the rRNAs from the pre-rRNA transcript. The 16-S and 23-S rRNAs are further processed at their 5′ and 3′ ends; this trimming requires the presence of specific ribosomal proteins and occurs during ribosome assembly.

In all eukaryotes, from yeast to mammals, pre-rRNA transcripts are processed in a manner similar to the prokaryotic pre-rRNA processing. Every 45-S (~13.7-kb) rRNA transcript includes a single copy of the 18-S, 5.8-S, and 28-S rRNAs (in eukaryotes, the 5-S rRNA is separately encoded). However, processing of the human rRNA is more complex. The pre-rRNA transcript is cleaved at 11 different sites to generate the mature 18-S, 5.8-S, and 28-S rRNAs. Processing occurs on a huge ribonucleoprotein complex, termed the **processome.** In addition to modifications by cleavage, the mature human rRNA contains 115 specific methyl-group modifications (in most of these, the methyl group is added not to nucleobase but to the backbone ribosyl-2′-hydroxyl group, yielding a 2′-O-methyl modification) and 95 specific uridine-to-pseudouridine (U-to-ψ) conversions. These modifications are introduced into the pre-rRNA through the interaction with individual small nucleolar RNA protein complexes (**snoRNPs,** pronounced "snorps"). Each of these snoRNPs contains a unique guide RNA (~60 to 300 nt in length) and from one to four protein molecules. Each snoRNP is specific for a single or at most a few individual modification sites. The **snoRNA** (small ribonuclear RNA) component of the snoRNPs contains highly conserved structural motifs that belong to two groups, either the C/D box or the H/ACA box, the latter containing two hairpin loops. These sequences direct binding of snoRNPs to sites in the pre-rRNA molecules through a complementary nucleotide stretch (~10 to 20 nucleotides). This correctly positions a methyl transferase (box C/D) or a pseudouridine synthase (box H/ACA) along the pre-rRNA for modification. The processome is a complex structure, containing more than 100 snoRNAs and more than 100 individual proteins.

In addition to the rRNA genes, tRNAs are also synthesized in precursor form. As many as seven individual tRNAs can be synthesized from a single pre-tRNA gene. Processing of the tRNAs from the pre-tRNAs requires RNase P, which cleaves each tRNA from the pre-tRNA by a single cleavage at its 5′ end. RNase P is ribonucleoprotein complex containing a 377-nucleotide RNA and a 20-kDa protein. The protein portion is not required for enzymatic activity (i.e., the RNA is catalytic by itself). Another enzyme, RNase D, trims away the extra 3′ nucleotides from the pre-tRNAs, leaving the invariant CCA that is found at the 3′ end of every tRNA. A few tRNAs also contain introns within their anticodon loops, which must be removed during processing.

Ribozymes

In some instances, RNAs have a catalytic activity similar to the type of activities previously ascribed only to proteins (i.e., ribonuclease activity). These unusual catalytic RNAs are known

ADVANCED CONCEPT BOX
THE RNA WORLD AND RIBOZYMES

Primordial organisms appeared on earth about 3.5 billion years ago. The mechanisms that describe this transition from no life to life are not understood. The central dogma of molecular biology states that "DNA makes RNA, makes protein." However, over the past few decades, a novel idea has emerged that suggests that DNA may not have been the original nucleic acid. Instead, it is currently believed that RNAs were the most primitive catalytic biopolymers to form on earth. There are several lines of evidence that support this hypothesis. First is the discovery of self-splicing RNA - that is, the self-removal of introns from pre-mRNAs by endogenous enzymatic activity. Second, the ribosome is a large molecular complex of RNA and protein; however, both structural and biochemical analysis of ribosomes reveals that the mechanism of protein synthesis is catalyzed by the rRNA and not the ribosomal proteins. Thus the earliest life-forms may have used RNA to both store genetic information and catalyze biochemical processes even before proteins developed. Then, early in life's history, a ribozyme that could copy or replicate RNA storage strands evolved. Later, a more stable information-storage system (DNA) and improved catalytic structures (proteins) evolved to yield our current life strategy.

as ribozymes. The substrate specificity of a ribozyme is determined by nucleotide base pairing between complementary sequences contained within the enzyme and the RNA substrate that it cleaves. Just like proteinaceous enzymes, the ribozyme is a catalyst that cleaves its substrate (RNA) at a specific site and then releases it, without itself being consumed in the reaction. Some RNA viruses and virus-like particles, such as hepatitis virus delta agent (HVD), utilize a rolling–circle replicative cycle that require ribozymes to cleave viral RNAs from the pre-RNA product.

Because sequences required for ribozyme activity have been identified, ribozymes have been designed that will cleave allele-specific RNAs. Recombinant ribozymes are being considered as possible therapeutic agents for diseases such as muscular dystrophy, Alzheimer's, Huntington's, and Parkinson's, which are caused by the inappropriate expression of mutated RNAs. Although studies in humans are still at an experimental stage, rats treated with ribozymes specific for the mitochondrial aldehyde dehydrogenase *(ALDH2)* gene exhibit a decrease in voluntary alcohol consumption.

Pre-mRNA processing

Prokaryotes rapidly synthesize their mRNAs and typically do not process or modify them; both the 5′ and the 3′ ends of prokaryotic mRNAs are naked and unprotected. Consequently, even newly synthesized mRNAs are rapidly degraded by normal cellular RNases. This is not a problem for rapidly growing organisms (bacteria) because they quickly alter the rate of RNA synthesis for protein production. After their immediate needs have been met, they subsequently degrade their mRNAs and reuse the ribonucleotides for the synthesis of other mRNAs. A typical half-life of prokaryotic mRNAs is about 3 min. In contrast, eukaryotes take special precautions to stably maintain their mRNAs for continued use. mRNA half-lives in eukaryotes range from a few minutes for some highly regulated transcription factors to as long as 30 h for some long-lived transcripts.

Eukaryotic mRNAs have longer half-lives than prokaryotic mRNAs because of protective modifications at their 5′ and 3′ ends

Eukaryotes have evolved methods to protect each end of their mRNAs. At the 5′ end, a unique structure termed a **5′-cap** is added. The cap consists of a **7-methylguanidine** residue that is attached in the *reverse orientation* to the first nucleotide of the mRNA - that is, by a 5′-to-5′ triphosphate linkage. Because the mRNA capping enzyme also interacts with the RNAPol II, the addition of the cap to the nascent mRNA occurs soon after the mRNA synthesis begins. Most cellular exo-RNases do not have the ability to hydrolyze this cap from the mRNA, so the 5′ end is protected from exo-5′-RNase activity. At the 3′ end of nearly all eukaryotic mRNAs (with the exception of histone mRNAs), a polyadenosine track (the **poly[A] tail**) is added as soon as the mRNA synthesis has concluded. The adenosine residues are not encoded by the DNA; instead, they are added by the action of poly(A) polymerase using ATP as a substrate. This poly(A) tail is frequently more than 250 nucleotides in length. Although it is still susceptible to the action of exo-3′-RNases, the presence of the poly(A) tail significantly reduces the turnover of mRNA, thereby increasing its lifetime. The presence of the poly(A) tail has historically been used to isolate mRNA from eukaryotic cells by affinity chromatography.

The spliceosome joins exons from pre-mRNA to form a mature mRNA

In the more complicated posttranscriptional processing of eukaryotic mRNAs, sequences called **introns** (intervening sequences) are removed from the primary transcript, pre-RNA, the major component of heterogeneous nuclear RNA (hnRNA). The remaining segments, termed **exons** (expressed sequences), are ligated to form a functional mRNA. This process involves a large complex of proteins and auxiliary RNAs called small nuclear RNAs (snRNAs; pronounced "snurps"), which interact to form a **spliceosome.** The function of the five snRNAs (U1, U2, U4, U5, U6) in the spliceosome is to help position reacting groups within the substrate mRNA molecule so that the introns can be removed and the appropriate exons can be spliced together (Table 21.3). The snRNAs accomplish this task by base pairing with sites on the mRNA that represent intron/exon boundaries.

Table 21.3 The function of small nuclear RNAs (snRNA) in the splicing of mRNAs

snRNA	Size	Function
U1	165 nt	Binds the 5′ exon/intron boundary
U2	185 nt	Binds the branch site on the intron
U4	145 nt	Helps assemble the spliceosome
U5	116 nt	Binds the 3′ intron/exon boundary
U6	106 nt	Displaces U1 after first rearrangement

The removal of an intron and rejoining of two exons can be considered to occur in three steps (Fig. 21.7). The first step involves the binding of the U1 snRNA to the exon/intron boundary at the 5′ end of the intron, along with the binding of the U2 snRNA to a target adenosine nucleotide, usually found about 30 nt upstream of the 3′ end of the intron. After binding of the U4/U5/U6 snRNP complex just upstream of the 5′ splice site, the intron loops back on itself, positioning the ends of the introns in the correct orientation. In this process, the U6 snRNP displaces the U1 snRNP from the mRNA. Subsequently, a transesterification reaction between the 2′-hydroxyl of the target adenosine and the phosphodiester bond of the intron's 5′-guanosine residue breaks the upstream splice site and forms a branched-chain structure in which the target adenosine has 2′-, 3′-, and 5′-phosphate groups. The looped structure of the intron is similar in appearance to a cowboy's **lariat**. After a subsequent physical rearrangement that releases the U4 snRNP, a second transesterification reaction ligates the 3′ end of exon 1 with the 5′ end of exon 2. The spliceosome then disassembles, releasing the lariat structure, which is degraded, and the mature mRNA is ready for further processing.

Alternative splicing produces multiple mRNAs from a single pre-mRNA transcript

Most eukaryotic mRNAs consist of multiple introns and multiple exons. If splicing were consistent, only a single mature mRNA would result from the pre-mRNAs. However, many eukaryotic genes undergo a process called **alternative splicing**, in which different mRNA regions are removed from the pre-mRNA, resulting in multiple mature mRNAs with different sequences. When these different mRNAs are translated, multiple protein isoforms are produced. In humans, almost 60% of pre-mRNAs give rise to multiple mature mRNAs after alternative splicing. About 80% of these alternatively spliced mRNAs result in alterations in the encoded proteins. Alternative splicing can result in insertion or deletion of amino acids in the protein sequence, shifts in reading frames, or even introduction of novel stop codons. Such alternative splicing can also add or remove mRNA sequences that can alter regulatory elements affecting translation, mRNA stability, or subcellular localization.

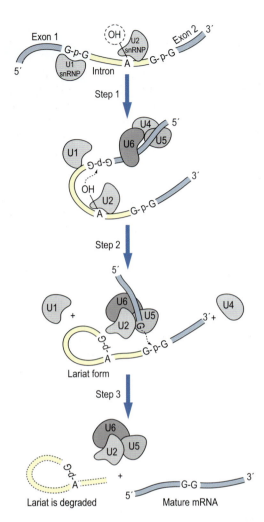

Fig. 21.7 **RNA splicing.** RNA splicing is a multistep process catalyzed by ribonucleoprotein complexes, "simplified" in this diagram. In a transesterification reaction, the phosphate bond of a guanosine residue at the 5' exon/intron boundary is broken and joined to the 2'-OH of an adenine residue located in the middle of the intron. In a later step, the phosphate bond at the 3' intron/exon boundary is first cleaved, and then the two exons are spliced together by reformation of a phospho-diester bond between the nucleotides at either end of the exons. The intron is eliminated in the form of a lariat structure, cyclized through a 2',3'5'-phosphorylated adenosine residue. N, any nucleotide.

Editosomes modify the nucleotide sequence of mature mRNAs

Finally, in some instances, mRNAs are posttranscriptionally modified by a large multiprotein complex termed the **editosome.** Several different editing mechanisms are involved. These include specific C-to-U modifications catalyzed by cytosine deaminases or A-to-I modifications catalyzed by adenosine deaminases; even deletion of single or multiple U residues to change the nucleotide sequence of the mRNA, often in the 3' untranslated region of the mRNA. These changes result in frameshifting and codon changes that produce different amino

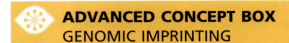

ADVANCED CONCEPT BOX
GENOMIC IMPRINTING

snoRNAs also function in genomic imprinting. Genomic imprinting is an epigenetic process that results in differential expression of maternal and paternal genes in a developing embryo. This process occurs in both mammals and plants because both of these groups of organisms share placental connections with their offspring. Specific genes are methylated during meiosis and thereby inactivated. This methylation occurs differentially in oocyte and spermatocyte development, thereby uniquely inactivating either the maternal or the paternal alleles during embryonic development. Genomic imprinting can affect a number of health risks in humans, including susceptibility to asthma, cancer, diabetes, obesity, and neurobehavioral disorders, such as Angelman and Prader–Willi syndromes. These syndromes are caused by deletion of the same 2.0-Mb domain (15q11-q13) of chromosome 15 that contains a cluster of imprinted genes. They are dissimilar disorders because the deleted region contains both paternally and maternally imprinted genes. These include the paternally expressed proteins (NDN, MKRN3, MAGEL2, SNURF-SNRPN) as well as C/D box snoRNAs and a single maternally expressed gene, ubiquitin ligase (*UBE3A*). Inheritance of the deletion of this imprinted region from either the father or the mother results in either Angelman or Prader–Willi syndrome. At least 83 genes in humans and more than 1300 genes in mice are known to be imprinted.

acid sequences in the protein and can also cause changes in levels of mRNA expression.

The snoRNAs that function in rRNA and tRNA modifications also function in the mRNA editing processes. The snoRNAs bind to the editing sites within the mRNAs and position the editosome with either cytosine deaminase or adenosine deaminase activity at the correct position to complete the modification.

SELECTIVE DEGRADATION OR INACTIVATION OF mRNA

Micro-RNAs, siRNA, RNAi, and RISC

Only 3% of the human genome encodes for mRNA exons - and therefore proteins - but almost 80% of the genome is transcribed. So what is this large amount of transcribed, noncoding RNAs within the cell, and what does it do? The DNA source of these noncoding RNAs was originally called "junk DNA," but more recent studies suggest that these sequences have significant functions in regulating the expression of normal cellular mRNAs.

One of the most unique classes of RNA consists of a group of uniquely small RNAs that bind to and affect normal gene expression within cells. These fall into two large categories:

miRNAs and siRNAs. Micro-RNAs (miRNA) are noncoding RNAs that are predicted to regulate large fractions (up to 30%) of all protein-coding genes in both plants and animals. This regulation of genes by miRNAs permits the cell to fine-tune the level of gene expression in itself. Small interfering RNAs (siRNA) are derived from double-stranded RNAs (dsRNA); they function in a manner similar to mi-RNAs to down-regulate gene expression.

miRNAs

Primary transcripts of miRNAs, pri-miRNA, are transcribed by RNAPol II from noncoding portions of the genome. The primary-miRNA genes contain natural inverted duplications that, upon transcription, are able to form multiple native hairpin folds within the pri-miRNAs (Fig. 21.8). These folds may encompass similar or different miRNAs. The authentic miRNAs are excised from the pri-miRNAs by a pair of RNase III–type proteins. The first of these proteins, termed **Drosha**,

is nuclear-localized and cleaves the pri-miRNAs into individual pre-miRNAs. Subsequently, after GTP-dependent transport from the nucleus, the pre-miRNA interacts in the cytoplasm with the second RNase III protein, Dicer. **Dicer** cleaves the pre-miRNA into very small (21- to 25-nt) fragments with 3′ overhanging ends. Further processing by phosphorylation results in a double-stranded miRNA duplex. This phosphory-lated duplex is unwound, producing a "guide strand" that is bound by the **Argonaute** protein (AGO) and a "passenger strand" that is degraded. The Argonaute (with bound guide strand) is then loaded into a multiprotein complex dubbed the **RNA-induced silencing complex**, or **RISC**. The RISC/ guide strand then acts as an RNA-targeting cofactor that scans cellular mRNAs for complementary sequences. Once a complementary sequence is identified and bound by the RISC/ guide-strand complex, the Argonaute protein activates and cleaves the target mRNA, resulting in down-regulation of gene expression.

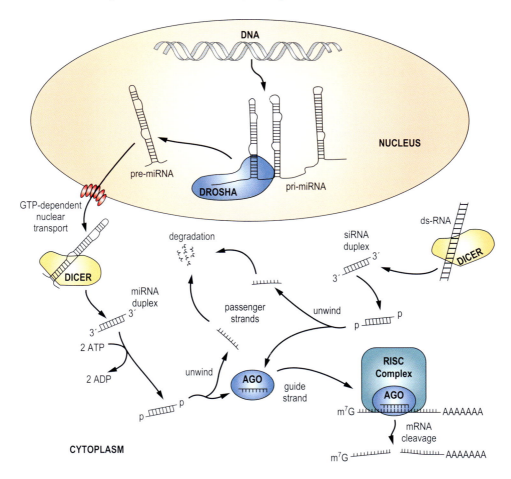

Fig. 21.8 **Synthesis and action of miRNAs and siRNAs.** In the nucleus, pri-miRNAs are synthesized from noncoding portions of the genomes. The pri-miRNAs are recognized by an RNase, Drosha, to cleave the primary miRNAs into pre-miRNAs. After export from the nucleus to the cytoplasm, a second RNase, Dicer, cleaves the small double-stranded fragments (21–25 nt) from the pre-miRNA. After phosphorylation, the miRNA duplex is unwound, and the guide strand is bound to the protein Argonaute (AGO). The Argonaute/guide complex is then loaded into the RNA-induced silencing complex (RISC). The RISC scans cellular mRNAs for sequences complementary to the guide strand. Any recognized mRNAs activate Argonaute, which cleaves those recognized mRNAs, downregulating gene expression. siRNAs are similarly processed but from double-stranded RNAs found in the cytoplasm and originally derived from viral RNAs.

The human genome may contain more than 900 miRNA sequences. Some of these target many different cellular genes (perhaps as many as 200 genes) and can therefore affect hundreds or thousands of different mRNAs. Some gene sequences contain multiple miRNA target sites and are therefore regulated by multiple miRNAs, suggesting complex regulatory networks coordinating gene expression. miRNAs regulate central metabolic processes such as adipocyte differentiation and insulin production, which are involved in the development of obesity and diabetes.

si-RNAs

Small interfering RNAs (siRNA) are part of the innate cellular immunity of cells that specifically targets RNA sequences for rapid degradation. This process is termed RNA interference (RNAi) or posttranscriptional gene silencing (PTGS). The siRNAs are derived from duplex RNAs introduced into the cell by viral infection rather than from the cellular genome. They are thought to have evolved as a defense against double-stranded forms of RNA viruses, but they also function as an endogenous mechanism for gene regulation during the development of eukaryotes.

This process begins when duplex RNA is recognized within cells by Dicer. As before, Dicer produces short duplex RNA fragments similar to miRNA duplex. After unwinding, the guide strand of the siRNA duplex is bound by Argonaute and functions to degrade expressed cellular mRNAs. During the innate cellular immune response, siRNAs and RISC function to degrade the replicative forms of many RNA viruses. This process has been widely used by researchers to down-regulate gene expression for functional studies on numerous genes of interest as well as for therapeutic options (see accompanying Advanced Concept Box).

Interferon activates additional pathways that inhibit proliferation of RNA viruses

RNA viruses pose a major challenge for eukaryotic cells. They generally form a double-stranded (ds) replicative intermediate during their life cycles, and this unique structure is not found in eukaryotic cells. In addition to recognition by Drosha and siRNAs, it can be recognized by other dsRNA-binding proteins and will subsequently trigger responses to limit viral infection. One of these mechanisms involves the **dsRNA-activated protein kinase R (PKR)**. When activated by binding dsRNA, PKR can phosphorylate and inactivate the protein translation factor, eIF2α, thereby down-regulating translation when dsRNA is present in the cell. Likewise, when activated by dsRNA, the enzyme 2′-5′-oligoadenylate synthase polymerizes ATP into a series of short nucleotides (**2′-5′-oligoadenylate, [2-5 A]** - different from the 5′–3′ structure found in normal RNA). The most active form is a trimer, pppA-2′-p-5′-A-2′-p - 5′-A. The accumulation of 2-5 A oligonucleotides inhibits viral (and host) protein translation by activating an endoribonuclease (RNase L) that indiscriminately degrades both mRNAs and rRNAs within the cell. Both genes, PKR and 2-5 A synthase, are induced by interferon, which is itself upregulated by viral infection. This results in an efficient amplification mechanism, leading to programmed cell death (**apoptosis**) to limit the growth and spread of the virus.

ADVANCED CONCEPT BOX
RNAI AS A THERAPEUTIC OPTION

Age-related macular degeneration (AMD) is the leading cause of blindness for the elderly in the developed world. AMD results from an atrophy of the macula in the retina. The result of atrophy is a loss of central vision, which can lead to the inability to read or even recognize faces of loved ones. The most severe type of AMD (the wet form) causes vision loss due to overgrowth of blood vessels (neovascularization) in the retinal choriocapillaris, which leads to blood and protein leakage beneath the macula if untreated. This eventually causes scarring and irreversible damage to the photoreceptors.

One mechanism that causes neovascularization is the aberrant expression of proangiogenic vascular endothelial growth factor (VEGF) in the retina, which results in blood vessel outgrowth. One approach to the treatment of AMD involves the injection of anti-VEGF antibodies (ranibizumab [Lucentis] or bevacizumab [Avastin]) directly into the vitreous humor of the eye. These antibodies bind to and inactivate VEGF, thereby reducing angiogenesis and prolonging eyesight. Recent studies using long-term drug-releasing technologies (polymer nanostructures) suggest that drug-releasing devices can be implanted into the vitreous humor and provide sustained release of the active agents for up to 12 months.

The ability of a cell to down-regulate specific mRNAs, coupled with the localized treatment area offered by the vitreous humor, make the VEGF gene an ideal candidate for RNAi-mediated down-regulation. Small RNA molecules complementary to VEGF mRNA are injected into the vitreous humor. When these molecules are taken into the cell, they function as siRNAs, causing degradation of VEGF mRNA and decreasing VEGF biosynthesis. Other siRNA studies are well under way. In 2016, at least 29 different clinical trials of RNAi drug candidates were in progress against 27 targets of many different diseases.

SUMMARY

The major products of transcription are the rRNAs, tRNAs, and mRNAs. These RNAs perform specific functions within a cell: mRNAs carry the genetic information from nuclear DNA to ribosomes for proteins synthesis; rRNAs interact with proteins to form ribosomes, the cellular machinery on which protein synthesis occurs; and tRNAs function as amino acid carriers that link (translate) the information stored in the mRNA nucleotide sequence to the amino acid sequence of proteins.

■ In eukaryotic cells, each of these RNA classes is produced by a different, specific RNA polymerase

ACTIVE LEARNING

1. Which commonly used antibiotics are directed at inhibition of bacterial RNA polymerase but do not affect the mammalian complex? Why are these drugs less effective against fungal infections?
2. Review the pathogenesis of systemic lupus erythematosus (SLE), an autoimmune disease in which antibodies to ribonucleoprotein particles are implicated in the development of chronic inflammation. The clinical presentation of SLE includes swelling of joints, fever > 100°F, hair loss, nose or mouth sores, and skin rash following sun exposure. Explain how each of these symptoms may result from SLE pathogenesis.
3. Review the pathogenesis of hemoglobin E/β-thalassemia. Understand how the Hb-E single-point mutation at codon 26 (β26; GAG → AAG) can result in reduced accumulation of the hemoglobin E transcript and result in β-thalassemia.

(RNAPol I, II, or III), whereas in bacterial cells, a single RNA polymerase synthesizes all three classes of RNA.

- The basic structures of rRNAs and tRNAs from eukaryotic and bacterial cells are similar. However, mRNAs from eukaryotic cells have a 5'-(m^{7}Gppp) cap and a 3'-poly(A) tail. Prokaryotic mRNA transcripts do not have these modifications on their 5' and 3' ends and can be polycistronic.
- Most, but not all, eukaryotic mRNAs undergo a process called splicing to be functional, whereas prokaryotic mRNAs are functional as soon as they are synthesized. Splicing involves the removal of intervening sequences called introns and rejoining of expressed sequences called exons to form a mature, functional mRNA.
- The process of transcription consists of three parts: initiation, elongation, and termination. Initiation involves the recognition and binding of promoter sequences by RNA polymerase and associated transcriptional cofactors. Elongation involves the selection of the appropriate nucleotide and formation of phosphodiester bridges between each nucleotide in an RNA molecule. Finally, termination involves the dissociation of the RNA polymerase from the DNA template. This is mediated by either RNA secondary structure or specific protein factors.
- Small RNA molecules, miRNAs, direct specific cleavage of mRNAs, downregulating the expression of genes or networks of genes.

FURTHER READING

Baralle, D., & Buratti, E. (2017). RNA splicing in human disease and in the clinic. *Clinical Science*, 131, 355–368.

Bobbin, M. L., & Rossi, J. J. (2016). RNA Interference (RNAi)-based therapeutics: Delivering on the promise? *Annual Review of Pharmacology and Toxicology*, 56, 103–122.

Chapman, C. G., & Pekow, J. (2015). The emerging role of miRNAs in inflammatory bowel disease: A review. *Therapeutic Advances in Gastroenterology*, 8, 4–22.

Li, Y., Sun, N., Lu, Z., et al. (2017). Prognostic alternative mRNA splicing signatures in non-small cell lung cancer. *Cancer Letters*, 393, 40–51.

Li, X. (2014). miR-375, a microRNA related to diabetes. *Gene*, 533, 1–4.

Mouillet, J.-F., Ouyang, Y., Coyne, C. B., et al. (2015). MicroRNAs in placental health and disease. *American Journal of Obstetrics and Gynecology*, 213(Suppl. 4), S163–S172.

Posthuma, C. C., Te Welthuis, A. J., & Snijder, E. J. (2017). Nidovirus RNA polymerases: Complex enzymes handling exceptional RNA genomes. *Virus Research*, 234, 58–73.

Smith, A., & Hung, D. (2017). The dilemma of diagnostic testing for Prader-Willi syndrome. *Translational Pediatrics*, 6, 46–56.

Wen, M. M. (2016). Getting miRNA therapeutics into the target cells for neurodegenerative diseases: A mini-review. *Frontiers in Molecular Neuroscience*, 9, 129.

Xu, Y., & Vakocm, C. R. (2017). Targeting cancer cells with BET bromodomain inhibitors. *Cold Spring Harbor Perspectives in Medicine*, 7(7), doi:10.1101/cshperspect.a026674.

RELEVANT WEBSITES

RNA polymerase:
   http://www.rcsb.org/pdb/101/motm.do?momID=40
   http://www.ncbi.nlm.nih.gov/books/NBK22085/
Spliceosome and alternative splicing:
   http://www.eurasnet.info/alternative-splicing/what-is-alternative-splicing/AS
micro-RNA and RNAi:
   http://www.sigmaaldrich.com/life-science/functional-genomics-and-rnai/mirna/learning-center/mirna-introduction.html
   http://www.youtube.com/watch?v=cK-OGB1_ELE
   http://www.youtube.com/watch?v=5YsTW5iOXro
   https://www.ibiology.org/genetics-and-gene-regulation/introduction-to-micrornas/
   http://www.youtube.com/watch?v=IOmHDBX4jQk
Macular degeneration:
   http://www.macular.org/what-macular-degeneration
   https://nei.nih.gov/health/maculardegen/armd_facts
The RNA world:
   https://www.ibiology.org/evolution/origin-of-life/

ABBREVIATIONS

dsRNA	Double stranded RNA
hnRNA	Hetergeneous nuclear RNA
kb	Kilobase
MDR	Multi-drug resistance
mRNA	Messenger RNA
miRNA	Micro-RNA
nt	Nucleotide
RISC	RNA-induced silencing complex
RNApol	RNA polymerase
rRNA	Ribosomal RNA
siRNA	Small interfering RNA
snoRNA	Small ribonuclear RNA
snoRNP	Small ribonuclear protein complex
tRNA	Transfer RNA
UAS	Upstream activation sequence
UTR	Untranslated region

Protein Synthesis and Turnover

Edel M. Hyland and Jeffrey R. Patton

LEARNING OBJECTIVES

After reading this chapter, you should be able to:

- Describe how various RNAs involved in protein synthesis interact to produce a polypeptide.
- Outline the structure and redundancy of the genetic code.
- Explain how proteins are targeted to specific subcellular organelles.
- Describe the major steps in synthesis and degradation of a cytosolic protein.

INTRODUCTION

Translation is the process by which the information encoded in an mRNA is translated into the primary structure of a protein

Protein synthesis or translation represents the culmination of the transfer of genetic information, stored as nucleotide bases in deoxyribonucleic acid (DNA), to protein molecules that are the major structural and functional components of living cells. It is during translation that this information, expressed as a specific nucleotide sequence in a messenger ribonucleic acid (mRNA) molecule, is used to direct the synthesis of a protein. The protein then folds into a three-dimensional structure that is defined, in large part, by its amino acid sequence. To translate an mRNA into protein, three main RNA components are necessary:

- Ribosomes, containing ribosomal RNA (rRNA)
- Messenger RNA (mRNA)
- Transfer RNA (tRNA)

The ribosome, composed of both rRNAs and numerous proteins, is the macromolecular machine on which all protein synthesis occurs. The information required to direct the synthesis of the primary sequence of the protein is contained in mRNA. The amino acids that are to be incorporated into the protein are enzymatically attached to specific tRNAs through a process called charging. The ribosome facilitates the interaction between the mRNA and the charged tRNA molecules so that the correct amino acid is incorporated into the growing polypeptide chain. The translation of mRNA begins

near the 5′ end of the template and moves toward the 3′ end, and proteins are synthesized starting with their amino-terminal ends. Therefore the 5′ end of the RNA encodes the amino-terminal end of the protein, and the 3′ end of the RNA encodes the carboxyl-terminal end of the protein.

This chapter begins with an introduction to the genetic code and the components needed for protein synthesis. This is followed by the presentation of the structure and function of the ribosome, detailing the process of translation by outlining the initiation, elongation, and termination of protein synthesis and the mechanism by which proteins are targeted to specific locations in the cell. After a discussion of posttranslational modifications of proteins, the chapter ends with a description of the role of a second macromolecular complex, the **proteasome,** in protein quality control and turnover.

THE GENETIC CODE

The genetic code is degenerate and not quite universal

The mRNA template for translation is composed of only four nucleotides - adenosine, A; cytidine, C; guanosine, G; and uridine, U - but it will encode a protein containing as many as 20 different amino acids. As such, there is not a one-to-one correspondence between nucleotide and amino acid sequence; instead, a series of three nucleotides in the mRNA, known as a **codon,** is required to specify each amino acid. When all combinations of four nucleotides are taken into account, three at a time, 64 possible codons result (Table 22.1). Three of these codons (UAA, UAG, UGA) are **stop codons,** used to signal the termination of protein synthesis; they do not specify an amino acid. The remaining 61 codons specify the 20 amino acids, which illustrates that the genetic code is **degenerate,** meaning that more than one codon can specify a specific amino acid. For example, codons GUU, GUC, GUA, and GUG all code for the amino acid valine. Indeed, all the amino acids, with the exception of methionine (AUG) and tryptophan (UGG), have more than one codon. The codon AUG, which specifies methionine, encodes methionine anywhere it appears in the RNA, but it also has a unique function in defining the starting point for protein synthesis in most mRNAs (see the following discussion for a few exceptions).

The genetic code as specified by the triplet nucleotides is, for the most part, the same for all organisms and is referred to as "universal." However, there are notable exceptions. In bacteria, for example, both GUG and UUG can be read as a

Table 22.1 The genetic code

First position	Second position				Third position
	G	A	C	U	
G	Gly	Glu	Ala	Val	G
	Gly	Glu	Ala	Val	A
	Gly	Asp	Ala	Val	C
	Gly	Asp	Ala	Val	U
A	Arg	Lys	Thr	Met	G
	Arg	Lys	Thr	Ile	A
	Ser	Asn	Thr	Ile	C
	Ser	Asn	Thr	Ile	U
C	Arg	Gln	Pro	Leu	G
	Arg	Gln	Pro	Leu	A
	Arg	His	Pro	Leu	C
	Arg	His	Pro	Leu	U
U	Trp	Stop	Ser	Leu	G
	Stop	Stop	Ser	Leu	A
	Cys	Tyr	Ser	Phe	C
	Cys	Tyr	Ser	Phe	U

The genetic code is degenerate, meaning more than one codon can code for a given amino acid, and in many cases, changing the nucleotide at the third position does not change the amino acid encoded. To find the sequence(s) of the codons that encode a particular amino acid, one simply finds the amino acid in the table and combines the nucleotide sequence for each position. For example, methionine (Met) is encoded by the sequence AUG. To find the amino acid that matches a codon sequence, reverse this process.

Table 22.2 Effect of mutations on protein synthesis

Description of change in gene sequence	mRNA sequence	Protein sequence	Result of change
Normal gene	AUG GGG AAU CUA UCA CCU GAU C ...	Met-Gly-Asn-Leu-Ser-Pro-Asp-...	Normal protein
Insertion of a **C**	AUG GG**C** GAA UCU AUC ACC UGA UC ...	Met-Gly-Glu-**Ser-Ile-Thr-Stop**	Frameshift leading to a premature stop
Deletion of an **A**	AUG GGG AAU CUA UCC CUG AUC ...	Met-Gly-Asn-Leu-Ser-**Leu-Ile**-...	Frameshift leading to a different sequence
Substitution **CG** for UC	AUG GGG AAU CUA **CG**A CCU GAU C ...	Met-Gly-Asn-Leu-**Arg**-Pro-Asp-...	Single amino acid substitution
Substitution **G** for A	AUG GGG AAU CU**G** UCA CCU GAU C ...	Met-Gly-Asn-Leu-Ser-Pro-Asp-...	No change (silent)
Substitution **G** for C	AUG GGG AAU CUA U**G**A CCU GAU C ...	Met-Gly-Asn-Leu-**Stop**	Premature stop

*Mutations in a gene are transcribed into the mRNA, and the resulting changes in the protein sequence are shown. Note that depending on the position of the mutation, single-nucleotide substitutions can result in **silent changes**, a change in a single amino acid (**missense**), or even premature termination (**nonsense**).*

methionine codon if they occur close to the 5′ end of the mRNA. There are also minor differences in the genetic code in mitochondrial DNA; for instance, in vertebrate, mitochondrial methionine is specified by additional codons - UGA, normally a stop codon, encodes tryptophan - and there are additional stop codons.

Another aspect of the genetic code is that once synthesis has initiated at the first AUG codon encoding methionine, each successive triplet from that start codon will be read in register without interruption until a stop codon is encountered. Thus the **reading frame** of the mRNA will be dictated by the start codon. Mutations that cause the addition or deletion of even single nucleotides will cause a shift in the reading frame, resulting in a protein with a different amino acid sequence after the mutation or a protein that is prematurely terminated if a stop codon is now in frame (**nonsense mutation;** Table 22.2).

THE MACHINERY OF PROTEIN SYNTHESIS

The ribosome is a multistep assembly line for protein synthesis

Ribosomes are the molecular machines that conduct protein synthesis. They consist of a small and a large subunit; each

CLINICAL BOX
SICKLE CELL ANEMIA: MUTATION OF THE GENETIC CODE

Sickle cell anemia is an example of a disease in which a single nucleotide change within the coding region of the gene for the β-chain of hemoglobin A, the major form of adult hemoglobin, yields an altered protein that has impaired function (see Chapter 5). The mutation that causes this disease is a single nucleotide change, whereby a glutamate codon GAG is changed to GUG, encoding valine. The polar glutamate residue is located on a surface of hemoglobin, which is exposed only in the deoxygenated state. Substitution of Glu with Val creates a hydrophobic surface that promotes the polymerization of deoxyhemoglobin molecules, leading to the formation of rod-shaped structures. This results in deformation of red blood cells, particularly in venous capillaries, altering and blocking blood flow. This example, whereby an amino acid with an acidic side chain is substituted for an amino acid with a nonpolar, hydrophobic side chain, is termed a **nonconservative change.** Conversely, the replacement of one amino acid by another with similar physical and chemical properties is termed **conservative** and is predicted to have less severe consequences on protein function (e.g., an Arg → Lys or Asp → Glu mutation).

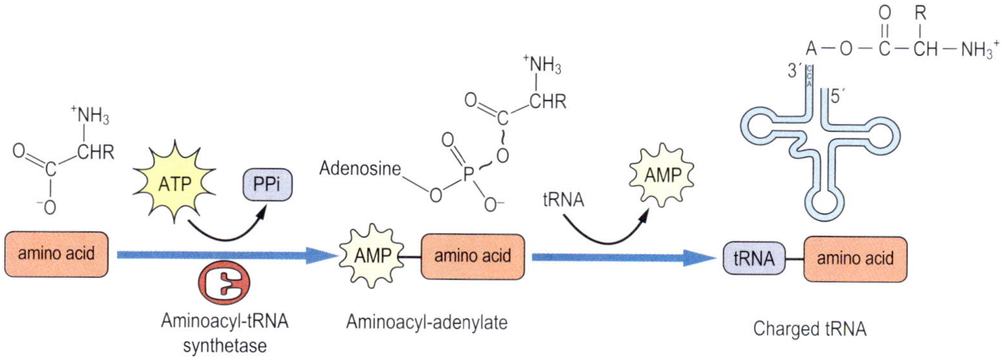

Fig. 22.1 **Activation of an amino acid and attachment to its cognate tRNA.** The amino acid must be activated by an aminoacyl-tRNA synthetase to form an aminoacyl-adenylate intermediate before its attachment to the 3′ (CCA) end of the tRNA. AMP, adenosine monophosphate; PPi, inorganic pyrophosphate.

is a ribonucleoprotein particle (approximately 1 : 1 ratio of rRNA to protein) containing a total of four species of RNA and 80 protein subunits. The association of these subunits forms three specific sites within the ribosome, which individual tRNAs occupy in a defined succession as they progress through the steps of protein synthesis. These sites are known as the **aminoacyl-tRNA, or A site**; the **peptidyl-tRNA, or P site**; and the **exit site, or E site**. The A site is where a donor tRNA molecule, charged with the appropriate amino acid, is positioned before that amino acid is incorporated into the growing polypeptide. The P site is the location in the ribosome that contains a tRNA molecule with the amino-terminal polypeptide of the newly synthesized protein still attached. The process of peptide bond formation takes place between the A and P sites. This process is catalyzed by a peptidyl transferase activity, which forms the peptide bond between the amino group of the amino acid in the A site and the carboxyl terminus of the nascent peptide attached to the tRNA in the P site. The E site is a third site of interaction between tRNA and mRNA on the ribosome, occupied by the deacylated tRNA after the peptide bond is formed but before it exits the ribosome. The pausing of the deacylated tRNA at the E site before exiting is important in maintaining the reading frame and assuring the fidelity of translation.

- A site - site occupied by donor aminoacyl-tRNA
- P site - site occupied by tRNA with growing peptide chain
- E site - site occupied by deacylated tRNA

Each amino acid has a specific synthetase that attaches it to all the tRNAs that encode it

Although there is a distinct tRNA molecule for most of the codons represented in Table 22.1, the structure of individual tRNAs is very similar (see Fig. 21.2). All tRNAs are between 73 and 93 nucleotides in length and have a similar "cloverleaf" secondary structure composed of four distinct base-paired stems and three loops. In its tertiary folded form, tRNAs adopt an L-like structure. The 3′ end of the tRNA molecule, or one end of the "L," is called the **acceptor stem**, where an enzyme called **aminoacyl-tRNA synthetase** catalyzes the addition of a specific amino acid, and the other end of the "L" contains the **anticodon loop**, which interacts with the mRNA. Aminoacyl-tRNA synthetases catalyze the formation of an ester bond linking the 3′ hydroxyl group of the adenosine nucleotide of the tRNA to the carboxyl group of the amino acid (Fig. 22.1). The attachment of an amino acid to a tRNA is a two-step reaction. The carboxyl group of the amino acid is first activated by reaction with adenosine triphosphate (ATP) to form an amino-acyladenylate intermediate, which is bound to the synthetase complex. The enzymology of activation of the carboxyl group of amino acids is similar to that for activation of fatty acids by thiokinase (Chapter 11), but rather than the transfer of the acyl group to the thiol group of coenzyme A, the aminoacyl group is transferred to the 3′-hydroxyl of the tRNA. The product is described as a **charged tRNA** molecule. At this point, it is ready to bind to the A site of the ribosome, where it will contribute its amino acid to the growing peptide chain at the B site. There is a unique synthetase enzyme specific for each of the 20 amino acids, and each synthetase will attach the correct amino acid to all the tRNAs that recognize the different codons specifying that amino acid.

Some flexibility in base pairing occurs at the 3′ base of the mRNA codon

Interaction of the charged tRNA with its cognate codon is accomplished by association of the anticodon loop in tRNA with the codon in mRNA through hydrogen bonding of complementary base pairs (Fig. 22.2). However, organisms do not typically have a unique tRNA to recognize each of the 64 codons. To deal with this, the base-pairing rules between tRNA and mRNA specifically at the third position (3′ end) of the codon deviate from those in DNA (Chapter 20). At this position, nonclassical base pairs can form between this nucleotide and the first base (5′ end) of the anticodon. The so-called **wobble**

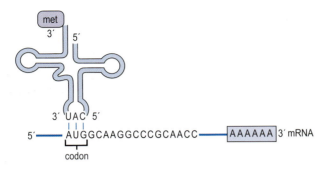

Fig. 22.2 **Interaction of charged tRNA with mRNA.** The interaction of a charged tRNA with an mRNA occurs by base pairing of complementary bases in the anticodon loop and the codon of the mRNA.

Table 22.3 Base-pairing possibilities between the third position or 3′ nucleotide of the mRNA codon and the first position or 5′ nucleotide of the tRNA anticodon

Codon, third or 3′ position (mRNA)	Anticodon, first or 5′ position (tRNA)
G	C
U	A
A or G	U
C or U	G
A or C or U	I

ADVANCED CONCEPT BOX
FIDELITY OF TRANSLATION

Aminoacyl-tRNA Synthetases Have Proofreading Ability

To preserve the unambiguous codon–amino acid correspondence dictated by the genetic code, the individual aminoacyl-tRNA synthetases are capable of identifying the small differences between each unique tRNA in order to pair the correct tRNA with its cognate amino acid. This discrimination is facilitated by specific hydrogen bonds between the enzyme and the correct tRNA. In addition, aminoacyl-tRNA synthetases have evolved the ability not only to discriminate between amino acids before they are attached to the appropriate tRNA but also to remove amino acids that are attached to the wrong tRNA via a proofreading step. These capabilities are accomplished by two specific sites in the enzyme that discriminate amino acids based on size. The first, the "synthetic site" where the tRNA acylation takes place, will accommodate both the cognate amino acid and the other smaller amino acids that retain similarity to the cognate. At the second "editing site," the enzymes will remove the misincorporated smaller amino acid because of the lack of hydrogen bonding interactions that only occur between the enzyme and the cognate amino acid. These discriminatory mechanisms combine to ensure the accurate transfer of information from mRNA to protein and contribute to the low error frequency of translation, which is only approximately 1 error in 10^3–10^4 polymerized amino acids.

hypothesis of codon–anticodon pairing allows a tRNA with an anticodon that is not perfectly complementary to the mRNA codon to recognize the sequence and allow for the incorporation of the amino acid into the growing peptide chain. For example, a guanine residue at the 5′ end of the anticodon can form a base pair with either a cytidine or a uridine residue in the 3′ end of the codon. Similarly, if the modified adenosine residue, inosine, occurs at the 5′ end of the anticodon, it can form a base pair with uridine, adenosine, or even cytidine at the 3′ end of the codon (Table 22.3). This imprecise pairing allows

a tRNA with the anticodon GAG to decode the CUU and CUC codons, both of which code for leucine. Therefore wobble pairing reduces the number of tRNAs needed to decode mRNA and provides a mechanistic rationale that accounts for the degeneracy of the genetic code, since degeneracy always occurs in the third residue of the codon.

How does the ribosome know where to begin protein synthesis?

The mRNA molecule carries the information that will be used to direct the synthesis of a protein's polypeptide chain, but how does the synthetic machinery know where to start - which nucleotide starts the first codon to be translated into protein? Most eukaryotic mRNAs contain regions both before and after the protein-coding region, called 5′ and 3′ **untranslated regions (UTR).** These sequences are important for mRNA stability and for determining the start site and regulating the rate of protein synthesis. In eukaryotic cells, the ribosome first binds to a 7-methylguanine "cap" structure (Chapter 21) at the 5′ end of the mRNA, then moves down the molecule, scanning the sequence until it encounters the first AUG codon (Fig. 22.3). This signals the ribosome to initiate protein synthesis, beginning with a methionine residue and stopping when it encounters one of the termination codons. On some viral and eukaryotic mRNAs, an alternative ribosome recruitment site, an **internal ribosome entry site** (IRES; Fig. 22.3), allows cap-independent initiation of translation.

Prokaryotic mRNA is different in numerous ways. First, it lacks a 5′ m^{7}G cap to facilitate ribosome binding. Second, prokaryotic mRNAs can be **polycistronic,** meaning that several polypeptides are encoded by a single mRNA, making it difficult for the ribosome to know where to begin protein synthesis. However, a sequence has been identified in most prokaryotic mRNAs that directs the ribosome to the beginning of each protein-coding region. This purine-rich sequence, known as the **Shine–Dalgarno (SD) sequence,** is complementary to a portion of the 16-S rRNA in the small bacterial ribosomal subunit (Fig. 22.3). Through the formation of hydrogen bonds, the ribosome is positioned at the start of each protein-coding region.

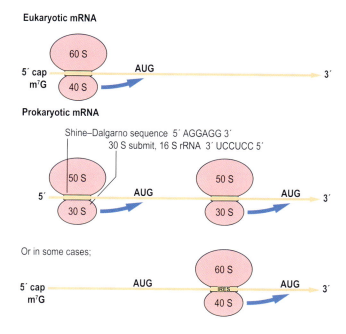

Eukaryotic mRNA

Prokaryotic mRNA

Shine–Dalgarno sequence 5′ AGGAGG 3′
30 S submit, 16 S rRNA 3′ UCCUCC 5′

Or in some cases;

Fig. 22.3 **Finding the protein-coding region.** The ribosome binds to the mRNA before locating the protein-coding region. (Top) Eukaryotic ribosomes bind to the 5′ cap of mRNAs and then move down the mRNA until they encounter the first AUG codon. (Middle) Bacterial ribosomes bind to a Shine–Dalgarno sequence complementary to a sequence in the ribosomal 16-S rRNA; Shine–Dalgarno sequences are located a short distance from the start of the protein-coding region. In contrast to eukaryotic mRNA, bacteria mRNA is polycistronic, with multiple initiation sites in the same mRNA. (Bottom) In some cases, particularly in viral mRNAs, eukaryotic ribosomes may bind internally at an internal ribosome entry site (IRES) and then move to the AUG. This cap-independent mechanism allows translation of viral mRNA when the translation of genomic RNA is inhibited by viral proteins.

THE PROCESS OF PROTEIN SYNTHESIS

Translation is a dynamic process that involves the interaction of mRNA, enzymes, tRNAs, translation factors, ribosomal proteins, and rRNAs

Translation is divided into three steps:

- Initiation
- Elongation
- Termination

Initiation

Synthesis of a protein is initiated at the first AUG (methionine) codon in the mRNA

In eukaryotes, the initiation of translation depends on the coordinated interaction of at least 12 eukaryotic initiation factors (eIF), mRNA, and the ribosome. Initially, a **ternary complex** is formed between eIF-2, GTP, and initiator methionine

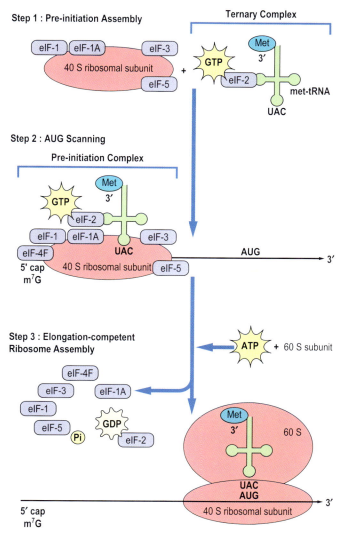

Fig. 22.4 **Initiation of protein synthesis in eukaryotic cells.** The 40-S ribosomal subunit with bound initiation factors eIF-1, eIF-1A, eIF-3, and eIF-5; mRNA with eIF-4F bound to the 5′ cap; and met-tRNA bound to eIF-2 are brought together. Once these components are assembled, the complex translocates to the AUG, scanning the mRNA sequence and hydrolyzing ATP in the process. The 60-S ribosomal subunit completes the initiation complex, and in the process, the initiation factors are released. Note that at initiation, the P site is occupied by the initiator met-tRNA, as shown in Fig. 22.5. GDP, guanosine diphosphate; eIF, eukaryotic initiation factor.

tRNA (Met-tRNAi) (Fig. 22.4) to deliver Met-tRNAi to the A site of the 40-S small ribosomal subunit. The **preinitiation complex** is then assembled on the 40-S ribosomal subunit by the interaction of the ternary complex with eIF-1, eIF-1A, eIF-3, and eIF-5. This preinitiation complex is directed to the 5′ end of the mRNA by interaction with the eIF-4F complex, made up of a preassembled 7-methyl guanosine cap-binding protein eIF-4E and other related eIF-4s. Using the energy of ATP hydrolysis, the complex scans the mRNA to locate the

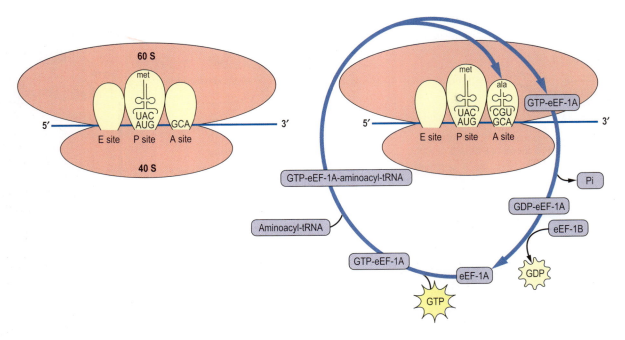

Fig. 22.5 **Recycling of elongation factor eEF-1A.** A charged tRNA molecule is brought to the A site of the initiation complex, with the aid of eEF-1A with bound GTP, to begin the process of elongation. The factor is released once GTP is hydrolyzed, and the process of recycling eEF-1A is aided by the exchange factor eEF-1B. Each successive amino acid addition requires that the correctly charged tRNA molecule be brought to the A site of the ribosome. ala, alanine; Pi, inorganic phosphate.

first AUG codon. Upon AUG recognition, the GTP bound to IF-2 is hydrolyzed, triggering the disassembly of all eIFs and the concomitant recruitment of the 60-S large ribosomal subunit. With the help of eIF-5B (not shown), the Met-tRNAi is correctly positioned into to the P site of the ribosome (Fig. 22.5) in preparation for the subsequent elongation phase. In prokaryotic cells, the process involves three initiation factors (IF-1, IF-2, and IF-3), and the initiation complex first forms just 5′ upstream from the coding region as a result of the interaction of 16-S rRNA in the small subunit with the Shine–Dalgarno sequence on the mRNA. N-formyl methionine (fmet), encoded by AUG, is the first amino acid in all bacterial proteins, instead of methionine.

Elongation

Factors involved in the elongation stage of protein synthesis are targets of some antibiotics

After initiation is complete, the process of translating the information in mRNA into a functional protein starts. The elongation cycle begins with the binding of a charged tRNA to the A site of the ribosome. In eukaryotic cells, the charged tRNA molecule is brought to the ribosome by the action of a GTP-bound elongation factor called eEF-1A (Fig. 22.5). Upon

 CLINICAL BOX
MISREGULATION OF TRANSLATION INITIATION IN HUMAN DISEASE

A Growing Number of Mutations in Proteins That Regulate the Initiation of Peptide Synthesis Are Linked to Disease

The control of translation is essential to fine-tune the levels of each protein in a cell in order to meet the cell's requirements. Altering the regulation of peptide synthesis can have detrimental effects. One such example is the discovery of mutations in the translation-initiation machinery that alter the level and function of the eukaryotic initiation factor 2 (eIF2B), causing rare but fatal neurological diseases, such as childhood ataxia with central nervous system hypomyelination (CACH) and vanishing white-matter leukoencephalopathy (VWM). Mutations in eIF2 and eIF2α kinase are also associated with acute myeloid leukemia and a rare form of infantile diabetes characterized by impaired development of pancreatic β-cells (Wolcott–Rallison syndrome). Alterations in eIF2 phosphorylation and eIF2α kinase are also observed in the brain in neurodegenerative diseases, including Alzheimer's and Parkinson's diseases. There is growing interest in the development of drug therapies to target the regulation of eukaryotic initiation factors to treat these and other diseases.

pairing of the tRNA anticodon with its cognate codon, GTP is hydrolyzed, and eEF-1A is released. For eEF-1A to be reused, it is regenerated by an elongation factor called eEF-1B, which promotes the replacement of GDP from eEF-1A with GTP so that it may bind to another charged tRNA molecule (see Fig. 22.5). Once the correctly charged tRNA molecule has been delivered to the A site of the ribosome, the **peptidyl transferase** activity of the ribosome catalyzes the formation of a peptide bond between the amino acid in the A site and the amino acid at the end of the growing peptide chain in the P site. The tRNA-peptide chain is now transiently bound to the A site (Fig. 22.6). With the help of eEF-2, the ribosome then translocates one codon down the mRNA (toward the 3′ end), resulting in the repositioning of the tRNA with the nascent peptide chain attached from the A site into the P site. This movement also causes the uncharged tRNA in the P site to reposition into the E site, resulting in a total of nine nucleotide pairs stabilizing the ribosome–mRNA–tRNA complex. This cycle is repeated for incorporation of the next amino acid (Fig. 22.6). The mechanics of this complex process are identical in prokaryotic cells, but the ribosomes and elongation factors are different, allowing for the development of antibiotics that selectively inhibit protein synthesis in bacteria (Table 22.4).

Termination

Termination of protein synthesis in both eukaryotic and bacterial cells is accomplished when the A site of the ribosome reaches one of the stop codons of the mRNA. Proteins called eukaryotic releasing factors (eRF) recognize these codons and cause the protein that is attached to the last tRNA molecule in the P site to be released (Fig. 22.7). This process is an energy-dependent reaction catalyzed by the hydrolysis of GTP, which transfers a water molecule to the end of the protein, thus releasing it from the tRNA in the P site. After release of the newly synthesized protein, the ribosomal subunits, tRNA, and mRNA dissociate from each other, setting the stage for the translation of another mRNA.

PROTEIN FOLDING AND ENDOPLASMIC RETICULUM (ER) STRESS

ER stress, the result of errors in protein folding, develops in many chronic conditions, including obesity, diabetes, and cancer

For a newly synthesized protein to become functionally active, it must be folded into a unique three-dimensional structure. Given that there are multiple possible conformations that a polypeptide can potentially adopt, proteins require the help of a class of proteins called **chaperones** to achieve their correct native structures. Chaperones promote the correct folding,

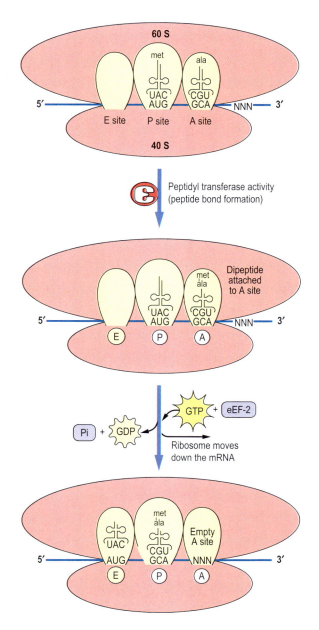

Fig. 22.6 **Peptide bond formation and translocation.** The formation of the peptide bond between each successive amino acid is catalyzed by peptidyl transferase. Once the peptide bond is formed, an elongation factor (eEF-2 in this case) will move the ribosome down one codon on the mRNA so that the A site is vacant and ready to receive the next charged tRNA. The E site is now occupied by the uncharged tRNA (met). NNN is the codon for the next amino acid.

assembly, and organization of proteins as well as macromolecular structures such as the nucleosome and electron-transport complexes. In the ER, chaperones bind to exposed hydrophobic regions of unfolded proteins, shielding these interactive surfaces and thus preventing misfolding and the formation of nonspecific aggregates. The chaperones promote the correct folding of newly synthesized proteins by cycles of

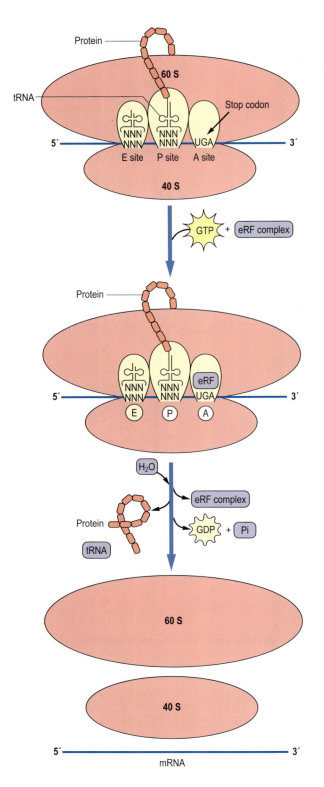

Fig. 22.7 **Termination of protein synthesis.** Termination of protein synthesis occurs when the A site is located over a termination codon. A releasing factor complex (eRF), with eRF-1 in the A site, will cause the completed protein to be released, and the ribosome, mRNA, and tRNA will dissociate from each other to begin another cycle of translation.

Table 22.4 Selected antibiotics that affect protein synthesis

Antibiotic	Target
Tetracycline	Bacterial ribosome A site
Streptomycin	Bacterial 30-S ribosome subunit
Erythromycin	Bacterial 50-S ribosome subunit
Chloramphenicol	Bacterial ribosome peptidyl transferase
Puromycin	Causes premature termination
Cycloheximide	Eukaryotic 80-S ribosome

Note that cycloheximide is toxic to humans.

CLINICAL BOX
A NONCOMPLIANT PATIENT WHO WAS PRESCRIBED AN ANTIBIOTIC

A young man being treated for a sinus infection returns to your clinic after 1 week, still complaining of sinus headaches and stuffiness. He explains that he began to feel better about 3 days after starting to take the antibiotic tetracycline, which you had prescribed. You inquire whether he continued to take the full dose of the drug even after he began to feel better. He reluctantly admits that as soon as he felt better, he stopped taking the drug. How do you explain to your patient that it is important that he takes the drug for as long as you prescribed it, even if he feels better after only a few days?

Comment

As a physician, you know that tetracycline is a broad-spectrum antibiotic that inhibits the protein synthetic machinery of the bacterial cell by binding to the A site of the ribosome (Table 22.4). You also know that if the drug is removed, protein synthesis can resume. If the drug is not taken for the entire period recommended, bacteria may begin to grow again, leading to the resurgence of the infection. Further, those bacteria that begin to grow after early termination of treatment are likely to be the most resistant to the drug. Because of the selection for more resistant mutant strains, the secondary infection is likely to be more difficult to control.

protein (substrate) binding and release, regulated by ATPase activity and specific cofactor proteins. **Heat shock proteins (HSP)** are a group of chaperone proteins that are expressed by cells in response to high temperature. However, HSPs assist in the refolding of denatured proteins, not only as a result of heat, but also in response to physical and chemical stresses.

When a misfolded protein is detected in the ER, the protein **GRP78/BiP** (78 KDa glucose-regulated protein/binding immunoglobulin protein) binds the unfolded protein and traps it in the ER, preventing its further transport and secretion.

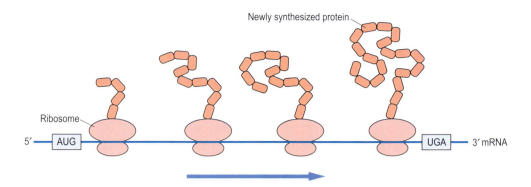

Fig. 22.8 **Protein synthesis on polysomes.** Proteins can be synthesized by several ribosomes bound to the same mRNA, forming a structure known as a polysome.

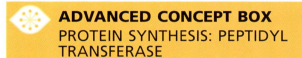

ADVANCED CONCEPT BOX
PROTEIN SYNTHESIS: PEPTIDYL TRANSFERASE

Peptidyl Transferase Is Not Your Typical Enzyme - It Is a Ribozyme

Peptidyl transferase is the activity responsible for peptide bond formation during protein synthesis. This enzyme activity catalyzes the reaction between the amino group of the aminoacyl-tRNA in the A site and the carboxyl carbon of the peptidyl-tRNA in the P site, forming a peptide bond from an ester bond. The activity is attributed to the ribosome, but the ribosomal proteins do not have the capacity to catalyze this reaction. Crystal structures of the ribosome have shown that the peptidyl-transferase activity is catalyzed by the 28-S RNA in the major subunit of rRNA. Although specific amino acids are important for positioning the tRNAs and stabilizing their interaction with the rRNA, the catalytic activity resides entirely in the rRNA.

The unfolded protein is then routed to the **ER-associated degradation (ERAD) pathway**, which facilitates export to the cytosol and proteasomal degradation of the misfolded protein (see below).

A condition known as **ER stress** develops if chaperone and ERAD activities are overwhelmed, leading to the accumulation of protein aggregates in the lumen of the ER. This might happen as a result of a protein mutation or a glycosyl transferase deficiency or inhibitor, such as tunicamycin (Fig. 17.11). ER stress activates the **unfolded protein response (UPR)** in a GRP78/BiP-dependent manner, which increases the expression of several chaperones and ERAD proteins. In addition, the protein PERK (protein kinase RNA-like ER kinase) is activated via oligomerization and autophosphorylation, and it phosphorylates eIF-2, inhibiting translation initiation (Fig. 22.4). This slows down the rate of protein synthesis and, if successful, restores homeostasis. However, if ER stress is too severe, apoptosis (Chapter 29) will be triggered to eliminate

the cell. A number of human diseases are characterized by ER stress and the UPR, including some forms of cystic fibrosis and retinitis pigmentosa. ER stress and the UPR also inhibit insulin signaling, causing insulin resistance, and play a role in the development of pathology in obesity and type 2 diabetes mellitus (Chapter 31).

PROTEIN TARGETING AND POSTTRANSLATIONAL MODIFICATIONS

Protein targeting

An mRNA can have several bound ribosomes at one time, and this is known as a **polyribosome or polysome** (Fig. 22.8). There are two classes of polysomes found in cells: mRNAs that encode proteins destined for the cytoplasm or nucleus are translated primarily on polysomes free in the cytoplasm, whereas mRNAs encoding membrane and secreted proteins are translated on polysomes attached to the ER. Regions of the ER studded with bound ribosomes are described as the **rough endoplasmic reticulum (RER)**.

Cellular fate of proteins is determined by their signal peptide sequences

Proteins that are destined for export, for insertion into membranes, or for specific cellular organelles such as the nucleus, lysosomes, or mitochondria are distinct from proteins that reside in the cytoplasm. The distinguishing characteristic of proteins targeted for these locations is that they contain a **signal sequence** of 20–30 amino acids, usually at the amino-terminal end of the protein. For secretory or membrane proteins, the signal sequence is recognized cotranslationally by a ribonucleoprotein complex known as the **signal recognition particle (SRP)**, which is composed of a small RNA and six proteins. By binding the signal sequence, the SRP halts translation of the remainder of the protein. This complex then

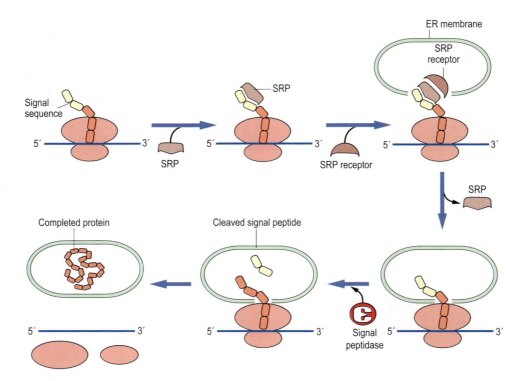

Fig. 22.9 **Protein synthesis on the endoplasmic reticulum.** The signal sequence of the protein being translated is bound to an SRP, and this complex is recognized by the SRP receptor on the endoplasmic reticulum (ER), where the signal sequence is inserted through the membrane. A signal peptidase typically removes the signal sequence, but not on every protein. Once synthesis of the protein is complete, the protein is inserted into the membranes or secreted.

targets the ribosome-bound mRNA with its nascent peptide to the ER membrane via an interaction with the SRP receptor, and the signal sequence is inserted through the membrane. Inside the ER, the SRP dissociates, and translation resumes with the polypeptide chain being moved, as it is synthesized, across the membrane into the interstitial space of the ER (Fig. 22.9). The protein is then transferred to the Golgi apparatus and then to its final destination.

In contrast to secretory and membrane proteins, mitochondrial and nucleoplasmic proteins are transported after translation is complete. In the case of proteins destined for the mitochondrion, they can have up to two unique signal sequences on their *N*-terminal ends, depending on whether they are destined for the mitochondrial matrix or the intermembrane space. Mitochondrial proteins must be unfolded before they can be transported through transporters in the inner and outer membranes (TIM and TOM; Fig. 8.3). In contrast, nuclear proteins have **nuclear localization signals** (NLS) located anywhere in the protein sequence but exposed on the three-dimensional protein surface. Nuclear proteins do not require unfolding before transport because nuclear pores are very large, open channels that can accommodate the recognition and transport of a protein in its native state. Certain glycoproteins targeted to the lysosome lack a classical amino acid signal sequence. Instead, they are substrates for

enzymes that add modified high-mannose oligosaccharide with terminal Man-6-P residues that serve as the targeting signal (Fig. 17.14).

Posttranslational modification

Most proteins require posttranslational modification before they become biologically active

The endoplasmic reticulum and Golgi apparatus are major sites of posttranslational modification of proteins. In the ER, an enzyme called **signal peptidase** removes the signal sequence from the amino-terminus of certain proteins, resulting in a mature protein that is 20–30 amino acids shorter than that encoded by the mRNA. In the ER and Golgi apparatus, carbohydrate side chains are added and modified at specific sites on the protein (Chapter 17). One of the common amino-terminal modifications of eukaryotic cells is the removal of the amino-terminal methionine residue that initiates protein synthesis. Finally, many proteins (e.g., the hormones insulin and glucagon) are synthesized as preproteins and proproteins that must be proteolytically cleaved to be active. The cleavage of a precursor to its biologically active form is usually accomplished by a specific protease and is a tightly regulated cellular event.

Proteasomes: Cellular machinery for protein turnover

Unlike DNA, damaged proteins are not repaired but degraded

Protein degradation is a complex process that is critical to biological regulation and quality control. There are a number of triggers that cause a protein to be degraded:

1. A protein has experienced gradual denaturation during normal environmental stress.
2. A protein has become inappropriately modified by an illegitimate reaction with reactive intracellular compounds, such as a metabolic intermediate, a reactive oxygen species, or a carbonyl compound (Chapters 29 and 42).
3. The protein's function is no longer required, and it needs to be removed. For example, proteins involved in signaling pathways or the cell cycle or those that act as transcription factors sometimes have a small window of time to function, and then they need to be rapidly removed to attenuate the response or signal. Some of these latter proteins have a characteristic amino acid sequence or N-terminal residues that promote their rapid turnover. For certain proteins, an internal **PEST (ProGluSerThr)** sequence signals their rapid degradation, and proteins with N-terminal arginine generally have short half-lives compared with proteins with N-terminal methionine.

The proteasome is a multicatalytic complex designed for degradation of cytosolic proteins

Because protein degradation is a destructive process, it must be sequestered within specific cellular organelles. Lysosomes, for example, ingest and degrade damaged mitochondria and other membranous organelles. However, most soluble cytoplasmic proteins are degraded in structures called **proteasomes.** The 26-S proteasome (Fig. 22.10) consists of two types of subunits: a 20-S multimeric, multicatalytic protease (MCP) and a 19-S ATPase. The proteasome is a barrel-shaped structure formed by a stack of four rings of seven homologous monomers, α-type subunits in the outer ends, and β-type subunits on the inner rings of the barrel. The proteolytic activity - three different types of threonine proteases - resides on β-subunits with active sites facing the inside of the barrel, thereby protecting cytoplasmic proteins from inappropriate degradation. The ATPase subunits are attached at either end of the barrel and act as gatekeepers, allowing only proteins destined for destruction to enter. The proteins are unfolded in a process that requires ATP and degraded by the protease activities to small peptides, six to nine amino acids in length, that are released into the cytoplasm for further degradation.

Ubiquitin targets proteins to the proteasome for degradation

Proteins destined for proteasomal destruction are covalently tagged with a chain of a highly conserved 76–amino acid

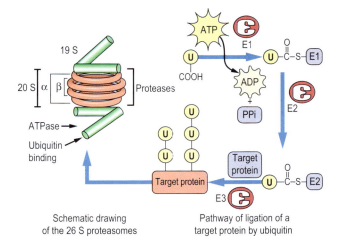

Schematic drawing of the 26 S proteasomes

Pathway of ligation of a target protein by ubiquitin

Fig. 22.10 **Structure of the proteasome and the role of ubiquitin (U) in protein turnover.** The proteasome shown on the left is a barrel-shaped structure. The 20-S multicatalytic protease in the middle rings of the barrel has protease activity on the inner face. The 19-S caps at each end of the barrel function to bind and release ubiquitin, have ATPase activity, and control access of proteins to the inside of the barrel for degradation. The ubiquitin cycle is involved in marking proteins for degradation by the proteasome. Ubiquitin is first activated as a thioester derivative by ubiquitin-activating enzyme E1; it is then transferred to ubiquitin-conjugating enzyme E2, then to a lysine residue on the target protein, catalyzed by ubiquitin-ligase E3, and finally polymerized into chains on target proteins. The longer the chain of polyubiquitin, the more susceptible the protein is to proteasomal degradation. Note that the drawing is not to scale; the proteasome is a 26-S macromolecular complex (≥2,000,000 Da); target proteins are smaller, and ubiquitin is less than 10,000 Da.

protein called **ubiquitin,** which is found in all cells. First, ubiquitin must be activated to fulfill its role (Fig. 22.10), which is accomplished by a ubiquitin-activating enzyme called E1. Activation occurs when E1 is attached via a thioester bond to the C-terminus of ubiquitin by ATP-driven formation of a ubiquitin–adenylate intermediate. The activated ubiquitin is then attached to a ubiquitin carrier protein, known as E2, by a thioester linkage. And finally, a ubiquitin protein ligase known as E3 transfers the ubiquitin from E2 to the target protein, forming an **isopeptide bond** between the carboxyl-terminus of ubiquitin and the ε-amino group of a lysine residue on a target protein. From this single ubiquitin monomer, a chain of ubiquitin is polymerized on target proteins (**polyubiquitination**), which is recognized by a ubiquitin-binding site on the 19-S subunit of the proteasome. Once bound, the polyubiquitinated protein enters the proteasome barrel, the ubiquitin is released by ubiquitinase activity, and ubiquitin is recycled to the cytosol for reuse.

The ubiquitin pathway leading to proteasomal degradation of proteins is complex and tightly regulated. Although the number of E1 enzymes is typically small, there are several E2 and many E3 proteins with different target specificities. There

ADVANCED CONCEPT BOX
INHIBITING THE PROTEASOME TO TREAT CANCER

Multiple myeloma (MM) is a cancer of plasma cells (B lymphocytes), which are normally found in bone and synthesize antibodies as part of the immune system (see Chapters 40 and 43). The unchecked growth of these plasma cells results in anemia, tumors in the bones, and a compromised immune response. One successful treatment option for patients with recurring MM is bortezomib, an inhibitor of protease activity in the proteasome. This drug improves the chances for survival of MM patients and increases the length of time before remission, especially when combined with other therapies such as radiation or additional chemotherapy. Bortezomib causes increased accumulation of unfolded proteins in the endoplasmic reticulum, inducing ER stress and apoptosis. Second-generation proteasome inhibitors targeting different parts of the complex are currently in clinical trials to treat different types of cancer as well as MM patients who are resistant to bortezomib.

ACTIVE LEARNING

1. Review the mechanism of action of various drugs that inhibit protein synthesis on the bacterial ribosome.
2. Describe the signal sequences that target proteins to the lysosome, the mitochondria, or the nucleus.
3. Discuss the role of the *N*-terminal amino acid as a factor regulating the rate of turnover of a cytoplasmic protein.
4. Explain how viruses take control of the cellular protein translation machinery during viral infections to favor the synthesis of viral proteins.

are six different ATPase activities associated with the 19-S subunit. These enzymatic activities are involved in the denaturation of ubiquitinated proteins and transporting the peptide chains into the core of the proteasome. All of these variations in components of the pathway provide a flexible and regulated pathway for protein turnover.

- Elongation is a stepwise addition of the individual amino acids to a growing peptide chain by the action of the ribozyme peptidyl transferase.
- Termination of protein synthesis occurs when the ribosome reaches a stop codon and releasing factors catalyze the release of the protein.
- After release, the newly synthesized proteins must be correctly folded with the help of ancillary proteins called chaperones, may be modified posttranslationally, and are targeted to specific subcellular compartments by signal sequences.
- Protein degradation by the macromolecular proteasome is a controlled mechanism by which a cell eliminates unwanted or damaged proteins.

SUMMARY

- Protein synthesis is the culmination of the transfer of genetic information from DNA to proteins. In this transfer, information must be translated from the four-nucleotide language of DNA and RNA to the 20–amino acid language of proteins.
- The genetic code, in which three nucleotides in mRNA (codon) specify an amino acid, represents the translation dictionary of the two languages.
- The tRNA molecule is the bridge between the sequence of the nucleotides in mRNA and the amino acids in protein. tRNAs accomplish their task by virtue of their anticodon loop, which interacts with specific codons on the mRNA and also with specific amino acids via their amino acid attachment sites located on the 3' ends of the molecules.
- The process of translation consists of three parts: initiation, elongation, and termination.
- Initiation involves the assembly of the ribosome and charged tRNA at the initiation codon (AUG) of the mRNA.

FURTHER READING

Bohnert, K. R., McMillan, J. D., & Kumar, A. (2017). Emerging roles of ER stress and unfolded protein response pathways in skeletal muscle health and disease. *Journal of Cellular Physiology, 9999*, 1–12.

Brar, G. A. (2016). Beyond the triplet code: Context cues transform translation. *Cell, 167*, 1681–1692.

Finley, D., Chen, X., & Walters, K. J. (2016). Gates, channels, and switches: Elements of the proteasome machine. *Trends in Biochemical Sciences, 41*, 77–93.

Gilda, J. E., & Gomes, A. V. (2017). Proteasome dysfunction in cardiomyopathies. *Journal of Physiology, 595*, 4051–4071.

McCaffrey, K., & Braakman, I. (2016). Protein quality control at the endoplasmic reticulum. *Essays in Biochemistry, 60*, 227–235.

Qi, L., Tsai, B., & Arvan, P. (2017). New insights into the physiological role of endoplasmic reticulum-associated degradation. *Trends in Cell Biology, 27*(6), 430–440.

Ramakrishnan, V. (2014). The ribosome emerges from a black box. *Cell, 159*, 979–984.

Śledź, P., & Baumeister, W. (2016). Structure-driven developments of 26S proteasome inhibitors. *Annual Review of Pharmacology Toxicology, 56*, 191–209.

Wehmer, M., & Sakata, E. (2016). Recent advances in the structural biology of the 26S proteasome. *International Journal of Biochemistry and Cell Biology, 79*, 437–442.

Yusupova, G., & Yusupov, M. (2014). High-resolution structure of the eukaryotic 80S ribosome. *Annual Review of Biochemistry, 83*, 467–486.

Zhang, J., & Ferré-D'Amaré, A. R. (2016). The tRNA elbow in structure, recognition and evolution. *Life (Basel), 6*(1), E3.

RELEVANT WEBSITES

Genetic code: http://www.ncbi.nlm.nih.gov/Taxonomy/Utils/wprintgc
 .cgi?mode = c
IRES: http://www.iresite.org
Proteasome: http://www.biology-pages.info/P/Proteasome.html
Ubiquitin: http://www.rcsb.org/pdb/101/motm.do?momID=60
Ribosome: http://www.weizmann.ac.il/sb/faculty_pages/Yonath/home.html
Translocation: http://rna.ucsc.edu/rnacenter/ribosome_movies.html

ABBREVIATIONS

eEF	Eukaryotic elongation factor
eIF	Eukaryotic initiation factor
eRF	Eukaryotic releasing factor complex
ERAD	ER-associated degradation pathway
HSP	Heat shock protein
IRES	Internal ribosomal entry site
PEST	ProGluSerThr degradation signal
MCP	Multicatalytic protease
RER	Rough endoplasmic reticulum
SRP	Signal recognition particle
UPR	Unfolded protein response
UTR	Untranslated region

Regulation of Gene Expression: Basic Mechanisms

Edel M. Hyland and Jeffrey R. Patton

After reading this chapter, you should be able to:

- Describe the general mechanisms of regulation of gene expression, with an emphasis on initiation of transcription.
- Describe the many levels at which gene expression may be controlled, using steroid-induced gene expression as a model.
- Explain how alternative mRNA splicing, alternate promoters for the start of mRNA synthesis, posttranscriptional editing of the mRNA, and the inhibition of protein synthesis by small RNAs can modulate the expression of a gene.
- Explain how the structure and packaging of chromatin can affect gene expression.
- Explain how genomic imprinting affects gene expression, depending on whether alleles are maternally or paternally inherited.

INTRODUCTION

Despite identical DNA in all cells, gene expression varies significantly with time and place in the body as well as sex

The study of genes and the mechanism whereby the information they hold is converted into proteins to carry out all cellular functions is the realm of molecular biology. Except for the erythrocyte, all cells in the body have the same DNA complement. However, in spite of this, there are significant differences between different cell types depending on the unique set of genes they express. One of the most fascinating aspects of molecular biology is the study of the mechanisms that control differential gene expression, both in time and in place, and the consequences if these control mechanisms are disrupted.

The goal of this chapter is to introduce the basic concepts involved in regulation of protein-coding genes and how these processes are involved in the causation of human disease. The basic mechanism of gene expression regulation will be described first, followed by a discussion of a specific gene regulation system to highlight various aspects of the basic mechanism. The chapter ends with a discussion of various ways in which the gene regulatory apparatus can be adapted to suit the needs of different tissues and situations.

BASIC MECHANISMS OF GENE EXPRESSION

Gene expression is regulated at several different steps

The control of gene expression in humans occurs principally at the level of transcription, the synthesis of mRNA. However, transcription is just the first step in the conversion of the genetic information encoded by a gene into the final processed gene product, and it has become increasingly clear that posttranscriptional events allow for exquisite control of gene expression. The sequence of events involved in the ultimate expression of a particular gene may be summarized as follows:

1. Initiation of transcription
2. Posttranscriptional processing the mRNA transcript
3. Transport of the processed mRNA to the cytoplasm
4. Translation of the processed mRNA into protein

At each of these steps, quality control checks dictate whether the cell proceeds to the next step or attenuates or halts the process. For instance, if the processing of the RNA is not correct or complete, the resulting mRNA would be useless and possibly destroyed. In addition, if the mRNA is not transported out of the nucleus, it will not be translated. Clearly, during the growth of a human embryo from a single fertilized ovum to a newborn infant, differences in the regulation of gene expression allow the differentiation of a single cell into many types of cells that develop tissue-specific characteristics. Such programmed events are common in all organisms, and the production of these phenotypic changes in cells - and thus the whole organism - are a result of changes in the expression of key genes. Although each cell type and stage of development relies on the expression of different subsets of genes, the regulatory mechanisms underlying these differences are available to basically all cells. Table 23.1 outlines some of the regulatory mechanisms in humans and most other eukaryotes at each stage of gene expression, along with their potential outcomes.

Gene transcription depends on key cis-acting DNA sequences in the region of the gene

For protein-coding genes, the goal of transcription is to convert the information held within the DNA of the gene into messenger RNA, which can then be used as a template for synthesis of the protein product of the gene. Therefore the enzyme that catalyzes the formation of mRNA, RNA polymerase II (RNAPol II), must be able to identify DNA sequences that mark the

Table 23.1 Regulator mechanisms in the control of gene expression and their outcomes

Process	Regulatory mechanism	Possible outcomes
Transcription of mRNA	Control of access to gene sequence by manipulating chromatin structure (condensed chromatin is a poor template for transcription)	(i) Temporal regulation of specific gene transcription (ii) Allele-specific transcription
	DNA methylation of promoter sequences to inhibit transcription	(i) Permanently shuts off transcription of specific promoter(s) (ii) Selection of alternative promoters giving different start sites
	Availability of correct *trans*-acting factors such as transcription factors and cofactors	(i) Tissue-/cell-specific transcription (ii) Temporal regulation of specific gene transcription
mRNA processing	Capping of mRNA 5′ end with *N*-7-methyl guanosine; addition of poly-adenosine (poly[A]) to 3′ end of most mRNA	(i) Stabilization of mRNA (ii) Recognition by factors that facilitate transport of mRNA to the cytoplasm (iii) Regulated initiation of mRNA translation to protein
	Removal of introns from mRNA splicing	(i) Alternative splicing, increases coding potential
	Sequences in 3′ untranslated regions (UTR) of mRNAs that can stabilize or mark the RNA for destruction	(i) Controls the half-life of an mRNA transcript
mRNA editing	Editing of mRNAs to change the coding sequence, changing an amino acid or creating a stop codon	(i) Alters amino acid sequence of protein (ii) Introduces a stop codon in mRNA, producing a truncated protein
Translation of mRNA	Availability of factors to transport mRNA to cytoplasm	(i) Temporal regulation of the initiation of translation (ii) Delivery of mRNA to specific regions of the cytoplasm, such as the ends of axons, for local translation
	Availability of factors needed for protein synthesis	(i) Temporal regulation of the initiation of translation (ii) Use of alternative start codons due to internal ribosome entry site (IRES)
	Production of miRNAs to decrease abundance of specific transcript	(i) Limited or no translation of transcript

beginning and end of a gene. In all organisms, RNAPol II does not accomplish this feat alone; regulated transcription requires the action of many other proteins that recognize particular DNA sequence elements that are associated with each gene. These DNA sequences are collectively called *cis*-acting regulatory elements because they are physically on the same molecule of DNA as the gene to be transcribed; **cis-acting sequences** include promoters, enhancers, and response elements. The proteins that recognize them are termed **trans-acting factors**.

A transcription unit encompasses more than just a gene

Classically, a protein-coding gene has been defined as a sequence of DNA that encodes all the information needed to make a functional protein. Historically, the belief was that one gene gives rise to one gene product, or protein. However, now it is clear that many functional products - different mRNA species or different protein products - may arise from a single region of transcribed DNA as a result of differences at the levels of transcription or posttranscription. Therefore there is now a tendency to refer to such "genes" instead as transcription units. The **transcription unit** encapsulates not only those parts of the gene classically regarded as the gene unit, such as the promoters, exons, and introns, but also the additional DNA sequence elements that modify the transcription process from the initiation of transcription to the final posttranscriptional

modifications. Fig. 23.1 illustrates our current understanding of the known sequence elements within a transcriptional unit that regulate the timing and extent of its expression. Each one of these sequence elements will be described in more detail in the following sections.

Promoters

Promoters are usually upstream of the transcription start point of a gene

Sequences that are relatively close to the start site of transcription of a gene and control its expression are collectively known as the promoter. In eukaryotes, promoters lie between a few hundred to a few thousand nucleotides of the start point and are referred to as **proximal promoters.** The promoter sequence acts as a basic recognition unit, signaling to RNAPol II that there is a gene that can be transcribed. Additionally, the promoter provides the information for RNAPol II to initiate RNA synthesis at the right place and using the correct strand of DNA as a template. The promoter also plays an important role in ensuring that mRNA is synthesized at the right time in the right cell. Because the promoter is critical to gene expression, it is often regarded as being part of the gene it controls; without it, the mRNA would not be made. However,

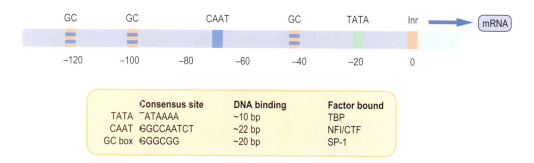

Fig. 23.1 **Idealized version of a transcription unit comprising various promoter elements.** Each transcription unit is composed of introns, exons, and untranslated regions (UTR) as well as distinct promoter elements that are classified as core, proximal, or distal, depending on their position relative to the transcriptional start site (TSS). The position of distal promoter elements is much less well defined and can be anywhere from 2 to 50 kb away from the TSS. Certain elements have consensus sequences that bind ubiquitous transcription-activating factors. Binding of transcription factors encompasses the consensus site and a variable number of anonymous adjacent nucleotides, depending on the promoter element. CTF, a member of a protein family whose members act as transcription factors; TBP, TATA-binding protein; NFI, nuclear factor I; SP-1, ubiquitous transcription factor.

given that promoters are typically upstream (5′) of the transcription start site, they are not transcribed into mRNA, although there are some documented exceptions to this rule. The exact structure of promoters varies from gene to gene within the same organism, but there are a number of key sequence elements that can be identified within promoters. These elements may be present in different combinations between different genes, and some elements may be present in one gene but absent in another.

The efficiency and specificity of gene expression are conferred by promoter elements

Although the nucleotide sequence immediately surrounding the start of transcription of a gene varies from gene to gene, the first nucleotide in the mRNA transcript tends to be adenosine, usually followed by a pyrimidine-rich sequence, termed the **initiator (Inr).** In general, it has the nucleotide sequence Py_2CAPy_5 (Py-pyrimidine base) and is found between positions −3 to +5 in relation to the starting point. In addition to Inr, most promoters possess a sequence known as the **TATA box** approximately 25 base pairs (bp) upstream from the start of transcription. The TATA box has an 8-bp consensus sequence that usually consists entirely of adenine-thymine (A-T) base pairs, although very rarely a guanine-cytosine (G-C) pair may be present. This sequence is important in the process of transcription because nucleotide substitutions that disrupt the TATA box result in a marked reduction in the efficiency of transcription. The positions of Inr and the TATA box relative to the start are relatively fixed, and together with the transcriptional start site (TSS) and RNA polymerase binding site are referred to as the **core promoter** (Fig. 23.1). However, it must be pointed out that there are many eukaryotic genes that do not have an identifiable TATA box, and for these genes, other sequences are essential for determining the start of transcription.

In addition to the TATA box, other commonly found *cis*-acting proximal promoter elements have been described. For example, the **CAAT box** is often found upstream of the TATA box, typically about 80 bp from the start of transcription. As in the case of the TATA box, it may be more important for its ability to increase the strength of the promoter signal rather than in controlling tissue- or time-specific expression of the gene. Another commonly noted promoter element is the **GC box**, a GC-rich sequence; multiple copies may be found in a single promoter region. Fig. 23.1 illustrates some of the common *cis*-acting elements seen within eukaryotic promoters.

Alternative promoters permit tissue or developmental stage–specific gene expression

Although it is clear that promoters are essential for gene expression to occur, a single promoter cannot direct the tissue specificity or developmental-stage specificity directing expression of a gene at different times and places. Some genes have evolved a series of promoters that can confer tissue-specific expression. In addition to the use of different promoters that are physically separated, each of the alternative promoters is often associated with its own first exon, and as a result, each mRNA and subsequent protein has a tissue-specific 5′ end and amino acid sequence. A good example of the use of alternative promoters in humans is the gene for dystrophin, the muscle protein that is deficient in Duchenne muscular dystrophy (see Chapter 37). This gene uses alternative promoters that give rise to brain-, muscle-, and retinal-specific proteins, all with differing N-terminal amino acid sequences.

Enhancers

Enhancers modulate the strength of gene expression in a cell

Although the promoter is essential for initiation of transcription, it is not necessarily alone in influencing the strength of transcription of a particular gene. Another group of *cis*-acting elements, known as **enhancers,** can regulate the level of

ADVANCED CONCEPT BOX
IDENTIFYING THE FUNCTION AND SPECIFICITY OF NUCLEOTIDE SEQUENCES

Consensus sequences are nucleotide sequences that contain unique core elements that identify the function and specificity of the sequence - for example, the TATA box. The sequence of the element may differ by a few nucleotides in different genes or in different species, but a core, or consensus, sequence is always present. In general, the differences do not influence the effectiveness of the sequence. These consensus sequences are deduced by comparing the promoters of the same genes from different species of eukaryotes, by comparing the promoter sequences from genes that bind the same transcription factor, or by experimentally determining the actual sequence of DNA that serves as the binding element for a transcription factor (see Fig. 23.1).

transcription of a gene, but unlike promoters, their position may vary widely with respect to the start point of transcription, and their orientation has no effect on their efficiency. **Enhancers** may lie upstream or downstream of the proximal promoter and are sometimes referred to as distal promoters. Many enhancers are important in conferring tissue-specific transcription, and in some instances, a nonspecific promoter may initiate transcription only in the presence of a tissue-specific enhancer. Alternatively, a tissue-specific promoter may initiate transcription but with a greatly increased efficiency in the presence of a nearby enhancer that is not tissue specific. In some genes - for example, immunoglobulin genes - enhancers may actually be present downstream of the start point of transcription, within an intron of the gene being actively transcribed.

Insulators

Insulators restrict the action of enhancers

Given that enhancer elements can be positioned at significant distances from a gene's proximal promoter, it was unclear how a given enhancer accurately targets the correct gene. Genetic elements, called **insulators,** were subsequently identified that act as boundary elements, allowing genes to maintain independent expression programs. These insulator elements are short DNA sequences that recruit *boundary element proteins,* preventing enhancers from influencing expression from an unintended neighboring promoter. Although the properties of insulator elements are well characterized, their precise mechanism of action is an active area of research; there is evidence that they work by altering the local structure of the DNA (e.g., by inducing the formation of loops).

Response elements

Response elements are binding sites for transcription factors and coordinately regulate expression of multiple genes (e.g., in response to hormonal or environmental stimuli)

Response elements (RE) are sequences that allow specific stimuli, such as steroid hormones (steroid-response element [SRE]), cyclic AMP (cyclic AMP–response element [CRE]), or insulin-like growth factor-1 (IGF-1, insulin response element [IRE]), to stimulate or repress gene expression. Response elements are part of promoters or enhancers, where they function as binding sites for specific transcription factors. Response elements are *cis*-acting sequences, typically 6–12 bases in length, and consensus sequences have been determined for those that are responsive to the same stimulus. A single gene may possess a number of different response elements, possibly having transcription stimulated by one stimulus and inhibited by another. Multiple genes may possess the same response element, and this facilitates coinduction or corepression of groups of genes, such as in response to a hormonal stimulus.

Transcription factors

Transcription factors are DNA-binding proteins that regulate gene expression

Promoters, enhancers, and response elements are sequence elements that are part of the gene; transcription factors are the proteins that recognize these sequences. Transcription factors are *trans*-acting factors because they are soluble proteins that can diffuse within the nucleus and act on multiple genes on different chromosomes. Unlike *cis*-acting sequences, they are not physically connected with the gene being transcribed. The human genome encodes approximately 2000 different transcription factors, representing more than 10% of all human genes.

Transcription factors can affect transcription directly by controlling the function of RNA polymerase or indirectly by affecting the chromatin structure

There are two main types of transcription factors: (1) general transcription factors and (2) sequence-specific transcription factors. General transcription factors are required for the expression of every gene. These transcription factors interact with RNA polymerase, forming the **initiation complex** that is required for the initiation of transcription. The general transcription factors will vary depending on the class of gene being transcribed, being generally different for RNA polymerase I, II, and III (Chapter 21). RNAPol II, for example, requires the general transcription factors TFIIA, B, D, E, F, and H.

Sequence-specific transcription factors are DNA-binding proteins that recognize specific nucleotide sequences and regulate gene expression (Fig. 23.2). These transcription factors can act positively to promote transcription or negatively to

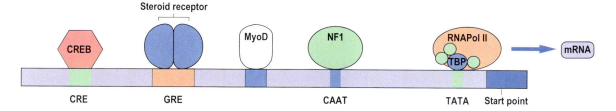

Fig. 23.2 **Regulation of gene expression by specific regulatory elements.** Binding of transcription factors to a steroid-response element modulates the rate of transcription of the message. Different elements have varying effects on the level of transcription, with some exerting greater effects than others, and they may also activate tissue-specific expression. CRE, cyclic AMP response element; CREB, CRE-binding protein; GRE, glucocorticoid response element; MyoD, muscle cell–specific transcription factor; NF1, nuclear factor 1. The proteins are shown in a linear array for convenience, but they interact physically with one another because of both their size and the folding of DNA.

promote gene silencing. The unique repertoire of transcription factors present in a cell at a given time will determine in large part which portion of the genome is transcribed into RNA. In eukaryotic cells, particularly mammalian cells, the RNA polymerases cannot recognize promoter sequences themselves. It is the task of the gene-specific factors to create a local environment that can successfully attract the general factors, which in turn attract the polymerase. However, there is emerging evidence that the RNA polymerase complex itself may also be important in the regulation of gene expression.

In addition, other proteins can bind to the sequence-specific transcription factors and modulate their function by repressing or activating gene expression; these factors are often called **coactivators** or **corepressors.** Thus the overall rate of RNA transcription from a gene is the result of the complex interplay of a multitude of transcription factors, coactivators, and corepressors. Because there are thousands of these factors in a cell, there is an almost unimaginably large number of combinations that can occur, and thus the control of gene expression can be very specific and very subtle.

There are many differences in transcriptional regulation between prokaryotes and eukaryotes. Gene structure is fundamentally different in prokaryotes because genes are typically organized into polycistronic operons, whereby one promoter sequence regulates the expression of multiple genes. Furthermore, in prokaryotes, the *cis*-elements that control the start site and, in general, the initiation of transcription are placed closer to the starting point. These *cis*-elements are fewer in number and are much less varied compared with those from eukaryotes, and distal promoter elements, such as enhancers, do not exist. In addition, there are fewer *trans*-acting factors that control gene expression, and for the most part in prokaryotes, genes are typically in the "on" state, with the *trans*-acting factors acting primarily as transcriptional repressors. Overall, gene expression regulation is much less complex in prokaryotes compared with eukaryotes.

Initiation of transcription requires binding of general transcription factors to DNA

For transcription to occur, transcription factors must bind to DNA. One of the first steps in transcription initiation is the recognition and binding of the TATA box sequence by a **TATA-binding protein (TBP).** For RNAPol II transcription initiation, TBP associates with a variety of other proteins to comprise the multisubunit general transcription factor **II D (TFIID,** or **TF$_{II}$D).** Binding of TBP to the TATA box has two effects: (1) It directs the positioning of the transcription apparatus at a fixed distance from the start point of transcription and thus allows RNAPol II to be positioned exactly at the site of initiation of transcription. (2) It distorts the DNA duplex, causing the DNA at that site to bend. Upon the recruitment of other general transcription factors and in the presence of ATP, the DNA at this site is partially unwound, exposing the correct DNA strand to the RNAPol II active site to be used as a template for DNA-templated RNA synthesis. This is termed **promoter opening.** Once transcription begins and the initial RNA:DNA hybrid is stabilized, many of the transcription factors required for binding and alignment of RNAPol II are released, and the polymerase travels along the DNA, forming the pre-mRNA transcript in a process named **promoter clearance.**

The function of transcription factors (TF) is controlled by intricate cellular-signal transduction networks that process external signals, such as stimulation by growth factors, hormones, and other extracellular cues, into changes in TF activities. Such changes are often conferred by phosphorylation, which can regulate the nuclear localization of TFs, their ability to bind to DNA, or their regulation of RNA polymerase activity. The presence of different TF-binding sites in a gene promoter further confers combinatorial regulation. This multilayered type of control ensures that gene transcription can be finely adjusted in a highly versatile way to specific cellular states and environmental requirements.

Transcription factors have highly conserved DNA-binding sites

The binding of transcription factors to DNA involves a relatively small area of the transcription factor protein, which comes into close contact with the major and/or minor groove of the DNA double helix to be transcribed. The regions of these proteins that contact the DNA are called DNA-binding domains, or motifs, and they are highly conserved between species. There is a variety of DNA-binding domains, some of which occur in multiple transcription factors or multiple times in the same factor. **Four common classes of DNA-binding domain are the following:**

1. Helix-turn-helix
2. Helix-loop-helix motifs
3. Zinc fingers (discussed later in the chapter)
4. Leucine zippers

Most known sequence-specific transcription factors contain at least one of these DNA-binding motifs, and proteins with unknown function that contain any of these motifs are likely to be transcription factors. The average transcription factor binds to a 10-nucleotide sequence of DNA and has 20 or more sites of contact between protein and DNA, which amplifies the strength and specificity of the interaction. There are an estimated 2000 transcription factors in the human genome, representing ~10% of genes, enabling sophisticated regulation of gene expression.

In addition to a DNA-binding domain, sequence-specific transcription factors also have a **transcription-regulatory domain** that is required for their ability to modulate transcription. This domain may function in a variety of ways. It may interact directly with the RNA polymerase–general transcription factor complex, it may have indirect effects via coactivators or corepressor proteins, or it may be involved in remodeling the chromatin (discussed later in the chapter) and so alter the ability of the promoter to recruit other transcription factors.

One way to characterize the interaction of a transcription factor with a particular DNA sequence is to use a technique termed the **electrophoretic mobility shift assay (EMSA**; see Fig. 23.3). This method has been used to aid in the purification of transcription factors, to identify them in complex mixtures (such as a cellular extract), to delineate the size of the binding site, and to estimate the strength of the interaction between the factor and the DNA sequence it recognizes.

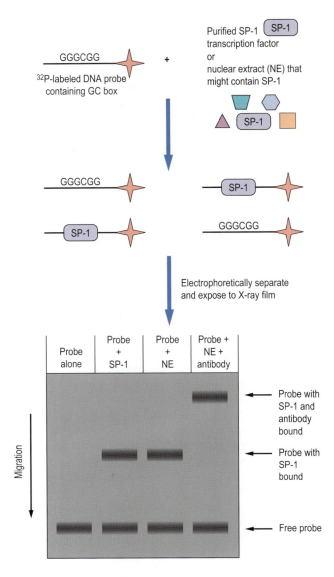

Fig. 23.3 **Electrophoretic mobility shift assay (EMSA).** The basic components of the EMSA method are included in the diagram. In this example, a DNA probe that is labeled with ^{32}P is first incubated either with the purified transcription factor SP-1 or with nuclear extract (NE) that contains SP-1 and is then subjected to native (nondenaturing) gel electrophoresis. If SP-1 binds to the probe, it has a slower mobility in the gel than the probe without protein bound (free probe). If an antibody to SP-1 is included in the reaction with NE, then the probe/anti-SP-1 antibody complex migrates even more slowly, confirming that the protein bound to the probe is indeed SP-1. EMSA can be used to help characterize any nucleic acid–protein interaction, including the interaction of RNA and proteins.

STEROID RECEPTORS

Steroid receptors possess many characteristics of transcription factors and provide a model for the role of zinc finger proteins in DNA binding

Steroid hormones have a broad range of functions in humans and are essential to normal life. They are derived from a common precursor, cholesterol, and thus share a similar structural backbone (Chapter 14). However, differences in hydroxylation of certain carbon atoms and aromatization of the steroid A-ring give rise to marked differences in biological effect. Steroids bring about their biological effects by binding to steroid-specific hormone receptors; these receptors are found in the cell cytoplasm and nucleus. For the type I (cytoplasmic) receptors, the steroid ligand induces structural changes that lead to dimerization of the receptor and exposure of a **nuclear localization signal (NLS)**; this signal, as well as dimerization, is commonly blocked by a heat shock protein that is released on steroid binding. The ligand–receptor complex now enters the nucleus, where it binds to DNA at the steroid-response element (SRE), alternatively called the **hormone-response element (HRE).** SREs may be found many kilobases upstream or downstream of the start of transcription. The steroid–receptor complex functions as a sequence-specific transcription factor, and binding of the complex to the SRE results in activation of the promoter and initiation of transcription (Fig. 23.4) or, in some cases, the repression of transcription. As might be expected, because of the large number of steroids found in humans, there are correspondingly large numbers of distinct steroid-receptor proteins, and each of these recognizes a consensus sequence, an SRE, in the region of a promoter.

The zinc finger motif

A zinc finger motif in steroid receptors binds to the steroid-response element in DNA

Central to the recognition of the SRE in the DNA, and to the binding of the receptor to it, is the presence of the so-called zinc finger region in the DNA-binding domain of the receptor molecule. Zinc fingers consist of a peptide loop with a zinc atom at the core of the loop. In the typical zinc finger, the loop comprises two cysteine and two histidine residues in highly conserved positions relative to each other, separated by a fixed number of intervening amino acids; the Cys and His residues are coordinated to the zinc ion. The zinc finger mediates the interaction between the steroid receptor molecule and the SRE in the major groove of the DNA double helix. Zinc finger motifs in DNA are generally organized as a series of tandem-repeat fingers; the number of repeats varies in different transcription factors. The precise structure of the steroid-receptor zinc finger differs from a consensus sequence (Fig. 23.5).

Zinc finger proteins recognize and bind to short **palindromic sequences** of DNA. Palindromes are DNA sequences that read the same (5′ to 3′) on the antiparallel strands - for example, 5′-GGATCC-3′, which reads the same 5′-to-3′ sequence on the complementary strand. The dimerization of the receptor and recognition of identical sequences on opposite strands strengthen the interaction between receptor and DNA and thus enhance the specificity of SRE recognition.

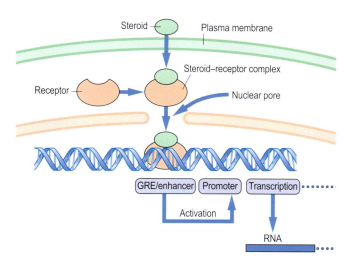

Fig. 23.4 **Regulation of gene transcription by glucocorticoids.** Steroids induce dimerization of receptor molecules that, in turn, bind to an enhancer, activating transcription of the gene. GRE, glucocorticoid-response element.

Organization of the steroid receptor

Steroid receptors are products of a highly conserved gene family

One central feature of all the steroid-receptor proteins is the similarity in organization of their receptor molecules. Each receptor has a DNA-binding domain, a transcription-activating domain, a steroid hormone–binding domain, and a dimerization domain. There are three striking features about the structure of the steroid-hormone receptors:

- The DNA-binding region always contains a highly conserved zinc finger region, which, if mutated, results in loss of function of the receptor.

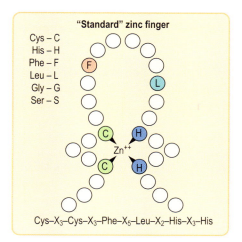

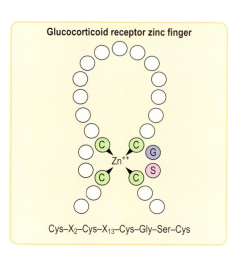

Fig. 23.5 **A "standard" zinc finger and a steroid-receptor zinc finger.** Zinc fingers are commonly occurring sequences that allow protein binding to double-stranded DNA. C, cysteine; G, glycine; S, serine; X, any intervening amino acid.

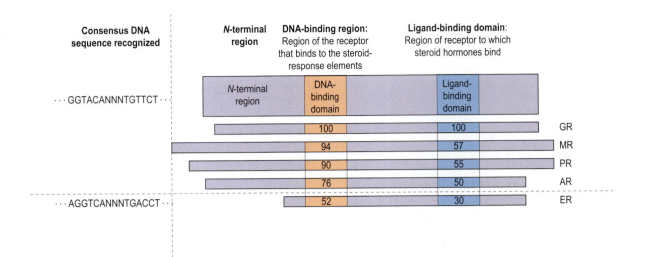

Consensus DNA sequence recognized	N-terminal region	DNA-binding region: Region of the receptor that binds to the steroid-response elements	Ligand-binding domain: Region of receptor to which steroid hormones bind	
···GGTACANNNTGTTCT···	N-terminal region	DNA-binding domain	Ligand-binding domain	
		100	100	GR
		94	57	MR
		90	55	PR
		76	50	AR
···AGGTCANNNTGACCT···		52	30	ER

Fig. 23.6 **Similarity between different steroid receptors.** The DNA-binding and hormone-binding regions of steroid receptors share a high degree of homology. The estrogen receptor is less similar to the glucocorticoid receptor than are the others. AR, androgen receptor; ER, estrogen receptor; GR, glucocorticoid receptor; MR, mineralocorticoid receptor; PR, progesterone receptor; NNN, any three nucleotides. Numbers denote percent amino acid homology to sequence in GR.

ADVANCED CONCEPT BOX
STEROID-RECEPTOR GENE FAMILY: THE THYROID HORMONE RECEPTORS

The steroid-receptor gene family, although large, is in fact only a subset of a much larger family of so-called nuclear receptors. All members of this family have the same basic structure as the steroid hormone receptors: a hypervariable N-terminal region, a highly conserved DNA-binding region, a variable hinge region, and a highly conserved ligand-binding domain (see Fig. 23.6). They are separated into two basic groups. **Type I (cytoplasmic) receptors** are a group of receptor proteins that form homodimers and bind specifically to steroid hormone–response elements only in the presence of their ligand, such as the glucocorticoid receptor. **Type II (nuclear) receptors** form homodimers that can bind to response elements in the absence of their ligand. The type II receptors include the thyroid hormone, vitamin D, and retinoic acid receptors.

▪ The DNA-binding regions of all the steroid-hormone receptors have a high degree of homology to one another.
▪ The steroid-binding regions show a high degree of homology to one another.

These common features have identified the steroid-receptor proteins as products of a gene family. It would appear that during the course of evolution, diversification of organisms has resulted in the need for different steroids with varied biological actions, and consequently, a single ancestral gene has undergone duplication and evolutionary change over millions of years, resulting in a group of related but slightly different receptors (Fig. 23.6).

ALTERNATIVE APPROACHES TO GENE REGULATION IN HUMANS

Promoter access

Chromatin structure affects access of transcription factors to genes and thereby affects gene expression

DNA in the cell nucleus is packaged into nucleosomes and higher-order structures in association with histones and other proteins forming chromatin (Chapter 20). Thus the promoters of some genes may not be readily accessible to transcription factors, even if the transcription factors themselves are present in the nucleus. It has become evident that the degree of packaging of promoter DNA and the presence, absence, and precise location of nucleosomes on a promoter influence the degree of access for both sequence-specific transcription factors and the RNAPol II complex associated with general transcription factors. Condensed chromatin, termed **heterochromatin**, where the DNA is tightly associated with the nucleosomes, is not a good template for transcription; chromatin remodeling (discussed later in the chapter) is required before transcription proceeds. **Euchromatin** is the term given to genomic regions that are only partially condensed into chromatin and typically, but not always, contain regions of active gene transcription. Remodeling may also be necessary in portions of euchromatin, depending on the cell or tissue, but the initial state of the chromatin is more accessible. Different regions of the genome will be packaged into heterochromatin and euchromatin depending on the cell type, allowing for regulation of gene expression at the level of DNA accessibility. Certain portions of chromosomes, such as centromeres and telomeres, are constitutively maintained in a heterochromatic state and are refractory to transcription.

Nucleosomes are dynamically altered during gene expression through the action of enzymes that modify and remodel them

The packaging of DNA into chromatin in eukaryotic cells has led to the evolution of regulatory mechanisms that control histone packaging and nucleosome stability and therefore the accessibility of DNA to the transcription machinery. Two classes of transcription factors exist that influence chromatin structure; they may either facilitate or repress transcription:

1. Those that alter the chemical makeup of chromatin by posttranslational modification of histone proteins
2. Those that utilize the energy from ATP hydrolysis to physically reposition nucleosomes relative to the underlying DNA

Histone proteins are substrates for enzymes that add and remove numerous chemical groups and small proteins (Table 23.2). The first histone modification identified was **histone acetylation,** the addition of an acetyl group from acetyl-CoA to the amino group of lysine residues, predominantly in the N-terminal domain of histone H3 and H4. Histones residues are also phosphorylated, methylated, and ubiquitinated, and many enzymes have been identified that catalyze the addition and removal of these modifications. The consequence of histone modifications is twofold. They can act directly by interfering with the histone:DNA interaction. For example, acetylation of lysine residues neutralizes their positive charge and weakens the histone:DNA interaction, making the underlying DNA more accessible. Second, histone modifications can act indirectly by serving as docking sites for the recruitment of other transcription factors to specific regions of the genome. For example, the methylation of histone H3 leads to the binding of a protein

HP-1 (heterochromatin protein-1) and associated factors, leading to increased condensation of DNA in this region. These two examples illustrate how different histone modifications can impact chromatin structure in contrasting ways and therefore have opposite effects on transcription. In general, histone acetylation correlates with active gene transcription, whereas histone methylation tends to cause gene silencing. However, it should be noted that there are examples that contradict this rule, and the effect of a given histone modification depends on the specific histone residue that is modified as well as the genomic context of the modified nucleosome.

Chromatin remodelers represent the second class of transcription factors affecting chromosome structure; they are ATP-dependent DNA translocases that are important for packaging the genome and regulating the accessibility of DNA in packaged regions. Transcription is influenced by chromatin remodelers in antagonistic ways: certain remodelers act to organize chromatin and restrict access to the transcription machinery, whereas others eject nucleosomes from *cis* regulatory sequences in promoters, thus promoting the activation of transcription. Certain remodelers are also essential to aid the progression of RNA polymerase along a gene during transcription elongation. Chromatin remodelers act in concert with histone modifications because many of the remodeling proteins contain histone modification–recognition domains that target them to specific genomic locations via a direct interaction with a modified histone. Taken together, it is evident that the dynamic interplay of chromatin structure, transcription factor, and cofactor binding is important in determining whether a gene is transcribed and how efficiently the RNA polymerase transcribes it.

Methylation of DNA regulates gene expression

Methylation is one of several epigenetic modifications of DNA; patterns of DNA methylation at birth affect risk for a number of age-related diseases

In multicellular eukaryotes, certain nucleotides, principally cytidine at the fifth position on the pyrimidine ring, can undergo enzymatic methylation without affecting Watson–Crick pairing. The methylated cytidine residues are usually found associated with a guanosine because the dinucleotide CpG - and in double-stranded DNA, the complementary cytidine - is also methylated, giving rise to a palindromic sequence:

5′ ^{m}CpG 3′
3′ GpC^{m} 5′

The presence of the methylated cytidine can be examined by susceptibility to restriction enzymes (Chapter 20) that cut DNA at sites containing specifically unmethylated CpG groups compared with other restriction enzymes that cut regardless of whether the CpG is methylated. In addition, a **bisulfite sequencing** technique that relies on the differential reactivity

Table 23.2 Examples of histone posttranslational modifications in humans

Transcriptional effect	Modification	Histone protein	Residue
Transcriptional repression	Arginine methylation	H3	Arg2
	Lysine methylation	H3	Lys9, Lys27
Transcriptional activation	Lysine methylation	H3	Lys4, Lys36, Lys79
		H4	Lys20
		H2B	Lys5
	Lysine acetylation	H3	Lys4, Lys14, Lys18, Lys23, Lys27
		H4	Lys5, Lys8, Lys12, Lys16, Lys20, Lys91
		H2A	Lys5, Lys9
		H2B	Lys5, Lys12, Lys20, Lys120
	Serine phosphorylation	H3	Ser10
		H4	Ser1

ADVANCED CONCEPT BOX
EPIGENETIC REGULATION OF GENE EXPRESSION

Methylation is one aspect of the study of **epigenetics**, a broad field that, in general, addresses alternative and heritable states of gene expression that rely on modifications of DNA and protein without alterations to the DNA sequence. Epigenetic control mechanisms include DNA methylation and histone modifications, and evidence suggests that these mechanisms can be directly influenced by an organism's environment. For example, the field of nutrigenomics asks how diet and nutritional factors regulate gene expression; early nutritional deprivation for a short time frame affects epigenetic mechanisms. Specifically, this deprivation can cause nutritional imprinting, generating chromatin states, which in certain individuals primes the gene-expression machinery for the development of diseases later in life. Thus the risk for age-related diseases, such as metabolic syndrome, obesity, atherosclerosis, diabetes, arthritis, and cancer, may be affected by diet and lifestyle factors during youth. The impact of epigenetic factors may change our approach to medical care, emphasizing the importance of preventive medicine and early intervention for control of age-related diseases because the starting point to disease susceptibility may happen many years before the onset of the first symptoms.

Cancer susceptibility and progression may also be predetermined by our epigenome. For example, hypermethylation of tumor-suppressor genes is commonly observed in human cancers. Drugs that inhibit DNA methyl transferases are being tested as a means to uncover these repressed genes for treatment of leukemias. Additionally, genes that negatively regulate cell growth are often repressed by the deacetylation of histones at these loci, creating a more compact, transcriptionally silent form of chromatin. **Histone deacetylase (HDAC) inhibitors** are being tested as therapeutic agents for the treatment of rapidly growing cancers, such as lymphomas.

ADVANCED CONCEPT BOX
CRISPR: EDITING THE GENOME

Clustered **r**egularly **i**nterspaced **s**hort **p**alindromic **r**epeats (CRISPR) are genetic loci that were originally described in bacterial genomes. The palindromic repeats are separated (interspersed) by unique sequences that comprise a DNA library derived from previous exposure to viruses. These gene clusters function together with CRISPR-associated system (cas) genes as part of the bacterial adaptive immune system. Upon infection by a virus, the CRISPR system will target and cleave complementary gene sequences in the viral DNA and inhibit its replication; a similar system targets foreign RNA.

Cas9, an RNA-guided DNA exonuclease, is a central component of CRISPR. Cas9 binds a highly structured CRISPR RNA (crRNA) that contains a short (~20 nucleotide) extension called a guide RNA (gRNA). Guide RNAs are derived from the interspersed DNA and are complementary to sequences in the viral genome. The guide RNA directs Cas9 to the target gene sequence with high precision, the viral genome is cleaved by a double strand break by Cas9, and the break is extended by Cas9 exonuclease activity - the infective agent has been destroyed.

CRISPR technology has revolutionized genome editing. Simply by engineering a guide RNA complementary to a specific DNA target and expressing Cas9 protein, CRISPR can be applied in many cellular contexts, including eukaryotic cells. Indeed, the CRISPR/Cas9 system has already been used to disrupt, or knock out, eukaryotic genes by introducing a double-strand break in what would become an exon in mRNA. Although the double-strand break by itself doesn't alter gene function, the process of repair by the cell, typically through nonhomologous end joining (see Chapter 20), introduces a modified DNA sequence at the site complementary to that surrounding the break. In this way, the sequence of the DNA is edited, and the gene function is permanently disrupted. In more sophisticated applications, the DNA cleavage and repair processes can be controlled to insert a modified DNA sequence, correcting a mutation in the genome.

CRISPR technology has been applied to cells in culture, stem cells, embryos, and even whole mammals. Currently, studies in animal models are promising, and although the Cas9 enzyme still makes occasional errors, CRISPR is being used in individual humans and in clinical studies. Depending on the success of these efforts, gene editing is likely to be directed at a wide range of genetic diseases; sickle cell anemia, cystic fibrosis, and cancer are prime candidates for initial studies.

of methyl cytidine can be used to precisely map the sites of methylation at single-base-pair resolution.

DNA methylation is carried out by a group of enzymes known as DNA-methyl transferases (DNMT), which are present in genomes from bacteria to humans. However, the extent to which an organism's genome is methylated varies widely. The human genome is largely methylated, and it has become clear that **methylation is generally associated with regions of DNA that are less actively transcribing RNA.** This is thought to be the result of both (a) the inability of certain transcription factors to bind methylated DNA and (b) the direct recruitment of histone-modification enzymes whose activity results in a more compacted, silent heterochromatin state. Although DNA methylation was once viewed as a permanent mark, it has become evident that demethylation of a gene at both its promoter and coding sequences permits initiation and optimal efficiency of transcription, respectively. In fact, regulation of the methylation state of promoters may be a more dynamic process than previously believed - for example, a

decreased methylation of certain gene promoters has been observed in muscle cells after exercise.

Many genes in humans (about 50%) have concentrated stretches of CG dinucleotides, so-called **CpG islands (CPI)**, in the region of their promoters. These CPIs are conspicuous in that they tend to be unmethylated and therefore permit the initiation of transcription at these loci. However, hypermethylation of specific CPIs has been detected in certain diseases, such as cancer, schizophrenia, and autism spectrum disorders. Furthermore, a link has recently been observed in humans between CPI hypermethylation and aging.

Alternative splicing of mRNA

Alternative splicing yields many variants of a protein from a single pre-mRNA

In Chapter 21, the concept of splicing the initial transcript, or pre-mRNA, was introduced. Most pre-mRNAs can be spliced in alternative ways, including or excluding different combinations of exons. In humans, more than 90% of multiexon genes are subject to alternative splicing. It is argued that alternative splicing is one mechanism to provide sufficient diversity among species to explain individual uniqueness, despite similarities in their gene complement. Because there are, on average, about seven exons per human gene, one pre-mRNA can give rise to many different versions of the mRNA and thus different final proteins, known as **isoforms.** These protein isoforms may differ by only a few amino acids or, alternatively, may have significant differences that confer different biological roles. For example, the inclusion or exclusion of a particular exon may affect where in the cell the protein is localized, whether a protein remains in the cell or is secreted, and whether there are specific isoforms in skeletal versus cardiac muscle. In some instances, alternative splicing produces a truncated protein isoform, known as a **dominant negative mutant protein,** which acts to inhibit the function of the full-length protein.

Alternative splicing is tightly regulated, so particular splice forms are typically present only in specific cells or tissues, at defined stages of development, or under well-defined conditions. For example, in the human brain, there is a family of cell-surface adhesion proteins, the **neurexins,** that mediate the complex network of interactions between approximately 10^{12} neurons. The neurexins are among the largest human genes, and hundreds, perhaps thousands, of neurexin isoforms are generated from only three genes by alternative promoters and splicing. These isoforms facilitate a diverse range of intercellular communications required for the development of sophisticated neural networks. The neurexins probably have an equally complex set of ligand isoforms, providing tremendous flexibility for reversible cellular interactions during the development of the central nervous system.

Editing of RNA at the posttranscriptional level

The editosome modifies the internal nucleotide sequence of mature mRNAs

RNA editing involves enzyme-mediated alteration of mature mRNAs before translation. This process, performed by **editosomes** (Chapter 21), may involve the insertion, deletion, or conversion of nucleotides in the RNA molecule. Like alternative splicing, the substitution of one nucleotide for another can result in tissue-specific differences in transcripts. For example, *APOB*, the gene for human apolipoprotein B (apoB), a component of low-density lipoprotein, encodes a 14.1-kb mRNA transcript in the liver and a 4536–amino acid protein product,

CLINICAL BOX
ALTERNATIVE SPLICING AND TISSUE-SPECIFIC EXPRESSION OF A GENE: A GIRL WITH A SWELLING ON THE NECK

A 17-year-old girl noticed a swelling on the left side of her neck. She was otherwise well, but both her mother and maternal uncle have had thyroid tumors removed. Blood was withdrawn and sent to the laboratory for measurement of calcitonin, a biomarker of medullary carcinoma. Calcitonin was greatly increased, and pathology of the excised thyroid mass confirmed the diagnosis of medullary carcinoma of the thyroid. This family has a genetic mutation causing the condition known as multiple endocrine neoplasia type IIA (MEN IIA). MEN IIA is an autosomal dominant cancer syndrome of high penetrance caused by a germline mutation in the RET protooncogene. About 5%–10% of cancers result from germline mutations, but additional somatic mutations are required for cancer to develop.

Comment
Expression of the calcitonin gene provides an example of how different mechanisms may regulate gene expression and give rise to tissue-specific gene products that have very different activities. The calcitonin gene consists of five exons and uses two alternative polyadenylation signaling sites. In the thyroid gland, the medullary C cells produce calcitonin by using one polyadenylation signaling site associated with exon 4 to transcribe a pre-mRNA comprising exons 1–4. The associated introns are spliced out, and the mRNA is translated to give calcitonin; elevated calcitonin is diagnostic for this condition. However, in neural tissue, a second polyadenylation signaling site next to exon 5 is used. This results in a pre-mRNA comprising all five exons and their intervening introns. This larger pre-mRNA is then spliced, and in addition to all of the introns, exon 4 is also spliced out, leaving an mRNA comprising exons 1–3 and 5, which is then translated into a potent vasodilator, calcitonin gene-related peptide (CGRP).

apoB100 (Chapter 33). However, in the small intestine, the mRNA is translated into a protein product called apoB48, which is 2152 amino acids long (~48% of 4536), those amino acids being identical to the first 2152 amino acids of apoB100. The difference in protein size occurs because, in the small intestine, nucleotide 6666 is "edited" by the deamination of a single cytidine residue, converting it to a uridine residue. The resulting change, from a glutamine to a stop codon, causes premature termination, yielding apoB48 in the intestine (Fig. 23.7).

In addition to this cytidine deaminase, there are other enzymes that modify mRNAs before translation, such as the **ADARs (adenosine deaminases acting on RNA).** ADAR1 catalyzes the deamination of adenosine to inosine residues in dsRNAs; the RNA editing is essential for the development of hematopoietic stem cells, and mutations in this enzyme in mice cause early embryonic death. ADAR2 modifies a neuronal glutamate receptor mRNA, which results in the change of a

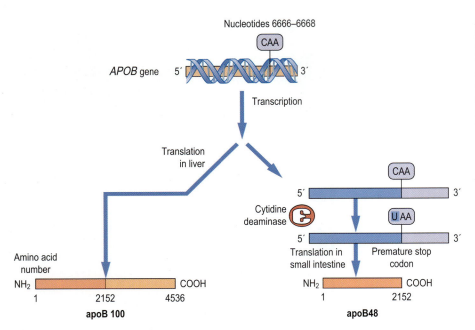

Nucleotides 6666–6668

Fig. 23.7 **RNA editing of the *APOB* gene in humans gives rise to tissue-specific transcripts.** In the small intestine, nucleotide 6666 of apoB mRNA is converted from a cytosine to uracil by the action of the enzyme cytidine deaminase. This change converts a glutamine codon in apoB100 mRNA to a premature stop codon, and when the mRNA is translated, the truncated product apoB48 is produced. (See also Chapter 33.)

single amino acid required for the function of the receptor; deficiency of this enzyme leads to seizures and neonatal death in mice.

RNA interference

RNA interference (RNAi), discussed in more detail in Chapter 21, is another way to control gene expression. At the heart of RNAi are very small noncoding RNAs, about 20–30 nucleotides long, known as micro-RNAs (miRNA). These are involved in the attenuation or repression of translation by binding to the 3′ UTR of an mRNA and recruiting factors that inhibit protein synthesis or by the destruction of the mRNA by an alternative pathway, e.g., an RNA-induced silencing complex (RISC) (see Chapter 21). During embryogenesis and in certain pathologic states, such as cancer, there are changes in the pattern of miRNA expression in cells, thereby changing gene expression in ways that might alter cell fate or favor cellular proliferation. RNAi holds promise in the treatment of human diseases where the inhibition of the expression of a gene product or the destruction of RNA would be therapeutic, such as in viral infections or cancer.

Preferential activation of one allele of a gene

Human genes are biallelic, but sometimes only one allele of the gene is expressed

The normal complement of human chromosomes comprises 22 pairs of autosomes, one from each parent, and two sex chromosomes. Genes located on each of the pairs of autosomes are therefore present in two copies: they are biallelic. Under normal circumstances, both genes are expressed without preference being given to either allele of the gene - that is, both the paternal and maternal copies of the gene can be expressed, unless there is a mutation in one allele that prevents this from occurring.

The situation with regard to sex chromosomes is slightly different. Sex chromosomes are of two types, X and Y, the X being substantially larger than the Y. Females have two X chromosomes, whereas males have one X and one Y chromosome. Although there are certain genes in common to both the X and Y chromosomes, there are also genes specific to the X chromosome and those only present on the Y chromosomes - for example, SRY, a sex-determining gene. Such genes are said to be monoallelic; they offer no choice as to which allele of the gene will be expressed.

Apart from the specific cases of monoallelic genes on sex chromosomes, all biallelic genes should be expressed. However, in humans, certain biallelic genes have been identified whereby only one allele - either maternal or paternal - is preferentially expressed, despite the fact that both alleles are functional genes and, in some cases, have the identical sequence. Three mechanisms have been identified in humans that restrict the expression of biallelic genes (Table 23.3). Genomic imprinting is true parent-specific expression, whereby either the maternal or the paternal allele is constitutively expressed, whereas the other allele remains permanently silent. In contrast, for X-chromosome inactivation and allelic exclusion, there is stochastic expression of either allele, resulting in different cells in the same individual expressing either the maternal or the paternal allele. Although there is no consensus regarding the mechanism that governs each type of allele-specific expression, epigenetic mechanisms play a key role.

CLINICAL BOX
IRON STATUS REGULATES TRANSLATION OF AN IRON CARRIER PROTEIN: A MAN WITH BREATHLESSNESS AND FATIGUE

A 57-year-old Caucasian male presented to his family doctor with breathlessness and fatigue. He noticed that his skin had become darker. Clinical evaluation indicated cardiac failure with impaired left ventricular function as a result of dilated cardiomyopathy, a low serum concentration of testosterone, and an elevated fasting concentration of glucose. Serum ferritin concentration was greatly increased, at > 300 μg/L, and the diagnosis of hereditary hemochromatosis was suspected. The man was treated by regular phlebotomy until his serum ferritin was < 20 μg/L (normal value 30–200 μg/L), at which point the phlebotomy interval was increased to maintain the serum ferritin concentration at < 50 μg/L.

Comment

In conditions of iron excess - for example, hemochromatosis - there is an increase in the synthesis of ferritin, an iron-binding and storage protein. Conversely, in conditions of iron deficiency, there is an increase in the synthesis of the transferrin-receptor protein, which is involved in the uptake of iron. In both cases,

the RNA molecules themselves are unchanged, and there is no change in the synthesis of the respective mRNAs. However, both the ferritin mRNA and the transferrin-receptor mRNA contain a specific sequence known as the iron-response element (IRE), a specific IRE-binding protein that can bind to mRNA. In iron deficiency, the IRE-binding protein binds the ferritin mRNA, prevents translation of ferritin, and binds the transferrin-receptor mRNA and prevents its degradation. Thus, in iron deficiency, ferritin concentrations are low, and transferrin-receptor concentrations are high. In states of iron excess, the reverse process occurs, and translation of ferritin mRNA increases, whereas transferrin-receptor mRNA undergoes degradation, serum ferritin concentrations are high, and transferrin-receptor concentrations are low (Fig. 23.8). About 10% of the US population carries the gene for hereditary hemochromatosis, but only homozygotes are affected with the disease. (See also the discussion of iron metabolism and hemochromatosis in Chapter 32.)

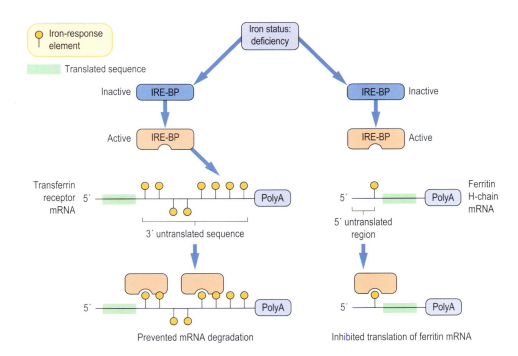

Fig. 23.8 **Regulation of mRNA translation by iron status.** The binding of a specific binding protein to the iron-response element (IRE) of the mRNA of iron-responsive genes can alter the translation of the mRNA into functioning proteins in different ways. When iron is deficient, the IRE-binding protein (IRE-BP) is activated and can bind to the 3′ end of the mRNA for the transferrin receptor. This prevents the degradation of the mRNA and thus increases the amount of transferrin receptor that can be made (*left*), thus increasing the amount of iron that the receptor can deliver to the cell. However, the IRE-BP also binds to the 5′ end of the ferritin mRNA and prevents its translation (*right*). Ferritin is a protein that sequesters and stores iron in the cytoplasm, and less is needed in times of iron deficiency. (See also Fig. 32.8.)

Table 23.3 Examples of types of restriction of biallelic genes in humans

Genomic imprinting	Parent-of-origin expression of specific (<100) autosomal genes established in germ cells. Imprinting may be tissue specific - monoallelic expression in some tissues, biallelic in others. Examples include insulin-like growth factor 2 (IGF-2) and Wilms' tumor susceptibility gene (WT1).
Allelic exclusion	Occurs specifically in B cells during the expression of immunoglobulin heavy and light chains, whereby only one allele is expressed at a given time to facilitate the production of a functional antibody. Once accomplished, expression of the allele that did *not* contribute to the functional antibody is permanently repressed.
X-chromosome inactivation (Lyonization)	Repression of transcription of the majority of genes on one X chromosome in all females, to account for gene dosage imbalance with males, who only have one X chromosome. The choice of which X chromosome is inactivated in each female cell is random.

For some genes, although two alleles exist in any particular cell, only one of these alleles is active. Hence the gene behaves as if it were monoallelic, although it is, in fact, biallelic.

ADVANCED CONCEPT BOX
X-CHROMOSOME INACTIVATION

Males have one X chromosome, whereas females have two. Thus, genes on the X chromosome are biallelic in females but monoallelic in males. To counteract this gene-dosage imbalance, in females, one of the X chromosomes in each cell is inactivated at an early stage of embryogenesis, shutting down the expression of the majority of its genes. This transcriptional repression is due primarily to the methylation of CpG islands on most of the genes on the inactivated chromosome. The inactivated X chromosome may be paternally or maternally derived, and which one is inactivated for a given cell is therefore random, but the descendants of that cell will have the same X inactivated. The inactivated X chromosome can still express a few genes, however, including XIST (inactive X–Xi-specific transcript), which codes for a noncoding RNA that is crucial in maintaining stable X inactivation. The inactivated X chromosome is reactivated during oogenesis in the female.

SUMMARY

- The control of gene expression involves both transcriptional and posttranscriptional events that regulate the expression of a gene in both time and place and in response to numerous developmental, hormonal, and stress signals.

ACTIVE LEARNING

1. How are steroid-response elements identified in the genome? Discuss the consequences of a mutation in an SRE versus a mutation in the SRE-binding protein. How does the zinc finger protein for the glucocorticoid receptor differ from that for the androgen or estrogen receptor?
2. What are the biochemical consequences of *APOB* gene editing in humans? Compare the effects of editing to introduce a substitution versus an insertion or deletion in an mRNA molecule.
3. Some genes have promoters that have no TATA box (TATA-less genes). Without this box, what determines where the RNAPol II complex will start transcription?
4. Compare the total number of genes with the number of translated proteins that may be synthesized by the human genome. Compare the concentration of transcription factors to the concentration of glycolytic enzymes in the cell.

- DNA sequences and DNA-binding proteins control gene expression. The DNA sequences include *cis*-acting promoters, such as the TATA box, and enhancers and response elements.
- The DNA-binding proteins are *trans*-acting transcription factors that bind with high specificity to these sequences and facilitate the binding and positioning of RNAPol II for the synthesis of pre-mRNA.
- Other factors that affect the conversion of genes to protein include access of the transcriptional apparatus to the gene, enzymatic modification of histones and nucleotides in the DNA, factors that affect alternative intron splicing, posttranscriptional editing of pre-mRNA, RNA interference, and restricted expression of biallelic genes.

FURTHER READING

Chery, J. (2016). RNA therapeutics: RNAi and antisense mechanisms and clinical applications. *Postdoc Journal*, *4*, 35–50.

Desiderio, A., Spinelli, R., Ciccarelli, M., et al. (2016). Epigenetics: Spotlight on type 2 diabetes and obesity. *Journal of Endocrinological Investigation*, *39*, 1095–1103.

Duarte, J. D. (2013). Epigenetics primer: Why the clinician should care about epigenetics. *Pharmacotherapy*, *33*, 1362–1368.

Jiang, F., & Doudna, J. A. (2017). CRISPR-Cas9 structures and mechanisms. *Annual Review of Biophysics*, *46*, 505–529.

Khyzha, N., Alizada, A., Wilson, M. D., et al. (2017). Epigenetics of atherosclerosis: Emerging mechanisms and methods. *Trends in Molecular Medicine*, *23*(4), 332–347.

Kuneš, J., Vaněčková, I., Mikulášková, B., et al. (2015). Epigenetics and a new look on metabolic syndrome. *Physiological Research*, *64*, 611–620.

Liscovitch-Brauer, N., Alon, S., Porath, H. T., et al. (2017). Trade-off between transcriptome plasticity and genome evolution in cephalopods. *Cell*, *169*, 191–202.

Oliveto, S., Mancino, M., Manfrini, N., et al. (2017). Role of microRNAs in translation regulation and cancer. *World Journal of Biological Chemistry*, *8*, 45–56.

Qin, J., Li, W., Gao, S. J., et al. (2017). KSHV microRNAs: Tricks of the devil. *Trends in Microbiology, 25,* 648–661.

Sabari, B. R., Zhang, D., Allis, C. D., et al. (2017). Metabolic regulation of gene expression through histone acylations. *Nature Reviews. Molecular Cell Biology, 18,* 90–101.

Salsman, J., & Dellaire, G. (2017). Precision genome editing in the CRISPR era. *Biochemistry and Cell Biology, 95,* 187–201.

Smith, N. C., & Matthews, J. M. (2016). Mechanisms of DNA-binding specificity and functional gene regulation by transcription factors. *Current Opinion in Structural Biology, 38,* 68–74.

RELEVANT WEBSITES

Catalog of genetic diseases: http://www.ncbi.nlm.nih.gov/omim

CRISPR:

　　https://www.youtube.com/watch?v=MnYppmstxIs

　　https://www.addgene.org/crispr/guide/

Epigenetics: http://learn.genetics.utah.edu/content/epigenetics/

Gene regulation: http://www.biology-pages.info/P/Promoter.html

RNA editing: http://dna.kdna.ucla.edu/rna/index.aspx

RNA interference: http://www.rnaiweb.com/

Steroid hormone receptors: http://www.biology-pages.info/S/SteroidREs.html

ABBREVIATIONS

ADAR	Adenosine deaminase acting on RNA
EMSA	Electrophoretic mobility shift assay
HRE	Hormone response element
Inr	Initiator
IRE	Iron response element
SRE	Steroid response element
TF	Transcription factor
TSS	Transcriptional start site

Genomics, Proteomics, and Metabolomics

Andrew R. Pitt and Walter Kolch

LEARNING OBJECTIVES

After reading this chapter, you should be able to:

- Describe what the terms genomics, transcriptomics, proteomics, and metabolomics mean.
- Discuss the differences between the -omics methods and their particular challenges.
- Give several examples of methods used in the various -omics technologies.
- Discuss biomarkers and their role in evidence-based medicine.

INTRODUCTION

Surprisingly, the 3 billion bases of the human genome only harbor and estimated 19,000–22,000 protein-coding genes. This is only about four times the number of genes of yeast, twice as many as the fruit fly *Drosophila melanogaster*, and less than many plants. However, the discovery of more than 1800 miRNAs - biologically active, short, non-protein-coding RNAs that are also transcribed from human DNA - demonstrates that genes are not the only biologically important parts of our DNA. The complexity of human biology can only be explained by the complex interactions of genes, miRNAs, proteins, and metabolites.

Many of the complex biological functions are generated by interactions among genes rather than by individual genes

Many of the complex biological functions that characterize humans are generated by **combinatorial interaction between genes,** rather than the now outdated dogma of each individual gene being responsible for a specific biological function. Most mammalian genes consist of multiple exons, which are the parts that eventually constitute the mature mRNA, and introns, which separate the exons and are removed from the primary transcript by splicing. Mammalian cells use **alternative splicing** and alternative gene promoters to produce four to six different mRNAs from a single gene, so the number of protein-coding mRNAs produced by gene transcription, the

transcriptome, may be as large as 100,000 (see Chapters 21 and 22).

Posttranslational modifications add further levels of complexity

This complexity is further augmented at the protein level by posttranslational modifications and targeted proteolysis that could generate an estimated 500,000–1,000,000 functionally different protein entities, which comprise the **proteome**. An estimated 10%–15% of these proteins function in metabolism, which collectively describes the processes used to provide energy and the basic low-molecular-weight building blocks of cells, such as amino acids, fatty acids, and sugars. It also includes the processes that metabolize exogenous substances such as drugs or environmental chemicals.

The human metabolome database currently contains about 42,000 entries. The real size of the **metabolome** is unknown because it increases with the number of environmental substances an organism is exposed to. The relationship between the different -omes is depicted in Fig. 24.1.

Studies of the genome, transcriptome, proteome, and metabolome pose different challenges

The genome and transcriptome consist entirely of the nucleic acids DNA and RNA, respectively. Their uniform physicochemical properties have enabled efficient and ever-cheaper methods for their amplification, synthesis, sequencing, and highly multiplexed analysis. The proteome and metabolome pose much more significant analytical challenges because they consist of molecules with widely differing physicochemical properties and abundance. For example, the concentration of proteins in human serum spans 12 orders of magnitude, and under normal conditions, genes are equally abundant and the genome is relatively static, whereas the transcriptome and proteome are dynamic and can change on a timescale of seconds in response to internal and external cues. The most pronounced dynamic responses may manifest themselves in the metabolome because it directly reflects the interactions between organism and environment. Thus complexity increases as we move from the genome to the transcriptome and on to the proteome and metabolome, whereas our detailed knowledge of the components decreases. The analysis of all -omics data requires large and sophisticated **bioinformatics** resources and has stimulated the development of **systems biology**, which uses mathematical and computational modeling to interpret the functional information about biological processes contained in these data.

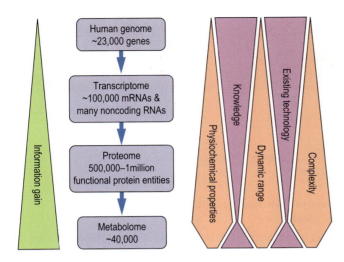

Fig. 24.1 **Relationship between the -omics.** Complexity, dynamic range and diversity in physicochemical properties increase as we move from genes to transcripts and proteins but may decrease again at the level of metabolites. This presents a huge technologic challenge but also represents a rich source of information gain, especially if the different -omics disciplines can be integrated into a common view.

GENOMICS

Genome analysis provides a way to predict the probability of a condition, but it does not provide information on whether and when this probability will manifest itself

The "whether and when" information is better gained from the transcriptome, proteome, and metabolome. They give a dynamic picture of the current state of an organism and lend themselves to monitoring of changes in that state (e.g., during disease progression or treatment). Thus the information provided by the -omics technologies is complementary, and their use for diagnostic purposes is mainly limited by the complexity of the equipment and analysis. Genomics and transcriptomics are making their way into the clinical laboratory and are poised to become part of routine diagnostics in the near future.

Many diseases have an inheritable genetic component

Many diseases are caused by genetic aberrations, and many more manifest a genetic predisposition or component. The Online Mendelian Inheritance in Man (OMIM) database lists more than 22,000 gene mutations that are associated with more than 7700 phenotypes that cause or predispose to disease. These numbers suggest that many diseases are caused by mutations in single genes and that many more have an inheritable genetic component. Thus the genome holds a rich source of information about our physiology and pathophysiology. We now have a broad arsenal of techniques for genome analysis at our disposal, allowing the detection of gross abnormalities down to single-nucleotide changes,

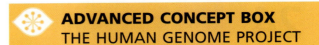

ADVANCED CONCEPT BOX
THE HUMAN GENOME PROJECT

The Human Genome Project (HGP) officially began in 1990 and culminated with the deposition of the completed sequence into public databases in 2003. However, in-depth analysis and interpretation will go on for much longer. The HGP was unique in several ways. It was the first global life science project, being coordinated by the Department of Energy and the National Institutes of Health (United States). The Wellcome Trust (United Kingdom) became a major partner in 1992, and further significant contributions were made by Japan, France, Germany, China, and other countries. More than 2800 scientists from 20 institutions around the world contributed to the paper describing the finished DNA sequence in 2004. This work was conducted on an industrial scale with industrial-style logistics and organization. In fact, the HGP received competition from Celera Genomics, a private company founded in 1998, and the first draft sequences of the human genome were published in two parallel papers in 2001. The HGP used a **"clone-by-clone" approach** where the genome was cloned first, and then these large clones were divided into smaller portions and sequenced. Celera followed a fundamentally different strategy, **shotgun sequencing,** where the whole genome was broken up into small pieces that can be sequenced directly, with the full sequence being assembled afterward. This approach is much faster but less reliable in producing continuous sequences, and it is much less able to mend gaps in the assembled sequence. The 2001 draft genomes estimated the existence of 30,000–35,000 genes. The refined HGP 2003 sequence confirmed 19,599 protein-coding genes and identified another 2188 DNA predicted genes, a surprisingly low number. They are contained in 2.85 billion nucleotides covering more than 99% of the euchromatin (i.e., gene-containing DNA). Many thousands of genomes have been sequenced since then, and the human reference genome is constantly updated. In 2016, using a combination of four approaches, a sequence with only 85 euchromatic gaps was published, compared with the 150,000 in the draft sequence, and the current sequences are extremely accurate. Genome sequences are accessible publicly through all major nucleotide databases. The rapidly falling cost of genome sequencing makes it affordable for widespread use in research and clinical diagnostics.

and these techniques are increasingly being used for clinical diagnostics.

Karyotyping, comparative genome hybridization (CGH), chromosomal microarray analysis (CMA), and fluorescence in situ hybridization (FISH)

Karyotyping assesses the general chromosomal architecture

Early successes of exploiting genome information for the diagnosis of human disease include the discovery of trisomy

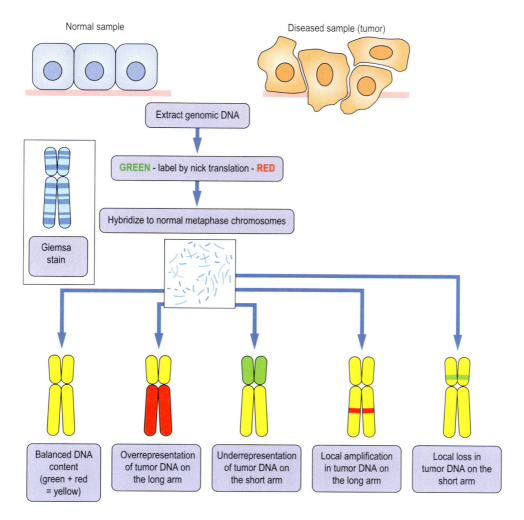

Fig. 24.2 **Principles of comparative genome hybridization (CGH).** Genomic DNA is isolated from a normal and a diseased sample (here, from a tumor) to be compared. The DNA is labeled by nick translation with green or red fluorescent dyes, then hybridized to a normal chromosome spread. If the DNA content between samples is balanced, equal amounts of the control (green) and tumor (red) DNA will hybridize, resulting in a yellow color. Global or local amplifications or losses of genetic material will reveal themselves by a color imba ance.

21 as the cause of **Down's syndrome** in 1959 and the discovery of the **Philadelphia chromosome** associated with **chronic myelogenous leukemia** (CML) in 1960. Since then, karyotyping has identified a large number of chromosomal aberrations, including amplifications, deletions, and translocations, especially in tumors. The method is based on simple staining of chromosome spreads by Giemsa or other stains that reveal a banding pattern characteristic for each chromosome that is visible through the light microscope. Although it only reveals crude information, such as number, shapes, and gross alterations of general chromosomal architecture, karyotyping is still a mainstay of clinical genetic analysis.

Comparative genome hybridization compares two genomes of interest

A refinement of karyotyping is **comparative genome hybridization (CGH),** which detects differences in copy number between test and reference chromosomal DNA. The principle of CGH is to compare two genomes of interest, usually a diseased against a normal control genome. The genomes that are to be compared are labeled with two different fluorescent dyes. The fluorescently labeled DNAs are then hybridized to a spread of normal chromosomes and evaluated by quantitative image analysis (Fig. 24.2). Because fluorescence has a large dynamic range (i.e., the relationship between fluorescence intensity and concentration of the probe is linear over a wide range), CGH can detect regional gains or losses in chromosomes with much higher accuracy and resolution than conventional karyotyping. Losses of 5–10 megabases (Mb) and amplifications of < 1 Mb are detectable by CGH, permitting the detection of chromosomal deletions and duplications. However, balanced changes, such as inversions or balanced translocations, escape detection because they do not change the copy number and hybridization intensity.

In chromosomal microarray analysis, the labeled DNA is hybridized to an array of oligonucleotides

Further improvements in resolution are afforded by **chromosomal microarray analysis (CMA)**. In this method, the labeled DNA is hybridized to an array of oligonucleotides. Modern oligonucleotide synthesis and array manufacturing can produce arrays containing many million oligonucleotides on chips the size of a microscope slide. By choosing the oligonucleotides so that they cover the region of interest to an equal extent, a very high resolution can be achieved, allowing the detection of copy-number changes at the level of 5–10 kb in the human genome. CMA is used in **prenatal screening for the detection of chromosomal defects**. Because the probe DNA can be amplified by polymerase chain reaction (PCR; Fig. 24.3), only minute amounts of starting material are required.

Fluorescence in situ hybridization can be used when the gene in question is known

If the gene of interest is known, the respective recombinant DNA can be labeled and used as a probe on chromosome spreads. This method, called **fluorescence in situ hybridization (FISH)**, can detect gene amplifications, deletions, and chromosomal translocations. With the use of different-colored fluorescent labels, several genes can be stained simultaneously.

Gene mutations can be studied by sequencing

Efforts to find individual disease genes were hampered by insufficient knowledge of the genome and by the lack of high-resolution mapping methods. This situation dramatically

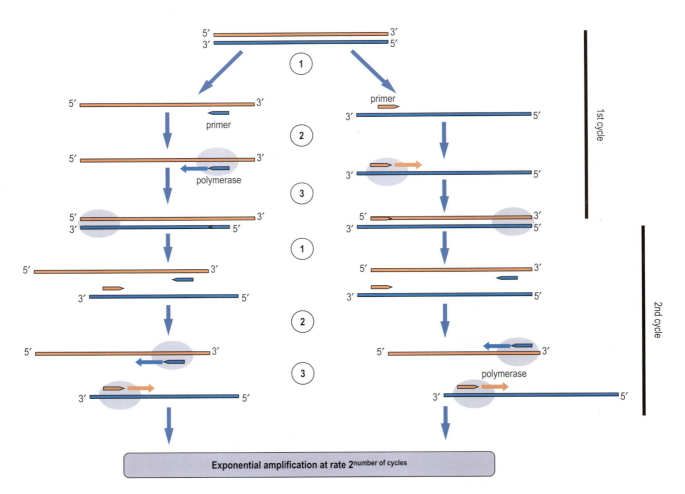

Exponential amplification at rate $2^{\text{number of cycles}}$

Fig. 24.3 **Polymerase chain reaction (PCR).** This method is widely used for the amplification of DNA and RNA. The nucleic acid template is heat-denatured, and specific primers are annealed by lowering the temperature **(step 1)**. The primers are extended using reverse transcriptase if the template is RNA, or a DNA polymerase if the template is DNA **(step 2)**. The result is a double-stranded product **(step 3),** which is heat-denatured so that the cycle can start again. Typically, between 25 and 35 cycles are used. The amplification is exponential, and hence PCR enables us to analyze minute amounts of DNA or RNA down to the single-cell level. The use of heat-stable and high-fidelity DNA polymerases permits amplification of fragments up to several thousand base pairs long. Many variations of PCR have been developed for a wide range of applications, such as molecular cloning, site-directed mutagenesis, generation of labeled probes for hybridization experiments, quantitation of RNA expression, DNA sequencing, genotyping, and many others.

changed with the completion of the human genome sequence in 2003 and the rapid development of novel technologies, called **next-generation sequencing (NGS),** which made sequencing both fast and affordable.

Four principles of DNA sequencing

There are four principles of DNA sequencing. (1) The **Maxam–Gilbert method** uses chemicals to cleave the DNA at specific bases and then separate the fragments by size on high-resolution gels, allowing the sequence to be read from the fragments. (2) **The Sanger method** uses a polymerase to synthesize DNA in the presence of small amounts of chain-terminating nucleotides (Fig. 24.4). These methods were the first successful DNA sequencing techniques. Although the former has become obsolete, the Sanger method is still widely used. (3) The extension of the complementary DNA strand is measured when a

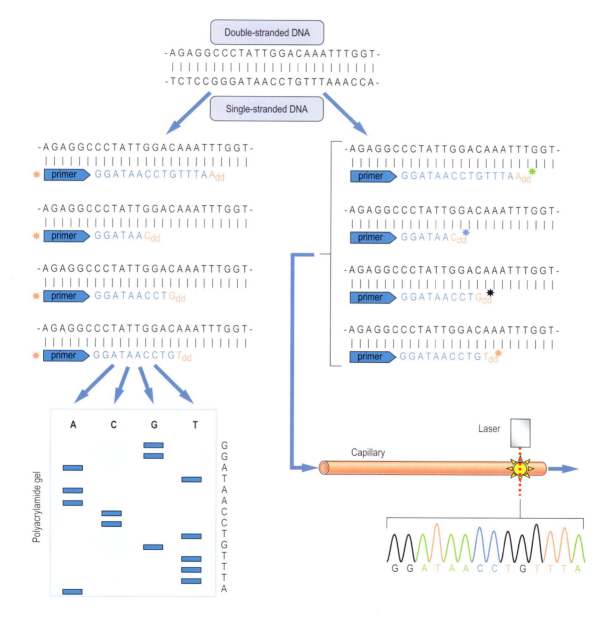

Fig. 24.4 DNA sequencing using Sanger's chain termination method. Double-stranded DNA is heat-denatured to generate single-stranded DNA. Primers (usually hexamers of random sequence) are annealed to generate random initiation sites for DNA synthesis, which is carried out in the presence of DNA polymerase, deoxynucleotides (dNTP), and small amounts of dideoxynucleotides (ddNTP). The ddNTPs lack the 3'-hydroxyl group that is required for DNA strand elongation. They terminate the synthesis, leading to fragments of different sizes, each ending in a specific nucleotide. These fragments can be separated by polyacrylamide gel electrophoresis, and the sequence is then read from the "ladder" of fragments on the gel. To visualize the fragments, either the DNA can be labeled by adding radioactive or fluorescent dNTPs or the primers can be labeled (as indicated in the figure) with a fluorescent dye. Using ddNTPs labeled with different dyes permits all four reactions being mixed together and separated by capillary electrophoresis. Online laser detection enables direct reading of the sequence. This "capillary DNA sequencing" gives longer reads than gels, permits multiplexing, and has high throughput. It was the method used for most of the sequencing in the Human Genome Project.

matching nucleotide is added. (4) The ligation of a synthetic oligonucleotide to the DNA target to be sequenced is monitored; this only occurs when a nucleotide pair in the oligonucleotide matches the sequence of the target DNA. Variations of these four methods are incorporated in NGS workflows.

There are several NGS methods using different ways to read the DNA sequence

All NGS methods share the principle of conducting many millions of parallel sequencing reactions in microscopic compartments on arrays, nanobeads, or via nanopores. These sequence pieces are assembled into complete genome sequences using sophisticated bioinformatics methods. Whereas the first human genome sequence cost $2.7 billion and took more than 10 years to complete, thanks to NGS, we can now sequence a human genome in a single day for ~$1000. Thus NGS has enabled the large-scale hunt for gene mutations by direct sequencing. Notable examples of such projects are the **Cancer Genome Projects** executed by the Wellcome Trust Sanger Centre in the United Kingdom and the US National Cancer Institute and the **100,000 Genomes Project** funded by the UK government. The aim of these projects is to establish a systematic map of mutations in disease and use this map for risk stratification, early diagnosis, and choice of the best treatment in patients, as well as potentially providing information on the underlying causes of disease that may lead to better therapies.

Single-nucleotide polymorphisms (SNP) are useful in identification and assessment of disease risk

Genomes in a population vary slightly by small changes, most often just involving single nucleotides, called **single-nucleotide polymorphisms (SNP)**. The most common way to examine SNPs is by direct sequencing or array-based methods. For the first method, DNA is usually amplified by PCR and then sequenced. For the second method, oligonucleotide arrays containing all possible permutations of SNPs are probed with genomic DNA, so successful hybridization only occurs when the DNA sequences match exactly.

Systematic SNP mapping has proved useful in studying genetic identity and inheritance and also in the identification and risk assessment of genetic diseases

The initial human genome sequences yielded approximately 2.5 million SNPs, whereas by 2016, nearly 550 million SNPs had been catalogued. **The International HapMap Project** systematically catalogues genetic variations based on large-scale SNP analysis in more than 1300 humans from 11 diverse ethnic origins.

Genome-wide association studies (GWAS) try to link the frequency of SNPs to disease risks

Although GWASs have discovered new genes involved in diseases such as Crohn's disease and age-related macular degeneration, the typically low risk associated with individual SNPs hampers such correlations, especially in multigenetic diseases. There is much debate on how feasible it is to overcome this limitation by examining very large cohorts.

Epigenetic changes are heritable traits not reflected in the DNA sequence

Although the genome as defined by its DNA sequence is commonly viewed as the hereditary material, there are also other heritable traits that are not reflected by changes in the DNA sequence

These traits are called epigenetic changes (see also Chapter 23). They comprise **histone modifications such as acetylation and methylation** that affect chromatin structure. Another modification is **methylation of the DNA** itself, which occurs at the N^5 position of cytosines, typically in the context of the sequence CpG. Methylation of CpG clusters, so-called CpG islands, in gene promoters can shut down the expression of a gene. These methylation patterns can be heritable by a poorly understood process called **genomic imprinting**.

Aberrations in gene methylation patterns can cause diseases and are common in human tumors, often serving to silence the expression of tumor-suppressor genes.

The most common methods to analyze DNA methylation rely on the fact that bisulfite converts cytosine residues into uracil but leaves 5-methylcytosine intact (Fig. 24.5). This change in the DNA sequence can be detected by several methods, including DNA sequencing of the treated versus untreated DNA, differential hybridization of oligonucleotides that specifically detect either the mutated or unchanged DNA, or array-based methods. The latter methods, similar to SNP analysis, also rely on differential hybridization to find bisulfite-induced changes in the DNA, but because millions of oligonucleotide probes may be displayed on an array, they are able to interrogate large numbers of methylation patterns simultaneously. The main limitations are the possibility that bisulfite modification may be incomplete, giving rise to false positives, and the severe general DNA degradation that occurs during the harsh conditions of bisulfite modification. Some new NGS methods can detect DNA methylation directly, and this will accelerate progress in epigenomics. **The epigenome is more variable between individuals than the genome.** Hence it will require a greater effort to map it systematically, but it also holds more individual information that can be useful at this time for designing personal medicine approaches.

Gene expression and transcriptomics

Genes represent the DNA sequences that correspond to functionally distinguishable units of inheritance. This definition goes back to experiments performed by Gregor Mendel, the father of genetics, in the 1860s, who showed that the color of pea

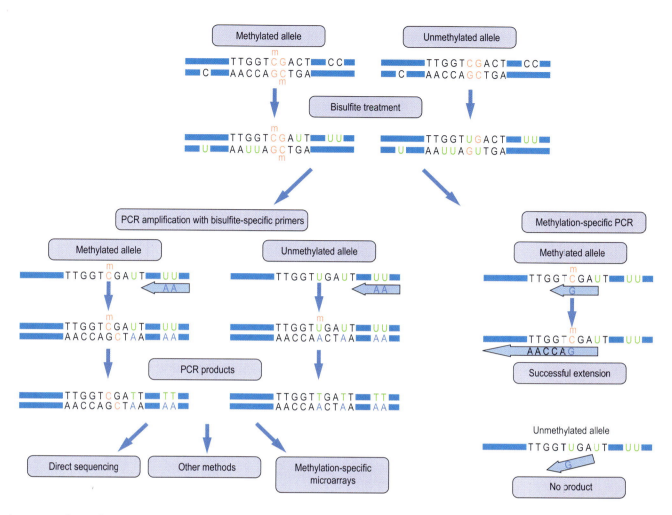

Fig. 24.5 **Analysis of DNA methylation.** DNA methylation typically occurs on cytosine in the context of "CpG islands" (colored orange), which are enriched in the promoter regions of genes. Bisulfite converts cytosine residues to uracil but leaves 5-methylcytosine residues unaffected. This causes changes in the DNA sequence that can be detected in various ways. Many methods use a polymerase chain reaction (PCR) amplification step with primers that will selectively hybridize to the modified DNA (left panel). The PCR products have characteristic sequence changes where the unmodified cytosine-guanosine base pairs are replaced by thymidine-adenosine, whereas the original sequence is maintained when the cytosine was methylated. There are many methods to analyze these PCR products. The most common are direct sequencing or hybridization to a microarray that contains oligonucleotides representing all permutations of the expected changes. Another common method is methylation-specific PCR (MSP), where the primer is designed so that it can only hybridize and extend if the cytosine was methylated and hence preserved during bisulfite treatment.

plants is inherited as discrete genetic units. About 100 years later, Marshall Nirenberg defined a simple relationship - that is, "Gene makes RNA, makes protein" - that anchored the concept that genes encode the information to make proteins, and RNA is the messenger that transports that information (hence the name mRNA). It has turned out that each step is highly regulated and diversified.

Humans possess about 20,000 protein-coding genes, each of which gives rise to an average of four to six mRNA transcripts generated by differential splicing, RNA editing, and alternative promoter usage. The transcriptome represents the complement of RNAs transcribed from the genome. However, the largest part of the transcriptome is not protein-coding genes but noncoding RNAs that fulfill structural and regulatory functions. The transcriptome is naturally more dynamic than the genome and may differ widely between different cell types, tissues, and conditions.

The translation of mRNAs into proteins (Chapter 22) is also a highly regulated process, so no direct general correlations between mRNA expression and protein concentrations can be drawn. **Protein-coding genes only constitute 1%–2% of the human genome sequence,** and the assumption that most transcripts originate from genes has recently been superseded by the discovery that more than 80% of the genome can be transcribed. Although some of these **noncoding RNAs** serve structural functions (e.g., as part of ribosomes), most

ADVANCED CONCEPT BOX
NONCODING RNAs ncRNA

Noncoding RNAs (ncRNA) is a summary name for RNAs that do not encode proteins. They comprise abundant species, such as transfer RNAs and ribosomal RNAs, which are involved in protein translation, and several ncRNAs function as molecular guides that participate in processes that require sequence-specific recognition, such as RNA splicing or telomere maintenance. However, the vast majority of ncRNAs seems to have regulatory functions in gene expression. The call to fame came with the award of the Nobel Prize to Andrew Fire and Craig Mello in 2006 for their discovery of RNA interference–gene silencing by double-stranded RNA. These **small interfering (si) RNAs** are part of an enzyme complex that targets and cleaves mRNAs with high specificity conferred by the siRNA sequence. siRNAs have now become a powerful tool in the arsenal of the molecular biologist to down-regulate the expression of selected mRNAs with high specificity and efficiency. **Micro-RNAs (miRNA)** are also small RNAs that are either transcribed under control of their own promoter or often also as part of introns in protein-coding genes. They originate from longer transcripts and are more extensively processed than siRNAs. Functionally, an important distinction is that **siRNAs are very specific**, requiring a perfect match to their targets, whereas **miRNAs have imperfect sequence recognition** and therefore act on a larger range of targets, often regulating whole sets of genes. Another difference is that siRNAs induce mRNA degradation, whereas miRNAs can also prevent mRNA translation. The human genome encodes more than 1800 miRNAs, which may regulate as much as 60% of genes, thus playing a major role in the control of gene expression. Due to their pleiotropic targeting, **miRNAs** can affect whole programs of gene expression, and aberrant miRNA expression has been implicated in many human diseases, including cancer, obesity, and cardiovascular disease. The discovery of **long noncoding RNAs (lncRNA)**, which are more than 200 nucleotides long and seem to have many different functions, extends the role of RNA even further. It appears that very little, if any, of the genome is "junk" as was commonly believed just 10 years ago.

regulate gene transcription, mRNA processing, mRNA stability, and protein translation. **Thus the largest part of the transcriptome seems dedicated to regulatory functions,** and these regulatory RNAs can even be transcribed from within protein-coding genes. Therefore the concept of what constitutes a gene will likely be revised over time.

Studying gene transcription by gene (micro)arrays and RNA sequencing

Methods for studying global transcription are now well established. The original methods relied on **gene (micro) arrays,** which contain several million DNA spots arranged on a slide in a defined order (Fig. 24.6). Modern arrays use synthetic oligonucleotides, which can be either prefabricated and deposited on the chip or synthesized directly on the chip surface. Usually several oligonucleotides are used per gene. They are carefully designed based on genome sequence information to represent unique sequences suitable for the unambiguous identification of specific RNA transcripts. Today's high-density arrays contain enough data points to survey the transcription of all human genes, map exon content, and splice variants of mRNAs; in tiling arrays, overlapping oligonucleotide sequences representing the entire genome are used. Noncoding RNAs such as siRNAs and miRNAs can also be included.

The arrays are hybridized with complementary RNA (cRNA) probes corresponding to the RNA transcripts isolated from the cells or tissues that are to be compared. The probes are made from isolated RNAs by copying them first into complementary DNA (cDNA) using reverse transcriptase, a polymerase that can synthesize DNA from RNA templates. The resulting cDNA is transcribed back into cRNA, as RNA hybridizes stronger to the DNA oligonucleotides on the array than cDNA would. During cRNA synthesis, modified nucleotides are incorporated that are labeled with fluorescent dyes or tags, such as biotin, which can easily be detected after hybridization of the cRNA probes to the array. After hybridization and washing off unbound probes, the array is scanned, and the hybridization intensities are compared using statistical and bioinformatic analyses. The results allow a relative quantitation of changes in transcript abundances between two samples or different time points. Thanks to a common convention for reporting microarray experiments, called minimal information for the annotation of microarray experiments (MIAME), array results from different experiments can be compared, and public gene-array databases are a valuable source for further analysis. Gene-array analysis is already being used for clinical applications. For instance, patterns of gene transcription in **breast cancers** have been developed into tests for assessing the risk of recurrence and the potential benefit of chemotherapy.

Transcriptome analysis is now most commonly performed by **direct sequencing** once the RNAs have been converted to cDNAs. The advances in rapid and cheap DNA sequencing methods permit every transcript to be sequenced multiple times. These **"deep sequencing" methods** not only unambiguously identify the transcripts and splice forms but also allow the direct counting of transcripts over the whole dynamic range of RNA expression, resulting in absolute transcript numbers rather than relative comparisons. These sequencing methods, dubbed **RNAseq,** have become the mainstay of transcriptomics, although array-based methods continue to be improved and still have value. RNAseq is rapid and captures all RNAs without any prior knowledge, so it is the best discovery tool. However, the RNA generally needs to be fragmented into shorter pieces, with the full sequence reconstructed after analysis, which adds to the complexity, and some data may be missing. Technology

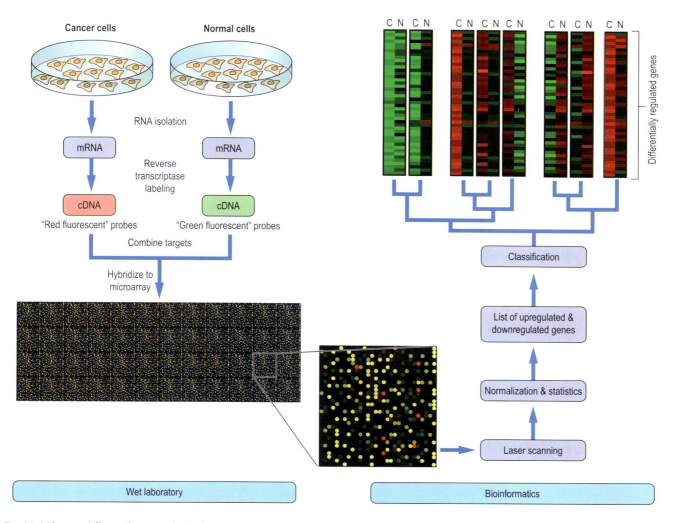

Fig. 24.6 **The workflow of a gene (micro)array experiment.** A two-color array experiment comparing normal and cancer cells is shown as an example. See text for details. A common way to display results is heat maps, where increasing intensities of reds and greens incicate up- and down-regulated genes, respectively, whereas black means no change. C, cancer cells; N, normal cells. The figure is modified from http://en.wikipedia.org/wiki/DNA_microarray.

is improving rapidly in this area, and with advances such as the nanopore systems, it may not be long before transcriptomes can be read on small USB-connected devices in the clinic.

ChIP-on-chip technique combines chromatin immunoprecipitation with microarray technology

Mapping of the occupancy of transcription-factor-binding sites can reveal which genes are likely to be regulated by these factors

Our ability to survey the transcription of all known human genes poses the question of which transcription factors (TF) are controlling the observed transcriptional patterns. The

human genome contains many thousands of binding sites for any given TF, but only a small fraction of these binding sites actually is occupied by TFs and involved in the regulation of gene transcription. Thus **the systematic mapping of the occupancy of TF-binding sites can reveal which genes are actually regulated by which TFs**. The techniques developed for this (Fig. 24.7) combine **chromatin immunoprecipitation (ChIP)** with **microarray technology (chip)** or DNA sequencing and are called **ChIP-on-chip or ChIP-seq**.

ChIP involves the covalent crosslinking of proteins to the DNA they are bound to by formaldehyde treatment of living cells. Then the DNA is purified and fragmented into small (0.2–1.0 kb) pieces by ultrasound sonication. These DNA fragments are isolated by immunoprecipitating the crosslinked protein with a specific antibody. The associated DNA is then eluted and identified by PCR with specific primers that amplify

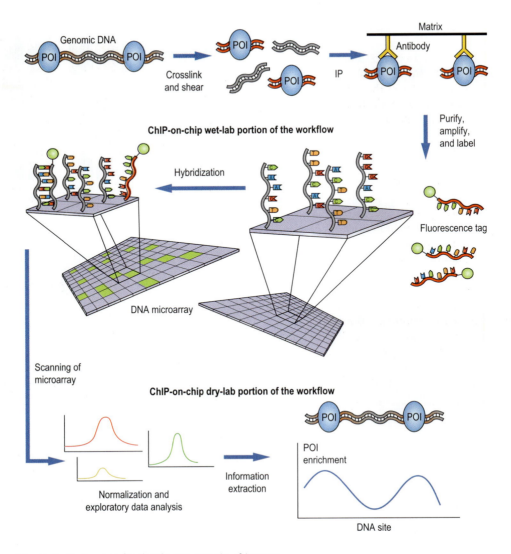

Fig. 24.7 **ChIP-on-chip analysis.** See text for details. POI, protein of interest.

the DNA region one wants to examine. This method assesses one binding site at a time and requires a hypothesis suggesting which site(s) should be examined. The identification of the associated DNA, however, can be massively multiplexed by using DNA microarrays for detection that represent the whole or large parts of the genome. Similarly, as discussed previously, as an alternative to gene microarrays, the associated DNA can be identified by sequencing.

ChIP-on-chip and ChIP-seq are powerful and informative techniques allowing the correlation of TF binding with transcriptional activity. **The ChIP techniques can be used to study any protein that interacts with DNA,** including proteins involved in DNA replication, DNA repair, and chromatin modification. Success is critically dependent on the quality and specificity of the antibodies used because the amounts of

coimmunoprecipitated DNA are very small, and there is no other separation step than the specificity provided by the antibody.

PROTEOMICS

Proteomics is the study of the protein complement of a cell, the protein equivalent of the transcriptome or genome

The word *proteome* was coined by Marc Wilkins in a talk in Siena in 1994. Wilkins defined the proteome as the protein complement of a cell, the protein equivalent of the transcriptome or genome. Since that time, the study of the proteome, called proteomics, has evolved along a number of different themes encompassing many areas of protein science.

Proteomics is possibly the most complex of all the -omics sciences but is also likely to be the most informative because proteins are the functional entities in the cell, and virtually no biological process takes place without the participation of a protein. Mapping the proteome will provide an understanding of how biology works and what goes wrong in disease as well as the ability to diagnose the disease and track its progression and response to therapy.

Initially, proteomics concentrated on cataloguing the proteins contained in an organelle, cell, tissue, or organism, validating the existence of the predicted genes in the genome in the process. This rapidly evolved into comparative proteomics, where the protein profiles from two or more samples are compared in order to identify quantitative differences that could be responsible for the observed phenotype - for example, from diseased versus healthy cells or looking at changes induced by hormone or drug treatment. Now, proteomics also includes the **study of posttranslational modifications** of individual proteins, the makeup and dynamics of **protein complexes,** the mapping of networks of **interactions between proteins,** and the identification of **biomarkers in disease.** Quantitative proteomics has become a robust tool, and even absolute quantification is relatively routine now.

Proteomics poses several challenges

It quickly became apparent that the complexity of the proteome would be a major obstacle to achieving Wilkins's initial ideal of looking at all the proteins in a cell or organism at the same time. Although the number of genes in an organism is not overwhelming, in eukaryotic systems, alternate splicing of genes and the posttranslational modifications (PTM) of proteins, such as the potential addition of more than 40 different covalently attached chemical groups (e.g., phosphorylation and glycosylation) means that there may be 10 or, in extreme cases, 1000 different protein species, all fairly similar, generated from each gene. The predicted 20,000 genes in the human genome could easily give rise to 500,000 or more individual protein species in the cell. In addition, there is a wide range of protein abundances in the cell, estimated to range from less than 10 to 500,000 or more molecules per cell, and a protein's function may depend on its abundance, PTMs, localization in the cell, and association with other proteins, and these may all change in seconds!

There is no protein equivalent of PCR that would allow for the amplification of protein sequences, so we are limited to the amount of protein that can be isolated from the sample

If the sample is small (e.g., a needle biopsy), a rare cell type such as tumor cells circulating in the blood, or an isolated signaling complex, ultrasensitive methods are needed to detect and analyze the proteins. It is only since the introduction of new methods in **mass spectrometry** in the mid-1990s

ADVANCED CONCEPT BOX
POSTTRANSLATIONAL MODIFICATIONS

During the process of transcription and translation and in the functioning of the cell, proteins can undergo a range of modifications. During transcription, introns are spliced out of the gene, and differential splicing of the gene can result in a number of different mRNAs being produced, and hence a number of proteins that differ markedly in their sequences can emerge from the same gene. After translation of the mRNA into protein, the protein can be "decorated" with a bewildering array of additional chemical groups covalently attached to it, many of which regulate the activity of the protein. Some examples are as follows:

- **The addition of fatty acids** to cysteine residues, which anchor the protein to a membrane.
- **Glycosylation:** the addition of complex oligosaccharides to an asparagine or serine residue, which is common in membrane proteins that have an extracellular component or are secreted. Many proteins involved in cell–cell recognition events are glycosylated, as are antibodies.
- **Phosphorylation:** the addition of a phosphate group to serine, threonine, tyrosine, or histidine residues. This is a modification that can be added or removed, allowing the system to respond very rapidly to a changing environment. It is fundamental to signaling events in the cell. It has been estimated that one-third of all eukaryotic proteins may undergo reversible phosphorylation.
- **Ubiquitination:** the addition of a polyubiquitin chain that targets the protein for destruction by the proteasome. Ubiquitination also can regulate enzyme activities and subcellular localization. Ubiquitin is itself a small protein.
- **Formation of disulfide bridges** between cysteine residues in the polypeptide backbone, which are close together in space once the protein is folded. These play a number of roles, including adding additional structural stability, especially for exported proteins, and sensing the redox balance in the cell.
- **Acetylation** of residues, most commonly the N-terminus of the protein or lysine. Acetylation of lysines on histones plays an important role in the gene transcription process, and drugs that target the proteins that acetylate or deacetylate histone are potential cancer therapeutics.
- **Proteolytic cleavage:** most proteins have the N-terminal methionine removed that results from the ATG initiation codon of gene translation. In some proteins, cleavage of the polypeptide chain occurs, such as in the activation of zymogens in the clotting cascade, or significant parts of the initial polypeptide chain are removed completely, for example, in the conversion of proinsulin into insulin.
- **Nonenzymatic modifications,** such as glycation, oxidation, carbonylation, deamidation and crosslinking (Chapter 42).

that an attempt could be made to analyze the proteome. The proteomes of simple eukaryotic species (e.g., yeast) have been deciphered in terms of identifying expressed proteins and many of their interactions. However, it is worth noting that even in the most comprehensive studies of this simple organism, 5% of the confidently predicted genes have still not been shown to give rise to proteins. The complement of human proteins expressed in many cell lines has been determined, including mapping of more than 35,000 PTMs (including around 24,000 phosphorylation sites), and in 2014, two papers published a draft of the "human proteome," but we are still far away from being able to identify all protein variants and PTMs.

Proteomics in medicine

Despite the challenges, proteomics has become a powerful tool for understanding fundamental biological processes

Like the other -omics technologies, proteomics makes it possible to discover new information about a biological problem without needing to have a clear understanding in advance of what might change. There are often more data generated from a good proteomics experiment than is reasonable, or possible, to follow up on.

Proteomics has been applied successfully to the study of basic biochemical changes in many different types of biological samples: cells, tissues, plasma, urine, cerebrospinal fluid, and even interstitial fluid collected by microdialysis

In cells isolated from cell culture, it is possible to investigate complex fundamental biological questions. Deciphering the mitogenic signaling cascades, which involve specific association of proteins in multiprotein complexes, and understanding how these can go wrong in cancer is one widely studied area. It is possible to gain information from biological fluids on the overall status of an organism because, for example, blood would have been in contact with every part of the body. Diseases at specific locations may eventually show up as changes in the protein content of the blood as leakage from the damaged tissue occurs. This area is now often described as **biomarker discovery.** Tissues are a more of a challenge. The heterogeneity of many tissues makes it difficult to compare tissue biopsies, which may contain differing amounts of connective tissue, vasculature, and so forth. Improvements in the sensitivity of analysis are now being overcome by allowing small amounts of material recovered from tissue-separation methods, such as laser capture microdissection or flow cytometry, to be used for the analysis. There is much effort being directed toward the ultimate challenge: the analysis of individual cells. This is valuable because current approaches average out changes in the analyzed sample, and we lose all information on natural heterogeneity in biology - for instance, a recorded 50% change in the level of a protein

could be 50% in all cells, or it could be 100% in 50% of the cells in the sample.

Main methods used in proteomics

Proteomics relies on the separation of complex mixtures of proteins or peptides, quantification of protein abundances, and identification of the proteins

This approach is multistep but modular, which is reflected in the many combinations of separation, quantitation, and identification. Here we focus on highlighting the principles rather than trying to be comprehensive.

Protein separation techniques

Strategies for protein separation are driven by the need to reduce the complexity - that is, the number of proteins being analyzed - while retaining as much information as possible on the functional context of the protein, which includes the subcellular localization of the protein, its incorporation in different protein complexes, and the huge variety of PTMs. No method can reconcile all these requirements. Therefore different methods have been developed that exploit the range of physicochemical properties of proteins (size, charge, hydrophobicity, PTMs, etc.) for separating complex mixtures (Fig. 24.8).

A classic protein-separation method is two-dimensional (2D) polyacrylamide gel electrophoresis (2DE, 2D-PAGE)

In 2D-PAGE, proteins are separated by isoelectric focusing according to their electrical charge in the first dimension and according to their size in the second dimension (see Fig. 2.15). Labeling the proteins with fluorescent dyes or using fluorescent stains makes the method quantitative, but protein spots have to be picked from the gels individually for subsequent identification by **mass spectrometry** (MS).

2D-PAGE is now rarely used and has been largely replaced by **high-performance liquid chromatography** (HPLC), which can be directly coupled to MS. Thus molecules eluting from the chromatographic column can be measured and identified in real time. Because MS-based identification works better with smaller molecules, for technical reasons, proteins are digested with proteases (usually trypsin) into small peptides before HPLC-MS analysis. HPLC separates proteins or peptides on the basis of different physicochemical properties, most commonly the charge of the molecule or its hydrophobicity, using ion-exchange or reversed-phase chromatography, respectively. This is achieved by having chemical groups attached to a particulate resin packed into a column and flowing a solution over this. Molecules will bind to the resin (the stationary phase) with differing affinities. Those with a high affinity will take longer to traverse the length of the column and hence will elute from the column at a later time. Molecules are

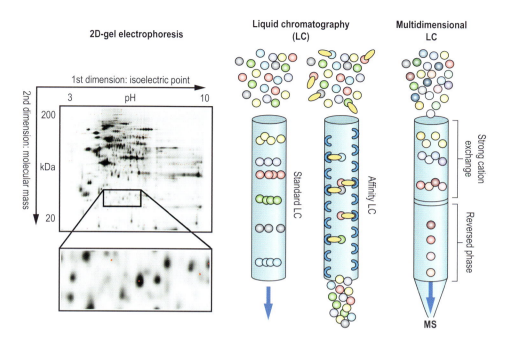

2D-gel electrophoresis

Liquid chromatography (LC)

Multidimensional LC

Fig. 24.8 **Protein- and peptide-separation techniques.** The **left panel** shows a two-dimensional (2D) gel where protein lysates were separated by isoelectric focusing in the first dimension and according to molecular weight in the second dimension. Protein spots were visualized with a fluorescent stain. The **middle panel** illustrates the principles of liquid chromatography (LC), where proteins or peptides are separated by differential physicochemical interactions with the resin as they flow through the column. A variation is affinity LC, where the resin is modified with an affinity group that retains molecules that selectively bind to these groups. The **right panel** demonstrates the setup for multidimensional LC, where a strong cation exchange column is directly coupled with a reversed-phase column, enabling a two-step separation by hydrophilicity and hydrophobicity. The eluate can be directly infused into a mass spectrometer for peptide identification.

therefore separated in time in the effluent that elutes off the column. Affinity chromatography uses specialized resins that strongly bind to certain chemical groups or biological epitopes and retain proteins carrying these groups. For instance, resins containing chelated Fe^{3+} or TiO_2 (**immobilized metal affinity chromatography** [IMAC]) bind phosphate and are used to select phosphorylated peptides. HPLC can also be carried out in two dimensions. Adding a **strong cation exchange (SCX) chromatography** step before IMAC removes many nonphosphorylated peptides, enhancing the enrichment of phosphopeptides in the IMAC step.

The first 2D liquid chromatography (LC) method with direct coupling of the two dimensions is called multidimensional protein identification technology (MudPIT)

In MudPIT the total protein content of the sample is first digested with trypsin, and the resulting peptides are fractionated by an SCX column, which separates peptides according to charge. Then the peptide fractions are further separated by reversed-phase LC and directly injected into the MS. Modern fast-scanning, high-resolution MS instruments coupled with high-resolution separation by HPLC now make it possible to dispense with the first dimension for all but the most complex samples. This method of MS-enabled, peptide-based protein identification is often referred to as **bottom-up or "shotgun" proteomics**. In **top-down proteomics,** intact proteins are isolated in an ion-trap mass spectrometer for fragmentation and protein identification.

Protein identification by mass spectrometry

Mass spectrometry is a technique used to determine the molecular masses of molecules in a sample

MS can also be used to select an individual component from the mixture, break up its chemical structure, and measure the masses of the fragments, which can then be used to determine the structure of the molecule. There are many different types of mass spectrometers available, but the underlying principles of mass spectrometry are relatively simple. The first step in the process is to generate charged molecules, ions, from the molecules in the sample. This is relatively easily achieved for many soluble biomolecules because their polar chemistry provides groups that are easily charged. For example, the addition of a proton (H^+) to amino terminal amino acid or the side-chain groups on the basic amino acids lysine, arginine, or histidine gives a positively charged molecule. When a charged molecule is placed in an electric field, it will be repelled by an

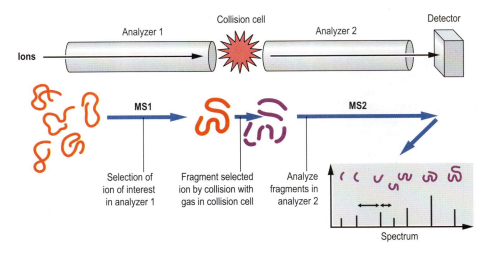

Fig. 24.9 **The basic principles of tandem mass spectrometry.** See text for details. MS, mass spectrometer.

electrode of like sign and attracted by an electrode of opposite sign, accelerating the molecule toward the electrode of opposite charge. Because the force is equal for all molecules, larger molecules will accelerate less than small molecules (force = mass × acceleration), so small molecules will acquire a higher velocity. This concept is utilized to determine the mass. For example, after the molecules have been accelerated, the time then taken for them to travel a certain distance can be measured and related to the mass. This is called **time-of-flight mass spectrometry**.

A tandem mass spectrometer is effectively two mass spectrometric analyzers joined together sequentially, with an area between them where molecules can be fragmented

The first analyzer is used to select one of the molecules from a mixture based on its molecular mass, which is then broken up into smaller parts, usually by collision with a small amount of gas in the intermediate region (called the collision cell). The fragments that are generated are then analyzed in the second mass spectrometer (Fig. 24.9). Because peptides tend to fragment at the peptide bond, the fragment peaks are separated by the masses of the different amino acids in the corresponding sequence. This result is, in principle, similar to the Sanger method of DNA sequencing (Chapter 2), allowing the peptide sequence to be deduced. However, in contrast to Sanger DNA sequencing, peptide fragmentation is not uniform, and the spectra usually only cover part of the sequence, leaving gaps and ambiguous sequence reconstruction. Further, MS measures and fragments peptides as they elute from the LC, resulting in abundant proteins being identified many times, whereas low-abundance proteins are overlooked if the MS is overwhelmed by a flow of abundant peptides. This is a main reason why protein or peptide prefractionation increases the number of successfully identified proteins. Finally, the **peptide sequence is predicted based on a statistical matching of observed masses against a virtual digest and peptide fragmentation of proteins in a database** (Fig. 24.10). With today's highly accurate MS and well-annotated databases, these computational sequence predictions are very reliable. Proteomics is intimately reliant on the quality and completeness of genome sequencing and the genome databases that are used to infer the sequence of encoded proteins.

To enable the targeted identification of specific proteins, a technique was developed, called selected-reaction monitoring (SRM) or multiple-reaction monitoring (MRM)

This method uses MS1 to select a peptide ion out of a mixture, then fragment it and select defined fragment masses for detection in MS2 (Fig. 24.11). A software protocol for MS1 peptide selection and MS2 fragment detection gives unique protein identifications based on the measurement of a few selected peptides. This is a powerful method to streamline the identification of proteins from complex samples by systematically monitoring only the most informative peptide fragmentations. The peptide atlas is a database of such informative fragments that greatly facilitates the systematic analysis of proteomes and subproteomes.

Quantitative mass spectrometry

MS can be made quantitative in a number of ways. If possible, samples can be grown in a selective medium that provides an essential amino acid in the natural form (the "light" form) or isotopically labeled with a stable isotope (e.g., ^{13}C or ^{2}H, the "heavy" form) that makes all of the peptides containing this amino acid appear heavier in the mass spectrometer. This is called the **stable isotope labeling with amino acids in cell culture** (SILAC) method, and it is one of the most widely used and robust of the labeling technologies (Fig. 24.12). The samples

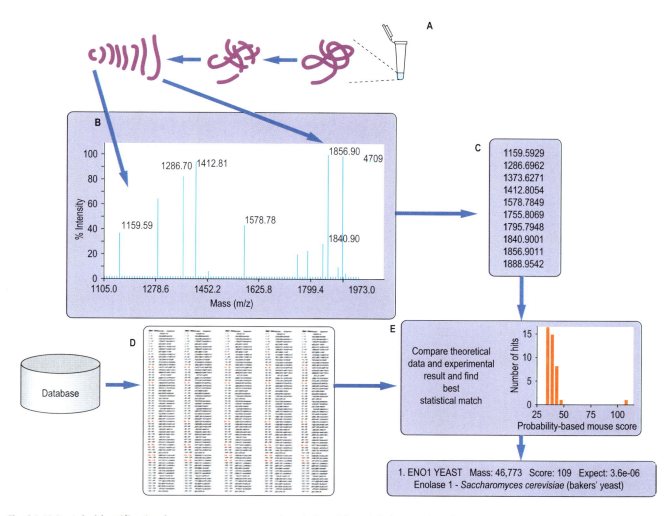

Fig. 24.10 **Protein identification by mass spectrometry.** A typical workflow: (A) The sample is digested with a specific protease, usually trypsin, to give a set of smaller peptides that will be unique to the protein. (B) The mass of a subset of the resulting peptides is measured using MS; in tandem MS, each peptide is fragmented, and the mass of the fragments is measured as well. (C) A list of the observed experimental masses is generated from the mass spectrum. (D) A database of protein sequences is theoretically digested (and fragmented in the case of tandem MS) *in silico,* and a set of tables of the expected peptides is generated. (E) The experimental data are compared with the theoretical digested database, and a statistical score of the fit of the experimental to theoretical data is generated, giving a "confidence" score that indicates the likelihood of correct identification.

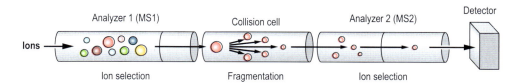

Fig. 24.11 **The principles of selected-reaction monitoring (SRM) or multiple-reaction monitoring (MRM) experiments.** See text for details.

are mixed together and analyzed using the shotgun approach. The ratios of "heavy" to the equivalent "light" peptides are used to determine the relative quantities of the protein from which they were derived.

Alternative methods include chemically reacting the proteins in the sample (e.g., using the **isotope-coded affinity tags**

[ICAT]) or the peptides after digestion of the sample (e.g., **in isobaric tags for relative and absolute quantitation [iTRAQ]**), with a "light" or equivalent isotopically labeled "heavy" chemical reagent, then mixing the samples and analyzing them as in the SILAC approach. Direct comparison of one-dimensional liquid chromatography (1D-LC) runs based

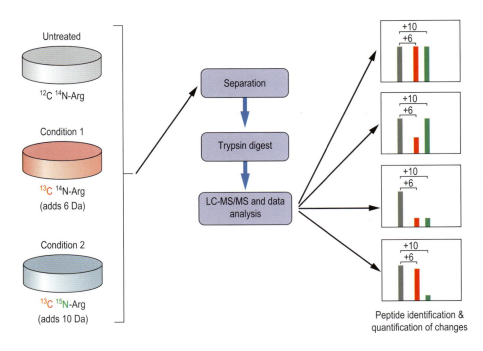

Fig. 24.12 **Stable isotope labeling with amino acids in cell culture (SILAC) for quantitative mass spectrometry.** See text for details.

on the normalized signal intensity without the need for labeling is also possible due to improvements in the reproducibility of LC and software. In addition, counting of peptide ions in the mass spectrometer has led to so-called **label-free quantitation methods** that are rapidly improving and soon may allow accurate quantification without the need to label cells or proteins. The advantage of these methodologies is that the analysis is easily automated and that approaches can be used to get information on proteins that do not work well with the 2D isoelectric focusing approach, such as membrane proteins, small proteins, and proteins with extreme pIs (e.g., histones). The disadvantage is that information on posttranslational modifications is usually lost, and digesting the sample generates a much more complex sample for the separation step.

Affinity capture methods for molecular interactions

A recent development in proteomics has been the use of small molecules immobilized on solid surfaces to enrich proteins that bind to the molecule. This has been used to screen for particular classes of proteins and to understand the effects of drugs. An example is the immobilization of low-selectivity kinase inhibitors on solid beads to affinity-enrich a large number of kinases (the "kinome") from a cell lysate. The lysate is passed over the beads, and proteins that interact with the immobilized drug bind to it. The proteins can then be selectively released by competing them off with soluble drug, then analyzed using standard proteomics techniques. This has been commercialized as *kinobeads*. The same method can be used for profiling the selectivity of drugs, where the proteins that bind identify the drug target along with any off-target binding of the drug that might be responsible for side effects. Medicinal chemistry can then be used to improve the drug, and the same approach can be used to determine if selectivity has been improved. Chemical probes have been developed that also allow the capture of other enzymes, such as ATPases, hydrolases, and proteases.

Non-MS-based technologies

Although MS remains a mainstay technique used for proteomics, various other methods are becoming established. **Protein microarrays** are conceptually similar to those used for transcriptomics. They come in three versions (Fig. 24.13). In the **reverse-phase protein array** (RPPA), lysates of cells or tissues are spotted on a microscope slide with a protein-friendly coating. These arrays are then probed with an antibody specific to a protein or a certain PTM. After washing to remove unbound antibodies, successful binding events are visualized by a secondary anti-antibody antibody, which carries a detectable label, usually a fluorescent dye. Thereby, a large number of samples or treatment conditions can be compared simultaneously. The success of this method is completely dependent on the specificity of the antibody, and it is constrained by the limited availability of high-quality mono-specific antibodies. In the **capture array,** antibodies are deposited onto the array, which then is incubated with a protein lysate. Detection of the captured proteins is by another antibody. Thus the overall specificity is the overlap between the specificities of the capturing and detecting antibodies, relaxing the requirement that each

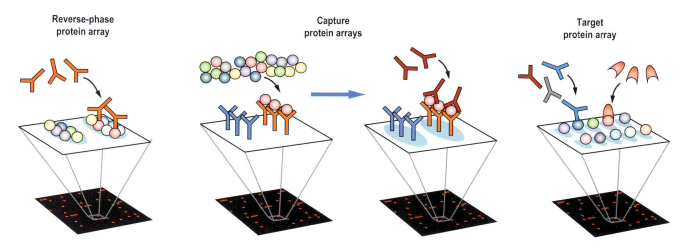

Reverse-phase protein array	Capture protein arrays	Target protein array

Fig. 24.13 **Protein (micro)arrays.** See text for details.

antibody should be absolutely specific. **Target arrays** contain a single species of purified protein in each spot. These arrays are used to find binding partners for specific proteins. They can be probed with another purified protein, with a cell extract, or with a mixture of antibodies (e.g., from patient sera) to determine whether a patient has antibodies against particular proteins. Protein microarrays can be used to quantify the amount of the protein present in a sample and thus lend themselves to clinical diagnostics.

The Human Protein Atlas aims to generate antibodies to every protein in the human proteome and use these to visualize proteins and their subcellular localization in healthy and diseased human tissues

In 2016, the HPA comprised more than 17,000 proteins - that is, more than 80% of gene products, if splice forms and other variants are neglected. Efforts to include protein variants and posttranslational modifications are under way. Thus the HPA is becoming a major resource for proteome analysis.

Microscopy has also become a tool that is frequently used in spatial proteomics to assess where proteins are localized in the cell and how this changes under different conditions. This has been enabled by the advances in the intracellular expression of proteins that are a fusion between the proteins of interest and green fluorescent protein (GFP) or its analogs. The cellular location of the protein can then be tracked by microscopy by following the fluorescent signal of the protein attached to it. There are now analogues of GFP that emit at a wide range of wavelengths, meaning that three or even four proteins can be followed in parallel.

METABOLOMICS

Metabolites are the small chemical molecules, such as sugars, amino acids, lipids, and nucleotides, present in a biological

ADVANCED CONCEPT BOX
NUCLEAR MAGNETIC RESONANCE SPECTROSCOPY

Nuclear magnetic resonance (NMR) spectroscopy gives useful structural information on molecules that can be used to identify them. Atomic nuclei behave like small magnets, so when they are put in a strong magnetic field, they align with the field. Application of an appropriate energy (radiofrequency electromagnetic radiation) causes the nuclei to flip and align with the field. They then return to their ground state once the field is turned off by flipping back, and as they do so, they emit specific frequencies of radiation. These can be recorded and plotted. Each nucleus in a molecule that has a unique environment will emit a unique frequency, and nuclei bonded together or close together in space will interact with adjacent nuclei (coupling), and this can also be measured. This rich information on the molecule allows the structural elements to be determined, and the amplitude of the signals can be used to quantify the amount of material with reasonable accuracy. This is very useful in **metabolomics.** The main limitation is that the NMR spectrum quickly becomes congested with information from a complex sample, so high resolution (coming from very strong magnetic fields) is required. Furthermore, the technique is relatively insensitive, having a limit of detection three to four orders of magnitude worse than mass spectrometry.

sample. The study of the metabolite complement of a sample is called **metabolomics,** whereas the quantitative measurement of the dynamic changes in the levels of metabolites as a result of a stimulus or other change is often referred to as **metabonomics.** The words *metabolomics* and *metabonomics* are often used interchangeably, although purists will claim that although both involve the multiparametric measurement of metabolites, metabonomics is dedicated to the analysis of dynamic changes in metabolite levels, whereas metabolomics focuses on identifying and quantifying the steady-state levels of intracellular metabolites. Metabolomics is the most commonly used generic term.

Metabolomics gives another level of information on a biological system

Metabolomics measures metabolite concentrations and provides information on the results of the activity of enzymes, which may not depend on the abundance of the protein alone because this may be modulated by the supply of substrates, the concentration of cofactors or products, and the effects of other small molecules or proteins that modulate the activity of the enzyme (effectors). In some ways, metabolomics may be easier to perform than proteomics. In the metabolome, there is an amplification of any changes that occur in the proteome because the enzymes will turn over many substrate molecules for each molecule of enzyme. The methods used to look for a metabolite in each organism will be the same because many of the metabolites will be identical, unlike proteins, whose sequences are much less conserved between organisms. Thus metabolic networks are more constrained, making them easier to follow.

However, the analysis of the metabolome is still complex because it is very dynamic; many metabolites give rise to a number of molecular species by forming adducts with different counterions or other metabolites. Molecules that do not come from the host but from foodstuffs, drugs, the environment, or even the microflora in the gut complicate the analysis greatly; the actual metabolome may be getting close to being as complicated as the proteome.

In a similar way, **lipidomics** has become a topic in its own right, studying the dynamic changes in lipids in diverse functions such as membranes, lipoproteins, and signaling molecules. In 2007 the Human Metabolome Project released the first draft of the human metabolome consisting of 2500 metabolites, 3500 food components, and 1200 drugs. Currently, there is information on approximately 20,000 metabolites, approximately 1600 drug and drug metabolites, 3100 toxins and environmental pollutants, and around 28,000 food components.

The most commonly used methods for investigating the metabolome are mass spectrometry, often coupled with LC, as used in proteomics, and **nuclear magnetic resonance (NMR) spectroscopy**. Identification of signals corresponding to specific metabolites can then be used to quantify these metabolites in a complex sample and see how they change.

Metabolomics can be broken down into a number of areas

- **Metabolic fingerprinting:** taking a "snapshot" of the metabolome of a system, generating a set of values for the intensity of a signal from a species, without necessarily knowing what that species is. Often there is no chromatographic separation of species. It is used for biomarker discovery.

- **Metabolite profiling:** generating a set of quantitative data on a number of metabolites, usually of known identity, over a range of conditions or times. It is used for metabolomics, metabonomics, and systems biology and biomarker discovery.

- **Metabolite target analysis:** measuring the concentration of a specific metabolite or small set of metabolites over a range of conditions or times.

Biomarkers

Biomarkers are markers that can be used in medicine for the early detection, diagnosis, staging, or prognosis of disease or for determination of the most effective therapy

A **biomarker** is generally defined as a marker that is specific for a particular state of a biological system. The markers may be metabolites, peptides, proteins, or any other biological molecule or measurements of physical properties (e.g., blood pressure). The importance of biomarkers is rapidly increasing because advances in personalized medicine require the detailed and objective characterization of patients afforded by biomarker analysis. Biomarkers can arise from the disease process itself or from the reaction of the body to the disease. Thus they can be found in body fluids and tissues. For ease of sample sourcing and patient compliance, most biomarker studies use urine or plasma, although saliva, interstitial fluid, nipple duct aspirates, and cerebrospinal fluid also have been used.

The most common methods for biomarker discovery have developed from those used in transcriptomics, proteomics, and metabolomics (i.e., gene arrays; mass spectrometry, often coupled with chromatography; and NMR spectroscopy)

Biomarker discovery is often done on small patient cohorts, but to be clinically useful, a robust statistical analysis of a large number of samples from healthy and sick individuals in well-controlled studies is required. Improvements in methods for statistical analysis, coupled with detection methods that can differentiate hundreds to tens of thousands of individual components in the complex sample, have improved the selectivity to the level where these aims are achievable. It is usually necessary to define a number of markers (i.e., a **biomarker panel**) that are indicative of a given disease to achieve selectivity rather than just detecting a general systemic response, such as the inflammatory response, or a closely related disease. In theory, it is not necessary to actually identify what the biomarker is, although doing so may give insight into the underlying biochemistry of the disease, and many regulatory authorities demand that the markers be identified before a method can be licensed. This may also allow subsequent development of cheaper and higher-throughput assays.

Some well-known examples of biomarkers are the measurement of blood glucose levels in diabetes, prostate-specific antigen for prostate cancer, and **HER-2** *or* **BRCA1/2** *genes in breast cancer*

Biomarker research can also elucidate disease mechanisms and further markers or potential drug targets. For example, using a 2D isoelectric focusing approach to determine which DNA repair pathways had been lost in **breast cancer** led to the discovery that cancers deficient in the *BRCA1/2* genes are sensitive to the inhibition of another DNA repair protein, poly(ADP-ribose) polymerase 1, known as PARP-1. Inhibitors of PARP-1 are showing promise in clinical trials for the treatment of *BRCA1/2*-deficient tumors.

Data analysis and interpretation by bioinformatics and systems biology

The -omics experiments can generate many gigabytes, even terabytes, of information. However, **data are not information, and information is not knowledge**. Making use of such data is fundamentally dependent on computational methods. **Bioinformatics** is the term used for computational methods for the extraction of useful information from the complex datasets generated from -omics experiments - for instance, generating quantitative data on gene transcription from next-generation sequencing or identifying proteins from the fragments generated in mass spectrometry. The annotation of these datasets, for instance, with protein function or localization, and the hierarchical organization of the data can be seen as static information. **Systems biology** takes this further and generates computational and mathematical models from our knowledge of biology and the refined data coming from bioinformatics analysis. These models are used to simulate biochemical and biological processes *in silico* (an expression meaning "performed on computers") and reveal how complex systems, such as intracellular signaling networks, actually work.

SUMMARY

- The -omics approaches hold a huge potential for the risk assessment, early detection, diagnosis, stratification, and tailored treatment of human diseases.
- The -omics technologies are being introduced into clinical practice, with genomics and transcriptomics leading the way. This is mainly because DNA and RNA have defined physicochemical properties that are amenable for amplification and the design of robust assay platforms compatible with the routines of clinical laboratories. For instance, PCR and DNA sequencing are used in forensic medicine to establish paternity and to determine the identity of DNA samples left at crime

ACTIVE LEARNING

1. What is a gene?
2. Whose genomes were sequenced in the Human Genome Project?
3. How does the information content increase when moving from genomics to transcriptomics, then proteomics and metabolomics?
4. Transcription factors represent about 20% of the proteins in the genome. Discuss the limitations of proteomics technology for quantifying changes in transcription factors and their extent of phosphorylation in response to hormonal stimuli.

scenes. Genetic tests for the diagnosis of gene mutations and inherited diseases are now in place.
- Transcriptomic-based microarray tests for breast cancer have been approved, and similar tests for other diseases are becoming available.
- Proteomics and metabolomics require specialized equipment and expertise, which are currently difficult to put into the routine clinical laboratory. However, their information content exceeds that of genomics, and with further progress in technology, their clinical applications will become a reality.

FURTHER READING

Adamski, J. (2016). Key elements of metabolomics in the study of biomarkers of diabetes. *Diabetologia*, 59, 2497–2502.

Aronson, J. K., & Ferner, R. E. (2017). Biomarkers - A General Review. *Current Protocols in Pharmacology*, 76, 9.23.1–9.23.17.

Corbo, C., Cevenini, A., & Salvatore, F. (2017). Biomarker discovery by proteomics-based approaches for early detection and personalized medicine in colorectal cancer. *Proteomics. Clinical Applications*, 11(5–6), doi:10.1002/prca.201600072.

Duarte, T. T., & Spencer, C. T. (2016). Personalized proteomics: The future of precision medicine. *Proteomes*, 4(4), 29.

Faria, S. S., Morris, C. F., Silva, A. R., et al. (2017). A timely shift from shotgun to targeted proteomics and how it can be groundbreaking for cancer research. *Frontiers in Oncology*, 7, 13.

Fu, S., Liu, X., Luo, M., et al. (2017). Proteogenomic studies on cancer drug resistance: Towards biomarker discovery and target identification. *Expert Review of Proteomics*, 14(4), 351–362.

Lima, A. R., Bastos, M. L., Carvalho, M., et al. (2016). Biomarker discovery in human prostate cancer: An update in metabolomics studies. *Translational Oncology*, 9, 357–370.

Matthews, H., Hanison, J., & Nirmalan, N. (2016). "Omics"-informed drug and biomarker discovery: Opportunities, challenges and future perspectives. *Proteomes*, 4(3), 28.

Mokou, M., Lygirou, V., Vlahou, A., et al. (2017). Proteomics in cardiovascular disease: Recent progress and clinical implication and implementation. *Expert Review of Proteomics*, 14, 117–136.

Newgard, C. B. (2017). Metabolomics and metabolic diseases: Where do we stand? *Cell Metabolism*, 25, 43–56.

O'Gorman, A., & Brennan, L. (2017). The role of metabolomics in determination of new dietary biomarkers. *The Proceedings of the Nutrition Society*, 1–8.

Walsh, A. M., Crispie, F., Claesson, M. J., et al. (2017). Translating omics to food microbiology. *Annual Review of Food Science and Technology*, 8, 113–134.

RELEVANT WEBSITES

The Human Genome Project: https://www.genome.gov/10001772/
The Cancer Genome Atlas: https://cancergenome.nih.gov/
The Human Protein Project: http://www.thehpp.org/
The Human Metabolome Database: http://www.hmdb.ca/
MicroRNA database: http://www.mirbase.org
Introduction to proteomics: https://www.unil.ch/paf/files/live/sites/paf/files/
　　shared/PAF/downloads/PROTEOMICS_INTRO.pdf
The Human Protein Atlas: http://www.proteinatlas.org/
Multi-organism peptide atlas: http://www.peptideatlas.org
Online Mendelian inheritance in man: https://www.omim.org/

ABBREVIATIONS

CGH	Comparative genome hybridization
ChIP	Chromatin immunoprecipitation
ChIPseq	Combination chromatin immunoprecipitation and RNAseq technology
ChIP-on-chip	Combination chromatin immunoprecipitation and microarray technology
CMA	Chromosomal microarray analysis
cDNA	Complementary DNA
cRNA	Complementary RNA
FISH	Fluorescence in situ hybridization
GWAS	Genome-wide association study
HGP	Human genome project
IMAC	Immobilized metal affinity chromatography
lncRNA	Long non-coding RNA
miRNA	MicroRNA
MRM	Multiple reaction monitoring
MS	Mass spectrometry
MudPIT	Multidimensional protein identification technology
ncRNA	Non-coding RNA
NGS	Next generation sequencing
PCR	Polymerase chain reaction
PTM	Posttranslational modification
RNAseq	Deep sequencing technology for transcriptome analysis
siRNA	Small interfering RNA
SNP	Single nucleotide polymorphism

Membrane Receptors and Signal Transduction

Ian P. Salt

INTRODUCTION

Cellular signals are processed by specific receptors, effector elements, and regulatory proteins

Cells sense, respond to, and integrate multiple, diverse signals from their environment. These signals can be hormones produced elsewhere from their site of action (**endocrine signaling**), signals generated locally to the target cell (**paracrine signaling**), signals from cells in physical contact with the target cell (**juxtacrine signaling**), or signals generated by the target cell itself (**autocrine signaling**). Hydrophobic signals and small molecules can cross the plasma membrane and exert their effects via receptors within the cell, whereas the majority of signals are hydrophilic, are not able to cross the lipid plasma membrane, and require specific cell-surface membrane receptors. In either case, signals are sensed and processed by **cellular signal transduction cassettes** that comprise specific receptors, effector signaling elements, and regulatory proteins. These signaling cassettes serve to detect, amplify, and integrate the diverse external signals to generate the appropriate cellular response (Fig. 25.1). Ultimately, signals can rapidly alter cellular processes such as metabolism or

exocytosis, and they alter transcription factor activity, leading to changes in target gene expression.

In this chapter, we first discuss how cell-surface receptors sense and transduce their specific signal by transmembrane coupling to effector enzyme systems, including generation of low-molecular-mass molecules termed second messengers. We then discuss the diversity of these second messengers and how they influence the activity of a range of key effector proteins that ultimately determine the obtained biological response.

TYPES OF HORMONE AND MONOAMINE RECEPTORS

Receptors for steroid hormones differ from those for polypeptide hormones and monoamines

Hormones are biochemical messengers that act to orchestrate the responses of different cells within a multicellular organism (Chapter 27). They are generally synthesized by specific tissues and secreted directly into the blood, which transports them to their target responsive organs. Hormone signaling can broadly be subdivided into two major classes:

- Steroid hormone signaling
- Polypeptide and monoamine hormone signaling.

Hormones achieve their biological effects by interacting with specific receptors to induce intracellular signaling cascades (Table 25.1).

Steroid hormones traverse cell membranes

Steroid hormones, such as glucocorticoids, mineralocorticoids, sex hormones, and vitamin D, are derived from cholesterol and are therefore hydrophobic. Thus they can traverse the plasma membrane of cells to initiate their responses via cytoplasmic steroid hormone receptors (Fig. 25.1). Steroid hormone receptors belong to a superfamily of cytoplasmic receptors called the **intracellular receptor superfamily,** members of which also transduce signals from other small hydrophobic signaling molecules such as tyrosine-derived thyroid hormones (e.g., thyroxine) and vitamin A–derived retinoids (e.g., retinoic acid).

Intracellular receptors for steroid and thyroid hormones and retinoids are transcription factors

The intracellular receptors for steroid/thyroid hormones and retinoids are **transcription factors;** they bind to regulatory

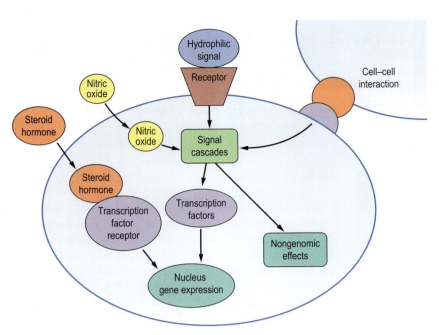

Fig. 25.1 **Mechanisms of cell signaling.**

Table 25.1 Classification of membrane receptors

Receptor class	Transmembrane-spanning domains	Intrinsic catalytic activity	Accessory coupling/regulatory molecules	Examples of receptor classes/ligands
G-protein–coupled receptors (serpentine receptors)	Multipass (seven transmembrane α-helices)	None	G-proteins	Glucagon α-Adrenergic, β-adrenergic (epinephrine) Muscarinic (acetylcholine) rhodopsin (vision) Chemokines (IL-8)
Ion-channel receptors (ligand-gated channels)	Multipass; generally form multimeric complexes	Ion-channel activity	None	Neurotransmitters Ions Nucleotides Inositol trisphosphate (IP$_3$)
Intrinsic tyrosine kinase receptors	Single-pass transmembrane domain but may be multimeric (e.g., insulin receptor)	Tyrosine kinase	None	Insulin Peptide growth factors (e.g., PDGF, FGF, NGF, EGF)
Tyrosine kinase–associated receptors	Single-pass transmembrane domain but generally form multimeric receptors	None	Some require ITAM/ITIM-containing proteins	Antigen receptors (ITAM-Src-related kinases) FcγR (ITIM–Src-related kinases) Leptin, IL-6 (Janus kinases)
Intrinsic tyrosine phosphatase receptors	Single-pass transmembrane domain	Tyrosine phosphatase	None	CD45-phosphatase receptor
Intrinsic serine/threonine kinase receptors	Single-pass transmembrane domain	Serine/threonine kinase	None	Transforming growth factor-β (TGF-β)
Intrinsic guanylate cyclase receptors	Single-pass transmembrane domain	Guanylyl cyclase (generates cGMP)	None	Atrial natriuretic protein (ANP)
Death-domain receptors	Single-pass transmembrane domain	None	Death-domain accessory proteins (TRADD, FADD, RIP, TRAFs)	Tumor necrosis factor-α (TNF-α) Fas

cGMP, cyclic guanosine monophosphate; FADD, Fas-associated death domain; FcγR, Fc-γ receptor (receptor for immunoglobulin G); IL, interleukin; ITAM/ITIM, immunoreceptor tyrosine activation/inhibition motif; RIP, receptor-interacting protein; Src, Src tyrosine kinase; TRADD, TNF-receptor-associated death domain; TRAFs, TNF-receptor-associated factors; PDGF, platelet-derived growth factor; FGF, fibroblast growth factor; EGF, epidermal growth factor; NGF, nerve growth factor; FGF, fibroblast growth factor; EGF, epidermal growth factor; NGF, nerve growth factor.

regions of the DNA of genes that are responsive to the particular steroid/thyroid hormone. Such "ligand binding" (ligation) induces a conformational change in the transcription factor that allows it to activate or repress gene induction. Although all the target cells have specific receptors for the individual hormones, they express distinct combinations of cell type–specific regulatory proteins that cooperate with the intracellular hormone receptor to dictate the precise repertoire of genes that are induced. Hence the hormones induce distinct sets of responses in different target cells (Chapter 23).

Polypeptide hormones act through membrane receptors

In contrast to the steroid hormones, polypeptide hormones cannot cross cell membranes and must initiate their effects on their target cells via specific cell **surface receptors** (Fig. 25.1). Binding to the specific cell-surface receptor causes a conformational change in that receptor that can engage **signaling cascades** in several different ways. Receptor binding can do the following:

- Regulate the production of low-molecular-mass signaling molecules, such as cyclic adenosine monophosphate (cAMP) or calcium, which are called **second messengers**
- Alter the intrinsic catalytic activity of the receptor
- Alter the recruitment of regulatory molecules to the receptor (Table 25.1)
- Alter other molecules that signal through membrane receptors

In addition to polypeptide hormones, a wide range of signaling molecules use transmembrane signal transduction cassettes to elicit their biological effects. Such signals include polypeptide growth factors, polypeptide signals that mediate inflammation and immunity (cytokines and chemokines), and small hydrophilic molecules (such as acetylcholine, catecholamines, purines, nucleotides, or inositol trisphosphate; Table 25.1).

Some low-molecular-mass signaling molecules traverse the cell membrane

Although most extracellular signals mediate their effects via receptor–ligand interaction of either cell-surface or cytoplasmic receptors, some low-molecular-mass signaling molecules are able to traverse the plasma membrane and directly modulate the activity of the catalytic domains of transmembrane receptors or cytoplasmic signal-transducing enzymes (Fig. 25.1). For example, nitric oxide (NO), which has a variety of functions, including the relaxation of vascular smooth muscle cells, can stimulate guanylyl cyclase, leading to the generation of the second messenger, cGMP. Patients with **angina pectoris** are treated with glyceryl trinitrate, which is converted to NO, resulting in relaxation of the blood vessels delivering oxygen and nutrients to the heart. The consequent improvement in oxygen delivery to the heart muscle eases the pain that was caused by inadequate blood flow to the heart.

RECEPTOR COUPLING TO INTRACELLULAR SIGNAL TRANSDUCTION

Membrane receptors couple to signaling pathways utilizing diverse mechanisms

Some membrane receptors - for example, the β-adrenergic receptors or the antigen receptors on lymphocytes - have no intrinsic catalytic activity and serve simply as specific recognition units. These receptors use a variety of mechanisms, including adaptor molecules or catalytically active regulatory molecules such as **G-proteins** (guanosine triphosphatases [GTPases], which hydrolyze GTP) to couple them to their effector signaling elements, which are generally enzymes (often called signaling enzymes or signal transducers), or ion channels (Fig. 25.2). In contrast, other receptors (e.g., the intrinsic tyrosine kinase receptors for insulin and many growth factors; the intrinsic serine kinase receptors for molecules such as transforming growth factor-β) have extracellular ligand-binding domains and cytoplasmic catalytic domains. After receptor ligation, these receptors can directly initiate their signaling cascades by phosphorylating and modulating the activities of target signal-transducing molecules (downstream signaling enzymes). These in turn propagate the growth factor signal by modulating the activity of further specific signal transducers or transcription factors, leading to gene induction (Chapter 23). Furthermore, sensory systems such as vision (Chapter 39), taste, and smell use similar mechanisms of cell-surface membrane receptor–coupled signal transduction (Table 25.1).

Some receptors possess intrinsic protein kinase activity

Ligand binding to many growth factor receptors stimulates protein kinase activity of an intracellular domain of the receptor complex. The activated receptor subsequently phosphorylates substrate proteins, in which the γ-phosphate from ATP is transferred to the side-chain hydroxyl groups on serine, threonine, or tyrosine residues. All receptor protein kinases are either specific serine/threonine kinases or tyrosine kinases, but never both. Furthermore, protein kinases phosphorylate substrates at specific serine, threonine, or tyrosine residues, depending on the sequence surrounding the site of phosphorylation. Upon ligand binding, receptor protein kinases often **autophosphorylate (self-phosphorylate)**. The introduction of the bulky charged phosphate moiety during autophosphorylation or onto other substrate proteins markedly alters the conformation of the protein, leading to changes in activity or acting as docking sites for other (adapter) proteins. Adapter proteins contain specific domains that recognize and bind to the phosphorylated proteins. Because receptor protein kinases often phosphorylate at several sites, this can lead to several different adapter proteins being recruited to the activated receptor complex. Subsequently, these adapter proteins can engage several different signaling pathways.

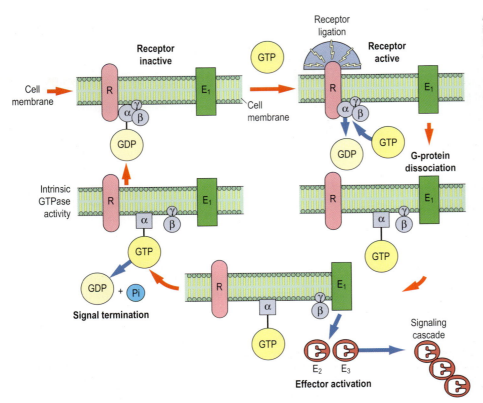

Fig. 25.2 Mechanism of G-protein signaling. In the inactive state, G-proteins exist as heterotrimers with GDP bound tightly to the α-subunit. None of the subunits are integral membrane proteins; however, the G-protein is anchored to the plasma membrane by lipid modification of the γ-subunits (prenylation) and some of the α-subunits (myristoylation in the $G_{i\alpha}$ family). Ligation of the receptor (R) drives exchange of GDP for GTP and induces a conformational change in Gα, which results in a decrease in its affinity both for the receptor and for the βγ-subunits, leading to dissociation of the receptor–G-protein complex. The activated Gα (GTP-bound) or the released βγ-subunits or both can then interact with one or more effectors, to generate intracellular second messengers that activate downstream signaling cascades. Signaling is terminated by the intrinsic GTPase activity of the α-subunit, which hydrolyzes GTP to GDP to allow reassociation of the inactive, heterotrimeric G-protein, Gαβγ.

The example of insulin signaling

An example of this is insulin signaling. Insulin binding to the insulin receptor (IR) causes activation and autophosphorylation of the intracellular tyrosine kinase domains. Adapter proteins including the insulin receptor substrate (IRS) proteins and Shc (Src-homology and collagen-like) proteins bind the phosphotyrosine residues on the IR. Next, IRSs are themselves phosphorylated by the IR on tyrosine residues, generating docking sites for the lipid kinase phosphatidylinositol 3′-kinase, which generates phosphatidylinositol 3,4,5-trisphosphate (PIP_3) at the plasma membrane. Newly formed PIP_3 recruits the serine/threonine protein kinase Akt to the plasma membrane, and Akt is subsequently phosphorylated and activated by other protein kinases (Fig. 25.3). Activation of Akt is the key signaling pathway by which insulin exerts the majority of its metabolic effects, including stimulation of glucose transport and suppression of gluconeogenesis (Chapter 31). Binding of Shc to the activated IR leads to recruitment of growth factor receptor-bound protein (Grb2) to Shc, which subsequently activates a guanine nucleotide exchange factor (SOS), which stimulates the small G-protein Ras, which initiates the protein kinase cascade in which several protein kinases phosphorylate each other in turn. Signaling through this pathway is associated with the mitogenic, growth-promoting actions of insulin. Therefore **ligand binding can initiate multiple signaling pathways with different cellular effects**.

Some membrane receptors are coupled to G-proteins

G-protein–coupled receptors (GPCR) comprise a superfamily of structurally related receptors for hormones, neurotransmitters, inflammatory mediators, proteinases, taste and odorant molecules, and light photons. A classic example of this class of receptors is the **β-adrenergic receptor** (for which the ligand is epinephrine) because its structure–function properties have been extensively studied with respect to its activation of signal transduction cascades. GPCRs are integral membrane proteins characterized by the seven transmembrane-spanning helices within their structure. They generally comprise an extracellular N-terminus, seven transmembrane-spanning α-helices (20–28 hydrophobic amino acids each), three extracellular and intracellular loops, and an intracellular C-terminal tail. Ligands, such as epinephrine, typically bind to the GPCR by sitting in a pocket formed by the transmembrane helices. GPCRs have no intrinsic catalytic domains; upon activation, they recruit G-proteins via their third cytoplasmic loop to couple to their signal transduction elements. GPCRs are often the target of drugs; indeed, it has been estimated that approximately 30% of all currently available therapeutics act on GPCRs. Furthermore, using the information gained by sequencing the human genome, it is apparent that there are many additional members of the GPCR family for which the signal has not yet been identified.

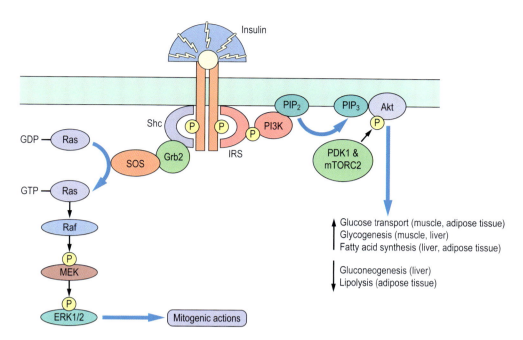

Fig. 25.3 Insulin signaling pathways. Insulin binding to the dimeric insulin receptor tyrosine kinase stimulates autophosphorylation of the receptor. The insulin receptor substrate (IRS) and Src-homology and collagen-like (Shc) adapter proteins bind to the phosphotyrosines on the insulin receptor. IRSs are subsequently phosphorylated by the insulin receptor, generating docking sites for phosphatidylinositol 3'-kinase (PI3K), which generates the phosphorylated lipid signaling molecule phosphatidylinositol 3,4,5-trisphosphate (PIP₃) from phosphatidylinositol 4,5-bisphosphate (PIP₂). PIP₃ recruits the serine/threonine protein kinase Akt to the plasma membrane, where Akt is phosphorylated and activated by phosphoinositide-dependent kinase 1 (PDK1) and the mammalian target of rapamycin complex 2 (mTORC2). Akt is essential for the metabolic effects of insulin in muscle (M), liver (L), and adipose tissue (A). Insulin receptor-bound Shc recruits growth factor receptor-bound protein 2 (Grb2), which is bound to the guanine nucleotide exchange factor Son of Sevenless (SOS). SOS catalyzes GDP–GTP exchange on the small G-protein Ras. The GTP-bound active Ras initiates a protein kinase cascade in which the protein kinase Raf phosphorylates and activates another protein kinase MEK, which subsequently phosphorylates and activates the protein kinases ERK1 and ERK2, which mediate many of the mitogenic actions of insulin. For more detail, see Chapter 31, Fig. 31.4.

G-proteins regulate a diverse range of biological processes

G-proteins constitute a group of regulatory molecules that are involved in the regulation of a diverse range of biological processes, including signal transduction, protein synthesis, intracellular trafficking (targeted delivery to the plasma membrane or intracellular organelles), and exocytosis, as well as cell movement, growth, proliferation, and differentiation. The G-protein superfamily predominantly comprises two major subfamilies: the small, monomeric Ras-like G-proteins and the heterotrimeric G-proteins. Heterotrimeric G-proteins regulate the transduction of transmembrane signals from cell-surface receptors to a variety of intracellular effectors, such as adenylyl cyclase, phospholipase C (PLC), cGMP-phosphodiesterase (PDE) and ion-channel effector systems. Heterotrimeric G-proteins consist of three subunits: α (39–46 kDa), β (37 kDa), and γ (8 kDa). In general, effector specificity is conferred by the α-subunit, which contains the GTP-binding site and an intrinsic GTPase activity. However, it is now widely accepted that βγ-complexes can also directly regulate effectors such as phospholipase A₂ (PLA₂), PLC-β isoforms, adenylyl cyclase, and ion

channels. Four major subfamilies of α-subunit genes have been identified on the basis of their cDNA homology and function: $G_s\alpha$, $G_i\alpha$, $G_{q/11}\alpha$, and $G_{12/13}\alpha$ (Table 25.2). Many of these Gα subunits have been shown to exhibit a broad pattern of expression in mammalian systems at the mRNA level, but it is also clear that certain α-subunits have a tissue-restricted profile of expression. Moreover, there is evidence of differential expression of α-subunits during cellular development.

G-proteins act as molecular switches

Heterotrimeric G-proteins regulate transmembrane signals by acting as molecular switches, linking cell-surface G-protein–coupled receptors to one or more downstream signaling molecules (Fig. 25.2). Ligation of a GPCR initiates an interaction with the inactive, GDP-bound heterotrimeric G-protein. This interaction drives the exchange of GDP for GTP, inducing a conformational change in Gα, which results in a decrease in its affinity for both the GPCR and the βγ-subunits, leading to dissociation of the GPCR–G-protein complex. The activated Gα (GTP-bound), released βγ-subunits, or both can then interact with one or more effectors to generate intracellular second messengers, which activate downstream signaling cascades. Signaling is terminated by the intrinsic GTPase activity of the

Table 25.2 Properties of mammalian G-protein α-subunits

G-protein subfamily	α subunit	Tissue distribution	Toxin substrate	Examples of effectors
$G_s\alpha$	$G_s\alpha$	Ubiquitous	Cholera toxin	Activates adenylyl cyclase ($G_s,G_{olf}\alpha$) K^+ channels ($G_s\alpha$) Src tyrosine kinases ($G_s\alpha$)
	$G_{olf}\alpha$	Olfactory neurons, central nervous system	Cholera toxin	
$G_i\alpha$	$G_i\alpha$	Ubiquitous	Pertussis toxin	Inhibits adenylyl cyclase ($G_i,G_o,G_z\alpha$) Activates K^+ channels ($G_i,G_o,G_z\alpha$) cGMP phosphodiesterase ($G_t\alpha$),
	$G_o\alpha$	Neuronal/neuroendocrine tissues	Pertussis toxin	
	$G_z\alpha$	Neurons, platelets	None	
	$G_t\alpha$	Retina	Pertussis toxin	
	$G_{gust}\alpha$	Taste buds	Pertussis toxin	
$G_{q/11}\alpha$	$G_q\alpha$	Ubiquitous	None	Activates PLC indirectly through activation of calcium channels Activates K^+ channels ($G_q\alpha$)
	$G_{11}\alpha$	Ubiquitous	None	
	$G_{14}\alpha$	Lung, kidney, liver, spleen, testis	None	
	$G_{16}\alpha$ ($G_{15}\alpha$ in mouse)	Hematopoietic cells	None	
$G_{12/13}\alpha$	$G_{12}\alpha$	Ubiquitous	None	Activates PLCε indirectly through activation of calcium channels Activates PLD Activates Rho GEF
	$G_{13}\alpha$	Ubiquitous	None	

cGMP, cyclic guanosine monophosphate; PLC, phospholipase C; PLD, phospholipase D; Rho GEF, Rho GTPase guanine nucleotide exchange factor.

✳ ADVANCED CONCEPT BOX
BACTERIAL TOXINS THAT TARGET G-PROTEINS CAUSE SEVERAL DISEASES

A variety of bacterial toxins exert their toxic effects by covalently modifying G-proteins and hence irreversibly modulating their function. For example, **cholera toxin** from *Vibrio cholerae* contains an enzyme (subunit A) that catalyzes the transfer of ADP-ribose from intracellular NAD^+ to the α-subunit of G_s; this modification prevents the hydrolysis of G_s-bound GTP, resulting in a constitutively (permanently) active form of the G-protein. The resulting prolonged increase in cAMP concentrations within the intestinal epithelial cells leads to PKA-mediated phosphorylation of Cl^- channels, causing a large efflux of electrolytes and water into the gut, which is responsible for the severe diarrhea that is characteristic of cholera. Enterotoxin action is initiated by specific binding of the B (binding) subunits of the cholera toxin (AB_5) to the oligosaccharide moiety of the monosialoganglioside, GM_1, on epithelial cells. A similar molecular mechanism has been attributed to the action of the **heat-labile enterotoxin,** labile toxin secreted by several strains of *Escherichia coli* responsible for "traveler's diarrhea."

In contrast, **pertussis toxin** (another AB_5 toxin) from *Bordetella pertussis*, the causative agent of whooping cough, catalyzes the ADP-ribosylation of $G_{i\alpha}$, which prevents $G_{i\alpha}$ from interacting with activated receptors. Hence, the G-protein is inactivated and cannot act to inhibit adenylyl cyclase, activate PLA_2 or PLC, open K^+ channels, or open and close Ca^{2+} channels, causing a generalized uncoupling of hormone receptors from their signaling cascades.

α-subunit, which hydrolyzes GTP to GDP to allow reassociation of the inactive heterotrimeric G-protein (Gαβγ).

SECOND MESSENGERS

Cyclic AMP (cAMP) is a key molecule in signal transduction

cAMP is a small molecule that has a key role in the regulation of intracellular signal transduction and is derived from ATP by the catalytic action of the signaling enzyme **adenylyl cyclase** (Fig. 25.4). This cyclization reaction involves the intramolecular attack of the 3′-OH group of the ribose unit on the α-phosphoryl group of ATP to form a phosphodiester bond. Hydrolysis of cAMP to 5′-AMP by specific cAMP phosphodiesterases terminates the cAMP signal.

Glucagon and β-adrenergic receptors are coupled to cAMP

Glucagon and β-adrenergic receptors are GPCRs that stimulate cAMP generation. The β-adrenergic hormone epinephrine induces the breakdown of glycogen to glucose-1-phosphate

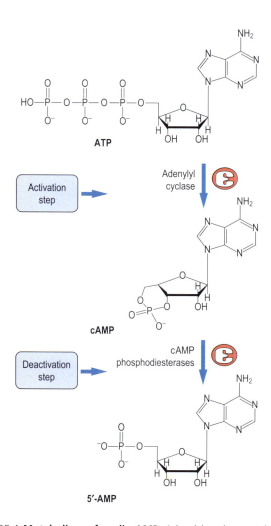

Fig. 25.4 **Metabolism of cyclic AMP.** Adenylyl cyclase catalyzes a cyclization reaction to produce the active cAMP, which is then deactivated by cAMP phosphodiesterases. cAMP, cyclic adenosine monophosphate.

in muscle and, to a lesser extent, in the liver. The breakdown of glycogen in the liver is predominantly stimulated by the polypeptide hormone glucagon, which is secreted by the pancreas when plasma glucose is low (Chapters 12 and 31). Binding of epinephrine or glucagon to the β-adrenergic or glucagon receptors, respectively, stimulates adenylyl cyclase activity in liver and muscle cells and stimulates glycogen breakdown, effects that can be mimicked by cell-permeant analogs of cAMP, such as dibutyryl cAMP in hepatocytes, highlighting the importance of cAMP.

Adenylyl cyclase is regulated by G-protein α-subunits

The β-adrenergic and glucagon receptors are coupled to adenylyl cyclase activation by the action of a specific form of the α-subunit of the G-protein, termed $G_s\alpha$. Although hydrolysis of GTP by the intrinsic GTPase of the $G_s\alpha$-subunit acts to switch off adenylyl cyclase activation, the hormone–GPCR

CLINICAL BOX
A CHILD WITH PREMATURE BREAST DEVELOPMENT: McCune–ALBRIGHT SYNDROME

A 3-year-old girl was brought to the hospital because her mother had been concerned about apparent breast development over the last 6 months and a spot of blood on her pants last week. On examination, she had Tanner Stage 3 breast development. On her trunk, she had three areas of brown skin pigmentation with ragged edges.

Comment

This child is suffering from McCune–Albright syndrome. She is likely to develop polyostotic fibrous dysplasia, with areas of thinning and sclerosis in her long bones, which may fracture. Other endocrinopathies include thyrotoxicosis, growth hormone hypersecretion, Cushing's syndrome (cortisol excess), and hyperparathyroidism. The cause is an activating missense mutation in the gene encoding the $G_s\alpha$-subunit of the G-protein that stimulates cyclic AMP formation. The problem presents following a somatic cell mutation with clinical features dependent on a mosaic distribution of aberrant cells. The incidence of the syndrome is 1 in 25,000.

CLINICAL BOX
FIBROBLAST GROWTH FACTOR RECEPTOR 3 AND ACHONDROPLASIA

Fibroblast growth factor (FGF) receptor 3 (FGFR3) is an intrinsic tyrosine kinase receptor with an important role in the regulation of bone growth. In chondrocytes (the cells that synthesize cartilage at the epiphyses of long bones), FGF binding to two FGFR3 monomers causes dimerization of the receptor, allowing the intracellular tyrosine kinase domains to transphosphorylate each other. This autophosphorylation of FGFR3 leads to activation of signaling pathways including the transcription factor, signal transducer and activator of transcription-1 (STAT1) and the small G-protein Ras, which subsequently activates the Raf–MEK–ERK protein kinase cascade. Activation of these pathways inhibits chondrocyte differentiation and proliferation. Thus FGFR3 stimulation suppresses long-bone growth because the reduced number of chondrocytes decreases the cartilage deposition that would normally serve as a template for osteoblasts to form bone by ossification.

Achondroplasia, characterized by short stature and macrocephaly, has an incidence of 1 in 15,000–40,000 newborns. The majority of people with achondroplasia have mutations in FGFR3 that increase its tyrosine kinase activity in the absence of FGF. As a consequence, chondrocyte proliferation and cartilage deposition are impaired, leading to a reduced length of the long bones.

complex must also be deactivated to return the cell to its resting, unstimulated state. In the case of β-adrenergic receptors, this receptor desensitization, which occurs after prolonged exposure to the hormone, involves phosphorylation of the C-terminal tail of the hormone-occupied β-adrenergic receptor by a kinase known as β-adrenergic receptor kinase. Other GPCRs, such as α_2-adrenergic receptors in smooth muscle, act to inhibit adenylyl cyclase and cAMP generation. In this case, receptors are coupled to a specific inhibitory form of the α-subunit of the G-protein, termed $G_i\alpha$ (Table 25.2), which inhibits adenylyl cyclase activity, reducing cAMP concentrations.

Signals can activate different receptor subtypes, with different consequences

Receptor subtypes are expressed in a tissue-specific manner for some signals, such as epinephrine and angiotensin II. These different receptor subtypes may couple in different ways; for example, epinephrine stimulates cAMP synthesis through $G_s\alpha$-coupled β-adrenergic receptors in skeletal muscle yet inhibits cAMP synthesis through $G_i\alpha$-coupled α_2-adrenergic receptors in smooth muscle. **Therefore the same signal can have differing effects on intracellular signaling cascades depending on the tissue being examined**.

Protein kinase A

cAMP transduces its effects on glycogen–glucose-1-phosphate interconversion by regulating a key signaling enzyme, protein kinase A (PKA), which phosphorylates target proteins on serine and threonine residues.

Protein kinase A binds cAMP and phosphorylates other enzymes

PKA is a multimeric enzyme comprising two regulatory (R) subunits and two catalytic (C) subunits: the R_2C_2 tetrameric form of PKA is inactive, but binding of four molecules of cAMP to the R-subunits leads to the release of catalytically active C-subunits, which can then phosphorylate and modulate the activity of two key enzymes, phosphorylase kinase and glycogen synthase (Fig. 25.5), which are involved in regulation of glycogen metabolism (Chapter 12).

Many other cellular responses can be mediated by the cAMP–PKA signaling cassette

PKA-mediated phosphorylation can regulate the activity of a number of ion channels, such as K^+, Cl^-, and Ca^{2+} channels, and that of phosphatases involved in the regulation of cellular signaling. In addition, translocation of activated PKA into the nucleus allows modulation of the activity of transcription factors such as the cAMP response element-binding protein (CREB) and the activation transcription factor (ATF) families, leading to either the induction or the repression of expression of specific genes (Fig. 25.5).

CLINICAL BOX
OREXIN RECEPTOR ANTAGONISTS - FROM ORPHAN G-PROTEIN COUPLED RECEPTOR TO TREATING INSOMNIA

Approximately 30% of drugs currently in clinical use target G-protein–coupled receptors (GPCR). Sequencing of the human genome identified more than 800 genes that encode members of the GPCR superfamily, yet it is not known what modulates approximately 140 of these GPCRs, which are termed "orphan GPCRs." Due to the involvement of GPCRs in regulation in a wide range of human physiology and pathophysiology, GPCRs are a popular therapeutic target for drug discovery, and there is great interest in the further characterization of the biology, structure, and potential therapeutic potential of orphan GPCRs. To understand the function of orphan GPCRs, their tissue distribution and subcellular localization have been studied, and the physiologic and behavioral phenotype of animal models that lack the orphan GPCR in question have been examined. Furthermore, potential ligands for orphan GPCRs have been identified by screening using cultured cells that are genetically manipulated to express high levels of the orphan GPCR in question and then using this as a "reporter system" to see whether the GPCR is influenced.

Two orphan GPCRs that were "deorphanized" in this way are the orexin receptors. Researchers screened fractions derived from tissue extracts against cell lines that each expressed 1 of more than 50 orphan GPCRs. They discovered several fractions from rat brain extracts that stimulated individual orphan GPCRs and then purified those fractions to determine the component that influenced the orphan GPCR. By doing this, they found two peptides that bound to the GPCRs and that these peptides stimulated feeding behavior when administered to rodents. They therefore named them orexin A and orexin B from the Greek word *orexis*, meaning "appetite," and deorphanized two GPCRs, orexin receptor-1 and orexin receptor-2. This led to significant research effort to understand the biology of these entirely novel peptides and their receptors. Intriguingly, mutations in orexin receptor-2 were found in dogs, which had a narcolepsy phenotype, and further research identified that a high proportion of people with narcolepsy had orexin deficiency. Narcolepsy is a disorder of the organization of the sleep–wake cycle, in which people exhibit excessive daytime sleepiness and cataplexy. As a consequence, efforts were made to identify orexin-receptor agonists to treat narcolepsy and orexin-receptor antagonists to treat insomnia. This work culminated in the approval of suvorexant as an orexin-receptor antagonist for the treatment of insomnia in the United States.

cAMP can stimulate cellular signaling independent of PKA

It has become clear that not all actions of cAMP are mediated by PKA. cAMP can also bind to Epacs (exchange proteins directly activated by cAMP), which are guanine-nucleotide-exchange factors for the Rap small GTPase. Epac activation

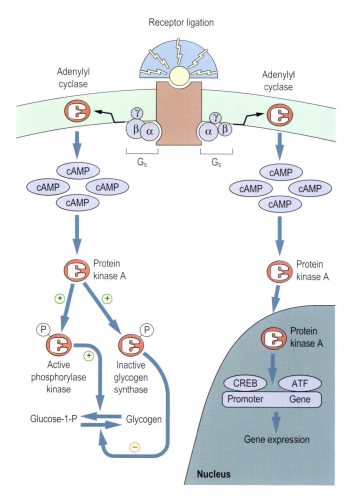

Fig. 25.5 **Protein kinase A (PKA) acts as a signaling enzyme for the second messenger, cAMP.** Binding of a stimulatory G-protein (G$_s$) to the hormone–receptor complex activates adenylyl cyclase, which catalyzes the production of cAMP. PKA is activated by binding four molecules of cAMP. Translocation of PKA into the nucleus modulates the activity of transcription factors such as CREB and ATF (see text), leading to induction or repression of gene expression. (See also Chapter 12.)

has been implicated in the antiinflammatory action of cAMP and in neuronal growth and development.

Signal cascades amplify signals initiated by receptor binding

The concentrations of hormones and other signals are often in the nanomolar (10^{-9} mol/L) or picomolar (10^{-12} mol/L) range. As a consequence, it is important that the signal is amplified. Multilayered signal transduction cascades cause substantial amplification of the original signal at each stage of the cascade, ensuring that binding of only a few hormone molecules leads to an appropriate biological response. For example, stimulation of glycogen breakdown by glucagon or epinephrine involves amplification of the signal at the level of G-proteins, adenylyl cyclase, PKA, and phosphorylase,

such that many glucose-1-phosphate molecules are released (Fig. 25.6).

Phosphodiesterases terminate the cAMP signal

Phosphodiesterases (PDE) terminate the cAMP signal by hydrolyzing cAMP to 5′-AMP (Fig. 25.4) and therefore play key roles in the regulation of various physiologic responses in many different cells and tissues. There are many different PDE isoforms that exhibit a tissue-specific pattern of expression and different selectivity for cAMP or cGMP. PDEs have been demonstrated to regulate platelet activation, vascular relaxation, cardiac muscle contraction, and inflammation. Selective inhibitors of PDEs have been used as therapeutic agents for **asthma** (methylxanthines), **erectile dysfunction** (sildenafil), and **heart failure** (milrinone). Milrinone is selective for the PDE$_3$ isoforms, which increases the force of contraction of the heart, presumably due to increased cAMP concentrations and PKA activity, leading to phosphorylation of cardiac calcium channels and a subsequent increase in intracellular calcium concentration.

Phospholipase-derived second messengers

Phospholipase C hydrolyzes the membrane phospholipid phosphatidylinositol 4,5-bisphosphate to generate two second messengers

GPCRs that are coupled to the G$_q$α subtype of the G-protein α-subunit stimulate the activity of **phospholipase C (PLC).** In addition, other types of membrane receptors - such as the vascular endothelial growth factor (VEGF) receptor, which has intrinsic tyrosine kinase activity - also are able to stimulate PLC. PLC catalyzes the hydrolysis of a minor phospholipid species, phosphatidylinositol 4,5-bisphosphate (PIP$_2$), which typically represents about 0.4% of total phospholipids in membranes, generating two second messengers: **inositol-1,4,5-trisphosphate** (IP$_3$) and **diacylglycerol** (DAG; Fig. 25.7). IP$_3$ is hydrophilic and mobilizes intracellular stores of calcium upon release into the cytosol. DAG is a lipid second messenger, which is anchored in the plasma membrane by virtue of its hydrophobic fatty acid side chains and activates a key family of signaling enzymes known as **protein kinase C (PKC).**

IP$_3$ stimulates intracellular calcium mobilization

Once synthesized from PIP$_2$, IP$_3$ binds to receptors found on the endoplasmic reticulum of all cells. IP$_3$ receptors are a family of related glycoproteins (molecular mass 250 kDa) comprising six transmembrane-spanning domains. The active receptor is expressed as a multimer of four IP$_3$ receptor molecules that acts as a **ligand-gated Ca^{2+} channel**. The tetrameric structure of the IP$_3$ receptor gives rise to cooperativity in Ca^{2+} channel activity. It has been estimated that stimulation with IP$_3$ causes transport of 20–30 calcium ions, revealing the amplification inherent in this signaling cascade. Consistent with the transient nature of the release of intracellular Ca^{2+} that is observed after hormone receptor ligation, cellular concentrations of IP$_3$ are

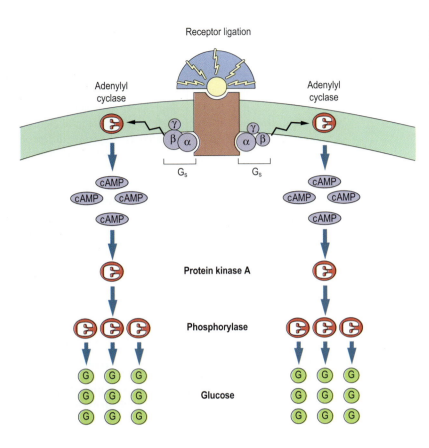

Receptor ligation

Adenylyl cyclase

Adenylyl cyclase

G_s G_s

cAMP

Protein kinase A

Phosphorylase

Glucose

Fig. 25.6 **Signal cascade induces amplification of hormone signal.** Each activated hormone–receptor complex can stimulate multiple G_s molecules. Each adenylyl cyclase can catalyze the generation of many cAMP molecules, and each protein kinase A can activate many phosphorylase molecules, leading to the breakdown of glycogen into many glucose-1-phosphate molecules as a result of glycogen degradation. (See also Chapter 12.)

rapidly returned to resting values (10 nmol/L) by more than one route of degradation (Fig. 25.7).

Signal transduction by Ca^{2+}

Ca^{2+} is a ubiquitous messenger with an important role in the transduction of signals leading to diverse cellular responses that include **cell motility changes, egg fertilization, neurotransmission, secretion, differentiation, and proliferation**. Cells expend considerable energy maintaining a Ca^{2+} concentration gradient such that the intracellular Ca^{2+} concentration in resting, unstimulated cells is of the order of 10^{-7} mol/L, whereas the extracellular Ca^{2+} concentration is approximately 10,000-fold greater, typically 10^{-3} mol/L. This steep gradient allows for rapid, abrupt, transient changes in Ca^{2+} concentration in response to signals. Ligand binding by a wide range of receptors leads to a PLC-mediated rapid (within seconds) and transient increase in intracellular Ca^{2+} concentration to the micromolar range (see also Chapter 4). The rapid changes in Ca^{2+} concentrations are very tightly regulated and utilize a variety of mechanisms involving cell compartmentalization. For example, intracellular Ca^{2+} concentrations can be lowered by **sequestration of Ca^{2+} into the endoplasmic reticulum** by Ca^{2+}-ATPases **or into the mitochondria** using the energy-driven electrochemical gradient. Alternatively, free Ca^{2+} can be **chelated** by Ca^{2+}-binding proteins such as calsequestrin.

Many downstream signaling events mediated by Ca^{2+} are modulated by a Ca^{2+}-sensing and binding protein, calmodulin

Calmodulin (CaM) is an abundant 17-kDa protein that contains a Ca^{2+}-binding structural motif called an EF hand motif (Fig. 25.8). CaM is composed of two similar globular domains joined by a long α-helix, with each globular lobe having two EF hand motifs. Binding of three to four calcium ions occurs when intracellular Ca^{2+} concentration increases to about 500 nmol/L, inducing a major conformational change that allows CaM to bind to and modify target proteins. Binding of several Ca^{2+} ions allows cooperativity in the activation of CaM, such that small changes in Ca^{2+} concentration cause large changes in the concentration of an active Ca^{2+}/CaM complex, providing amplification of the original hormone signal.

Calmodulin has a wide range of target effectors

CaM has a wide range of target effectors, including **NO synthase (NOS)**, which stimulates NO synthesis in response to Ca^{2+}-mobilizing signals, and **Ca^{2+}/CaM-dependent protein kinases,** which phosphorylate serine-threonine residues on proteins to regulate a variety of processes. For example, the broad-specificity kinase Ca^{2+}/CaM-kinase II is involved in the regulation of fuel metabolism, ion permeability, neurotransmitter biology, and muscle contraction. CaM also serves as a permanent regulatory subunit of phosphorylase kinase and

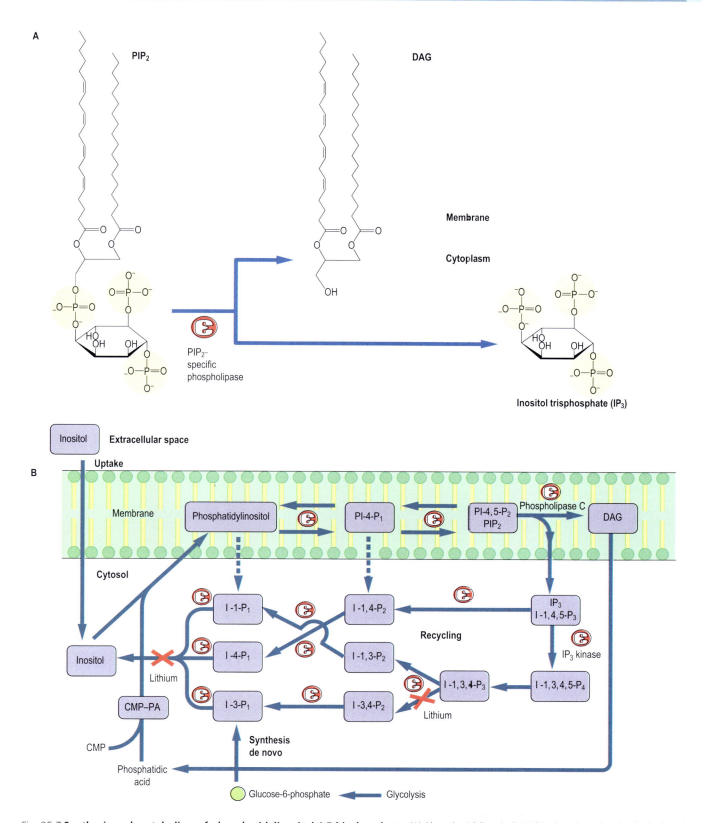

Fig. 25.7 **Synthesis and metabolism of phosphatidylinositol 4,5-bisphosphate.** (A) Phosphatidylinositol 4,5-bisphosphate (PIP$_2$) is hydrolyzed by a PIP$_2$-specific PLC to generate two second messengers: Inositol-1,4,5-P$_3$ (IP$_3$) and DAG IP$_3$ are released into the cytosol and have been shown to mobilize intracellular stores of calcium. DAG is a lipid second messenger that is anchored in the plasma membrane and activates PKCs. (B) PIP$_2$ is generated from phosphatidylinositol by phosphatidylinositol 4-kinase and phosphatidylinositol 5-kinase. IP$_3$ is degraded by (i) the sequential action of phosphatases converting Inositol-1,4,5-P$_3$ to inositol, and (ii) an IP$_3$ kinase, which generates inositol-1,3,4,5-P$_4$, which is in turn sequentially degraded to inositol by inositol phosphate-specific phosphatases, some of which are inhibited by lithium. DAG, diacylglycerol; PA, phosphatidic acid; CMP-PA, cytosine monophosphate-phosphatidic acid.

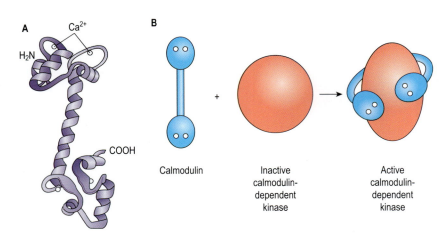

Fig. 25.8 **Calmodulin.** (A) Structure of calmodulin. (B) Binding of calcium induces a conformational change, allowing calmodulin to bind to and modify the activity of target signaling enzymes.

Table 25.3 The protein kinase C (PKC) superfamily

	Conventional PKCs			Novel PKCs				Atypical PKCs	
	α	β	γ	δ	ε	η	θ	λ (ι in mouse)	ζ
Ca^{2+}-sensitive	Yes	Yes	Yes	No	No	No	No	No	No
DAG-sensitive	Yes	Yes	Yes	Yes	Yes	Yes	Yes	No	No

may also regulate certain adenylyl cyclase isoforms and cAMP-specific PDEs, permitting "cross-talk" between cAMP- and Ca^{2+}-dependent signaling pathways.

Diacylglycerol activates protein kinase C

DAG fulfills its second messenger role by activating DAG-sensitive protein kinase C (PKC) isoforms, which phosphorylate a wide range of target signal transduction proteins on serine or threonine residues. PKCs are a superfamily of related kinases that have different activation requirements (Table 25.3) and exhibit tissue-specific expression. Nevertheless, all these enzymes comprise two major domains: an N-terminal regulatory domain and a C-terminal catalytic kinase domain. The regulatory domain contains a "pseudosubstrate" sequence that resembles the consensus phosphorylation site in PKC substrates. In the absence of activating cofactors (Ca^{2+}, phospholipid, DAG), this pseudosubstrate sequence interacts with the substrate-binding pocket in the catalytic domain and represses PKC activity. Binding of activating cofactors reduces the affinity of this interaction and induces a conformational change in the PKC, stimulating PKC activity. Consistent with the fact that the activator/cofactor, DAG, is anchored in the membranes, PKC activation is generally associated with translocation from the cytosol to the plasma membrane or nuclear membranes.

Other phospholipases hydrolyze phosphatidylcholine or phosphatidylethanolamine, generating a range of lipid second messengers

Additional receptor-coupled lipid signaling pathways have been identified involving hydrolysis of phosphatidylcholine or phosphatidylethanolamine, which can give rise to DAG and

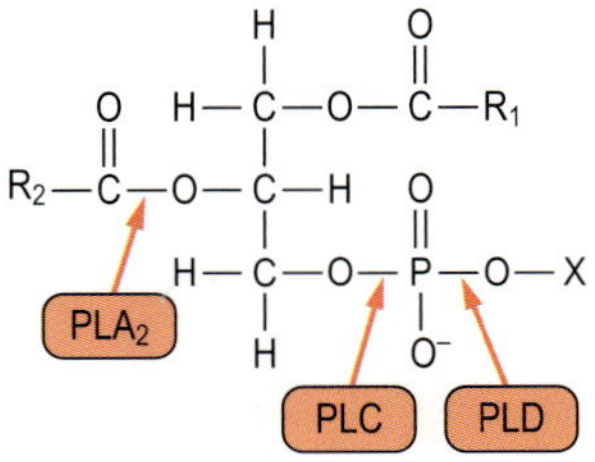

Fig. 25.9 **Sites of action of phospholipases.** Hydrolysis of phosphatidylcholine or phosphatidylethanolamine by phospholipase A_2 (PLA_2) results in the production of lysophosphatidylcholine or lysophosphatidylethanolamine and a fatty acid. Hydrolysis by phospholipase C (PLC) results in the synthesis of DAG and phosphocholine or phosphoethanolamine. Hydrolysis of phosphatidylcholine or phosphatidylethanolamine by phospholipase D (PLD) results in the production of phosphatidic acid and choline or ethanolamine. R1, R2, fatty acyl chains; X, choline/ethanolamine.

other biologically active lipids (Fig. 25.9) in response to a wide range of growth factors and mitogens. **Phosphatidylcholine comprises about 40% of total cellular phospholipids**. It can be hydrolyzed by distinct phospholipases, generating a diversity of lipid second messengers, including fatty acids such as arachidonic acid (generated by PLA_2) as well as different species of DAG (generated by PLC) and phosphatidic acid (generated by phospholipase D [PLD]). Hormone-stimulated phosphatidylethanolamine-PLD activities have also been reported. Some hormones or growth factors can stimulate only one or other of these phospholipases, but other ligands can stimulate all these pathways after binding to their specific receptors.

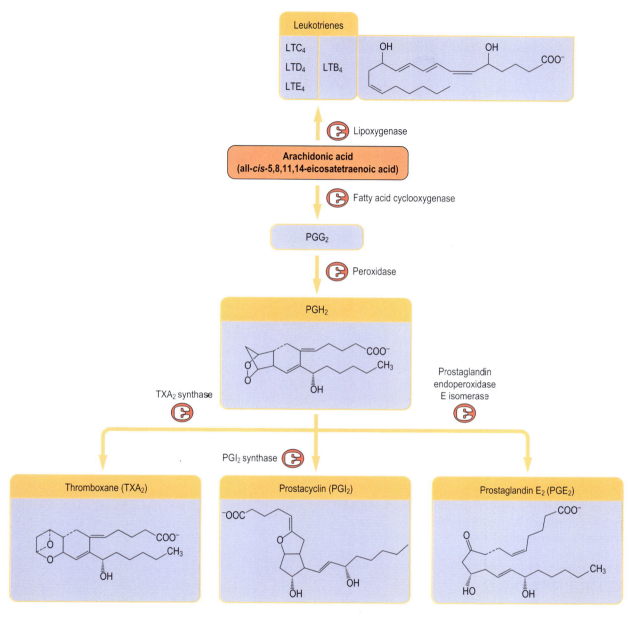

Fig. 25.10 **Synthesis of eicosanoids.** Eicosanoids are primarily derived from arachidonic acid. Leukotrienes (LT) are synthesized via a lipoxygenase-dependent pathway, whereas prostaglandins (PG), prostacyclins, and thromboxanes (TX) arise from cyclooxygenase-dependent routes.

Arachidonic acid is a second messenger regulating phospholipases and protein kinases

Arachidonic acid is a C-20 polyunsaturated fatty acid containing four double bonds. Increased arachidonic acid synthesis has been demonstrated to regulate several signaling enzymes, including PLC and conventional PKC isoforms. Furthermore, arachidonic acid is a key inflammatory intermediate. Arachidonic acid is synthesized by several PLA_2 enzymes, including cytosolic PLA_2, that can be regulated by Ca^{2+} and phosphorylation by protein kinases and secreted PLA_2, largely responsible for the inflammatory actions of arachidonic acid.

Arachidonic acid is the precursor of eicosanoids

As a key inflammatory mediator, arachidonic acid is the major precursor of the group of molecules termed **eicosanoids**, which encompass **prostaglandins, prostacyclins, thromboxanes, and leukotrienes.** Eicosanoids signal via GPCRs and have a wide variety of biological activities, including modulation of vascular smooth muscle contraction, platelet aggregation, gastric acid secretion, salt and water balance, and pain and inflammatory responses. Prostaglandins, prostacyclins, and thromboxanes are synthesized in membranes from arachidonic acid by the successive actions of several enzymes, starting with cyclooxygenase (Fig. 25.10).

Stockert, J. A., & Devi, L. A. (2015). Advancements in therapeutically targeting orphan GPCRs. *Frontiers in Pharmacology*, 6, 10.

ACTIVE LEARNING

1. Compare and contrast a receptor for a polypeptide hormone and for a steroid.
2. Describe the mechanism of G-protein signaling.
3. Give an example of a receptor possessing protein kinase activity and the components of its signaling cascade.
4. Comment on the diversity of phospholipase enzymes.
5. Describe the termination mechanism of cAMP activation.

RELEVANT WEBSITES

Science magazine's signal transduction knowledge environment: http://www.stke.org
Kimball's biology pages: http://www.biology-pages.info/C/CellSignaling.html
Cell signaling pathway maps: http://www.cellsignal.com/reference/pathway/index.html

SUMMARY

■ Cells specifically respond to the multiple environmental signals via signal transduction cassettes, which comprise specific cell-surface membrane receptors, effector signaling systems (e.g., adenylyl cyclase, phospholipases, ion channels), and regulatory proteins (e.g., G-proteins, protein kinases).

■ These signal transduction cassettes serve to detect, amplify, and integrate diverse external signals to generate the appropriate cellular response.

■ Receptors can have intrinsic enzyme activity (e.g., protein kinase, protein phosphatase, ion-channel activity) or are coupled to proteins that stimulate the cytosolic generation of low-molecular-mass molecules, termed second messengers (e.g., cAMP, IP_3, DAG, Ca^{2+}), which mediate their signaling functions by regulating key signaling proteins.

■ The specificity of a particular response can be further heightened by the variety of available phospholipase-signaling activities (PLC, PLD, and PLA_2), which can generate a diverse array of lipid second messengers.

FURTHER READING

Fredholm, B. B., Hökfelt, T., & Milligan, G. (2007). G-protein-coupled receptors: An update. *Acta Physiologica*, 190, 3–7.

Halls, M. L., & Cooper, D. M. (2011). Regulation by Ca^{2+}-signaling pathways of adenylyl cyclases. *Cold Spring Harbor Perspectives in Biology*, 3, a004143.

Houslay, M. D. (2010). Underpinning compartmentalized cAMP signaling through targeted cAMP breakdown. *Trends in Biochemical Sciences*, 35, 91–100.

Jastrzebska, B. (2013). GPCR: G protein complexes: The fundamental signaling assembly. *Amino Acids*, 45, 1303–1314.

Leslie, C. C. (2015). Cytosolic phospholipase A2: Physiological function and role in disease. *Journal of Lipid Research*, 56, 1386–1402.

Leto, D., & Saltiel, A. R. (2012). Regulation of glucose transport by insulin: Traffic control of GLUT4. *Nature Reviews. Molecular Cell Biology*, 13, 383–396.

Michel, T., & Vanhoutte, P. M. (2010). Cellular signaling and NO production. *Pflugers Archiv: European Journal of Physiology*, 459, 807–816.

Osborne, J. K., Zaganjor, E., & Cobb, M. H. (2012). Signal control through Raf: In sickness and in health. *Cell Research*, 22, 14–22.

Parekh, A. B. (2011). Decoding cytosolic Ca^{2+} oscillations. *Trends in Biochemical Sciences*, 36, 78–87.

Smith, W. L. (2008). Nutritionally essential fatty acids and biologically indispensable cyclooxygenases. *Trends in Biochemical Sciences*, 33, 27–37.

ABBREVIATIONS

Akt	Protein kinase
ATF	Activation transcription factor
cAMP	Cyclic adenosine monophosphate
cGMP	Cyclic guanosine monophosphate
CaM	Calmodulin
CMP-PA	Cytosine monophosphate-phosphatidic acid
CREB	cAMP response element-binding protein
DAG	Diacylglycerol
EGF	Epidermal growth factor
Epacs	Exchange proteins directly activated by cAMP
ERK	Extracellular signal-regulated kinases
FADD	Fas-associated death domain
FcγR	Fc-γ receptor (receptor for immunoglobulin G)
FGF	Fibroblast growth factor
FGFR3	Fibroblast growth factor receptor 3
GPCR	G-protein coupled receptor
Grb2	Growth factor receptor-bound protein 2
GTPase	Guanosine triphosphatase
IP_3	Inositol-1,4,5-trisphosphate
IR	Insulin receptor
IRS	Insulin receptor substrate
ITAM/ITIM	Immunoreceptor tyrosine activation/inhibition motif
LT	Leukotriene
mTORC2	Mammalian target of rapamycin complex 2
MEK	Mitogen-activated protein kinase
NGF	Nerve growth factor
NO	Nitric oxide
NOS	Nitric oxide synthase
PA	Phosphatidic acid
PDE	Phosphodiesterase
PDGF	Platelet-derived growth factor
PDK1	Phosphoinositide-dependent kinase 1
PG	Prostaglandins
PI3K	Phosphatidylinositol 3′-kinase
PIP_2	Phosphatidylinositol 4,5-bisphosphate
PIP_3	Phosphatidylinositol 3,4,5-trisphosphate
PK	Protein kinase: PKA, PKC
PL	Phospholipase: PLA_2, PLC, PLC-β, PLD
Raf	Family of serine/threonine kinases

Rap	Small GTPase
Ras	Small monomeric G-protein
Rho GEF	Rho GTPase guanine nucleotice exchange factor
RIP	Receptor-interacting protein
Shc	Src-homology and collagen-like adapter proteins
Src	Tyrosine kinase

SOS	Son of Sevenless, guanine nucleotide exchange factor
STAT1	Signal transducer and activator of transcription-1
TRADD	TNF-receptor-associated death domain
TRAFs	TNF-receptor-associated factors
TX	Thromboxanes
VEGF	Vascular endothelial growth factor

LEARNING OBJECTIVES

After reading this chapter, you should be able to:

- Outline the criteria that need to be met before a molecule can be classified as a neurotransmitter.
- Identify the major neurotransmitter types, and be aware that some molecules have neurotransmitter properties but cannot in the strictest sense be classified as neurotransmitters.
- Explain the generation of action potentials, appreciate how neurotransmitters can be excitatory or inhibitory, and summarize the process whereby a neurotransmitter is released from the presynaptic cell.
- Describe the different neurotransmitter receptors and their general mode of action.
- Describe the major biochemical pathways for neurotransmitter synthesis and degradation.
- Identify some clinical disorders that can arise as a result of disruption of neurotransmitter metabolism.

INTRODUCTION

Neurotransmitters are molecules that act as chemical signals between nerve cells

Nerve cells communicate with each other and with target tissues by secreting chemical messengers called neurotransmitters. This chapter describes the various classes of neurotransmitters and how they interact with their target cells. It discusses their effects on the body, how alterations in their signaling may cause disease, and how pharmacologic manipulation of their concentrations may be used therapeutically. Traditionally, for a molecule to be labeled as a neurotransmitter, a number of criteria have to be met:

- Synthesis of the molecule occurs within the neuron (i.e., all biosynthetic enzymes, substrates, cofactors, and so on must be present for de novo synthesis).
- Storage of the molecule occurs within the nerve ending before release (e.g., in synaptic vesicles).
- Release of the molecule from the presynaptic ending occurs in response to an appropriate stimulus, such as an action potential.

- There is binding and recognition of the putative neurotransmitter molecule on the postsynaptic target cell.
- Mechanisms exist for the inactivation and termination of the biological activity of the neurotransmitter.

Rigorous adherence to these criteria means that some molecules that are involved in the cross talk between neurons are not classified as neurotransmitters in the strict sense. Thus nitric oxide (NO), adenosine, neurosteroids, and polyamines, among others, are often termed **neuromodulators** rather than neurotransmitters.

A **classification of neurotransmitters** based on chemical composition is shown in Table 26.1. Many are derived from simple compounds, such as amino acids (Table 26.2), but peptides are also now known to be extremely important. The principal transmitters in the peripheral nervous system are norepinephrine and acetylcholine (ACh; Fig. 26.1).

Several transmitters may be found in one nerve

An early dogma of nerve function held that one nerve contained one transmitter. This is now known to be an oversimplification, and combinations of transmitters are the rule. The pattern of cellular transmitters may characterize a particular functional role, but details of this also remain unclear. A major low-molecular-weight transmitter such as an amine is often present, along with several peptides, an amino acid, and a purine. Sometimes there may even be more than one possible transmitter in a particular vesicle, as is believed to be the case for adenosine triphosphate (ATP) and norepinephrine in sympathetic nerves. In some cases, the intensity of stimulation may control which transmitter is released, with peptides often requiring greater levels of stimulus. Furthermore, different transmitters may have a different timescale of action. Sympathetic nerves are good examples of nerves for which this is the case: it is believed that ATP causes their rapid excitation, whereas norepinephrine and the neuromodulator neuropeptide Y (NPY) cause a slower phase of action. In some tissues, NPY on its own may be able to produce a very slow excitation.

NEUROTRANSMISSION

Action potentials are caused by changes in ion flows across cell membranes

The signal carried by a nerve cell reflects an abrupt change in the voltage potential difference across the cell membrane. The normal **resting potential** difference is a few millivolts,

Table 26.1 Classification of neurotransmitters

Group	Examples
Amines	Acetylcholine (ACh), norepinephrine, epinephrine, dopamine, 5-HT
Amino acids	Glutamate, GABA
Purines	ATP, adenosine
Gases	Nitric oxide
Peptides	Endorphins, tachykinins, many others

5-HT, 5-hydroxytryptamine; GABA, γ-amino butyric acid.
Neurotransmitters can be classified in several ways. The scheme shown relies on chemical similarities. All except the peptides are synthesized at the nerve ending and packaged into vesicles there; peptides are synthesized in the cell body and transported down the axon.

Table 26.2 Neurotransmitters of low molecular weight

Compound	Precursor	Site of production
Amino acids		
Glutamate		Central nervous system (CNS)
Aspartate		CNS
Glycine		Spinal cord
Amino acid derivatives		
GABA	Glutamate	CNS
Histamine	Histidine	Hypothalamus
Norepinephrine	Tyrosine	Sympathetic nerves, CNS
Epinephrine	Tyrosine	Adrenal medulla, a few CNS nerves
Dopamine	Tyrosine	CNS
Serotonin	Tryptophan	CNS, enterochromaffin gut cells, enteric nerves
Purine derivatives		
ATP		Sensory, enteric, sympathetic nerves
Adenosine	ATP	CNS, peripheral nerves
Gas		
Nitric oxide	Arginine	Genitourinary tract, CNS
Miscellaneous		
Acetylcholine	Choline	Parasympathetic nerves, CNS

Many neurotransmitters are simple compounds, often derived from common amino acids.

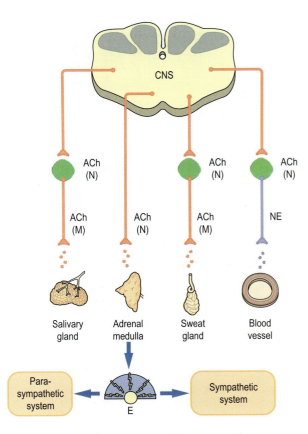

Fig. 26.1 **Transmitters in the autonomic nervous system. Catechol-amines and acetylcholine (ACh)** are transmitters in the **sympathetic** and **parasympathetic** nervous systems. **Preganglionic** nerves all release ACh, which binds to **nicotinic (N) receptors.** Most **postganglionic** sympathetic nerves release norepinephrine (NE), whereas postganglionic parasympathetic nerves release ACh, which acts at **muscarinic (M) receptors.** Adrenal glands release epinephrine **(E)**. Motor neurons release ACh, which acts at distinct nicotinic receptors.

with the **inside of the cell being negative,** and is caused by an imbalance of ions across the plasma membrane: the concentration of K^+ ion is much greater inside cells than outside, whereas the opposite is true for Na^+ ion. This difference is maintained by the action of the **Na^+/K^+-ATPase** (Chapter 35). Only those ions to which the membrane is permeable can affect the potential, as they can come to an electrochemical steady state under the combined influence of concentration and voltage differences. Because the membrane in all resting cells is comparatively permeable to K^+ as a result of the presence of voltage-independent (leakage) K^+ channels, this ion largely controls the resting potential.

A change in voltage that tends to drive the resting potential toward zero from the normal negative voltage is known as a depolarization, whereas a process that increases the negative potential is called hyperpolarization

So far, this picture is common to all cells. However, nerve cells contain voltage-dependent sodium channels that open very

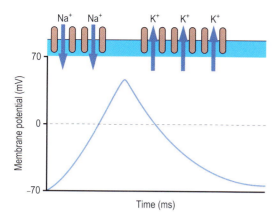

Fig. 26.2 **Generation of action potential.** Action potential is formed as follows: At the start of an action potential, the membrane is at its resting potential of about −70 mV. This is maintained by voltage-independent K⁺ channels. When an impulse is initiated by a signal from a neurotransmitter, voltage-dependent Na⁺ channels open. These allow inflow of Na⁺ ions, which alter the membrane potential to positive values. The Na⁺ channels then close, and K⁺ channels, called delayed rectifier channels, open to restore the initial balance of ions and the negative membrane potential.

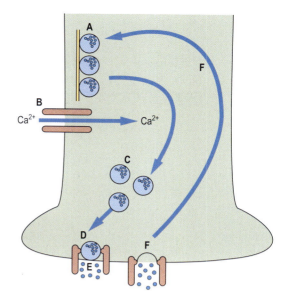

Fig. 26.3 **Release of neurotransmitters.** Neurotransmitters are released from vesicles at the synaptic membrane. (A) In the resting state, vesicles are attached to microtubules. (B) When an action potential is received, calcium channels open. (C) Vesicles move to the plasma membrane, then (D) bind to a complex of docking proteins. (E) Neurotransmitter is released, and (F) vesicles are recycled.

rapidly when a depolarizing change in voltage is applied. When they open, they allow the inward passage of huge numbers of Na⁺ ions from the extracellular fluid (Fig. 26.2), which swamps the resting voltage and drives the membrane potential to positive values. This reversal of voltage is the **action potential.** Almost immediately afterward, the sodium channels close, and so-called delayed potassium channels open. These restore the normal resting balance of ions across the membrane, and after a short refractory period, the cell can conduct another action potential. Meanwhile, the action potential has spread by electrical conductance to the next segment of nerve membrane, and the entire cycle starts again.

Neurotransmitters alter the activity of various ion channels to cause changes in the membrane potential

Excitatory neurotransmitters cause a **depolarizing** change in voltage, in which case an action potential is more likely to occur. In contrast, **inhibitory** transmitters **hyperpolarize** the membrane, and an action potential is then less likely to occur.

Neurotransmitters act at synapses

Neurotransmitters are released into the space between cells at a specialized area known as a synapse (Fig. 26.3). In the simplest case, they diffuse from the presynaptic membrane across the synaptic space, or cleft, and bind to receptors at the postsynaptic membrane. However, many neurons, particularly those containing amines, have several varicosities along the axon, containing transmitter. These varicosities may not be close to any neighboring cell, so transmitter released from them has the possibility of affecting many neurons. Nerves innervating smooth muscle are commonly of this kind.

When the action potential arrives at the end of the axon, the change in voltage opens calcium channels. Calcium entry is essential for mobilization of vesicles containing transmitter and for their eventual fusion with the synaptic membrane and release through it.

Because transmitters are released from vesicles, impulses arrive at the postsynaptic cell in individual packets, or quanta. At the neuromuscular junction between nerves and skeletal muscle cells, a large number of vesicles are discharged at a time, and a single impulse may therefore be enough to stimulate contraction of the muscle cell. The number of vesicles released at synapses between neurons, however, is much smaller; consequently, the recipient cell will be stimulated only if the total algebraic sum of the various positive and negative stimuli exceeds its threshold. As each cell in the brain receives input from a huge number of neurons, this implies that there is a far greater capability for the fine control of responses in the central nervous system (CNS) than there is at the neuromuscular junction.

Receptors

Neurotransmitters act by binding to specific receptors and opening or closing ion channels

There are several mechanisms by which receptors for excitatory neurotransmitters can cause the propagation of an action

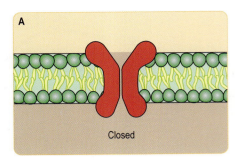
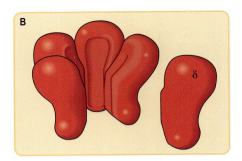
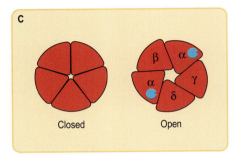
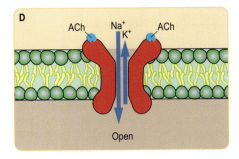

Fig. 26.4 **Mechanism of action of ionotropic receptors.** Ionotropic receptors directly open ion channels (in fact, they are themselves ion channels). The best-studied example is the nicotinic ACh receptor. This is a transmembrane protein (A) consisting of five nonidentical subunits (B), each one passing right through the membrane. The subunits surround a pore (C) that selectively allows certain ions through when it is opened by a ligand (D).

potential in a postsynaptic neuron. Directly or indirectly, they cause changes in ion flow across the membrane until the potential reaches the critical point, or threshold, for initiation of an action potential. Receptors that directly control the opening of an ion channel are called **ionotropic,** whereas **metabotropic** receptors cause changes in second-messenger systems, which in turn alter the function of channels that are separate from the receptor.

Ionotropic receptors (ion channels)

Ionotropic receptors contain an ion channel within their structure (Fig. 26.4; see also Chapter 4). Examples include the **nicotinic ACh receptor** and some glutamate and γ-**amino butyric acid (GABA) receptors.** These are transmembrane proteins, with several subunits, usually five, surrounding a pore through the membrane. Each subunit has four transmembrane regions. When the ligand binds, there is a change in the three-dimensional structure of the complex, which allows the flow of ions through it. The effect on membrane potential depends on the particular ions that are allowed to pass: the nicotinic ACh receptor is comparatively nonspecific toward sodium and potassium and causes depolarization, whereas the GABA$_A$ receptor is a chloride channel and causes hyperpolarization.

Metabotropic receptors

All known metabotropic receptors are coupled to G-proteins

Metabotropic receptors are coupled to second-messenger pathways and act more slowly than ionotropic receptors. All known metabotropic receptors are coupled to **G-proteins** (Chapter 25) and, like hormone receptors, have seven transmembrane regions. Typically, they then couple either to adenylate cyclase, altering the production of cyclic adenosine monophosphate (cAMP) or to the phosphatidyl inositol pathway, which alters calcium fluxes. Ion channels that are separate from the receptor are then usually modified by phosphorylation. For instance, the β-adrenergic receptor, which responds to norepinephrine and epinephrine (Chapter 25) causes an increase in cAMP, which stimulates a kinase to phosphorylate and activate a calcium channel. Some of the muscarinic class of ACh receptors have similar effects on K$^+$ channels.

Regulation of neurotransmitters

The action of transmitters must be halted by their removal from the synaptic cleft

When transmitters have served their function, they must be removed from the synaptic space. Simple diffusion is probably the major mechanism of removal of neuropeptides. Enzymes such as **acetylcholinesterase,** which cleaves ACh, may destroy any remaining transmitter. Surplus transmitters may also be taken back up into the presynaptic neuron for reuse, and this is a major route of removal for catecholamines and amino acids. Interference with uptake causes an increase in the concentration of transmitter in the synaptic space; this often has useful therapeutic consequences.

Concentrations of neurotransmitters may be manipulated

The effects of neurotransmitters can be altered by changing their effective concentrations or the number of receptors. Concentrations can be altered by

- changing the rate of synthesis,
- altering the rate of release at the synapse,
- blocking reuptake, or
- blocking degradation.

Changes in the number of receptors may be involved in long-term adaptations to the administration of drugs.

CLASSES OF NEUROTRANSMITTERS

Amino acids

It has been particularly difficult to prove that amino acids are true neurotransmitters; they are present in high concentrations because of their other metabolic roles, and therefore simple measurement of their concentrations did not provide conclusive evidence. Pharmacologic studies of responses to different analogues and the cloning of specific receptors finally provided the proof.

Glutamate

Glutamate is the most important excitatory transmitter in the CNS

Glutamate acts on both ionotropic and metabotropic receptors. Clinically, the receptor characterized in vitro by **N-methyl-D-aspartate (NMDA)** binding is particularly important (Fig. 26.5).

The hippocampus (Fig. 26.6) is an area of the limbic system of the brain that is involved in emotion and memory. Certain synaptic pathways there become more active when chronically stimulated, a phenomenon known as long-term potentiation. This represents a possible model of how memory is laid down, and it requires activation of the NMDA receptor and the consequent influx of calcium.

Glutamate is recycled by high-affinity transporters into both neurons and glial cells. The glial cells convert it into glutamine, which then diffuses back into the neuron. Mitochondrial glutaminase in the neuron regenerates glutamate for reuse.

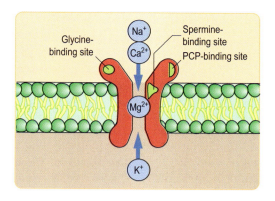

Fig. 26.5 **The NMDA glutamate receptor.** The glutamate receptor that binds *N*-methyl-D-aspartate (NMDA) is complex. This receptor is clinically important because it may cause damage to neurons after stroke (excitotoxicity). It contains several modulatory binding sites, so it may be possible to develop drugs that could alter its function. Glycine is an obligatory cofactor, as are polyamines such as spermine. Magnesium physiologically blocks the channel at the resting potential, so the channel can open only when the cell has been partially depolarized by a separate stimulus. It therefore causes a prolongation of the excitation. This receptor also binds phencyclidine (PCP). Because this drug of abuse can cause psychotic symptoms, it is possible that dysfunction of pathways involving NMDA receptors causes some of the symptoms of schizophrenia.

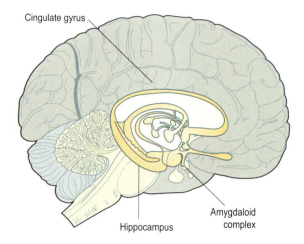

Fig. 26.6 **Limbic system.** The limbic system of the brain is involved in emotions and memory. It consists of various areas surrounding the upper brain stem, including the hippocampus, the amygdaloid body, and the cingulate gyrus. Removal of the hippocampus prevents the laying down of short-term memory, whereas intact amygdaloid function is required for the emotion of fear.

Glutamate and excitotoxicity

Extracellular glutamate concentration is increased after **trauma** and **stroke,** during severe convulsions, and in some organic brain diseases such as **Huntington's chorea, AIDS-related dementia**, and **Parkinson's disease.** This is because of the release of glutamate from damaged cells and damage to the glutamate uptake pathways.

Excess glutamate is toxic to nerve cells

The activation of NMDA receptor allows calcium entry into cells. This activates various proteases, which in turn initiate the pathway of programmed cell death or **apoptosis** (see Chapter 28). There may, in addition, be changes in other ionotropic glutamate receptors that also cause aberrant calcium uptake. Uptake of sodium ions is also implicated and causes swelling of cells. Activation of NMDA receptors also increases the production of nitric oxide, which may in itself be toxic. Cell death in some models of excitotoxicity can be prevented by inhibitors of nitric oxide production, but the mechanism of toxicity is not clear.

Attempts are being made to develop drugs to inhibit NMDA activation and suppress excitotoxicity. The hope is that damage caused by stroke can be limited or even reversed. Unfortunately, many of the drugs have side effects because they bind to the phencyclidine-binding site and have unpleasant psychologic effects such as paranoia and delusions.

γ-Amino butyric acid (GABA)

GABA is synthesized from glutamate by the enzyme glutamate decarboxylase

GABA (Fig. 26.7) is the major inhibitory transmitter in the brain. There are two known GABA receptors: the $GABA_A$ receptor is ionotropic, and the $GABA_B$ receptor is metabotropic. The $GABA_A$ receptor consists of five subunits that arise from several gene families, giving an enormous number of potential receptors with different binding affinities. This receptor is the target for several useful therapeutic drugs. **Benzodiazepines** bind to it and cause a potentiation of the response to endogenous GABA; these drugs reduce anxiety and also cause muscle relaxation. **Barbiturates** also bind to the GABA receptor and stimulate it directly in the absence of GABA; because of this lack of dependence on an endogenous ligand, they are more likely to cause toxic side effects in overdose.

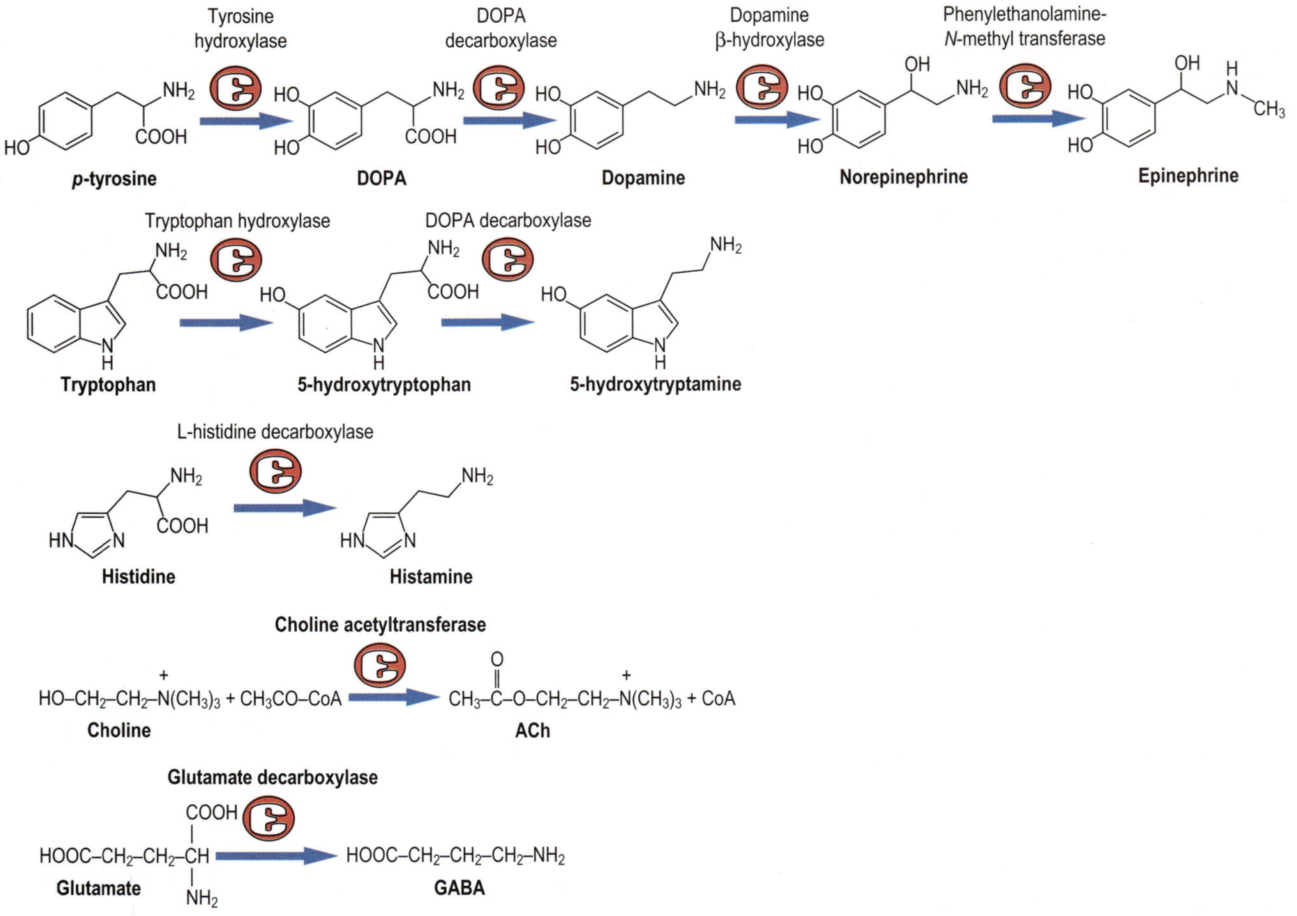

Fig. 26.7 **Synthesis of neurotransmitters and their precursors.** The amino acid tyrosine is the precursor of dopamine, norepinephrine, and epinephrine. Tryptophan is the precursor of serotonin (5-hydroxytryptamine), and histamine derives from the amino acid histidine. Choline, an amino alcohol, is the precursor of acetylcholine, and the common amino acid glutamic acid is the precursor of the GABA. Note that DOPA decarboxylase is also known as aromatic L-amino acid decarboxylase, AADC.

Glycine acts as an inhibitory neurotransmitter in the spinal cord and brain stem but also has excitatory effects in the cortex. Glycine levels are regulated by the glycine cleavage system (GCS), a complex of four proteins that break down glycine to ammonia and carbon dioxide. The GCS is present in high levels in liver, brain, and placental tissue. Defects in the GCS result in elevated plasma and cerebrospinal fluid (CSF) levels of glycine and cause glycine encephalopathy, also known as nonketotic hyperglycinemia (NKH). In glycine encephalopathy, CSF levels of glycine are disproportionately raised compared to plasma, and it is thought that the pathophysiology is primarily due to the effects of high glycine in the brain. Glycine encephalopathy typically presents with neurological symptoms including hypotonia, seizures, mental retardation, and brain malformations. It is usually a severe, early-onset disease with poor prognosis, although milder, later-onset phenotypes do exist, depending on the precise mutation. Currently, there is no effective medication.

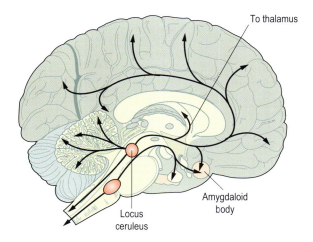

Fig. 26.8 **Norepinephrine neurons in the central nervous system (CNS).** Norepinephrine-containing neurons arise in the locus ceruleus in the brain stem and are distributed throughout the cortex.

Glycine

Glycine is primarily found in inhibitory interneurons in the spinal cord, where it blocks impulses traveling down the cord in motor neurons to stimulate skeletal muscle. The glycine receptor on motor neurons is ionotropic and is blocked by strychnine; motor impulses can then be passed without negative control, which accounts for the rigidity and convulsions caused by this toxin.

Catecholamines

Norepinephrine, epinephrine, and dopamine, known as catecholamines, are all derived from the amino acid tyrosine (Fig. 26.7). In common with other compounds containing amino groups, such as serotonin, they are also known as **biogenic amines.** Nerves that release catecholamines have varicosities along the axon, instead of a single area of release at the end. Transmitter is released from the varicosities and diffuses through the extracellular space until it finds a receptor. This allows it to affect a wide area of tissue, and these compounds are believed to have a general modulatory effect on overall brain functions such as mood and arousal.

Norepinephrine and epinephrine

Norepinephrine (also known as noradrenaline) is a major transmitter in the sympathetic nervous system

Sympathetic nerves arise in the spinal cord and run to ganglia situated close to the cord, from which postganglionic nerves run to the target tissues. Norepinephrine (Figs 26.1 and 26.7)

A 50-year-old man had been suffering from depression for some years. His condition was treated with tranylcypromine, an inhibitor of monoamine oxidase types A and B. He developed a severe, throbbing headache, and his blood pressure was found to be 200/110 mmHg. The only unusual occurrence had been that he had attended a cocktail party the previous evening, at which he ate cheese snacks and drank several glasses of red wine.

Comment
The patient was experiencing a hypertensive crisis caused by an interaction between the food he had eaten and the drug he was treated with, a monoamine oxidase (MAO) inhibitor. This drug inhibits the main enzyme that catabolizes catecholamines. Several foods, including cheese, pickled herring, and red wine, contain an amine called tyramine, which is similar in structure to natural amine transmitters and is also broken down by MAO. If this enzyme is not functional, the concentrations of tyramine increase, and it starts to act as a neurotransmitter. This can cause a hypertensive crisis, as it did in this patient.

is the transmitter for these postganglionic nerves, whereas the transmitter at the intermediate ganglia is ACh. Stimulation of these nerves is responsible for various features of the "fight-or-flight" response, such as stimulation of the heart rate, sweating, vasoconstriction in the skin, and bronchodilation.

There are also norepinephrine-containing neurons in the CNS, largely in the brain stem (Fig. 26.8). Their axons extend in a wide network throughout the cortex and alter the overall state of alertness or attention. The stimulatory effects of **amphetamines** are caused by their close chemical similarity to catecholamines.

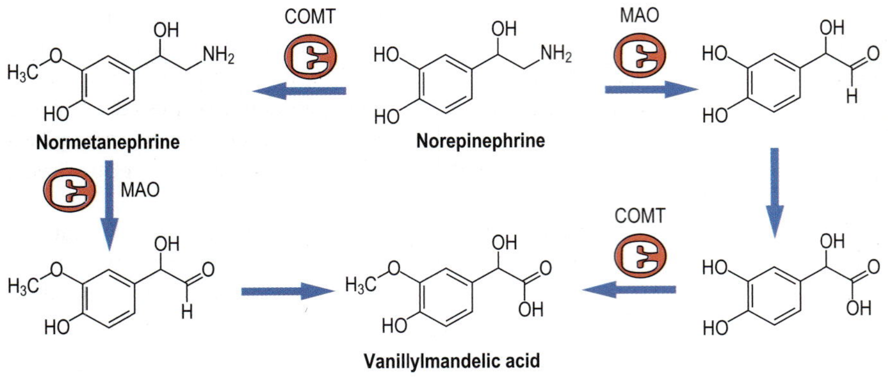

Normetanephrine

Norepinephrine

Vanillylmandelic acid

Fig. 26.9 **Catabolism of catecholamines.** Catecholamines are degraded by oxidation of the amino group by the enzyme mono-amine oxidase (MAO) and by methylation by catecholamine-*O*-methyltransferase (COMT). The pathway shown is for norepinephrine, but the pathways for epinephrine, dopamine, and 5-HT are analogous.

Epinephrine (also known as adrenaline) is produced by the adrenal medulla under the influence of ACh-containing nerves, analogous to the sympathetic preganglionic nerves

Epinephrine is more active than norepinephrine on the heart and lungs, causes redirection of blood from the skin to skeletal muscle, and has important stimulatory effects on glycogen metabolism in the liver. In response to epinephrine, a sudden extra supply of glucose is delivered to muscle, the heart and lungs work harder to pump oxygen around the circulation, and the body is then prepared to run or to defend itself (Chapter 31). Epinephrine is not essential for life, however, as it is possible to remove the adrenal medulla without serious consequences.

The receptors for norepinephrine and epinephrine are called **adrenoceptors**. They are divided into α- and β-receptor classes and subclasses on the basis of their pharmacology. Epinephrine acts on all classes of the receptors, but norepinephrine is more specific for α-receptors. **β-Blockers**, such as atenolol, are used to treat **hypertension** and chest pain (angina) in **ischemic heart disease** because they antagonize the stimulatory effects of catecholamines on the heart. Nonspecific **α-blockers** have limited use, although the more specific $β_1$-blockers, such as prazosin, and $α_2$-blockers, such as clonidine, can be used to treat **hypertension**. Certain subclasses of β-receptors are found in particular tissues; for instance, the $β_2$-receptor is present in the lung, and **$β_2$-receptor agonists** such as salbutamol are therefore used to produce bronchial dilatation in asthma without stimulating the $β_1$-receptor in the heart.

Norepinephrine is taken up into cells by a high-affinity transporter and catabolized by the enzyme monoamine oxidase (MAO). Further oxidation and methylation by catechol-amine-*O*-methyltransferase (COMT) convert the products to **metanephrines and vanillylmandelic acid** (4-hydroxy-3-methoxymandelic acid) (Fig. 26.9), which can be measured in the urine as indices of the function of the adrenal medulla. They are particularly increased in patients who have the tumor of the adrenal medulla known as pheochromocytoma. This tumor causes hypertension because of the vasoconstrictor action of the catecholamines it produces.

✿ ADVANCED CONCEPT BOX

DEPRESSION AS A DISEASE OF AMINE NEUROTRANSMITTERS: THE ANTIDEPRESSANTS

Monoamine oxidase (MAO) inhibitors prevent the catabolism of catecholamines and serotonin. They therefore increase the concentrations of these compounds at the synapse and increase the action of the transmitters. Compounds with this property are **antidepressants**. Reserpine, an antihypertensive drug that depletes catecholamines, caused depression and is no longer in use. These findings gave rise to the "amine theory of depression," which states that depression is caused by a relative deficiency of amine neurotransmitters at central synapses and predicts that drugs that increase amine concentrations should improve the symptoms of the condition.

In support of this theory, tricyclic antidepressants inhibit the transport of both norepinephrine and serotonin into neurons, thereby increasing the concentration of amines in the synaptic cleft. **Selective serotonin reuptake inhibitors (SSRI),** such as fluoxetine (Prozac), are also highly effective **antidepressants.** However, because the symptoms of depression do not resolve for several days after treatment is started, it is likely that long-term adaptations of concentrations of transmitters and their receptors are at least as important as acute changes in amine concentrations in the synaptic cleft.

This role of monoamines in depression is undoubtedly an oversimplification. Thus, cocaine is also an effective reuptake inhibitor but is not an antidepressant, and amphetamines both block reuptake and cause the release of catecholamines from nerve terminals, but they cause mania rather than relief of depression.

Dopamine

Dopamine is both an intermediate in the synthesis of norepinephrine and a neurotransmitter

Dopamine is a major transmitter in nerves that interconnect the nuclei of the basal ganglia in the brain and control voluntary movement (Fig. 26.10). Damage to these nerves causes

CLINICAL BOX
A 56-YEAR-OLD WOMAN PRESENTED WITH SEVERE HYPERTENSION: PHEOCHROMOCYTOMA

A 56-year-old woman presented with severe hypertension. She suffered from attacks of sweating, headaches, and palpitations. Her high blood pressure had not responded to treatment with an angiotensin-converting enzyme inhibitor and a diuretic. A sample of urine was taken for measurement of catecholamines and metabolites. The rate of excretion of norepinephrine was 1500 nmol/24 h (253 mg/24 h; reference range <900 nmol/24 h, <152 mg/24 h), that of epinephrine 620 nmol/24 h (113 mg/24 h; reference range <230 nmol/24 h, <42 mg/24 h), and that of vanillylmandelic acid 60 mmol/24 h (11.9 mg/24 h; reference range <35.5 mmol/24 h <7.0 mg/24 h).

Comment
The patient had a pheochromocytoma, which is a tumor of the adrenal medulla that secretes catecholamines. Both norepinephrine and epinephrine may be secreted; norepinephrine causes hypertension by activating α_1-adrenoceptors on vascular smooth muscle, and epinephrine increases heart rate by activating β_1-adrenoceptors in the heart muscle. Hypertension may be paroxysmal and severe, leading to stroke or heart failure.

Diagnosis is made by measuring catecholamines in plasma or urine or their metabolites, such as metanephrines and vanillylmandelic acid in urine. The tumor is usually localized by radiologic techniques such as nuclear magnetic resonance (NMR) or computed tomography (CT) scanning.

Although this is a rare cause of hypertension, comprising only about 1% of cases, it is very important to remember it because the condition is dangerous and often amenable to surgical cure.

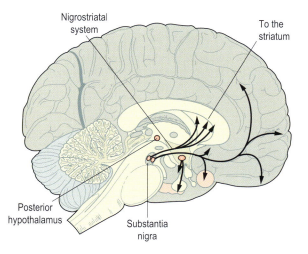

Fig. 26.10 **Dopamine in the nigrostriatal tract.** Nerves containing dopamine run in well-defined tracts. One of the most important tracts, the nigrostriatal, connects the substantia nigra in the midbrain with the basal ganglia below the cortex. Damage to this causes Parkinson's disease, with the loss of fine control of movement.

Parkinson's disease, which is characterized by tremor and difficulties in initiating and controlling movement. Dopamine is also found in pathways affecting the limbic systems of the brain, which are involved in emotional responses and memory. Defects in dopaminergic systems are implicated in **schizophrenia** because many antipsychotic drugs used to treat this disease have been found to bind to dopamine receptors.

In the periphery, dopamine causes vasodilatation, and it is therefore used clinically to stimulate renal blood flow and is important in the treatment of **renal failure**. The catabolism of dopamine is comparable to norepinephrine. However, the major metabolite formed is **homovanillic acid (HVA)**.

Serotonin (5-hydroxytryptamine)

Serotonin, also called 5-hydroxytryptamine (5-HT), is derived from tryptophan

Serotonin biosynthesis has a number of biochemical similarities to dopamine synthesis. Thus tryptophan hydroxylase, like tyrosine hydroxylase, displays a cofactor requirement for tetrahydrobiopterin (BH_4; see below). Furthermore, 5-hydroxytryptophan

CLINICAL BOX
TYROSINE HYDROXYLASE AND AROMATIC AMINO ACID DECARBOXYLASE DEFICIENCIES: INHERITED CAUSES OF IMPAIRED BIOGENIC AMINE METABOLISM

Tyrosine hydroxylase catalyzes the first step in dopamine biosynthesis, and inherited disorders affecting the activity of this enzyme result in brain dopamine deficiency. A number of clinical phenotypes have been described and include a progressive gait disorder and infantile parkinsonism. Treatment of tyrosine hydroxylase deficiency is by the administration of L-dopa. In order to prevent the decarboxylation of L-dopa to dopamine in the blood (by peripheral aromatic amino acid decarboxylase, AADC), an inhibitor (which does not affect the activity of the brain AADC) is given at the same time as the L-dopa. Such inhibition optimizes the transport of L-dopa across the blood–brain barrier. Within the brain, AADC can then convert the L-dopa to dopamine.

AADC catalyzes the conversion of L-dopa to dopamine and 5-hydroxytryptophan to serotonin. Consequently, an inborn error of metabolism affecting the activity of this enzyme results in a brain deficiency of both dopamine and serotonin. Patients with AADC deficiency have a clinical picture that includes a severe movement disorder, abnormal eye movements, and neurologic impairment. Treatment of AADC deficiency consists of preventing the degradation of any dopamine and serotonin that may be produced by residual AADC activity (i.e., by the use of monoamine oxidase inhibitors). In addition, dopamine agonists such as pergolide and bromocriptine are used to "mimic" the effects of dopamine.

CLINICAL BOX
LOSS OF ACTIVITY OF A DOPAMINE TRANSPORTER LEADS TO A CLINICAL PICTURE SUGGESTIVE OF A DOPAMINE DEFICIENCY STATE

Dopamine released into the synaptic cleft is taken back, via the dopamine transporter (DAT; SLC6A3), into presynaptic neurons, where it can be recycled. Autosomal recessive mutations are now documented that affect the DAT. This results in an intracellular neuronal dopamine deficiency and a marked increase in extracellular levels of the neurotransmitter. This excess dopamine is metabolized to **homovanillic acid (HVA)** via nonneuronal monoamine oxidase and catechol-*O*-methyltransferase. A markedly elevated cerebrospinal fluid (CSF) concentration of HVA is a strong indicator of DAT deficiency. Serum prolactin may also be elevated in this disorder. Clinically, patients with DAT mutations can present with parkinsonism-dystonia, associated with an eye movement disorder and pyramidal tract features. Currently, there is not an adequate treatment.

ADVANCED CONCEPT BOX
SECONDARY FACTORS MIMICKING NEUROTRANSMITTER DISORDERS

As more genetic mutations in neurometabolic/neurodegenerative disorders are being characterized, it is becoming apparent that these can have secondary negative effects on neurotransmission. Examples include **mitochondrial impairment** and a resultant loss of brain ATP availability. This in turn may limit packaging of neurotransmitters, such as dopamine, into vesicles, leading to accelerated catabolism. Loss of **lysosomal function** is also reported to impair monoamine neurotransmitter metabolism, although the exact mechanism for this is not yet known. However, neuronal mitochondrial recycling (mitophagy) is dependent on lysosomal function. Consequently, mitochondrial function may again be compromised, leading to increased neurotransmitter catabolism. It is of note that mutations affecting either mitochondrial or lysosomal metabolism are associated with parkinsonism, which is a dopamine-deficiency state.

CLINICAL TEST BOX
SERUM HORMONE CONCENTRATION CAN POINT TO CENTRAL NEUROTRANSMITTER DEFICIENCY: PROLACTIN AND DOPAMINE

Hypothalamic dopamine is an inhibitor of the release of **prolactin** from the pituitary. Consequently, a profound deficiency of central dopamine can lead to elevations in the concentration of serum prolactin. However, critical to the use of this peripheral biomarker is the adoption of appropriate age-related reference intervals because, for instance, the serum prolactin concentration declines markedly during the first year of life. Although serum prolactin may not be elevated in all cases of central dopamine deficiency, documented elevations have been noted in the inherited disorders of tetrahydrobiopterin metabolism and in tyrosine hydroxylase and aromatic amino acid decarboxylase deficiency states. Furthermore, correction of the central dopamine deficit can be accompanied by a lowering of the serum prolactin concentration, thereby enabling the monitoring of treatment efficacy.

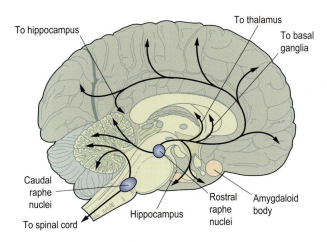

Fig. 26.11 **Serotoninergic nerves in the central nervous system (CNS).** Serotonin-containing nerves arise in the raphe nuclei, part of the reticular formation in the upper brain stem. In common with those containing norepinephrine, they are distributed widely.

in so-called vegetative behaviors such as feeding, sexual behavior, and temperature control.

Acetylcholine

Acetylcholine (ACh) is the transmitter of the parasympathetic autonomic nervous system and of the sympathetic ganglia (Fig. 26.1)

Stimulation of the parasympathetic system produces effects that are broadly opposite to those of the sympathetic system, such as slowing of the heart rate, bronchoconstriction, and

is converted to serotonin by dopa decarboxylase (also known as aromatic amino acid decarboxylase) (Fig. 26.7).

Serotoninergic neurons are concentrated in the raphe nuclei in the upper brain stem (Fig. 26.11) but project up to the cerebral cortex and down to the spinal cord. They are more active when subjects are awake than when they are asleep, and serotonin may control the degree of responsiveness of motor neurons in the spinal cord. In addition, it is implicated

Multiple receptors have been isolated for dopamine and serotonin. Not all those that have been cloned have been shown to be functional, but the possible relevance in terms of drug development is obvious. In some cases, specific manipulation of particular receptors can be exploited therapeutically.

There are five known dopamine receptors, falling into two main groups (**D$_1$-like**: D$_1$ and D$_5$; and **D$_2$-like**: D$_2$, D$_3$, and D$_4$) that differ in their signaling pathways. D$_1$ receptors increase the production of cAMP, whereas D$_2$ receptors inhibit it. Antipsychotic drugs such as phenothiazines and haloperidol tend to inhibit D$_2$-like receptors, suggesting that excessive dopamine activity may be important in causing the symptoms of schizophrenia.

The D$_2$ receptor is a major receptor in the nerves that interconnect the basal ganglia. Because it is known that destruction of these nerves causes **Parkinson's disease**, it is not surprising that antipsychotic drugs that inhibit the D$_2$ receptor tend to have the side effect of causing abnormal movements. Drugs, such as clozapine that bind preferentially to the D$_4$ receptor appear to be free of such side effects, although that particular drug also binds to several other receptors.

More than a dozen **serotonin (5-HT) receptors** have been isolated using molecular biology techniques. They have been divided into classes and subclasses on the basis of their pharmacologic properties and their structures. Most are metabotropic, although the 5-HT$_3$ receptor is ionotropic and mediates a fast signal in the enteric nervous system. The 5-HT$_{1A}$ receptor is found on many presynaptic neurons, where it acts as an autoreceptor to inhibit the release of 5-HT.

In general, increasing the brain concentration of 5-HT appears to increase **anxiety**, whereas reducing its concentration is helpful in treating the condition. The antidepressant buspirone acts as an agonist at 5-HT$_{1A}$ receptors and presumably causes a decrease in production of 5-HT. In addition to its effects on the D$_4$ dopamine receptor, clozapine binds strongly to the 5-HT$_{2A}$ receptor, and it may be that a combination of a high level of 5-HT$_{2A}$ antagonism and low D$_2$-binding activity is desirable for drugs that can be used to treat schizophrenia with the minimum frequency of side effects. The 5-HT$_3$ blocker ondansetron is an antiemetic and is extensively used to prevent vomiting during chemotherapy. Migraine can be treated with sumatriptan, a 5-HT$_{1D}$ agonist.

The central role of 5-HT in controlling brain function and the huge number of associated receptors suggest that it may be possible to tailor a large number of drugs to treat specific disorders and that pharmacologic manipulation of the function of the nervous system is probably still in its infancy.

A 60-year-old man complained of attacks of flushing, associated with an increased heart rate. He also had troublesome diarrhea and abdominal pain, and he had lost weight. The symptoms suggested a diagnosis of carcinoid syndrome caused by excessive secretion of serotonin and other metabolically active compounds from a tumor. To confirm this, a urine sample was taken for measurement of **5-hydroxyindoleacetic acid (5-HIAA),** the major metabolite of 5-HT; the concentration was found to be 120 mmol/24 h (23 mg/24 h; reference range 10–52 mmol/24 h, 3–14 mg/24 h).

Comment
The patient had carcinoid syndrome, which is caused by tumors of enterochromaffin cells, usually originating in the ileum, that have metastasized to the liver. These cells are related to the catecholamine-producing chromaffin cells in the adrenal medulla and convert tryptophan to serotonin (5-HT). Serotonin itself is believed to cause diarrhea, but other mediators, such as histamine and bradykinin, may be more important in the flushing attacks. The **urinary concentration of 5-HIAA** provides a useful diagnostic test and can be used to monitor the response of the cancer to treatment.

ACh is synthesized from choline by the enzyme choline acetyl transferase. After it is secreted into the synaptic cleft, it is largely broken down by acetylcholinesterase. The remainder is taken back up into the nerve cell by transporters similar to those for amines.

There are two main classes of ACh receptors: **nicotinic** and **muscarinic** (see Chapter 39, Fig. 39.3). Both respond to ACh but can be distinguished by their associated agonists and antagonists; they are quite different structurally and differ in their mechanisms of action.

- **Nicotinic receptors are ionotropic.** They bind nicotine and are found on ganglia and at the neuromuscular junction. When ACh or nicotine binds, a pore opens, which allows both Na$^+$ and K$^+$ to pass through. Because the action of the ligand on the channel is direct, the action is rapid.
- **Muscarinic receptors, responding to the fungal toxin muscarine, are metabotropic.** They are much more widespread in the brain than are nicotinic receptors, and are also the major receptors found on smooth muscle and glands innervated by parasympathetic nerves. **Atropine** specifically inhibits these receptors. There are several separate muscarinic receptors, differing in their tissue distribution and signaling pathways. As yet, no clear pattern has emerged as to their specific functions.

stimulation of intestinal smooth muscle. ACh also acts at neuromuscular junctions, where motor nerves contact skeletal muscle cells and cause them to contract. Apart from these roles, ACh may be involved in learning and memory, as neurons containing this transmitter also exist in the brain.

CLINICAL BOX
A WOMAN WITH OCCASIONAL DOUBLE VISION AND A CHANGE IN HER VOICE: MYASTHENIA GRAVIS

A 35-year-old woman noticed that she had difficulty in keeping her eyes open. She also had periods of double vision when her voice was indistinct and nasal, and she had difficulty swallowing. Her physician suspected myasthenia, a disease of nerve–muscle conduction. The serum titer of **antiacetylcholine receptor** antibodies was measured and found to be elevated.

Comment
The patient was suffering from myasthenia gravis. This is a disease that manifests itself as weakness of voluntary muscles and is corrected by treatment with acetylcholinesterase inhibitors. It is caused by **autoantibodies directed against the nicotinic acetylcholine receptor,** which circulate in serum. Because of these autoantibodies, transmission of nerve impulses to muscle is much less efficient than normal.

Drugs that inhibit acetylcholinesterase increase the concentration of acetylcholine in the synaptic space, which compensates for the reduced number of receptors. Improvement in nerve–muscle conduction in response to edrophonium can be used as a diagnostic test but requires several precautions; long-acting acetylcholinesterase inhibitors such as pyridostigmine can be used to treat the disease, but corticosteroids are often effective.

Clinically, ACh agonists, in common with acetylcholinesterase inhibitors, are used to treat **glaucoma,** an eye disease characterized by high intraocular pressure, by increasing the tone of the muscles of accommodation of the eye. They are also used to stimulate intestinal function after surgery. On the other hand, when acetylcholinesterase is inhibited by **organophosphate insecticides** or **nerve gases,** a toxic syndrome is caused by the resulting excess of ACh. There may be diarrhea, increased secretory activity of several glands, and bronchoconstriction. This syndrome can be antagonized by atropine, although longer-term treatment involves the use of drugs that can remove the insecticide from the enzyme, such as pralidoxime.

Nitric oxide gas

In autonomic and enteric nerves, nitric oxide (NO) is produced from arginine by the tetrahydrobiopterin-dependent nitric oxide synthases

NO has a number of attributed physiologic functions, including relaxation of both vascular and intestinal smooth muscle and the possible regulation of mitochondrial energy production. Furthermore, within the brain, NO may have a role in memory formation. However, excessive NO formation has been implicated in the neurodegenerative process associated with **Parkinson's** and **Alzheimer's** diseases. Although the exact mechanism whereby excessive NO causes neuronal death is not known, a growing body of evidence suggests that irreversible damage to the mitochondrial electron transport chain may be an important factor.

NO is not stored in vesicles but released directly into the extracellular space

Consequently, NO does not, in the strictest sense, meet all the current criteria to be labeled as a neurotransmitter. NO itself diffuses comparatively easily between cells, and it binds directly to heme groups in the enzyme guanylate cyclase, stimulating the production of cyclic guanosine monophosphate.

Other small molecules

ATP and other purine-containing molecules derived from it are now known to have transmitter functions

ATP is present in synaptic vesicles of sympathetic nerves, along with norepinephrine, and is responsible for rapid excitatory potentials in smooth muscle. Adenosine receptors are widespread in the brain and in vascular tissue. Adenosine is largely inhibitory in the CNS, and inhibition of adenosine receptors is believed to underlie the stimulatory effects of **caffeine.**

The study of histamine in nerves is complicated by the large amounts that are present in mast cells

Histamine is found in a small number of neurons, mainly in the hypothalamus, although their projections are widespread throughout the brain. It has been shown to control the release of pituitary hormones, arousal, and food intake. **Antihistamines** designed to control **allergies** caused by release from mast cells act on the H_1 receptor and tend to be sedative, suggesting that other central functions also probably exist. The **histamine receptor in the stomach** is of the H_2 class; therefore the H_2 inhibitors, such as **cimetidine** and **ranitidine,** that are used to treat peptic ulcers have no effect on allergy.

Peptides

Many peptides act as neurotransmitters

It is an open question whether all the peptides that have been described are really true neurotransmitters. Nevertheless, more than 50 small peptides have now been shown to influence neural function. All known peptide receptors are metabotropic and coupled to G-proteins (Chapter 25), so they act comparatively slowly. There are no specific uptake pathways or degradative enzymes, and the main route of disposal is simple diffusion followed by cleavage by a number of peptidases in the extracellular fluid. This allows a peptide to affect a number of neurons before it is finally degraded.

Vasoactive intestinal peptide (VIP) is one of many peptides that affect the function of the intestine through the enteric nervous system. It was originally described as a gut hormone that affected blood flow and fluid secretion, but it is now known to be an important enteric neuropeptide, inhibiting smooth muscle contraction. It also causes vasodilatation in several secretory glands, and it potentiates stimulation by ACh.

Many neuropeptides belong to a multigene family

The **opioid peptides** and opioid receptors provide a good example of a multigene family. They are the endogenous ligands for opiate analgesics such as morphine and codeine. The control of pain is complex, and opioid peptides and receptors are found both in the spinal cord and in the brain itself. There are at least three genes that code for these peptides, and each contains the sequences for several active molecules:

- **Proopiomelanocortin** contains β-endorphin, which binds to opiate μ-receptors, and also adrenocorticotropic hormone (ACTH) and the melanocyte-stimulating hormones (MSH), which are pituitary hormones (Chapter 27).
- **Proenkephalin A** contains the sequences for Met- and Leu-enkephalins, which bind to δ-receptors and are involved in pain regulation at local levels in the brain and spinal cord.
- **Prodynorphin** contains sequences for dynorphin and several other peptides, which bind to the κ-class of receptors.

Opiates affect pleasure pathways in the brain, which explains their euphoriant effects, and they also have side effects, such as respiratory depression, that limit their use. In excess, they cause contraction of the muscles of the eye, resulting in "pinpoint" pupils. It has been shown that **endorphins** are released after strenuous exercise, giving the so-called **"jogger's high."** It is hoped that increased knowledge of the specific opioid receptors and neural opioid pathways will allow the development of analgesics with fewer side effects and less likelihood of abuse.

Substance P is another example of a member of a multigene family, known as the tachykinin family. It is present in afferent fibers of sensory nerves and transmits signals in response to pain. It is also involved in so-called neurogenic inflammation stimulated by nerve impulses and is an important neurotransmitter in the intestine.

Neuropeptides can act as neuromodulators

Some peptides do act as true neurotransmitters, but they also have many other actions. They often alter the action of other transmitters, acting as neuromodulators, but have no action of their own. For instance, VIP enhances the effect of ACh on salivary gland secretion in cat submandibular glands (glands located under the jawbone) by causing vasodilatation and potentiating the cholinergic component. NPY causes inhibition of the release of norepinephrine at autonomic nerve terminals, acting at presynaptic autoreceptors, and potentiates the action of norepinephrine in certain arteries while having only weak actions itself. Opioid peptides also are capable of modulating neurotransmitter release.

SUMMARY

- Neurons communicate at synapses by means of neurotransmitters.
- A large number of compounds, whether of low molecular weight, such as the biogenic amines, or larger peptides, can act as neurotransmitters.

ACTIVE LEARNING

1. Does nitric oxide meet all the criteria to be defined as a true neurotransmitter?
2. Explain how a neurotransmitter such as serotonin can have so many diverse effects within the central nervous system.
3. Explain how neurotransmitters can be excitatory or inhibitory.
4. What neurotransmitter types are likely to become deficient in the brain of a patient with an inborn error affecting tyrosine hydroxylase, aromatic amino acid decarboxylase, and tetra-hydrobiopterin metabolism?
5. Discuss the factors that need to be considered when establishing a diagnostic method for disorders of dopamine and serotonin metabolism.
6. Explain the concept of ionotropic and metabotropic receptors.

- Neurotransmitters act on specific receptors, and there is normally more than one receptor for each neurotransmitter.
- The presence of several transmitters in the same nerves and the identification of multiple receptors suggest that there is a high degree of flexibility and complexity in the signals that can be produced in the nervous system.

FURTHER READING

Aitkenhead, H., & Heales, S. J. (2013). Establishment of paediatric age-related reference intervals for serum prolactin to aid in the diagnosis of neurometabolic conditions affecting dopamine metabolism. *Annals of Clinical Biochemistry, 50,* 156–158.

Clayton, P. T. (2006). B6-responsive disorders: A model of vitamin dependency. *Journal of Inherited Metabolic Disease, 29,* 317–326.

De la Fuente, C., Burke, D., Eaton, S., et al. (2017). Inhibition of neuronal mitochondrial complex I or lysosomal glucocerebrosidase is associated with increased dopamine and serotonin turnover. *Neurochemistry International.* doi:10.1016/J.neuroint.2017.02.013.

Kurian, M. A., Zhen, J., Meyer, E., et al. (2011). Clinical and molecular characterisation of hereditary dopamine transporter deficiency syndrome: An observational cohort and experimental study. *The Lancet. Neurology, 10,* 54–56.

Lam, A. A. J., Hyland, K., & Heales, S. J. R. (2007). Tetrahydrobiopterin availability, nitric oxide metabolism and glutathione status in the hph-1 mouse: Implications for the pathogenesis and treatment of tetrahydrobiopterin deficiency states. *Journal of Inherited Metabolic Disease, 30,* 256–262.

Ng, J., Papandreou, A., Heales, S. J., et al. (2015). Monoamine neurotransmitter disorders – clinical advances and future perspectives. *Nature Reviews. Neurology, 11*(10), 567–584.

RELEVANT WEBSITES

AADC Research Trust: http://www.aadcresearch.org

Databases of pediatric neurotransmitter disorders (PNDs): http://www.BioPKU.org

PND Association, an organization representing children and families who are affected by a pediatric neurotransmitter disease: http://www.pndassoc.org

ABBREVIATIONS

AADC	Aromatic amino acid decarboxylase
ACh	Acetylcholine
ACTH	Adrenocorticotropic hormone
ATP	Adenosine triphosphate
BH4	Tetrahydrobiopterin
cAMP	Cyclic adenosine monophosphate
CNS	Central nervous system
COMT	Catecholamine-*O*-methyltransferase
CT	Computed tomography scanning
DAT	Dopamine transporter
GABA	γ-amino butyric acid
GCS	Glycine cleavage systems
5-HIAA	5-hydroxyindoleacetic acid
5-HT	5-hydroxytryptamine, serotonin
HVA	Homovanillic acid
MAO	Monoamine oxidase
MSH	Melanocyte-stimulating hormone
NKH	Non-ketotic hyperglycinemia
NMDA	N-methyl-D-aspartate
NMR	Nuclear magnetic resonance
NO	Nitric oxide
NPY	Neuropeptide Y
PCP	Phencyclidine
PLP	Pyridox(am)ine-5'-phosphate oxidase
PNPO	Pyridoxal phosphate
VIP	Vasoactive intestinal peptide

Biochemical Endocrinology

David Church and Robert Semple

INTRODUCTION

Regulation of cellular processes is required to maintain the body's equilibrium in the presence of an ever-changing environment. The hypothalamus integrates the nervous system with the endocrine system to mediate the adaptive process. The nervous system acts rapidly through reflexes and motor actions for "fight-or-flight" responses that may require a reaction to threats within seconds. The endocrine system instigates change over seconds to days or weeks, and it may alter processes such as cellular metabolism, growth, and sexual function. Dysregulation of these mechanisms may lead to disruption of the body's homeostasis and, ultimately, to disease.

HORMONES

There are endocrine, paracrine, and autocrine hormones

Hormones are chemical messengers produced by specialized secretory cells that interact with target cell receptors, initiating a response. Classically, **endocrine hormones** (e.g., cortisol, insulin, and prolactin) are those messengers transported in the blood to a target distant from the site of secretion, whereas **paracrine hormones** (e.g., neurotransmitters and growth factors) exert their action locally at the site of secretion. Furthermore, when hormones act on the cells of their synthetic origin, they are described as **autocrine hormones** (e.g., IL-2 in activated lymphocytes). These can influence their own hormonogenesis.

Classification of hormones

Structurally, hormones may be modified amino acids, peptides, glycoproteins, or steroids

Hormones may be classified according to their structure as (1) modified amino acids, (2) peptides, (3) glycoproteins, or (4) steroids. **Modified amino acids** are chemically among the simplest hormones (Table 27.1). Examples include thyroxine, which is present in plasma mostly bound to plasma proteins (in particular, thyroid-binding globulin, TBG), and catecholamines such as epinephrine (adrenaline) and norepinephrine (noradrenaline), which circulate as free hormones. **Peptide** hormones range in size from simple tripeptides (e.g., thyrotropin-releasing hormone, TRH) to complex **glycoproteins** (e.g., luteinizing hormone, LH). Smaller peptide hormones are often synthesized from larger polypeptide precursors, or prohormones, that undergo posttranslational cleavage by proteolytic enzymes, leading to secretion of bioactive hormone from the endocrine gland. An example of this is insulin, which is produced with a connecting peptide (C-peptide) as a result of the proteolytic cleavage of proinsulin by endopeptidases (Chapter 31). Many amine-like and peptide hormones interact with cell-surface receptors to initiate a "second-messenger" response. These rely on a cascade of post-activation phosphorylation events that, in turn, alter enzyme activity and gene expression (Chapter 25). **Steroid** hormones are derived from cholesterol, are hydrophobic, and are present in plasma principally bound to proteins, with the unbound ("free") hormone bioavailable to apply its action (Chapters 14 and 40). The total hormone concentration is affected by changes in the amount of carrier protein, such as cortisol for patients taking the oral contraceptive pill. Steroid hormones interact with intracellular receptors after passive diffusion across cellular lipid bilayers. The search for new hormones continues, and there are many putative

Table 27.1 Chemical derivation of hormones

Tyrosine derivatives	Thyroxine
	Triiodothyronine
	Epinephrine (adrenaline)
	Norepinephrine (noradrenaline)
Peptides	Thyrotropin-releasing hormone
	Corticotropin-releasing hormone
	Adrenocorticotropic hormone
	Gonadotropin-releasing hormone
	Growth hormone–releasing hormone
	Ghrelin
	Growth hormone
	Somatostatin
	Insulin
	Insulin-like growth factor-1 (IGF-1)
	Prolactin
Glycoproteins	Thyroid-stimulating hormone
	Follicle-stimulating hormone
	Luteinizing hormone
	Inhibin
Hormones derived from cholesterol	Cortisol
	Testosterone
	Androstenedione
	Dehydroepiandrosterone
	Estradiol
	Progesterone
	Aldosterone

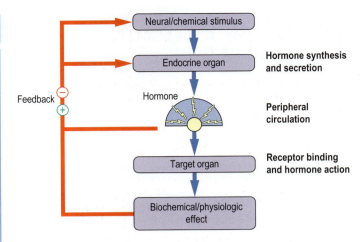

Fig. 27.1 **Basic endocrine processes.** The feedback regulation of hormone action is a classic example of self-regulation, and feedback loops can operate at different levels of the endocrine system.

Regulation of hormone production

Hormone systems are typically controlled by feedback mechanisms

Negative feedback describes inhibition of hormone production resulting from the hormone itself or as a response to the action of the hormone and is the most common form of feedback in systems of homeostasis. An example is the effect of **thyroxine (T4) and triiodothyronine (T3)** on the hypothalamus and pituitary. Negative feedback mechanisms do not exist without external influence; if they did, then hormonogenesis would remain constant. Indeed, many endocrine organs, particularly those that are under hypothalamic control, exhibit rhythmicity, which is influenced by neuronal input. **Positive feedback** describes the stimulation of hormone production resulting from the hormone itself or as a response to the action of the hormone. This is rarer, and examples include the secretion of LH in the female menstrual cycle, where the hormone concentrations quickly increase before ovulation.

Hormone degradation and clearance

The inactivation of hormones is key to their function as controllers of homeostasis

Decreased secretion is one mechanism to reduce plasma concentrations; however, there may be persistence of action until the hormone is adequately cleared from the circulation. Hormone degradation may occur in the blood, in organs such as the liver or kidneys, or in target tissue itself after receptor-mediated internalization. The clearance of hormones varies widely, from minutes (insulin), to hours (glucocorticoids), to days (T4). Clearance can also alter in disease states, such as the delayed clearance of insulin that may be observed in liver disease.

receptors for yet-undiscovered hormones that have been identified by virtue of sequence homology. These putative receptor-encoding genes are a focus of search for possible drug targets for pharmaceutical research.

Principles of hormone action

Endocrine systems exhibit core general properties: (1) release of hormones in response to a stimulus, (2) transport of the hormone to the target tissue, (3) hormone stimulation of cell receptors, (4) feedback regulation of hormone secretion (Fig. 27.1), and (5) clearance of hormones.

LABORATORY ASSESSMENT OF HORMONE ACTION

Measurement of hormones in blood and fluids (e.g., urine and saliva) forms part of the assessment of hormone action and endocrine axes

Measurement of hormones in blood and fluids (e.g., urine and saliva) forms part of the assessment of hormone action and endocrine axes, with diagnostic criteria for common endocrine disorders usually based on measurement of hormones under standardized conditions. Hormone values are continuous variables with reference limits or action limits developed with reference to clinical correlations used to guide clinicians on how to manage results. Correct clinical interpretation of endocrine results requires an appreciation of the clinical scenario in addition to the hormone measurement and related biochemical results. Individual values can have very different connotations, depending on the clinical context - critically, an endocrine result may be abnormal even if it is within provided reference limits. An example of this is parathyroid hormone (PTH), which may be within the reference limits and yet be abnormal (i.e., not suppressed) in the face of hypercalcemia. Another example is serum cortisol; interpretation requires knowledge of the timing of the sample and whether the patient is taking medication, such as the oral contraceptive pill or exogenous glucocorticoids. Laboratory investigation can identify patients not only with clinical disease but also individuals whose results are consistent with "subclinical" disorders that may require monitoring or treatment in their own right.

Most commonly, it is the **hormone** of interest that will be measured in blood as part of the endocrine assessment. However, it may be appropriate either technically (e.g., due to issues with measurement or analyte stability) or physiologically (e.g., due to rapid fluctuations in levels where a single time-point measurement may be misleading) to measure **upstream trophic hormones** (e.g., 25-hydroxy vitamin D) or **downstream metabolites** (e.g., urine metanephrines). Measurement of more than one hormone may be required to assess the hormone axis completely, to discriminate autonomous hormone hypersecretion from secondary hormone elevation, or to distinguish hormone insufficiency from appropriate secretory suppression.

Hormone day profiles, stimulation tests, and suppression tests

Isolated measurements of hormones that exhibit circadian rhythm, such as cortisol and growth hormone are of limited value

Isolated measurements of hormones that exhibit circadian rhythm are of limited value because, in addition to the inter-individual variation, intra-individual variation complicates interpretation of single values. Endocrinologists can use, for example, comparisons of day and night cortisol concentrations to assess diurnal variation, and in individuals with adrenal insufficiency, a cortisol day profile may be employed to help confirm adequate hydrocortisone replacement. Hormone **stimulation** and **suppression** tests (Table 27.2) are used to identify hypo- and hypersecretion of hormones, respectively. Here, hormones are measured in the steady state and again after administration of an appropriate pharmacologic or physiologic challenge. Stimulating the endocrine gland aims to elicit a high secretory response yielding information about the functional reserve of the gland in question, and clinical action limits are developed by correlation of biochemical testing results with

Table 27.2 Examples of commonly used dynamic function tests

Endocrine axis	Stimulus	Measurement	Rationale/use
Hypothalamo–pituitary–adrenal cortex	Synthetic adrenocorticotropic hormone	Cortisol	Tests functional integrity of adrenal gland, which is dependent on trophic actions of adrenocorticotropic hormone
Hypothalamo–pituitary–adrenal cortex	Insulin-induced hypoglycemia	Cortisol	Severe hypoglycemia mimics stress to test the hypothalamus robustly
Hypothalamo–pituitary–thyroid	Thyroid releasing hormone (TRH)	Thyroid-stimulating hormone	The pattern of thyroid-stimulating hormone release after TRH stimulation can give useful information in the diagnosis of central hypothyroidism
Hypothalamo–pituitary–growth hormone	Insulin-induced hypoglycemia	Growth hormone	To test for growth hormone deficiency; baseline pulsatility of growth hormone is overcome by applying a strong stimulus to its release
Hypothalamo–pituitary–growth hormone	Oral glucose load	Growth hormone	Failure of suppression of growth hormone by glucose is used in the diagnosis of acromegaly

clinical outcomes. Conversely, using an agent known to suppress secretion of a hormone allows identification of autonomous secretion (such as by an adenoma) that demonstrates normal physiologic (negative) feedback. Metabolic stimulations of endocrine glands used in clinical practice include oral glucose tolerance testing to assess pancreatic beta cell insulin secretion and insulin-induced hypoglycemia to assess the pituitary-adrenal axis.

Endocrine laboratory

In the clinical laboratory, hormone levels in blood and urine are usually measured using immunoassay or mass spectrometry (MS)

Immunoassay utilizes antibodies to bind the hormone of interest and generate a signal that is then compared with calibrators of known hormone value to determine the hormone concentration in the sample. MS is useful for specific measurement of certain hormones (e.g., testosterone) and relies on the characteristic mass-to-charge ratio of ionized compounds (and their fragments) for identification and measurement. Accurate hormone measurement depends on the specificity of an assay to measure the hormone of interest and discriminate it from other compounds. To limit deterioration in sample quality before analysis, specific sample preparation (e.g., addition of preservative to plasma) and/or collection requirements (e.g., urgent centrifugation) may be necessary for endocrine tests.

CAUSES OF ENDOCRINE DISEASE

Autoimmunity and neoplasia

Loss of functioning endocrine tissue may be the result of destruction due to autoimmunity or neoplasia

Endocrine autoimmunity may be organ specific or, as in autoimmune polyendocrine syndromes, may affect clusters of glands. Serum endocrine organ-specific antibodies can be detected in autoimmune endocrinopathy and may be used to predict future disease. Typically, autoimmunity is associated with hypofunction of the gland; however, in Graves' disease, hyperthyroidism occurs in the presence of antibodies that stimulate the thyroid-stimulating hormone (TSH) receptor.

Endocrine neoplastic disease may be benign or malignant

Benign adenomas may be found incidentally on imaging (often called "incidentalomas"); however, they may also cause disease through autonomous hypersecretion of hormones and may damage neighboring endocrine tissues through mass effects, especially in enclosed anatomical spaces such as the pituitary fossa. Malignancies in endocrine glands may be primary or due to metastases.

Exogenous hormone administration

Hormone therapy may result in clinical problems attributable to excess hormone administration, loss of physiologic pulsatility, or loss of diurnal rhythm

When glucocorticoid therapy is used for antiinflammatory or immunosuppressant purposes, a consequence of clinical improvement in the principal medical complaint (e.g., autoimmune or inflammatory disease) may commonly be Cushing syndrome, discussed in more detail later in the chapter. Occult self-administration of exogenous hormones may also mimic endogenous hypersecretion. Examples include the surreptitious use of excess prescribed thyroxine to aid weight loss, which can have an adverse effect on cardiac function and bone density, or recreational use of anabolic steroids (e.g., testosterone) to increase muscle mass or enhance athletic performance.

THE HYPOTHALAMUS AND THE PITUITARY GLAND

Structure

The **hypothalamus** occupies the forebrain adjacent to the third ventricle and is connected to the pituitary gland by the hypophyseal stalk (Fig. 27.2).

The pituitary is a pea-sized gland encased in a bony cavity of the skull called the *sella turcica*. It is divided into two embryologically and physiologically distinct components, the **anterior pituitary** (adenohypophysis) and the **posterior**

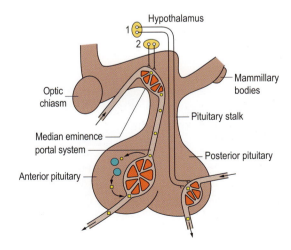

Fig. 27.2 **Basic outline of anatomical links between the hypothalamus and pituitary.** Hormones of the posterior pituitary are synthesized and packaged in the supraoptic and paraventricular nuclei of the hypothalamus (1), transported along axons, and stored in the posterior pituitary before release into the circulation. The anterior pituitary hormones are synthesized in the arcuate and various other hypothalamic nuclei (2) and transported to the median eminence; from there, the hormones travel to the anterior pituitary via a portal venous system.

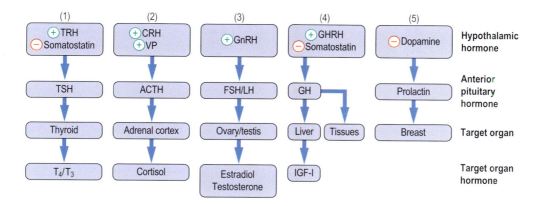

Fig. 27.3 **Hypothalamo–anterior–pituitary regulatory target organ axes.** The hypothalamo–anterior–pituitary regulatory system comprises five parallel endocrine axes, regulating the biosynthesis and release of the following: (1) thyroid hormone, (2) glucocorticoids, (3) sex steroids, (4) growth hormone, and (5) prolactin. T4, thyroxine; T3, triiodothyronine; GNRH, growth hormone–releasing hormone; GnRH, gonadotrophin-releasing hormone; IGF-1, insulin-like growth factor 1; ACTH, adrenocorticotrophic hormone; FSH, follicle-stimulating hormone; LH, luteinizing hormone; TSH, thyrotropin-releasing hormone; CRH, corticotrophin-releasing hormone; TSH, thyroid-stimulating hormone; VP, vasopressin; (+) indicates stimulatory action; (–) indicates inhibitory action.

pituitary (neurohypophysis). The anterior pituitary originates embryologically from oral cavity ectoderm (Rathke's pouch) and comprises secretory glandular tissue. It is a target organ for hypothalamic hormones and receives blood via hypophyseal portal vessels that link it with the hypothalamus. The posterior pituitary, which consists largely of neurons, develops embryologically from the brain and is connected to the hypothalamus. Cell bodies of specialized neurons are present in the paraventricular and supraoptic nuclei of the hypothalamus, and these cell bodies synthesize and package hormones that are transported along axons to the posterior pituitary, where they are released into the blood via their terminals.

Hypothalamic regulation of the pituitary

Both the anterior and posterior pituitary are under the influence of the hypothalamus

The hypothalamus receives synaptic inputs from different higher centers of the brain and receives peripheral signals across the blood–brain barrier.

Both the anterior and posterior pituitary are under the influence of the hypothalamus. The hypothalamus acts to orchestrate many endocrine and neural processes. The hypothalamic-pituitary networks controlling downstream target organs are described individually as **axes**.

Anterior pituitary

The hypothalamus secretes hormones that may stimulate or inhibit the release of hormones from the anterior pituitary

The hypothalamus secretes hormones that are transported in the hypophyseal portal blood that may stimulate or inhibit

Table 27.3 Clinical conditions resulting from pituitary hormone disorders

Hormone	Excess	Deficiency
Adrenocorticotropic hormone	Cushing disease	Secondary hypoadrenalism
Thyroid-stimulating hormone	Secondary hyperthyroidism	Secondary hypothyroidism
Follicle-stimulating hormone / luteinizing hormone	Precocious puberty	Secondary hypogonadism
Growth hormone	Gigantism/acromegaly	Short stature in children
Prolactin	Galactorrhea/impotence (men), infertility (women)	None

the release of hormones from the anterior pituitary and are termed *releasing* or *inhibiting* hormones, respectively. Pituitary hormones and the downstream target organ products can regulate the hypothalamus through negative feedback inhibition (Fig. 27.3).

Six well-described peptide hormones are secreted from the anterior pituitary. These are adrenocorticotropic hormone (ACTH), thyroid-stimulating hormone (TSH), follicle-stimulating hormone (FSH), LH, prolactin, and growth hormone (GH). ACTH, TSH, and FSH/LH are considered **"trophic"** hormones for target endocrine organs (i.e., adrenals, thyroid, and gonads, respectively), and they augment the amount and biological half-life of the downstream hormones produced. GH is a trophic hormone (stimulating hepatic production of insulin-like growth factor-1 [IGF-1]) that also has direct metabolic effects. Prolactin is not a trophic hormone. Excess or deficiency of pituitary hormone(s) results in endocrine disease (Table 27.3).

Posterior pituitary

Oxytocin *and* vasopressin *are two peptide hormones synthesized in the cell bodies of the hypothalamic neurons that are subsequently secreted by the posterior pituitary*

Oxytocin stimulates smooth muscle contraction in the uterus and breast, functioning in childbirth and breastfeeding, respectively. It is released in response to stimulation of mechanoreceptors in the breast with suckling. Synthetic oxytocin may be used to induce labor or to control uterine bleeding after childbirth. Vasopressin (VP), also known as antidiuretic hormone (ADH), is critical to homeostatic control of extracellular fluid tonicity, and its function is described in detail in Chapter 35. The vasopressor response is related to how its name was derived, although it is less significant physiologically. Human VP is referred to as arginine vasopressin (AVP) due to the presence of the amino acid arginine at position 8 of the nonapeptide.

THYROID FUNCTION: THE HYPOTHALAMIC–PITUITARY–THYROID AXIS

Thyrotropin-releasing hormone (TRH)

TRH *(also known as thyreoliberin), a tripeptide synthesized in the peptidergic hypothalamic nuclei and transported to the anterior pituitary via the portal circulation, stimulates TSH synthesis and secretion.*

Secretion is stimulated by TRH binding to G protein–coupled receptors on the pituitary thyrotrope cell membrane that are linked to phospholipase C (Chapter 25). There is an increase in intracellular inositol triphosphate (IP_3) that leads to the release of intracellular calcium, which in turn results in secretion of TSH. The number of TRH receptors on the thyrotropes is regulated by the concentration of both TRH itself and of the thyroid hormones.

Thyroid-stimulating hormone (TSH)

TSH *is a glycoprotein heterodimer consisting of an α- and β-subunit and is about 15% carbohydrate by weight*

The α-subunit has an identical structure to other glycoprotein hormones (LH, FSH, human chorionic gonadotropin [hCG]); however, the β-subunit is specific to TSH. TSH production is regulated by the stimulatory action of TRH and the inhibition of T4 and T3. The secretion of TSH is both pulsatile and circadian, and it has a plasma half-life of approximately 1 h. The receptor for TSH is part of the rhodopsin-like G protein–coupled receptor family and is present on the basolateral membrane of follicular cells of the thyroid. TSH binds to an extracellular domain with high affinity and acts via a G protein. Actions of TSH include the stimulation of uptake of iodide into thyroid follicular epithelium, thyroglobulin (Tg) synthesis and secretion, iodination of Tg tyrosine residues, and T4 and T3 secretion into the circulation.

Thyroxine (T4) and triiodothyronine (T3)

The thyroid consists of spherical follicles comprising a single layer of cuboidal epithelial cells surrounding the follicle lumen, which are filled with homogeneous colloid composed of proteins such as Tg, a tyrosine-rich colloidal-binding glycoprotein. Tg is a dimeric molecule containing 115–123 tyrosine residues that is produced in the thyroid cells and secreted into colloid. Tg is glycosylated and then secreted into the follicular lumen, where the tyrosine residues are iodinated.

Iodide ions are actively pumped against a gradient into the follicular epithelium and then pass into thyroid follicles, where they are oxidized to iodine molecules. Oxidation of iodide is catalyzed by the enzyme thyroid peroxidase (TPO) on the inner aspect of the thyrocyte. Iodine combines with tyrosine attached to Tg, and monoiodotyrosine (MIT) and diiodotyrosine (DIT) are produced. The follicular cells of the thyroid glands are the secretory units for the bioactive hormones, thyroxine (DIT + DIT), also known as T4, and, in lesser amounts, triiodothyronine (MIT + DIT), also known as T3, which are stored in colloid until released into the bloodstream (Fig. 27.4). Synthesized thyroid hormones are secreted into the capillary network that surrounds the thyroid follicles. The thyroid may also convert some T4 by deiodination to a product that is generally considered biologically inactive, known as "reverse T3" (rT3). The thyroid also secretes small amounts of reverse T3 (rT3) and the T4/T3 precursors monoiodotyrosine (MIT) and diiodotyrosine (DIT). Iodine recovered by the deiodination of MIT and DIT is reused by the thyroid gland for additional hormone synthesis.

T4 accounts for 80%–95% of thyroid hormones produced by the thyroid gland. Most T3 (>80%) is formed by the 5′ deiodination of T4 by deiodinases (Fig. 27.5) present in peripheral tissues such the liver, kidneys, and skeletal muscle and the central nervous system rather than by direct thyroid secretion. T3 has about five times the potency of T4; therefore T4 is generally considered as a prohormone. There is a large plasma pool of T4, which has a slow turnover in contrast to T3, which is mainly intracellular and has a faster turnover rate. rT3 is produced by 3′ deiodination of T4 (Fig. 27.5) and is a mechanism by which T3 production from T4 can be controlled.

Although free hormones are secreted by the thyroid, T4 and T3 are relatively lipophilic and mainly bound to protein in plasma, with more than 99% of both hormones attached to TBG and albumin (the latter having highest T4 binding capacity) and transthyretin. Although measured total T4 ("free" plus bound) concentrations are approximately 40 times those

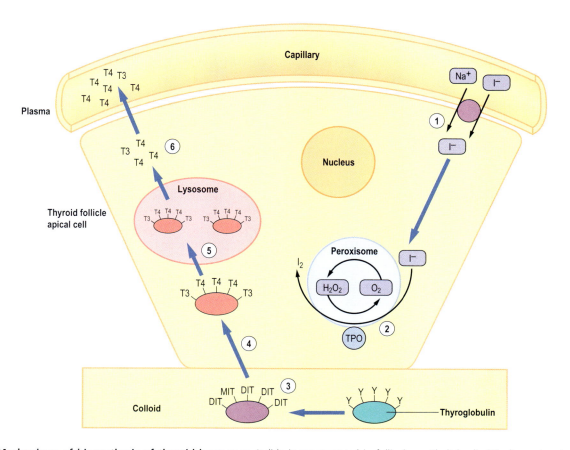

Fig. 27.4 **Mechanisms of biosynthesis of thyroid hormones.** Iodide is concentrated in follicular epithelial cells (1) after entry via a sodium iodide symporter, before (2) oxidation by thyroid peroxidase (TPO) in the peroxisome to iodine. At the plasma membrane adjacent to the follicular lumen (3), conversion of tyrosyl (Y) residues on the surface of the thyroid glycoprotein thyroglobulin to either monoiodotyrosine (MIT) or diiodotyrosine (DIT) occurs. Coupling of iodinated tyrosine residues to form either T4 (DIT+DIT) or T3 (MIT+DIT) then occurs. Thyroglobulin is exocytosed (4) and hydrolyzed (5) in lysosomes to release free T4 and free T3. The thyroid hormones are transported to the plasma membrane and released into the bloodstream.

Fig. 27.5 **Structures of the thyroid hormones thyroxine (T4), triiodothyronine (T3), and reverse T3 (rT3).**

of T3, due to the difference in the protein binding, the free T4 (fT4) concentration is only 4 times that of free T3 (fT3). Conversion of T4 to T3 is conserved over a wide range of T4 concentrations. Circulating total thyroid hormone levels depend on plasma binding protein concentrations, and it is the free hormones (fT4; fT3) that are bioactive and measured in routine clinical practice. The principal clearance mechanisms of thyroid hormones are tissue metabolism and hepatic conjugation, with some additional excretion in the urine, although this is restricted by protein binding. Conjugated thyroid hormones (with sulfate and glucuronic acid) are excreted in the bile, passing into the intestine, where some of the iodine is reabsorbed by enterohepatic circulation.

Actions of thyroid hormones

The physiologic effects of thyroid hormones can be divided into the metabolic and the developmental

Metabolic effects of thyroid hormones

Thyroid hormones increase metabolic rate, with increased oxygen consumption and heat production

There is an increase in the metabolism of carbohydrates, free fatty acids, and protein. Heart rate and cardiac output are increased, and gastrointestinal motility is stimulated. Bile acid formation is increased, leading to an increase in fecal excretion of cholesterol derivatives, thereby decreasing circulating cholesterol concentrations.

Developmental effects of thyroid hormones

The thyroid hormones have a critical effect on normal skeletal and central nervous system development

Little T4 or T3 transfers to the fetal circulation from the maternal circulation, and the functional fetal thyroid gland (from around 10 weeks' gestation) is required for normal growth and development.

Mechanism of action of thyroid hormones

Thyroid hormones exert their effects via nuclear receptors.

Two receptor isoforms are encoded by the thyroid hormone receptor alpha (*THRA)* gene and undergo alternative splicing: *TRα1* is mainly expressed in bone, the heart, skeletal muscle, the central nervous system, and the gastrointestinal tract, whereas *TRα2* (non-T3-binding) is expressed in tissues such as the testis and brain. A further two receptor isoforms that differ in their amino-terminal region are encoded by the thyroid hormone receptor beta (*THRB*) gene: *TRβ1* is mainly expressed in kidney, liver, and thyroid, and *TRβ2* is involved in auditory and visual development. Thyroid receptors bind to short, repeated sequences of DNA known as thyroid-response elements. Binding to the receptor leads to alteration of transcription of specific thyroid-responsive genes and protein synthesis.

Disorders of thyroid function

Hyperthyroidism

Hyperthyroidism, *also described as an "overactive thyroid," is the excessive production and secretion of thyroid hormones and is caused by a number of conditions (Table 27.4)*

The term "thyrotoxicosis" is used to describe the clinical hypermetabolic state due to excess thyroid hormone activity. The most common cause of hyperthyroidism is **Graves' disease,** an autoimmune disorder involving the production of TSH-stimulating IgG antibodies. The patient may present with a diffusely enlarged thyroid **(goiter)** and symptoms of hyperthyroidism; serum anti-TSH receptor antibodies can also be measured by the clinical laboratory. Thyrotoxicosis may also be caused by thyroid nodules **("toxic multinodular goiter")** or by solitary toxic thyroid nodules that do not respond

Table 27.4 Hyperthyroidism
Common causes
Graves' disease - autoimmune disease with stimulatory thyroid-stimulating hormone–receptor antibodies and diffuse thyroid hyperplasia   Toxic multinodular goiter - multiple thyroid nodules secreting thyroid hormones (Plummer disease)   Solitary toxic adenoma - single thyroid nodule autonomously producing thyroid hormones
Less common causes
Subacute (de Quervain) thyroiditis - inflammatory thyroiditis leading to release of thyroid hormones   Drugs - excess exogenous thyroid hormone administration; amiodarone (may also produce hypothyroidism)   Ectopic thyroid tissue (e.g., functional thyroid cancer metastases; struma ovarii)
Symptoms
Weight loss (with normal/increased appetite)   Palpitations   Anxiety   Heat intolerance   Sweating/greasy skin   Diarrhea   Oligomenorrhea
Signs
Tachycardia/atrial fibrillation   Tremor   Eyelid lag and/or retraction   Goiter/nodule/nodules (cause-dependent)

to the usual negative feedback mechanisms and secrete thyroid hormones autonomously. In primary hyperthyroidism, serum TSH is below the reference limit, and fT4, fT3, or both are raised. Treatment of hyperthyroidism is based on antithyroid drugs, radioiodine ablation, and surgical resection or combinations of these.

CLINICAL BOX
HYPERTHYROIDISM AND TSH RECEPTOR–STIMULATING ANTIBODIES

A 31-year-old woman presented with nervousness, a "racing heartbeat," chronic tiredness, and itchiness. Over recent months, her dress size had reduced, but she had not deliberately lost weight. On examination, she had a fine symmetrical tremor of her outstretched hands, and her palms were clammy. She had tachycardia (heart rate of 114/min and regular), and there were marks on her legs consistent with her scratching. There was a mild diffuse enlargement of the thyroid (goiter) and a bruit, or audible murmur, over the gland.

Serum TSH was suppressed (<0.05 mU/L; reference range 0.35–4.5 mU/L), and fT4 was raised (52 pmol/L [4.0 ng/dL]; reference range 9–21 pmol/L [0.7–1.6 ng/dL]), as was fT3 at 18 pmol/L (1168 pg/dL; reference range 2.6–6.5 pmol/L [162–422 pg/dL]). Serum anti-TSH-receptor antibodies were detected.

Comment
Graves' disease is autoimmune thyroid disease characterized by hyperthyroidism due to direct stimulation of the thyroid epithelial cells by TSH receptor–stimulating antibodies. Additional clinical features can include diffuse thyroid enlargement and systemic features such as ophthalmopathy and dermopathy. Clinicians utilize nuclear medicine imaging (where thyroid update of a radionucleotide is studied, e.g., technetium-99m or iodine 123) and measurement of serum anti-TSH receptor antibodies. Assays that are designed to detect anti-TSH receptor antibodies by their ability to compete for binding of TSH receptor with a TSH ligand (e.g., TSH or monoclonal anti-TSHR antibody) will be unable to discriminate stimulating from nonstimulating (neutral or inhibiting) antibodies. Advances have been made to detect antibodies that bind epitopes on the N-terminal section of the human TSH receptor. It is these antibodies that cause stimulation rather than those antibodies that bind the C-terminal residues that block receptor activity. Until recently, assays specific to stimulating TSH receptor antibodies could only be measured by bioassays; however, there are new automated immunoassays becoming available to clinical laboratories with specificity for the stimulating antibodies, which may be better at discriminating Graves' from other forms of hyperthyroidism.

Hypothyroidism

Hypothyroidism, *also described as an "underactive thyroid," is thyroid hormone deficiency*

Clinical features range from mild and nonspecific to life-threatening (Table 27.5). Hypothyroidism may be identified

Table 27.5 Hypothyroidism

Common causes

Atrophic hypothyroidism - diffuse lymphocytic infiltrate
Hashimoto thyroiditis - chronic autoimmune thyroiditis with lymphocytic/plasma cell infiltrate

Less common causes

Iodine deficiency (common worldwide)
Iatrogenic - post-surgery, anti-thyroid agents (e.g., carbimazole, radioactive iodine treatment), other drugs (e.g., amiodarone, lithium)
Hypopituitarism (rare) - pituitary tumors, postpartum ischemic necrosis (Sheehan syndrome)

Symptoms

Tiredness, lethargy
Intolerance to cold
Weight gain
Constipation
Menorrhagia
Poor cognition
Dry skin and hair

Signs

Bradycardia
Nonpitting edema
Slow relaxation of tendon reflexes
Peripheral neuropathy

after laboratory investigation for secondary causes of, for example, infertility or hypercholesterolemia. **Myxedema** is a term used for severe hypothyroidism and the accumulation of mucopolysaccharides in the skin and subcutaneous tissues. Myxedema coma can present after chronic untreated severe hypothyroidism as decreased mental acuity, hypothermia, bradycardia, and unconsciousness. **Iodine deficiency** is the most common cause of goitrous hypothyroidism worldwide, and the resultant increase in TSH has a trophic effect to cause the enlargement of the thyroid. Iodine deficiency can result in restricted growth in utero and during childhood. Iodine-containing drugs (e.g., amiodarone) can lead to iodine overload, resulting in inhibition of thyroid hormone production (Wolff–Chaikoff effect). In contrast to iodine deficiency, primary atrophic hypothyroidism is nongoitrous because there is tissue atrophy despite high TSH concentrations.

Primary hypothyroidism, where TSH is above and fT4 concentrations below their respective reference limits, is treated with thyroid hormone replacement, usually with daily oral levothyroxine (T4). Although fT4 concentrations respond quickly to T4 replacement, TSH levels can take 6 or more weeks to reach a new steady state. Primary hypothyroidism is more common in individuals with autoimmune diseases (e.g., type 1 diabetes; celiac disease) and may occur as part of multiple autoimmune endocrinopathies (autoimmune polyendocrine syndromes). **Secondary hypothyroidism** is rare; however, it may occur in patients with pituitary pathology. Secondary hypothyroidism, demonstrated biochemically, is a TSH below or at the lower end of the reference limit and a disproportionately low fT4; it is rare and mainly a consequence of pituitary tumors.

Congenital hypothyroidism is rare and may occur as the result of complete absence of thyroid tissue, of disorders of thyroid hormone synthesis, or as a result of congenital TSH deficiency. TSH resistance in humans due to genetic defects in both $TR\alpha$ and $TR\beta$ has been identified, although resistance to thyroid hormones due to a $TR\beta$ mutation (RTHβ) is far more common. RTHβ is characterized by elevated serum thyroid hormone levels in the absence of TSH suppression, and presentations range from asymptomatic to thyrotoxicosis. Individuals with resistance to thyroid hormones due to a TRβ mutation (RTHβ) may have a normal or slightly raised TSH and low/low-normal fT4 (and decreased fT4/fT3 ratio), and most usually have no abnormal characteristics at birth but may later go on to display features of hypothyroidism. Neonatal screening programs for primary hypothyroidism exist in much of the developing world; however, TSH may be measured in isolation; thus secondary hypothyroidism may not be identified.

Laboratory investigations of thyroid function

Serum TSH is typically used as a first-line screen for thyroid disease; an fT4 may also be requested if there is a strong clinical suspicion of thyroid disease or if there is an indication to consider pituitary disease

If the TSH concentration is low or high, then fT4 should be measured, and the assay of fT4 may be automatically performed by the clinical laboratory after the detection of abnormal TSH concentrations. Some basic interpretations of thyroid function test results are given in (Table 27.6).

Primary thyroid disease describes an abnormality in thyroid hormone production due to pathology in the thyroid itself. A raised fT4 and fT3 with a TSH below the reference limit (suppressed) is consistent with primary hyperthyroidism. In the context of a low TSH and an fT4 within the reference limit (in a patient without known thyroid disease), an fT3 measurement

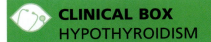

CLINICAL BOX
HYPOTHYROIDISM

A 64-year-old woman presented with extreme tiredness and becoming mentally less alert, resulting in her finding it difficult to do her job as a librarian. She had been suffering intolerance to cold, wearing extra clothing compared with her work colleagues. On further questioning, she had suffered constipation for some months. Her sister had an "underactive thyroid." On examination, she was overweight and had dry skin, a puffy face, a slow heart rate (54 beats/min and regular); her thyroid gland was not palpable.

TSH was raised (80 mU/L; reference range 0.35–4.5 mU/L), and fT4 was low (5 pmol/L; reference range 9–21 pmol/L [0.7–1.6 ng/dL]).

Comment

The onset of hypothyroidism can be insidious, and the clinical features are fairly nonspecific. The elevated TSH with low fT4 is consistent with a primary thyroid disorder. Follow-up blood tests were positive for antithyroid peroxidase antibodies. The diagnosis of lymphocytic thyroiditis (Hashimoto thyroiditis) was made.

ADVANCED CONCEPT BOX
IGSF1 AND CENTRAL HYPOTHYROIDISM

Immunoglobulin superfamily member 1 (*IGSF1*) is a highly polymorphic gene located on the X chromosome and encodes a membrane glycoprotein. Mutations in *IGSF1* have been recently identified as a cause of secondary ("central") hypothyroidism. Affected males present with secondary hypothyroidism, either in isolation, or in combination with hypoprolactinemia and adult macroorchidism. Although a role for *IGSF1* in hypothalamic and pituitary physiology is supported by studies of cellular expression and sequelae of *IGSF1* deficiency, its function is not completely understood. Higher concentrations of FSH compared with LH in serum may suggest that the macroorchidism may be due to excess hypothalamic TRH (which increases FSH and not LH in a GnRH-independent fashion [Schoenmakers et al., 2015]).

Table 27.6 Thyroid function test interpretation

		Plasma free thyroxine (fT4)		
		Above reference range	**Within reference range**	**Below reference range**
Plasma thyroid-stimulating hormone (TSH)	**Above reference limit**	Secondary hyperthyroidism ("TSH-oma") - very rare	Subclinical/compensated hypothyroidism	Primary hypothyroidism; sick euthyroid syndrome (recovery phase)
	Within reference limit	Thyroid hormone resistance	Euthyroidism	Sick euthyroid syndrome; secondary hypothyroidism (pituitary failure)
	Below reference limit	Primary hyperthyroidism	Sick euthyroid syndrome; "T3-toxicosis" (raised free triiodothyronine [fT3])	Secondary hypothyroidism (pituitary failure)

is indicated to identify "T3 toxicosis." In this situation, serum fT3 concentration is raised, leading to suppression of TSH, and may occur in some patients with a solitary toxic adenoma, multiple thyroid nodules, or in early Graves' disease.

A low fT4 with a raised TSH is consistent with primary hypothyroidism. It is noteworthy that T4-to-T3 conversion may be preserved in hypothyroidism, and thus fT3 concentrations may be within reference limits. In secondary hypothyroidism, fT4 concentrations are low; however, TSH levels may be low or within the reference range (TSH is insufficient to raise fT4).

Subclinical hyper- and hypothyroidism broadly describe a low or high TSH concentration, respectively, in the context of fT4 and fT3 within reference limits. It is noteworthy that some patients may experience thyroid symptoms with thyroid hormones at the extremes of, but within, reference limits, and a decision to treat should consider the clinical presentation. Clinical states of **euthyroid hypothyroxinemia** may occur in nonthyroidal illness and is termed "sick euthyroid syndrome." Decreased peripheral conversion of T4 to T3 (with a corresponding increase in rT3) may occur in early nonthyroidal illness, and TSH may decrease. During recovery from severe illness, TSH may rise. It is therefore advisable to interpret thyroid function tests with caution during acute or severe illness and to avoid testing unless clinically indicated.

THE HYPOTHALAMIC–PITUITARY–ADRENAL AXIS

Corticotropin-releasing hormone (CRH)

Corticotropin-releasing hormone (CRH, corticoliberin) is a 41–amino acid peptide synthesized by the hypothalamic paraventricular nuclei. It is secreted into the hypophyseal portal blood and acts via G protein–coupled receptors on pituitary corticotrope cells. Activation of an adenosine 3′,5′-cyclic monophosphate (cAMP) messenger system leads to stimulation of ACTH synthesis and secretion. The release of CRH is both episodic and circadian, and it promotes a circadian rhythm of ACTH production. CRH and ACTH are under the influence of negative feedback from circulating cortisol.

Adrenocorticotropic hormone (ACTH)

ACTH (also termed corticotropin) is a 39–amino acid polypeptide that is synthesized from a 241–amino acid precursor molecule, pro-opiomelanocortin (POMC)

The cleavage of POMC also gives rise to other hormones, including melanocyte stimulating hormone (MSH) and endorphin (see also Chapter 32). ACTH is released from the anterior pituitary gland, and secretion is pulsatile and exhibits diurnal rhythm. A trough serum concentration is reached at midnight, with a rapid increase in concentration at approximately 3 a.m., to reach a peak at around 8 a.m. with a subsequent decline thereafter. ACTH secretion is also increased by stress, either psychologic or physical (e.g., exercise, illness, trauma, hypoglycemia). Its secretion is inhibited by negative feedback from cortisol. Therefore lack of cortisol production, such as in adrenal failure or after adrenalectomy, leads to an increase in plasma ACTH concentrations. Conversely, cortisol excess, either via endogenous overproduction or exogenous administration, leads to a reduction in plasma ACTH. Negative feedback by cortisol can act at both the hypothalamic and pituitary level, with fast feedback or slow feedback. The former alters hypothalamic CRH release, and the latter follows decreased synthesis of CRH plus suppression of POMC gene transcription, resulting in decreased ACTH synthesis.

ACTH circulates unbound in plasma, and its half-life is approximately 10 min

ACTH acts on the adrenal cortex via interaction with cell surface G protein–coupled receptors, leading to stimulation of cAMP production. The resultant acute rise in adrenal cortical synthesis of cortisol happens within 3 min, largely due to stimulation of cholesterol esterase in adrenal cells, resulting in hydrolysis of cholesterol esters to free fatty acids and cholesterol. Longer-term effects of ACTH (hours to days) include increased transcription of genes encoding steroidogenic enzymes. Low ACTH, such as in suppression due to exogenous glucocorticoids, causes atrophy of the adrenal cortex, and in cases of significantly prolonged suppression, it can take days to weeks to recover a functional hypothalamic–pituitary–adrenal axis.

Anatomy and biochemistry of the adrenal gland

The adrenal glands are paired bodies, one situated at the upper pole of each kidney. The glands consist of an outer cortex surrounding the central medulla, each region being embryologically and functionally distinct.

The cortex consists of three zones that are distinguishable histologically: the zona reticularis (adjacent to the adrenal medulla), the zona fasciculata, and the zona glomerulosa (outer layer; Fig. 27.6). Conversion of cholesterol to pregnenolone is the initial rate-limiting step in steroidogenesis and occurs in the mitochondria (Chapter 14). Pregnenolone is the steroid precursor from which adrenal androgens (zona reticularis), glucocorticoids (zone fasciculata), and mineralocorticoids (zona glomerulosa) are synthesized. A simplified scheme of steroidogenesis is shown in (Fig. 27.7). The zona glomerulosa is under the control of the renin–angiotensin system; however, the zona fasciculata and zona reticularis are under the influence of ACTH. This is an important consideration when investigating adrenal disease, which can affect both glucocorticoid and mineralocorticoid synthesis, and pituitary disease that results typically only in glucocorticoid deficiency.

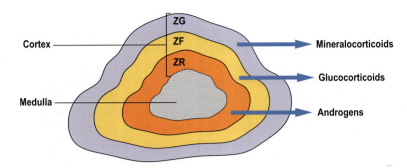

Fig. 27.6 **Adrenal structure.** Zones of the adrenal cortex are shown with their respective hormones indicated. The central region of the adrenal, the adrenal medulla, is regulated by preganglionic sympathetic nerves, the activity of which stimulates adrenal secretion of catecholamines (epinephrine, norepinephrine; see Chapter 26). ZG, zona glomerulosa; ZF, zona fasciculata; ZR, zona reticularis.

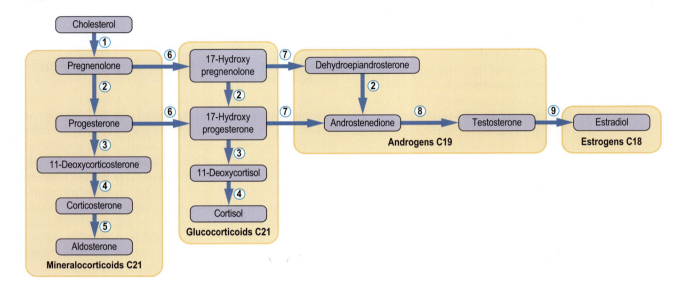

Fig. 27.7 **Summary of steroid hormone biosynthesis.** (1) cholesterol 20,22-desmolase; (2) 3β-hydroxysteroid dehydrogenase/Δα4,5 isomerase; (3) 21β-hydroxylase; (4) 11β-hydroxylase; (5) aldosterone synthase; (6) 17α-hydroxylase; (7) 17,20-lyase/desmolase; (8) 17β-hydroxysteroid dehydrogenase; (9) aromatase (Chapter 14).

Biosynthesis of cortisol

Cortisol, a steroid hormone and the major glucocorticoid synthesized and secreted by the human adrenal cortex, is synthesized and released as required

The principal physiologic stimulus for cortisol synthesis and secretion is ACTH. Cortisol secretion has a diurnal rhythm that is reflected in plasma concentrations; the level at 4 p.m. through midnight is some 75% or less than the 8 a.m. level. Random blood sample collections for cortisol measurement can be a challenge to interpret and can have limited value in the diagnosis of hyper-and hyposecretion. Approximately 95% of plasma cortisol is bound to protein, mainly cortisol-binding globulin (CBG, also known as transcortin). The remaining cortisol is unbound in plasma, and this "free" cortisol is excreted unchanged in urine. Increases in plasma cortisol concentrations lead to an increase in the proportion of free cortisol in plasma. This is because CBG-binding of cortisol is nearly saturated as physiologic concentrations of cortisol, and increases in cortisol secretion are reflected in a disproportionate increase in the amount of free cortisol in urine. Cortisol has a half-life of approximately 100 min and is metabolized in the liver and other organs. Inactivation is mainly due to the reduction of the double bond between the C_4 and C_5 atoms. There are further reduction and conjugation steps before metabolites are excreted in urine.

Actions of cortisol

There are four broad areas of cortisol action: negative feedback to the hypothalamus and anterior pituitary, metabolic homeostasis, fluid/electrolyte homeostasis, and antiinflammatory/immunosuppressive effects

The principal metabolic action of cortisol is on carbohydrate and protein metabolism. Cortisol has a significant effect on glucose homeostasis, as the name "glucocorticoid" suggests

(Chapter 31). It acts both on peripheral tissues to decrease uptake and utilization of glucose and on nuclear receptors to increase gluconeogenesis (glucose production from noncarbohydrate substrates), with a net action to increase blood glucose. Glycogen synthesis and storage is also stimulated. Cortisol has the effect of reducing extrahepatic cellular protein, such as in muscle, by suppressing RNA and protein synthesis. In cortisol excess, muscle breakdown may be sufficient to cause muscle weakness, as seen in Cushing syndrome. The converse occurs in the liver, where hepatic delivery of amino acids allows increased protein synthesis and gluconeogenesis. Cortisol has a permissive effect on growth hormone, glucagon, and catecholamines (i.e., cortisol is required for these hormones to exert maximum effect). High-dose glucocorticoids decrease GH secretion, inhibit growth, and also decrease TSH release.

Cortisol has multiple actions in adipose tissue, acting to induce lipogenic genes and adipose endocrine function

Although cortisol is generally cited as a lipolytic hormone, experimental evidence is conflicting, and results differ with glucocorticoid concentration and animal model used. Indeed, chronic cortisol exposure of human adipose tissue has been shown to increase the activity of the genes involved with lipogenesis and lipolysis simultaneously. Excess systemic cortisol in humans' results in an increase in central (particularly visceral) adiposity and wasting of peripheral adipose tissue, which can be clinically identified (see following discussion of Cushing syndrome).

Cortisol has a weak mineralocorticoid action, and the mineralocorticoid receptor binds aldosterone and cortisol with equal affinity

The total plasma molar concentration of cortisol is around 1000 times higher than the mineralocorticoid aldosterone. However, target cells for aldosterone express 11-β-hydroxysteroid dehydrogenase, which acts to convert cortisol to cortisone, the latter having only a low affinity for the mineralocorticoid receptor. This conversion allows aldosterone to bind to the mineralocorticoid receptor. Cortisol influences bone metabolism, and it induces a tendency toward negative calcium balance by increasing gastrointestinal calcium absorption and increasing renal excretion. Exogenous glucocorticoid therapy can result in rapid bone density loss, resulting in osteoporosis. Central to this process is increased bone resorption and apoptosis of osteoblasts and osteocytes; decreased function of osteoblasts also contributes.

The immune system is modulated by cortisol through effects on leucocyte events, cytokine production, and blood vessel proliferation, and the antiinflammatory properties of glucocorticoids are utilized therapeutically to treat a broad range of inflammatory and autoimmune diseases. Glucocorticoids reduce vasodilation, having a permissive effect on vasodilators such as catecholamines.

Disorders of cortisol secretion

Adrenal hypofunction

Adrenocortical insufficiency may be due to primary adrenal pathology or secondary to anterior pituitary failure to produce ACTH

The most common form of adrenal insufficiency follows exogenous glucocorticoid therapy, which exerts negative feedback on the secretion of CRF and ACTH. Administration of exogenous glucocorticoids also can result in suppression of CRF and ACTH, leading to reduced stimulation of the adrenals and, consequently, adrenal gland atrophy. After the cessation of long-term glucocorticoid therapy, adrenal gland secretion of cortisol may take months to return to normal. Therefore patients on long-term glucocorticoid therapy are at risk of adrenal insufficiency if exogenous steroids are stopped abruptly.

CLINICAL BOX
ACUTE GLUCOCORTICOID WITHDRAWAL

A 47-year-old man presented to the emergency department with persistent nausea, vomiting, lethargy, and generalized abdominal pain after a bout of food poisoning. He had been able to drink some fluids but had been unable to keep food or his tablets down. He had a history of chronic severe asthma that was recently well controlled with inhalers and long-term oral glucocorticoids. On examination, there was a mild bilateral wheeze in his lungs; his abdomen was soft and nontender, and bowel sounds were present. His blood pressure was 115/65 mmHg lying down. Venous blood glucose was 3.8 mmol/L 68 mg/dL (4–6 mmol/L; 72–109 mg/dL). The patient was administered hydrocortisone and fluids intravenously and made a full recovery.

Comment

This presentation is an **acute hypoadrenalism** following sudden withdrawal of glucocorticoid therapy. Due to long-term exogenous glucocorticoid use, patients can have adrenal atrophy (due to lack of ACTH production). Stress can precipitate an adrenal crisis in patients who are unable to mount an adequate cortisol response, and "sick-day rules" are taught so that individuals can increase their dose of steroids during periods of illness.

Primary adrenal insufficiency

Primary adrenocortical insufficiency (also known as "Addison's disease") is a failure of the adrenal cortex

A failure of the adrenal cortex may follow autoimmune destruction of the gland (the commonest cause in the developed world), neoplastic invasion (e.g., metastases from lung, breast, or renal carcinoma), amyloid infiltration, hemochromatosis, hemorrhage, infections such as tuberculosis (the commonest cause worldwide), or cytomegalovirus (in immunocompromised individuals). Adrenal glands can also be resected during surgery.

The identification of cortisol deficiency can be clinically challenging, particularly in the early stages of the disease, because some common presenting features are nonspecific (Table 27.7)

Plasma cortisol and ACTH results must be carefully interpreted, and timing of samples considered (see the previous section "Laboratory Assessment of Hormone Action"). Most clinical features are related to insufficient glucocorticoid (cortisol) and mineralocorticoid (aldosterone) production for normal health. Biochemically, the lack of mineralocorticoid activity

Table 27.7 Primary adrenocortical insufficiency

Common causes

Long-term exogenous glucocorticoid administration
Autoimmune adrenalitis
Tuberculosis

Less common causes

Malignancy (metastases)
Amyloidosis
Hemochromatosis
Hemorrhage
Infection
Adrenalectomy

Symptoms

Fatigue, lethargy
Generalized weakness
Anorexia
Dizziness (postural hypotension)
Pigmentation
Nonspecific abdominal pain, nausea, vomiting
Weight loss
Hypoglycemia

Signs

Pigmentation (palmar creases, buccal mucosa)
Postural hypotension

(see Chapter 35) ultimately results in low serum sodium, high potassium concentrations, and metabolic acidosis. The adrenal glands fail to elicit an appropriate increase in cortisol release in response to administration of synthetic ACTH (Synacthen; Fig. 27.8). Baseline plasma ACTH concentrations are high, reflecting a physiologic response to lack of cortisol. The increased production of ACTH can result in skin pigmentation as ACTH is derived from the cleavage of POMC, which is also a precursor for melanocyte-stimulating hormone (MSH). Lifelong glucocorticoid replacement, commonly in conjunction with mineralocorticoid replacement, is necessary in what is otherwise a life-threatening condition, and glucocorticoid therapy must be increased during times of acute illness to mimic the endogenous stress response in those with functional glands. Adequate replacement of cortisol is assessed clinically by measurement of plasma ACTH and by serial measurements of serum cortisol (a cortisol "day curve"), ensuring the optimal balance between adequate treatment dosing and limitation of the risk of over replacement. Mineralocorticoid activity is assessed by measuring plasma renin and aldosterone (see Chapter 35), with increased renin and decreased aldosterone being consistent with adrenal insufficiency.

Autoimmune adrenal disease can occur as part of a cluster of autoimmune diseases (such as type 1 diabetes and hyper- or hypothyroidism) presenting in the same patient. These other disorders may be undiagnosed and can affect the clinical presentation and biochemical profile. Addison's disease without hypothyroidism can present in association with a raised TSH that resolves after glucocorticoid replacement therapy. This is important to appreciate because treatment with thyroxine can exacerbate the features of hypoadrenalism.

Adrenal insufficiency may result from genetic conditions caused by defects in steroid biosynthesis

In congenital adrenal hyperplasia (CAH), cortisol deficiency leads to increased ACTH secretion by the pituitary, resulting in adrenal hyperplasia (due to ACTH stimulation) and a rise in steroid precursors. Deficiency of 21-hydroxylase is the most common enzyme defect in CAH and patients typically present

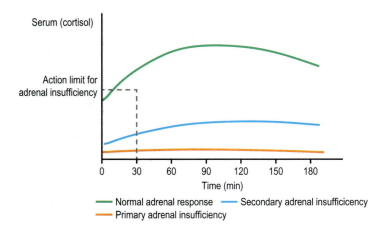

Fig. 27.8 **Serum cortisol response to ACTH stimulation testing.** Concentrations below the 30-min threshold indicated are consistent with adrenal insufficiency. The diminished cortisol response in secondary adrenal insufficiency is due to adrenal atrophy.

in the neonatal period with ambiguous genitalia in genetic females (excess 17-hydroxyprogesterone [17-OHP] is converted to androgens) and, in the presence of near-complete loss of enzyme activity, a hyperkalemic hyponatremic "salt-losing crisis" (cortisol and aldosterone deficiency presenting as acute hypoadrenalism) during the second or third week of life (see also Chapter 14 and clinical box on p. 185). Diagnosis of the condition involves measuring high serum concentrations of 17-OHP (Fig. 27.7). Screening for deficiency of 21-hydroxylase can be performed in the neonatal period by measurement of dry blood spot ("Guthrie card") 17-OHP concentration. Rarely, presentation is delayed until after puberty ("late-onset" 21-hydroxylase deficiency), and female patients present with clinical features such as hirsutism, menstrual irregularity, or infertility. CAH resulting from 11β-hydroxylase deficiency results in marked virilization in genetic females; however, mineralocorticoid action is maintained due to increased 11-deoxycorticosterone, and a salt-losing crisis does not occur. Deficiency of 17α-hydroxylase results in loss of androgens as well as cortisol synthesis and can cause ambiguous genitalia in genetic males or sexual infantilism in genetic females, with hypertension due to excess mineralocorticoid.

A rare inherited cause of adrenal insufficiency is X-linked **adrenoleukodystrophy** caused by a defect of peroxisomes. Failure of the breakdown of fatty acids in cells leads to accumulation of very long–chain fatty acids in blood and damage to the adrenal glands and myelin. Although patients typically present after the first few years of life, some patients may not present until adulthood. The most common and severe form of the disease manifests as progressive neurologic deterioration in childhood. For other forms of adrenoleukodystrophy, there is a wide range of clinical severity, and adrenal involvement may precede or follow neurologic symptoms.

Secondary adrenal insufficiency

Isolated deficiencies of CRH and ACTH are rare and typically present with other hypothalamic or pituitary hormone insufficiency. Aldosterone secretion is not ACTH dependent and negates significant renal salt wasting, although hypotension can still occur as the lack of cortisol reduces the activity of catecholamines on arteriolar smooth muscle.

Adrenal hyperfunction

Hypercortisolism

Cushing syndrome is the clinical presentation of hypercortisolism-which is most commonly iatrogenic, caused by use of exogenous glucocorticoid therapy (e.g., prednisolone, dexamethasone) (Table 27.8)

However, Cushing syndrome may also be due to primary or secondary hyperfunction. A **pituitary corticotrope adenoma** accounts for 70% of cases (**"Cushing disease"**), an **adrenal adenoma** accounts for 15%, with remaining causes including adrenal hyperplasia, due to genetic abnormalities or ectopic ACTH secretion associated with some tumors (e.g., small-cell

Table 27.8 Cushing syndrome

Causes

Adrenocorticotropic hormone (ACTH) dependent

Pituitary hypersecretion of ACTH and bilateral adrenal hyperplasia (Cushing disease)
Ectopic ACTH secretion (e.g., small cell carcinoma of the lung carcinoid tumors)
Iatrogenic (ACTH administration)

ACTH independent

Iatrogenic (exogenous glucocorticoid therapy)
Adrenal adenoma
Adrenal carcinoma
ACTH-independent macronodular adrenal hyperplasia

Clinical features

Obesity and weight gain
Facial plethora
Truncal obesity ("moon face," dorsocervical fat pad)
Plethora
Thin skin
Easy bruising, slow wound healing
Reduced libido
Menstrual irregularity, hirsutism
Abdominal striae
Proximal muscle weakness
Psychiatric disturbance (depression, euphoria, mania)
Erectile dysfunction

Associated features

Osteopenia/osteoporosis
Hypertension
Glucose intolerance
Nephrolithiasis

lung cancer, bronchial carcinoid tumors, medullary carcinoma of the thyroid, and thymic carcinoid).

The clinical manifestations of chronic endogenous hypercortisolemia vary from mild, nonspecific symptoms to weight gain, depression, proximal muscle wasting, and remodeling of adipose tissue (increase in central adiposity, moon face, dorsocervical fat pad ["buffalo hump"], supraclavicular fat), plethora, thin skin, bruising, slow wound healing, and abdominal striae. Associated metabolic consequences of hypercortisolemia include osteoporosis (with fractures), hypertension, and impaired glucose tolerance or diabetes. Cortisol excess may suppress the hypothalamic axis, resulting in erectile dysfunction in men and irregular menses in women. Some patients can present with symptoms that fluctuate because of variations in cortisol secretion in a state described as "cyclical" Cushing syndrome. Ectopic ACTH-dependent Cushing syndrome may present after a much shorter duration of illness, with profound hypercortisolism and hypokalemia (significant hypercortisolemia is associated with hypokalemia alkalosis).

Diagnosis of Cushing syndrome

Broadly, there are two stages to establishing the laboratory diagnosis of Cushing syndrome: confirming autonomous hypersecretion of cortisol and determining whether cortisol secretion is ACTH dependent or independent

Random serum cortisol measurements have limited utility in the diagnosis of Cushing syndrome due to the pronounced circadian rhythm and considerable biological variability of cortisol, and a 9 a.m. cortisol within the reference range does not exclude the diagnosis. To confirm the presence of hyper-cortisolemia, a **24-h urine free cortisol (UFC)** is typically used, overcoming the challenge of diurnal variation. The diagnostic utility of urine collections for biochemistry testing is affected by how well the collection is performed, and an incomplete collection or collecting urine for more than 24 h will affect the result. This test may be used as a screening tool, with further investigations performed depending on the results of this test and the pretest clinical suspicion. To deter-mine *autonomous* hypersecretion, additional investigations that are commonly employed are dexamethasone suppression testing to look for normal negative feedback suppression of cortisol production and testing of unstressed midnight cortisol to assess circadian rhythm. Both are usually lost in Cushing syndrome. Administration of the synthetic glucocorticoid dexamethasone (**"overnight dexamethasone suppression test"** [ONDST]) leads to suppression of ACTH in normal individuals. In the ONDST, dexamethasone is taken orally between 11 p.m. and midnight, and a serum cortisol measurement is taken at 9 a.m. the following morning. Dexamethasone is used as the ACTH/cortisol suppressor because dexamethasone does not cross-react in clinical cortisol immunoassays (therefore only endogenous cortisol is detected). Failure to suppress cortisol production at 9 a.m. is indicative of Cushing syndrome. Limita-tions of the ONDST include patient failure to take the dexa-methasone as directed or the use of medications that induce the CYP3A4 enzyme, thus increasing metabolism of dexa-methasone (e.g., phenytoin, rifampicin) or increase "total" cortisol by increased CBG (e.g., exogenous estrogens). In the **low-dose dexamethasone suppression test**, dexamethasone is administered at 6-h intervals for 48 h, starting at 9 a.m. on day 1, with serum cortisol measurement performed at 9 a.m. on day 3, 6 h after the last dexamethasone dose.

Loss of or altered diurnal variation of cortisol secretion is an early observation in Cushing syndrome and can be estab-lished by measurement of a **midnight cortisol concentra-tion,** when levels are physiologically at their lowest. This can be done during inpatient admission, although stress to the patient must be minimized to prevent stress-induced hyper-cortisolemia. An alternative is the measurement of a late night salivary free cortisol. Salivary cortisol has practical benefits because it negates the requirement for admission, and sample stability means that the salivary swab can simply be stored in a refrigerator before sending to the laboratory.

Measurement of plasma ACTH in the presence of hypercortisolemia is used to determine whether cortisol production is ACTH-driven rather than autonomous

Lack of suppression of ACTH suggests ACTH of pituitary or ectopic source, the latter often producing extremely high concentrations. At this stage, appropriate imaging is employed to identify the lesion and guide management. This may include pituitary magnetic resonance imaging (MRI) for Cushing disease; adrenal computerized tomography (CT)/MRI for adrenal adenoma/carcinoma; and, where indicated, CT chest/abdomen, whole-body scintigraphy, or positron-emission tomography (PET) to look for the site of production of ACTH/cortisol excess. When first-line laboratory investigations and imaging do not clearly distinguish between Cushing disease and ectopic ACTH-dependent Cushing syndrome, a bilateral inferior petrosal sinus sampling (with comparison of ACTH concentra-tions with those of peripheral blood) can be used to localize autonomously secreting lesions. In **ACTH-independent Cushing syndrome,** adrenal venous sampling can be used to compare the serum cortisol from the right with the left adrenal vein. Definitive treatment of an adenomatous lesion is usually surgical, and when surgery is not possible, the use of drugs to suppress cortisol production can help reduce a patient's symptoms. Metyrapone is a therapeutic agent that inhibits 11β-hydroxylation in cortisol (and to a lesser extent aldosterone) biosynthesis. There follows the desired fall in cortisol levels, and an increase in ACTH is observed by decreasing the negative

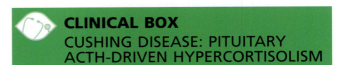

CLINICAL BOX
CUSHING DISEASE: PITUITARY ACTH-DRIVEN HYPERCORTISOLISM

A 42-year-old woman presented with fatigue, depression, weight gain, and irregular menstrual bleeding for several months. She complained of difficulty climbing stairs and recently noted that she bruised easily on her arms. She had a medical history of type 2 diabetes and mild hypertension, which was being moni-tored. Urinary free cortisol (UFC) was 1064 nmol/24 h (34 μg/dL; reference range < 250 nmol/24h [<9 μg/dL]). Baseline ACTH concentration was 120 ng/L (reference range < 80 ng/L), and 9 a.m. serum cortisol concentration was 580 nmol/L (21 μg/dL) following 1 mg oral dexamethasone (reference range < 50 nmol/L [<1.8 μg/dL]).

Comment

This woman has clinical features consistent with Cushing syn-drome. Biochemistry investigations showed increased cortisol production (confirmed by raised UFC) that failed to suppress appropriately with dexamethasone. The unsuppressed ACTH supports ACTH-driven hypercortisolemia that may be due to a pituitary adenoma (most likely) or ectopic ACTH secretion from an occult neoplasm. In this case, magnetic resonance imaging revealed a tumor of the pituitary.

feedback to the pituitary. Consequently, 11-deoxycortisol (Fig. 27.7) is released into the circulation, metabolized by the liver, and renally excreted. When monitoring patients taking this medication, it is important to note that the increased amounts of precursors of cortisol may cross-react (i.e., be measured as "cortisol") in the cortisol immunoassay, and results may not reflect treatment response. Specific measurement of cortisol can be undertaken by mass spectrometry in specialist clinical laboratories.

Hyperaldosteronism

Primary hyperaldosteronism is autonomous hypersecretion of aldosterone (i.e., independent of the renin–angiotensin–aldosterone system [Chapter 35], resulting in sodium and water retention and suppressed renin production

Patients are typically asymptomatic and present with hypertension that may be difficult to control. Some patients may present with sequelae of **hypokalemia.** Biochemistry results show a suppressed renin with raised aldosterone concentrations, typically associated with hypokalemia (due to excessive renal excretion), a normal or raised sodium, and metabolic alkalosis. Caution must be taken when interpreting renin and aldosterone results in patients taking antihypertensive medications (e.g., beta blockers or angiotensin-converting enzyme inhibitors) because these can affect aldosterone secretion. In approximately two-thirds of patients, primary hyperaldosteronism is caused by a **solitary aldosterone-producing adenoma (Conn's syndrome)**; in one-third of patients, it is caused by bilateral diffuse adrenocortical hyperplasia. Glucocorticoid-suppressible hyperaldosteronism is a rare inherited cause of primary hyperaldosteronism in which aldosterone is under the influence of ACTH.

THE HYPOTHALAMO–PITUITARY– GONADAL AXIS

Gonadotropin-releasing hormone (GnRH)

GnRH is essential for secretion of FSH and LH

Gonadotropin-releasing hormone (GnRH) is a decapeptide synthesized within the arcuate nucleus of the medial basal and the medial preoptic area of the hypothalamus and is essential for secretion of FSH and LH. GnRH is transported down the axons of specialized neurons and released into the portal circulation that surrounds the anterior pituitary. The GnRH receptor is a member of the rhodopsin-like G protein–coupled receptor superfamily and has a transmembrane domain. GnRH binding results in a receptor conformational change and activation of intracellular signaling pathways, with downstream transcription of multiple target cell genes. GnRH secretion is highly pulsatile, and release stimulates

synthesis of both FSH and LH expression. GnRH release is active during the neonatal period, followed by a dormant stage during infancy until the onset of puberty that is heralded by GnRH pulses, which increase in frequency and amplitude. The resulting increase in gonadotropin levels stimulate the previously dormant ovaries or testes. Exactly what triggers the onset of puberty is not known, but there are several lines of evidence suggesting that this is largely determined centrally. The hypothalamic neuropeptides **kisspeptin,** a potent secretagogue of GnRH, and **neurokinin B,** which has an important role in kisspeptin and gonadotropin release, have been identified as critical components of the central mechanism determining puberty onset.

Administration of long-acting GnRH agonists (e.g., leuprolide, buserelin, and goserelin) cause continuous GnRH stimulation and thus down-regulation of GnRH receptors, thereby inhibiting gonadotropin secretion. This exploits negative feedback for therapeutic purposes. Such agonists are used as therapy to treat prostate cancer (reducing testosterone and dihydrotestosterone and therefore cancer growth). GnRH agonists can also be used in women to treat estrogen-dependent conditions such as endometriosis or menorrhagia.

Follicle-stimulating hormone (FSH) and luteinizing hormone (LH)

The pituitary gland produces the gonadotropins FSH and LH, critical to gonadal reproductive function in both males and females

FSH and LH (together with TSH and hCG) are glycoprotein hormones that are composed of non-covalently-bound peptide α- and β-subunits. They share structural homology, having an identical α-subunit, but with a hormone-specific β-subunit. Gonadotropin release is stimulated by GnRH, and the pulse frequency and amplitude controls FSH and LH synthesis and secretion. An outline of hypothalamo–pituitary–gonadal axes in the male and female is shown in Fig. 27.9. LH receptors are present on Leydig cells of the testis and thecal cells of the ovary. Both FSH and LH receptors are located on plasma membranes of Sertoli cells of the testis and granulosa cells of the ovary.

Action of gonadotropins on the testes

In males, LH stimulates testosterone secretion by Leydig cells of the testes, acting via a membrane-associated G protein–coupled receptor, resulting in a downstream increase in cAMP and activation of the cAMP-dependent intracellular protein kinase A pathway (Chapter 25). FSH, in cooperation with intratubular testosterone, promotes spermatogenesis in the seminiferous tubule. Testosterone (and estradiol produced from testosterone) provides negative feedback to GnRH and LH secretion.

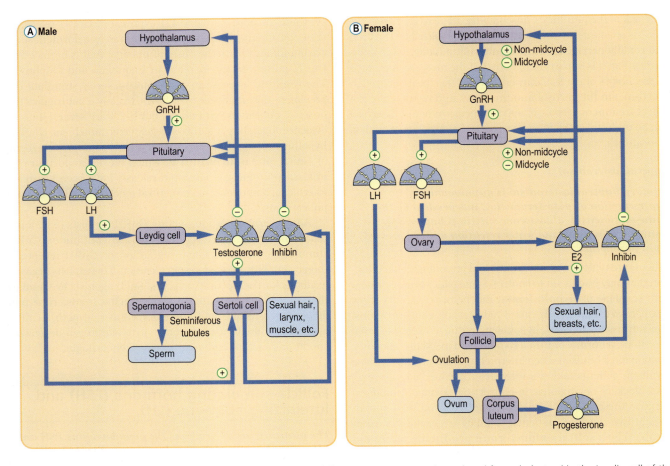

Fig. 27.9 **Control of the hypothalamic–pituitary–gonadal axes.** (A) In men, testosterone is produced from cholesterol in the Leydig cell of the testis in response to LH stimulation. Testosterone and FSH support spermatogenesis. (B) In women, estradiol (E2) is produced by the granulosa cell of the ovary and developing follicle after feedback stimulation. E2 feedback is mainly negative, but in midcycle, there is positive E2 central feedback culminating in the surge of LH that causes ovulation. Progesterone is secreted by the resultant corpus luteum.

Androgens

Biochemical actions of testosterone in the male

Testosterone is an anabolic hormone and increases muscle mass by stimulating protein synthesis (Fig. 27.10)

During embryonic development, testosterone produced by testicular cells that ultimately develop into Leydig cells induces the development of the Wolffian duct. However, unlike after birth, when testosterone production is under the influence of the hypothalamic–pituitary system, the embryonic testes are controlled by hCG.

Not all testosterone originates from the testes, with approximately 5% being produced by the adrenal gland. During adrenarche, the adrenal glands synthesize weak androgens, particularly androstenedione, dehydroepiandrosterone (DHEA), and dehydroepiandrosterone sulfate (DHEAS). These androgens are metabolized to testosterone and dihydrotestosterone (DHT) and stimulate axillary and pubic hair growth.

Testosterone deficiency in males

Endocrine failure of the testes may be primary, due to trauma or inflammation of the testes, for example, or secondary, due to a failure of the hypothalamus or pituitary

Indeed, the gonadotropes are among the anterior pituitary cell types more sensitive to damage (e.g., due to compression from an adenoma within the bony constraints of the sella turcica), and consequently, **gonadal failure is often the earliest manifestation** of pituitary failure. **Secondary hypogonadism** ("hypothalamic hypogonadism") may be congenital (e.g., Kallmann syndrome) or acquired (e.g., infiltrative lesions of the pituitary and hypothalamus). It can occur in response to severe weight loss (e.g., anorexia nervosa) or physiologic stress (e.g., severe burns), when it is an energy-sparing maneuver, or can be associated with Cushing disease or chronic opioid use.

During the investigation of suspected testosterone deficiency, measurement of testosterone by the clinical laboratory (by

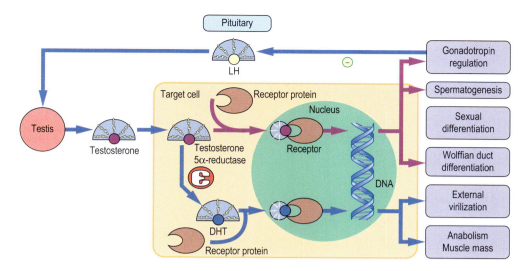

Fig. 27.10 **Mechanism of action of testosterone.** Testosterone from the testis enters a target cell and binds to the androgen receptor, either directly or after conversion to 5α-dihydrotestosterone (DHT). Actions mediated by testosterone are indicated with purple lines; those mediated by DHT are shown by blue lines.

immunoassay) typically quantifies circulating total testosterone (protein-bound and free forms). Approximately 97% of plasma testosterone is bound to sex hormone–binding globulin (SHBG) and, to a lesser degree, to albumin and other proteins in circulation. Measurement of free testosterone is challenging, but there are free-testosterone estimation formulae that take into consideration serum albumin, SHBG, and testosterone concentrations. In males, serum testosterone levels show circadian variation, with the highest levels in the morning and the lowest levels in the late afternoon. Such intra-individual variation in testosterone levels can be approximately 35%.

Gonadal dysgenesis in the male

Klinefelter syndrome, which is most commonly caused by the acquisition of one extra copy of the X chromosome in each cell (karyotype 47, XXY), has a prevalence of 1 in 500–1000 of all phenotypic males

Additional copies of genes on the X chromosome interfere with normal male sexual development and cause varying degrees of hypogonadism. The classical manifestations of Klinefelter include eunuchoidism (hypogonadism with incomplete sexual maturation), gynecomastia (abnormal benign proliferation of male breast glandular tissue), microorchidism (small testes), and azoospermia (absence of viable spermatozoa in the semen), although some individuals have few or no associated signs and symptoms. The FSH is elevated, and LH is usually elevated, but the Leydig cells do not respond normally, and plasma testosterone may be subnormal. Some individuals with features of Klinefelter syndrome may have more than one extra X chromosome, mosaicisms, or 46 chromosomes (karyotype 46 XY), with translocation of the male sex-determining region of chromosome Y onto the X chromosome.

Androgen excess in the male

Hyperandrogenism due to testicular androgen excess may cause precocious puberty

Precocious puberty is a rare condition that may result from early activation of the normal hypothalamo–pituitary–gonadal axis or a gain-of-function mutation in the LH or kisspeptin receptor. Androgen excess may also be due to a tumor secreting androgen or hCG. Adrenal androgen excess may cause hirsutism in children, but in the adult male, it may not cause overt clinical manifestations. Exogenous androgen administration, such as for the purpose of enhancing athletic performance or muscular hypertrophy, may lead to side effects such as prostate abnormalities, cholestatic jaundice, changes in libido, suppression of spermatogenesis, gynecomastia, polycythemia, hypertension, hirsutism, male-pattern baldness, and acne. Excess adrenal androgen secretion also may be associated with Cushing syndrome.

Actions of FSH and LH on the ovary

In the mature female, there are cyclic changes in the hypothalamic–pituitary–gonadal axis orchestrated by the GnRH pulse generator

Unlike the mature male, in whom steroidogenesis is continuous, in the mature female, there are cyclic changes in the hypothalamic–pituitary–gonadal axis orchestrated by the GnRH pulse generator. After puberty, the human ovaries contain approximately 400,000 primordial follicles, each containing an oocyte in an arrested state, with no further gametes formed postnatally. Primordial follicles begin hormone-independent growth and maturation before the start of the menstrual cycle, but only at the start of the cycle, when they have acquired the

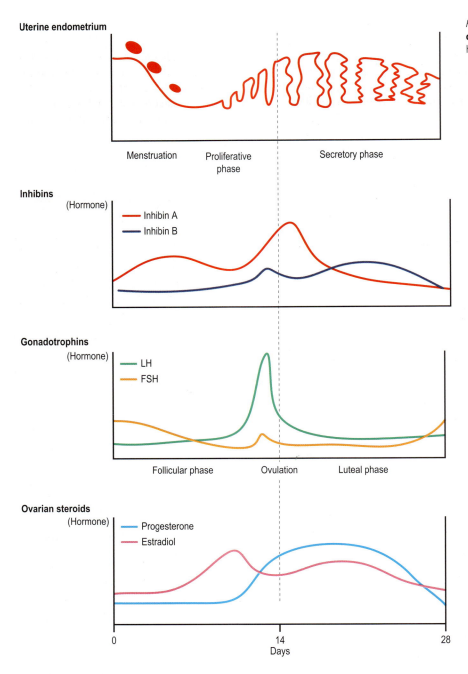

Uterine endometrium

Menstruation   Proliferative phase   Secretory phase

Inhibins
(Hormone)
— Inhibin A
— Inhibin B

Gonadotrophins
(Hormone)
— LH
— FSH

Follicular phase   Ovulation   Luteal phase

Ovarian steroids
(Hormone)
— Progesterone
— Estradiol

0   14   28
Days

Fig. 27.11 **Hormone and endometrial changes during the menstrual cycle.** LH, luteinizing hormone; FSH, follicle-stimulating hormone.

capacity to respond to FSH, are a few follicles preserved from atresia. During the follicular phase, rising FSH concentrations stimulate estradiol synthesis (Fig. 27.11) and granulosa cell proliferation. Additional FSH receptors and new LH receptors are synthesized on granulosa cells under the influence of FSH. As estradiol rises, FSH secretion is suppressed, and this combination plays an important role in the selection of a dominant follicle for further development, while nondominant follicles undergo atresia. Under the influence of estradiol, maturation of the dominant follicle continues, uterine endometrial growth is stimulated, and there is more LH secretion from the pituitary. Positive feedback in the dominant follicle resulting in increasing

estradiol causes the negative feedback for estrogen to switch to positive feedback, initiating an LH surge. LH binds to receptors on the dominant follicle, and this culminates in the release of a mature ovum from the ovary approximately 9 h after the LH peak.

After ovulation, the ruptured follicle transforms into the corpus luteum, which secretes progesterone and estradiol to sustain the oocyte and stimulate the preparation of estrogen-primed endometrium for implantation of a fertilized ovum. During this period, known as the luteal phase, the progesterone acts to prevent another LH surge by the secreted estrogen. In the investigation of infertility in women, measurement of serum progesterone at concentrations normal for the luteal phase can provide evidence that ovulation has occurred. In the absence of fertilization, corpus luteum function declines, progesterone and estradiol concentrations fall, and follicular development proceeds for the following cycle. Subsequent vascular changes in the endometrium lead to tissue involution and menstruation.

Inhibin and the ovary

Granulosa cells secrete inhibin, a heterodimeric glycoprotein composed of an α-subunit linked by a disulfide bridge to one of two homologous β-subunits

Inhibin B (α-βB), produced by pre-antral and small antral follicles, is highest during the mid-follicular phase (Fig. 27.11) and has a role with estradiol to suppress synthesis and secretion of FSH, assuring dominant follicle selection. Declining inhibin A (α-βA) levels during the late luteal phase, after a peak during the mid-luteal phase, are suggested to be the predominant regulator of rising FSH concentration during the transition between the luteal and follicular phase.

Gonadotropins and pregnancy

After successful implantation of a fertilized ovum, maintenance of the corpus luteum and progesterone production is vital to ensure progression of development

hCG, which exhibits homology with LH, secreted by the gestational trophoblast, maintains the corpus luteum until around week 9 of pregnancy, at which time the trophoblast itself can produce sufficient progesterone. hCG may be detected in urine and blood from 1–2 weeks after fertilization. Measurement of hCG in urine and/or blood is used clinically to **confirm pregnancy,** and in early pregnancy, serial serum measurements can be taken to help assess early pregnancy viability, when approximate doubling of hCG levels every 48 h may be expected. An hCG level that is low and/or falls over time may indicate miscarriage or nonviable uterine gestation, and levels that remain static or increase slowly may indicate an ectopic (tubal) pregnancy. Higher-than-expected levels can indicate multiple gestations or a molar pregnancy. Blood tests are supported by clinical assessment and ultrasound examination. As the placenta becomes the principal site of progesterone production, hCG is required to maintain progesterone synthesis by the syncytiotrophoblast; hCG levels peak at around 7 weeks' gestation and then decrease to achieve a steady-state level for the rest of the pregnancy.

Gonadotropins and menopause

Ovarian follicles become depleted of oocytes after 30–40 years of ovulatory cycles, and normal pregnancy is no longer possible

When menstruation ceases permanently due to the loss of ovarian follicular activity, this is termed menopause, or the climacteric. At this time, circulating estrogens become reduced, and with the lack of negative feedback, FSH and LH concentrations rise accordingly and remain high relative to the concentrations measured during the normal menstrual cycle. Long-term postmenopausal estrogen deficiency is known to increase the rate of bone loss, resulting in osteoporosis, and with altered lipoprotein metabolism, there is an increased risk of cardiovascular disease.

CLINICAL BOX
INVESTIGATION OF SECONDARY AMENORRHEA

A 22-year-old woman presented to primary care complaining of lethargy and not having had a period for several months. She was a university student and was anxiously working toward her final exams. Her food intake over the past few weeks had been reduced. Previously her menstrual bleeds were regular, after starting around the age of 12. Physical examination was unremarkable, and BP was 110/60 mmHg.

Comment
Secondary amenorrhea may be defined as the absence of menstruation in women with previously normal and regular menses or in women with previous oligomenorrhea. Although there is no general consensus on defined time periods, there is agreement to evaluate after 3–6 months in a patient with previously normal menstruation. The differential diagnosis in this patient includes pregnancy, secondary hypogonadism (e.g., due to anorexia nervosa or excessive exercise), polycystic ovarian syndrome (a complex endocrine disorder that can present with oligomenorrhea or amenorrhea; other clinical features include hirsutism and acne [due to excess androgens] and multiple cysts in the ovary), and primary hypothyroidism. **Pregnancy (absent cyclic LH release) should be excluded first** as a cause of secondary amenorrhea in any female patient of reproductive age. This can usually be performed in primary care using a urine hCG test.

Estrogens and progesterone: Actions of steroid hormones in the female

Aside from their role in the menstrual cycle, the female sex steroids have additional roles

Plasma estrogen, concentrations of which are low before puberty, promotes the development of some female secondary sexual characteristics, and in the adult female, both estrogen and progesterone support breast function. Progesterone is responsible for the rise in body temperature during the luteal phase of the menstrual cycle (around 1–2 days after ovulation), and decreases in progesterone secretion may contribute to premenstrual changes in mood.

THE GROWTH HORMONE AXIS

GH secretion by the anterior pituitary is regulated by two hypothalamic hormones: growth hormone–releasing hormone (GHRH), which stimulates GH release, and somatostatin, which inhibits GH release.

Growth hormone–releasing hormone (GHRH)

GHRH is a 44–amino acid peptide synthesized in the arcuate and ventromedial hypothalamic nuclei of the hypothalamus

GHRH is secreted episodically, binds to GHRH receptors on pituitary somatotrope cells, and activates both adenylyl cyclase and intracellular calcium–calmodulin systems to stimulate GH transcription and secretion. GHRH synthesis and secretion is under negative feedback control from GH and IGF-1.

Ghrelin is a 28–amino acid peptide hormone with a fatty acid chain that is also a potent inducer of GH secretion

Originally isolated from the stomach, ghrelin has since been identified in the gastrointestinal tract, pancreas, adrenal cortex, and ovary. In addition to its function in energy balance (Chapter 32), ghrelin binds to the growth hormone secretagogue receptor and appears to act synergistically with GHRH to modulate GH secretion.

Somatostatin

Somatostatin (sometimes referred to as growth hormone–inhibiting hormone [GHIH]) is synthesized in the paraventricular and ventromedial nuclei of the hypothalamus

Somatostatin is found as two isoforms, one of 14 and one of 28 amino acids, both produced by the cleavage of the same 116–amino acid gene product, and both are active in inhibiting GH secretion. Somatostatin acts on the hypothalamo–pituitary axis and also the gastrointestinal tract. In addition to inhibiting GH release, TSH secretion from the anterior pituitary is also inhibited. Somatostatin binds to G protein–coupled transmembrane receptors that are linked to adenylyl cyclase, and a decrease in cAMP production occurs on receptor activation.

Somatostatin suppresses the release of the gastrointestinal hormones gastrin, cholecystokinin, vasoactive intestinal peptide (VIP), gastric inhibitory polypeptide, insulin, and glucagon

Somatostatin analogs are used therapeutically to inhibit GH secretion in patients with GH excess and can be used in the treatment of secretory neuroendocrine tumors, such as in carcinoid syndrome, VIPomas, and glucagonomas, and are also used to inhibit exocrine pancreas secretions after pancreatic surgery.

Growth hormone (GH)

GH release is episodic and under the influence of the hypothalamus, with approximately two-thirds of total 24-h GH secretion occurring at night

The human growth hormone (hGH) cluster contains five genes: one, *hGH-N*, is principally expressed in pituitary somatotropes, and the remaining four genes (the chorionic somatomammotropin genes, *hCS-L*, *hCS-A*, and *hCS-B*, and *hGH-V*) are expressed selectively by the placenta. The GH secreted by the anterior pituitary is a heterogeneous mixture as a consequence of posttranslational modifications, such as glycosylation, and peripheral metabolism. This is relevant to the measurement of GH because there are multiple variants of GH in plasma that may be detected to different extents in any given GH assay, including monomeric isoforms, homo- and hetero-polymers, fragments, and complexes with other molecules, in addition to the effect of GH binding to protein (up to 50% GH is protein bound).

GH is synthesized by the somatotropic cells of the anterior pituitary and stored within granules

GH release is episodic and under the influence of the hypothalamus, with approximately two-thirds of total 24-h GH secretion occurring at night. Surges may occur at other times, such as after meals, but plasma concentrations are typically lower during the day. Consequently, plasma GH may be below GH immunoassay quantitation limits in normal health, without necessarily indicating GH deficiency. Overall, GH concentrations are highest in adolescents and lowest in old age. Different stimuli, such as physical stress (e.g., exercise, hypoglycemia), psychologic stress, and increases in circulating amino acids (e.g., arginine and leucine) stimulate GH secretion, whereas glucose and fatty acids suppress GH release. Hormone modulators of GH secretion include TRH, glucocorticoids, testosterone, and estrogens that act at the level of the hypothalamus and pituitary. At peak plasma concentrations, GH amounts can be 100-fold greater than baseline, and therefore reference limits are of limited use, although levels to rule out GH excess and deficiency are applied to the relevant suppression and stimulation tests, respectively. Multiple plasma measurements may be taken over a 24-h period to provide information on the pattern and amount of GH secretion, but the task is often impractical.

The **GH transmembrane receptor** is expressed as a monomer; however, it functions as a constitutive dimer, with the ligand–receptor complex made up of one GH molecule and two GH receptors (homodimer). GH binding results in structural changes to the complex, and kinases below the cell membrane are able to activate each other by transphosphorylation initiating intracellular signaling cascades, leading to transcription of many enzymes, hormones, and growth factors, including IGF-1 (Chapter 28).

The overall action of GH is to promote growth of bone, cartilage, and soft tissue

GH is an anabolic hormone and has the net effect of positive nitrogen balance and phosphate balance. The diversity of GH

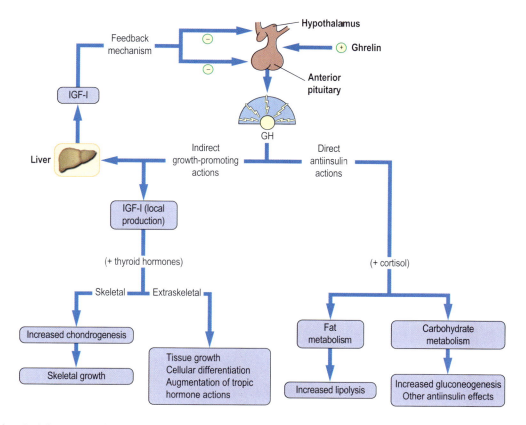

Fig. 27.12 **Biochemical functions of growth hormone.** These can be divided into direct actions on lipid and carbohydrate metabolism and indirect actions on protein synthesis and cell proliferation.

action makes it challenging to integrate all its functions. It can therefore be convenient to divide the functions into direct and indirect (Fig. 27.12). Direct actions of GH are on lipid, carbohydrate, and protein metabolism. During hypoglycemia, GH stimulates lipolysis, induces peripheral insulin resistance, and stimulates uptake of nonesterified fatty acids by muscle. Indirect actions of GH are mediated by IGF-1, and these actions include the promotion of chondrocyte proliferation and the synthesis of cartilage matrix in skeletal tissues. IGF-1 has been shown to increase glucose oxidation in adipose tissue and stimulate glucose and amino acid transport into the heart and diaphragmatic muscle.

Insulin-like growth factor-1 (IGF-1)

Measurement of IGF-1 has clinical utility as an indicator of integrated GH activity

IGF-1 is a 70–amino acid peptide that is secreted mostly by the liver and then transported to target tissues, acting as an endocrine hormone, although some IGF-1 is secreted by other cells and acts as a paracrine hormone, such as in cartilaginous tissue. IGF-1 has an A and B chain connected by disulfide bonds and shares homology with insulin. This structural similarity

may explain the ability of IGF-1 to bind (with low affinity) to the insulin receptor. Although circulating concentrations of IGF-1 are much higher than those of insulin, in contrast to insulin, which is unbound in circulation, 99% of IGF-1 is complexed with a series of IGF-binding proteins (IGFBP) that moderate bioavailability. Approximately 80% of circulating IGF-1 in humans is transported by IGFBP-3 in a complex of one molecule of IGF-1, one molecule of IGFBP-3, and one molecule of acid labile subunit. The relative affinities of insulin and IGF-1 for their respective receptors results in little cross-stimulation in normal physiology, although in pathologic situations, it is possible for insulin to have some IGF-1 activity, and vice versa. This has implications for states of severe insulin resistance, where some clinical features have been attributed to IGF-1, such as darkened, thickened patches of skin (acanthosis nigricans).

Measurement of IGF-1 has clinical utility as an indicator of integrated GH activity. Plasma concentrations of IGF-1 increase during childhood and reach adult levels around the time of puberty. The reference limits for IGF-1 in adults aged 20–60 years is relatively constant, and IGF-1 concentrations fall after the sixth decade of life. IGF-1 concentrations are expected to be increased in patients with GH excess and reduced in GH deficiency and in restricted growth states, such as chronic nutritional deficiency.

ADVANCED CONCEPT BOX
BIG IGF-2 AND HYPOINSULINEMIC HYPOGLYCEMIA

Unlike IGF-1, which is a principal regulator of postnatal growth, insulin-like growth factor-2 (IGF-2) plays an important role in normal fetal development and placental function, promoting cell proliferation and survival. **Non–islet cell tumor hypoglycemia (NICTH)** is a rare paraneoplastic disorder where hypoglycemia is induced by incompletely processed IGF-2 precursors that are released by tumors. The high-molecular-weight ("big") IGF-2, which has a potent glucose-lowering action, favors existence as a binary complex with IGFBP-3 and the complex is believed to have the ability to cross the endothelial barrier. The net physiologic effects are to inhibit glucose output from the liver, increase peripheral uptake of glucose, and inhibit GH, glucagon (counter-regulatory hormones), and ketone production. Hypoglycemia is associated with a suppressed insulin / C-peptide (see Chapter 31), a suppressed IGF-1, IGF-2 within reference limit or raised, raised IGF-2:IGF-1 ratio, and the presence of the secreting tumor (Bodnar, Acevedo, & Pietropaolo, 2014).

Table 27.9 Growth hormone excess
Causes
Pituitary adenoma Ectopic growth hormone Growth hormone–releasing hormone-secreting tumor
Clinical features
Tall stature (children/adolescents) Coarsening of facial features - prominent supraorbital ridge, prognathism, widely spaced teeth, macroglossia Soft tissue swelling in larynx - snoring, obstructive sleep apnea Acral enlargement (excessive hand growth - "spade-like" hands, increased ring size; excessive foot growth - increased shoe size) Hyperhidrosis (excessive sweating) Arthralgia Carpal tunnel syndrome Impaired glucose tolerance or diabetes mellitus (increased gluconeogenesis and decreased peripheral glucose uptake) Hypertension; left/biventricular hypertrophy; cardiac failure Local compression symptoms - headache, visual field defect

Clinical disorders of GH secretion

Clinically significant GH excess or deficiency is relatively uncommon and can be difficult to diagnose

The absence of a sensitive and specific reference range for GH means that laboratory diagnosis requires the study of the dynamics of GH secretion or the use of a relevant dynamic function test. Basal IGF-1 can serve as a screening test and can be used in the diagnosis of GH deficiency or excess because concentrations correlate with GH secretion over the preceding 24 h. However, in approximately 25% of individuals with GH excess, IGF-1 is within reference limits. Therefore in individuals with a normal IGF-1 concentration where the clinical suspicion is high, further investigation is necessary. In Laron syndrome (or Laron-type dwarfism), GH concentrations are high, yet IGF-1 concentrations are low; this is an autosomal recessive condition caused by a defect in the growth hormone receptor.

Growth hormone deficiency

Childhood GH deficiency is a possible cause for short stature

Severe congenital GH deficiency can present with hypoglycemia and hyperbilirubinemia in the neonatal period or growth failure during the first year of life. Childhood GH deficiency is a possible cause for short stature and failure to meet centile targets for growth. Auxologic parameters are used to identify patients to investigate for GH deficiency, including height and height velocity. Treatment involves the regular injection of recombinant hGH, which is synthesized using recombinant DNA technology. Adults with a definite cause for GH deficiency (e.g.,

hypopituitarism) are also candidates for GH replacement, where it can sometimes improve quality of life.

Growth hormone excess

Excess GH secretion is most commonly due to a pituitary tumor

Excess GH secretion is most commonly due to an autonomously secreting pituitary tumor, although GHRH-secreting tumors in the hypothalamus and ectopic GHRH production are possible (Table 27.9). Prolonged exposure to GH excess results in overgrowth of the skeleton and soft tissue. In childhood and before the fusion of the epiphyseal growth plates, GH excess manifests as gigantism, characterized by excessive linear growth. In adult GH excess, acromegaly, there is soft tissue and bone overgrowth, but linear bone growth is not possible. Signs may develop insidiously, leading to a delay before a diagnosis is made. Classically, GH excess is diagnosed using an oral glucose tolerance test by demonstrating lack of inhibition of GH release after the glucose load. Paradoxically, some individuals with acromegaly display a rise in GH in response to glucose. Lack of GH suppression is not specific for acromegaly and may occur in diabetes, hepatic disease, and renal disease, and so the serum IGF-1 concentration should be used in conjunction with the oral glucose tolerance test (OGTT) result. More than 95% of cases of acromegaly are caused by a GH-secreting pituitary adenoma arising from somatotrope cells, and these most commonly occur sporadically and in isolation. Pituitary tumors can be identified using MRI, for which transsphenoidal surgery is the preferred treatment option, although long-acting somatostatin analogs (e.g., octreotide, lanreotide) and radiotherapy can also be effective. Pegvisomant, a genetically modified analog of human growth hormone, is a selective growth hormone receptor antagonist used in the treatment of acromegaly in patients with inadequate response after pituitary surgery, radiation, or treatment with somatostatin analogs. Acromegaly is associated with an increased risk of certain tumors, with colorectal cancer being among the best documented, although it is the cardiovascular complications that are the leading cause of death.

THE PROLACTIN AXIS

Prolactin and dopamine

Prolactin is a 198–amino acid polypeptide hormone secreted solely by lactotrope cells of the anterior pituitary

The principal physiologic role of prolactin is during pregnancy, when prolactin initiates and sustains lactation. As a hormone, it is unusual because its secretion is under tonic inhibitory control by the hypothalamus, and it is not regulated by negative feedback from its target tissue. The inhibitor is the molecule **dopamine** that is secreted by tuberoinfundibular neurons into the portal circulation and binds to a G protein–coupled receptor inhibiting adenylyl cyclase and phospholipase C (Chapter 26). In the absence of dopamine, prolactin secretion is autonomous. Some peptides, such as TRH, VIP, oxytocin, and serotonin, may stimulate secretion, but they are not considered physiologically important. The secretion of prolactin is pulsatile, and serum concentrations can rise during pregnancy and can also increase during stress, such as with physical exertion, and hypoglycemia.

Dopamine stimulates D2 receptors to inhibit adenylyl cyclase and thereby inhibit prolactin synthesis and secretion

Lactotrope cells increase in number during pregnancy as serum prolactin increases and peaks at term; concentrations then decrease in the absence of breastfeeding after birth and after around 3 months with continued breastfeeding. Mechanical stimulation of the nipple during breastfeeding promotes secretion of prolactin to help milk production. Raised prolactin during breastfeeding can have contraceptive action by inhibiting GnRH secretion from the hypothalamus, thereby limiting gonadotropin production and inhibiting ovulation and menstruation. The only clinical manifestation of a low prolactin is loss of ability to lactate.

Disorders of prolactin secretion

Pathologic hyperprolactinemia

Extreme hyperprolactinemia is highly suggestive of a prolactinoma in patients not taking antidopaminergic drugs

Hypersecretion of prolactin by lactotrope cells may be due to an autonomous prolactin-secreting tumor (insensitive to dopamine inhibition), loss of dopamine inhibition (e.g., compression

Table 27.10 Hyperprolactinemia

Causes

Physiologic - pregnancy/breastfeeding
Drugs (e.g., phenothiazine, haloperidol)
Prolactinoma - macro- or macroprolactinoma
Pituitary stalk compression
Hypothalamic disease (e.g., craniopharyngioma)
Hypothyroidism

Symptoms

Female: Menstrual irregularity, infertility
Male: Erectile dysfunction, galactorrhea
Compression effects (e.g., bilateral temporal hemianopia)

of pituitary stalk by nonfunctioning adenoma), or use of antidopaminergic drugs (e.g., classic antipsychotic medications, such as phenothiazines). Extreme hyperprolactinemia is highly suggestive of a prolactinoma in patients not taking antidopaminergic drugs. The diagnosis is more challenging with patients taking antidopaminergic medication because serum prolactin concentrations can be comparable to the high levels measured in patients with a prolactinoma. Hyperprolactinemia can present in females with menstrual irregularities and in men or women with **infertility** or **galactorrhea.** A list of clinical features is given in Table 27.10. Once a prolactinoma is identified, treatment options include a long-acting dopamine agonist such as bromocriptine or cabergoline, use of which decreases prolactin secretion and almost invariably shrinks large tumors. In some individuals, drugs can be stopped and hyperprolactinemia does not recur. Transsphenoidal surgery may be required for resistant tumors, particularly where such tumors cause compression (e.g., of optic chiasm, causing a visual defect).

Macroprolactin is prolactin bound to antibody circulating as a complex and may be detected by some prolactin assays resulting in a high measured serum prolactin concentration

These complexes, however, are biologically inactive yet can still be detected by immunoassay. Laboratory techniques such as polyethylene glycol precipitation (to precipitate prolactin bound to antibody) and gel filtration chromatography (to separate antibody-bound prolactin from unbound prolactin; Fig. 27.13) are used to identify this entity.

ENDOCRINE SYSTEMS NOT CONSIDERED IN THIS CHAPTER

There are other endocrine systems that are not considered in this chapter, although they are governed by the same general principles. Some of these systems are described in other chapters in this book as part of the physiologic function of the hormones.

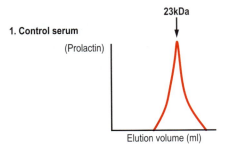

1. Control serum

(Prolactin)

23kDa

Elution volume (ml)

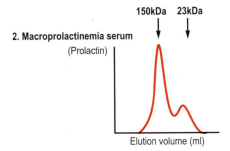

2. Macroprolactinemia serum

(Prolactin)

150kDa   23kDa

Elution volume (ml)

3. Chromatography separating prolactin species according to size

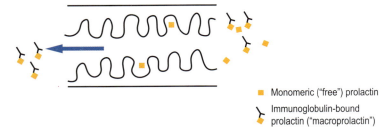

■ Monomeric ("free") prolactin

Immunoglobulin-bound
prolactin ("macroprolactin")

Fig. 27.13 **Gel filtration chromatography of (1) control and (2) macroprolactinemia serum.** Prolactin is measured in eluted chromatography buffer. Prolactin species are separated according to size: smaller molecules flow more slowly through the column because they can access pores in the gel material inaccessible to larger molecules. Control serum generates one peak consistent with monomeric prolactin (23 kDa); macroprolactinemia serum generates two peaks consistent with both monomeric prolactin (23 kDa) and macroprolactin (150 kDa) being present.

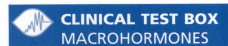

CLINICAL TEST BOX
MACROHORMONES

Macrohormones are hormones bound to immunoglobulin in a circulating complex that may still be detected by hormone assay. Macrocomplexes have been described for many hormones, including LH, FSH, TSH, hCG, and insulin, although **macroprolactin** is the best characterized. Size separation of prolactin species using gel filtration chromatography (Fig. 27.13) has shown three prolactin forms: monomeric (MW 23 kDa), big (MW 50–60 kDa), and big-big (>150 kDa). Where there are normal concentrations of bioactive monomeric prolactin, increased concentrations of big-big prolactin that give rise to hyperprolactinemia is termed "macroprolactinemia," and it has been reported in up to one in four patients with hyperprolactinemia. It is important to identify macroprolactin to avoid overinvestigation and even misdiagnosis of patients with a reported raised serum prolactin concentration. Laboratory techniques currently used to screen for hormone–antibody complexes include immunoprecipitation with polyethylene glycol, which works by volume exclusion and precipitation of the complexes once protein solubility is exceeded.

ADVANCED CONCEPT BOX
NONCLASSIC ENDOCRINE ORGANS

Apart from classic ductless endocrine glands, many tissues are now known to be active endocrinologically (termed "nonclassic" because hormone production is not their primary function). New understanding of these hormones has helped to explain certain physiologic and pathologic processes, and measurement of these hormones can help clinical diagnosis of certain conditions. Examples of nonclassic endocrine hormones include the following: (1) the production of **leptin** from white adipose tissue and leptin released from the stomach, which together play a role in the control system for energy balance in humans (Chapter 32); (2) the production of **fibroblast growth factor (FGF-23)** by osteocytes (which decreases the renal reabsorption and increases excretion of phosphate) - mutations in the FGF-23 gene can lead to increased activity, and FGF-23 may be produced ectopically by some tumors resulting in hypophosphatemia; (3) the production of **hCG** by the developing placenta, along with progesterone, placental growth hormone, and human placental lactogen, which have defined roles in pregnancy; (4) production of **brain natriuretic peptide (BNP)** by cardiac ventricles in humans, which acts to decrease systemic vascular resistance - BNP and its prohormone, NT-proBNP, are measured in the diagnosis and assessment of severity of heart failure; and (5) the production of **glucagon-like peptide-1 (GLP-1)**, which decreases blood glucose in a glucose-dependent manner by enhancing insulin secretion by intestinal enteroendocrine L-cells.

ACTIVE LEARNING

1. Trace the two-way flow of signaling between the hypothalamus and the ovaries during the menstrual cycle, and describe how the female hormones change during pregnancy.
2. Describe how GH, cortisol, and insulin interact to regulate lipid and carbohydrate metabolism.

endocrine gland (primary) or from hypo-/hyperfunction of the pituitary (secondary).

■ Laboratory diagnosis of endocrine disorders depends on the measurement of hormones, and secretion of hormones can be pulsatile (e.g., growth hormone), circadian (e.g., cortisol, testosterone), or infradian (rhythms over periods longer than 24 h, e.g., FSH, LH), thus limiting the utility of "random" sampling; careful attention must often be paid to the timing of the sample, and it is preferable, and sometimes necessary, to use an appropriate provocation test for which action limits are available.

Thus the reader is referred to Chapter 31 for **carbohydrate homeostasis** and to Chapter 35 for **water and electrolyte balance and the control of blood pressure.** The intracellular systems through which hormones exert their effects are described in Chapter 25.

SUMMARY

■ The endocrine system is a collection of glands that produces hormones, a structurally diverse group of chemical messengers that regulate and coordinate whole-body metabolism, growth, reproduction, and responses to external stimuli.
■ The hypothalamo–anterior–pituitary axis is a critical link between the brain and endocrine glands and orchestrates the synthesis and action of thyroid hormones, glucocorticoids, sex steroids, growth hormone, and prolactin.
■ Feedback mechanisms are an important regulator of endocrine systems, and both overactivity and underactivity of these systems can produce clinical syndromes; measurement of blood levels of target and pituitary hormones can help determine whether endocrine dysfunction originates from a peripheral

FURTHER READING

Antonelli, A., Ferrari, S. M., Corrado, A., et al. (2015). Autoimmune thyroid disorders. *Autoimmunity Reviews, 14,* 174–180.

Bodnar, T. W., Acevedo, M. J., & Pietropaolo, M. (2014). Management of non-islet-cell tumor hypoglycemia: A clinical review. *The Journal of Clinical Endocrinology and Metabolism, 99*(3), 713–722.

Brandão Neto, R. A., & de Carvalho, J. F. (2014). Diagnosis and classification of Addison's disease (autoimmune adrenalitis). *Autoimmunity Reviews, 13,* 408–411.

Chaker, L., Bianco, A. C., Jonklaas, J., et al. (2017). Hypothyroidism. *Lancet.* doi:10.1016/S0140-6736(17)30703-1, pii: S0140-6736(17)30703-1.2017. (Epub ahead of print).

Clemmons, D. R. (2010). Clinical laboratory indices in the treatment of acromegaly. *Clinica Chimica Acta, 412,* 403–409.

Cooper, D. S., & Biondi, B. (2012). Subclinical thyroid disease. *Lancet, 379,* 1142–1154.

De Leo, S., Lee, S. Y., & Braverman, L. E. (2016). Hyperthyroidism. *Lancet, 388,* 906–918.

Fahie-Wilson, M., & Smith, T. P. (2013). Determination of prolactin: The macroprolactin problem. *Best Practice and Research. Clinical Endocrinology and Metabolism, 27,* 725–742.

Henderson, J. (2005). Ernest Starling and 'Hormones': An historical commentary. *The Journal of Endocrinology, 184,* 5–10.

Higham, C. E., Johannsson, G., & Shalet, S. M. (2016). Hypopituitarism. *Lancet, 388,* 2403–2415.

Höybye, C. & Christiansen, J. S. (2015). Growth hormone replacement in adults: Current standards and new perspectives. *Best Practice and Research. Clinical Endocrinology and Metabolism, 29,* 115–123.

Koulouri, O., Moran, C., Halsall, D., et al. (2013). Pitfalls in the measurement and interpretation of thyroid function tests. *Best Practice and Research. Clinical Endocrinology and Metabolism, 27,* 745–762.

Loriaux, D. L. (2017). Diagnosis and differential diagnosis of Cushing's syndrome. *The New England Journal of Medicine, 376,* 1451–1459.

Melmed, S. (2006). Medical progress: Acromegaly. *The New England Journal of Medicine, 355,* 2558–2573.

Melmed, S., Casanueva, F. F., Hoffman, A. R., et al. (2011). Diagnosis and treatment of hyperprolactinemia: An Endocrine Society clinical practice guideline. *The Journal of Clinical Endocrinology and Metabolism, 96,* 273–288.

Molitch, M. E. (2017). Diagnosis and treatment of pituitary adenomas: A review. *JAMA: The Journal of the American Medical Association, 317,* 516–524.

Schoenmakers, N., Alatzoglou, K. S., Chatterjee, V. K., et al. (2015). Recent advances in central congenital hypothyroidism. *The Journal of Endocrinology, 227,* R51–R57.

Semple, R. K., & Topaloglu, A. K. (2010). The recent genetics of hypogonadotrophic hypogonadism: Novel insights and new questions. *Clinical Endocrinology, 72,* 427–435.

Smith, T. J., & Hegedüs, L. (2016). Graves' disease. *The New England Journal of Medicine, 375,* 1552–1565.

Vilar, L., Vilar, C. F., Lyra, R., et al. (2017). Acromegaly: Clinical features at diagnosis. *Pituitary, 20,* 22–32.

RELEVANT WEBSITES

Cushing's Support & Research Association: http://www.CSRF.net
Endotext: http://www.endotext.org
National Institute of Diabetes and Digestive and Kidney Diseases:
     http://www.endocrine.niddk.nih.gov/
Pituitary Network Association: http://www.pituitary.org
The Endocrine Society: http://www.endocrine.org/
Thyroid disease manager: http://www.thyroidmanager.org

MORE CLINICAL CASES

Please refer to Appendix 2 for more cases relevant to this chapter.

ABBREVIATIONS

α-βA	Inhibin A
α-Bb	Inhibin B
ACTH	Adrenocorticotropic hormone
ADH	Antidiuretic hormone
AVP	Arginine vasopressin
CAH	Congenital adrenal hyperplasia
cAMP	Adenosine 3′,5′-cyclic monophosphate
CBG	Cortisol-binding globulin (also known as transcortin)
CRH	Corticotropin-releasing hormone
CT	Computerized tomography
DHEA	Dehydroepiandrosterone
DHEAS	Dehydroepiandrosterone sulfate
DHT	Dihydrotestosterone
DIT	Diiodotyrosine
fT3 and fT4	Free T3 and free T4
GH	Growth hormone
GHRH	Growth hormone–releasing hormone
GnRH	Gonadotropin-releasing hormone
hCG	Human chorionic gonadotropin
hGH	Human growth hormone
hCS-A, hCS-B, hCS-L, and hGH-V	Human somatomammotropin (GH) genes
IGF-1	Insulin-like growth factor-1
IGFBP	IGF-binding proteins
LH	Luteinizing hormone
MIT	Monoiodotyrosine
MS	Mass spectrometry
MRI	Magnetic resonance imaging
MSH	Melanocyte stimulating hormone
17-OHP	17-hydroxyprogesterone
OGTT	Oral glucose tolerance test
ONDST	Overnight dexamethasone suppression test
POMC	Pro-opiomelanocortin
rT3	Reverse T3
SHBG	Sex hormone–binding globulin
T3	Triiodothyronine
T4	Thyroxine
Tg	Thyroglobulin
THRB	Thyroid hormone receptor beta gene
TPO	Thyroid peroxidase
TRH	Thyrotropin-releasing hormone
TSH	Thyroid-stimulating hormone
UFC	24-h urine free cortisol
VP	Vasopressin
ZF	Zona fasciculata
ZG	Zona glomerulosa
ZR	Zona reticularis

Cellular Homeostasis: Cell Growth and Cancer

Alison M. Michie, Verica Paunovic, and Margaret M. Harnett

LEARNING OBJECTIVES

After reading this chapter, you should be able to:

- Define the stages of the mammalian cell cycle.
- Outline how the cell cycle is regulated by cyclins and cyclin-dependent kinases.
- Describe the molecular events that enable growth factors to regulate cellular proliferation.
- Discuss different mechanisms that enable cells to cease proliferation or die.
- Explain the cellular and molecular events that define apoptosis and autophagy.
- Outline some experimental techniques that enable elucidation of cellular growth, proliferation, and death.
- Explain how subversion of normal physiologic growth can lead to the development of tumors.
- Distinguish between oncogenes and tumor-suppressor genes, and describe their role in tumor progression/suppression.

INTRODUCTION

Development and survival of multicellular organisms such as human beings are reliant on the appropriate regulation of growth, differentiation, and death of individual cell types to maintain the integrity of the organism

Although cells have evolved a complex program of control mechanisms to deter replication of damaged cells and to enable repair, if the growth control mechanisms become damaged, this can lead to the development of cancer. The majority of cells in an adult are not dividing. However, under certain conditions, such as tissue repair and senescence, regulated growth and proliferation are promoted. Thus, as cells die, either by senescence or as a result of tissue damage, they must be replaced in a strictly regulated manner. Cellular homeostasis maintains organ integrity through controlled cell survival, proliferation, and cell death to ensure that healthy cells, unlike cancerous (transformed) cells, generally stop dividing when they contact neighboring cells.

Research in transformed cancerous cells has highlighted important mechanisms that regulate cellular growth and cell division in normal cells

Through investigation of genetic alterations in cancer cells, it has been possible to identify a large number of genes that are critical for the regulation of normal cell proliferation. It is perhaps unsurprising to find that molecular mechanisms that favor cell survival and proliferation processes are commonly upregulated in human cancers. Mutated proliferative genes are called **oncogenes** (cancer-causing genes), the normal cellular counterparts of which are called **protooncogenes.** Protooncogenes are predominantly signal transducers that act to regulate normal cell growth and division; aberrant regulation of these processes leads to cellular transformation. Conversely, the proteins involved in suppressing proliferation, or **tumor-suppressor genes**, are generally inhibited during oncogenesis, leading to uncontrolled proliferation. Exploring the role of these proteins under normal physiologic conditions can assist in the understanding of how they can be subverted when they become dysregulated during oncogenesis.

CELL CYCLE

Individual cells multiply by duplicating their contents and then dividing into two daughter cells

Cell division is tightly controlled by a complex mechanism known as cell cycle. The duration of cell cycle varies between organisms as well as between cell types within a single organism. In mammals, for example, it can last from minutes to years. However, in immortalized cell lines, which are widely used as experimental model systems, one round of cell cycle is typically completed within 24 h.

In recent years, extensive research of the cell cycle has defined a number of key control points

Traditionally, the cell cycle is divided into several phases (Fig. 28.1). **Mitosis (M phase)** is the stage of cell division, which is usually completed within an hour. The remainder of the cell cycle, during which cells prepare for division and duplicate DNA, is referred to as **interphase.** Nuclear DNA replication occurs in the **synthesis (S) phase** of interphase. The period between M and S phase is called **G1 phase,** and the interval between S and M phase is called **G2 phase.** During G1 and G2 phases, cells use several checkpoints to ensure that

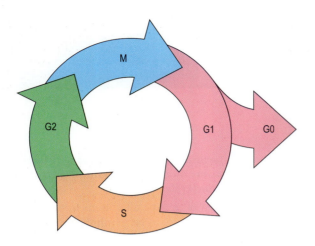

Fig. 28.1 **The phases of the cell cycle.** The cell cycle is divided into interphase and mitotic phase. In interphase, composed of G1, S, and G2 phases, cells grow, prepare for division, and duplicate their DNA. Mitosis is the stage of cell division into two daughter cells. M, mitosis; S, synthetic phase of interphase; G1, interval between M and S phases; G2, interval between S and M phases; G0, resting, or quiescent, phase.

appropriate cellular growth and accurate DNA synthesis occur before cell division, thus preventing the incorporation of mutated DNA into daughter cells. The duration of an individual cell cycle varies enormously, and most of this variability can be attributed to the different length of the G1 phase. This is due to the fact that some cells, which are not stimulated to duplicate their DNA, can enter into the specialized form of G1 phase, called **G0 phase**.

The G0 phase is a form of the resting state, or quiescence, in which cells reside until they receive appropriate signals - for example, from growth factors - stimulating them to re-enter and progress through the cell cycle

In mammals, the time required for a cell to transit from the beginning of S phase through mitosis is typically 12–24 h, irrespective of the duration of G1 phase. Thus, the majority of variation in proliferation rates observed between different cell types is due to the amount of time spent in the G0/G1 phase. In conditions that favor cell growth, the total ribonucleic acid (RNA) and protein content of the cell increases continuously, except in M phase, when the chromosomes are too condensed to enable transcription to occur.

Of note, the majority of cells in the human body have either irreversibly withdrawn from the cell cycle into a terminally differentiated state (neurons, myocytes, or surface epithelial cells of skin and mucosa) or are in the reversible quiescent G0 phase (stem cells, glial cells, hepatocytes, or thyroid follicular cells). Only a minority of cells are normally actively cycling, and these cells are located mainly in the stem/transit compartments of self-renewing tissues, which include the bone marrow and epithelia.

REGULATION OF CELL PROLIFERATION AND GROWTH: GROWTH FACTORS

Cells of a multicellular organism have to receive positive signals in order to grow and divide

Many of these signals are in the form of **polypeptide hormones** (e.g., insulin), **growth factors** (e.g., epidermal growth factor [EGF]), or **cytokines** (e.g., interleukins IL-1 to IL-36). These growth factors bind to specific cell-surface receptors, initiating an intricate network of intracellular signaling cascades that counteract negative regulatory controls present in resting cells to block cell-cycle progression and division.

In most cell types, proliferation is controlled by signals generated from a specific combination of growth factors rather than stimulation by a single growth factor

In this way, a relatively small number of growth factors can selectively regulate the proliferation of many cell types. In addition, some of the factors may induce cell growth without providing a signal for division. Indeed, neurons in the G0 phase of the cell cycle grow very large without dividing. Although proliferating cells can stop growing when they are deprived of growth factors, they progress through the cell cycle until they reach the point in the G1 phase at which they can enter G0 phase (the resting state) or undergo senescence.

Growth factors bind to specific cell-surface receptors

Growth factors bind to specific cell-surface receptors expressed on effector cells, which are generally transmembrane proteins with a growth factor (or ligand)–binding domain and cytoplasmic protein tyrosine kinase (PTK) domain (see also Chapter 25). There are about 50 known growth factors, of which platelet-derived growth factor (PDGF) was the first identified. The growth and proliferative responses associated with PDGF binding are prototypic for many growth factors, and these responses include the following:

- Immediate increase in intracellular Ca^{2+} levels - indicating the initiation of transmembrane signaling.
- Reorganization of actin stress fibers - to comply with anchorage dependence of cell attachment, a requirement for cell cycle progression.
- Activation and/or nuclear translocation of transcription factors that bind to regulatory regions of the DNA that encode genes responsive to a specific growth factor. These genes are referred to as **immediate early genes**, which usually code for transcription factors themselves that mediate expression of components of the cell-cycle machinery, such as cyclins.
- DNA synthesis and cell division.

Growth factors selectively initiate signaling cascades

Individual growth factors activate distinct cohorts of signaling molecules and transcription factors that in turn induce a unique

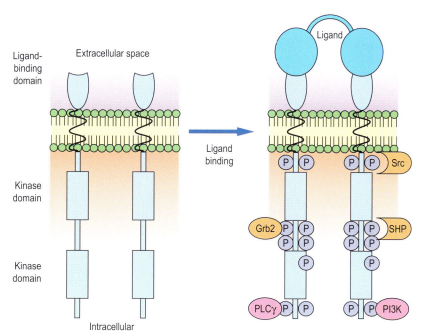

Fig. 28.2 **Activation of growth factor receptors by ligand binding and recruitment of signaling molecules.** The binding of growth factors such as PDGF and EGF to their receptors causes receptor dimerization and activation of the tyrosine kinase, intrinsic to the receptor cytoplasmic domains. This leads to tyrosine phosphorylation of the dimerized receptors at specific sites within the cytoplasmic domains by the process of transphosphorylation. The phosphorylation events create docking sites that enable protein–protein interactions between the receptor and downstream signaling components such as PLC-γ, protein tyrosine kinase Src, tyrosine phosphatase SHP, PI3K, and adapter molecules like Grb2, which, in the latter case, in turn recruits the Ras/MAPK pathway. PLC-γ, phospholipase Cγ; PI3K, phosphatidylinositol 3-kinase; Grb2, growth factor receptor–bound protein 2; SHP, SH2 domain-containing phosphatase.

repertoire of gene expression. In this way, specific growth factors initiate characteristic differential responses that have a unique impact on cell behavior (see also Chapter 25).

Growth factors selectively initiate signaling cascades by binding to their receptors

The binding to a receptor causes receptor dimerization or oligomerization and activation of the intracellular tyrosine kinase domain, which in turn mediates receptor transphosphorylation at specific amino acids within the cytoplasmic domain. The phosphorylated region of the receptor is then able to act as a **"docking site"** for the binding of specific transducer proteins, thus enabling protein–protein interactions (Fig. 28.2). This in turn leads to the recruitment and activation of additional signaling molecules such as enzymes and **adapter molecules,** which mediate the propagation of the intracellular signaling cascade from the surface of plasma membrane inside the cell. Transphosphorylation of receptor cytoplasmic domains creates a **scaffold for binding of signal transduction elements** such as phospholipase Cγ(PLC-γ), GTPase-activating proteins (GAP), nonreceptor PTKs (designated Src, Fyn, Abl), phosphotyrosine phosphatases (PTPases), and adapter molecules (Shc, Grb2) via their phosphotyrosine recognition domains.

Epidermal growth factor receptor (EGFR) signaling

Upon ligand binding, the EGFR activates signals through Ras/Raf/MAPK- and PI3K/Akt/mTor-mediated signaling cascades

EGFR can be bound and activated by a number of ligands, including EGF and transforming growth factor-α (TGF-α).

Ligation of the EGFR leads to the recruitment and activation of the *Src* family of PTKs, which catalyze phosphorylation of PLC-γ, leading to the activation of this enzyme. Activated PLC-γ then catalyzes the hydrolysis of phosphatidylinositol 4,5-bisphosphate (PIP$_2$) to generate the intracellular second messengers inositol 1,4,5-trisphosphate (IP$_3$) and diacylglycerol (DAG). IP$_3$ stimulates the release of Ca^{2+} from intracellular stores (mainly endoplasmic reticulum [ER]), and DAG activates members of an important signal transducer family of proteins, the protein kinase C (PKC) family. Ligation of the EGFR also induces activation of a lipid-modifying enzyme, phosphatidylinositol 3-kinase (PI3K). This enzyme mediates phosphorylation of PIP$_2$, generating the lipid second messenger phosphatidylinositol 3,4,5-trisphosphate (PIP$_3$), which can also contribute to the activation of selected members of the PKC family (Fig. 28.3). Moreover, PIP$_3$ can activate another kinase referred to as PIP$_3$-dependent kinase (PDK1) or serve as a docking site for proteins that contain pleckstrin homology (PH) domains.

Signaling cascade involving Ras GTPase is important in regulating cell division

A quarter of all tumors have constitutively active mutations in the signaling component Ras, which is critical for the transmission of proliferation and differentiation signals from the extracellular receptors to the nucleus. Ras, a GTPase, is constitutively attached to the plasma membrane via a post-translational modification involving the addition of a lipophilic farnesyl group. Ligation of the EGFR recruits Ras by its binding to the adaptor protein Grb2. Ras cycles between an active GTP-bound and inactive GDP-bound form (Fig. 28.3). Its intrinsic catalytic activity is low, and it is enhanced by binding to a GTPase-activating protein (GAP). GDP/GTP exchange is

✦ ADVANCED CONCEPT BOX
PROTEIN TYROSINE KINASES

Role in Signal Transduction

Protein tyrosine kinases (PTK) are enzymes that transfer the γ-phosphate group of ATP to tyrosine residues on target substrate proteins. The term *protein tyrosine kinase* is a generic term for a large superfamily of enzymes that includes both transmembrane-spanning receptors with an intrinsic tyrosine kinase activity in their cytoplasmic domains (e.g., some growth factor receptors) and a wide range of nonreceptor or cytoplasmic tyrosine kinase subfamilies, such as the Src, Abl, Syk, Tec, or Janus kinase (JAK) families (see also Chapter 25).

Tyrosine phosphorylation is a covalent modification that provides a rapid and reversible (by the action of protein tyrosine phosphatases) mechanism of changing the enzymatic activity of target proteins or modifying these proteins so that they can act as adapters to recruit other signaling molecules.

For example, tyrosine phosphorylation of receptors or signaling molecules creates "docking sites" that enable protein–protein interactions via specific domains, such as those referred to as SH2 domains of other signaling transducers. SH2 stands for Src-homology region 2, from the cytoplasmic Src tyrosine kinase, in which this domain was first characterized. SH2 domains contain approximately 100 amino acids and specifically recognize a phosphotyrosine in the context of the three amino acids immediately C-terminal to that phosphotyrosine.

Role in the Regulation of Cellular Proliferation, Survival, and Differentiation

PTKs play a critical role in the regulation of cellular proliferation, survival, and differentiation, and the importance of these regulatory events is highlighted by the defects that are observed upon dysregulation of genes encoding PTKs. Indeed, dysregulated expression of growth factor receptors carrying intrinsic PTK activity can lead to the constitutive activation of the Ras/Raf/MEK/ERK and Ras/PI3K/Akt/mTor signaling pathways, leading to enhanced cell growth, survival, and proliferation and a subversion of molecular events that regulate apoptosis, events that are dysregulated in cancer. Mutations have been identified in PDGFR, EGFR, and in other receptor tyrosine kinases such as c-Kit and Flt3 in specific cancer types. Indeed, **mutations in the EGFR family of receptors are responsible for 30% of all epithelial cancers, including lung and brain cancers.**

Nonreceptor tyrosine kinases also play critical roles in cellular responses, with mutations leading to a loss in kinase activity, resulting in serious **abnormalities in B- and T-lymphocyte development**. For example, loss of expression/activity of ZAP-70, a PTK that is essential for antigen-dependent T-cell activation, can lead to **severe combined immunodeficiency (SCID)** due to a lack of T-cell effector function during an immune challenge. Similarly, **X-linked agammaglobulinemia**, an immunodeficiency caused by a lack of IgG antibody production, occurs as a result of loss-of-function mutations of Btk, a PTK that is important for B-cell effector functions.

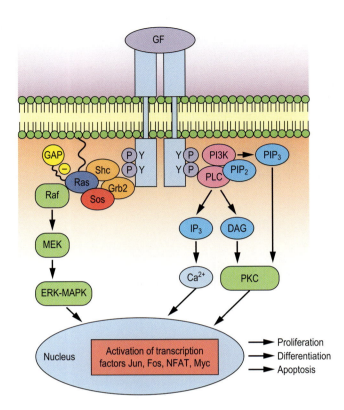

Fig. 28.3 Activation of the Ras–ERK–MAPK and PKC signaling cascades upon growth factor binding. Growth factor signals activated at the plasma membrane as a result of ligand binding can regulate gene transcription, cell-cycle progression, proliferation, differentiation, or apoptosis. Growth factor receptor signals activate signals to recruit the adapter molecules such as Grb2 and Shc, which in turn lead to the activation of ERK–MAPK and PI3K/Akt and PKC pathways. Ras is anchored in the plasma membrane and recruited to the activated growth factor receptor via interaction with the Grb2–Sos complex. Receptor-stimulated GTP/GDP exchange, required for Ras activation, is promoted by Sos, whereas GAP inactivates Ras by stimulating its intrinsic GTPase activity. Ras couples growth factor receptors to the MAPK signaling cascade via stimulation of the intermediary kinases Raf and MEK. MAPK translocates into the nucleus and phosphorylates key transcription factors involved in the regulation of DNA synthesis and cell division, such as Jun and Fos (which dimerize to form AP1), NFAT, and Myc. These regulate the induction of components of the cell cycle machinery that controls cell-cycle progression and identify the need for DNA repair. If DNA damage is detected, the cell cycle is arrested, and if the damage is too great, then apoptosis is induced. GF, growth factor; DAG, diacylglycerol; GAP, GTPase-activating protein; IP_3, inositol 1,4,5-trisphosphate; MAPK, mitogen-activated protein kinase; PI3K, phosphatidylinositol 3-kinase; PIP_2, phosphoinositol 4,5-bisphosphate; PIP_3, phosphoinositol 3,4,5-trisphosphate; PKC, protein kinase C; PLC, phospholipase C; Shc, Src homology and collagen domain protein; Sos, Son of Sevenless.

promoted by binding to a guanine nucleotide exchange factor, called Sos, which returns Ras to an active state. One of the main functions of active Ras is to act as an allosteric regulator of the mitogen-activated protein kinase (MAPK) signaling cascade. Ras transduces signals from EGFR via activation of two intermediary kinases, Raf and MEK kinase. MEK is a kinase that activates MAPK, specifically the two isoforms extracellular-signal regulated kinase (ERK) 1 and 2, by mediating dual-specificity phosphorylation of tyrosine and threonine residues within their Thr-Glu-Tyr (TEY) activation motif. Upon activation, they translocate into the nucleus and phosphorylate (on serine and threonine) key transcription factors responsible for regulating genes controlling DNA synthesis and cell division (Fig. 28.3; compare this to the insulin signaling described in Chapter 31).

mTORC-1 and mTORC-2 complexes integrate mitogen and nutrient signals

In addition to regulating selective members of the PKC family, PI3K is also responsible for activating PDK1, which in turn activates Akt. This enzyme mediates the activity of mechanistic target of rapamycin (mTor), a serine/threonine protein kinase. mTor can participate in two distinct signaling complexes, mTORC-1 and mTORC-2, integrating mitogen and nutrient signals to promote cell survival, growth, and proliferation. PI3K/Akt activation by receptor ligation leads to phosphorylation of the tuberous sclerosis protein 1/2 (TSC1/2), resulting in mTORC-1 activation. The best-characterized downstream effectors of mTORC-1 are translational regulators within the protein synthesis pathway, initiation factor 4E (eIF4E)-binding protein 1 (4E-BP1), and ribosomal S6 kinase 1 (S6K1), which are stimulated by mTORC1-mediated phosphorylation (Fig. 28.4).

Although the signaling pathways just described are linear, a significant amount of cross-talk occurs among these cascade elements

For example, the ERK-MAPK signaling cascade is capable of regulating mTORC-1 by activating the kinase RSK1, which in turn phosphorylates and inhibits TSC1/2, thus resulting in activation of mTORC-1. Examples such as this illustrate the complexity that exists in intracellular signaling pathways downstream of receptors. Indeed, cross-talk highlights how a mutation in a single signaling component can impact a wide array of biological responses within a single cell.

Cytokine receptor signaling

Cytokines are growth factors that mainly coordinate the development of hematopoietic cells and the immune response, although they also have multiple effects on non-hematopoietic cell types

Similar to growth factors, cytokines also exert their effects on cells by binding to cellsurface receptors. There are multiple classes of cytokine receptors, of which many belong to the **hematopoietic receptor** superfamily. These are transmembrane glycoprotein receptors, characterized by conserved

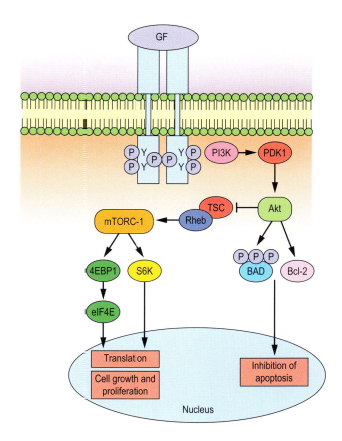

Fig. 28.4 **Growth factor stimulation of mTor signaling.** Growth factor signals activated at the plasma membrane as a result of ligand binding can result in the recruitment of PI3K, thus activating PDK1/Akt, which enhances protein synthesis via mTOR (which is the catalytic subunit of the mTORC-1 protein complex shown), thereby contributing to cell cycle progression. It also inhibits apoptosis by increasing the expression of cyclins and antiapoptotic Bcl-2 family members. In addition, Akt inhibits apoptosis by mediating hyperphosphorylation of proapoptotic BAD, leading to the stabilization of mitochondria. See text for more details. GF, growth factor; PI3K, phosphatidylinositol 3-kinase; PDK1, PIP$_3$-dependent kinase; mTOR, mechanistic target of rapamycin; BAD, Bcl-2-associated death promoter; TSC, tuberous sclerosis complex; Rheb, Ras homologue enriched in brain; eIF4E, eukaryotic initiation factor 4E; S6K1, ribosomal S6 kinase 1; 4E-BP1, eIF4E-binding protein 1.

extracellular ligand-binding domains, which contain characteristic cysteine pairs and a pentapeptide motif WSXWS (tryptophan-serine-X-tryptophan-serine, where X is any amino acid). Many consist of multisubunit receptors that contain a unique ligand-binding subunit that gives specificity, along with a common signal transducer subunit that is often shared by several related cytokines. Sharing of the signal-transducing subunit gives the basis for classification of cytokines into distinct subfamilies and helps explain the severe immunodeficiencies that result from naturally occurring defects in these receptors.

Janus kinases (JAK) link the hematopoietic receptors with the downstream signaling and gene transcription

In contrast to growth factor receptors, **cytokine receptors do not possess an intrinsic catalytic activity.** However, members of a family of cytosolic PTKs, called Janus kinases (JAK), are essential for linking the hematopoietic receptors with the downstream signaling and gene transcription. Thus, after ligand engagement with the receptor, JAKs associate with the receptors by binding to the conserved regions near the transmembrane domain. Upon cytokine binding, which causes receptor oligomerization, JAKs become phosphorylated and activated to mediate phosphorylation of their downstream targets, which are transcription factors called signal transducer and activators (STATs; Fig. 28.5). In unstimulated cells, STATs are found in the cytoplasm in monomeric forms. Cytokine stimulation leads to JAK-mediated STAT phosphorylation and dimerization. STAT dimers then translocate to the nucleus, where they mediate transcription of the target genes by binding to their specific DNA sequences. Recently, growth factors such as EGF and PDGF have also been shown to induce activation of JAK/STAT pathways; therefore **JAK/STAT signaling may be a universal mechanism utilized by growth factors to regulate gene induction and cellular responses.** Moreover, most cytokines, in common with classic growth factors, can signal through PLC, PI3K, and Ras-MAPK signaling cascades.

The finding that mutation of a JAK family member, JAK3, resulted in **severe combined immunodeficiency (SCID)** suggested that JAK3 may be a good therapeutic target for the development of novel immunosuppressants. Indeed, the JAK3 inhibitor tofacitinib is used as an immunosuppressant to prevent **organ transplant rejection** as well as autoimmune diseases such as **psoriasis, psoriatic arthritis, inflammatory bowel syndrome,** and **rheumatoid arthritis.** Moreover, JAK3 inhibitors are potential **antitumor therapeutics** for cancers exhibiting increased JAK3 activity, such as **acute myeloid leukemia (AML)** and **colorectal** and **lung cancers.**

REGULATION OF THE CELL CYCLE

Cyclin-dependent kinase (CDK) family and cyclins regulate cell-cycle transition points

As cells progress through the cell cycle in response to growth factor stimulation, they must pass through three switch-like transition/restriction points, positioned at the G1/S phase boundary and at the entry and exit of M phase. Master regulators of these transition points include members of the cyclin-dependent kinase (CDK) family of serine/threonine kinases and a family of proteins known as cyclins.

CDKs are expressed as heterodimers comprising a protein kinase subunit and a regulatory cyclin subunit. Their activity is tightly regulated by different mechanisms, including the phosphorylation status of the kinase subunit, levels of cyclins, and/or interaction with inhibitory proteins (CDKI) that block their catalytic activity. Whereas CDK expression levels are relatively constant throughout the cell cycle, the expression levels of cyclins are strictly controlled at both the mRNA and protein level (transcriptional and translational control). Indeed, cyclins were originally defined as proteins that were specifically degraded during every mitosis.

The traditional model of the cell cycle states that a specific cyclin–CDK partner drives distinct parts of the cell cycle: D-type cyclins and CDK4/6 regulate the events in early G1 phase, cyclin E-CDK2 triggers S phase, cyclin A-CDK2 and cyclin A-CDK1 regulate the completion of the S phase, and cyclin B-CDK1 controls mitosis (Fig. 28.6).

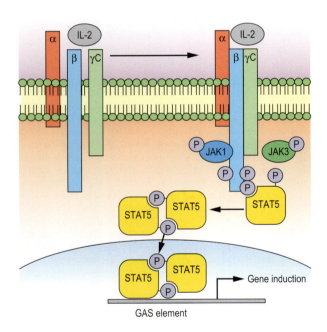

Fig. 28.5 **Cytokine receptor signaling: IL-2 receptor.** The receptor is composed of the IL-2 receptor α-chain (IL-2Rα), IL-2/15Rβ, and the common cytokine-receptor γ-chain (γc). Binding of IL-2 to the α-subunit causes association of this subunit with β- and γ-subunits, thus forming a stable heterotrimer. JAK molecules associate with β-subunit (JAK1) and γc-subunit (JAK3) and phosphorylate themselves and key tyrosine residues within β- and γc-intracellular domains, thus enabling STAT5 recruitment and phosphorylation. Phosphorylated STAT5 molecules dissociate from the receptors and form dimers, which rapidly translocate into the nucleus and act as transcription factors, binding to GAS elements. Different JAKs and STATs can be utilized to achieve the specific response of individual cytokines. These pathways control transcription, cell growth, proliferation, and survival. JAK, Janus kinase; STAT, signal transducer and activator of transcription; GAS, gamma interferon activation site.

Mitogenesis

Mitogenic signals activated by growth factors exert their effects between the onset of the G1 phase and a point late in the G1 phase, called the restriction point

The key event for initiation of the cell cycle in the G1 phase is the phosphorylation of **retinoblastoma protein** (Rb) at various residues. Rb controls the expression of genes that commit cells that have reached restriction point late in the G1 phase to enter the S phase (DNA synthesis) of the cell cycle. In

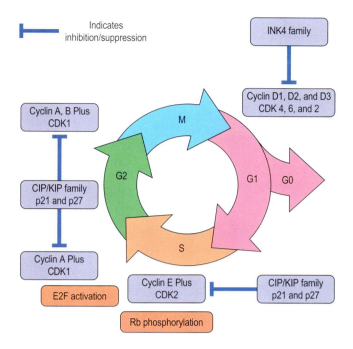

Fig. 28.6 **Regulation of cell-cycle phases.** The cell cycle is divided into interphase and mitotic phase. In interphase, composed of G1, S, and G2 phases, cells grow, prepare for division, and duplicate their DNA. Mitosis is the stage of cell division into two daughter cells. Progression through the cell cycle is regulated by interplay between specific cyclin–CDK partners and their inhibitors. Cyclin expression, particularly of those controlling G1 and S phase, is regulated by growth factor signaling. INK4 family members inhibit cyclin D–specific CDKs (CDK4 and 6), whereas the CIP/KIP family inhibits all CDKs. M, mitosis; S, synthetic phase of interphase; G1, interval between M and S phases; G2, interval between S and M phases; G0, resting, or quiescent, phase; CDK, cyclin-dependent kinase; CDKI, CDK inhibitor; E2F, transcription factor; Rb, retinoblastoma protein; INK4, inhibitors of CDK4 family.

the early G1 phase, Rb molecules are in a hypophosphorylated state. This allows them to bind and repress the DNA-binding activity of the main regulators of the G1/S phase transition, members of E2F family of transcription factors, thus inhibiting cell cycle progression (Fig. 28.6). Additional molecules that play an important role at this stage are **histone deacetylases** and **chromatin remodeling complexes** that epigenetically regulate gene transcription. Stimulation with growth factors and/or mitogens affects the entry into the cell cycle by triggering the expression and/or activation of **protooncogenes,** such as *Ras* and *Myc*, which results in the induction of expression of cyclins from the D-type family (D1, D2, and/or D3), followed by the cyclins from E-type family (E1 and E2). The D-type cyclins partner with CDK4/6 and stimulate their activity, whereas E-type cyclins increase the kinase activity of CDK2. These cyclin-CDK partners modulate the phosphorylation state of Rb by converting it from the hypophosphorylated to the hyperphosphorylated state, thus inactivating Rb and promoting the release of E2F from the Rb inhibitory complex. Free E2F proteins mediate gene transcription, the products of which are important for entry into the S phase and beyond, such

Pioneering studies assessing cells at different stages of the cell cycle using classical biochemical approaches, such as overexpression of kinase-dead CDK mutants and selective pharmacologic CDK inhibitors, revealed the preferred cyclin–CDK partners, leading to the formulation of the traditional model of the cell cycle. However, results from recent genetic studies employing specific deletions of cyclins and CDKs in mice and yeast indicate that this model should be revised. Mouse embryos are viable in the absence of CDK2, CDK4, or CDK6, indicating that these CDKs have redundant functions and are dispensable for controlling cell proliferation. The absence of these CDKs, however, affects the proliferation and/or differentiation of some specific cell types:

- CDK2 knockout mice survive to up to 2 years of age, but they are sterile, indicating an absolute requirement for CDK2 during meiosis.
- CDK4 controls proliferation/differentiation of pancreatic β-cells, and pituitary hormone–producing cells.
- CDK6 regulates proliferation/differentiation of some hematopoietic cells.
- CDK1 is essential for driving the cell cycle in most cell types, at least until halfway through gestation.

From these studies, a new model has emerged, referred to as the **minimal threshold model.** In this model, either CDK1 or CDK2 coupled with cyclin A or E is sufficient to control interphase, whereas CDK1 coupled with cyclin B drives cells into mitosis. The differences in activity of the same cyclin–CDK complexes in interphase and mitosis may be attributed not only to the substrate specificity but also to the different localization within the cell and higher activity threshold for mitosis than for interphase. In addition to being regulated by binding of cyclins, CDK activation is also modulated by phosphorylation. CDK-activating complex (CAK), composed of CDK7, cyclin H, and MAT1 (ménage a trois), mediates phosphorylation/activation of CDK1, CDK2, CDK4, and CDK6 when bound to their cyclin partners. Moreover, CAK plays a role in gene transcription as a part of TFIIH, which is a general transcription factor. In this context, CAK phosphorylates the RNA polymerase I large subunit C-terminal domain (CTD). This event is part of the process of promoter clearance and progression from the preinitiation to the initiation phase of transcription.

as A- and B-type cyclins (Fig. 28.6). From this point onward, cell-cycle progression is independent of growth factors.

When E-type cyclins are degraded, CDK2 binds to the A-type cyclins, and these complexes phosphorylate many protein targets necessary for the proper completion and exit from the S phase. At the end of the S phase, A-type cyclins also associate with CDK1, and these complexes share substrates with cyclin A-CDK2. The importance of the existence of both cyclin A-CDK2 and cyclin A-CDK1 complexes is still not clear.

Nevertheless, during the G2 phase, A-type cyclins are degraded by ubiquitin-mediated proteolysis, and B-type cyclins are synthesized and interact with CDK1. It is estimated that cyclin B-CDK1 complexes phosphorylate more than 70 target proteins, which are important mediators of both regulatory and structural processes (chromosomal condensation, fragmentation of the Golgi network, and breakdown of the nuclear envelope) during G2/M transition. Finally, the inactivation of cyclin B-CDK1 complexes is necessary for the exit from mitosis. This is achieved by the ubiquitin-labeling and subsequent proteasomal degradation of B-type cyclins regulated by the anaphase-promoting complex (APC). The main phosphatase that mediates return to interphase after mitosis is a form of protein phosphatase-2A (PP2A), whose activity is increased after degradation of the mitotic cyclins.

Monitoring for DNA damage

Molecular checkpoints that mediate appropriate progression through the cell cycle sense problems that may occur during DNA synthesis and chromosome segregation

The ultimate role of these checkpoints is to inhibit cyclin–CDK activity and thus delay or arrest cell division. During replication, DNA is less condensed and therefore protected to a lesser degree from the attack of exogenous and endogenous genotoxic agents, which may cause DNA damage.

In the case of damage occurring, the DNA damage checkpoints sense alterations and activate signaling pathways that mediate DNA repair

If the damage is beyond repair, they induce apoptosis. The core molecules of the DNA damage checkpoint are **sensor kinases,** ataxia-telangiectasia mutated (ATM) and ataxia-telangiectasia Rad3-related (ATR) - which detect double-strand breaks and replication stress, respectively - and **checkpoint kinases,** CHK1 and CHK2, which relay the signals from the sensor kinases. These molecules prevent G1/S and G2/M phase transitions by inhibiting the CDK activity through increasing the expression of CDK inhibitor (CDKI) protein, p21 via p53 protein stabilization, and/or inhibiting the CDK activator Cdc25phosphatases.

The tumor-suppressor protein p53 is predominantly a DNA-damage-sensing protein that monitors DNA damage throughout the cell cycle

If DNA damage is detected, ATM and, subsequently, CHK2 kinases are activated, an action that contributes to the stabilization of p53 and thus enables the induction of DNA repair mechanisms. One role of p53 is to act as a transcription factor, increasing the expression of the CDKI p21 (*WAF1*gene). In turn, p21 inhibits cyclin D–CDK4 complexes, preventing Rb phosphorylation and thus promoting Rb/E2F binding and suppression of E2F-mediated gene transcription. Moreover, type-E cyclin–CDK2 complexes are inhibited, enabling cell-cycle arrest at the G1/S transition. This allows the cell time to repair the DNA damage, thus preventing the incorporation of mutated genetic material into daughter cells. However, if the DNA damage is beyond repair, p53-dependent programmed cell death by **apoptosis** is triggered.

A p53-independent pathway involving the INK4 family of proteins can also induce cell-cycle arrest in the G1 phase in response to DNA damage

These proteins, including p16 (INK4A), p15 (INK4B), p18 (INK4C), and p19 (INK4D), mediate cell-cycle arrest by binding to CDK4/6 or their binding partner, cyclin D, thereby inactivating the cyclin D–CDK4/6 complexes. Another important checkpoint is the spindle assembly checkpoint (SAC), which ensures proper alignment and segregation of chromosomes in the metaphase of mitosis. The SAC signal is generated by the presence of unattached or improperly attached kinetochores (protein complexes on chromatids that mediate attachment to the mitotic spindle), ultimately leading to inhibition of the APC and thus preventing the onset of anaphase.

Defects in the DNA damage checkpoints allow accumulation of DNA alterations, contributing to **genomic instability,** whereas defective SAC may lead to the unequal segregation of the genetic material among the daughter cells, thus creating **chromosomal aberrations.** Both genomic instability and chromosomal aberrations are major causes of cell transformation and oncogenesis.

CLINICAL BOX
ATAXIA TELANGIECTASIA

Ataxia telangiectasia is a rare autosomal recessive disease caused by mutations in the ataxia-telangiectasia mutated *(ATM)* gene. Patients with this disease have the following symptoms and signs: an unsteady gait, telangiectasia, skin pigmentation, infertility, immune deficiencies, and increased incidence of cancer, especially lymphoreticular tumors.

Comment
ATM is a serine/threonine protein kinase involved in the induction of a DNA damage checkpoint in response to ionizing radiation, anticancer treatment, or programmed DNA breaks during meiosis. Ataxia telangiectasia cells exhibit chromosomal instability, hypersensitivity to reagents that induce DNA strand breaks and defects in the G1/G2 phases, and altered regulation of p53 and p21 expression. ATM is constitutively expressed during the cell cycle and is involved in induction of p53-mediated cell-cycle arrest and/or apoptosis. In ataxia telangiectasia, cells with mutated ATM **cannot properly activate p53** and hence induce cell-cycle arrest or apoptosis in response to ionizing radiation. When p53 is also mutated, the cell cycle is not adequately regulated, which further increases the risk of tumor formation as a result of the accumulation of mutations.

CELL DEATH

Cell death is a fundamentally important part of a cell's life cycle, and appropriate regulation of this process is critical to maintaining the homeostatic regulation of a multicellular organism

Cell death may be accidental or programmed, initiated and executed through distinct biochemical pathways. **Programmed** cell death (PCD) is genetically regulated, and its role is to remove superfluous, damaged, or mutated cells. For many years, apoptosis was a synonym for PCD; however, this concept is changing due to the recent findings identifying different modes of controlled cell death.

Both initiation and execution of cell death are complex processes, with scientists classifying the various forms of cell death on the basis of morphologic and/or biochemical features as the most common criteria. According to morphologic criteria, cell death can be classified as follows:

- **Apoptosis** - the rounding up of the cell, retraction of pseudopods, reduction of cellular and nuclear volume (pycnosis), chromatin condensation and fragmentation (karyorrhexis), plasma membrane blebbing, formation of apoptotic bodies, and engulfment by resident phagocytes in vivo.
- **Necrosis or necrotic cell death** - an enlargement of the cell volume, swelling of the organelles and plasma-membrane bursting, with concomitant loss of the intracellular content. Necrosis is often considered to be an accidental and uncontrollable form of cell death that occurs after severe insult to the cell. However, recent research has shown that necrosis can be controlled and initiated through specific signaling pathways involving RIP1 serine/threonine kinase. This type of necrosis is called **necrosis-like PCD** or necroptosis, and it has been observed in cancer cells, proliferating cells that have suffered DNA damage, and cells infected with certain viruses (such as *Vaccinia*).
- **Autophagic cell death** (ACD; autophagy) - massive vacuolization of the cytoplasm, accumulation of the double membrane autophagic vacuoles, without chromatin condensation and little or no uptake by phagocytes in vivo. ACD is often confused with PCD accompanied by autophagy instead of the death mediated by the process of autophagy. Therefore, the term ACD should be used only when cell death is executed by the mere autophagy processes without involving apoptosis or necrosis. Thus far, this type of PCD has been identified in mammalian cells when apoptosis is defective or blocked and in *Drosophila* salivary glands.

Apoptosis

Apoptosis is initiated and executed through either perturbation of intracellular homeostasis by intrinsic (mitochondrial) or extrinsic (e.g., Fas, TNFR) pathways

For both of these pathways, two families of proteins are considered quintessential regulators: cysteine proteases called **caspases** and the **B-cell lymphoma protein 2 (Bcl-2)–related family members,** which interact to modulate life-versus-death decisions (Fig. 28.7). However, there is a growing body of evidence for other PCD pathways that sense stress and damage in other cellular organelles (such as ER and lysosomes) and result in the initiation of death programs. These programs can occur in association with, or independently of, the intrinsic mitochondrial pathway.

Caspases

Caspases are cysteine proteases with aspartate substrate specificity

They are synthesized as inactive proenzymes (zymogens) referred to as procaspases. According to their role in the death pathways, caspases can be categorized as initiator or effector caspases.

Initiator caspases (caspase-2, -8, -9, -10) are synthesized as monomers, and when the cell receives a death signal, they undergo activation, resulting from proximity-induced conformational changes and dimerization within multimeric complexes, as well as autoproteolytic cleavage, which induces full enzymatic activity. Once cleaved/activated, caspases mediate proteolytic cleavage of other caspases in the death pathway cascade.

Effector caspase proenzymes are expressed as pre-formed dimers, which are activated by the direct proteolytic attack of initiator caspases. These effectors then execute the cell death program by cleaving many vital cellular proteins (such as lamins, gelsolin), inducing cell-cycle arrest, and disabling the initiation of homeostatic and repair mechanisms. Collectively, these events lead to detachment of the cell from its surrounding tissue, dismantling structural components, and ultimately flagging the phosphatidylserine (PS) "eat-me" signal for phagocytosis. Overexpression of active caspases is sufficient to induce cellular apoptosis.

IAP gene family: its main function is to inhibit apoptosis

The inhibitor of apoptosis (IAP) gene family, coding for nine family members (X-linked IAP, cIAP1, cIAP2, melanoma IAP, IAP-like protein, neuronal apoptosis inhibitory protein, survivin, livin, and apollon), is evolutionarily conserved from *Drosophila* through to humans. The main function of this gene family is, as its name indicates, to inhibit apoptosis by either directly blocking caspases and/or activating survival pathways via NFκB function. For example, XIAP inhibits caspase-3, -7, and -9 by direct binding to the active pocket of caspase-3 and -7, whereas in the case of caspase-9, it prevents the dimerization necessary for full activation. In contrast, cIAP1 and cIAP2 are positive regulators of both canonical and noncanonical pathways of NFκB activation. Survivin, in addition to inhibiting apoptosis, plays a role in cell-cycle progression by blocking the activity of caspase-3, thus preserving the integrity of p21 within the survivin–caspase-3–p21 complex and by mediating proper chromosome segregation as a part of the complex that binds chromosomes to kinetochores. It is not surprising, therefore, that IAP family members can contribute to tumor cell survival, cell invasion, and metastasis in many human cancers. Interestingly, loss of cIAP1/cIAP2 is implicated in the development of **multiple myeloma.**

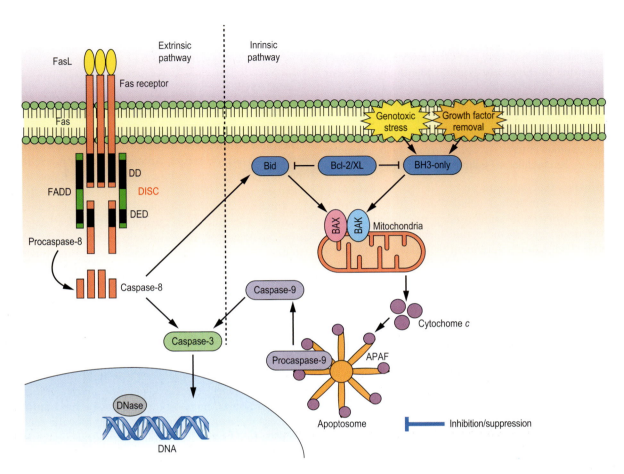

Fig. 28.7 **Regulation of apoptosis.** Two main modes of apoptosis are induced through the ligation of death receptors, such as Fas, by growth factor deprivation or genotoxic stress. Fas receptor ligation induces the extrinsic death pathway; the main initiator caspase is caspase-8. FasL binding causes receptor trimerization and formation of a macromolecular structure called DISC, which acts as a platform for caspase-8 activation. When activated, caspase-8 may directly cleave and activate effector caspase-3, or it may cleave the BH-3-only protein Bid, which acts directly on mitochondria, thus feeding into the second death pathway, referred to as an intrinsic pathway. This pathway is initiated by the upregulation or activation of BH-3-only family members, which relieve the inhibition mediated by Bcl-2/xL, thus allowing formation of the Bax/Bak pore in the mitochondrial outer membrane. This causes leakage of cytochrome C into cytoplasm, where it forms the apoptosome with APAF-1 and procaspase-9. The apoptosome is a platform for caspase-9 activation, which, when cleaved, adopts active conformation and can cleave effector caspase-3. Active caspase-3 then mediates bulk proteolysis either by activating other hydrolases or by directly cleaving structural components. APAF1, apoptotic protease activating factor 1; DISC, death-inducing signaling complex; Bid, BH-3-interacting-domain death agonist; BAX, Bcl2-associated X protein; BAK, Bcl-2 homologous antagonist/killer; APAF-1, apoptotic protease activating factor 1; FADD, FAS-associated death domain protein; DD, death domain; DED, death effector domain.

The Bcl-2 gene family is composed of structurally related proteins that form homo- or heterodimers and act as positive or negative regulators of apoptosis

The *Bcl-2* gene was initially discovered in a follicular B-cell lymphoma as a protein that is constitutively expressed due to a t(14;18) chromosome translocation, which placed the *Bcl-2* gene under the control of the immunoglobulin (Ig) heavy-chain promoter. *Bcl-2* family members have traditionally been classified into three groups: prosurvival family members (Bcl-2, Bcl-xL, Bcl-W, Mcl-1), proapoptotic BAX/BAK family, and proapoptotic BH-3-only proteins (BIM, BID, PUMA, NOXA, BAD, BIK). Whereas Bcl-2 function involves preserving the integrity of the outer mitochondrial membrane, proapoptotic

family members BAX and BAK are responsible for inducing mitochondrial outer-membrane permeabilization and subsequent release of apoptotic mediators (such as cytochrome *c*), leading to effector caspase activation. Bcl-2 and Bcl-xL prevent apoptosis induction by inhibiting BAX and BAK, whereas BH-3-only family members prevent this inhibition by a direct binding to Bcl-2 and other antiapoptotic family members (Fig. 28.7).

There are alternative routes to apoptosis

The rupture of lysosomal membranes causes release and activation of **lysosomal proteases** (i.e., cathepsins), which either mediate direct proteolytic cleavage of cellular components or activation of the intrinsic pathway. Endoplasmic reticulum (ER) stress is generally caused by the accumulation of unfolded proteins in the lumen, giving rise to the unfolded protein response or irregular intracellular Ca^{2+} flux. These perturbations usually induce apoptosis through the intrinsic pathway. Accumulation of unfolded or misfolded protein aggregates is associated with many neurodegenerative disorders, including **Alzheimer's, Huntington's**, and **Parkinson's diseases.** For example, amyloid-β-protein aggregates and mutations in the ER-associated presenilin 1 have been associated with the development of familial Alzheimer's disease. Interestingly, all these pathways may cross-talk and perform complex death programs in both the morphologic and the biochemical sense.

ADVANCED CONCEPT BOX
INTRINSIC AND EXTRINSIC DEATH PATHWAY

The extrinsic apoptotic pathway is activated by the engagement of death receptors such as TNF family members (Fas, TNFR, TRAIL, or TWEAK). For example, binding of homotrimeric FasL to Fas causes receptor oligomerization and assembly of an intracellular "death-inducing signaling complex" (DISC). DISC contains procaspase-8, its adaptor/activator Fas-associated death domain (FADD), and its modulator cFLIP. Activation of caspase-8 occurs first by conformational change, which enables full enzymatic activity, and then by auto-proteolytic cleavage of the procaspase form. Cleaved caspase-8 molecules then leave the DISC and gain access to downstream targets, which include either effector caspases, such as caspase-3 and -7, or proapoptotic Bcl-2 family member BH3-interacting-domain death agonist (Bid). Cleaved Bid then feeds into the intrinsic pathway to amplify the death signal (Fig. 28.7).

The intrinsic apoptotic pathway is also referred to as a Bcl-2-regulated pathway due to the complex interplay between the pro- and antiapoptotic Bcl-2 family members, which determines cell fate. It is usually activated by developmental cues, viral infections, DNA damage, growth factor deprivation, or other cytotoxic insults. These stress conditions increase the expression of BH3-only family members or, alternatively, their posttranslational activation, depending on the context of death induction. Activated proapoptotic Bcl-2 family members relieve the inhibition of Bcl2-associated X protein (BAX) and Bcl-2 homologous antagonist/killer (BAK) at the pores of the outer mitochondrial membrane, enabling cytochrome c release from the mitochondrial intermembrane space into the cytoplasm. Cytoplasmic cytochrome C then binds to apoptotic protease activating factor 1 (APAF1), allowing the formation of an apoptosome, which serves as a platform for caspase-9 activation (Fig. 28.7). Active caspase-9 then cleaves caspase-3 and/or -7, which in turn mediates bulk proteolysis of vital cellular proteins, activates DNases, and orchestrates the demolition of the cell.

Autophagy

Autophagy is a process that degrades cellular components, in which a part of cytoplasm is engulfed by a specific membrane and the contents are degraded by lysosomal enzymes

Autophagy is a highly regulated stepwise homeostatic process that plays a role in the turnover of long-lived or damaged proteins and in the elimination of defective organelles such as mitochondria (mitophagy) or ER (reticulophagy; Fig. 28.8). In addition to being associated with cell death, autophagy also enables cells to survive starvation in circumstances of decreased availability of extra- and intracellular nutrients. In this case, autophagy induces catabolic processes, which generate metabolic substrates from "self"-components, thus allowing cells to meet their bioenergetic needs and initiate so-called adaptive protein synthesis in the time of scarcity. The main regulators of autophagy are members of the autophagy-related gene *(ATG)* family, composed of 31 genes to date. Since their initial discovery in *Saccharomyces cerevisiae*, orthologues (genes in different species that evolved from a common ancestral gene) have been identified in mammals, indicating this gene family is conserved from yeast.

Autophagy is induced by a variety of stress stimuli, including nutrient and energy stress as well as hypoxia, oxidative stress, infections, ER stress, and mitochondrial damage

All of these stresses induce distinct signaling pathways that regulate autophagy. A characteristic signaling event that induces autophagy as a result of nutrient deprivation is the inhibition of **mTORC-1** signaling and/or **5'AMP-activated protein kinase (AMPK)** activation. The process of autophagy involves the formation of a membrane structure, termed a phagophore (most likely by de novo synthesis), which encases part of the cytoplasm or a whole organelle, forming a double-membrane structure called the autophagosome. The autophagosome can then fuse with an endosome, creating an amphisome. Subsequently, these structures fuse with a lysosome, generating an autolysosome where acid hydrolases break down the inner membrane and the cargo. Digested macromolecule building blocks are then recycled back into the cytoplasm through protein channels referred to as permeases (Fig. 28.8).

Apart from its roles in the maintenance of cell homeostasis, autophagy plays a role in both innate and adaptive immunity. For example, autophagy is used to eliminate intracellular bacteria such as *Streptococcus pyogenes* and *Mycobacterium tuberculosis*. Moreover, the Epstein–Barr virus nuclear antigen 1 (EBNA1) is processed through an autophagic pathway and loaded on MHC class II molecules for presentation to the CD4[+] T lymphocytes (Chapter 43).

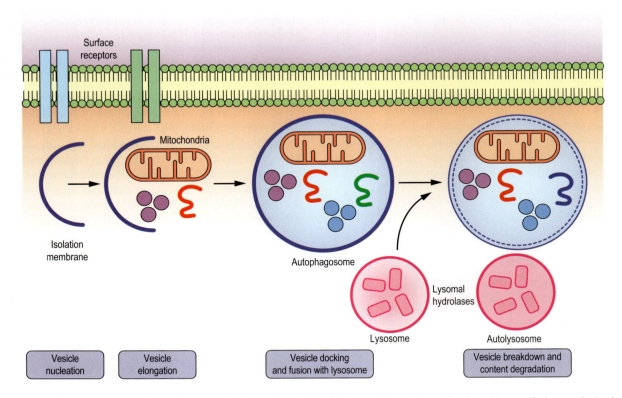

Fig. 28.8 **Autophagy.** The process of autophagy starts by formation of the isolation membrane (phagophore), which engulfs damaged mitochondria and/or misfolded proteins and forms the double-membraned vesicle autophagosome (autophagic vacuole). Autophagosomes then mature and fuse with lysosomes, thus creating autolysosomes, in which the inner membrane of the autophagosome and its luminal content are degraded by the action of lysosomal acid hydrolases, such as cathepsins.

 EXPERIMENTAL TECHNIQUE BOX
ANALYSIS OF CELL-CYCLE PROGRESSION, APOPTOSIS, AND AUTOPHAGY

Apoptosis is a complex and dynamic process with many distinct features that have enabled the development of experimental techniques for the detection of discrete stages through which dying cells pass on the way to death: plasma membrane asymmetry leading to extracellular expression of phosphatidylserine (PS), changes in mitochondrial membrane potential (MMP), and caspase activity as indicated by the presence of cleaved caspase and DNA content can all be detected by flow cytometry combined with the appropriate fluorescent staining. **Flow cytometry** is a quantitative technique that measures fluorescence at the single-cell level within a sample of cells in suspension. In addition, **laser-scanning cytometry (LSC)** allows both quantification and imaging in a slide-based format, enabling similar fluorescent apoptosis analyses not only of cells but also within tissues.

Cell proliferation can be measured using carboxy-fluorescein-diacetate succinimidyl ester (CFDA SE) staining of cells whose two acetate side chains render it highly membrane permeable. When the molecules of CFDA SE enter the cell, the acetate groups are cleaved by cellular esterases, converting them into a fluorescent CFSE form, which exit the cell at a slower rate. At the same time, the succinimydil moiety binds to free amino groups of a range of amine-containing molecules, some of which have a short half-life or get transported out of the cell. However, a sufficient number of long-lived amines are labeled with CFSE, such as cytoskeletal proteins, enabling the tracking of cells in vivo for weeks. Fluorescence intensity of CFSE-stained cells is proportional to the CFSE concentration used and the duration of staining. When stained cells are stimulated to divide, CFSE is partitioned equally among the daughter cells. This phenomenon can be detected by flow cytometry. The decrease in brightness of fluorescence is observed as distinct peaks with halving median fluorescent values, enabling analysis of division progression with division numbers defined by gates set around each peak.

DNA content increases during S phase from diploid chromosomal DNA in G0/G1 phase to tetraploid at G2/M before returning to diploid again after M phase. During apoptosis, DNA is fragmented by the action of DNA endonucleases, creating a population of cells that exhibit a subdiploid content. Therefore, both cell cycle and apoptosis can be detected by measuring the DNA content of cells. The most commonly used fluorescent staining protocols for assessing DNA content are staining with propidium iodide (PI) or with 4′-6′-diamidino-2-phenylindole (DAPI). PI is DNA-intercalating

EXPERIMENTAL TECHNIQUE BOX - CONT'D
ANALYSIS OF CELL-CYCLE PROGRESSION, APOPTOSIS, AND AUTOPHAGY

dye; therefore the extent of binding, measured by the fluorescence emitted, is indicative of the total DNA content. DAPI works in a similar manner except that the dye molecules preferentially bind to the A-T base pairs. Indeed, staining cells fixed on a slide with DAPI and analyzing with an LSC enables cell-cycle progression to be determined by virtue of DAPI maximum pixel value (chromatin condensation) along the x-axis and the DAPI integral value (DNA content) along the y-axis. Apoptotic (AP) cells exhibit low (sub G1) DNA content. LSC analysis enables images of individual cells at distinct stages of the cell cycle to be viewed. Another commonly used method for assessing DNA content, in the context of DNA synthesis (indicative of the progress through S phase), is pulsing the cells with bromodeoxyuridine (BrdU), which is incorporated into DNA instead of thymidine during DNA synthesis. The quantity of incorporated BrdU is often measured by flow cytometry using anti-BrdU antibodies coupled to fluorescent dyes.

DNA fragmentation can also be measured by the TUNEL assay, in which DNA fragments are labeled with fluorescent dyes. This

technique employs the ability of the enzyme terminal deoxynucleotidyl transferase (TdT) to add biotin labeled nucleotide, such as dUTP, to the ends of DNA fragments. Subsequently, these fragments are visualized by binding of the biotin ligand, streptavidin, coupled with fluorescent dyes. The simplest way to detect DNA fragmentation is separating fragments by agarose gel electrophoresis, which enables visualization of "DNA ladders."

Autophagy is also a dynamic and complex process. Over the years, several techniques have been developed to detect different steps of autophagy. For example, an accumulation of autophagosomes can be visualized using either electron microscopy or flow cytometry / fluorescent microscopy to detect increases in fluorescence of acidotropic dyes, such as acridine orange or lysotracker red, or by assaying the conversion of a form of microtuble-associated protein 1A/1B-light chain 3 (LC3-1) to the phosphatidylethanolamine (PE)-modified form (LC3-II) by Western blotting or immunofluorescence.

CLINICAL BOX
DEREGULATED APOPTOSIS AND AUTOPHAGY CAN CAUSE DISTINCT PATHOLOGIC CONDITIONS

Deregulated Apoptosis
Excessive apoptosis is linked to **neurodegenerative diseases** and **immunodeficiency,** whereas evasion of apoptosis is an important contributor to **oncogenesis** and the development of **autoimmune diseases.** Mutations (deletions/additions of one or a few nucleotides in the coding exons or splice sites) in the death receptor Fas lead to a defect in Fas-mediated apoptosis, which results in increased survival of activated lymphocytes, causing autoimmune lymphoproliferative syndrome (ALPS). This rare inherited disorder usually presents in early childhood. Patients with ALPS have lymphadenopathy, splenomegaly, and autoimmune cytopenias and have increased risk for development of lymphomas. Mutation of Fas or deletion of the Bcl-2 family member Bim in mice causes systemic lupus erythematosus–like (SLE-like) disease, whereas chromosomal translocation of the Bcl-2 to the Ig heavy-chain locus (t[14;18]) results in the constitutive expression of Bcl-2, leading to the development of follicular lymphoma. Consistent with this,

aberrant expression and function of Bcl-2 family members are also implicated in the development of autoimmune diseases and cancer.

Deregulated Autophagy
Perturbations in induction and execution of autophagy may also lead to a series of disorders and diseases. Monoallelic deletions of BECN1/ATG are tumorigenic in mice, and a decrease in expression of Beclin 1 is observed in **human breast carcinoma.** Loss-of-function mutations in the Pink1 and Parkin genes, which are regulators of mitophagy, are linked to familial Parkinson's disease in humans. Similar to the common neurodegenerative diseases are **lysosomal storage disorders,** which include more than 40 genetic conditions, most of which are linked to the deficiency of lysosomal hydrolases. Reduced or impaired function of these enzymes leads to the accumulation of otherwise degraded macromolecules, whereas **Huntington's and Parkinson's diseases** are associated with accumulation of a mutant form of protein α-synuclein.

CANCER

Cells that develop mutations affecting normal regulation of the cell cycle are able to undergo unchecked proliferation, resulting in a loss of homeostatic regulation and the development of a tumor or neoplasm

As long as neoplastic cells remain as an intact tumor, the tumor is considered **benign.** However, if further mutations allow such tumor cells to invade and colonize other tissues,

creating widespread secondary tumors, or **metastases,** the tumor is described as **malignant** and classified as a **cancer.** Each cancer is derived from a single cell that has undergone some germline mutation that allows it to outgrow its surrounding cells; by the time they are first detected, tumors typically contain a billion cells. Cancers are classified according to the tissue and cell type that they are derived from: those from epithelial cells are **carcinomas,** those from connective tissue or muscle cells are termed **sarcomas,** and those from the hematopoietic system are called **leukemias/lymphomas.**

About 90% of human cancers are carcinomas, the five most common being those of the **breast, prostate, lung, bowel, and malignant melanoma**.

In the majority of cases, a single mutation is not sufficient to convert a healthy cell to a cancer cell; several rare mutations have to occur together

Mutations in DNA occur spontaneously at a rate of 10^{-6} mutations per gene, per cell division (even more in the presence of mutagens). Because approximately 10^{16} cell divisions occur in the human body over an average lifetime, every human gene is likely to undergo mutation on about 10^{10} occasions. Clearly, then, a single mutation is not normally sufficient to convert a healthy cell to a cancer cell; several rare mutations have to occur together, as demonstrated by epidemiologic studies showing that for any given cancer, the incidence increases exponentially with age. It has been estimated that three to seven independent mutations are usually required, with leukemias apparently needing the fewest mutations and carcinomas the most.

Mutations need to occur in the appropriate cells to enable the neoplasm to develop, indicating that cell context has an important bearing on the type of cancer that subsequently develops

In addition to developing cancer-promoting mutations, the cell in which a mutation occurs must then be permissive to being a cancer-initiating cell. This relates to the cellular context in which an oncogene is expressed and the properties bestowed upon a cancer cell by expression of a particular oncogene. In order to become oncogenic and promote cancer cell growth, the cell must possess self-renewal capacity. If oncogene expression occurs in a stem cell, then oncogene expression could inhibit the negative regulatory networks in place that would ordinarily stop cell growth and proliferation, thus generating a **cancer stem cell.** Cancers such as **chronic myeloid leukemia (CML)** and **acute myeloid leukemia (AML)** can arise from mutations in stem cells. However, it is not essential for the cell of origin of individual cancers to arise from stem cells. Indeed, cancers can arise in committed progenitor cells, but they require mutations that enable those cells to undergo self-renewal, therefore providing a cellular source for cancer.

Mutations that lead to the expression of established oncogenes do not necessarily lead to the development of cancer if they occur in nonsusceptible cells

For example, the Philadelphia chromosome (t[9;22]) contains a gene derived from two genes on different chromosomes, which fuse after the exchange of fragments (translocation) between chromosome 9 and 22. This gene generates a fusion protein BCR-Abl, encoding a constitutively active form of the PTK c-Abl (the causative mutation in the development of >95% CML cases), which is detected at a very low level in circulating peripheral blood cells isolated from around 30% of healthy individuals. Studies have demonstrated that expression of BCR-Abl alone does not confer self-renewal properties on

committed progenitor cells, indicating that secondary mutations are required to make committed progenitor cells cancerous. This finding suggests that the expression of oncogenes such as BCR-Abl within a stem-cell environment can enable it to hardwire into the initiation of the neoplastic program.

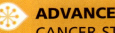

ADVANCED CONCEPT BOX
CANCER STEM CELLS

Although cells within tumors all share similar genetic aberrations responsible for their growth, the tumors are composed of multiple different cell types, differing in morphology and cell surface markers. In this way, tumors bear broad characteristics similar to those of normal tissue. Analysis of the proliferation rates of the distinct tumor cells revealed that although the majority of cells cycled at a fast rate, there was a small population of cells that proliferated at a slower rate. This latter population was capable of remaining dormant, or quiescent, for weeks. Two mutually exclusive models were generated to explain this behavior. In the **stochastic model** of cancer development, tumor cells are biologically homogeneous; however, influences from intrinsic and extrinsic microenvironmental factors induce heterogeneity within the tumor, randomly influencing the properties of the cells with regard to morphology, proliferation rate, and the ability of the cells to form new tumors. Conversely, in the **hierarchy model,** as seen in normal tissue, only a distinct cellular subset, or cancer stem cell (CSC), is capable of generating new tumors (self-renewal), whereas the CSC progeny proliferate to make up the majority of the tumor bulk but are unable to self-renew. This model indicates that CSCs develop stem cell–like properties but should not imply that CSCs only arise from normal stem cells. Indeed, studies from leukemias have established that some mutations are capable of promoting self-renewal in progenitor cells, thus bestowing these cells with this critical stem cell property, which is essential for its capacity to maintain tumor growth. Thus far, CSCs have been identified in leukemias (CML, ALL, AML) and brain, breast, prostate, skin, and colon cancers.

Comment

The finding that CSCs, or cancer-initiating cells, possess stem cell properties has posed a problem with regard to therapeutic intervention. Normal stem cells (and CSCs) are quiescent, are long-lived, and self-renew. This makes CSCs difficult to remove because the majority of therapies target actively proliferating cells. Although this will remove the bulk of the tumor, the root of the tumor, or the CSC, remains, resulting in tumor regrowth, or relapse. For this reason, it has become critically important to elucidate the differences between normal stem cells and CSCs to enable the development of therapies that specifically target CSCs, thus removing the root of the cancer. To complicate matters further, due to subversion of cell-cycle regulatory checkpoints in CSCs, a feature of these cells is genetic instability. In this dynamic background, it is possible for the cancer clone to evolve, a process known as **clonal evolution,** leading to the outgrowth of a more aggressive cancer clone that can thrive and potentially be resistant to novel therapies, hence the **requirement for second- and third-line therapies.**

Although genetic mutations are common and expected, with loss of function in p53, PTEN, and Rb and gain of function with Ras, genome sequencing has also identified mutations in "unexpected" genes in individual cancers. For example, the *Notch* gene is mutated to form a constitutively active Notch protein and is linked to the generation of around 50% of T-lymphocyte–acute lymphoblastic leukemia (T-ALL) cases. However, activating mutations in *Notch1* have also been identified in B-lineage diseases, including chronic lymphocytic leukemia (CLL) and mantle cell lymphoma (MCL). Interestingly, an inactivating mutation of Notch has recently been identified in head and neck squamous cell carcinoma, indicating that whereas in hematopoietic lineages Notch acts as a tumor promoter, it can behave as a tumor suppressor in squamous cell carcinogenesis.

Alterations in gene expression have also been identified as a mechanism for tumor development/promotion. Indeed, expression patterns of specific PKC isoforms are dysregulated, possibly through alterations in the epigenetic regulation of gene expression, in a number of cancers. In particular, PKCα is upregulated in breast, gastric, prostate, and brain cancers, suggesting that it contributes to tumorigenesis. Moreover, PKCα expression levels have also been linked with the aggressiveness and invasive capacity of breast cancer cells. However, PKCα expression is downregulated in epidermal, pancreatic, and colon cancers and CLL, suggesting that PKCα can also function as a tumor suppressor. Taken together, these findings indicate that the cell in which the mutation or modulation of expression of a protein occurs has a direct bearing on whether cancer formation is a likely outcome.

Tumor promoters: Oncogenes

Mutations that lead to uncontrolled proliferation of cancer cells can result either from disruption of the control of normal cell division or, alternatively, from a reduction in the normal processes of terminal differentiation or apoptosis. This distinction is reflected by the two major groups of genes targeted for mutation in cancer: **oncogenes** and **tumor-suppressor genes**.

Oncogenes were first identified as viral genes that infect normal cells and transform them into tumor cells

The Rous sarcoma virus, which is a retrovirus that causes connective tissue tumors in chickens, infects and transforms fibroblast cells grown in cell culture. The transformed cells outgrow the normal cells and exhibit a number of growth abnormalities, such as a loss of cell contact-mediated inhibition of growth and loss of anchorage dependence of growth. In addition, the cells have a rounded appearance and can proliferate in the absence of growth factors. Moreover, the cells are immortal, do not senesce, and can induce tumor formation when injected into a suitable animal host, confirming their capacity for self-renewal.

The key to understanding cell transformation lies in the mutation of a normal cellular gene that controls cell growth

The use of mutant Rous sarcoma viruses that, despite multiplying normally, had lost the ability to transform host cells showed that it was the *Src* gene that was responsible for such cell transformation. The breakthrough in our understanding of how this single gene could transform cells in culture came when it became apparent that the viral oncogene was a mutated homologue of a normal cellular gene. This gene is now called the c-*Src* protooncogene and has been identified as a PTK signal transducer involved in the normal control of cell growth. Because expression of this gene is not essential to the survival of the retrovirus, it is likely that *Src* was accidentally incorporated by the virus from a previous host genome and was mutated during this process. Indeed, in the Rous sarcoma virus, the introns normally present in c-*Src* are spliced out, and there are a number of mutations causing amino acid substitutions, resulting in a constitutively (independently of metabolic conditions) active PTK.

Cell transformation can, however, also result from oncogenes that are not constitutively activated but, rather, are overexpressed in an abnormally high number of copies as a consequence of the gene being under the control of powerful promoters or enhancers in the viral genome. Alternatively, for retroviruses, DNA copies of the viral RNA can be inserted into the host genome at or near sites of protooncogenes (insertional mutation), causing abnormal activation of these protooncogenes. In this situation, the altered genome is inherited by all progeny of the original host cell.

Most human tumors are nonviral in origin and arise from spontaneous or induced mutations

Approximately 85% of human tumors arise as a result of point or deletion mutations. These mutations may be spontaneous or induced by carcinogens or radiation, resulting in overexpression or hyperactivity of the protooncogenes. *Ras*, which is mutated to a constitutively activated form in approximately 25% of all tumors, appears to exert many, if not all, of its effects by upregulating cyclin D expression and, hence, promoting cell-cycle progression. Cyclin D upregulation results from activation of the MAPK cascade by *Ras* and induction of the transcription factor AP-1.

Whole-exome/genome sequencing of individual patients, utilized to determine the specific mutational landscape within cancer subtypes, has enabled links to be established between seemingly diverse cancers that result from similar genetic mutations

Of note, a B-Raf^{V600E} mutation was found to be present in nearly all **hairy cell leukemia** (HCL) patients assessed. B-Raf^{V600E} is oncogenic in a number of tumors, including melanoma, encoding active B-Raf kinase leading to the constitutive

CLINICAL BOX
mTOR IN CANCER AND METABOLIC DISORDERS

Because of its vital role in regulating cell proliferation/survival and its intricate relationship with the PI3K pathway, components of the mTOR pathway are often dysfunctional in many types of cancers and metabolic disorders. **Tuberous sclerosis complex (TSC)** is an autosomal dominant genetic disorder that occurs as a result of inactivating mutations within the *Tsc1* or *Tsc2* genes. TSC is characterized by multiple benign tumors such as angiofibroma of the skin, lymphangioleiomyoma of the lungs, renal angiomyolipoma, and astrocytoma of the brain.

In the context of the mTORC-1 axis, *Tsc1/2* serve as a relay center for tumor microenvironmental cues. Under normal circumstances, hypoxia (via Hif1α), DNA damage (via p53), and nutrient deprivation (via LKB1 transcription factor) activate *Tsc1/2* to regulate mTORC-1, thus controlling biosynthetic processes. These pathways are inactivated during tumorigenesis, usually by the cooperative action of oncogenic PI3K/PDK1 and Ras/MAPK pathways to reduce *Tsc1/2* activity. Upregulation of mTORC-1 signaling leads to overactivated protein and lipid biosynthesis, which supports the bioenergetic needs of energy-demanding proliferating tumor cells. Enhanced protein synthesis often promotes increased expression of cell-cycle regulators such as cyclin D1 and cyclin E, whereas constitutively active Akt contributes to the inactivation of cell-cycle inhibitors p27 and p21. The role of mTORC-2 in tumorigenesis is still not well defined; however, part of the mTORC-2 complex called Rictor is overexpressed in many *gliomas*. Higher expression promotes mTORC-2 complex assembly and activation, enabling increased cell proliferation and invasion. These events suggest that cancer could be considered a metabolic disorder.

Moreover, mTOR pathway dysregulation contributes to the development of metabolic disorders such as **obesity, nonalcoholic fatty liver, and type 2 diabetes mellitus**. For example, in the hypothalamus, leptin relays signals via mTORC-1 for the reduction in food intake. Overactivation of mTORC-1 due to a high-fat diet may promote obesity by favoring resistance to the leptin-induced anorexia signals, thus promoting hyperphagia. Moreover, increased activation of mTORC-1 promotes adipogenesis and adipose tissue expansion; inhibits insulin signaling in the skeletal muscles, liver, and pancreas by promoting insulin resistance; and contributes to the induction of apoptosis in pancreatic β-cells by exhausting the homeostatic process of β-cell compensation (see Chapters 31 and 32).

activation of the MEK/ERK signaling pathway. This mutation has a major impact on the cell cycle. Interestingly, now that the *B-Raf*^{V600E} mutation has been identified as a causal/driver event of HCL, it presents the opportunity for targeted therapies, specifically inhibiting active *B-Raf*, which would otherwise have not been considered for the treatment of HCL. Identification of specific driver mutations in a particular cancer cell opens up the possibility of treating patients with a therapy targeted toward that mutation.

Karyotyping of tumor cells has also shown that chromosomal translocation can bring oncogenes under the control of an inappropriate promoter. For example, in **Burkitt's lymphoma**, overexpression of the *Myc* gene occurs through its translocation into the vicinity of an Ig locus. Because *Myc* normally acts as a nuclear proliferative signal, overexpression of *Myc* induces the cell to divide, even under conditions that would normally dictate growth arrest.

Tumor-suppressor genes: Subversion of the cell cycle

Mutations in tumor-suppressor genes are recessive, and mutations in both copies of the gene are thus usually required for transformation. Because it is difficult to identify the loss of function of a single gene in a cell, much of the initial information relating to tumor-suppressor genes was obtained by studying a range of inherited cancer syndromes (Table 28.1).

p53: Guardian of the genome

The protein p53 plays a critical role in regulating the G1/S phase transition of the cell cycle and monitoring for DNA damage, and it becomes activated upon sensing damage, stress, and oncogenic signals to induce cell-cycle arrest and/or death. Therefore it is perhaps unsurprising that p53 function is commonly disrupted in cancer cells. This can either be directly through inactivating mutations of p53 function, abrogating its transcriptional activity, or by dysregulating pathways responsible for p53 activation. The importance of p53 is highlighted in individuals who only have one functional copy of the *p53* gene. People with this syndrome, called **Li–Fraumeni syndrome,** are predisposed to develop a wide range of tumors, including sarcomas; carcinomas of the lung, breast, larynx, and colon; brain tumors; and leukemias. This syndrome is rare, and tumor cells in affected patients exhibit defects in both copies of *p53*. Deletion of *p53*, in addition to allowing uncontrolled cell-cycle progression, also permits replication of damaged DNA, leading to further carcinogenic mutations or gene amplification.

Phosphatase and Tensin homologue (PTEN)

The tumor suppressor PTEN is one of the most commonly inactivated proteins in sporadic cancer

As described previously, PI3K-mediated signaling pathways are activated in response to a multitude of growth factor stimuli, resulting in the promotion of cell growth, survival, and proliferation. The main protein responsible for attenuating PI3K activity and downstream pathways is the dual-specificity protein and lipid phosphatase PTEN. It reverses the activity

Table 28.1 Selected inherited cancer syndromes

Syndrome	Cancer	Gene product
Li–Fraumeni	Sarcomas; adrenocortical carcinomas of breast, lung, and larynx; colon and brain tumors; leukemias	p53: transcription factor, DNA damage and stress
Familial retinoblastoma	Retinoblastoma, osteosarcoma	Rb1: cell-cycle and transcriptional regulation
Familial adenomatous polyposis (FAP)	Colorectal cancer; colorectal adenomas, duodenal and gastric tumors, jaw osteomas and desmoid tumors (Gardner syndrome), medulloblastoma (Turcot syndrome)	APC: regulation of β-catenin, microtubule binding
Wiedmann–Beckwith syndrome	Wilms' tumor, organomegaly, hemihypertrophy, hepatoblastoma, adrenocortical cancer	p57/KIP2: cell-cycle regulator
PTEN hamartoma tumor syndrome	Benign tumors: breast, thyroid, colorectal, endometrial, and kidney cancers	PTEN: protein and lipid phosphatase, regulating Akt kinase and cell cycle
Neurofibromatosis type 1 (NF1)	Neurofibrosarcoma, AML, brain tumors	GTP-ase activating protein (GAP) for Ras
Hereditary papillary renal cancer	Renal cancer	MET receptor for HGF
Familial melanoma	Melanoma, pancreatic cancer, dysplastic nevi, atypical moles	p16 (CDK): inhibitor of cyclin-dependent kinase (CDK4/6)

AML, acute myeloid leukemia; HGF, hepatocyte growth factor; KIP2, 57-kDa inhibitor of cyclin–CDK complexes.

CLINICAL BOX
SPECIFIC MUTATIONS THAT DEFINE A CANCER THERAPY

In the majority of cases, a number of mutations are required in to order to change a healthy cell into a cancer cell. One possible exception to this rule is **chronic myeloid leukemia (CML),** which in 95% of cases develops as a result of a translocation between chromosomes 9 and 22 (t[9;22]), leading to the development of the Philadelphia chromosome in the hemato-poietic stem cell compartment. This type of translocation can also be found in 255–30% of acute lymphoblastic leukemia (ALL) cases and a minority of acute myeloid leukemia (AML) cases. The translocation forms a fusion between the breakpoint cluster regions (*BCR*) and the Abl PTK gene (*ABL*), resulting in the constitutive expression of fusion protein BCR-Abl, which exhibits enhanced PTK activity. Because Abl regulates a number of proteins involved with the cell cycle, the result is that BCR-Abl expression increases cell division, leading to an overproduction of myeloid-lineage cells. Moreover, BCR-Abl inhibits DNA repair mechanisms, leading to genomic instability, which enables cells to accumulate several additional mutations that precipitate disease progression. This transforms the disease from the chronic phase that is stable for several years to the acute / blast crisis phase.

Comment
BCR-Abl was one of the first proteins for which drugs were designed specifically to antagonize the signal transducer of interest, a so-called targeted therapy. Imatinib (Glivec) is a tyrosine kinase inhibitor (TKI) developed to specifically inhibit the Abl kinase activity. Although it was unable to completely eradicate the CML cells, it reduced their proliferation rate and delayed the onset of blast crisis. Although imatinib is an important drug for the treatment of the majority of CML patients, a small percentage of patients are resistant or develop resistance to imatinib treatment, possibly due to acquired mutations within BCR-Abl, which has led to the development of second-line (e.g., dasatinib and nilotinib) and third-line (ponatinib) therapies for CML. Of note, TKI therapies to date have been unsuccessful at eradicating the CML CSCs; therefore there is a risk of relapse in TKI-treated patients if the therapy is withdrawn or if the patients develop chemoresistance.

of PI3K by dephosphorylating PIP$_3$. The tumor suppressor PTEN is one of the most commonly inactivated proteins in sporadic cancer, resulting in sustained PI3K/Akt signaling and uncontrolled cell survival and proliferation. Mutations in PTEN have been identified in a wide range of cancers, **including breast, thyroid, prostate, and brain cancers.** Interestingly, individuals with inherited germline mutations in PTEN, known as PTEN **hamartoma tumor syndrome,** develop benign tumors associated with breast, thyroid, colorectal, endometrial, and kidney tissue. However, these patients also carry an elevated lifetime risk of developing malignant cancers in these tissues. The increased susceptibility to cancer in cells carrying germline PTEN mutations underlines the importance of this protein as a tumor suppressor.

ACTIVE LEARNING

1. How is progression through the cell cycle regulated?
2. Outline experimental assays that can be used to quantitate cell viability and proliferation.
3. Describe, with reference to specific examples, how growth factor receptor ligation mediates cellular proliferation.
4. Contrast the distinct mechanisms by which a cell can undergo cell death.
5. Explain, with specific examples, how selected mutations within normal growth signals can give rise to a cancerous phenotype in human cells.
6. Define the cancer stem cell theory, and explain how this theory may influence the design of future cancer therapies.

SUMMARY

- Most protooncogenes and tumorsuppressor genes have a function associated with signal transduction, mimicking the effects of persistent mitogenic stimulation and thereby uncoupling cells from normal external controls.
- These signaling pathways converge on the machinery that controls the transition of the cell through the G1 phase and prevent cell-cycle exit.
- Additional genes, many of which are targeted by cancer-specific chromosomal translocations and epigenetic regulation, lead to aberrant cell-fate decisions that would normally induce apoptosis. The two tumor-suppressor proteins, PTEN and p53, which have key roles in determining cell-cycle progression and apoptosis, and the genes coding for these proteins, are most frequently disrupted in cancer cells.

FURTHER READING

Chiara Maiuri, M., Zalckvar, E., Kimchi, A., et al. (2007). Self-eating and self-killing: Crosstalk between autophagy and apoptosis. *Nature Reviews. Molecular Cell Biology, 8,* 741–752.

Dick, J. E. (2008). Stem cell concepts renew cancer research. *Blood, 112,* 4793–4807.

Hollander, M. C., Blumenthal, G. M., & Dennis, P. A. (2011). PTEN loss in the continuum of common cancers, rare syndromes and mouse models. *Nature Reviews Cancer, 11,* 289–301.

Hotchkiss, R. S., Strasser, A., McDunn, J. E., et al. (2009). Cell Death. *The New England Journal of Medicine, 361,* 157–183.

Laplante, M., & Sabatini, D. M. (2012). mTOR signaling in growth control and disease. *Cell, 149,* 274–293.

Levine, A. J., & Oren, M. (2009). The first 30 years of p53: Growing ever more complex. *Nature Reviews Cancer, 9,* 749–758.

Malumbres, M., & Barbacid, M. (2009). Cell cycle, CDKs and cancer: A changing paradigm. *Nature Reviews Cancer, 9,* 153–166.

Taylor, R. C., Cullen, S. P., & Martin, S. J. (2008). Apoptosis: Controlled demolition at the cellular level. *Nature Reviews Molecular Cell Biology, 9,* 231–241.

RELEVANT WEBSITES

Wiley Essential for Life Sciences - Citable reviews in life sciences: http://www.els.net/

Kimball's Biology Pages: http://users.rcn.com/jkimball.ma.ultranet/BiologyPages/

KEGG - Human cell cycle: http://www.genome.jp/kegg/pathway/hsa/hsa04110.html

ABBREVIATIONS

Abl	Nonreceptor PTK
ACD	Autophagic cell death (autophagy)
ALL	Acute lymphoblastic leukemia
ALPS	Autoimmune lymphoproliferative syndrome
AML	Acute myeloid leukemia
AMPK	5'AMP-activated protein kinase
AP-1	Transcription factor
APAF1	Apoptotic protease activating factor 1
APC	Anaphase-promoting complex
ATG	Autophagy-related gene
ATM	Ataxia-telangiectasia mutated, checkpoint kinase
ATR	Ataxia-telangiectasia Rad3–related checkpoint kinase, CHK1 and CHK2
BAD	Bcl-2-associated death promoter
Bak	Bcl-2 homologous antagonist/killer
BAX	Bcl-2-associated X protein
Bcl-2	B-cell lymphoma protein 2; Bcl-2 family members include prosurvival family members (Bcl-2, Bcl-xL, Bcl-W, Mcl-1); proapoptotic BAX/BAK family, and proapoptotic BH-3-only proteins (BIM, Bid, PUMA, NOXA, BAD, BIK)
BCR	Breakpoint cluster region
BH-3	Interacting-domain death agonist
BrdU	Bromodeoxyuridine
Btk	A protein tyrosine kinase
CAK	CDK-activating complex, composed of CDK7, cyclin H, and MAT1 (ménage a trois)
CDK	Cyclin-dependent kinase
CDKIs	Cyclin-dependent kinase inhibitory proteins
CFDA SE	Carboxy-fluoresceindiacetate succinimidyl ester
cFLIP	Modulator of FADD, Fas-associated death domain
CHK1	CHK2, checkpoint kinases
CLL	Chronic lymphocytic leukemia
CML	Chronic myeloid leukemia
CSC	Cancer stem cell
CTD	C-terminal domain
DAG	Diacylglycerol
DAPI	4'-6'-diamidino-2-phenylindole
DD	Death domain
DED	Death effector domain
DISC	Death-inducing signaling complex
4E-BP1	eIF4E-binding protein 1

E2F	Family of transcription factors
EBNA1	The Epstein–Barr virus nuclear antigen 1
eIF4E	Eukaryotic initiation factor 4E
EGF	Epidermal growth factor
EGFR	Epidermal growth factor receptor
ER	Endoplasmic reticulum
ERK 1 and 2	Extracellular-signal regulated kinases; two isoforms of MEK kinase that activate MAPK
FADD	Fas-associated death domain; Fas, death receptor, TNF family member
Fyn	Nonreceptor PTK
FasL	Fas ligand
G0	Resting, or quiescent, phase
G1	Interval between M and S phases
G2	Interval between S and M phases
GAPs	GTPase-activating protein
GAS	Gamma interferon activation site
Grb2	Growth factor receptor-bound protein 2, adapter molecule
HCL	Hairy cell leukemia
HGF	Hepatocyte growth factor
Ig	Immunoglobulin
IAP	Inhibitor of apoptosis gene family
IL-2	Interleukin 2 INK (4A,4B,4C, 4D) proteins mediating cycle arrest, inhibitors of CDK4 family (also known as p16, p15, p18, and p19, respectively)
IP$_3$	Inositol 1,4,5-trisphosphate
JAK	Janus kinase
KIT	Tyrosine kinase 3 genes
KIP2	57-kDa inhibitor of cyclin–CDK complexes
LC3	Microtubule-associated protein light chain 3
LSC	Laser-scanning cytometry
M	Mitosis
MCL	Mantle cell lymphoma
MMP	Mitochondrial membrane potential
MAPK	Mitogen-activated protein kinase
MEK	A kinase that activates MAPK; two isoforms, extracellular-signal regulated kinase (ERK) 1 and 2
mTOR	Mechanistic target of rapamycin a serine/ threonine protein kinase
mTORC-1 and mTORC-2	mTor complexes
Myc	Transcription factor
NFAT	Transcription factor
p53	Tumor-suppressor protein
PCD	Programmed cell death
PDGF	Platelet-derived growth factor
PDK1	PIP$_3$-dependent kinase
PE	Phosphatidylethanolamine
PH	Pleckstrin homology domains
PI	Propidium iodide
PI3K	Phosphatidylinositol 3-kinase
PIP$_2$	Phosphatidylinositol 4,5-bisphosphate
PIP$_3$	Phosphatidylinositol 3,4,5-trisphosphate
PP2A	Protein phosphatase-2A
PKC	Protein kinase C
PLC-γ	Phospholipase Cγ
PS	Phosphatidylserine
PTK	Protein tyrosine kinase domain
PTEN	Phosphatase and TENsin homologue
PTPase	Phosphotyrosine phosphatase
Ras	A GTPase
Rb	Retinoblastoma protein
Rheb	Ras homologue enriched in brain
Rictor	mTORC-2 complex
RIP1	Serine/threonine kinase
RNA	Ribonucleic acid
RSK1	A kinase
S	Synthetic phase of interphase
S6K1	Ribosomal S6 kinase 1
SAC	Spindle assembly checkpoint
SCID	Severe combined immunodeficiency
SH2	Src-homology region 2, from the cytoplasmic
Shc	Adapter molecule
SHP	SH2 domain-containing phosphatase
Sos	Son of Sevenless, guanine nucleotide exchange factor
Src	Homology and collagen domain protein, a nonreceptor PTK
STATs	Signal transducer and activators, transcription factors
T-ALL	T lymphocyte–acute lymphoblastic leukemia
TdT	Terminal deoxynucleotidyl transferase
TFIIH	General transcription factor
TKI	Tyrosine kinase inhibitor
TGF-a	Transforming growth factor-a
TNFR	Death receptor, TNF family member
TRAIL	Death receptors, TNF family member
TSC	Tuberous sclerosis complex
TSC1/2	Janus kinases (JAK)
TSC1/2	Tuberous sclerosis protein 1/2
TWEAK	Death receptor, TNF family member
UVRAG	UV radiation resistance–associated gene protein
ZAP-70	PTK that is essential for antigen-dependent T-cell activation

Aging

John W. Baynes

INTRODUCTION

Aging may be defined as the time-dependent deterioration in function of an organism

Although it has broad-based physiologic effects, aging is fundamentally the result of changes in cellular structure and function, biochemistry, and metabolism (Table 29.1). The result of aging, even healthy aging, is increased susceptibility to disease and increased probability of death - the endpoint of aging. However, aging is not a disease. Diseases affect a fraction of the population; aging affects all of us, whether it is programmed or stochastic.

With the aging of the population, gerontology and geriatric medicine are becoming increasingly important. This chapter presents an overview of the biochemical and physiologic changes associated with aging in general and with the aging of specific organ systems. It includes a review of current theories on aging (there are several theories, and in general, the more theories there are, the less we really understand about something) and concludes with a discussion of the relationship between cancer and aging and an update on approaches to lifespan extension.

Aging of complex systems

Excluding genetic defects, childhood disease, and accidents, humans survive until about age 50 with limited maintenance requirements or risk of death; then we become increasingly frail, and our death rate increases with time, reaching a maximum at about age 76. Our lifespan is affected by our genetics and our environmental exposure, and death is usually attributable to the failure of a critical organ system (cardiovascular, renal, pulmonary, etc.). The capacity of these interdependent physiologic systems usually declines as a linear function of age, leading to an exponential increase in the age-specific death rate (Fig. 29.1). Historically, improvements in health care and environment have resulted in **"rectangularization" of the survival curve** - our mean lifespan has increased but without a significant effect on our maximum lifespan (see Fig. 29.1A).

The Hayflick limit: Replicative senescence

The replicative capacity of cells decreases with age

Differentiated cells from animals undergo only a limited number of cell divisions (population doublings) in tissue culture, unless they become transformed to cancer cells by mutation or infection with certain viruses. The number of potential cell divisions is greater in longer-lived animals, suggesting a relationship between cell-division potential and longevity. Human neonatal fibroblasts will divide up to 70 times, then enter a nondividing, senescent state, whereas fibroblasts from mice, which have shorter lifespans, undergo about 20 cell divisions in vitro. Cells from younger donors have a greater replicative capacity and a greater number of cell divisions in cell culture, but the number of dividing cells decreases with age. This limited doubling capacity, described by Dr. Leonard Hayflick, is known as the **Hayflick limit.** The relevance of the Hayflick limit to human aging is still debated - certainly, human cells retain some replicative capacity, even at advanced age, and major tissues, such as muscle and nerve, are largely postmitotic (i.e., not actively dividing). However, changes in the metabolism of senescent cells, including decreased responsiveness to hormones and the decline in their synthetic and degradative capacities (e.g., in the immunologic and reticuloendothelial systems), may affect our adaptability and susceptibility to stress and age-related diseases, placing limits on our lifespan.

Table 29.1 Decline in biochemical and physiologic systems with age

Biochemical	Physiologic
Basal metabolic rate	Lung expansion volume
Protein turnover	Renal filtration capacity (glomerular)
Glucose tolerance	Renal concentration capacity (tubular)
Reproductive capacity	Cardiovascular performance
Telomere shortening	Musculoskeletal system
Oxidative phosphorylation	Nerve conduction velocity
	Endocrine and exocrine systems
	Immunologic defenses
	Sensory systems (vision, audition)

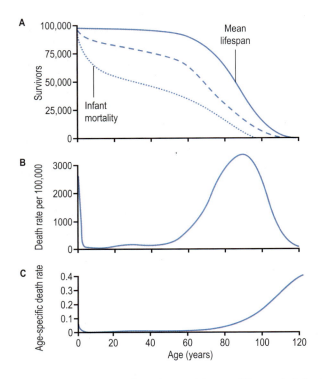

Fig. 29.1 **Survival curve and death rate.** (A) **Mean lifespan** is defined as the age at which 50% of a population survives (or has died). The negative slope of the survival curve reaches a maximum at the mean lifespan, which was 84 years (average of both sexes) in Japan in 2015. The dotted line describes a survival curve in the third world, where infant mortality and disease significantly decrease mean lifespan. The dashed line describes the survival curve for the United States in the early part of the 20th century. (B) The **death rate** reaches a maximum at the mean lifespan. (C) The **age-specific death rate**, defined as the number of deaths per time at a given age (e.g., deaths per 100,000 persons of a specific age per year) increases exponentially with age. The lifespan, or maximum lifespan potential (MLSP), is defined as the maximum age attainable by a member of the population, which is about 120 years for humans.

Mathematical models of aging

In poikilotherms, the rate of aging is correlated with temperature, physical activity, and metabolic rate

In the early 19th century, Gompertz observed that the age-specific death rate of humans increased exponentially after 35 years of age and that human survival curves could be modeled by what is now known as the **Gompertz equation** (Fig. 29.2):

$$m_t = Ae^{\alpha t}$$

The term m_t is the age-specific death rate at age t; α is the slope, the effect of time on the death rate; and A, the *y*-axis intercept, is the death rate at birth. The Gompertz–Makeham equation

$$m(t) = Ae^{\alpha t} + B$$

adds a constant, B, to correct for the age-independent death rate (e.g., as a result of infant mortality or accidents) and provides a better fit to actuarial data.

The Gompertz plots in Fig. 29.2 illustrate the time-dependent changes in the death rate for three different species of vertebrates and for flies raised at different temperatures. Shorter-lived mammals have a greater age-adjusted rate of death (α = slope), whereas the death rate for poikilotherms varies with ambient temperature - flies live longer when grown at lower temperatures. This observation has been interpreted as evidence for the **rate-of-living** or **wear-and-tear** theories of aging. Flies, being more active at higher temperatures, consume more energy, wear out, and die more rapidly. Flies that are restrained (e.g., in a matchbox rather than a large carboy) also live longer, wingless flies live longer, and male flies, segregated from females, also live longer. In each case - in small enclosures, without wings, and in the absence of the opposite sex - male flies are less active, have lower basal metabolic rates, and have longer mean and maximum lifespans. None of these strategies for lifespan extension is applicable to humans.

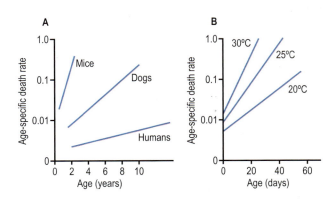

Fig. 29.2 **Gompertz plots for humans and other species.** (A) Humans and other vertebrates. (B) Flies raised at various temperatures (adapted from the work of Professor RS Sohal).

THEORIES OF AGING

Theories of aging can be divided into two general categories: Biological and chemical

Biological theories of aging treat aging as a genetically controlled event, determined by the programmed expression or repression of genetic information. Aging and death are seen as the orchestrated endstage of birth, growth, maturation, and reproduction. **Apoptosis** (programmed cell death) and thymic involution are examples of genetically programmed events at the level of cells and organs, and the decline in the immunologic, neuroendocrine, and reproductive systems may be seen, in a broader context, as evidence for the action of a biological clock affecting the integrated functions of an organism. Biological theories attribute differences in lifespan to interspecies differences in genetics but also provide an explanation for the observation that there is a genetic component to longevity within a species (e.g., in families with a history of longevity). Differences in lifespan among species are also closely correlated with the efficiency of DNA repair mechanisms. Longer-lived species have more efficient DNA repair processes (Fig. 29.3). Numerous diseases of accelerated aging **(progeria)** also illustrate the importance of genetics and maintenance of the integrity of the genome during aging.

Chemical theories of aging treat it as a somatic process resulting from cumulative damage to biomolecules. At one extreme, the **error-catastrophe theory** proposes that aging is the result of cumulative errors in the machinery for replication, repair, transcription, and translation of genetic information. Eventually, errors in critical enzymes, such as DNA and RNA polymerases or enzymes involved in the synthesis and turnover of proteins, gradually affect the fidelity of expression of genetic information and permit the accumulation of altered proteins. The propagation of errors and resultant accumulation of dysfunctional macromolecules lead eventually to the collapse of the system. Consistent with this theory, increasing amounts of immunologically detectable, but denatured or modified, functionally inactive enzymes accumulate in cells as a function of age.

More general chemical theories treat aging as the result of chronic, cumulative chemical (nonenzymatic) modification, insults, or damage to all biomolecules (Table 29.2). Like rust or corrosion, the accumulation of damage with age gradually affects function. This damage is most apparent in long-lived tissue proteins, such as lens crystallins and extracellular collagens, which accumulate a wide range of chemical modifications with age. These proteins gradually brown with age as a result of the formation of conjugated compounds with absorbance in the yellow-red region of the spectrum (Fig. 29.4); in the lens, they act as a filter, contributing to the loss of color vision with age. Highly modified crystallins, the major protein in the lens, gradually precipitate, leading to the development of cataracts. Chemical damage to the integrity of the genome also occurs, but cumulative damage to DNA is more difficult

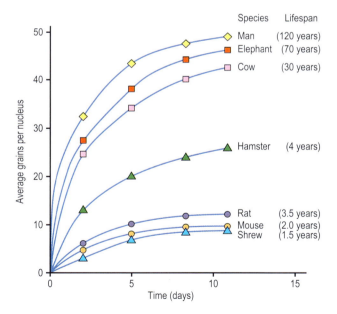

Fig. 29.3 **Relationship between DNA repair activity and longevity.** Fibroblasts from various species were irradiated briefly, forming thymine dimers and thymine glycol (Chapter 20; Chapter 42). The oxidized bases were removed and replaced by excision repair. DNA repair was assessed by the rate of incorporation of a [³H]thymidine tracer into DNA by autoradiography (adapted from Hart, R.W., & Setlow, R. B. [1974]. Correlation between deoxyribonucleic acid excision-repair and life-span in a number of mammalian species. *Proceedings of the National Academy of Sciences, 71,* 2169–2173).

Table 29.2 Age-dependent chemical changes in biomolecules		
Protein modification	**DNA modification and mutation**	**Other**
Crosslinking	Oxidation	Lipofuscin
Oxidation	Depurination	Inactive enzymes
Deamidation	Substitutions	
D-aspartate	Insertions and deletions	
Protein carbonyls	Inversions and transpositions	
Glycoxidation		
Lipoxidation		

Long-lived proteins, such as lens crystallins and tissue collagens, accumulate damage with age. Modification and crosslinking of proteins occur as a result of nonoxidative (deamidation, racemization) or oxidative (protein carbonyls) mechanisms or by reactions of proteins with products of carbohydrate or lipid peroxidation (glycoxidation, lipoxidation). Damage to DNA is often silent - that is, modified forms of nucleotides may not accumulate, but the damage increases in the form of mutations resulting from errors in repair.

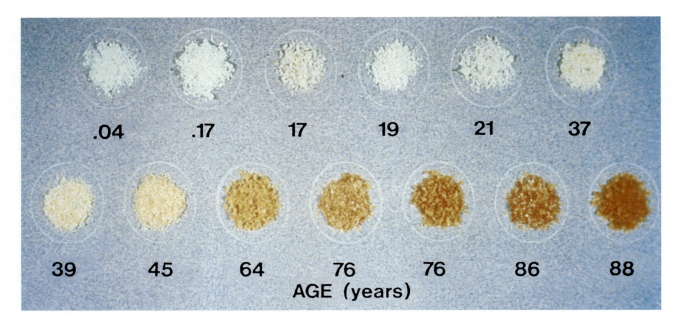

Fig. 29.4 **Changes in costal cartilage with age.** Browning is a characteristic feature of the aging of proteins, not just in the lens, which is exposed to sunlight, but also in tissue collagens throughout the body. Crosslinking of proteins also increases with browning. Crosslinking contributes to the gradual insolubilization of lens protein with age. Crosslinking of articular and vascular collagens decreases the resilience of vertebral disks and compliance of the vascular wall with age. These changes in extracellular proteins are similar to changes induced by reaction of carbohydrates and lipids with protein during the cooking of foods, a process known as the **Maillard or browning reaction.** At one level, humans have been described as low-temperature ovens, operating at 37°C, with long cooking cycles (≈75 years). Many of the Maillard reaction products detected in the crust of bread and pretzels have been identified in human crystallins and collagens, and they increase with age. (See also discussion of diabetic complications in Chapter 31.)

to quantify because of the efficiency of repair processes that excise and repair modified nucleotides. As noted in Table 29.2, there are a number of silent consequences of DNA damage. This damage is primarily endogenous but is enhanced by xenobiotic and environmental agents.

Organ system theories of aging incorporate various aspects of the theories just described. These theories attribute aging to the failure of integrative systems, such as the immunologic, neurologic, endocrine, or circulatory systems. Although they do not assign a specific cause, these theories integrate biological and chemical theories, acknowledging both genetic and environmental contributions to aging.

The free-radical theory of aging

The free-radical theory of aging is the most widely accepted theory of aging

The **free-radical theory of aging** (FRTA) treats aging as the result of cumulative oxidative damage to biomolecules: DNA, RNA, protein, lipids, and glycoconjugates. From the viewpoint of the FRTA, longer-lived organisms have lower rates of production of **reactive oxygen species** (**ROS**; Chapter 42), better antioxidant defenses, and more efficient repair or turnover processes. Although it is a chemical theory, the FRTA does not ignore the importance of genetics and biology in limiting the production of ROS or the role of antioxidant and repair mechanisms. It also interfaces with other theories of aging, such as the rate-of-living theory (because the rate of generation of ROS is a function of the overall rate and/or extent of oxygen consumption) and the crosslinkage theory (because some products of ROS damage crosslink proteins, contributing, for example, to the decrease in vascular elasticity with age). Finally, as a chemical hypothesis, the FRTA does not exclude cumulative chemical damage, independent of ROS, such as racemization and deamidation of amino acids, but focuses on ROS as the primary source of damage and the fundamental cause of aging.

The FRTA is supported by the inverse correlation between the basal metabolic rate (rate of oxygen consumption per unit weight) and maximum lifespan of mammals and by evidence of increased oxidative damage to proteins with age. Protein carbonyl groups, such as glutamic and aminoadipic acid semialdehyde, formed by oxidative deamination of arginine and lysine, respectively, are formed in proteins exposed to ROS. The steady-state level of **protein carbonyls** in intracellular proteins increases logarithmically with age and at a rate inversely proportional to the lifespan of species. Protein carbonyls are also much higher in fibroblasts from patients with progeria (accelerated aging; e.g., Werner's or Hutchinson–Gilford syndromes), compared with age-matched subjects. Similar concentrations of protein carbonyls are also present in tissues of old rats and elderly humans, supporting

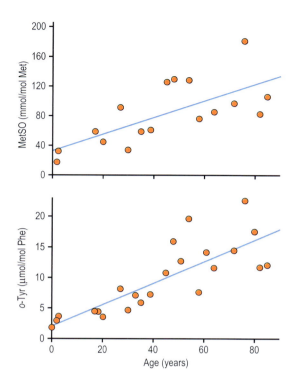

Fig. 29.5 **Accumulation of amino acid oxidation products in human skin collagen with age.** Methionine is oxidized to methionine sulfoxide (MetSO) by HOCl or H_2O_2; *ortho*-tyrosine is a product of hydroxyl radical addition to phenylalanine (Phe). Despite a 100-fold difference in their rate of accumulation in collagen, levels of MetSO and *o*-tyrosine correlate strongly with one another, indicating that multiple ROS contribute to oxidative damage to proteins (adapted from Wells-Knecht, M. C., et al. [1997]. Age-dependent accumulation of *ortho*-tyrosine and methionine sulfoxide in human skin collagen is not increased in diabetes: Evidence against a generalized increase in oxidative stress in diabetes. *Journal of Clinical Investigation, 100,* 839–846).

the argument that similar changes occur at old age in a range of organisms, regardless of the difference in their lifespans.

Fig. 29.5 illustrates the accumulation of two relatively stable amino acid oxidation products in human skin collagen: **methionine sulfoxide** and **ortho-tyrosine.** These compounds are formed by different mechanisms involving different ROS (Chapter 42) and are present at significantly different concentrations in skin collagen but increase in concert with age. Other amino acid modifications that accumulate in skin collagen with age include **advanced glycoxidation and lipoxidation end products (AGE/ALE),** such as N^{ε}-(carboxymethyl)lysine (CML), pentosidine (Fig. 29.6), and D-aspartate.

D-aspartate is a nonoxidative modification of protein that is formed by spontaneous, age-dependent racemization of L-aspartate, the natural form of the amino acid in protein. The more rapid turnover of skin collagen, compared with articular collagen, yields a lower rate of accumulation of D-aspartate in skin collagen with age and also explains the lower rates of accumulation of AGE/ALEs in skin versus articular collagen. AGE/ALEs are even higher in lens crystallins,

which have the slowest rate of turnover among proteins in the body. **Deamidation** of asparagine and glutamine is another nonoxidative chemical modification that increases with age in proteins; it has been described primarily in intracellular proteins.

The rate of accumulation of these modifications depends on the rate of turnover of the collagens (Fig. 29.7) and is accelerated by hyperglycemia and hyperlipidemia in diabetes and atherosclerosis. The increase in AGE/ALEs and oxidative crosslinking of collagen is thought to impair the turnover and contribute to the thickening of basement membranes with age. Increased age-adjusted levels of AGE/ALEs in collagen are implicated in the pathogenesis of complications of diabetes and atherosclerosis. These products are also increased together in the brain in various neurodegenerative diseases, including Alzheimer's, Parkinson's disease, and Creutzfeldt–Jakob (prion) diseases.

The age pigment **lipofuscin** is a less well-characterized but characteristic biomarker of aging. It accumulates in the form of fluorescent granules, derived from lysosomes, in the cytoplasm of postmitotic cells at a rate that is inversely related to species lifespan. It is considered the accumulated, indigestible debris of reactions between lipid peroxides and proteins. Lipofuscin may account for 10%–15% of the volume of cardiac muscle and neuronal cells at an advanced age, and its rate of deposition in cardiac myocytes in cell culture is accelerated by growth under hyperoxic conditions. In flies, the rate of accumulation of lipofuscin varies directly with ambient temperature and activity and inversely with lifespan, consistent with the effects of these variables on lifespan (see Fig. 29.2B).

In summary, a wide range of chemical modifications, both oxidative and nonoxidative, can accumulate in proteins with age. Although attention is often focused on modification of protein, the real damage from free radicals and oxidative stress is at the level of the genome; if the DNA is not repaired correctly, the cell will die, its capacity may be impaired, or the damage will be propagated. Damage to DNA accumulates not in the form of modified nucleic acids but as chemically "silent" errors in repair - insertions, deletions, substitutions, transpositions, and inversions of DNA sequences - that affect the expression and structure of proteins. Because repair is fairly efficient in humans compared with other animals, and the composition of DNA does not change on repair, mutations in DNA are not observable in tissues by conventional analytic techniques. However, the presence of oxidized pyrimidines and purines in urine (see Fig. 42.6) provides evidence of chronic oxidative damage to the genome.

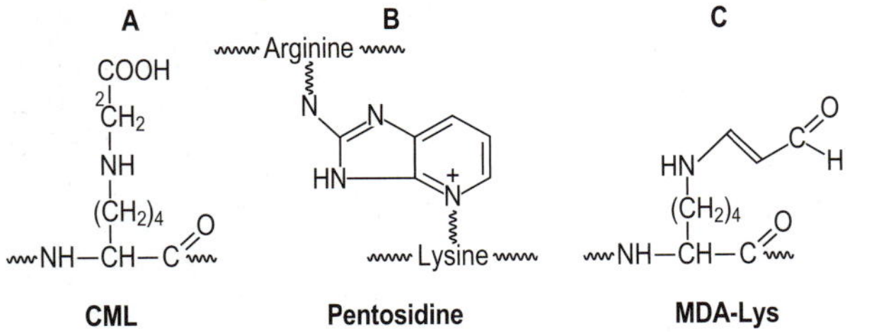

Mitochondrial theories of aging

Mitochondrial DNA is particularly susceptible to oxidative damage

Mitochondrial theories of aging are a blend of biological and chemical theories, treating aging as the result of chemical damage to mitochondrial DNA (mtDNA). Mitochondria contain proteins specified by both nuclear and mitochondrial DNA, but only 13 mitochondrial proteins are encoded by mitochondrial DNA. Although this may seem trivial, these 13 proteins

Fig. 29.6 **Structure of major advanced glycoxidation and lipoxidation end products (AGE/ALE).** (A) The AGE/ALE, N^ε-(carboxymethyl)lysine (CML), which is formed during both carbohydrate and lipid peroxidation reactions. (B) The AGE pentosidine, a fluorescent crosslink in proteins. (C) The ALE malondialdehyde-lysine (MDA-Lys), a reactive ALE that may proceed to form aminoenimine (RNHCH=CHCH=NR) crosslinks in proteins.

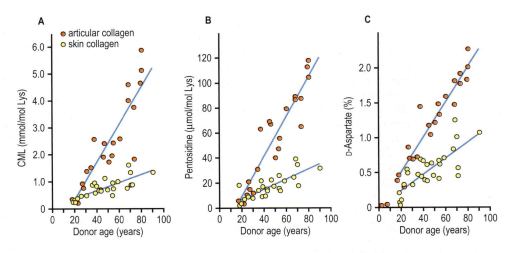

Fig. 29.7 **Accumulation of advanced glycoxidation and lipoxidation end products (AGE/ALE) and D-aspartate in articular and skin collagens with age.** N^ε-(carboxymethyl)lysine (CML) is formed by oxidative mechanisms from glycated proteins or reaction of glucose, ascorbate or lipid peroxidation products with protein. The fluorescent crosslink pentosidine is formed by oxidative reaction of glucose or ascorbate with proteins. D-Aspartate is formed nonoxidatively by racemization of L-aspartate residues in protein. Tissue levels of oxidative and nonoxidative biomarkers correlate with one another, and differences in their rates of accumulation in articular and skin collagen result from differences in rates of turnover of these collagens (adapted from Verzijl, N., et al. [2000]. Effect of collagen turnover on the accumulation of advanced glycation end products. *Journal of Biological Chemistry, 275,* 39027–39031).

CLINICAL BOX
BIOMARKERS OF OXIDATIVE STRESS AND AGING

Advanced glycoxidation and lipoxidation end products (AGE/ALE) are formed by reaction of proteins with products of oxidation of carbohydrates and lipids (see Fig. 29.6). Some compounds, such as N^ε-(carboxymethyl)lysine (CML), may be formed from either carbohydrates or lipids; others, such as pentosidine, are formed only from carbohydrates; and others, such as the malondialdehyde adduct to lysine, are formed exclusively from lipids. Carbohydrate sources of AGEs include glucose, ascorbate, and glycolytic intermediates; ALEs are derived from oxidation of polyunsaturated fatty acids in phospholipids. Lysine, histidine, and cysteine residues are the major sites of AGE/ALE formation in protein. More than 30 different AGE/ALEs have been detected in tissue proteins, and many of these are known to increase with age. AGE/ALEs are useful biomarkers of the aging of proteins and their exposure to oxidative stress.

CLINICAL BOX
ALZHEIMER'S DISEASE: OXIDATIVE STRESS IN NEURODEGENERATIVE DISEASE

Alzheimer's disease (AD) is the most common form of progressive cognitive deterioration in the elderly. It is characterized microscopically by the appearance of **neurofibrillary tangles** and senile plaques in cortical regions of the brain. The tangles are localized inside neurons and are rich in τ (tau) protein, which is derived from microtubules; it is hyperphosphorylated and polyubiquitinated. Plaques are extracellular aggregates, localized around amyloid deposits, formed from insoluble peptides derived from a family of **amyloid precursor proteins.** AD affects primarily cholinergic neurons, and drugs that inhibit the degradation of acetylcholine within synapses are a mainstay of therapy. A similar approach is used for preservation of dopamine in dopaminergic neurons in Parkinson's disease (i.e., by inhibiting the degradative enzyme monoamine oxidase).

Several studies have shown that both AGEs and ALEs are increased in tangles and plaques in the brain of AD patients compared with age-matched controls. Other indicators of generalized oxidative stress in the AD brain include increased levels of protein carbonyls, nitrotyrosine, and 8-OH-deoxyguanosine, all detected by immunohistochemical methods. The amyloid protein is toxic to neurons in cell culture and catalyzes oxidative stress and inflammatory responses in glial cells. Significant quantities of decompartmentalized redox-active iron, a catalyst of Fenton reactions (Chapter 42), are also detectable histologically in the AD brain and can be removed reversibly (in vitro) by treatment with chelators, such as desferrioxamine - heme iron is resistant to this treatment, indicating that the iron is free iron and potentially catalytically active in generation of ROS via Fenton reactions. Based on these and other data, oxidative stress is strongly implicated in the development and/or progression of AD, and chelators are being evaluated clinically for the treatment of AD.

ADVANCED CONCEPT BOX
AGING OF THE CIRCULATORY SYSTEM

The **extracellular matrix** of the aorta and major arteries becomes thicker and more highly crosslinked with age, contributing to both the decrease in elasticity and the ability of the endothelium to dilate blood vessels in response to physical and chemical stimuli. These changes occur naturally with age, independent of pathology, but may account for the increase in cardiovascular risk in the elderly. AGEs and ALEs are implicated in the crosslinking of the vascular extracellular matrix, explaining the age-adjusted increase in arterial crosslinking in diabetes and dyslipidemia. Increases in AGE/ALEs and protein crosslinking are also implicated in the altered filtration properties of the renal glomerular basement membrane in diabetes.

include essential subunits of the three proton pumps and ATP synthase. mtDNA is especially sensitive to mutations: mitochondria are the major site of ROS production in the cell (see Fig. 42.4), mtDNA is not protected by a sheath of histones, and mitochondria have limited capacity for DNA repair.

Mitochondrial diseases commonly involve defects of energy metabolism, including the pyruvate dehydrogenase complex, pyruvate carboxylase, electron transport complexes, ATP synthase, and enzymes of ubiquinone biosynthesis. These defects can be caused by mutations in both nuclear and mitochondrial DNA, but mtDNA suffers many more mutations than nuclear DNA. Such defects often result in the accumulation of lactic acid because of impaired oxidative phosphorylation, and they may cause cell death, especially in skeletal (myopathies) and cardiac muscles (cardiomyopathies) and the central nervous system (encephalopathies), all of which are heavily dependent on oxidative metabolism. The number of mitochondria and multiple copies of the mitochondrial genome in the cell provide some protection against mitochondrial dysfunction as a result of mutation, but the loss of fully functional mitochondria, and sometimes the number of mitochondria, is a characteristic feature of aging.

GENETIC MODELS OF INCREASED LIFESPAN

The effect of genetics on longevity is readily apparent in animal models

Different strains of mice vary by more than twofold in lifespan, and there are also significant differences in the lifespan of male and female mice of the same strain raised under identical conditions. Deficiencies in some hormones or defects in their receptors or postreceptor signaling pathways have a significant effect on mouse lifespan. Profound effects are observed in Ames and Snell dwarf mice. These mice have different pituitary

ADVANCED CONCEPT BOX
TELOMERES: A CLOCK OF AGING

Telomeres are the repetitive sequences at the ends of chromosomal DNA, typically thousands of copies of short, highly redundant, repetitive DNA - TTAGGG in humans (Chapter 20). DNA polymerase requires a double-stranded template for replication; RNA primers at the 5'-end of the template serve to initiate DNA synthesis. However, at the extreme ends of the chromosomes, DNA synthesis is restricted because there are no sequences further upstream for DNA primase engagement. Therefore each round of chromosome replication results in chromosome shortening. The enzyme telomerase is a reverse transcriptase containing an RNA with a sequence complementary to the telomere DNA. It functions to maintain the length of telomeres at the 3'-end of chromosomes. Telomerase is found in fetal tissues, in adult germ cells, and in tumor cells, but the somatic cells of multicellular organisms lack telomerase activity. This has led to the hypothesis that shortening of the telomere may contribute to the Hayflick limit and is involved in aging of multicellular organisms. Increased expression of telomerase in human cells results in elongated telomeres and an increase in the longevity of those cells by at least 20 cell doublings. Cells from individuals with progeria also have short telomeres. In contrast, cancer cells, which are immortal, express active telomerase activity. All of these observations suggest that the decrease in telomere length is associated with cellular senescence and aging. Knockout mice, in which the telomerase gene has been deleted, have chromosomes lacking detectable telomeres. These mice have high frequencies of aneuploidy and chromosomal abnormalities. The disease autosomal dyskeratosis congenita features a mutation in the telomerase locus, with the inability of somatic cells to reconstitute their telomeres, and hence loss of epidermis and hematopoietic marrow. This disease has many of the characteristics of accelerated aging.

ADVANCED CONCEPT BOX
AGING OF MUSCLE: DAMAGE TO MITOCHONDRIAL DNA

Old age is characterized by a general decrease in skeletal muscle mass **(sarcopenia)** and strength as a result of a decrease in both the number of motoneurons and the number and size of myofibers. The fiber loss is accompanied by an increase in interstitial, fibrous connective tissue and a reduction in capillary density, which limits the blood supply. The decrease in muscle mass and strength contributes to frailty and increased risk of mortality. The loss of skeletal muscle mass may also contribute to glucose intolerance in the elderly as a result of the decreasing mass of tissue available to take up glucose from the blood.

One of the major changes in muscle biochemistry with age is an increase in the number of muscle cells with mitochondria deficient in cytochrome oxidase, which limits the muscle's ability to do work. As mitochondria become less efficient in oxidizing NADH, they become more reduced, and the accumulation of partially reduced ubiquinone (semiquinone) promotes the reduction of molecular oxygen, leading to increased superoxide production in older mitochondria (see Chapter 42). Under these conditions, when oxidative phosphorylation is impaired, cells appear to generate ATP primarily by glycolysis. NADH is also oxidized extramitochondrially, primarily by NADH oxidases in the plasma membrane, which produces hydrogen peroxide but no ATP.

$$\text{NADH oxidases: } NADH + H^+ + O_2 \rightarrow NAD^+ + H_2O_2$$

These changes are observed in both cardiac and skeletal muscle and appear to result from major random deletions in mitochondrial DNA (25%–75% of total mtDNA), which are then amplified by clonal expansion, leading to fiber atrophy and breakage. The muscle fiber is only as strong as its weakest link, so small regions of fiber loss affect overall muscle capacity. Fortunately, sarcopenia can be delayed and partially reversed by resistance exercise, thus the emphasis on regular exercise among the elderly.

defects, both resulting in negligible secretion of growth hormone (GH; stimulates IGF-1 secretion by liver), thyroid-stimulating hormone, and prolactin (see Chapter 27). Their body weights are decreased as young adults by about 35% compared with littermates, and their maximum lifespan is increased by about 45%, but oddly, they become obese with age. Similar effects on weight and lifespan are observed in mice with defects in GH or IGF-1 receptors or signal transduction. Many of these strains are fragile: Ames and Snell dwarfs are hypothyroid, hypoglycemic, and hypoinsulinemic and have low body temperature; they have impaired reproductive capacity, are more susceptible to infection, and require special housing conditions to maintain body temperature - but they live longer! Treatment of hypothyroidism in Snell dwarfs resulted in a restoration of a near-normal lifespan, whereas hypophysectomy of young rats increased their maximum lifespan by 15%–20%. Thus three hormones that have a profound effect on metabolism and growth (**growth hormone, IGF-1 [and insulin], and thyroxine**) also have profound effects on lifespan.

In humans, the most significant genetic determinant of lifespan is sex: women live 5%–7% longer than men. Genetics accounts for an estimated 20%–50% of the remaining variance in mean lifespan, with the other 50%–80% being attributed to environment and random developmental variations. It was estimated (in 2008) that there are at least 30 genes that have a significant effect on human lifespan. The cross-breeding of human populations and the many allelic combinations of these genes may obscure effects seen in inbred strains of worms or rodents. However, there is a recent report that Ashkenazi Jews who live past age 95 have a higher frequency of mutations in the gene for the IGF-1 receptor (IGF-1R). There are other genes or gene products that are associated with increased longevity in humans (e.g., variants in ApoE, ApoC3, and CETP). However, these genes seem to increase mean lifespan, probably by modulating the cardiovascular effects of dietary cholesterol, rather than cause an increase in maximum lifespan.

ANTIAGING INTERVENTIONS: WHAT WORKS AND WHAT DOESN'T

Antioxidant supplements

Antioxidant supplements may improve health but do not increase lifespan

Based on the FRTA, it seems reasonable to speculate that antioxidant supplementation should have an effect on longevity. In fact, however, there is no rigorous, reproducible experimental evidence that antioxidant supplements have any effect on the maximum lifespan of humans or other vertebrates. At the same time, antioxidant supplements, most of which include vitamins, may improve health, particularly in persons with vitamin deficiencies. Thus the effects of antioxidant therapy on mean (and healthy) lifespan are not unexpected. Failure to affect the maximum lifespan may result from the fact that there are so many mechanisms for production and control of free radicals and inhibiting or reversing damage to biomolecules. Many of these processes depend on the activity of enzymes that detoxify ROS or regenerate endogenous antioxidants. These enzymes, such as superoxide dismutase, catalase and gluta-thione peroxidase (Chapter 42), are induced in response to oxidative stress and may also be repressed during times of low oxidative stress. Thus the body may respond to maintain a homeostatic balance between prooxidant and antioxidant forces (see Fig. 42.2), countering efforts to enhance antioxidant defenses. This response may be essential, for example, to maintaining effective bactericidal activity during the respiratory burst accompanying phagocytosis.

Calorie restriction

Caloric restriction is the only regimen known to increase lifespan in animals

Calorie restriction (CR) is the only intervention that con-sistently extends maximum lifespan in a variety of species, including mammals, fish, flies, worms, and yeast. Reduc-tion in total caloric intake is the essential feature of this intervention - that is, the beneficial, life-extending effects are observed whenever CR is applied and regardless of dietary composition, although early and prolonged intervention will result in more impressive effects. As shown in Fig. 29.8, CR leads to a significant increase in both the mean and maximum lifespan of laboratory rats, equivalent to extending human lifespan to about 180 years. Calorie-restricted rats have fewer muscle fibers lacking in cytochrome oxidase and decreased levels of deletions in muscle mitochondrial DNA. CR mice also have lower levels of inducible genes for hepatic detoxification, DNA repair, and response to oxidative stress, sug-gesting a lower rate of oxidative stress and damage to proteins and DNA.

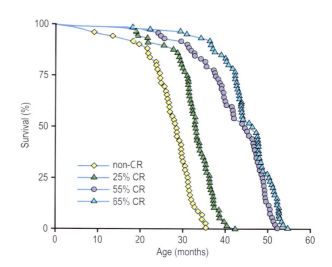

Fig. 29.8 **Calorie restriction (CR) extends longevity of mice.** The non-CR group received food ad libitum. Other groups were restricted by 25%, 55%, and 65% of the ad lib diet, starting at 1 month of age (adapted from Weindruch, R., et al. [1986]. Retardation of aging in mice by dietary restriction. *Journal of Nutrition, 116,* 651–654).

Caloric restriction delays the onset of age-related diseases, including cancer

CR is the most potent, broad-acting cancer-prevention regimen in rodents. It is argued that the extension of maximum lifespan by CR is achieved by delaying the onset of cancer (Fig. 29.9). Long-lived animals are more efficient in protecting their genome and thereby delaying the onset of cancer, but CR may limit damage even more, preserving the integrity of the genome and thereby leading to a longer lifespan. Although long-term CR has not been tested in humans, obesity, at the opposite end of the weight spectrum, is a proinflammatory state and is a risk factor for cancer in humans.

In CR experiments, it has been difficult to differentiate between the effects of dietary restriction on energy expenditure (rate of living) versus the reduction in body weight or adipose tissue mass that accompanies dietary restriction. FIRKO (adipose tissue [fat] insulin receptor knockout) mice have a 15%–25% decrease in body mass, largely because of a 50% decrease in fat mass. However, these mice consume identical amounts of food per day as control littermates - actually more than the control animals when normalized to their body weight. They also have a 20% increase in lifespan, suggesting that the decrease in body or fat mass is more important than caloric intake in determining maximum lifespan potential. In another study, overexpression of the gluconeogenic enzyme PEPCK in skeletal muscle produced a leaner mouse, with 50% of body weight and 10% of fat mass, compared with controls. These mice were seven times as active and ate 60% more than control mice, but they lived longer and had longer reproductive life. Overall, the decrease in body weight or adiposity during CR, rather than the decrease in food consumption, appears to have the greater effect on lifespan extension. One general outcome from these dietary and genetic experiments is that mitochondrial

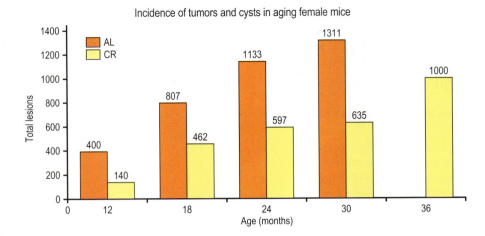

Incidence of tumors and cysts in aging female mice

Fig. 29.9 **Effect of calorie restriction (CR) on the development of tumors in mice.** More than 1000 mice, 50:50 male and female, from four different genotypes were divided into two groups, one fed ad libitum (AL) and the other receiving 60% of the caloric intake of the control group (CR), but with comparable intake of vitamins, minerals, and micronutrients. Cohorts of animals were sacrificed at specified times, and total lesions (tumors plus cysts) were measured. At 24 months, 51% of AL and 13% of CR mice had tumors. Note the absence of tumors in control (AL) mice at 36 months - all of the control mice are dead! CR extended the mean and maximum lifespan of the mice and also delayed the onset of cancer (adapted from Bronson, R. T., & Lipman, R. D. [1991]. Reduction in rate of occurrence of age related lesions in dietary restricted laboratory mice. *Growth, Development, and Aging, 55,* 169–184).

 ADVANCED CONCEPT BOX
SIRTUINS: SILENT INFORMATION REGULATORS AND MEDIATORS OF THE EFFECTS OF CALORIC RESTRICTION

Sirtuins are a family of NAD^+-dependent protein deacetylases; different isozymes are found in the nucleus and cytosolic and mitochondrial compartments. Sirtuins work on a wide range of protein substrates, including histones, regulatory enzymes, and DNA repair systems, and stimulate mitochondrial biogenesis and oxidative metabolism. Sirtuins were originally shown to extend the lifespan of yeast, *C. elegans,* and *Drosophila.* Sirtuin expression is increased in muscle and adipose tissue during caloric restriction in mice, overexpression of sirtuins mimics the effects of caloric restriction on mouse lifespan, and knockout of sirtuins blocks lifespan extension in mice. Mechanistically, the increase in the $NAD^+/NADH$ ratio observed during caloric restriction appears to both induce sirtuin expression and also provide increased substrate, NAD^+. Sirtuins are induced in eukaryotes by small molecules, such as **resveratrol** and quercetin, stimulating interest in the development of pharmaceutical approaches to lifespan extension.

efficiency, measured as lower rates of ROS/ATP production, appears to be an important determinant of longevity.

Studies on CR in longer-lived primate species have been under way since the 1980s. From these studies, there is clear evidence that monkeys on CR are more active and younger in appearance, have better insulin sensitivity and plasma lipid profiles and decreased risk for diabetes, have better overall cardiovascular and renal health, experience less age-related sarcopenia and brain atrophy, and have decreased risk for

cancer, compared with age-matched normally fed animals. However, the evidence of lifespan extension is weak and still controversial (Fig. 29.10). Even if CR can be shown to extend lifespan in monkeys, it is unlikely that humans will be able to adopt the strict dietary control required for this regimen. However, similar improvements in health have been observed in shorter-term studies with humans (i.e., improvement in fasting glucose, insulin sensitivity, and plasma lipid profile, along with decreased blood pressure, compared with a matched control group). Understanding the biological mechanisms of the effects of CR may lead to alternative strategies that mimic CR and possibly extend the healthy lifespan of humans.

SUMMARY

- Aging is characterized by a gradual decline in the capacity of physiologic systems, leading eventually to failure of a critical system, then death.
- At the biochemical level, aging is considered the result of chronic chemical modification of all classes of biomolecules.
- According to the free-radical theory of aging, ROS are the primary culprits, causing alterations in the sequence of DNA (mutations) and structure of proteins. Longevity is achieved by developing efficient systems to limit and/or repair chemical damage.
- Caloric restriction is, at present, the only widely applicable mechanism for delaying aging and extending the mean, healthy, and maximum lifespan of species.
- CR appears to work, in part, by inhibiting the production of ROS and limiting damage to

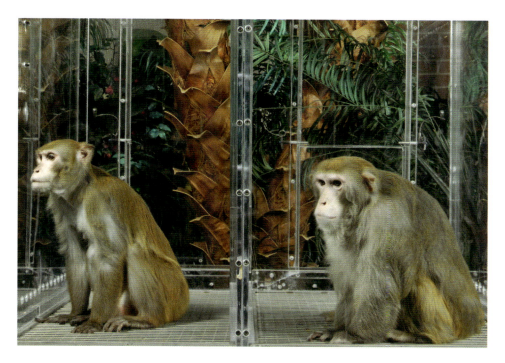

Fig. 29.10 **Effects of calorie restriction in primates.** The animal on the left was raised with calorie restriction, whereas that on the right was fed a normal diet. A study from the University of Wisconsin in 2009 concluded that calorie restriction extended the lifespan of rhesus monkeys, whereas another by the US National Institutes of Health in 2012, also with rhesus monkeys, concluded there was no effect. Studies with other primate species are still in progress, so the issue is not fully resolved; however, it is clear in all studies that calorie restriction produces a healthier phenotype, with fewer age-related chronic diseases and decreased risk for cancer (with permission from the National Institutes of Health).

biomolecules, delaying many of the characteristic features of aging, including cancer. Sirtuins have been identified as possible mediators of the effects of caloric restriction.

ACTIVE LEARNING

1. Discuss the nature of protein carbonyls and lipofuscin and their relevance to aging.
2. Discuss the relative importance of chemical damage to protein and DNA during aging.
3. Review recent literature on mouse genetic models of mammalian aging, and discuss the relationship between growth rate, obesity, calorie restriction, and aging in the mouse.
4. Nearly a dozen genes have been identified that, when mutated, extend the lifespan of animals. Why are the wild-type genes preserved in the gene pool?
5. Discuss the evidence that caloric restriction increases the mean, healthy, and maximum lifespan of primates.

FURTHER READING

Bhullar, K. S., & Hubbard, B. P. (2015). Lifespan and healthspan extension by resveratrol. *Biochimica et Biophysica Acta, 1852,* 1209–1218.

Carrero, D., Soria-Valles, C., & López-Otín, C. (2016). Hallmarks of progeroid syndromes: Lessons from mice and reprogrammed cells. *Disease Models and Mechanisms, 9,* 719–735.

Carvalho, A. N., Firuzi, O., Garra, M. J., et al. (2017). Oxidative stress and antioxidants in neurological diseases: Is there still hope? *Current Drug Targets, 18,* 705–718.

da Costa, J. P., Vitorino, R., Silva, G. M., et al. (2016). A synopsis on aging: Theories, mechanisms and future prospects. *Ageing Research Reviews, 29,* 90–112.

Michan, S. (2014). Calorie restriction and NAD/sirtuin counteract the hallmarks of aging. *Frontiers in Bioscience, Landmark Edition, 19,* 1300–1319.

Most, J., Tosti, V., Redman, L. M., et al. (2017). Calorie restriction in humans: An update. *Ageing Research Reviews, 39,* 36–45. doi:10.1016/j.arr.2016.08.005.

Pinto, M., & Moraes, C. T. (2015). Mechanisms linking mtDNA damage and aging. *Free Radical Biology and Medicine, 85,* 250–258.

Reeg, S., & Grune, T. (2015). Protein oxidation in aging: Does it play a role in aging progression? *Antioxidants and Redox Signaling, 23,* 239–255.

RELEVANT WEBSITES

Aging resources and links:
http://www.pathguy.com/lectures/aging.htm
http://www.benbest.com/lifeext/aging.html
Caloric restriction: http://www.crsociety.org
Caloric restriction and longevity in primates: http://www.iflscience.com/health-and-medicine/caloric-restriction-increases-lifespan-monkeys/
Progeria: http://www.progeria-research.org/index.html

ABBREVIATIONS

AD	Alzheimer's disease
AGE	Advanced glycation end-product
AL	Ad libitum
ALE	Advanced lipoxidation end-product
ApoE	Apolipoprotein E
ApoC3	Apolipoprotein C3
CETP	Cholesterol ester transfer protein
CML	Ne-(carboxymethyl)lysine **N.B.** superscript epsilon
CR	Calorie restriction
FIRKO	Adipose tissue (fat) insulin receptor knockout
FRTA	Free radical theory of aging
GH	Growth hormone
IGF	Insulin-like growth factor
MetSO	Methionine sulfoxide
MSLP	Maximum lifespan potential
mtDNA	Mitochondrial DNA
o-Tyr	*Ortho*-Tyrosine
ROS	Reactive oxygen species

Digestion and Absorption of Nutrients: The Gastrointestinal Tract

Marek H. Dominiczak and Matthew Priest

LEARNING OBJECTIVES

After reading this chapter, you should be able to:

- Describe the stages of digestion.
- Discuss mechanisms involved in the absorption of nutrients.
- Discuss the role of digestive enzymes.
- Discuss digestion of the main classes of nutrients: carbohydrates, proteins, and fats.
- Identify compounds arising from the digestion of carbohydrates, proteins, and fats that become substrates for further metabolism.

INTRODUCTION

All organisms require sources of energy and other materials to enable function and growth. Their survival depends on the ability to extract and assimilate these resources from the ingested food. The gastrointestinal (GI) tract and the organs functionally associated with it are responsible for digestion and absorption of food. The intestinal epithelium and the tight junctions between enterocytes form the most important barrier between the organism and its external environment. This barrier has selective absorption and secretion capacities and also may become a scene of immune or autoimmune response.

Digestion is the process by which food is broken down into components simple enough to be absorbed in the intestine. **Absorption** is the uptake of the products of digestion by intestinal cells (enterocytes) from the gut lumen and their delivery to blood or lymph. Digestion and absorption of nutrients are closely linked to and are regulated by the nervous system, hormones, and paracrine factors. The physical presence of food particles in the GI tract also stimulates these processes.

Absorption and secretion of ions, such as sodium, chloride potassium, and bicarbonate, and the absorption of water are also essential functions of the GI tract. Therefore many clinical problems associated with digestion and absorption are closely linked to fluid and electrolyte disorders (Chapter 35).

Impairment of digestion and absorption results in maldigestion and malabsorption syndromes, respectively. **Maldigestion** denotes impaired breakdown of nutrients to their absorbable products. **Malabsorption** is the defective absorption, uptake, and transport of (adequately digested) nutrients.

The key clinical signs of signs of malabsorption and/or maldigestion are **diarrhea, steatorrhea** (presence of excess fat in stools), and **loss of weight**. Children may present with **failure to thrive**. Whereas acute diarrhea carries a risk of rapid dehydration and electrolyte depletion, chronic diarrhea is associated with progressive malnutrition. According to data from the World Health Organization (WHO; 2015), diarrheal disease is the eighth leading cause of death worldwide (see Further Reading). Malabsorption and maldigestion may also develop as consequences of surgical intervention, such as gastrectomy, small bowel resection, or colectomy.

The overall function of the GI tract is to break down food into components that can be absorbed and utilized by the body (Fig. 30.1) and then to excrete the nonabsorbable material. Its different anatomical segments have specific functions relating to digestion and absorption:

- The mouth, stomach, and duodenum deal with the initial process of mixing ingested food and initiating digestion.
- In the duodenum, bile and pancreatic secretions enter through the common bile duct.
- The small intestine is the main digestive area: in the jejunum, digestive processes continue and absorption is initiated; it continues in the ileum.
- The large intestine (cecum, colon, and rectum; primarily the colon) is involved in the reabsorption and secretion of electrolytes and water.

WATER AND ELECTROLYTE HANDLING IN THE GASTROINTESTINAL TRACT

Handling of electrolytes and water by the GI tract is one of its main functions

Handling of electrolytes and water by the GI tract includes not only absorption and secretion but also cell volume maintenance, and it affects cell proliferation and differentiation as well as apoptosis and carcinogenesis.

A large volume of fluid is secreted and reabsorbed by the GI tract

In a 24-h period, around 10.0 L of fluid enters and leaves the GI tract. One liter of saliva, containing electrolytes, protein,

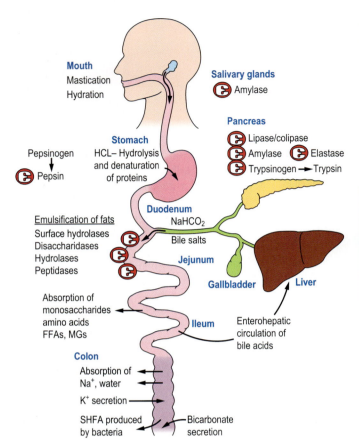

Fig. 30.1 **The gastrointestinal tract.** Digestion and absorption of nutrients require the integrated function of several organs. Mixing of food and initiation of digestion take place in the mouth and in the stomach. The absorptive processes start in the jejunum. However, most nutrients are absorbed in the ileum. The large intestine is involved in the absorption of water and electrolytes and participates in the recirculation of the bile acids to the liver. A large amount of fluid (approximately 10 L) passes through the GI tract every day. FFA, free fatty acids.

and mucus, is secreted per day. The average daily water intake is about 2.0 L, and intestinal secretions total about 7.0 L. Most of this fluid is reabsorbed by the small intestine. The colon absorbs around 90% of the fluid that passes through it, and only about 150–250 mL of water is normally excreted in the stool.

Electrolytes are secreted by the salivary glands, stomach, and pancreas

Several secretory processes take place in the GI tract. The salivary glands, stomach, and pancreas secrete digestive enzymes in the form of inactive zymogens. Secretion of hydrogen ion occurs in the stomach. Secretion of the bicarbonate ion takes place throughout the GI tract, with particularly large amounts present in the pancreatic juice. Potassium secretion occurs predominantly in the colon and is regulated by aldosterone.

Impaired intestinal function leads to potentially serious disorders of fluid–electrolyte and acid–base balance

Diseases of the GI tract and surgical removal of segments of small and large intestine carry a risk of major water and electrolyte disorders. Before treatment for cholera was known, a person with fulminant diarrhea caused by *Vibrio cholerae* infection could die of dehydration within hours. Severe acidosis due to bicarbonate loss can also be a feature of bowel disease (Chapter 36).

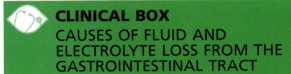

CLINICAL BOX
CAUSES OF FLUID AND ELECTROLYTE LOSS FROM THE GASTROINTESTINAL TRACT

Prolonged **vomiting** causes loss of water, hydrogen and chloride ions, and a further loss of potassium due to the body's compensatory mechanisms. **Diarrhea** may be caused by increased intestinal secretion due to, for instance, inflammation, or it may be caused by malabsorption of nutrients. Severe diarrhea that leads to the loss of alkaline intestinal contents may result in dehydration and metabolic acidosis. It also results in the loss of sodium, potassium, and other minerals. Patients with a short gut syndrome resulting from extensive small bowel resection - for example, in Crohn's disease - may develop severe fluid balance problems due to the inability to reabsorb water.

Mechanisms of water and electrolyte transport in the intestine

Sodium-potassium ATPase is the driving force for transport processes in the enterocytes

Enterocytes possess an array of transporters and ion channels (Fig. 30.2). The sodium-potassium ATPase, described in more detail in Chapter 35, is located on the basolateral membrane (the "blood side") and transports sodium ion outside the cell in exchange for potassium ion ($3Na^+$ to every $2K^+$ ions). This creates a sodium concentration gradient and hyperpolarizes the membrane, increasing intracellular negative potential and driving the passive transport systems (and consequently transcellular ion transport). Moreover, transport of sodium (and chloride) is accompanied by passive transport of water, which is both paracellular, through the tight junctions, and transcellular, utilizing membrane water transporters, the aquaporins.

Sodium cotransporters are a common mode of intestinal transport

Sodium cotransporters transport the sodium ion together with another molecule (Fig. 30.2A). For instance, glucose is absorbed together with sodium by the sodium-glucose cotransporter present in the luminal membrane, known as sodium/glucose linked transport-1(**SGLT-1**). Glucose is subsequently extruded

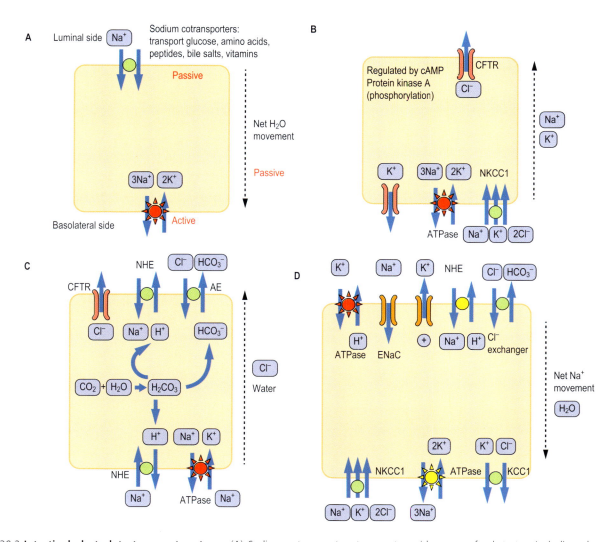

Fig. 30.2 **Intestinal electrolyte transport systems.** (A) Sodium cotransporters transport a wide range of substrates, including glucose. Low intracellular sodium concentration, and therefore a steep gradient between extracellular and intracellular Na$^+$ concentration, is created by the Na$^+$/K$^+$ ATPase located in the basolateral membrane. (B) CFTR transporter secretes chloride ion and is regulated by the cAMP-PKA signaling cascade. Sodium and potassium may also be secreted as counterions. Note the potassium "leak" channel in the basolateral membrane. The NKCC1 transporter supplies chloride to the cell. (C) Electroneutral sodium absorption and the secretion of bicarbonate. (D) Electrogenic sodium absorption and potassium secretion in the distal colon. Transporters marked **yellow** are regulated by **aldosterone** in the distal colon. See text for details. CFTR, cystic fibrosis transmembrane conductance regulator; NHE, sodium/hydrogen exchanger; ENaC, epithelial sodium channel; AE, anion exchanger (chloride/bicarbonate exchanger); NKCC1, Na$^+$ K$^+$ Cl$^-$ cotransporter; KCC1, K$^+$ Cl$^-$ cotransporter.

into plasma at the basolateral membrane by the **GLUT2** transporter. The discovery that the cellular transport of sodium and glucose is linked had enormous clinical consequences. During a cholera epidemic in Manila in the late 1960s, researchers observed that dehydrated patients with diarrhea did not absorb oral sodium chloride well during attempts at oral rehydration. However, when glucose was also provided, water and electrolyte absorption improved. This observation led to the formulation of the **WHO oral rehydration solution**, which subsequently saved the lives of millions of children affected by severe diarrhea worldwide (see Further Reading).

Other modes of sodium transport include electroneutral and electrogenic transport

Electroneutral sodium transport is through the sodium/hydrogen exchanger (**NHE**) and usually links with chloride transport via the AE chloride/bicarbonate exchanger (Fig. 30.2C). The exchangers are present on both luminal and basolateral membranes. This type of transport handles most of the sodium chloride reabsorption in the colon.

The electrogenic absorption of sodium occurs through the epithelial sodium channels (**ENaCs**, also known as amiloride-sensitive sodium channels), which are present on the luminal side of the epithelium (Fig. 30.2D). ENaCs are regulated by aldosterone and are particularly important in the distal colon. The absorbed Na$^+$ is followed by Cl$^-$ moving through a chloride channel. Aldosterone also upregulates the Na$^+$/K$^+$-ATPase.

Chloride transport: Cystic fibrosis transmembrane conductance regulator (CFTR)

Luminal secretion of chloride occurs via the CFTR (Fig. 30.2B). CFTR is a single-polypeptide membrane ion channel. It is also present in the epithelia of the lung and sweat glands. Its function is controlled by the G-protein–cAMP-protein kinase A (PKA) signaling cascade (Chapter 25). Because CFTR is activated by cAMP, chloride secretion can be activated by prostaglandin E$_2$ (PGE$_2$), serotonin, as well as the cholera toxin and the *Escherichia coli* heat-stable enterotoxin. The loss-of-function mutations of CFTR lead to **cystic fibrosis,** where chloride transport is impaired or inhibited. CFTR also has regulatory function: its phosphorylation inhibits the NHE exchanger, thus decreasing Na$^+$ absorption. Interestingly, CFTR is also able to transport chloride in the opposite direction, aiding chloride reabsorption. Basolateral Cl$^-$ uptake occurs through the Na$^+$K$^+$Cl$^-$ cotransporter (NKCC1) and through chloride/bicarbonate exchangers.

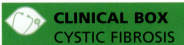

CLINICAL BOX
CYSTIC FIBROSIS

Cystic fibrosis, a monogenic autosomal recessive disorder, involves inhibition of chloride transport due to the absence of the CFTR. Different mutations of the *CFTR* gene lead to either complete absence of the transporter or impairment in its functionality.

The prevalence of CF is 1:3000 live births in the United States and Northern Europe. In the United States, cystic fibrosis is a leading cause of **malabsorption.** It manifests itself predominantly in childhood. The main problems are usually respiratory. Chloride secretion is decreased, and the Na$^+$ reabsorption is accelerated. This results in decreased hydration of epithelial secretions. In the respiratory tract, there is **decreased hydration of the airway mucus** and thus failure of its clearance, with ensuing bacterial infections. Gastrointestinal problems include **meconium ileus** and **intestinal obstruction.** The absence of the CFTR also affects the functioning of the Cl$^-$/HCO$_3^-$ exchanger (and thus the passive secretion of Na$^+$) in the pancreas - this results in impaired endocrine and exocrine function. Thickened biliary secretions may be a cause of focal **biliary cirrhosis** and **chronic cholelithiasis.** There also is impairment of mucus secretion in the colonic crypts, with enhanced Na$^+$ reabsorption through Na$^+$ channels and Na$^+$/H$^+$ transporters.

Potassium absorption and potassium secretion in the colon are aided by different potassium channels

Potassium absorption is mediated by **H$^+$/K$^+$ ATPases** present in the luminal membrane. Conversely, basolateral potassium

transport is by potassium channels and the K$^+$ and Cl$^-$ cotransporter (**KCC1**). Both luminal and basolateral K$^+$ channels are necessary to hyperpolarize the membrane to establish a driving force for the ENaC transporter. K$^+$ secretion through luminal K$^+$ channels parallels the Cl$^-$ secretion through CFTR and is similarly stimulated by cAMP, cGMP, and protein kinase C (PKC). Expression of luminal K$^+$ channels is also stimulated by aldosterone and glucocorticoids.

Reabsorption of short-chain fatty acids occurs together with bicarbonate secretion

The colon reabsorbs short-chain fatty acids (SCFA) derived from bacterial fermentation of fiber, and this is combined with the secretion of bicarbonate. Thus bicarbonate is secreted using the luminal anion exchangers SCFA/HCO$_3^-$ or Cl$^-$/HCO$_3^-$.

Aquaporins control colonic water reabsorption

Water reabsorption in the colon is mediated by ion channels known as aquaporins (AQPs; Chapter 35). AQP1, 3, and 4 are located on basolateral membranes, and AQP8 is located on luminal membranes.

Intestinal secretions differ in their pH

Hydrogen ion concentration varies widely in different parts of the GI tract. This facilitates digestive process and is also important for tissue protection in the stomach and intestine. Saliva secreted into the mouth is alkaline due to its bicarbonate content. In contrast, the contents of the stomach are strongly acidic, but the mucus protecting its walls is alkaline. Thus although the parietal cells of the stomach secrete large amounts of hydrogen ion, principally through the action of the luminal H$^+$/K$^+$-ATPase, the gastric surface cells secrete mucus containing bicarbonate ion, employing the Cl$^-$/HCO$_3^-$ exchanger. On entry to the duodenum, the acidic content of the stomach is neutralized by the strongly alkaline pancreatic secretions.

COMPONENTS OF DIGESTION

Chewing breaks the food down. The addition of saliva in the mouth begins the digestive process and acts as lubrication to facilitate swallowing. The food is then moved into the esophagus by a process driven by the esophageal reflex. As it transfers into the **stomach**, it is broken down into smaller particles. The presence of the digest triggers peristalsis, which further helps mixing and stimulates digestive secretions. Major stimuli to peristalsis are mediated through the parasympathetic nervous system. Absorption of nutrients depends on the rate of transit; thus increased motility may lead to inappropriately rapid transit and therefore malabsorption.

The stomach and intestine are lined by epithelium, which has an invaginated surface that greatly increases its absorptive area. The **small intestine** is lined by enterocytes arranged in intestinal **villi.** In addition, each cell contains **microvilli.** The total absorptive surface area of the intestine is approximately 250 m², roughly the area of a junior basketball court. **Celiac disease** (gluten sensitive enteropathy) causes inflammation of the small intestine and atrophy of the villi, significantly reducing this surface area, resulting in malabsorption.

ADVANCED CONCEPT BOX
DIGESTIVE FUNCTION OF THE STOMACH

There are different cell types in the mucosal wall of the stomach, each performing different digestive functions. Cells called "chief cells" secrete **pepsinogen,** which is a precursor of **pepsin.** Pepsinogen is activated to pepsin in the acidic environment of the stomach lumen. Parietal cells generate **hydrogen ions** through the action of carbonic anhydrase and then pump them into the lumen by an ATP-dependent proton pump on the luminal membrane. The H⁺ secretion is dependent on the parallel export of K⁺ through luminal K⁺ channels.

Parietal cell activity is stimulated by the action of **histamine** acting on H₂ receptors produced by histamine-secreting cells. The hormone **gastrin** is secreted by G cells and is triggered by food entering the stomach. Stomach cells also secrete **intrinsic factor (IF),** which facilitates absorption of vitamin B₁₂ in the intestine (Chapter 7). Last, but not least, epithelial cells secrete alkaline mucus, which protects the stomach lining from the effects of the strong acid.

Damage to the lining of the stomach or duodenum leads to **ulceration;** in the majority of cases, this is associated with infection with *Helicobacter pylori* in the stomach. Treatment of acid-related symptoms, such as **dyspepsia** or **gastroesophageal reflux,** can be achieved with **antacids,** which simply neutralize the pH; **H₂ antagonists** (e.g., cimetidine or ranitidine), which prevent histamine release; or **proton pump inhibitors** (e.g., omeprazole), which block H⁺ secretion by the parietal cells. Treatment of *H. pylori* with a combination of acid suppression and antibiotics will usually result in ulcer healing.

Digestion is a sequential series of processes

In the course of digestion, the carbohydrates, proteins, and fats contained in the food are broken into absorbable products. Some ingested material, such as complex carbohydrates of plant origin, is indigestible and constitutes fiber.

There are a number of stages that occur in a sequence, allowing contribution of the fluid content, pH, emulsifying agents, and enzymes. This requires the concerted secretory action of the salivary glands, liver and gallbladder, pancreas, and intestinal mucosa. The processes involved are outlined in Fig. 30.1 and can be summarized as follows:

- Lubrication and homogenization of food with fluids secreted by glands of the intestinal tract
- Secretion of enzymes that break down macromolecules to a mixture of oligomers, dimers, and monomers

- Secretion of hydrogen ion and bicarbonate within different parts of the GI tract to optimize the conditions for enzymic hydrolysis
- Secretion of bile acids to emulsify dietary lipid, facilitating enzymic hydrolysis and absorption
- Further hydrolysis of oligomers and dimers by membrane-bound enzymes
- Specific uptake of digested material into enterocytes and its transfer to blood or lymph
- Recycling of bile acids and absorption of the SCFAs produced by colonic bacteria
- Reabsorption of water and electrolytes

There is considerable functional reserve in all aspects of digestion and absorption

A considerable impairment of structure and/or function needs to be present before signs and symptoms of GI maldigestion or malabsorption occur. Minor functional loss may go unnoticed, allowing pathology to progress for some time before being diagnosed. For example, pancreatic disease manifests itself only after 90% of the pancreatic function is destroyed. Each of the organs involved in digestion and absorption has the capacity to increase its activity several-fold; this adds to the reserve capacity.

Note also that digestion of a particular nutrient takes place at several points in the GI tract. Lipids, carbohydrates, and proteins can be digested at multiple locations. Therefore disruption of digestive mechanisms at a single point is unlikely to result in a complete inability to digest a nutrient group (Fig. 30.3).

The GI tract can also accommodate loss of function of one constituent organ. For example, if the stomach is surgically

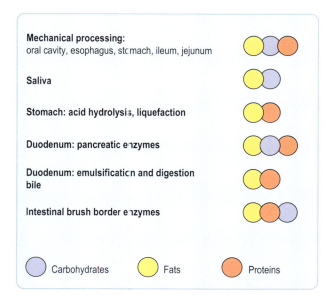

Fig. 30.3 **Digestion as a multiorgan process.** Because each of the main groups of nutrients (carbohydrates, proteins, and fats) undergoes digestion at multiple points, there is a considerable spare capacity and resilience in the system.

removed, the pancreas and small intestine can compensate for the loss of gastric digestion. In pancreatic disease, lingual lipases can accommodate some loss of pancreatic lipase.

Digestive enzymes and zymogens

Most digestive enzymes are secreted as inactive precursors

With the exception of salivary amylase and lingual (associated with the tongue) lipases, digestive enzymes are secreted into the gut lumen as inactive precursors, zymogens (Chapter 6). The process of secretion of digestive enzymes is similar in the salivary glands, gastric mucosa, and pancreas. These organs contain specialized cells for the synthesis, packaging, and transport of zymogen granules to the cell surface and then to the intestinal lumen. These secretions are termed **exocrine** (i.e., "secreting to the outside"), as opposed to the endocrine secretion of hormones.

Enzymes involved in the digestion of protein (proteases) and fat (lipase: phospholipase A_2) are synthesized as inactive zymogens and are only activated on their release to the gut lumen. In general, these enzymes, once in their active forms, can activate their own precursors. Activation of the precursors can also occur by change in pH (e.g., pepsinogen is converted into pepsin in the stomach at pH below 4.0) or by the action of specific enteropeptidases bound to the mucosal membrane of the duodenum (Fig. 30.1).

All digestive enzymes are hydrolases

The products of hydrolysis are oligomers, dimers, and monomers of parent macromolecules. Thus carbohydrates are hydrolyzed into a mixture of disaccharides and monosaccharides. Proteins are broken down to a mixture of di- and tripeptides and amino acids. Lipids are broken down to a mixture of fatty acids, glycerol, and mono- and diacylglycerols (Fig. 30.4).

DIGESTION AND ABSORPTION OF CARBOHYDRATES

Dietary carbohydrates enter the GI tract as mono-, di-, and polysaccharides

Dietary carbohydrates consist of mainly plant and animal starches - polysaccharides (starches), the disaccharides sucrose and lactose, and the monosaccharides (Fig. 30.5). **Monosaccharides** include glucose, fructose, and galactose, either present in the diet or generated by digestion of di- and polysaccharides. Lactose, for instance, is a **disaccharide** derived from dairy products and is hydrolyzed to the monosaccharides glucose and galactose by lactase and β-galactosidase. The sugar monomers are then absorbed from the GI tract.

Disaccharides and polysaccharides require hydrolytic cleavage into monosaccharides before absorption

Disaccharides are broken down by membrane-bound disaccharidases present on the mucosal surface in the intestine. Glycogen and starch require additional hydrolytic capacity of amylase found in the secretions of the salivary glands and pancreas (Fig. 30.6).

Starch is a plant polysaccharide, and glycogen is its animal equivalent. Both contain a mixture of linear chains of glucose molecules linked by α-1,4-glycosidic bonds (amylose) and by branched glucose chains with α-1,6 linkages (amylopectin). Glycogen has more branched structure than starch. Digestion of these polysaccharides is promoted by the endosaccharidases and amylase.

The products of hydrolysis of starch are the disaccharide maltose, the trisaccharide maltotriose, and a branched unit termed the α-limit dextrin. They are further hydrolyzed by enzymes bound to the enterocytes, yielding the monosaccharide glucose (Fig. 30.7A).

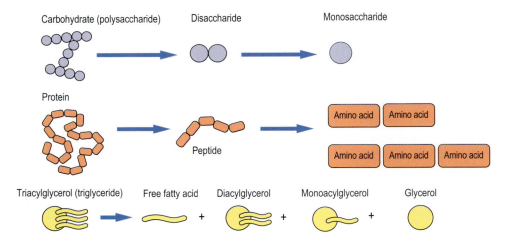

Fig. 30.4 **Digestion of dietary polymers.** The common denominator between the handling of different groups of nutrients is the breakdown of nutrient polymers into monomers. Thus polysaccharides are digested to yield di- and monosaccharides, and the proteins are digested into component amino acids. Fat (predominantly triacylglycerols) is digested to mono- and diacylacylglycerols.

Carbohydrate	Food source	Structure
Starch (amylose) [plant]	Potatoes, rice, bread, onions	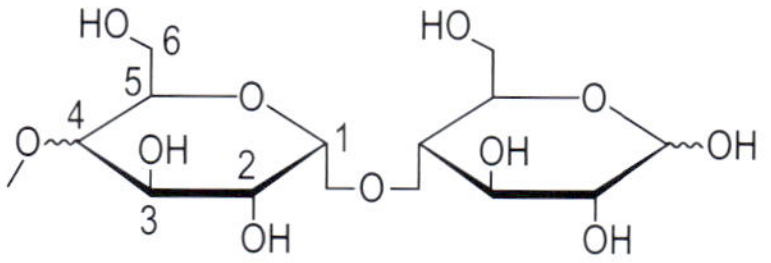
Amylopectin (glycogen) [plant, animal]	Potatoes, rice, bread, muscle, liver	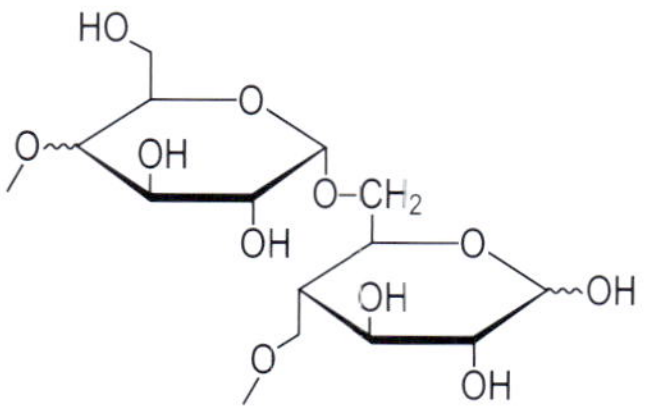
Sucrose	Desserts, sweets, table sugar	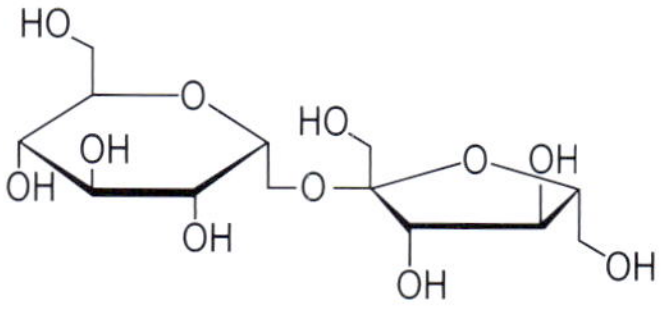
Lactose	Milk	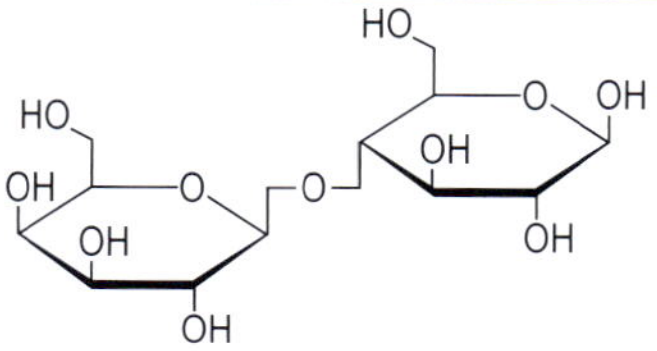
Fructose	Fruits, honey	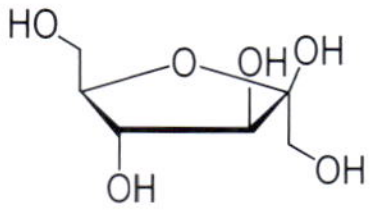
Glucose	Fruits, honey	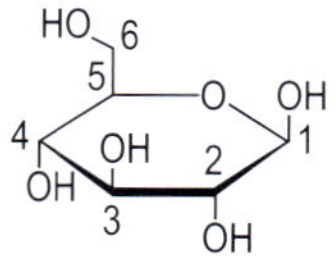

Fig. 30.5 **Key dietary carbohydrates.** Starch and amylopectin are polysaccharides. Only two component sugar molecules are shown for each to illustrate their intermolecular linkages. Sucrose and lactose are the most common disaccharides, and fructose and glucose the most common monosaccharides. Refer to the glucose molecule in the bottom row for standard numbering of carbon atoms.

Dietary disaccharides such as lactose, sucrose, and trehalose (a disaccharide made up of two glucose molecules joined by an α-1,1 linkage) are hydrolyzed to their constituent monosaccharides by specific **disaccharidases** attached to brush-border membrane in the small intestine. Catalytic domains of these enzymes project into the gut lumen, and their non-catalytic, structural domain(s) are attached to the enterocyte membrane.

Disaccharidases are inducible, with the exception of lactase

The greater the amount of a disaccharide, such as sucrose, that is present in the diet or produced by digestion, the greater is the amount of the relevant specific disaccharidase (e.g., sucrase) produced by the enterocytes. The rate-limiting step in the absorption of dietary disaccharides is the transport of

the resultant monosaccharides. Lactase, however, is a noninducible brush-border disaccharidase, and therefore the rate-limiting factor in lactose absorption is its hydrolysis.

Active and passive transport systems transfer monosaccharides across the brush-border membrane

The process of digestion results in a large increase in the number of osmotically active monosaccharide particles within the gut lumen. This leads to water being drawn into the lumen from the GI tract mucosa and vascular compartment. Increased brush-border hydrolysis increases the osmotic load, whereas increased monosaccharide transport across the brush border enterocyte decreases it. For most oligo- and disaccharidases, the transport of the resulting monomers is rate limiting. As concentrations of monomeric sugars (and, consequently, osmolality) increase in the gut lumen, there is a compensatory

ADVANCED CONCEPT BOX
ROLE OF AMYLASE, α-GLUCOSIDASES, AND ISOMALTASE IN POLYSACCHARIDE DIGESTION

During eating, homogenization of food occurs by chewing. It is aided by contractions of the stomach wall muscles and gastric folds. One consequence of this is that dietary polysaccharides become hydrated. This is necessary for the action of **amylase,** which is specific for internal α-1,4-glycosidic linkages and not the α-1,6 linkages. Amylase also does not act on α-1,4 linkages of glycosyl residues serving as branching units. Thus the cleaved units formed by its action are the disaccharide maltose, the trisaccharide maltotriose, and an oligosaccharide with one or more α-1,6 branches and containing on average eight glycosyl units, termed the "α-limit dextrin." These compounds are further cleaved to glucose by **oligosaccharidase** and **α-glucosidase,** the latter removing single glucose residues from α-1,4-linked oligosaccharides (including maltose). A **sucrase–isomaltase** complex is secreted as a single-polypeptide precursor molecule and is activated into two separate enzymes, one of which (isomaltase) is responsible for the hydrolytic cleavage of α-1,6-glycosidic bonds. Thus the final product of digestion of starches is glucose. Amylase occurs free in the lumen, whereas α-glucosidases and **isomaltase** are attached to the membrane of the enterocyte.

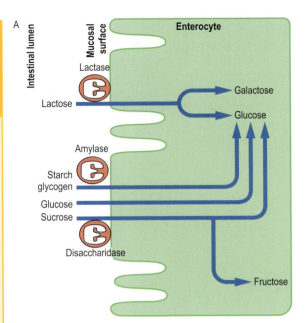

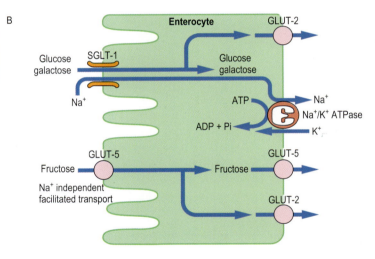

Fig. 30.7 Digestion and absorption of dietary carbohydrates. (A) Monosaccharides are released as a result of hydrolysis of the polysaccharides. Preliminary digestion occurs in the gut lumen, and the final stage takes place on the mucosal surface. Note that intestinal digestion of starch involves pancreatic amylase. (B) Links between absorption of monosaccharides and sodium and their relationship to the activity of Na+/K+-ATPase.

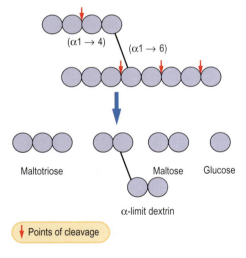

Fig. 30.6 Hydrolytic cleavage of polysaccharides. Polysaccharides and disaccharides are digested by enzymatic hydrolysis. The arrows illustrate points of cleavage and the type of hydrolyzed bond. Note that α-limit dextrin still contains both α-1,4 and α-1,6 bonds.

decrease in the activity of brush-border disaccharidases. This controls the osmotic load and prevents excessive fluid shifts.

Glucose, fructose, and galactose are the primary monosaccharides generated by digestion of dietary carbohydrates

Absorption of these sugars and other minor monosaccharides occurs by means of specific carrier-mediated mechanisms (Fig.

30.7B), shows saturation kinetics, and can be specifically inhibited. In addition, all monosaccharides may cross the brush-border membrane by simple diffusion, although this is extremely slow.

There are at least two carrier-mediated transport mechanisms for monosaccharides

At the brush-border membrane, both glucose and galactose are transported by the SGLT-1. This membrane-linked protein binds with glucose (or galactose) and Na+ at separate sites and

CLINICAL BOX
TYPES OF DIARRHEA

Diarrhea can be caused by the nonabsorbable solutes present in the gut (osmotic diarrhea), by the failure to either digest or absorb nutrients, and also by the secretory agonists (secretory diarrhea).

Osmotic diarrhea may be caused by malabsorption, digestive enzyme deficiencies, or short bowel and inflammatory diseases.

Secretory diarrhea may be caused by infections, by malabsorption of bile salts or fat, or by endocrine causes such as carcinoid syndrome or Zollinger–Ellison syndrome.

Absorption can be impaired, and secretion increased, in conditions that lead to the inflammation of the bowel (**inflammatory diarrhea**). The main causes of chronic inflammatory diarrhea are Crohn's disease and ulcerative colitis. Characteristically, secretory diarrhea, but not osmotic, persists on fasting.

The nature of diarrhea will vary depending on the area of the gastrointestinal tract involved. Ulcerative colitis only affects the large bowel and rarely causes malabsorption, although patients may develop anemia due to blood loss and a low-albumin state due to chronic inflammation and protein loss. Crohn's disease can affect any part of the gastrointestinal tract and is more likely to cause malabsorption due to small bowel inflammation or the formation of fistulae between different areas of the bowel.

CLINICAL BOX A
BOY WITH ABDOMINAL DISCOMFORT, BLOATING, AND DIARRHEA: LACTOSE INTOLERANCE

A 15-year-old African American boy came to the United Kingdom on an exchange visit for 2 months. After 2 weeks in the United Kingdom, he complained of abdominal discomfort, a feeling of being bloated, increased passage of urine, and more recently, the development of diarrhea. His only change in diet noted at the time was the introduction of milk. He had developed a considerable liking for milk and was consuming 1–2 large cartons per day. A lactose tolerance test was performed, whereby the young man was given 50 g lactose in an aqueous vehicle to drink. Plasma glucose levels did not rise by more than 1 mmol/L (18 mg/dL) over the next 2 h, with sampling at 30-min intervals. A diagnosis of lactose intolerance was made.

Comment

Lactose intolerance results from acquired lactase deficiency. Lactase activity decreases with increasing age in children, but the extent of the decline in activity is genetically determined and demonstrates ethnic variation. Lactase deficiency in the adult black population varies from 45% to 95%. If symptoms of malabsorption occur after the introduction of milk to adult diets, the diagnosis of acquired lactase deficiency should be considered. The diagnosis is made by challenging the small bowel with lactose and monitoring the rise in plasma glucose. An increase of more than 1.7 mmol/L (30 mg/dL) is considered normal. A rise of less than 1.1 mmol/L (20 mg/dL) is diagnostic of lactase deficiency. A rise of 1.1–1.7 mmol/L (20–30 mg/dL) is inconclusive.

transports both into the enterocyte cytosol. Na^+ is transported down its concentration gradient (the concentration within the gut lumen is higher than the intracellular concentration) and carries glucose along *against* the glucose concentration gradient. This transport is linked to Na^+/K^+-ATPase. Therefore it is an indirect active transport.

Fructose is transported across the brush-border membrane by sodium-independent facilitated diffusion involving the membrane-associated glucose transporter GLUT-5 present on the brush-border side of the enterocyte, and GLUT-2, which transfers monosaccharides out of the enterocyte into the circulation (Chapter 4).

An incomplete digestion of carbohydrates (the components of fiber) leads to their conversion to short-chain fatty acids (acetate, propionate, butyrate) by the colonic bacteria.

DIGESTION AND ABSORPTION OF LIPIDS

Approximately 90% of fat in the diet is **triacylglycerols (TGs; also termed triglycerides)**. The remainder consists of cholesterol, cholesteryl esters, phospholipids, and nonesterified fatty acids (NEFA).

Fats need to be emulsified before digestion

The hydrophobic nature of fats prevents the access of water-soluble digestive enzymes. Furthermore, fat globules present only a limited surface area for enzyme action. These issues are overcome by the emulsification process. The change in the physical nature of lipids begins in the stomach: the core body temperature helps liquefy dietary lipids, and the peristaltic movements of the stomach facilitate the formation of a lipid emulsion. The emulsification process is also aided by the acid-stable salivary and gastric lipases. Initially, the rate of hydrolysis is slow because of the separate aqueous and lipid phases and limited lipid–water interface. However, once hydrolysis begins, the water-immiscible TGs are degraded to fatty acids, which act as surfactants. They confer a hydrophilic surface to lipid droplets and break them down into smaller particles, thus increasing the lipid–water interface and facilitating hydrolysis. The lipid phase disperses throughout the aqueous phase as an emulsion. Dietary phospholipids, fatty acids, and monoacyl glycerols also act as surfactants.

Bile salts and pancreatic enzymes act on the lipid emulsion in the duodenum

The lipid emulsion passes from the stomach into the duodenum, where further digestion occurs, driven by enzymes secreted by the pancreas. Solubilization is aided by the release of

CLINICAL BOX
A YOUNG MAN WITH WEIGHT LOSS, DIARRHEA, ABDOMINAL BLOATING, AND ANEMIA: CELIAC DISEASE

A 22-year-old man presented with a history of weight loss, diarrhea, abdominal bloating, and anemia. He described his stools as pale and bulky. Laboratory features included hemoglobin of 90 g/L (9 g/dL; reference range 130–180 g/L; 13–18 g/dL). Biopsy of his small bowel demonstrated villous atrophy, with increased intraepithelial lymphocytes. A diagnosis of gluten-induced enteropathy (celiac disease) was made. All wheat products were removed from the patient's diet, and the symptoms resolved.

Comment
Celiac disease is an autoimmune condition precipitated by sensitivity to gluten resulting in inflammation of the small bowel mucosa. Gluten is a storage protein of wheat, barley, and rye. It is actually a mixture of proteins, which includes the gliadins (the alcohol-soluble fraction of gluten) and glutelins. The gliadins pass through the intestinal barrier during, for instance, infections, triggering the immune response. The inflammatory reaction ensues. The result is villous atrophy and hyperplasia of the crypts. Because the absorptive surface is markedly reduced, the resulting malabsorption can be severe.

Circulating antibodies to wheat gluten and its fractions are frequently present in cases of celiac disease. The diagnosis involves duodenal biopsy and testing the response to a gluten-free diet. The autoantibodies tested for are **tissue transglutaminase antibodies** (transglutaminase is an enzyme that deamidates gliadin in the intestinal wall), antiendomysial antibodies, and antigliadin antibodies. Celiac disease is common, affecting approximately 1 in 200 Caucasians, but is underdiagnosed, often being labeled as irritable bowel syndrome.

For hematology reference values, refer to Appendix 1.

ADVANCED CONCEPT BOX
SHORT-CHAIN FATTY ACIDS ARE PRODUCED IN THE LARGE BOWEL FROM UNDIGESTED CARBOHYDRATES

Decreased absorption of dietary starch leads to the bacterial production of short-chain fatty acids (SCFA) by the colonic bacteria.

SCFAs can be produced from fermentable oligosaccharides, disaccharides, monosaccharides, and polyols (known as FODMAP). Animal studies showed the presence of the short-chain fatty acid receptor 2 (FFA2), a G-protein-coupled receptor present on intestinal endocrine cells. Binding of SCFA releases serotonin, leading to the increase in intestinal motility.

The use of a low-FODMAP diet is increasingly recognized as beneficial in the management of some gastrointestinal disorders, particularly irritable bowel syndrome.

bile salts from the gallbladder, stimulated by the hormone cholecystokinin.

The major enzyme secreted by the pancreas is **pancreatic lipase**. Lipase remains inactive in the presence of bile salts normally secreted into the small intestine. This inhibition is overcome by the concomitant secretion of **colipase** by the pancreas. Colipase binds to both the water–lipid interface and the pancreatic lipase, simultaneously anchoring and activating the enzyme. As shown in Fig. 30.8, only a small proportion of dietary TGs becomes completely hydrolyzed to glycerol and fatty acids. The pancreatic lipase produces mainly **2-monoacyl glycerols** (2-MAG), which are absorbed into enterocytes.

Bile salts are essential for solubilizing lipids during the digestive process

Bile acids (which are bile salts at the alkaline pH of the intestine) act as detergents and reversibly form lipid aggregates, micelles. Micelles are considerably smaller than lipid emulsion droplets. The micelles transport the lipids to the brush border of the enterocyte.

Absorption of lipids into the epithelial cells lining the small intestine occurs by diffusion through the plasma membrane. Almost all the fatty acids and 2-MAGs are absorbed because both are water soluble. Water-insoluble lipids are

CLINICAL BOX
AN ALCOHOLIC MAN WITH CENTRAL ABDOMINAL PAIN: PANCREATITIS

A 56-year-old man with a long history of alcohol abuse presented with chronic central abdominal pain, weight loss, and diarrhea. He described his bowel motions as pale, greasy, and difficult to flush away. The abdominal radiograph revealed epigastric calcification in the area of the pancreas, and computed tomography (CT) scanning revealed an atrophic calcified pancreas. The stool sample sent for fecal elastase quantification revealed this to be significantly reduced. Treatment was initiated with pancreatic enzyme supplements, resulting in resolution of his diarrhea and weight gain.

Comment
Acute pancreatitis is a serious and life-threatening illness caused by gallstones blocking the pancreatic duct, by alcohol abuse, or more rarely by drugs such as azathioprine, viruses such as mumps, or hypertriglyceridemia. Patients present with severe abdominal pain, nausea, and vomiting. The most important biochemical marker of pancreatitis is an **increased serum amylase**. Increased activity of lipase and a decrease in serum calcium can also occur.

Chronic pancreatitis is a consequence of long-term inflammation and leads to malnutrition and **steatorrhea** due to loss of exocrine function - this can be demonstrated by finding reduced levels of fecal elastase in stool samples. It is also associated with failure of endocrine pancreatic function, leading to hyperglycemia and secondary diabetes.

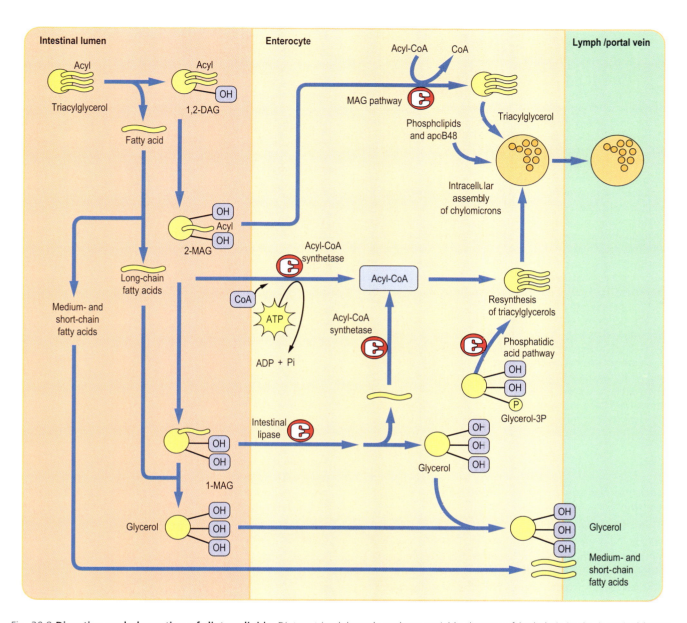

Fig. 30.8 **Digestion and absorption of dietary lipids.** Dietary triacylglycerols undergo variable degrees of hydrolysis in the intestinal lumen. Medium- and short-chain fatty acids are absorbed into the portal blood. However, long-chain fatty acids are resynthesized into TG within enterocytes. Fatty acids are activated by acetyl-CoA before the synthesis of acylglycerols can take place. Because enterocytes do not possess glycerol kinase, the formation of glycerol phosphate requires the presence of glucose. The resynthesized TGs are incorporated into chylomicrons. TG, triacylglycerol; DAG, diacylglycerol; MAG, monoacylglycerol; CoA, coenzyme A. Reproduced from Dominiczak MH. Medical Biochemistry Flash Cards. London: Elsevier, 2012, Card 38.

poorly absorbed: for instance, only 30%–40% of dietary cholesterol is absorbed. The secreted bile salts pass into the ileum, where they are reabsorbed and transferred back to the liver through the enterohepatic circulation (Chapter 14).

The fate of fatty acids depends on their chain length

Medium- and short-chain fatty acids (less than 10 carbon atoms) pass directly through the enterocytes into the hepatic portal system. In contrast, fatty acids containing more than

12 carbon atoms bind to a fatty acid–binding protein within the cell and are transferred to the rough endoplasmic reticulum for resynthesis into TGs. The glycerol required for this process is obtained from the absorbed 2-MAGs (the MG pathway; Fig. 30.8), from the hydrolysis of 1-MAG (which yields free glycerol), or from the glycerol-3-phosphate obtained from glycolysis (the phosphatidic acid pathway). Glycerol produced in the intestinal lumen is not used in the enterocyte for TG synthesis and passes directly to the portal vein.

The pancreas has two distinct functional roles: an **exocrine** function (i.e., secretion of digestive enzymes via the pancreatic duct) and an **endocrine** function (i.e., secretion of insulin, glucagon and other hormones by the islets of Langerhans; Chapter 31). These hormones are responsible for glycemic control and aspects of gastrointestinal function.

Exocrine secretions flow into the pancreatic duct, which empties into the duodenum along with the common bile duct from the liver and the gallbladder. Food entering the duodenum stimulates the secretion of **cholecystokinin**, and this in turn stimulates pancreatic enzyme production and secretion. The acidity of the stomach contents entering the duodenum stimulates the release of another hormone, **secretin**, which triggers the secretion of bicarbonate-rich pancreatic fluid, which neutralizes the acidity in the duodenum.

The pancreas secretes enzymes that digest carbohydrates, lipids, and proteins. Pancreatic **amylase** digests carbohydrates to oligo- and monosaccharides; **lipase** digests triacylglycerols; **cholesteryl esterase** yields free cholesterol and fatty acids; and finally, **proteases and peptidases** break down proteins and peptides. To prevent the powerful proteases from breaking down the pancreas itself (autodigestion), they are secreted as proenzymes and are activated in the intestinal lumen.

Triacylglycerol synthesis requires activation of fatty acids

All absorbed long-chain fatty acids are reutilized to form TGs before being transferred to chylomicrons. Fatty acid activation is accomplished by the acyl-CoA synthase. Chylomicrons are assembled within the rough endoplasmic reticulum before being released by exocytosis into the intercellular space. They leave the intestine via lymph (Chapter 33).

DIGESTION AND ABSORPTION OF PROTEINS

The gut receives 70–100 g dietary and 35–200 g endogenous proteins per day. The endogenous proteins, mostly enzymes, are either secreted into the gut or shed from the epithelium. Digestion and absorption of proteins are extremely efficient: of this large load, only 1–2 g of nitrogen, equivalent to 6–12 g of protein, are lost in the feces daily.

Proteins are hydrolyzed by peptidases

Peptide bonds are hydrolyzed by peptidases. Hydrolases can either cleave internal peptide bonds (**endopeptidases**) or cleave off one amino acid at a time from the either end of a molecule (**exopeptidases**). Exopeptidases that remove amino acids from amino terminus are **aminopeptidases**, and those

removing amino acids from the carboxy terminus of the polypeptide are **carboxypeptidases**. Endopeptidases break down large polypeptides into smaller oligopeptides, which can subsequently be acted upon by the exopeptidases to produce amino acids and di- and tripeptides, the final products of protein digestion, which are absorbed by the enterocytes. Depending on the source of the peptidases, protein digestion can be divided into gastric, pancreatic, and intestinal phases (Fig. 30.9).

Protein digestion begins in the stomach

In the stomach, the HCl reduces the pH to 1–2, with consequent denaturation of dietary proteins. Denaturation unfolds polypeptide chains, making proteins more accessible to proteases. In addition, chief cells of the gastric mucosa secrete pepsin. It is released as an inactive precursor, pepsinogen, and is activated by either an intramolecular reaction (autoactivation) at pH below 5.0 or active pepsin. At pH above 2.0, the liberated peptide remains bound to pepsin and acts as an inhibitor of its activity. This inhibition is removed by either a decrease in pH below 2.0 or further pepsin action. The products of digestion of proteins by pepsin are large peptide fragments and some free amino acids. They stimulate cholecystokinin release in the duodenum, which in turn triggers the release of the main digestive enzymes by the pancreas as well as the contraction of the gallbladder to release bile.

Proteolytic enzymes are released from the pancreas as inactive zymogens

A duodenal enteropeptidase converts trypsinogen to active trypsin. This enzyme is then capable of autoactivation. It also activates all other pancreatic zymogens (chymotrypsin, elastase, and carboxypeptidases A and B). Trypsin activity is controlled within the pancreas and pancreatic ducts by a low-molecular-weight inhibitory peptide.

Pancreatic proteases cleave peptide bonds in different locations in a protein

Trypsin cleaves proteins at arginine and lysine residues, **chymotrypsin** at aromatic amino acids, and **elastase** at hydrophobic amino acids. The combined effect is to produce an abundance of free amino acids and low-molecular-weight peptides of two to eight amino acids in length. Alongside protease secretion, the pancreas also produces copious amounts of **sodium bicarbonate**. This neutralizes the stomach contents as it passes into the duodenum, thus promoting pancreatic protease activity.

Final digestion of peptides depends on peptidases present in small intestine

Final digestion of oligopeptides and dipeptides is carried out in the small intestine by membrane-bound endopeptidases, dipeptidases, and aminopeptidases. The end products are free amino acids and di- and tripeptides. They are absorbed across the enterocyte membrane by specific carrier-mediated transport. Within the enterocyte, di- and tripeptides are hydrolyzed to their constituent amino acids. The final step is the transfer of free amino acids out of the enterocyte into the portal blood.

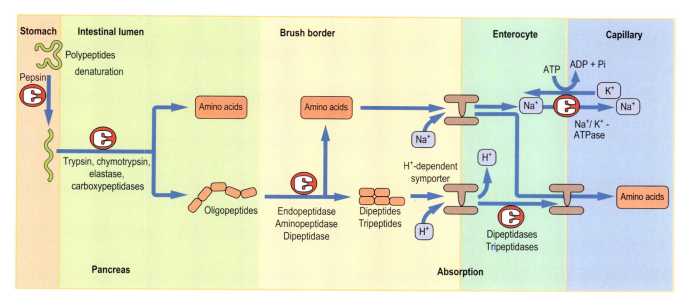

Fig. 30.9 **Digestion and absorption of dietary proteins.** The preliminary stage, protein denaturation, takes place in the stomach. Subsequently, peptide bonds between amino acids are hydrolyzed by endo- and exopeptidases. Free amino acids and di- and tripeptides are absorbed using specific transport systems located in the enterocyte membrane.

CLINICAL BOX
DIAGNOSTIC APPROACHES TO MALABSORPTION

Malabsorption can be caused by cystic fibrosis or deficiencies in lactase or other specific digestive enzymes. The most common cause of carbohydrate malabsorption is lactose deficiency. Pancreatic insufficiency is also an important cause, as is an inadequate amount of bile. Malabsorption can also result from the damage to the intestinal wall by, for instance, lymphoma, inflammatory bowel disease, or radiotherapy. Important causes are surgical interventions: gastrectomy, pancreatectomy, and resection of large fragments of the small bowel.

Rare endocrine causes include Zollinger–Ellison syndrome and abetalipoproteinemia (a rare disorder of lipoprotein metabolism in which chylomicron assembly is impaired).

The signs of malabsorption are **chronic diarrhea, anemia, steatorrhea, loss of weight**, and, in children, **failure to thrive**. Its complications result from the inadequate intake of nutrients, vitamins, or trace metals (Chapter 7).

Diagnosis of malabsorption syndromes involves the conventional hematology and biochemistry tests and testing for active inflammatory processes (C-reactive protein) as well as stool culture and stool biochemical analysis for elastase (assessing pancreatic exocrine function, calprotectin (assessing intestinal inflammation), and α-1-antitrypsin (assessing for protein loss). Specialist tests include testing for vitamin deficiencies. Imaging-based investigations such as abdominal ultrasound and CT scan can be performed, and portions of the upper and lower GI tract can be visualized through endoscopy. Biopsies can be taken from the stomach, duodenum, and small bowel.

The hydrogen breath tests are used in the diagnosis of carbohydrate malabsorption. Older tests for malabsorption include the xylose absorption test and lactose absorption test.

ADVANCED CONCEPT BOX
ACTIVE TRANSPORT OF AMINO ACIDS INTO INTESTINAL EPITHELIAL CELLS

Mechanisms of active transport of amino acids and di- or tripeptides into intestinal epithelial cells are similar to those described for glucose. At the brush-border membrane, Na^+-dependent symporters mediating amino acid uptake are linked to ATP-dependent pumping out of Na^+ at the basolateral membrane. A similar H^+-dependent symporter is present on the brush-border surface for di- and tripeptide transport into the cell. Na^+-independent transporters are present on the basolateral surface, allowing facilitated transport of amino acids into the portal vein. At least six specific symporter systems have been identified for the uptake of L-amino acids from the intestinal lumen:

- Neutral amino acid symporter for amino acids with short or polar side chains (Ser, Thr, Ala)
- Neutral amino acid symporter for aromatic or hydrophobic side chains (Phe, Tyr, Met, Val, Leu, Ileu)
- Imino acid symporter (Pro, OH-Pro)
- Basic amino acid symporter (Lys, Arg, Cys)
- Acidic amino acid symporter (Asp, Glu)
- β-amino acid symporter (β-Ala, Tau)

These transport systems are also present in the renal tubules, and defects in their molecular structure can lead to disease (e.g., **Hartnup disease,** an inherited disorder with defects of intestinal amino acid absorption and urinary loss of neutral amino acids).

SUMMARY

■ Digestion is a series of processes that prepare food for absorption.

■ Digestion and absorption of foods make the metabolic fuels available to the organism.

■ Carbohydrates are digested to simple sugars.

■ Fats are hydrolyzed to di- and monoglycerides.

■ Proteins are hydrolyzed to di- and tripeptides and free amino acids.

■ Defects in these mechanisms result in a variety of malabsorption and food intolerance syndromes.

ACTIVE LEARNING

1. Describe the process of digestion of starch.
2. Discuss the possible complications of persistent vomiting.
3. Which hormones aid digestion?
4. List the secretory products of the stomach.
5. Outline the mechanisms of sugar transport in the small intestine.
6. What is the role of micelles in the digestion of fat?

FURTHER READING

Ayling, R. M. (2012). New faecal tests in gastroenterology. *Annals of Clinical Biochemistry, 49,* 44–54.

Baumgart, D. C., & Sandborn, W. J. (2012). Crohn's disease. *Lancet, 380,* 1590–1605.

Chatchu, U., & Bhatnagar, S. (2013). Diarrhoea in children: Identifying the cause and burden. *Lancet, 382,* 184–185.

Di Sabatino, A., & Corazza, R. G. (2009). Coeliac disease. *Lancet, 373,* 1480–1493.

Harris, J. B., LaRocque, R. C., Qadri, F., et al. (2012). Cholera. *Lancet, 379,* 2466–2476.

Lankisch, P. G., Apte, M., & Banks, P. A. (2015). Acute pancreatitis. *Lancet, 386,* 85–96.

Kalla, R., Ventham, N. T., Satsangi, J., et al. (2014). Crohn's disease. *BMJ (Clinical Research Ed.), 349,* g6670.

Kunzelmann, K., & Mall, M. (2002). Electrolyte transport in the mammalian colon: Mechanisms and implications for disease. *Physiological Reviews, 82,* 245–289.

Malfertheiner, P., Chan, F. K. L., & McColl, K. E. L. (2009). Peptic ulcer disease. *Lancet, 374,* 1449–1461.

Ordas, I., Eckmann, L., Talamini, M., et al. (2012). Ulcerative colitis. *Lancet, 380,* 1606–1619.

RELEVANT WEBSITES

Diarrhoea: Why children are still dying and what can be done (WHO, 2009): http://www.who.int/maternal_child_adolescent/documents/9789241598415/en/index.html

Lab Tests Online - Malabsorption: http://labtestsonline.org/understanding/conditions/malabsorption/

UNICEF, Technical Bulletin No. 9 - New formulation of oral rehydration salts (ORS) with reduced osmolarity: https://www.unicef.org/supply/files/Oral_Rehydration_Salts(ORS)_.pdf

ABBREVIATIONS

AE	Anion exchanger (chloride/bicarbonate exchanger)
CFTR	Cystic fibrosis transmembrane conductance regulator
DAG	Diacylglycerol
ENaC	Epithelial sodium channel
GI	Gastrointestinal (tract)
GLUT	Glucose transporter
KCC1	K^+ and Cl^- cotransporter
MAG	Monoacylglycerol
NEFA	Nonesterified fatty acid
NHE	Sodium/hydrogen exchanger
NKCC1	Na^+ K^+ and Cl^- cotransporter
PGE$_2$	Prostaglandin E$_2$
PKA	Protein kinase A
PKC	Protein kinase C
SCFA	Short-chain fatty acid
SGLT-1	Sodium/glucose-linked transport-1
TG	Triacylglycerols (also triglycerides)

CHAPTER

31

Glucose Homeostasis and Fuel Metabolism: Diabetes Mellitus

Marek H. Dominiczak

LEARNING OBJECTIVES

After reading this chapter, you should be able to:

- Characterize main energy substrates (metabolic fuels).
- Outline the actions of insulin and glucagon.
- Compare and contrast metabolism in the fasting and postprandial state.
- Describe the metabolic response to injury, and compare it with metabolism in diabetes.
- Characterize type 1 and type 2 diabetes mellitus.
- Explain the basis of laboratory tests relevant to fuel metabolism and to monitoring of diabetes.

INTRODUCTION

Continuous provision of energy is essential to maintain life. This chapter describes metabolism of compounds known as energy substrates or metabolic fuels. It also discusses the most common metabolic disease, diabetes mellitus.

The most important energy substrates are glucose and fatty acids

After ingestion of food, the excess of glucose and fatty acids is stored, to be released again in case of need, thus providing continuous energy supply. First, a limited amount of glucose is stored as glycogen. Further excess is converted to fatty acids, the ultimate long-term energy-storage material. The caloric value of fat (9 kcal/g; 37 kJ/g) is higher than that of either carbohydrates (4 kcal/g; 17 kJ/g) or proteins (4 kcal/g), and therefore its storage is more efficient.

Controlled release of energy substrates from stores safeguards the energy supply both in the short term (i.e., between meals) and during prolonged fasting. In extreme circumstances, stored energy can ensure survival for months. The main pathways of fuel metabolism and the key metabolites are listed in Table 31.1.

Metabolism is geared toward safeguarding continuous glucose supply; glucose is being stored as glycogen and can also be synthesized from non-carbohydrate compounds

The reason why glucose is such an essential fuel is that in normal circumstances, it is the only fuel used by the brain.

Glucose is also the preferred fuel for muscle use during the initial stages of exercise. The amount of glucose present in the extracellular fluid is only about 20 g (1 oz), the equivalent of 80 kcal (335 kJ), and its concentration is maintained within a narrow range. This is backed up by the emergency store of glycogen in the liver (approximately 75 g; 2.5 oz) and in muscle (400 g; 1 lb), altogether equivalent to about 1900 kcal (7955 kJ).

When glucose concentration in the extracellular fluid decreases, it is first replenished from the liver glycogen, which can sustain glucose supply for approximately 16 h. During prolonged fasting or extreme exercise, another mechanism comes into play: the synthesis of glucose from noncarbohydrate compounds, known as **gluconeogenesis**.

The main substrates for gluconeogenesis are **lactate** derived from anaerobic glycolysis, **alanine** from the amino acids released during the breakdown of muscle protein, and **glycerol** from the breakdown of triacylglycerols in the adipose tissue (Chapter 12).

Fatty acids are the primary energy source during prolonged fasting and prolonged exercise; large amounts of fatty acids are stored as triacylglycerols

Fat is stored in the adipose tissue as esters of glycerol and fatty acids (triacylglycerols [TG], also termed triglycerides). In contrast to glucose, there is virtually unlimited capacity for fat storage. A 70-kg (154-lb) man will store approximately 15 kg (33 lb) of fat. This is equivalent to more than 130,000 kcal (544,300 kJ). In extreme circumstances, people can fast for as long as 60–90 days; obese persons may survive for more than a year without food.

Amino acids become a fuel after conversion to glucose

Amino acids are primarily used for the synthesis of body proteins. Excess amino acids taken in food are converted to carbohydrates. However, when energy needs increase (i.e., during prolonged fast, illness, or injury), body proteins are degraded, and the released amino acids are converted into glucose through gluconeogenesis.

Organs and tissues differ in their handling of fuels

The **brain** uses approximately 20% of all oxygen consumed by the body. Glucose is normally its only fuel. However, during starvation, the brain adapts to the use of **ketone bodies** as an alternative energy source.

Gluconeogenesis occurs primarily in the **liver** and, during prolonged fast, in **the kidneys**.

443

Table 31.1 Principal anabolic and catabolic pathways

Pathway	Main substrates	End products
Anabolic		
Gluconeogenesis	Lactate, alanine, glycerol	Glucose
Glycogen synthesis	Glucose-1-phosphate	Glycogen
Protein synthesis	Amino acids	Proteins
Fatty acid synthesis	Acetyl-CoA	Fatty acids
Lipogenesis	Glycerol, fatty acids	Triacylglycerols (triglycerides)
Catabolic		
Glycolysis	Glucose	Pyruvate, ATP
Tricarboxylic acid cycle	Pyruvate	$NADH + H^+$, $FADH_2$ CO_2, H_2O, ATP
Glycogenolysis	Glycogen	Glucose-1-phosphate, glucose
Pentose phosphate pathway	Glucose-6-phosphate	$NADPH + H^+$, Pentose sugars, CO_2
Fatty acid oxidation	Fatty acids	Acetyl-CoA CO_2, H_2O, ATP (ketone bodies)
Lipolysis	Triglycerides	Glycerol, fatty acids
Proteolysis	Proteins	Amino acids, glucose

Note that metabolites such as pyruvate and acetyl-CoA are common to several pathways. Note also which pathways generate reducing equivalents (NADH, NADPH, and FADH$_2$), which are substrates for the mitochondrial respiratory chain.

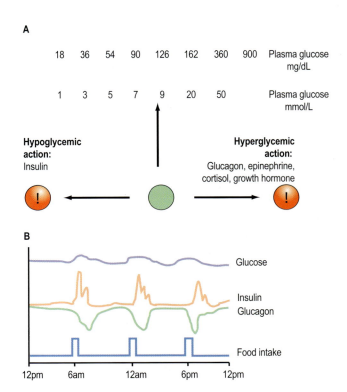

A

18	36	54	90	126	162	360	900	Plasma glucose mg/dL
1	3	5	7	9	20	50		Plasma glucose mmol/L

Hypoglycemic action:
Insulin

Hyperglycemic action:
Glucagon, epinephrine, cortisol, growth hormone

B

Glucose

Insulin

Glucagon

Food intake

12pm 6am 12am 6pm 12pm

Fig. 31.1 **Hormonal control of glucose homeostasis.** (A) Plasma-glucose concentration reflects the balance between the hypoglycemic (glucose-lowering) action of insulin and the hyperglycemic (glucose-increasing) action of the antiinsulin hormones. (B) Daily patterns of insulin and glucagon secretion and corresponding plasma glucose concentrations. Plasma glucose concentration is maintained within a narrow range throughout the day. Note suppression of glucagon secretion when insulin is released in response to a meal. To obtain glucose concentrations in mg/dL, multiply the value in mmol/L by 18.

Muscle uses both glucose and fatty acids as energy sources. During short-term exercise, the preferred substrate is glucose. However, at rest and during prolonged exercise, the main energy source is fatty acids (Chapter 37). Note that although the myocytes contain glycogen, they can only use it for their own energy needs; they cannot release glucose into circulation because they lack the enzyme glucose-6-phosphatase. Muscle contributes to gluconeogenesis by releasing lactate and, when needed, alanine. Both are transported to the liver.

GLUCOSE HOMEOSTASIS

The glucose concentration in **plasma** reflects the balance between, on the one hand, its dietary intake or its endogenous production (glycogenolysis and gluconeogenesis) and, on the other, its tissue utilization in glycolysis, the pentose phosphate pathway, and the tricarboxylic acid (TCA) cycle, and its storage (glycogenogenesis) (see also Chapter 12). In the fasting state, a person weighing 70 kg (154 lb) metabolizes glucose at a rate of approximately 200 g/24 h.

Insulin and the counterregulatory hormones control fuel metabolism

Glucose homeostasis is controlled, on the one hand, by the anabolic hormone **insulin** and, on the other, by a set of catabolic hormones **(glucagon, catecholamines, cortisol, and growth hormone)**, also known as counterregulatory hormones (Fig. 31.1). Insulin and glucagon are secreted from the pancreatic islets of Langerhans. Insulin is secreted by β cells (approximately 70% of all islet cells) and glucagon by the α cells. The **molar ratio of insulin to glucagon** at any given time is the key determinant of the pattern of fuel metabolism.

Pancreatic islets also secrete other hormones, such as somatostatin or amylin.

Insulin

Insulin was discovered in 1921–1922 by Frederick Banting, Charles Best, and John Macleod, all working in Toronto (see Further Reading). In 1979, it came to prominence again,

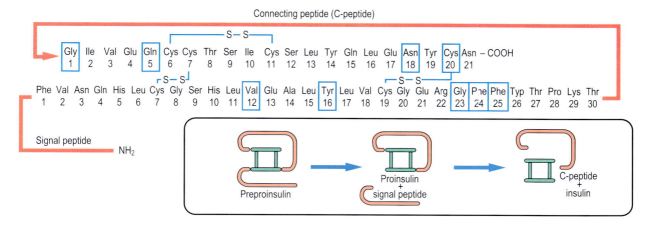

Fig. 31.2 **Insulin.** The insulin molecule consists of two polypeptide chains joined by two disulfide bridges. The third bridge is internal to the β-chain. Insulin is synthesized as a longer peptide, preproinsulin, which is cleaved into the signal peptide and proinsulin. Before being secreted from the β cell, proinsulin is split further into the C-peptide and insulin. Boxes drawn around amino acid residues indicate the amino acid involved in the binding of insulin to its receptor.

becoming the first recombinant human protein produced commercially. Its molecule consists of two peptide chains (alpha chain and beta chain) linked by two disulfide bonds. The molecular weight of insulin is 5500 Da. Insulin is synthesized in the rough endoplasmic reticulum of the pancreatic β-cells and is packaged into the secretory vesicles in the Golgi apparatus. The precursor of insulin is the single-chain molecule preproinsulin. First, a 24–amino acid signal sequence is cleaved from preproinsulin by a peptidase, yielding proinsulin. Proinsulin is then split by endopeptidases into insulin and C-peptide (Fig. 31.2), both of which are released from the cell in equimolar amounts. Clinical laboratories exploit this for the assessment of the β-cell function in patients treated with insulin. In such persons, endogenous insulin cannot be measured directly because the administered insulin would interfere in the assay. However, because C-peptide is present in the same molar concentration as native insulin, it serves as a marker of β-cell function.

Insulin secretion is controlled by glucose metabolism in the β-cell

The β cell takes up glucose using the membrane transporter GLUT-2 (Chapter 4). On entering the cell, glucose is phosphorylated by glucokinase and enters glycolysis. As glucose metabolism is stimulated, the ATP/ADP ratio in the cell increases. This closes the ATP-sensitive potassium channels in the cell membrane, decreasing potassium efflux and depolarizing the cell. This in turn opens the L-type calcium channels, allowing calcium ions to enter the cell. This activates Ca^{2+}-dependent proteins that cause the release of secretory granules containing insulin. The ensuing release of insulin is known as the first phase of insulin secretion (Fig. 31.3; compare this with the neurosecretory granules, Chapter 26). The second phase of insulin secretion involves the synthesis of new insulin and responds to signals such as an increase in the concentration of the cytosolic long-chain acyl-CoA. The loss of the first phase of secretion is an early sign of islet cell damage. Note that

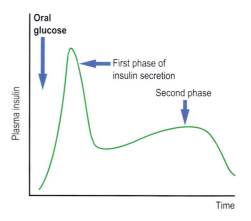

Fig. 31.3 **Insulin secretion.** Note the two phases of insulin secretion. Glucose is the most important stimulator of insulin secretion. Other stimulators are some of the amino acids (arginine, lysine, branched-chain amino acids), stimulation of the vagus nerve, and the hormones secreted by the gut (incretins).

amino acids, such as leucine, arginine, and lysine, also stimulate insulin secretion.

Insulin acts through a membrane receptor that triggers multiple intracellular signaling pathways; intracellular insulin signaling occurs through complex cascades of phosphorylation reactions

The event initiating insulin action is its binding to the membrane receptor. The insulin receptor has a high degree of homology with the receptor for insulin growth factor-1 (IGF1). In fact, both insulin and IGF1 interact with these two receptors, albeit with differing affinities.

The receptor is a four-subunit protein spanning the cell membrane. The beta subunit of the receptor has tyrosine kinase activity. The binding of insulin causes the receptor to phosphorylate itself (autophosphorylate). Phosphorylation induces a conformational change that enables recruitment of several proteins known as the insulin receptor substrates (IRS1–6). Phosphorylated IRS in turn bind other sets of proteins, which channel the signal into two main cascades, the IRS-PI3K-Akt cascade and GRB2-SOS-Ras-MAPK cascade (Fig. 31.4; compare Fig. 25.3). Other signaling pathways also exist, such as the PI3K- independent pathway, which contributes to the stimulation of cellular glucose transport.

The IRS-PI3K-Akt signaling pathway controls the metabolic effects of insulin

IRS proteins recruit adaptor proteins, which phosphorylate the phosphatidylinositol 3-kinase (PI3K). Activation of PI3K generates a lipid-based messenger, phosphatidylinositol -3,4,5-triphosphate (PIP$_3$; Chapter 25). It activates the 3'-phosphoinositide-dependent kinase 1 (PDK1), which in turn phosphorylates the Akt kinase, a key serine-threonine kinase belonging to the AGC protein kinase family (it is also called protein kinase B [PKB]).

Activation of Akt is enhanced by a complex designated mTORC2, which contains mTOR kinase. The Akt pathway regulates glycolysis, glyconeogenesis, and lipogenesis and suppresses glycogenolysis. Other Akt substrates include glycogen synthase kinase 3 and the transcription factors belonging to the forkhead box O (FOXO) family, which control the endogenous glucose production in the liver and play a role in lipogenesis and gluconeogenesis, as well as proteins involved in cell-cycle regulation, apoptosis, and survival. They also affect differentiation of the beta cells. Akt phosphorylation leads to the exclusion of FOXO from the nucleus and inhibition of their activity. Conversely, decreased FOXO phosphorylation leads to insulin resistance.

This pathway also involves the activation of some isoforms of protein kinase C (PKC), known as atypical PKCs, such as PKC λε, which regulate glucose transport.

The GRB2-SOS-Ras-MAPK signaling pathway has mitogenic effects

The GRB2-SOS-Ras-MAPK pathway is initiated by binding of Shc protein to the receptor. Shc recruits docking protein Grb2, which forms a complex with Son of Sevenless protein (SoS). The complex activates the Ras GTPase, which in turn phosphorylates the Raf kinase. Raf, through more intermediaries, activates MAP kinases ERK 1 and ERK2. MAP kinases phosphorylate

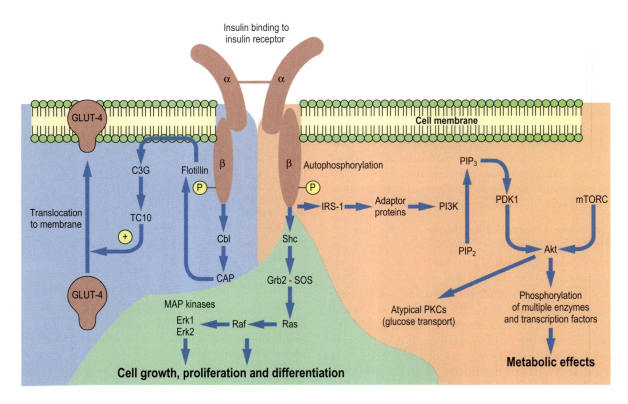

Fig. 31.4 **Insulin signaling.** Insulin-signaling cascades transfer the signal from the insulin molecule to its target molecules such as regulatory enzymes and the membrane-glucose transporter GLUT-4. The IRS-1-PI3K-Akt pathway mediates the main metabolic effects of insulin and affects glucose transport through activation of atypical PKCs. The PI3K-independent pathway affects translocation of the GLUT-4 transporter to the cell membrane. The GRB2-SOS-Ras-MAPK pathway mediates mitogenic effects: cell growth proliferation and differentiation. CAP, Cbl-associated protein; Cbl, adaptor protein in insulin signaling pathway; **C3G, guanyl nucleotide exchange factor;** Erk, extracellular signal-regulated kinase; Grb2, adaptor protein; IRS-1, insulin receptor substrate 1; **TC-10, a G-protein;** Shc, protein participating in signaling pathways. Also, a domain of certain signal transduction proteins, mTORC, protein complex containing mTOR kinase; PDK, phosphoinositide-dependent kinase; PI3K, phosphoinositol-3-kinase; PIP$_2$, phosphatidylinositol -4,5-bisphosphate; PIP$_3$, phosphatidylinositol -3,4,5-trisphosphate; PKC, protein kinase C; Ras, a GTPase; Raf, a protein kinase; SOS, son-of-sevenless protein. See text for detailed explanation.

a range of substrates involved in cell growth, proliferation, and differentiation.

The PI3K-independent pathway stimulates glucose transport

Glucose transport can also be activated through the **PI3K-independent pathway**, where the insulin receptor phosphorylates the Cbl protein that binds to Cbl-associated protein (CAP). CAP in turn binds to flotillin, a protein associated with lipid rafts in the cell membrane. Flotillin docks guanyl nucleotide exchange factor (C3G). This activates the G-protein called TC-10, which participates in the translocation of the **GLUT-4 transporter** in adipocytes to the cell membrane.

Termination of the insulin signal involves phosphatases such as the phosphotyrosine phosphatase 1B.

Metabolic effects of insulin

In general, insulin stimulates the anabolic pathways and suppresses the catabolic pathways. It acts mainly on three tissues:

the liver, adipose tissue, and skeletal muscle (Fig. 31.5). In the fasting state, the liver is the main target of insulin action. After a meal, though, the main targets become muscle and adipose tissue; for instance, after glucose infusion, skeletal muscle is responsible for about 80% of glucose disposal.

In the liver, insulin stimulates glycolysis and glycogen synthesis. Note that glucose transport in the liver is insulin independent. Insulin also stimulates the synthesis of long-chain fatty acids and lipogenesis (the synthesis of triacylglycerols). In addition, it promotes the assembly of the very-low-density lipoproteins (VLDL), which transport lipids from the liver to peripheral cells. Insulin also induces the **endothelial** lipoprotein lipase, an enzyme that liberates triacylglycerols from the chylomicrons and the VLDL (Chapter 33). At the same time, insulin suppresses gluconeogenesis and lipolysis.

In the adipose tissue, insulin stimulates triacylglycerol synthesis using glycerol-3-phosphate and fatty acids as substrates.

In muscle, it stimulates glucose transport, glucose metabolism, glycogen synthesis, and also uptake of amino acids and protein synthesis.

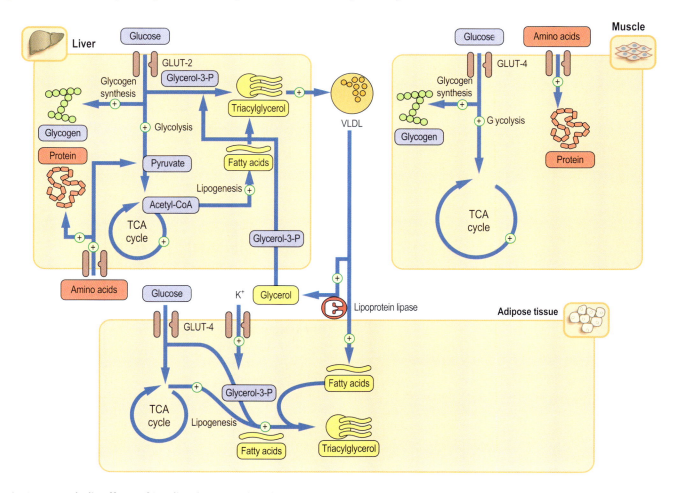

Fig. 31.5 **Metabolic effects of insulin.** The principal insulin target tissues are liver, muscle, and adipose tissue. Insulin affects carbohydrate, lipid, and protein metabolism. Insulin also promotes cellular potassium uptake. The plus sign indicates pathways stimulated by insulin. Note that in most instances, insulin also inhibits the opposite processes. Glucose transport in muscle and adipose tissue is mediated by the GLUT-4 transporter and is insulin dependent. On the other hand, GLUT-2 present in the liver is insulin independent.

Insulin stimulates glucose transport across the cell membrane

Insulin-dependent glucose entry into cells is mediated by proteins known as glucose transporters (Chapter 4). The GLUT-4 transporter controls glucose uptake in the skeletal muscle and adipocytes. It cycles between the endosomes and membrane. In an unstimulated cell, no more than 10% of GLUT-4 molecules are present in the plasma membrane. In humans, insulin doubles the GLUT-4 recruitment to cell membranes. However, fatty acids attenuate its expression. Importantly, muscle contraction during exercise increases expression of the GLUT-4 independently of insulin.

Insulin resistance: A key concept in glucose homeostasis

Insulin resistance is a condition in which a given dose of insulin produces less-than-expected cellular response. The concept of insulin resistance is crucial to understanding the pathogenesis of type 2 diabetes.

In the liver, insulin resistance results in an increase in VLDL production. It also causes an increased fibrinogen synthesis and increased plasminogen activator inhibitor 1 (PAI-1), leading to a procoagulant status. In muscle, glucose uptake decreases. In the adipose tissue, there is an overproduction of free fatty acids and changes in the adipokine secretion pattern, a decrease in adiponectin, and an increase in resistin (Chapter 32).

> ### ✦ ADVANCED CONCEPT BOX
> ### ASSESSMENT OF INSULIN RESISTANCE
>
> Insulin resistance is currently assessed mostly for research purposes. This can be done using a method known as the **hyperinsulinemic euglycemic clamp:** Insulin is infused at a constant rate together with variable amounts of glucose. The rate of glucose infusion is adjusted to keep plasma glucose concentration at 5.0–5.5 mmol/L (90–99 mg/dL). When a steady state is attained, the rate of glucose infusion is equal to the peripheral glucose uptake, and this reflects insulin sensitivity/resistance.

The most important cause of insulin resistance is defective insulin signaling (Table 31.2)

Insulin resistance can be caused by compromised insulin binding to its receptor - for instance, due to a very rare mutation in the insulin receptor gene or the presence of antireceptor autoantibodies. The most important causes, however, are defects in the insulin signaling pathways. When the IRS-PI3K-Akt pathway does not operate normally, the cellular translocation of the GLUT-4 transporter, and consequently glucose transport, is impaired in adipocytes (but not in the skeletal muscle). This has been observed in both in obesity and in diabetes.

Table 31.2 Sites of insulin resistance

Site of resistance	Possible defect	Comment
Prereceptor	Insulin receptor antibodies, abnormal molecule	Rare
Receptor	Decreased number or affinity of insulin receptors	Not significant in diabetes
Postreceptor	Defects in signal transduction: defective tyrosine phosphorylation, mutations in genes coding for IRS-1, phosphatidylinositol-3'-kinase, defective translocation of GLUT-4 to cell membrane, elevated concentration of fatty acids	Postreceptor resistance is the most common type of insulin resistance

Insulin resistance is associated with variants of genes coding for IRS-1 and PI3K. It can also be induced by excess fatty acids. Accumulation of triacylglycerols in liver and muscle (steatosis), seen in patients with high plasma triacylglycerol concentrations, also contributes to insulin resistance. FOXO transcription factors seem to play a key role in this. They normally switch liver metabolism from glucose utilization to glucose production during fasting. In their absence, fasting does not induce glucose-6-phosphatase and does not suppress glucokinase; therefore instead of glucose production, glucose carbons are directed toward lipogenesis. This leads to increased VLDL production and accumulation of triacylglycerols in the liver - and thus liver steatosis. Collectively, untoward phenomena linked to fatty acid excess are known as **lipotoxicity.** Hyperglycemia can also attenuate the insulin signal **(glucotoxicity)**.

GLUCAGON AND OTHER ANTIINSULIN HORMONES

Glucagon and other antiinsulin (counterregulatory) hormones increase plasma glucose concentration by stimulating glycogenolysis and gluconeogenesis

Glucagon acts on the liver. There are no glucagon receptors on muscle cells; muscle glycogenolysis is stimulated by another antiinsulin hormone, epinephrine.

Glucagon is a single-chain, 29–amino acid peptide, with a molecular weight of 3485 Da. It mobilizes fuel reserves to maintain plasma glucose concentration between meals. It stimulates glycogenolysis, gluconeogenesis, the oxidation of the fatty acids, and ketogenesis (Table 31.3). In parallel, it inhibits glycolysis, glycogen synthesis, and the synthesis of triacylglycerols (Fig. 31.6).

Glucagon binds to its own membrane receptor (Chapter 12), which signals through the membrane-associated G proteins

Table 31.3 Reciprocal effects of insulin and glucagon on key enzymes of gluconeogenesis

Enzyme	Effect of glucagon	Effect of insulin
Glucose-6-phosphatase (Glc-6-Pase)	Induction	Repression
Fructose-1,6-biphosphatase (Fru-1,6-BPase)	Induction	Repression
Phosphoenolpyruvate carboxykinase (PEPCK)	Induction	Repression

On a high-carbohydrate diet, *insulin induces transcription of genes coding for glycolytic enzymes glucokinase, phosphofructokinase (PFK), pyruvate kinase (PK), and glycogen synthase. At the same time, it represses the key enzymes of gluconeogenesis, pyruvate carboxylase (PC), PEPCK, Fru-1,6-BPase, and Glc-6-Pase. Glucagon effects oppose those of insulin.* ***On a high-fat diet,*** *glucagon represses the synthesis of glucokinase, PFK-1, and PK and induces the transcription of PEPCK, Fru-6-Pase, and Glc-6-Pase.*

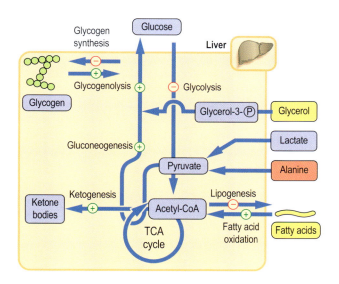

Fig. 31.6 **Metabolic effects of glucagon.** Glucagon mobilizes glucose from every available source. It also increases lipolysis and ketogenesis from acetyl-CoA. Glucagon actions are confined to the liver.

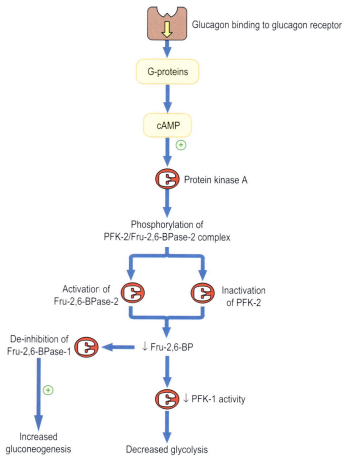

Fig. 31.7 **Regulation of glycolysis and gluconeogenesis by phosphofructokinase.** Glucagon regulates gluconeogenesis by controlling the bifunctional enzyme that slows the activity of **phosphofructokinase-2** (PFK-2) and **fructose 2,6-biphosphatase-2** (Fru-2,6-BPase-2). Glucagon binds to its membrane receptor and signals through G-proteins and adenylate cyclase, generating cAMP. cAMP in turn activates protein kinase A. Subsequently, this kinase phosphorylates the **PFK-2:Fru-2, 6-BPase complex.** Phosphorylation activates the bisphosphatase, which degrades Fru-2,6-BP, and lowering of Fru-2,6-BP reverses the inhibition of another enzyme, Fru-2,6-BPase-1, in the main pathway of gluconeogenesis. Thus **gluconeogenesis is stimulated**. Ingeniously, decrease in Fru-2,6-BP activity has a reciprocal inhibitory effect on the key glycolytic enzyme, phosphofructokinase (PFK-1). Thus **glycolysis is inhibited**.

and the cAMP cascade. First, the glucagon–receptor complex causes binding of guanosine 5′-triphosphate (GTP) to a G-protein complex (Chapter 25). This leads to the dissociation of G-protein subunits. One of these subunits (Gα) activates the adenylate cyclase, which in turn converts ATP to cAMP. cAMP activates cAMP-dependent protein kinase (protein kinase A), which controls the key steps in carbohydrate and lipid metabolism through phosphorylation of regulatory enzymes (Figs. 31.6, 31.7, and 31.8).

Epinephrine acts on liver and muscle

Epinephrine (adrenaline) is the key hormone responsible for stress-related hyperglycemia. Its metabolic effects are similar to those of glucagon: it inhibits glycolysis and lipogenesis, and it stimulates gluconeogenesis. It acts through the α- and β-adrenergic (mainly the β₂) receptors (Fig. 12.5). These receptors, similarly to the glucagon receptor, use the cAMP signaling cascade.

INCRETIN HORMONES

Incretin hormones are secreted by the gut and potentiate insulin secretion

Plasma insulin response to oral glucose is greater than that to intravenous infusion. **Gastrointestinal hormones,** such

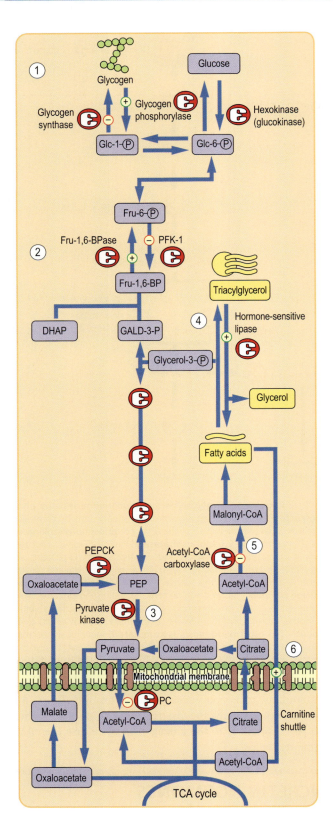

Fig. 31.8 Phosphorylation of key enzymes controlled by glucagon and epinephrine regulates carbohydrate and lipid metabolism. Phosphorylation usually stimulates enzymes in the catabolic pathways and inhibits enzymes in the anabolic pathways. **Glycogen metabolism:** glycogen phosphorylase is activated, and glycogen synthase is inactivated. This promotes glycogen breakdown (1). **Gluconeogenesis:** Fru-2,6-BPase-2 is activated, and PFK-2 is inhibited. This decreases Fru-2,6-BP formation and in turn inhibits PFK-1 (glycolysis) and stimulates FBPase (gluconeogenesis) (2). **Glycolysis:** normally, Fru-1,6-BP also allosterically activates pyruvate kinase downstream in the glycolytic pathway. Because its formation is decreased, glycolysis slows down (3). **Lipolysis:** phosphorylation stimulates hormone-sensitive lipase-stimulating lipolysis (release of fatty acids from triglycerides) (4). **Fatty acid oxidation:** phosphorylation inhibits acetyl-CoA carboxylase, inhibiting the generation of malonyl-CoA (5). Malonyl-CoA normally inhibits carnitine-palmitoyl transferase-1. Lack of malonyl-CoA disinhibits it (6), facilitating the entry of fatty acids into mitochondria. This stimulates lipid oxidation. DHAP, dihydroxyacetone phosphate; GALD-3-P, glyceraldehyde-3-phosphate; PEP, phosphoenolpyruvate.

as **glucagon-like peptide-1** (GLP-1), the **glucose-dependent insulinotropic peptide** (also known as gastric inhibitory peptide [GIP]), cholecystokinin, and vasoactive intestinal peptide (VIP), potentiate insulin secretion. They are secreted after ingestion of foods. This is known as **the incretin effect**.

GLP-1 is secreted in the intestinal mucosa, mostly in the distal ileum and colon. GLP-1 secretion increases rapidly after a meal. In the presence of elevated glucose concentration, GLP-1 increases insulin secretion and decreases glucagon secretion, thus decreasing endogenous glucose production. GLP-1 also decreases gastric emptying and increases feelings of satiety.

GIP is a 42–amino acid molecule synthesized in the duodenum and jejunum. GLP-1 and GIP act through G-protein-coupled receptors. The GLP-1 receptor is present in the α cells and β cells in the pancreatic islets and in the peripheral tissues. GLP-1 and GIP are inactivated by **dipeptidyl peptidase-4** (DPP-4).

THE FEED–FAST CYCLE

Human metabolism oscillates between the fed state and the fasting state; the molar ratio of insulin to glucagon in plasma depends on which pattern of metabolism is present

The **fed state** (also called the absorptive, or postprandial, state) occurs during a meal and for several hours thereafter. Its key characteristic is the high insulin and low glucagon concentration (a high insulin-to-glucagon ratio).

The opposite of the fed state is the **fasting state**. Fasting for 6–12 h is called the **postabsorptive state**. Fasting that lasts longer than 12 h is termed "**prolonged fasting," or starvation**. It is characterized by the low insulin and high glucagon concentration (a low insulin-to-glucagon ratio).

Insulin and glucagon switch genes on and off during feed–fast cycle

Insulin regulates the synthesis of key enzymes by controlling the activity of the FOXO transcription factors (so called because they have a helix-turn-helix structure with two additional loops). Two such transcription factors, forkhead box protein 1 (FOXO1) and FOXA2 (also known as HNF-3B), are essential for switching anabolism to catabolism.

FOXO1 promotes gluconeogenesis in the liver in the fasted state. FOXO1 and its coactivators stimulate gluconeogenesis by activating genes that code for the rate-limiting enzymes phosphoenolpyruvate carboxykinase (PEPCK) and glucose-6-phosphatase (Glc-6-Pase). FOXA2 regulates fatty acid oxidation.

They are both inactivated by kinases in the IRS-1/PI3K/Akt pathway. This inhibits hepatic gluconeogenesis.

Glucagon, conversely, induces gluconeogenic enzymes. Another forkhead transcription factor, FOXA2, regulates fat breakdown in the fasting state by inducing genes encoding enzymes of glycolysis, fatty acid oxidation, and ketogenesis. This increases plasma concentrations of free fatty acids, ketone bodies, and triacylglycerols, and it decreases the liver content of triacylglycerol. Insulin phosphorylates and inhibits FOXA2. The reciprocal effects of insulin and glucagon on main metabolic pathways are illustrated in Figs. 31.7 and 31.8.

Metabolism in the fed state

Metabolism in fed state is geared toward energy production and storage

A meal stimulates insulin release and inhibits glucagon secretion. This affects metabolism in the liver, adipose tissue, and muscle (Fig. 31.9). Glucose utilization by the brain remains unchanged. There is an increase in glucose uptake in the insulin-dependent tissues, principally in the skeletal muscle. Glucose oxidation and glycogen synthesis are stimulated, and lipid oxidation is inhibited. Glucose taken up by the liver is phosphorylated by glucokinase, yielding glucose-6-phosphate (Glc-6-P). Excess glucose is directed into the pentose phosphate pathway, generating $NADPH + H^+$, which is used in biosynthetic pathways that require reductions, such as synthesis of fatty acids and cholesterol. Further, oxidative glucose metabolism provides acetyl-CoA, which is a substrate for fatty acid synthesis.

Triacylglycerols absorbed in the intestine are transported in chylomicrons to peripheral tissues, where they are hydrolyzed to glycerol and free fatty acids by lipoprotein lipase (Chapter 33). In muscle, the released fatty acids are used as fuel. In the adipose tissue, they are reassembled into triacylglycerols and stored. Such reassembly requires glycerol, which is provided by glycolysis (triose phosphate being reduced to glycerol-3-phosphate).

Synthesis of fatty acids increases in the liver and adipose tissue. There is also stimulation of amino acid uptake and protein synthesis and a decrease in protein degradation in the liver, muscle, and adipose tissue.

Metabolism in the fasting state

Liver switches from a glucose-utilizing to a glucose-producing organ

During fasting (Fig. 31.10), the liver transforms from a glucose-utilizing to a glucose-producing organ. There is a decrease in glycogen synthesis and an increase in glycogenolysis. After an overnight fast, a steady state is reached, with hepatic glucose production becoming equal to peripheral glucose uptake. The key to this is two enzymes controlled by FOXO transcription factors: Glc-6-Pase and glucokinase. **Fasting induces Glc-6-Pase and suppresses glucokinase.**

The three key substrates for gluconeogenesis are lactate, alanine, and glycerol

In the fasting state, the muscle and adipose tissue together use only 20% of all available glucose. As much as 80% of all glucose is taken up by insulin-independent tissues. Of this, 50% goes to the brain and 20% to erythrocytes.

After a 12-h fast, 65%–75% of synthesized glucose is still derived from glycogen; the rest comes from gluconeogenesis. The contribution of gluconeogenesis increases with the duration of the fast. Muscle facilitates gluconeogenesis by releasing lactate, which is taken up by the liver and oxidized to pyruvate, which then enters gluconeogenesis. The newly synthesized glucose is released from the liver and returns to the skeletal muscle. This closes the loop known as the glucose-lactate or **Cori cycle** (Fig. 31.11).

Low insulin also stimulates muscle proteolysis and thus the release of amino acids, primarily alanine and glutamine. Alanine is taken up by the liver and converted to pyruvate. This **glucose–alanine cycle** parallels the Cori cycle.

The third gluconeogenic substrate, glycerol, is released during the hydrolysis of triacylglycerols (lipolysis) by the hormone-sensitive lipase, which is stimulated by glucagon.

Prolonged fasting (starvation)

Prolonged fasting is a chronic low-insulin, high-glucagon state (Fig. 31.12). Free fatty acids now become the major energy substrate. The β-oxidation of fatty acids liberated from triacylglycerols generates acetyl-CoA, which would normally enter the TCA cycle. However, because the ongoing gluconeogenesis depletes oxaloacetate (also a TCA cycle metabolite), the activity of the TCA cycle (Chapter 10) actually decreases. This causes accumulation of acetyl-CoA and channels it into ketogenesis. Ketogenesis yields acetoacetate, hydroxybutyrate, and the product of spontaneous decarboxylation of acetoacetate, acetone. The products of ketogenesis are collectively known as **ketone bodies**. During prolonged fasting, the concentration

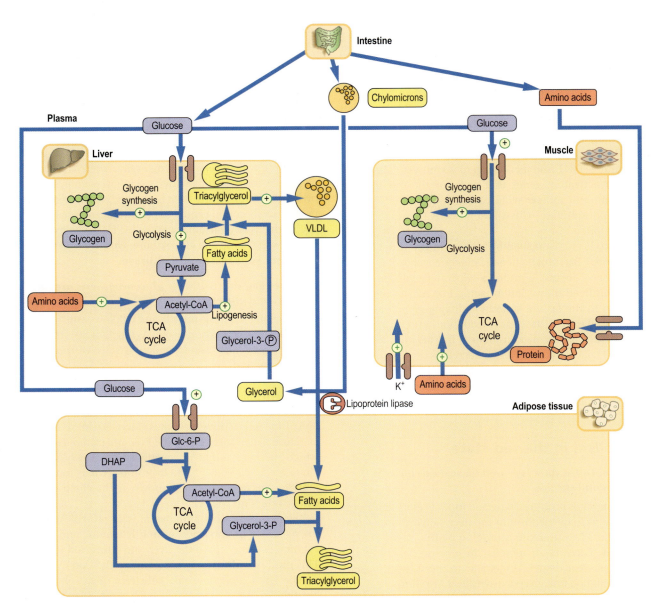

Fig. 31.9 **Metabolism in the fed (postprandial) state.** Carbohydrates, amino acids, and fats are absorbed in the intestine, and insulin secretion is stimulated. Insulin directs metabolism toward storage and synthesis (anabolism). **In the liver**, glucose is taken up by the GLUT-2 transporter and is channeled into glycolysis and glycogen synthesis. Aerobic glycolysis supplies acetyl-CoA, a key substrate for fatty acid synthesis. Fatty acids are subsequently esterified by glycolysis-derived glycerol, forming triacylglycerols in a process known as lipogenesis. Triacylglycerols are packaged into VLDL for transport to peripheral tissues. **In muscle**, glycogen synthesis, amino acid uptake, and protein synthesis are stimulated. **In the adipose tissue**, VLDL triacylglycerols are hydrolyzed, and fatty acids are taken up by cells. Triacylglycerols are resynthesized intracellularly, becoming storage material. DHAP, dihydroxyacetone phosphate; Glc-6-P, glucose-6-phosphate.

of ketone bodies in plasma increases. They can be used as energy substrates not only by cardiac and skeletal muscle but, during prolonged fasting, also by the brain.

To protect body proteins during starvation, the use of proteins as gluconeogenic substrates is minimized by almost total dependence on fat as an energy source (Fig. 31.12). The Cori cycle also helps decrease the requirement for endogenous glucose. Further, the number of the GLUT-4 transporters in the adipose tissue and muscle decreases, decreasing glucose uptake. The brain adapts by using ketone bodies as fuel. These mechanisms also "save" glucose. Finally, the concentration of

thyroid hormones decreases during starvation; this lowers the metabolic rate.

Metabolic response to stress

The metabolic response to stress mobilizes energy substrates from all available sources; during stress, metabolism is driven by the antiinsulin hormones

The metabolic response to stress is triggered by "fight-or-flight" situations and also by trauma, burns, surgery, and infection.

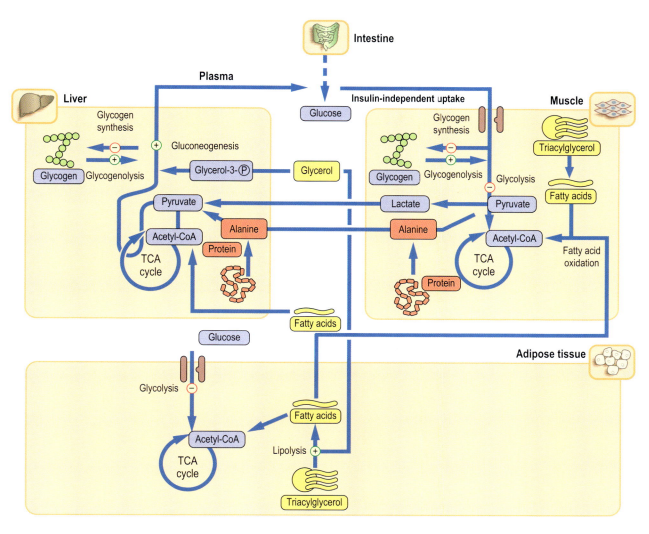

Fig. 31.10 **Metabolism after an overnight fast (postabsorptive state).** In postabsorptive state, liver metabolism changes from glucose utilization to glucose production (through gluconeogenesis). Glucagon also stimulates glycogenolysis and inhibits glycolysis. The substrates for gluconeogenesis are **alanine, lactate, and glycerol**. Alanine and lactate are transported to the liver from muscle. Glucose uptake by the muscle and adipose tissue decreases. Hydrolysis of triacylglycerols (lipolysis) and subsequent fatty acid oxidation are stimulated.

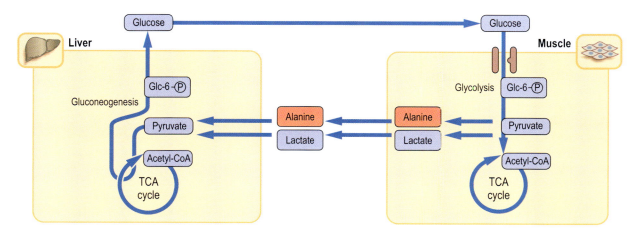

Fig. 31.11 **Cori cycle and glucose–alanine cycle.** The Cori cycle, also known as the glucose–lactate cycle, allows recycling of lactate back to glucose. Alanine is derived mostly from muscle proteolysis.

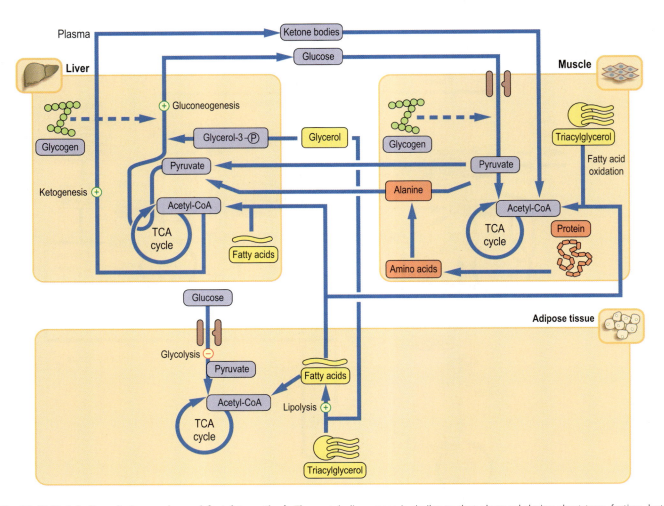

Fig. 31.12 **Metabolism during prolonged fast (starvation).** The metabolic pattern is similar to that observed during short-term fasting, but adaptive responses are in operation. At this stage, glycogen stores are depleted, and the supply of metabolic fuels depends on gluconeogenesis and lipolysis. Ketone bodies generated from large amounts of acetyl-CoA generated by fatty acid oxidation become an important energy source for muscle and the brain. Importantly, decreased demand for glucose (and thus gluconeogenesis) in turn decreases the demand for alanine, "sparing" muscle proteins.

It is associated with increased activity of the sympathetic nervous system and is driven by the antiinsulin hormones: catecholamines, primarily epinephrine; glucagon; and cortisol. The anabolic pathways (glycogen synthesis, lipogenesis) are suppressed, and the catabolic pathways (glycogenolysis, lipolysis, and proteolysis) are stimulated; thus the provision of metabolic fuels is maximized. Insulin-independent peripheral glucose uptake increases (Fig. 31.13). There is also early vasoconstriction to limit possible blood loss. There is also fever, increased heart rate (tachycardia), increased respiratory rate (tachypnea), and leukocytosis.

   The priority is to provide glucose for the brain; thus epinephrine and glucagon stimulate glycogenolysis and gluconeogenesis. In addition, decreased peripheral uptake of glucose makes more of it available to the brain. Later, the metabolic rate increases, and fatty acids become the major source of energy. Because the amino acids needed for gluconeogenesis are supplied from muscle; the nitrogen balance becomes negative within 2–3 days after injury.

The stress response includes insulin resistance

Insulin-dependent transport of glucose decreases under the influence of the glucocorticoids. Glucocorticoids also facilitate stimulation of gluconeogenesis by glucagon and catecholamines by inducing genes coding for the glucose-6-phosphatase and PEPCK (Table 31.3). Insulin-independent glucose uptake also increases, particularly in muscle, mediated by tumor necrosis factor α (TNF-α) and cytokines such as interleukin-1 (IL-1; Chapter 28). TNF-α also stimulates glycogen breakdown in muscle. Another interleukin, IL-6, helps induce PEPCK, stimulates lipolysis in the adipose tissue, and contributes to muscle proteolysis. Finally, there is increased lactate production.

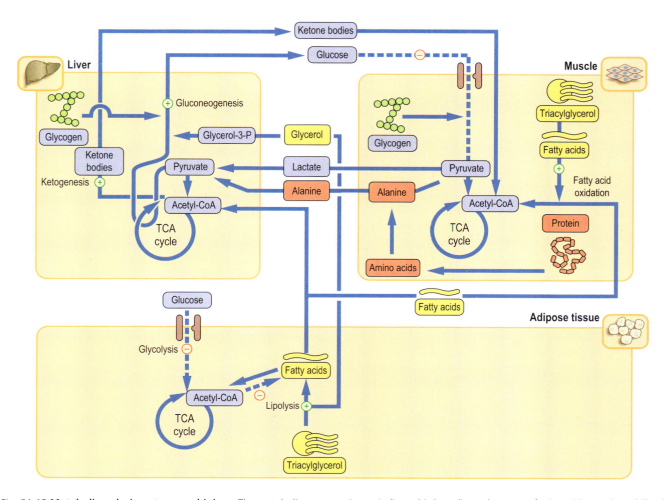

Fig. 31.13 **Metabolism during stress and injury.** The metabolic response is catabolic and is broadly analogous to fasting. Glucose is mobilized from all available sources. Here epinephrine plays a key role and, together with glucagon, inhibits insulin secretion. Stress also induces peripheral insulin resistance, further sparing glucose. Energy is provided from glucose, fatty acids, and protein catabolism.

CLINICAL BOX
STRESS RESPONSE AFFECTS RESULTS OF LABORATORY TESTS

Metabolic response to stress affects results of common laboratory measurements. Hyperglycemia is a common finding. Therefore, during stress, mild hyperglycemia should not be confused with diabetes mellitus. Also, infection, trauma, and injury are associated with the acute-phase response, which stimulates synthesis of a range of proteins, such as α_1-antitrypsin, C-reactive protein (CRP), haptoglobin, α_1-acid glycoprotein, complement, and others. Conversely, albumin synthesis is suppressed. Measurements of CRP are essential in monitoring treatment in patients with severe infections (Chapter 40).

CLINICAL BOX
A WOMAN WITH CHEST PAIN AND ELEVATED PLASMA GLUCOSE CONCENTRATION: A STRESS-INDUCED HYPERGLYCEMIA

A 66-year-old woman was admitted to the cardiology ward with chest pain. Myocardial infarction was diagnosed on the basis of EKG and increased plasma troponin concentration. She was successfully treated with thrombolysis. At that time, her random plasma glucose concentration was 10.5 mmol/L (189 mg/dL). The next day, the fasting blood glucose was only slightly raised at 7.5 mmol/L (117 mg/dL). Normal fasting plasma glucose is 4.0–6.0 mmol/L (72–109 mg/dL).

Comment
Major stress associated with myocardial infarction is associated with the counterregulatory hormone response, and this leads to the elevation of blood glucose concentration. Caution is needed in the interpretation of raised fasting plasma glucose in the context of acute illness. A glucose tolerance test should not be performed during acute illness. Measuring the glycated hemoglobin (HbA$_{1c}$) would help exclude diabetes.

DIABETES MELLITUS

The prevalence of diabetes mellitus has been increasing worldwide. There were 108 million diabetic individuals in 1980 and 422 million in 2014 (see Further Reading). This increase is linked to lifestyles that include an excess of high-energy foods combined with little physical exercise and the consequent obesity. The susceptibility to diabetes is a combined effect of genetic and environmental influences, the latter including the fetal metabolic environment and nutrition in the early years.

Diabetes is a disorder of fuel metabolism characterized by hyperglycemia and (later) by vascular damage

The two major components of diabetes mellitus are hyperglycemia and vascular complications. There are **four main forms of diabetes mellitus** (Table 31.4). Type 1 diabetes (T1D) constitutes 5%–10% of all cases of diabetes, and type 2 diabetes (T2D) comprises 90%–95% of all cases. The prevalence of gestational diabetes mellitus (GDM) is 1%–14% in different populations. Secondary diabetes is relatively rare.

In the long term, diabetes leads to changes in the walls of small and large arteries (**microangiopathy** and **macroangiopathy**, respectively). When microangiopathy occurs in the kidney (diabetic **nephropathy**), it may lead to kidney failure. Microangiopathy developing in the retina (diabetic **retinopathy**) may cause blindness, and that affecting the peripheral nervous system (diabetic **neuropathy**) leads to impairment of autonomic nerve function. Diabetic patients also develop lens opacities (**cataracts**). Diabetes is the main cause of blindness in the Western world and one of the main causes of kidney failure.

In addition, diabetic macroangiopathy is associated with a two to three times greater risk of **myocardial infarction** compared with nondiabetic individuals. When macroangiopathy affects peripheral arteries, it leads to **diabetic peripheral vascular disease** and to foot ulceration (diabetes remains a major cause of **lower limb amputations**). Cardiovascular disease is the most prevalent complication of diabetes and is the cause of death in more than 80% persons with T2D.

Type 1 diabetes is an autoimmune disease

T1D usually develops in people younger than 35 years, with peak incidence at approximately 12 years; 50%–60% of patients are now younger than 16–18 years at presentation. T1D is caused by autoimmune destruction of the pancreatic β cells. Its precipitating cause remains unclear; it could be a viral infection such as congenital rubella, environmental toxins, or foods. The autoimmune reaction could also be initiated by the cytokine response to infection.

Persons with T1D are prone to the development of ketoacidosis and are dependent on insulin treatment. Development of symptomatic disease may happen quickly, and a young person not known to have diabetes may present with ketoacidosis.

Susceptibility to type 1 diabetes is inherited

The concordance rate for T1D in monozygotic twins is 30%–40%. There are at least 20 regions of the genome associated with T1D. Susceptibility genes are located on chromosome 6 in the major histocompatibility complex (MHC; Chapter 43). Approximately 50% of the genetic susceptibility to diabetes resides in the HLA (IDDM1) genes: HLA genotypes DR and DQ and, to a lesser extent, in other loci known as IDDM2 (*insulin-VNTR*) and IDDM12 (*CTLA-4*). Both genes imparting risk (*DR3/4, DQA1*0301-DQB1*0302* and *DQA1*0501-DQB1*0201*) and genes imparting protection (*DQA1*0102-DQB1*0602*) have been identified within the HLA complex. Interestingly, this region also contains susceptibility genes associated with other autoimmune diseases; this means that patients with T1D are more susceptible to other autoimmune disorders, such as Graves' disease, Addison's disease, and celiac disease.

Altogether, about 50 genes are currently associated with type 1 diabetes.

In addition to inflammatory infiltration of the islets resulting from the abnormal T-cell response (Chapter 43), some patients demonstrate an abnormal B-cell response and thus circulating antibodies against various β-cell proteins. The autoantibodies may appear years before diagnosis and might be directed against

Table 31.4 Classification of diabetes mellitus

Syndrome	Comments
Type 1	Autoimmune destruction of β cells
Type 2	Impairment of β cells: B-cell inability to compensate for insulin resistance
Other types	Genetic defects of β cells (e.g., mutations of glucokinase gene) Rare insulin resistance syndromes
	Diseases of exocrine pancreas Endocrine diseases (acromegaly, Cushing's syndrome) Drugs and chemical-induced diabetes, infections (e.g., mumps)
	Rare syndromes characterized by the presence of antireceptor antibodies Diabetes accompanying other genetic diseases (e.g., Down syndrome)
Gestational diabetes	Glucose intolerance with onset or first diagnosis in pregnancy (Note that diabetes diagnosed at the first antenatal visit is regarded as overt diabetes, not gestational)

In older literature, type 1 diabetes was described as insulin-dependent diabetes (IDDM) and type 2 as noninsulin-dependent diabetes (NIDDM), or maturity-onset diabetes.

insulin, glutamic acid decarboxylase (GAD), protein tyrosine phosphatase, and islet antigens.

Type 2 diabetes develops when β cells fail to compensate for existing insulin resistance

T2D usually develops in obese patients who are more than 40 years old. In recent years, however, it has been increasingly observed in younger people. The two main contributory factors are the impairment of pancreatic β-cell function and peripheral insulin resistance.

Most of the discovered T2D susceptibility genes are linked to the β-cell function. If insulin resistance develops, β cells respond to the need for more insulin by proliferation and hypertrophy. Diabetes develops when such compensation becomes insufficient. Once metabolism becomes dysregulated, β cells can be further damaged by excess glucose (glucotoxicity) and fatty acids (lipotoxicity). Other factors that contribute to the development of diabetes are increased glucagon secretion, reduced incretin response, and reduced adiponectin in adipose tissue.

Genetic predisposition and obesity are the most important risk factors for type 2 diabetes

The two most important risk factors for T2D are family history and obesity. Obesity induces peripheral insulin resistance. The β cells compensate for this by increasing insulin secretion: hyperinsulinemia with normal glucose concentration develops. When compensation becomes insufficient, plasma glucose concentration increases slightly on fasting (this is defined as impaired fasting glucose [IFG]) or in response to glucose load (defined as impaired glucose tolerance [IGT]). Further impairment of insulin secretion leads to overt T2D.

Thus IFG and IGT signify **the risk of diabetes in the future** (IGT is also associated with an increased risk of cardiovascular disease).

Heritability of type 2 diabetes is greater than 50%

Monozygotic twins are approximately 70% concordant with respect to T2D, and dizygotic twins are 20%–30% concordant. First-degree relatives of persons with T2D have a 40% chance of developing the disease.

Population testing identified six genes associated with T2D. They include the one coding for peroxisome proliferator-activated receptor gamma (PPAR-γ). Another gene coding for the IRS-1 is associated with an impaired peripheral response to insulin. The gene coding for a potassium channel KCNJ11 affects insulin secretion. Its mutation causes a rare form of neonatal diabetes. The *WFS1* gene codes for wolframin, a protein detected in patients with a syndrome including both diabetes insipidus and juvenile diabetes as well as deafness and optic atrophy. Other genes are associated with forms of monogenic diabetes (MODY; see discussion below).

More than 80 loci associated with T2D have been identified, and a similar number of loci were linked to the so-called glycemic traits (i.e., glucose, insulin HbA1c, and proinsulin concentrations).

ADVANCED CONCEPTS BOX
MATURITY-ONSET DIABETES OF THE YOUNG (MODY) IS A RARE FORM OF TYPE 2 DIABETES

MODY develops before the age of 25 years and is characterized by persistent C-peptide secretion and a clear pattern of inheritance. It results from mutations of at least six different genes; among them are the one coding for glucokinase (affecting β-cell sensing of glucose and causing MODY2) and for transcription factors HNF1A, which causes MODY3 and HNF1B, which causes MODY5. There is also a mitochondrial DNA mutation that leads to impaired oxidative phosphorylation and causes the so-called mitochondrial diabetes.

MODY-associated genes give an insight into the genetic factors affecting response to treatment. In contrast to MODY types caused by the transcription factor mutations, MODY2 responds to diet, and these patients do not require insulin. Patients with HNF1A mutations respond to sulfonylurea drugs.

Table 31.5 Comparison of type 1 and type 2 diabetes

	Type 1	Type 2
Onset	Usually less than 20 years of age	Usually more than 40 years of age
Insulin synthesis	Absent: immune destruction of β-cells	Preserved: combination of insulin resistance and impaired β-cell function
Plasma insulin concentration	Low or zero	Low, normal, or high
Genetic susceptibility	Yes	Yes
Islet cell antibodies at diagnosis	Yes	No
Obesity	Uncommon	Common
Ketoacidosis	Yes	Rare, but can be precipitated by major metabolic stress
Treatment	Insulin	Hypoglycemic drugs and (if severe) insulin

DCCT, Diabetes Control and Complications Trial; IFCC, International Federation of Clinical Chemistry and Laboratory Medicine.

In type 2 diabetes, ketoacidosis is rare

Patients with T2D may develop microvascular complications as in T1D, but the main problems are the macrovascular complications, which eventually lead to coronary heart disease, peripheral vascular disease, and stroke. T1D and T2D are compared in Table 31.5.

Metabolism in diabetes

In poorly controlled diabetes, metabolic decompensation leads to ketoacidosis

In type 1 diabetes, because of lack of insulin, glucose cannot enter insulin-dependent cells such as adipocytes and myocytes. Lack of insulin means that metabolism, by default, enters the glucagon-controlled mode. Glycolysis and lipogenesis are inhibited, whereas glycogenolysis, lipolysis, ketogenesis, and gluconeogenesis are stimulated (Fig. 31.14). The liver turns into a glucose-producing organ. This, combined with impaired glucose transport into cells, leads to fasting hyperglycemia.

When plasma glucose concentration exceeds renal capacity for reabsorption, glucose appears in urine. Because glucose is osmotically active, its excretion is accompanied by increased water loss (osmotic diuresis). Poorly controlled diabetic patients pass large volumes of urine (**polyuria**) and drink an excessive amount of fluids (**polydipsia**). Fluid loss eventually leads to dehydration (Chapter 35). In parallel to the disturbed water balance, lipolysis generates an excess of acetyl-CoA, which is channeled into ketogenesis. The concentration of ketone bodies in plasma increases (**ketonemia**), and they are excreted in the urine (**ketonuria**). In some patients, acetone can be smelled on the breath. Overproduction of acetoacetic and β-hydroxybutyric acids increases the blood hydrogen-ion concentration (the blood pH decreases). This form of metabolic acidosis (Chapter 36) is known as the **diabetic ketoacidosis** (Fig. 31.15).

Key features of diabetic ketoacidosis are hyperglycemia, ketonuria, dehydration, and metabolic acidosis

Diabetic ketoacidosis may develop quickly, sometimes even after just a single missed dose of insulin. Ketoacidosis develops predominantly in persons with T1D who have no, or very little, insulin in plasma and, consequently, a very low ratio of insulin-to-glucagon concentration. It is rare in T2D, although it may occur after a major stress, such as myocardial infarction. Untreated ketoacidosis is life-threatening.

There are substantial similarities between metabolism in starvation and in diabetes; this is why diabetes was once described as "starvation in the midst of plenty." However, whereas fasting leads to only moderate ketonemia, in diabetes, large amounts of ketone bodies may accumulate.

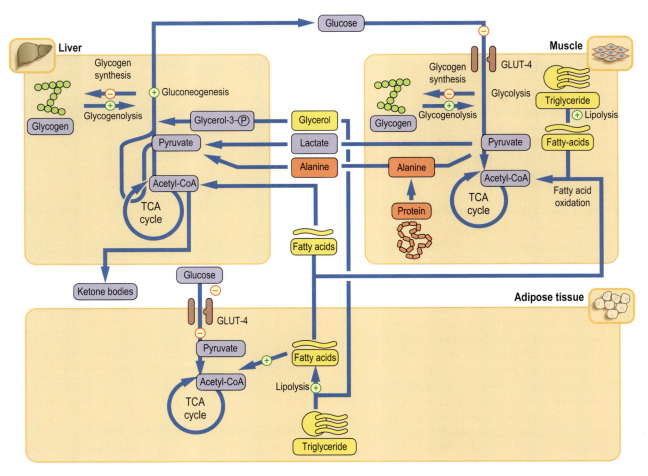

Fig. 31.14 **Metabolism in diabetes mellitus.** There is a decreased ability of tissues to use glucose because of lack of insulin, defective insulin action, or both. Hyperglycemia results from both impaired tissue uptake of glucose and its increased production in liver gluconeogenesis. Excess of fatty acids is available to the liver, but the TCA cycle is less efficient due to oxaloacetate being used for gluconeogenesis. This results in the accumulation of acetyl-CoA and its further conversion into ketone bodies.

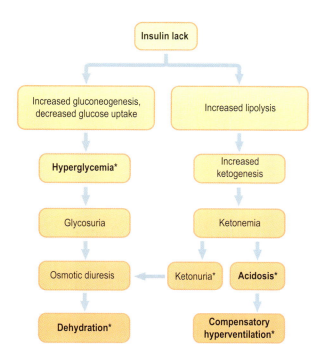

Fig. 31.15 **Diabetic ketoacidosis.** The clinical picture of ketoacidosis is a consequence of the lack of insulin; resulting hyperglycemia and its complications, such as osmotic diuresis and dehydration; and increased lipolysis and ketogenesis leading to ketonemia and acidosis. Treatment of ketoacidosis is devised to combat these problems and includes insulin infusion, rehydration, and potassium supplementation. *Indicates the most important clinical and laboratory findings.

CLINICAL BOX

A 15-YEAR-OLD GIRL ADMITTED CONFUSED AND WITH BREATH SMELLING OF ACETONE: DIABETIC KETOACIDOSIS

A 15-year-old girl never known to have diabetes was admitted to the accident and emergency department. She was confused, and her breath smelled of acetone. She had signs of dehydration, with reduced tissue turgor and dry tongue. She also had rapid, pauseless respirations. Her blood glucose was 18.0 mmol/L (324 mg/dL), and ketones were present in the urine. Her serum potassium concentration was 4.9 mmol/L (normal 3.5–5.0 mmol/L), and her arterial blood pH was 7.20 (normal 7.37–7.44; H^+ concentration 63 nmol/L; normal 35–45).

Comment

This is a typical (if unexpected in this case) presentation of diabetic ketoacidosis. Note that a substantial proportion of children present with ketoacidosis at the time of diagnosis of diabetes. Hyperventilation is a compensatory response to acidosis (see Chapter 36). Diabetic ketoacidosis is a medical emergency. This patient received an intravenous infusion containing physiologic saline with potassium supplements to replace lost fluid and potassium as well as an infusion of insulin.

Diabetes, obesity, and hypertension are linked with cardiovascular disease

Obesity, insulin resistance, and glucose intolerance (or diabetes) may be accompanied by dyslipidemia (Chapter 33) and arterial hypertension. Such cluster of conditions has been described as the **metabolic syndrome**. It is associated with low-grade inflammation affecting the vasculature, with an increased tendency to thrombosis (the hypercoagulable state; Chapter 41). Most importantly, it imparts an increased risk of cardiovascular disease.

Increasingly, there is the realization that diabetes mellitus and cardiovascular disease may have what some researchers call "common soil." The various links between obesity, diabetes, and atherosclerosis are illustrated in Fig. 31.16.

CLINICAL BOX

A 56-YEAR-OLD MAN WITH EFFORT-RELATED CHEST DISCOMFORT: DIABETES AND ISCHEMIC HEART DISEASE

A 56-year-old man was referred to the cardiology outpatient clinic for investigation of chest discomfort that he felt when climbing steep hills and when he was stressed or excited. The patient was 170 cm tall and weighed 102 kg (224 lb). His blood pressure was 160/98 mmHg (upper limit of normal 140/90 mmHg), triglyceride concentration was 4 mmol/L (364 mg/dL; desirable level, 1.7 mmol/L, 148 mg/dL), and fasting plasma glucose was 6.5 mmol/L (117 mg/dL). His resting EKG was normal, but an ischemic pattern was observed during exercise testing.

Comment

This obese man presented with arterial hypertension, hypertriglyceridemia, and impaired fasting glucose. The impaired fasting glucose observed in this case was due to peripheral insulin resistance. Such a cluster of abnormalities is known as the metabolic syndrome and carries increased risk of coronary heart disease.

Late vascular complications of diabetes mellitus

Oxidative stress, advanced glycation (glycoxidation) end products, and activity of the polyol pathway contribute to the development of complications

Glucose is toxic in excess. In the presence of transition metals such as copper or iron, it undergoes auto-oxidation, generating reactive oxygen species (ROS; Chapter 42). Glucose also attaches nonenzymatically to lysine and valine residues on proteins in a process known as protein glycation (Fig. 31.17). When glucose interacts with a protein, it forms glucose-protein adducts in the process known as nonenzymatic glycation. The most widely studied of these is the **glycated hemoglobin** (also known as hemoglobin A_{1c} [HbA_{1c}]). Other proteins such as albumin, collagen, and apolipoprotein B may also undergo glycation. Glycation may change the function of affected protein; for

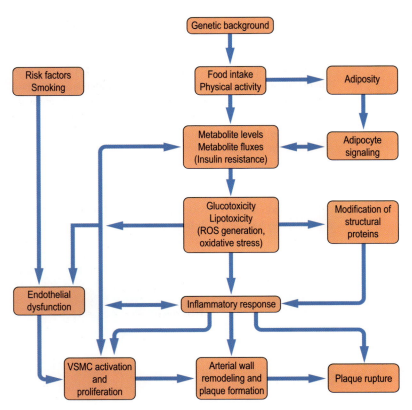

Fig. 31.16 **Obesity, glucose intolerance, diabetes, and atherosclerosis.** The endocrine activity of adipose tissue associated with obesity contributes to insulin resistance, glucose intolerance, and type 2 diabetes. Low-grade inflammation and increased oxidative stress can be induced both by obesity and by the classic cardiovascular risk factors and lead to endothelial damage. Once diabetes is present, protein glycation and formation of the advanced glycation end products further contribute to vascular damage.

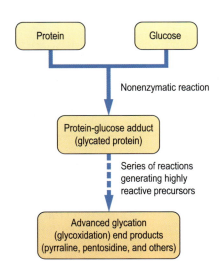

Fig. 31.17 **Modification of proteins by glucose: protein glycation and formation of the advanced glycation (glycoxidation) end products.** Nonenzymatic, concentration-dependent glycation reaction between glucose and protein leads to the formation of glucose adducts known as the Amadori products. Their presence modifies the structure and function of affected proteins. Glycated proteins are substrates for the formation of the advanced glycation (glycoxidation) end products (AGE). In addition, the triose phosphates generated by glycolysis and the increased activity of the polyol pathway generate precursors of AGE, such as methylglyoxal and 3-deoxyglucosone.

example, glycation of apolipoprotein B inhibits cellular uptake of LDL particles.

Glycated proteins may undergo further oxidation and chemical rearrangements of glycated structures that lead to the formation of a family of compounds known as **advanced glycation (or glycoxidation) end products** (AGE). Some of these compounds, such as 3-deoxyglucosone, possess very chemically active carbonyl groups. Some of the AGE are actually protein crosslinks, forming, for instance, on collagen or myelin and decreasing the elasticity of these proteins. AGE accumulation is part of the aging process, but it accelerates in the presence of hyperglycemia. AGE bind to their membrane receptors on endothelial cells, generating oxidative stress, which damages endothelium and stimulates proinflammatory pathways involving the activation of the transcription factor NFκB, which controls the expression of cytokines such as TNF-α, IL-1α, and IL-6. Formation of AGE is a factor in the development of the microvascular complications of diabetes and in atherogenesis. Importantly, AGE may also be involved in the pathogenesis of other age-related diseases, such as Alzheimer's disease.

A further source of increased oxidative stress is the respiratory chain. Hyperglycemia increases the amount of proton donors within the mitochondria, leading to an increased electrochemical potential difference across the inner mitochondrial membrane and, consequently, to increased ROS generation by the respiratory chain (Chapter 42). ROS generated during hyperglycemia deactivate nitric oxide (NO) generated by the endothelial cells from arginine, thus impairing endothelium-dependent relaxation of vascular smooth muscle cells. ROS also interfere with signaling cascades, affecting, for instance, activation of PKC.

Increased activity of the polyol pathway is associated with diabetic neuropathy and ocular cataracts

Hyperglycemia alters the cellular redox state, increasing the NADH/NAD$^+$ ratio and decreasing NADPH/NADP$^+$. This directs glucose into the **polyol pathway**, where it is reduced

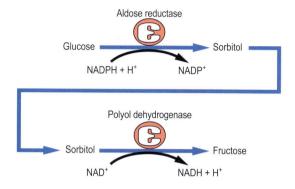

Fig. 31.18 The polyol pathway. The polyol pathway contributes to the development of diabetic neuropathy. It may be inhibited by inhibitors of its rate-limiting enzyme, aldose reductase.

to sorbitol by aldose reductase (Fig. 31.18). Aldose reductase and NO synthase compete for the available NADPH. Sorbitol is further oxidized to fructose by sorbitol dehydrogenase.

Aldose reductase has a high K_m for glucose; therefore the polyol pathway is not very active at normal glucose concentrations. However, during hyperglycemia, when glucose concentration in insulin-independent tissues (such as red blood cells, nerve, and lens) increases, the pathway activates. The problem is that, similarly to glucose, sorbitol is osmotically active. Therefore its accumulation in the ocular tissue contributes to the development of diabetic cataracts. In the nerve tissue, a high concentration of sorbitol decreases cellular uptake of another alcohol, myoinositol, inhibiting the membrane Na$^+$/K$^+$-ATPase and thus affecting nerve function. Accumulation of sorbitol, hypoxia, and reduced nerve blood flow all contribute to the development of diabetic neuropathy. Processes that contribute to the long-term diabetic complications are summarized in Fig. 31.19.

HYPOGLYCEMIA

Low blood glucose (hypoglycemia) is defined as blood glucose concentration below 4 mmol/L (72 mg/dL). Low plasma glucose stimulates the sympathetic nervous system. Epinephrine and glucagon are released, initiating the stress response. This

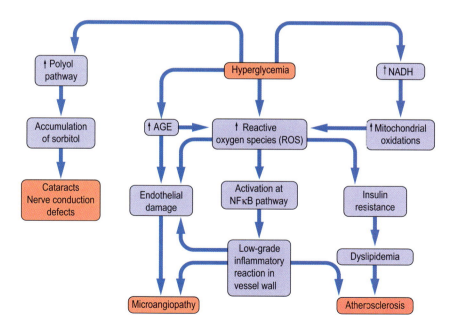

Fig. 31.19 Vascular complications of diabetes mellitus. Poor glycemic control is associated with the development of microvascular complications in type 1 and type 2 diabetes and with increased cardiovascular risk (the latter particularly in type 2 diabetes). Oxidative stress, protein glycation, and formation of advanced glycation end products (AGE) are the most important candidate mechanisms of development of microvascular complications. Hyperglycemia stimulates generation of the reactive oxygen species (ROS) through an increase in the flow of reductive equivalents through the respiratory chain and increased formation of AGE. ROS toxicity causes structural and functional damage to proteins and stimulates inflammatory phenomena induced through, for instance, the proinflammatory NFκB pathway. ROS damage endothelium and interfere with insulin signaling, contributing to insulin resistance. The low-grade inflammation and insulin resistance are particularly important in atherogenesis, contributing to macrovascular disease (Chapter 33). Note that increased oxidative stress and low-grade chronic inflammation have also been observed in obesity.

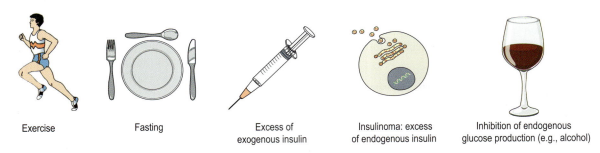

Exercise   Fasting   Excess of   Insulinoma: excess   Inhibition of endogenous
                                    exogenous insulin   of endogenous insulin   glucose production (e.g., alcohol)

Fig. 31.20 **Hypoglycemia.** Hypoglycemia is plasma glucose concentration below 4 mmol/L (72 mg/dL). Severe hypoglycemia is glucose concentration below 2.5 mmol/L (45 mg/dL). Hypoglycemia may result from decreased supply of glucose or from an increased insulin secretion. It also results from increased utilization of glucose by tissues during exercise.

manifests as sweating, tremor, tachycardia, and a feeling of hunger. Decreased glucose supply to the nervous system (neuroglycopenia) **compromises the function of the brain.** The affected person becomes confused and may lose consciousness (this usually happens when glucose concentration falls below 2.5 mmol/L [45 mg/dL]). Profound hypoglycemia can be fatal.

Hypoglycemia in healthy individuals may occur during exercise, after a period of fasting, or as a result of drinking alcohol and is usually mild. Alcohol increases the intracellular NADH/NAD$^+$ ratio; this favors conversion of pyruvate to lactate and reduces the amount of pyruvate available for gluconeogenesis.

Hypoglycemia may also occur when there is an insufficient amount of counterregulatory hormones to balance the effects of insulin; this happens in adrenal insufficiency (Chapter 27). Another endocrine cause of hypoglycemia is a rare tumor of the β cells, insulinoma, which may secrete large amounts of insulin. Glycogen storage diseases (Chapter 12) are a rare cause of hypoglycemia in childhood. The causes of hypoglycemia are summarized in Fig. 31.20.

Hypoglycemia is the most common acute complication of diabetes

It is worth remembering that hypoglycemia, not ketoacidosis, is the most common acute complication of diabetes. It can occur in both T1D and T2D. It results from an imbalance among insulin dose, dietary carbohydrate supply, and physical activity. Thus it may occur after taking too much insulin or after missing a meal. Because exercise increases the insulin-independent tissue glucose uptake, diabetic patients, to avoid hypoglycemia, need to decrease their insulin dose before strenuous exercise. Mild hypoglycemia can usually be treated by taking a sweet drink or eating a few lumps of sugar. Severe hypoglycemia, however, is a medical emergency that requires treatment with intravenous glucose or intramuscular injection of glucagon. Note that, unfortunately, the better the diabetic control achieved during treatment, the greater the risk of hypoglycemia.

CLINICAL BOX
A 12-YEAR-OLD DIABETIC BOY WHO LOST CONSCIOUSNESS ON THE PLAYING FIELD: HYPOGLYCEMIA

A 12-year-old diabetic boy was playing with his friends. He received his normal insulin injection in the morning but continued playing through the lunch hour without a meal. He became increasingly confused and finally lost consciousness. He was immediately given an injection of glucagon from the emergency kit his father carried, and he recovered within minutes.

Comment

Severe hypoglycemia is a medical emergency. An immediate improvement after glucagon injection confirms that this boy's symptoms were caused by hypoglycemia, resulting from the combination of the administration of exogenous insulin and insufficient food intake. Recovery from hypoglycemia was due to the action of glucagon. In the hospital, hypoglycemic patients who cannot eat or drink are usually treated with an intravenous dose of high-concentration glucose. An intramuscular glucagon injection is an emergency measure that can be applied at home.

LABORATORY ASSESSMENT OF FUEL METABOLISM

Diagnosis and monitoring of patients with diabetes mellitus

The key diagnostic tests for diabetes are measurements of plasma glucose and glycated hemoglobin concentration

Some diabetic patients have no clinical symptoms at all. In these individuals, the diagnosis is made solely on the basis of laboratory results (Table 31.6).

Measurement of plasma glucose concentration is interpreted in relation to the feed–fast cycle. The best time to assess

Table 31.6 Diagnostic criteria for diabetes mellitus and glucose intolerance

Condition	Diagnostic criteria (mmol/L)	Diagnostic criteria (mg/dL)
Normal fasting plasma glucose	Below 6.1	Below 110
Impaired fasting glucose (IFG)	Equal or above 5.6 but below 7.0	Equal or above 100 but below 126
Impaired glucose tolerance (IGT)	Plasma glucose during oral glucose tolerance test (OGTT), 2 h after 75-g load 7.8 or above, but below 11.1	Plasma glucose during OGTT, 2 h after 75-g load 140 or above, but below 200
Prediabetes	HbA1c 5.7%–6.4% (39–46 mmol/mol)	
Diabetes mellitus*		
Criterion 1	Random plasma glucose 11.1 or above[†]	Random plasma glucose 200 or above[†]
Criterion 2	Fasting plasma glucose 7.0 or above	Fasting plasma glucose 126 or above
Criterion 3	2-h value during 75-g OGTT 11.1 or above	2-h value during 75-g OGTT 200 or above
Criterion 4	HbA$_{1c}$ equal or above 48 mmol/mol (6.5%)	

*If one of the criteria is fulfilled, diagnosis is provisional. Diagnosis needs to be confirmed the next day using a different criterion.
[†]If accompanied by symptoms (polyuria, polydipsia, unexplained weight loss). These are the criteria proposed by the American Diabetes Association.

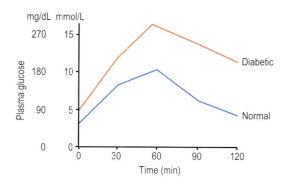

Fig. 31.21 **Oral glucose tolerance test (OGTT).** The principle of the test is the measurement of plasma-glucose concentration before and after a standard (75-g) oral glucose load. Glucose concentration increases, achieving a peak between 30 and 60 min after the load. It should return to near-fasting values after 2 h. Note the higher plasma-glucose values at all time points in a diabetic patient.

carbohydrate metabolism is after an 8- to 12-h fast (Fig. 31.10), when fuel metabolism reaches a steady state.

The measurements that are diagnostic for diabetes are the **fasting glucose** concentration (no caloric intake for approximately 8–12 h) and the concentration measured 2 h after oral ingestion of a standard amount of glucose.

Glucose concentration measured irrespective of the meal times is known as the **random plasma glucose.** It is useful for the diagnosis of hypoglycemia or severe hyperglycemia, but it is less helpful in assessing the significance of a mild hyperglycemia.

A continuum exists between normal, prediabetic, and diabetic states

When interpreting glucose concentration, a clinician wants to know whether it is normal **(normoglycemia),** too high **(hyperglycemia),** or too low **(hypoglycemia).** Further interpretation of glycemia includes the diagnosis, or exclusion, of diabetes and identification of the intermediate (prediabetic) conditions.

Fasting plasma glucose in an individual is remarkably stable. Impaired fasting glucose (IFG) and impaired glucose tolerance (IGT) are regarded as **prediabetic states**. The American Diabetes Association (ADA) recommends the diagnosis of IFG, whereas the World Health Organization (WHO) recommends a diagnosis of IGT, and this is accepted in Europe.

Persons with plasma glucose above the diagnostic cutoff points for diabetes mellitus are at an increased a risk of microvascular complications. IGT is also associated with increased cardiovascular risk, whereas IFG is just a risk factor for the future development of overt diabetes.

Normally, the fasting plasma glucose concentration should remain below 6.1 mmol/L (110 mg/dL). IGT is characterized by a normal fasting level but an elevated concentration 2 h after glucose load. IFG is defined as intermediate fasting plasma glucose (higher than 6.0 mmol/L but lower than 7.0 mmol/L [126 mg/dL]). **Fasting plasma glucose of 7.0 mmol/L (126 mg/dL) or above, if confirmed, is diagnostic for diabetes.** Laboratory diagnosis of diabetes is summarized in Table 31.6

Oral glucose tolerance test (OGTT) assesses blood glucose response to a carbohydrate load

The WHO recommendation is that the OGTT is performed on all individuals whose fasting plasma glucose falls in the IFG category. OGTT must be performed under standard conditions. The patient should attend in the morning after an approximately 10-h fast. To avoid stress- or exercise-related changes in plasma glucose, the person should sit throughout the test. The test should not be performed during or immediately after an acute illness. During the test, fasting plasma glucose is measured first. The patient is then given a standard quantity of glucose to drink (75 g in 300 mL of water), and plasma glucose concentration is measured again after 120 min (Fig. 31.21). In some protocols, glucose is measured after 20, 60, and

120 min. Normally, plasma glucose should reach peak concentration after approximately 60 min and should return to a near-fasting state within 120 min. If it remains above 11.1 mmol/L (200 mg/dL/min) in the 120-min sample, diabetes is diagnosed, even if the fasting blood glucose was normal. Nondiabetic fasting blood glucose with a post-load concentration between 6.1 and 7.8 mmol/L (100 mg/dL) signifies IGT.

The glycated hemoglobin (HbA₁c) concentration reflects average concentration of plasma glucose

The average plasma glucose concentration over a period of time is clinically relevant because it is related to the risk of development of late complications of diabetes. Assessing average glycemia by performing multiple plasma glucose measurements is cumbersome. Glycated hemoglobin (hemoglobin A_{1c} [HbA_{1c}]) is a better test for this purpose. HbA_{1c} forms in the blood erythrocytes at a rate proportional to the prevailing glucose concentration. Because the glycation reaction is irreversible, the formed HbA_{1c} remains in the circulation for the entire life of an erythrocyte. Thus its concentration reflects the average

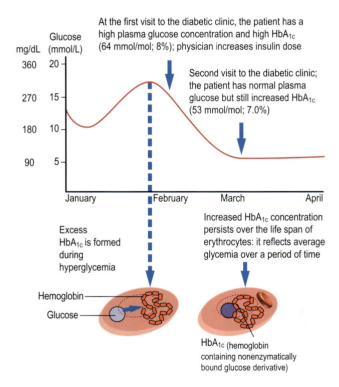

At the first visit to the diabetic clinic, the patient has a high plasma glucose concentration and high HbA_{1c} (64 mmol/mol; 8%); physician increases insulin dose

Second visit to the diabetic clinic; the patient has normal plasma glucose but still increased HbA_{1c} (53 mmol/mol; 7.0%)

Excess HbA_{1c} is formed during hyperglycemia

Increased HbA_{1c} concentration persists over the life span of erythrocytes: it reflects average glycemia over a period of time

Hemoglobin

Glucose

HbA_{1c} (hemoglobin containing nonenzymatically bound glucose derivative)

Fig. 31.22 The use of glycated hemoglobin (hemoglobinA₁c, HbA₁c) in the diagnosis and monitoring of diabetes. HbA_{1c} is hemoglobin A posttranslationally modified by a nonenzymatic glycation. The degree of glycation is proportional to hemoglobin's exposure to glucose during the life span of the erythrocyte. Measurements of HbA_{1c} are used for diagnosis of diabetes and for monitoring of the glycemic control. Introduction of a new reference method for the HbA_{1c} resulted in the change of units from the traditional (%) to mmol/mol. The conversion formulas are available (Table 31.6). To obtain glucose concentrations in mg/dL, multiply by 18.

concentration of plasma glucose (Fig. 31.22) over the 8–12 weeks preceding HbA_{1c} measurement. The exact time period it reflects is difficult to calculate precisely because at any time, plasma contains populations of erythrocytes of different age. Values such as 3–6 and 4–8 weeks have also been reported in the literature. Exposure to glucose over 30 days before measurement contributes approximately 50% to observed changes in HbA_{1c}. Note that HbA_{1c} concentration may be affected by anemia and the presence of hemoglobin variants.

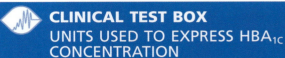

CLINICAL TEST BOX
UNITS USED TO EXPRESS HBA₁c CONCENTRATION

In the United States, HbA_{1c} measurements are reported as a percentage of total hemoglobin. Recently, a reference method capable of measuring the absolute amount of HbA_{1c} has been introduced in Europe. The new method is based on the cleavage of the N-terminal hexapeptide from the β-chain of HbA_{1c} by an endopeptidase and subsequent separation and quantification by mass spectrometry or capillary electrophoresis. The units employed are mmol/mol. The values obtained by one method can be converted into the other units using a conversion formula (see Appendix 1 and Table 31.7).

HbA₁c is used to diagnose diabetes and to monitor glycemic control

Guidelines developed by the ADA (2012) and WHO (2011) take the HbA_{1c} level of 48 mmol/L (6.5%) or above as diagnostic for diabetes. HbA_{1c} is also used in clinical practice to set targets for treatment. The ADA recommends that in a diabetic patient, one should aim to achieve a concentration below 7% (53 mmol/mol, normal level being below 6%). In some patients, particularly in young children and the elderly, this may be difficult because of the risk of hypoglycemia. The treatment goals must be adjusted to minimize such risk.

Table 31.7 Equivalent units of measurement for glycated hemoglobin (HbA₁c) measured using the traditional (DCCT) method and the newer reference method (IFCC)

DCCT units (%)	IFCC units (mmol/mol)
5	31
6	42
7	53
10	86

DCCT, Diabetes Control and Complications Trial; IFCC, International Federation of Clinical Chemistry and Laboratory Medicine.

Reprinted with permission from Misra S, Hancock M, Meeran K, Dornhorst A, Oliver NS. HbA1c: an old friend in new clothes. Lancet 377:1476–1477, 2011.

CLINICAL BOX
A BOY WHO DID NOT LIKE DIABETES TREATMENT: DISCREPANT GLUCOSE AND HBA₁c RESULTS

A 15-year-old insulin-dependent boy visited a diabetic clinic for a routine check-up. He told his doctor that he had followed all the dietary advice and never missed insulin injections. Although his random blood glucose was 6.0 mmol/L (108 mg/dL), the HbA₁c concentration was 86 mmol/mol (11%; adequate control: below 53 mmol/mol, 7%). He had no glycosuria or ketonuria.

Comment
Blood and urine glucose results indicate good control of this boy's diabetes at the time of measurement, but the HbA₁c level suggests poor control over the last 3–6 weeks. The probability is that he only complied with treatment days before he was due to come to the clinic. This is not uncommon in adolescents, who find it hard to accept the necessity to adjust their lifestyles to demanding diabetes treatment. Measurement of HbA₁c identifies diabetic patients who do not comply with treatment.

Urine glucose is not a diagnostic test for diabetes

At its normal plasma concentration, no glucose appears in the urine. The threshold for urinary glucose reabsorption is the plasma concentration of approximately 10.0 mmol/L (180 mg/dL). At higher concentrations, the reabsorptive capacity of the renal tubular transport system is exceeded, and glucose appears in the urine (this is known as glucosuria). Note that a healthy person may have a low renal glucose threshold and thus show glucosuria at nondiabetic blood glucose levels. Therefore diabetes cannot be diagnosed on the basis of urine testing alone.

Ketone bodies in the urine of a diabetic person signify metabolic decompensation

A high concentration of ketones in the urine (ketonuria) reflects a high rate of lipid oxidation. Mild ketonuria may occur in healthy individuals during prolonged fasting or to individuals who are on a high-fat diet. In a diabetic patient, **ketonuria is an important sign of metabolic decompensation** and requires active treatment.

Urinary albumin excretion is important in the assessment of diabetic nephropathy

Development of diabetic nephropathy can be predicted by detecting minute amounts of albumin in the urine (**micro-albuminuria**). To do this, laboratories employ a method that is more sensitive than the one used for the measurement of albumin in the plasma. The test is positive if more than 200 mg of albumin is excreted in the urine over 24 h. Urine protein above 300 mg/day signifies overt proteinuria. In diabetic patients, plasma urea (BUN) and creatinine concentrations are also routinely checked (Chapter 35).

Increased plasma lactate indicates inadequate tissue oxygenation

A high plasma lactate level indicates increased anaerobic metabolism and is a marker of inadequate tissue oxygenation (hypoxia; Chapter 5). In extreme situations, such as cardiac arrest, this causes severe (lactic) acidosis. In diabetes, measurements of plasma lactate are important in rare instances of hyperglycemic nonketotic coma, a life-threatening condition where very high plasma glucose levels and extreme dehydration occur in the absence of ketoacidosis.

ADVANCED CONCEPTS BOX
DIABETIC PATIENTS NEED REGULAR FOLLOW-UP

During a periodic assessment of a diabetic patient, the physician would check blood glucose and HbA₁c concentrations to assess glycemic control. She would perform an eye examination (looking for signs of retinopathy) and neurologic examination (looking for signs of neuropathy). She would also arrange to measure urea (BUN) and creatinine in plasma and microalbumin/protein in the urine (to determine the presence or assess the risk of nephropathy) as well as plasma lipids. She would check the blood pressure and assess the overall risk of cardiovascular disease (Chapter 33).

TREATING DIABETES

Keeping glycemia close to normal prevents development of diabetic complications

The goal of treating diabetes is the **prevention of its acute and chronic complications.** Maintaining good glycemic control is the fundamental tenet of diabetes care. Two major clinical trials, the Diabetic Control and Complications Trial (DCCT) in T1D and the UK Prospective Diabetes Study (UKPDS) in T2D, confirmed that microvascular complications are linked to the severity of hyperglycemia (see Further Reading). There is also strong evidence that concomitant management of cardiovascular risk, including treatment of hypertension and dyslipidemia, is optimal for the prevention of long-term complications.

Lifestyle modification is the mainstay of diabetes prevention and treatment

Diet and exercise are the key lifestyle measures in the management of diabetes mellitus. They underpin all drug treatments and also are essential preventive measures. Deterioration of glucose tolerance can be slowed down or, occasionally, reversed by weight reduction and exercise. Thus the presence of IFG or IGT should be regarded as a **strong signal for an individual to review his or her lifestyle to** minimize the chance of progress to overt diabetes. The Diabetes Prevention Program study demonstrated a 58% decrease in the development of T2D after lifestyle interventions involving diet and exercise (see Further Reading). Unfortunately, glycemia can be controlled by lifestyle measures alone in less than 20% of all diabetic patients.

Patients with type 1 diabetes are treated with insulin

Treatment with insulin is absolutely necessary in T1D. Available preparations of insulin differ in the duration of their action. The "classic" short-acting insulin is human regular insulin, the intermediate-acting insulins are the Isophane and Lente insulins, and the long-acting is Ultralente. Currently used analogs of human insulin are insulin lispro and insulin aspart (rapid acting) and insulin detemir and insulin glargine (slow acting).

Standard insulin treatment protocols involve daily subcutaneous injections throughout life

Insulin regimens need to be devised while taking into account a patient's preprandial glucose concentrations, carbohydrate intake, levels of anticipated exercise, and ability to respond to hypoglycemia (see Further Reading). Usually they consist of two subcutaneous injections of intermediate-acting insulin per day or a mixture of a short-acting and intermediate-acting insulin. The so-called basal-bolus approach involves insulin glargine or detemir used as the basal component and insulin lispro or aspart as boluses added before meals. The greatest challenge of insulin treatment is replicating normal daily patterns of insulin secretion with insulin injections. Multiple injections of short-acting insulin are used in patients where glycemia is particularly difficult to control. Rarely, a constant subcutaneous insulin infusion (CSII) is required; this is delivered by a portable pump programmed to increase the delivery rate at mealtimes or a pump that senses the plasma glucose concentration.

Emergency treatment of diabetic ketoacidosis includes intravenous insulin, rehydration, and potassium supplementation

Emergency treatment of diabetic ketoacidosis addresses five issues: insulin lack, dehydration, potassium depletion, acidosis,

and the primary cause of the metabolic decompensation. Insulin infusion is required to reverse metabolic effect of the excess of antiinsulin hormones, and fluids are infused to treat dehydration. These fluids normally contain potassium to prevent hypokalemia associated with shift of potassium into cells caused by insulin. Such treatment is usually sufficient to control the accompanying metabolic acidosis. However, when acidosis is severe, infusion of an alkalinizing solution (sodium bicarbonate) may also be required. The primary cause, such as infection, must also be treated.

Patients with type 2 diabetes are treated with oral hypoglycemic drugs, but some may also require insulin

In T2D patients, insulin synthesis is at least partly preserved; they can be treated with hypoglycemic drugs. However, if adequate control cannot be achieved, they do require insulin. Each year, 5%–10% of patients treated with hypoglycemic drugs need to commence treatment with insulin.

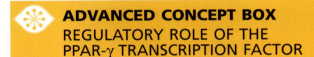

ADVANCED CONCEPT BOX
REGULATORY ROLE OF THE PPAR-γ TRANSCRIPTION FACTOR

Peroxisome proliferator-activated receptors (PPAR) are ligand-activated nuclear receptors belonging to the steroid receptor family. Binding of a ligand induces a conformational change that allows a PPAR to form a heterodimer with another receptor, such as the retinoid X receptor (RXR). PPAR may also bind small molecules, coactivators, or corepressors. The complex then binds to response elements in gene promoters (Fig. 31.23).

There are three types of PPARs: **PPAR-α,** which is discussed in Chapter 33; **PPAR-γ;** and **PPAR-β**. PPAR-γ is predominantly expressed in adipose tissue but also in the muscle, liver, intestine, and heart. It is activated by polyunsaturated fatty acids and by components of the oxidized LDL. It regulates carbohydrate and fatty acid metabolism, inducing, among others, genes coding for lipoprotein lipase (LPL), GLUT-4 glucose transporter, and glucokinase. It also induces the ABCA1 transporter, increasing the transfer of cholesterol from cells to the HDL (Chapter 14). It inhibits macrophage activation and the production of cytokines, such as tumor necrosis factor (TNF-α), interferon-γ, and interleukin-1 (IL-1). PPAR-γ is a target of **thiazolidinediones,** drugs that are used to treat T2D.

Antidiabetic drugs

Currently used oral hypoglycemic drugs target the three processes: insulin secretion, tissue insulin sensitivity, and absorption and digestion of carbohydrates.

Biguanides and thiazolidinediones sensitize the peripheral tissues to insulin

Metformin, a biguanide, is currently the most common oral treatment in T2D. It reduces hepatic gluconeogenesis. It inhibits

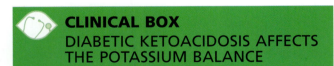

CLINICAL BOX
DIABETIC KETOACIDOSIS AFFECTS THE POTASSIUM BALANCE

Insulin increases cellular potassium uptake, and the lack of insulin leads to the release of potassium from cells. Because uncontrolled diabetes is also accompanied by osmotic diuresis, the released potassium is excreted in urine. As a result, **most patients admitted with ketoacidosis are potassium depleted** but, paradoxically, might have a normal or raised plasma potassium concentration. When exogenous insulin is given to such patients, it stimulates the entry of potassium into cells and can lead to an abrupt lowering of plasma potassium and severe **hypokalemia**. Hypokalemia is dangerous because of its effects on the cardiac muscle. Thus, except for patients with very high plasma concentrations, potassium needs to be given during treatment of diabetic ketoacidosis (see also Chapters 35 and 36).

glycogenolysis by inhibiting glucose-6-phosphatase. It decreases fatty acid and triglyceride synthesis, increases fatty acid oxidation, and increases peripheral insulin sensitivity. Metformin increases insulin-dependent glucose uptake in the skeletal muscle. Metformin has mitochondrial actions: it inhibits complex 1 of the respiratory chain. This increases the cellular AMP/ATP ratio, and through this, it may activate AMPK (Chapter 32) and glucose uptake in the skeletal muscle. Metformin also reduces weight.

Very rarely, metformin can precipitate lactic acidosis by its effect on the complex 1 of the mitochondria. Inhibiting complex 1 increases the ratio of NADH to NAD. This inhibits pyruvate dehydrogenase and leads to the accumulation of pyruvate, the excess of which can be converted into lactate. Patients with impaired renal function, severe sepsis, hypovolemia, and severe heart failure are at the greatest risk.

Thiazolidinediones, such as pioglitazone, improve peripheral glucose utilization and insulin sensitivity. They are ligands of the PPAR-γ transcription factor (Fig. 31.23) in the adipose tissue and, to a lesser extent, in muscle. PPAR-γ activation increases transcription of genes responsible for glucose and lipid metabolism, such as the lipoprotein lipase, acyl-CoA synthase, and the GLUT-4 transporter. Thiazolidinediones also activate the IRS-PI3K-Akt signaling pathway. They promote the expansion of subcutaneous adipose tissue, reduce lipolysis, and reduce adipose tissue inflammation.

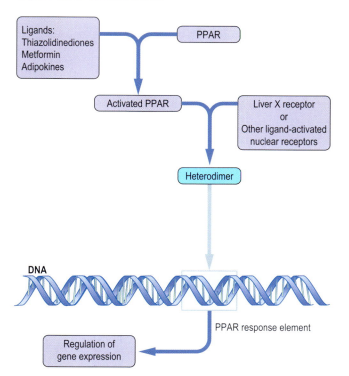

Fig. 31.23 **Transcriptional regulation by peroxisome proliferator-activated receptors (PPAR).** PPARs are activated by metabolites and drugs. They form heterodimer complexes with other nuclear receptors. Resulting complexes bind to the PPAR response elements in gene promoters, regulating gene expression.

The group of drugs known as **glitazars** is currently being tested; these agents stimulate both PPAR-α and PPAR-γ; therefore, apart from thiazolidinedione-like action, they may influence lipid metabolism by raising the HDL and decreasing the plasma triglyceride concentration (Chapter 33).

Sulfonylureas, meglitinides, and drugs affecting the incretin system stimulate insulin secretion

Sulfonylureas bind to a receptor in the plasma membrane of the pancreatic β-cells. The receptor contains the ATP-sensitive potassium channel. Binding of the drug closes the channel, depolarizes the membrane, and opens the calcium channel. Increasing intracellular cytoplasmic calcium concentration stimulates the release of insulin. Hypoglycemia is an important side effect of sulfonylurea treatment. **Meglitinides** are rapid-acting drugs that increase insulin secretion. They target the K-ATP channel similarly to the sulfonylureas.

Pramlintide, an analog of the β-cell hormone islet amyloid polypeptide, slows down gastric emptying, promotes satiety, and inhibits glucagon secretion. It is used as an adjunct to insulin treatment.

GLP-1 receptor agonists and DPP-4 inhibitors affect the incretin system

GLP-1 receptor agonists, such as exenatide or liraglutide, increase insulin secretion. They act via the cAMP–PKA pathway and potentiate insulin secretion induced by raised glucose. Endogenous GLP-1 can also be increased by using DPP-4 inhibitors such as sitagliptin, which prevents GLP-1 degradation and thus increases its effect.

Acarbose decreases the availability of glucose

Acarbose is an inhibitor of intestinal α-glucosidase, an enzyme that digests complex sugars. It delays intestinal absorption of glucose.

Sodium-glucose cotransporter 2 (SGLT2) inhibitors decrease glucose reabsorption in the kidney

SGLT2 is a membrane transporter that reabsorbs glucose in the renal proximal tubule. SGLT2 inhibitors such as canagliflozin improve the control of glucose by increasing urinary glucose excretion.

Bariatric surgery is used as an option for diabetes treatment in severely obese people

There are several surgical options that may involve gastric banding, gastric bypass, and resection or transposition of parts of the small intestine. Patients who undergo these procedures require careful long-term monitoring.

SUMMARY

- Glucose homeostasis involves the liver, adipose tissue, skeletal muscle, and pancreas.

■ The organism alternates between the fed and fasting state. Metabolite concentrations in blood change during the feed–fast cycle and are influenced by stress and disease. Therefore interpretation of metabolite levels needs to be related to mealtimes and to the overall clinical condition of the patient.

■ Measurement of plasma glucose concentration is part of a routine assessment of every patient admitted to the hospital. The measurements of plasma glucose and glycated hemoglobin (HbA_{1c}) are used for diabetes diagnosis and monitoring of glycemic control. In diabetic patients, measurements of plasma and urine glucose, urinary ketones, and HbA_{1c} and tests of renal function, including microalbuminuria, are performed.

■ Type 1 diabetes mellitus is an autoimmune disease caused by the destruction of pancreatic β-cells.

■ Type 2 diabetes results from the inability of functionally impaired β-cells to compensate for peripheral insulin resistance. Type 2 diabetes is strongly associated with obesity.

■ Short-term complications of diabetes include hypoglycemia and ketoacidosis. Long-term complications include diabetic retinopathy, nephropathy, and neuropathy and increased risk of cardiovascular disease linked to diabetic macroangiopathy.

ACTIVE LEARNING

1. Describe how insulin causes an increase in cellular glucose uptake.
2. What are the antiinsulin hormones?
3. What is the role of the incretin system in glucose homeostasis?
4. Why would a nondiabetic patient brought to the emergency unit with extensive burns have an increased plasma glucose concentration? Describe the patient's metabolic state.
5. You have asked a patient to come to the outpatient clinic to have plasma triglycerides tested. The patient asks whether he needs to be fasting that day. Provide an answer, and explain your reasoning.
6. Do people with impaired glucose tolerance develop long-term vascular complications?
7. What do obesity and diabetes mellitus have in common?

FURTHER READING

American Diabetic Association. (2015). Approaches to glycaemic treatment. *Diabetes Care, 38*(Suppl. 1), S41–S48.

Atkinson, M. A., Eisenbarth, G. S., & Michels, A. W. (2014). Type 1 diabetes. *Lancet, 383*, 69–82.

Bliss, M. (1983). *The discovery of insulin*. Edinburgh: Paul Harris Publishing.

Bluestone, J. A., Herold, K., & Eisenbarth, G. (2010). Genetics, pathogenesis and clinical interventions in type 1 diabetes. *Nature, 464*, 1293–1300.

Boucher, J., Kleinridders, A., & Kahn, C. R. (2014). Insulin receptor signaling in normal and insulin-resistant states. *Cold Spring Harbor Perspectives in Biology, 6*, 1–22.

Diabetes Control and Complications Trial (DCCT) Research Group. (1993). The effect of intensive treatment of diabetes on the development and progression of long-term complications in insulin-dependent diabetes mellitus. *The New England Journal of Medicine, 329*, 977–986.

Diabetes Prevention Program Research Group. (2002). Reduction in the incidence of type 2 diabetes with lifestyle intervention or metformin. *The New England Journal of Medicine, 24*, 387–388.

Dominiczak, M. H. (2003). Obesity, glucose intolerance and diabetes and their links to cardiovascular disease. Implications for laboratory medicine. *Clinical Chemistry and Laboratory Medicine, 41*, 1266–1278.

Kahn, S. E., Cooper, M. E., & Del Prato, S. (2014). Pathophysiology and treatment of type 2 diabetes: Perspectives on the past, present, and future. *Lancet, 383*, 1068–1083.

Mohlke, K. L., & Boehnke, M. (2015). Recent advances in understanding the genetic architecture of type 2 diabetes. *Human Molecular Genetics, 24*, R85–R92.

Pociot, F., & Lernmark, Å. (2016). Genetic risk factors for type 1 diabetes mellitus. *Lancet, 387*, 2331–2339.

Pajvani, U. B., & Accili, D. (2015). The new biology of diabetes. *Diabetologia, 58*, 2459–2468.

Stern, M. P. (1995). Diabetes and cardiovascular disease. The "common soil" hypothesis. *Diabetes, 44*, 369–374.

UK Prospective Diabetes Study (UKPDS) Group. (1998). Intensive blood-glucose control with sulphonylureas or insulin compared with conventional treatment and risk of complications in patients with type 2 diabetes (UKPDS 33). *Lancet, 352*, 837–853.

Zimmet, P., Alberti, K. G. M. M., & Shaw, J. (2001). Global and societal implications of the diabetes epidemic. *Nature, 414*, 782–787.

RELEVANT WEBSITES

American Diabetes Association - Type 1 Diabetes: http://www.diabetes.org/diabetes-basics/type-1/

American Diabetes Association - Type 2 Diabetes: http://www.diabetes.org/diabetes-basics/type-2/

Diabetes.co.uk - The Global Diabetes Community: http://www.diabetes.co.uk/index.html

IDF Diabetes Atlas, 8th ed.: http://www.diabetesatlas.org/resources/2017-atlas.html

Definition and Diagnosis of Diabetes Mellitus and Intermediate Hyperglycemia. Report of a WHO/IDF Consultation: http://www.who.int/diabetes/publications/diagnosis_diabetes2006/en/

WHO - Diabetes, Fact Sheet. (2016): http://www.who.int/mediacentre/factsheets/fs312/en/

WHO Consultation. Abbreviated Report. Use of Glycated Haemoglobin (HbA1c) in the Diagnosis of Diabetes Mellitus: http://www.who.int/diabetes/publications/report-hba1c_2011.pdf

ABBREVIATIONS

ABCA1	Transporter involved transfer of cholesterol from cells to the HDL
ADA	American Diabetes Association
AGE	Advanced glycation (glycoxidation) end products
AMPK	AMP-dependent protein kinase
BUN	Blood urea nitrogen
C3G	Guanyl nucleotide exchange factor
CAP	Cbl-associated protein
Cbl	Adaptor protein in insulin signaling pathway
CRP	C-reactive protein

DCCT	Diabetes Control and Complications Trial	mTORC2	Protein complex containing mTOR kinase
DHAP	Dihydroxyacetone phosphate	NIDDM	Noninsulin-dependent diabetes
DPP-4	Dipeptidyl peptidase-4	OGTT	Oral glucose tolerance test
FOXA2	Transcription factor, also known as HNF-3B	PAI-1	Plasminogen activator inhibitor 1
FOXO	Forkhead box O proteins; transcription factors belonging to the forkhead family (contains proteins designated FOXA to FOXR)	PC	Pyruvate carboxylase
		PDK1	3'-phosphoinositide-dependent kinase 1
		PEP	Phosphoenolpyruvate
		PEPCK	Phosphoenolpyruvate carboxykinase
Fru-1,6-BPase	Fructose 1,6-biphosphatase	PFK	Phosphofructokinase
Fru-2,6-BP	Fructose 2,6-biphosphate	PFK-2	Phosphofructokinase-2 phosphatidylinositol 3-kinase (PI3K).
Fru-2,6-BPase-2	Fructose 2,6-biphosphatase-2		
GAD	Glutamic acid decarboxylase	PI3K	Phosphatidylinositol 3-kinase
GALD-3-P	Glyceraldehyde-3-phosphate	PIP_3	Phosphatidylinositol -3,4,5-trisphosphate
GDM	Gestational diabetes mellitus	PK	Pyruvate kinase
GIP	Gastric inhibitory peptide	PKC	Protein kinase C
Glc-6-P	Glucose-6-phosphate	PPAR	Peroxisome proliferator-activated receptor
Glc-6-Pase	Glucose-6-phosphatase	Raf	Protein kinase
GLP-1	Glucagon-like peptide-1	Raf kinase	MAP kinase
GLUT-2	Glucose transporter	Ras	GTPase
Grb2	Adaptor protein in signal transduction pathways	Ras/MAP	Kinase pathway to the Shc protein
		ROS	Reactive oxygen species
HbA_{1c}	Hemoglobin A_{1c}, glycated hemoglobin	RXR	Retinoid X receptor
HDL	High-density lipoproteins	Shc	Protein participating in signaling pathways; also, a domain of certain signal transduction proteins
HNF1A, HNF1B	Transcription factor		
IDDM	Insulin-dependent diabetes		
IFCC	International Federation of Clinical Chemistry and Laboratory Medicine.	SoS	Son of Sevenless protein
		T1D	Type 1 diabetes mellitus
IFG	Impaired fasting glucose	T2D	Type 2 diabetes mellitus
IGT	Impaired glucose tolerance	TG	Triacylglycerol
IL-1, IL-6	Interleukins	TC-10	A G-protein
IRS 1–4	Insulin receptor substrates	TCA cycle	Tricarboxylic acid cycle
LPL	Lipoprotein lipase	TNF-α	Tumor necrosis factor α
MAP	Mitogen-activated protein **kinase**	UKPDS	UK Prospective Diabetes Study
MEK	MAP kinase	VIP	Vasoactive intestinal peptide
MHC	Major histocompatibility complex	VLDL	Very-low-density lipoproteins
MODY	Maturity-onset diabetes of the young	WHO	World Health Organization

32

Nutrients and Diets

Marek H. Dominiczak and Jennifer Logue

LEARNING OBJECTIVES

After reading this chapter, you should be able to:

- Describe mechanisms controlling food intake.
- Describe the role of AMP-activated kinase in maintaining cellular energy balance.
- Identify the main categories of nutrients and essential nutrients within these categories.
- Relate your knowledge of energy metabolism to current nutritional recommendations.
- Characterize malnutrition and obesity.
- Discuss nutritional assessment.

INTRODUCTION

Nutrition is an essential interaction of the organism with the environment. It underpins health and affects susceptibility to disease; both malnutrition and obesity are associated with health risks. Nutritional deficiencies at the extremes of age are particularly important.

Nutritional status is determined by biological, psychologic, and social factors

The factors that determine the nutritional status of an individual are the genetic background, the environment, the phase of the life cycle, the level of physical activity, and the presence or absence of illness (Fig. 32.1). Nutritional status is also affected by the availability of food, its palatability, and its variety. Nutritional deficiencies may result from dietary inadequacies or from genetically determined metabolic errors.

Basic definitions

Diet is the total of all the foods and drinks ingested by an individual. The **food, or foodstuff,** is the particular food that is ingested. **Nutrients** are chemically defined components of food required by the body.

MAIN CLASSES OF NUTRIENTS

The main nutrients are **carbohydrates** (including fiber), **fats, proteins, minerals, and vitamins**. Carbohydrates, proteins,

CLINICAL BOX
THE ABC OF EMERGENCY TREATMENT

Eating and drinking, like breathing, link a living organism with its environment. To survive, we need **oxygen, water, and nutrients.** One can exist without oxygen for minutes only. Without water, the survival time is days. With these two supplied, a human can survive without food for between 60 and 90 days.

These considerations determine the urgency of treatment in critical situations. Reestablishment of oxygen supply and circulating volume is the first priority **(the ABCs of resuscitation: airway, breathing, circulation).** Repletion of lost fluids and electrolytes is also necessary within hours to days, depending on the state of the patient. Provision of other nutrients becomes important as soon as the life-saving measures have been taken. The rule of thumb is that patients unable to eat would need nutritional support if they have been (or will be) unable to take food for more than 7 days. This period is shorter in hypercatabolic patients, such as those with severe burns or sepsis.

fat, fiber, and some minerals are macronutrients. Vitamins and trace metals are **micronutrients** (Chapter 7). The caloric values of the main nutrients are given in Table 32.1. The functions of nutrients are summarized in Fig. 32.2.

Carbohydrates

Carbohydrates and fats are the main **energy sources**. Dietary carbohydrates include refined carbohydrates, such as the sucrose in sweets, drinks, and fruit juices, and complex carbohydrates, such as the starch present in grains and potatoes. **Fiber** is carbohydrate that is indigestible by the human gut, such as cellulose, hemicellulose, lignin, pectin, and β-glucan. Fiber is present in unprocessed cereals, legumes, vegetables, and fruits. Its main role is to regulate gut motility and transit.

The glycemic index and glycemic load provide quantitative and qualitative insight into the handling of carbohydrate-containing foods

The glycemic index (GI) is the system of ranking of the carbohydrate-containing foods according to the degree of increase in blood glucose that takes place after their ingestion. The procedure that underpins the ranking is similar to the oral glucose tolerance test. The effect of a standard dose (25 or 50 g) of a particular

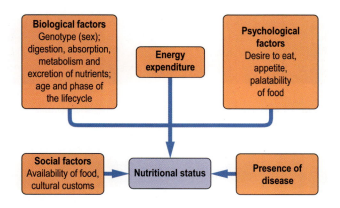

Fig. 32.1 **Factors that determine nutritional status.**

food on plasma glucose concentration is tested and compared with the reference nutrient (e.g. glucose). The comparison is based on the ratio of the area under the curve (AUC) for the tested nutrient and glucose.

$$GI = (AUC\ tested\ nutrient/AUC\ glucose) \times 100$$

The GI is expressed on a scale of 1 to 100 (low GI is 0–55, moderate 56–69, and high >69). Foods that are rapidly absorbed and digested have a high GI. Slower absorption and digestion yield low GI. The GI is affected by the nature of food, the type of starch, and also by the cooking method (e.g., the GI of lightly cooked spaghetti will have GI lower than that cooked for a longer period). The **low-GI foods** control postprandial glycemia and insulinemia and are beneficial for people with diabetes and better for weight control. Note that low-GI foods tend to be high in fat and low in carbohydrate and fiber.

The derivative of the GI is the **glycemic load (GL)**. It translates the qualitative information contained in the GI into

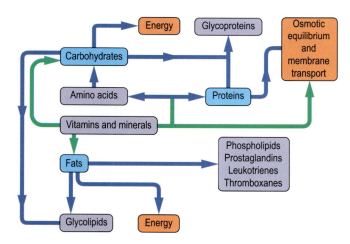

Fig. 32.2 **The functions of nutrients.** All main classes of nutrients can be used to produce energy, and all contribute to the synthesis of more complex compounds. The main role of vitamins and other micronutrients is participation in enzymatic reactions as cofactors or components of enzyme prosthetic groups. Minerals are essential for the maintenance of membrane potential, osmotic equilibrium, and bone structure.

Table 32.1 Caloric content of nutrients

Nutrient	Energy kJ/g	kcal/g
Starch	17	4
Glucose	17	4
Fat	37	9
Protein	17	4
Alcohol	30	7

Caloric content of nutrients (1 kJ = 239 cal; 1 kcal = 4.184 kJ).

data that can be used to calculate the carbohydrate content of a given portion of food.

$$GL = GI/100 \times CHO\ (grams\ per\ serving)$$

High-GI foods are digested rapidly and stimulate the craving/reward areas of the brain. Metabolically, these carbohydrates are also strong stimulators of hepatic lipogenesis and promote visceral fat deposition through insulin-mediated pathways and SREB1c transcription factor program. Thus the idea that eating carbohydrates avoids fat deposition in tissues is a falsity.

Proteins

Proteins provide cell structure and are responsible for many of the cell's functions, communications, and signaling. They serve as the "last resort" energy substrate: catabolic states are typically associated with release amino acids from muscle, and thus with **muscle wasting.** Due to the different composition of animal and plant proteins, eating no animal products at all may lead to nutrient deficiencies, such as those of vitamin B_{12}, calcium, iron, and zinc. Protein requirements change during the life cycle (Table 32.2).

Table 32.2 Daily protein requirements

Age	Males (g/day)	Females (g/day)
0–3 months	12.5	12.5
10–12 months	14.9	14.9
4–6 years	19.7	19.7
15–18 years	55.2	45
19–50 years	55.5	45
>50 years	53.3	46.5

Fats

Fats are the most important nutrients used for **energy storage.** Lipids also provide thermal insulation and are essential components of biological membranes (see also Chapter 4). Fatty acids may also serve as **signaling molecules.**

Long-chain fatty acids are not soluble in water, but short- (C-4 - C-6) and medium-chain fatty acids (C-8 - C-10) are. Short- and medium-chain fatty acids are transported in plasma bound to albumin, whereas the long-chain fatty acids are transported in chylomicrons.

Fats are divided into saturated and unsaturated (the latter being either mono- or polyunsaturated)

The most common saturated fatty acid is palmitic acid (C-16). Others are stearic (C-18), myristic (C-14), and lauric (C-12). All animal fats (beef fat, butterfat, lard) are highly saturated. Saturated fats are also present in palm oil, cocoa butter, and coconut oil.

Oleic acid (ω-9) is the only significant dietary monounsaturated fatty acid

Monounsaturated fatty acids are present in all animal and vegetable fats. Olive oil is a particularly rich source of mono-unsaturated fats. Monounsaturated *trans* fatty acids (Fig. 32.3), the isomers of the *cis*-oleic acid, are by-products of the hydrogenation process of liquid vegetable oils. Consumption of *trans* fatty acids are associated with increased risk of coronary disease.

Polyunsaturated fatty acids include ω-3 and ω-6 acids

The ω-3 fatty acids are α-linolenic (ω-3, C-18:3, $\Delta^{9,12,15}$), eicosapentaenoic (ω-3, C-20:5, $\Delta^{5,8,11,14,17}$), and docosahexaenoic (ω-3, C-22:6, $\Delta^{4,7,10,13,16,19}$) acids. They are present primarily in fish, shellfish, and phytoplankton, and also in some vegetable oils such as olive, safflower, corn, sunflower, and soybean oil, as well as in leafy vegetables.

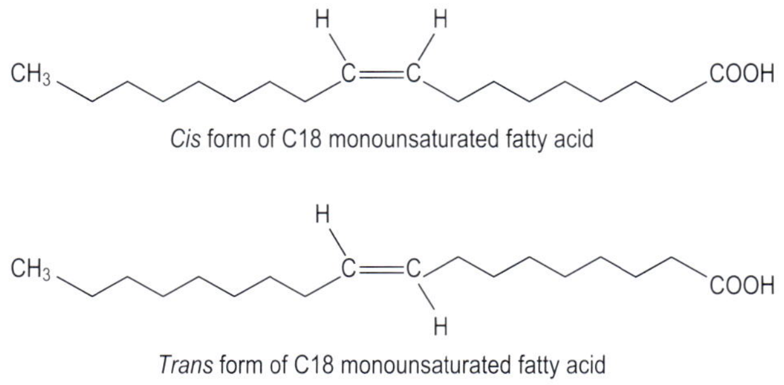

Cis form of C18 monounsaturated fatty acid

Trans form of C18 monounsaturated fatty acid

Fig. 32.3 **An example of a *cis*- and *trans*-monounsaturated fatty acid (18-carbon oleic acid).** *Trans* fatty acids are produced during hydrogenation of liquid vegetable oils.

The ω-6 acids are arachidonic acid (ω-6, C-20:4, $\Delta^{5,8,11,14}$) and its precursor, linoleic acid (ω-6, C-18:2, $\Delta^{9,12}$). The ω-6 fatty acids are present in soybean and canola oils and in fish oils (particularly in fatty fish such as salmon, sardines, and pilchards).

ESSENTIAL NUTRIENTS

Essential (limiting) nutrients are these that cannot be synthesized in the human body

Essential nutrients include essential amino acids, essential fatty acids (EFA), and some vitamins and trace elements. Note that carbohydrates are not essential nutrients.

Some plant proteins are relatively deficient in essential amino acids, whereas animal proteins usually contain a balanced mixture

Essential amino acids are phenylalanine (tyrosine can be synthesized from phenylalanine); the branched-chain amino acids valine, leucine, isoleucine, threonine, and methionine; and lysine (Chapter 15).

Essential fatty acids (EFA) are linoleic acid and α-linolenic acid

Arachidonic acid, eicosapentaenoic acid, and docosahexaenoic acid can be made in limited amounts from EFA; however, they also become essential when EFAs are deficient.

Vitamins and trace metals are important for the catalysis of chemical reactions

Vitamins and trace metals act as coenzymes and form functionally important prosthetic groups of enzymes. They are discussed in detail in Chapter 7.

HEALTHY EATING

Current dietary recommendations for general population focus on a balanced diet

Current recommendations stress the **balanced diet.** Recent dietary concepts depart from the focus on a particular nutrient (e.g., cholesterol or fat) and place emphasis on the type of foods and on dietary patterns (see Further Reading).

High intake of fruit and vegetables is unequivocally recommended. Nonstarchy vegetables are preferred to starchy ones because of the high GI value of some starchy foods, such as white potatoes. Minimally processed whole grains are probably the healthiest type of carbohydrates (as opposed to, for example, white bread or white rice). Restriction of carbohydrate foods such as refined grains, certain potatoes, sugar-sweetened beverages (SSB), and sweets is recommended.

Moderate intake of dairy products is recommended. Dairy products are a major source of calcium and vitamin A. Lower-fat options are available if calorie restriction is an issue. Fish,

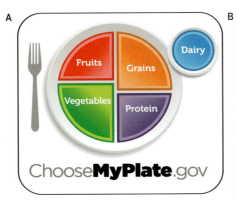

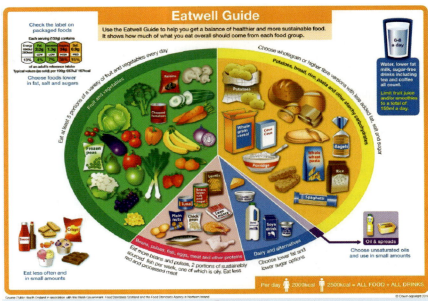

Fig. 32.4 **Healthy eating recommendations.**
A. My Plate illustrates the dietary recommendations of the US Department of Agriculture. B. The Eatwell Guide has been developed by Public Health England in association with the Welsh Government, Food Standards Scotland, and the Food Standards Agency in Northern Ireland.

poultry, legumes and nuts, and yogurt are regarded as healthy sources of proteins.

Vegetable cooking oils such as olive and canola oil are regarded as healthy fats, as opposed to saturated fats and particularly the *trans* fats.

Foods that should be consumed in lesser amounts are red meats, processed (sodium-preserved) meats, and foods that are rich in added sugars, salt, and *trans* fatty acids. Sodium restriction and moderation in alcohol consumption are recommended. Finally, a healthy diet should be combined with an **active lifestyle.**

The reader is referred to the Further Reading section for recommendations relevant to specific medical conditions. *MyPlate,* shown in Fig. 32.4A, contains the dietary recommendations of the US Department of Agriculture, which superseded the well-known food pyramid. The alternative, called the Healthy Eating Plate, has been recommended by the Harvard School of Public Health. The Eatwell Guide, shown in Figure 32.4B is the recommendation developed by the National Health Service in the United Kingdom.

REGULATION OF FOOD INTAKE

Food intake is controlled by hunger (a desire to eat) and appetite (a desire for a particular food)

Main centers regulating appetite are located in the hypothalamic arcuate and paraventricular nuclei in the central nervous system (CNS). In humans, the arcuate nucleus area is known as the infundibular nucleus. The brain regulates energy homeostasis and is also the primary regulator of body weight (Fig. 32.5). Signals controlling energy intake originate from adipose tissue and are sent to the CNS. These signals are mediated by the adipokine **leptin** (see following discussion) and by insulin. In response, the brain sends signals through a complex network of neuropeptides. These regulate appetite and hunger. The neurons in the arcuate nucleus express two neuropeptides: anabolic **neuropeptide Y (NPY)** and catabolic **proopiomelanocortin (POMC).** POMC is cleaved, yielding melanocortins such as α-MSH that decrease food intake. On the other hand, NPY expression increases when adipose tissue is depleted and when there is a decrease in leptin. NPY links to neurons expressing melanin-concentrating hormone (MCH) and orexins A and B. They, in turn, are involved in the control of food intake by acting on brainstem neurons. These neurons connect with the brain cortex (the satiety center) to promote hunger and to stimulate yet another set of hormones, such as **thyroliberin (TRH)** and **corticoliberin (CRH).** TRH increases thermogenesis and food intake, whereas CRH decreases food intake and, through the sympathetic activity, increases energy expenditure. Further signals that control food intake are conveyed by gastrointestinal peptides such as **glucagon, cholecystokinin, glucagon-like peptide, amylin, and peptide YY. Ghrelin,** secreted by the stomach, stimulates NPY-expressing neurons. It is the only known appetite-stimulating peptide. Gastric stretch also affects food intake. Finally, **hypoglycemia** decreases the activity of the satiety center.

The hypothalamus and brainstem translate the information about energy balance into eating behavior

This involves the **endogenous cannabinoid system.** Endocannabinoids are compounds synthesized from membrane phospholipids. They include Δ⁹-tetrahydrocannabinol and anandamide formed as a result of hydrolysis of *N*-arachidonylphosphatidyl ethanolamine by phospholipase D. Endocannabinoids are released at the synapses and bind to the synaptic receptors called CB1. The receptors are present in the CNS and also in

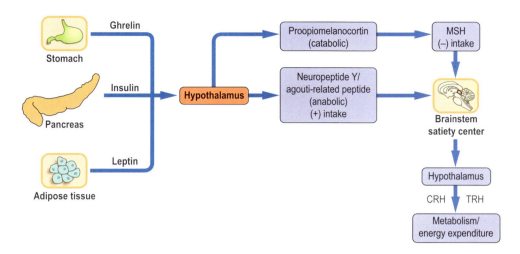

Fig. 32.5 **Regulation of food intake.** Regulation of food intake is accomplished by signals generated in the adipose tissue, pancreas, stomach, and brain. The hypothalamus translates signals related to the energy balance into eating behavior through secretion of a range of neuropeptides. The (+) sign means action leading to increase in appetite and food intake, and the (−) sign means those leading to a decrease. CRH, corticoliberin; TRH, thyroliberin; MSH, melanocyte-stimulating hormone.

the gut, adipose tissue, the liver, muscle, and the pancreas. They are coupled to G proteins and adenylate cyclase, and they also regulate potassium and calcium channels. The binding of endocannabinoids to the receptors modulates the release of neurotransmitters such as GABA, noradrenaline, glutamate, and serotonin (Chapter 26). Hypothalamic levels of endocannabinoids increase during food deprivation.

ENERGY BALANCE

Adipose tissue is an active endocrine organ

Adipose tissue, far from being an inert depot of storage fat, is an active endocrine organ (Fig. 32.6). Its products are known as adipokines. This endocrine activity influences the development of obesity and conditions such as insulin resistance. The two major adipokines secreted by the adipose tissue are **leptin** and **adiponectin.**

Leptin regulates adipose tissue mass and responds to the energy status

Leptin is a 16k-Da protein. Its secretion is linked to the adipose tissue mass and to the size of adipocytes. Acting in the CNS, it **decreases food intake.** It also acts on skeletal muscle, the liver, adipose tissue, and the pancreas. Leptin gene expression is regulated by food intake, energy status, hormones, and the presence of inflammation. It affects metabolism by stimulating fatty acid oxidation and by decreasing lipogenesis. Importantly, it also decreases ectopic deposition of fat in liver or muscle.

Leptin signals through a membrane receptor that has an extracellular binding domain and an intracellular tail. Its signaling pathways involve the Janus kinase / signal transducer and activator of transcription (JAK/STAT;

Chapter 25). Mitogen-activated protein kinase (MAPK) and phosphatidyl-inositol 3′ kinase (PI3K) are also involved, as is the AMP-activated kinase (AMPK; see following discussion).

Adiponectin increases insulin sensitivity; its lack leads to insulin resistance

Adiponectin is a 244–amino acid protein possessing a structural homology with collagens type VIII and X and with complement factor C1q. Adiponectin stimulates glucose utilization in muscle and increases fatty acid oxidation in muscle and the liver, thus increasing insulin sensitivity. It also decreases hepatic glucose production. Low adiponectin levels are linked with insulin resistance and with hepatic steatosis. Adiponectin downregulates secretion of proinflammatory cytokines interleukin 6 and 8 (IL-6 and IL-8) and monocyte chemoattractant protein-1 (MCP-1).

Physical training increases adiponectin expression and upregulates its receptors in the skeletal muscle. Conversely, its concentration decreases in obesity and in type 2 diabetes. Low levels of adiponectin are also associated with low-grade inflammation, oxidative stress, and endothelial dysfunction. Adiponectin receptors activate the AMPK, p38 mitogen-activated protein kinase, and PPARα, which in turn regulates fatty acid metabolism (Chapter 31).

Adipose tissue also secretes proinflammatory cytokines

In obese individuals, adipocytes secrete monocyte attractant protein-1 (MCP-1) and thus are able to recruit monocytes to adipose tissue. These transform into resident macrophages able to secrete proinflammatory cytokines tumor necrosis factor α (TNF-α) and IL-6 (Fig. 32.6). TNF-α is highly expressed in obese animals and humans, and it also induces insulin resistance and type 2 diabetes. TNF-α activates the proinflammatory NFκB pathway.

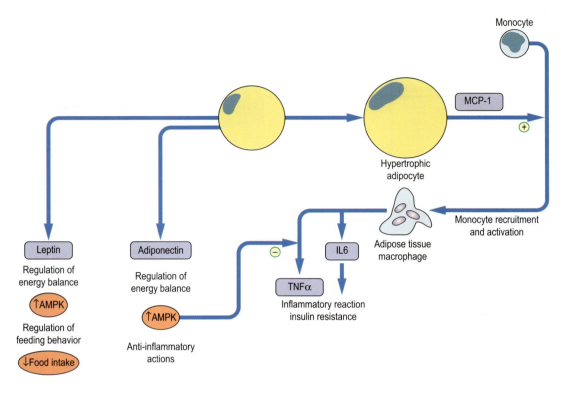

Fig. 32.6 **Endocrine activity of the adipose tissue in obesity.** Adipocytes secrete a range of adipokines (leptin and adiponectin are shown here) that regulate energy balance and eating behavior. In obese individuals, adipocytes secrete chemokine MCP-1, which recruits monocytes to the adipose tissue. After transformation, they become adipose tissue macrophages able to incite inflammatory reaction through secretion of proinflammatory cytokines such as TNF-α and IL-6. Note the antiinflammatory actions of adiponectin. AMPK, AMP-activated kinase; CNS, central nervous system; IL, interleukin; MCP-1, monocyte chemoattractant protein 1; TNF-α, tumor necrosis factor α.

ADVANCED CONCEPT BOX
ADIPOSE TISSUE AND DISEASE

Adipose tissue can be stored in three distinct depots in the body: **subcutaneous** fat under the skin; **visceral** fat within the abdominal cavity; and **ectopic** fat (the latter being, for example, the cardiac fat pad, the excess deposition in the liver itself, and in myocytes). The distribution of fat in a person depends on sex and ethnicity, combined with family history. For example, women are classically thought of as "pear-shaped," with large subcutaneous adipose stores on their hips and thighs, whereas men are "apple-shaped," with rounded abdomens due to excess visceral fat in the abdominal cavity. People of South Asian, Chinese, and Japanese descent are also generally more prone to depositing excess visceral rather than subcutaneous fat.

Subcutaneous fat is generally benign; it serves as an energy store. Health problems related to subcutaneous fat deposition are mainly mechanical when a person gets so large that he or she cannot function normally. Visceral fat, however, is an active endocrine organ that produces a number of mediators, including interleukin 6, that lead to accelerated atherogenesis and premature cardiovascular disease and facilitate the development of type 2 diabetes. It also promotes a procoagulant state (Chapter 41) by secreting plasminogen activator inhibitor 1 (PAI-1), which inhibits fibrin degradation.

One of the major problems associated with visceral adiposity is the **nonalcoholic fatty liver disease (NAFLD)**. This is due to excess fatty acids being deposited in the liver. It leads to hepatic insulin resistance and is a risk factor for type 2 diabetes, and it can also lead to hepatitis and cirrhosis of the liver.

Ectopic fat pads are less well understood. The main fat pads associated with disease are the cardiac fat pad and the pharyngeal fat pad. The cardiac fat pad is thought to have several characteristics that can mediate cardiac disease. The first is simple mechanical obstruction of the heart, which impairs cardiac function. There is also the possibility that these cells also release procoagulant and inflammatory mediators having a local effect on cells. There will also be toxic lipid accumulation in cardiac myocytes. The pharyngeal fat pad is associated with obstructive sleep apnea; in this condition, the pharynx is obstructed during sleep, leading to episodes of hypoxia and apnea (temporary cessation of breathing). People with this condition have very poor sleep quality and are at a high risk of developing cardiovascular disease, including hypertension. It is not known whether the pharyngeal fat pad has effects beyond obstructing the pharynx.

Visceral and ectopic fat is preferentially depleted during weight loss. This means that a person may not have to return to a "normal" weight in order to substantially decrease visceral and ectopic fat and the health risks these types of fat pose.

CLINICAL BOX
A 46-YEAR-OLD MAN WITH HYPERTRIGLYCERIDEMIA AND FATTY LIVER: CENTRAL OBESITY

Mr. C. is a 45-year-old man of South Asian descent. He has recently been gaining weight - "middle-age spread," as he puts it. This weight gain is concentrated in the abdominal area. His wife is concerned because his father had type 2 diabetes and died from a myocardial infarction at age 60, so she insists that he goes to the doctor for a checkup. He attends the doctor and has blood samples taken; these show moderately raised total cholesterol, high triglyceride concentration, and low HDL-cholesterol. He has impaired fasting glucose, and his liver function tests show a small rise in his transaminases. The liver ultrasound is consistent with intrahepatic fat deposition (fatty liver).

Comment.
The combination of Mr. C.'s sex, ethnicity, and family history has predisposed him to gain weight centrally rather than evenly through his body subcutaneously. This central obesity is due to fat within his abdominal cavity known as visceral fat. This fat is deposited around his liver and pancreas and increases his risk of developing type 2 diabetes. His plasma glucose is raised, but he is not yet at the level classified as diabetes (Chapter 31). There is a degree of inflammation in his liver due to the layer of fat across it, and this can later lead to liver cirrhosis, although rarely.

AMP-stimulated kinase (AMPK) is a cellular energy sensor

AMPK is a serine-threonine kinase. It is a heterotrimer encoded by three genes; it has a catalytic subunit α and two regulatory subunits, β and γ. It is activated by phosphorylation by a kinase known as LKB1, which is a tumor-suppressor molecule. The principal activator of the AMPK is a cellular accumulation of 5'-AMP and the increase of the ratio of 5'-AMP/ATP. AMP is generated in the myokinase (adenylate kinase) reaction:

$$ADP + ADP \rightleftharpoons ATP + AMP$$

A high 5'-AMP concentration induces allosteric changes facilitating phosphorylation of the AMPK catalytic subunit. A high creatine/phosphocreatine ratio also activates the enzyme.

AMPK stimulates energy-producing (catabolic) pathways and suppresses energy-utilizing (anabolic) ones.

Activated AMPK phosphorylates and inactivates acetyl-CoA carboxylase (ACC), the key enzyme in fatty acid synthesis; glycerol-3-phosphate acyltransferase, a triglyceride-synthesizing enzyme; and HMG CoA reductase, the rate-limiting enzyme in the cholesterol-synthesis pathway. Its effect on ACC is mediated through the suppression of SREBP-1c transcription factor (Chapter 14).

Inactivation of acetyl-CoA carboxylase leads to a decrease in malonyl-CoA concentration, disinhibition of carnitine

ADVANCED CONCEPT BOX
mTOR KINASE: CENTRAL REGULATOR OF CELL GROWTH AND PROLIFERATION

The mammalian target of rapamycin (mTOR) is a serine/threonine kinase. It constitutes a central component of the key insulin-stimulated pathway that controls cell growth and proliferation.

The pathway is controlled upstream by growth factors (IGFR and EGFR, among others) and also insulin-receptor substrates (IRS1/IRS2), some amino acids, and glucose. mTOR lies downstream from Akt kinase in the PI3K-Akt signaling pathway and is phosphorylated by Akt (Chapter 31).

mTOR, in turn, forms two complexes known as mTOR complex-1 (mTORC1) and mTOR complex 2 (mTORC2). Activated mTORC1 and mTORC2 phosphorylate and activate a range of transcription factors. These two complexes control the size and shape of the cell, respectively. mTORC1 also controls autophagy, by which cells break down their own organelles (Chapter 28). AMPK suppresses mTORC1 by blocking its ability to phosphorylate downstream substrates.

palmitoyl transferase 1, and consequent facilitation of fatty acid transport into mitochondria. Decreased fatty acid synthesis prevents lipid accumulation in tissues.

Thus in the liver, AMPK inhibits lipogenesis and cholesterol synthesis. AMPK is activated during exercise and enables muscle-contraction-stimulated glucose transport as well as fatty acid oxidation.

The AMPK in the skeletal muscle, the liver, and adipose tissue is stimulated by leptin and adiponectin. It is also activated by metformin, a commonly used antidiabetic drug.

AMPK also inhibits mTOR kinase (see the Advanced Concepts Box), thus affecting cell growth and proliferation. It affects cellular polarity and the cytoskeleton by acting on proteins involved in microtubule assembly. The effects of AMPK activation are summarized in Fig. 32.7.

ENERGY EXPENDITURE

Total daily energy expenditure is a sum of the basal metabolic rate, the thermic effect of food, and the energy used up during physical activity. Energy expenditure can be measured by direct calorimetry, which relies on measurements of heat production. Indirect calorimetry is based on the measurement of the oxygen consumption rate (VO_2). The ratio of VCO_2 to VO_2 is known as the respiratory exchange rate (RER), or respiratory quotient. For carbohydrates, RER = 1.0; for fat, RER = 0.7.

Basal metabolic rate is the energy expenditure required to maintain body function at complete rest

Basal metabolic rate (BMR) depends on sex, age, and body weight. At rest, energy is required for membrane transport

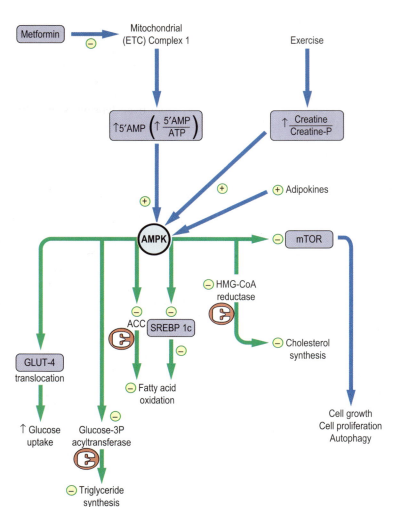

Fig. 32.7 **Outline of actions of AMP-activated kinase (AMPK).** AMPK responds to changes in cellular energy levels. Its main stimulator is the increase in 5′-AMP and an increased 5′-AMP/ATP ratio, which signal low cellular energy level. The effect of AMPK activation is inhibition of anabolic (energy-utilizing) pathways, such as lipogenesis and cholesterol synthesis, and stimulation of catabolic (energy-generating) pathways, such as fatty acid oxidation. Note the effect of exercise and the antidiabetic drug metformin on AMPK activity. See text for details. ACC, acetyl-CoA carboxylase; FFA, free fatty acid.

(30% of the total); for protein synthesis and degradation (30%); and for maintaining temperature, physical activity, and growth. Certain organs use particularly high amounts of energy: in a 70-kg person, brain metabolism constitutes approximately 20% of basal metabolic demand; liver, 25%; and muscle, 25%. Conversely, in very-low-birth-weight babies, the brain is responsible for as much as 60% of the BMR, the liver for 20%, and muscle for only 5%.

In health, physical activity is the most important changeable component of energy expenditure

The level of physical activity is normally expressed as metabolic equivalents of task (MET). Metabolism is dependent on the mass of the individual both at rest and during activity. METs use a reference value for resting metabolism of 1 kcal/kg/h, and activities use its multiples. This allows the intensity and energy expenditure to be compared between people of different weight. Examples of the energy expenditure associated with different activities are given in Table 32.3. Energy requirements also depend on sex and age (Table 32.4).

	Table 32.3 Energy expenditure
Energy expenditure	**Example of activity**
1.3	Watching TV, reading, writing
2.0	Dressing and undressing, making bed, walking slowly
2.3	Washing dishes, ironing
2.5	Dusting and cleaning, cooking
4.5	Cleaning windows, golf, carpentry
6.5	Jogging, digging, shoveling
8.0	Climbing stairs, cycling, football, skiing

Energy expenditure is expressed as metabolic equivalents of task (METs; i.e., multiples of the expenditure at complete rest).

Table 32.4 Estimated average daily requirements (EAR) for energy for selected age and sex groups

Age	EAR, kcal/day (mJ) Males	Females
1–2 months*	526 (2.2)	478 (2.0)
7–12 months	694 (2.9)	646 (2.7)
6 years	1577 (6.6)	1482 (6.2)
14 years	2629 (11.0)	2342 (9.8)
25–34 years	2749 (11.5)	2175 (8.1)
75+ years	2294 (9.6)	1840 (7.7)

*Based on EAR for breastfed infants.
Data from Dietary Reference Values for Energy; Scientific Advisory Committee on Nutrition 2011, London: TSO 2012.

NUTRIGENOMICS

Individual response to nutrients is also determined by genetics, although it seems that environmental factors are dominant. Genes influence the digestion and absorption of nutrients, as well as their metabolism and excretion. Perceptions such as taste or satiety are also, to an extent, genetically determined. This has consequences for nutritional guidelines: because the gene pool varies between populations, optimal nutritional guidelines should be population specific rather than general. Nutrigenomics, analogously to pharmacogenomics, aims to exploit the knowledge accumulated by the Human Genome Project, and technologies that enable the monitoring of the expression of a large number of genes, to devise individual dietary treatments customized to genetic background. Metabolomics, the monitoring of metabolic response patterns to nutrients, offers further opportunities to determine individual nutrition profiles (Chapter 24).

Genotype influences plasma concentrations of nutrients

An example of the genotype effect on nutrient intake is the response of plasma cholesterol concentration to its dietary content. Approximately 50% of individual variation in plasma cholesterol is genetically determined. Response to a cholesterol-containing diet is associated with the apoprotein E (apoE) genotype (Chapter 33). It exists in several isoforms coded by alleles designated ε2, ε3, and ε4. It has been observed that plasma cholesterol concentration increases on a low-fat/high-cholesterol diet in people with the E4/4 but not E2/2 phenotype.

There are many examples of nutrients affecting gene expression. For instance, the activities of key hepatic enzymes differ in persons remaining on a long-term high-fat diet

compared with a high-carbohydrate diet. Further, dietary cholesterol affects the activity of HMG-CoA reductase. Polyunsaturated fatty acids inhibit the expression of fatty acid synthase, and ω-3 fatty acids reduce mRNA coding for the platelet-derived growth factor (PDGF) and the inflammatory cytokine IL-1. In essential hypertension, sensitivity to dietary salt is controlled, at least to an extent, by the angiotensinogen gene variants. Only 50% of patients are sensitive to salt intake: 30%–60% of blood pressure variation is genotype related.

NUTRITION, LIFE CYCLE, AND METABOLIC ADAPTATION

Demand for nutrients is affected by both physiology and disease. **Pregnancy, lactation, and growth** (in particular, the intensive growth **in utero**, growth during infancy, and the adolescent growth spurt) are the three most important physiologic states associated with increased demand for nutrients.

Pregnancy is an example of metabolic adaptation termed expansive adaptation

The body of the mother adapts to carrying the fetus and supplying it with nutrients. Around the time of conception, the mother's body prepares for the metabolic demands of the fetus. In early pregnancy, the mother sets up the "supply capacity," and later in pregnancy, such supply takes place. Ninety percent of fetal weight is gained between the 20th and 40th weeks of pregnancy, and the steepest growth is established between the 24th and 36th weeks. The total amount of energy stored during pregnancy is about 70,000 kcal (293,090 kJ), amounting to approximately 10 kg of weight.

Nutrient intake changes during the life cycle

After delivery, there is a transition from feeding through the placenta to breastfeeding, and then the baby gradually adapts to a free diet. Up to the **breastfeeding stage,** nutrition is controlled by substrates, and the infant is entirely dependent on the mother for nutrition. Later, growth hormone assumes a major role in directing development. At **school age,** new eating and activity patterns emerge as a child learns to be independent from his or her parents. This continues during **adolescence.** At this stage, sex hormones begin to play a prominent developmental role. In **adulthood,** muscle mass increases between 20 and 30 years of age, and at that point, the level of physical activity stabilizes. Thereafter, muscle mass starts to decline, and the fat mass starts to increase. This accelerates after the age of 60. Bone mass also declines with age.

When nutrients are in short supply, either because of increased nutritional need or reduced availability of food, the so-called **reductive adaptation** takes place: the metabolic rate falls, and the desire to eat decreases. This limits weight loss.

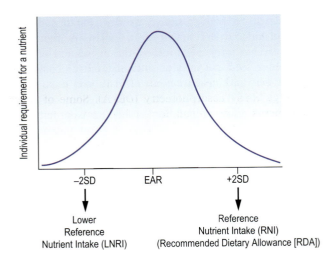

Fig. 32.8 **Dietary Reference Intakes (Recommended Daily Allowance [RDA]): related concepts.** Whereas the Estimated Average Requirement (EAR) reflects the intake adequate for half of a population, the Recommended Nutritional Intake (RNI) or RDA values represent adequate intake for the great majority of individuals. Note that RDA is used in the US and RNI and LNRI in the United Kingdom. SD, standard deviation.

ASSESSING NUTRITION

Dietary intake is not easy to assess

Available data are based on population surveys, which are sometimes incomplete. Sets of values derived from these describe suggested minimal, average, and adequate intakes of particular nutrients. Different values are used in different countries, and there has been a degree of confusion and overlap between various definitions. Currently, estimates of nutrient intake are based on the Dietary Reference Intakes (DRI) developed by the Food and Nutrition Board (FNB) at the Institute of Medicine (IOM) of the National Academies in the United States. They constitute the sets of values describing the intake of nutrients in a given population (Fig. 32.8).

Assessing the nutritional status of an individual

Nutritional assessment includes dietary habits and dietary history, a range of body (anthropometric) measurements, and biochemical and hematologic laboratory tests. Because there is no single definitive marker of nutritional status, assessment relies on the interpretation of a range of variables.

Dietary history should include more than the details of food intake

Dietary habits include meal patterns and the amount and composition of food. Individual diet is determined by biological, psychologic, sociologic, and cultural factors. Biological factors

ADVANCED CONCEPT BOX
DEFINITIONS IN NUTRITION SCIENCE

The definitions in the following list are used by the Food and Nutrition Board of the Institute of Medicine (IOM) of the National Academies in the United States. The definitions used in the United Kingdom are also mentioned. The requirements are described by the **Dietary Reference Intakes (DRI)**, which are as follows:

- **Estimated Average Requirement (EAR):** average daily nutrient intake estimated to meet the requirement of half of the healthy individuals in a particular gender group at a particular stage of life. The EAR is complemented by the RDI, AI, and UL values listed next.
- **Recommended Dietary Allowance (RDA; in the United Kingdom, the Reference Nutrient Intake [RNI]):** It describes the average daily nutrient intake level sufficient to meet the nutrient requirement of nearly all (97%–98%) healthy individuals. The *Lower Reference Nutrient Intake (LNRI),* used in the United Kingdom, is the daily intake observed at the low end of intake distribution in a population (about 2%). If intake falls below this, a deficiency may occur.
- **Adequate Intake (AI):** recommended average daily nutrient intake based on estimates of nutrient intake by a group of healthy people that are assumed to be adequate - used when an RDA cannot be determined.
- **Tolerable Upper Intake Level (UL):** highest average daily intake likely to pose no health risk to almost all individuals in a particular gender group at a particular stage of life. As intake increases above the UL, the risk of adverse effects increases.

Note that DRIs are intended for healthy people, and a DRI established for any one nutrient presupposes that requirements for other ones are being met.

involved are the state of the systems responsible for the intake, digestion, absorption, and metabolism of nutrients. Enzyme deficiencies, such as that of lactase (Chapter 30), cause impaired absorption of foodstuffs (in this case, milk). Psychologic factors also play a role in determining food intake; eating disorders such as anorexia nervosa and bulimia nervosa may lead to severe malnutrition. Sociologic factors include availability and price of food and societal measures taken to improve diets - for instance, school meals or subsidized meals for the elderly or disabled persons. Cultural factors determine eating patterns and the type of preferred foodstuffs. All these are important considerations when taking the dietary history. Individual food intake can be assessed more formally by food frequency questionnaires, 24-h dietary recalls, and food records and also by direct analysis of foods and by metabolic balance studies.

Simplified assessment of nutritional status

The Malnutrition Universal Screening Tool (MUST) has been introduced by the British Association for Parenteral and Enteral

Nutrition (BAPEN) to enable fast assessment of nutritional state in adults. It is a five-step method of identifying individuals at risk (Fig. 32.9).

Another method of nutritional assessment is the Mini Nutritional Assessment (MNA; see Further Reading) developed for the nutritional assessment of the elderly.

Body weight and the body mass index

Body weight in relation to height is the most commonly used measurement in nutritional assessment. The relationship between the two is expressed as the body mass index (BMI), calculated according to the following formula:

(3) $$BMI = weight\,(kg)/height\,(cm)^2$$

The BMI is used to categorize nutritional status, as shown in Table 32.5. Note that between ages 2 and 20 BMI needs to be interpreted in relation to age and sex. As mentioned previously, it should not be used as a sole/definitive indication of the nutritional status.

Other measurements used in nutritional assessment are the **waist-to-hip ratio**, the **mid-arm circumference**, and the **skinfold thickness** measured with carefully calibrated calipers. The waist circumference correlates with the amount of visceral fat and is used in the diagnosis of metabolic syndrome (Chapter 31). More detailed analysis includes the assessment of total body water, analysis of body bioelectrical impedance, and measurements of lean body mass using dual-energy X-ray absorptiometry (DEXA). Some of these measurements allow calculation of body fat content and composition. Functional measurements such as grip strength or peak expiratory flow are also relevant to the nutritional assessment.

Biochemical markers of nutritional status

Urinary nitrogen excretion helps assess nitrogen balance

Nitrogen balance relates to body protein requirements. It is the difference between the intake of nitrogen and its excretion. Positive nitrogen balance means that the intake exceeds loss. Negative nitrogen balance signifies that the loss exceeds intake. The 24-h urinary nitrogen excretion is an estimate of the quantity of proteins metabolized by the body. Ninety percent of the excreted nitrogen appears in the urine (80% of this as urea). The rest is excreted in the stool, hair, and sweat. Nitrogen excretion adjusts to protein intake over 2–4 days. Measurement of urinary nitrogen (or urea) excretion is the most reliable way of assessing daily protein requirements. However, it is now rarely used outside the research setting. Age-related protein requirements are listed in Table 32.2. As a guide, most people require 1.0–1.2 g protein/kg body weight/day.

Specific plasma proteins are used as markers of nutritional status

The concentration of a protein in plasma may reflect the nutritional status over a period in relation to its half-life. Proteins most commonly used for this purpose are **albumin** and **transthyretin** (prealbumin). Many studies confirm the link between liver albumin synthesis (albumin half-life is approximately 20 days; Chapter 40) and the nutritional status. Transthyretin, which has a half-life of 2 days, has also been used in nutritional assessment. It is synthesized in the liver and forms a complex with retinal-binding protein in plasma.

The interpretation of plasma concentrations of nutritionally relevant proteins is often not easy because they are not exclusively determined by the state of nutrition. For instance, plasma albumin concentration also depends on the state of **hydration;** it decreases in overhydrated patients (Chapter 35). In addition, albumin and transthyretin are affected by the **acute-phase response** (Chapter 40). Thus in critically ill patients, albumin is not a useful marker of nutritional state.

Full assessment involves measurements of vitamins and trace metals

This is particularly important in patients who remain on long-term parenteral nutrition.

Table 32.5 Nutritional status in relation to the body mass index (BMI) in adults - WHO criteria

Classification	BMI (kg/m²)	
	Principal cutoff points	Additional cutoff points
Underweight	<18.50	<18.50
Severe thinness	<16.00	<16.00
Moderate thinness	16.00–16.99	16.00–16.99
Mild thinness	17.00–18.49	17.00–18.49
Normal range	18.50–24.99	18.50–22.99 / 23.00–24.99
Overweight	≥25.00	≥25.00
Pre-obese	25.00–29.99	25.00–27.49 / 27.50–29.99
Obese	≥30.00	≥30.00
Obese class I	30.00–34.99	30.00–32.49 / 32.50–34.99
Obese class II	35.00–39.99	35.00–37.49 / 37.50–39.99
Obese class III	≥40.00	≥40.00

Source: http://apps.who.int/bmi/index.jsp?introPage=intro_3.html (accessed March 2017).

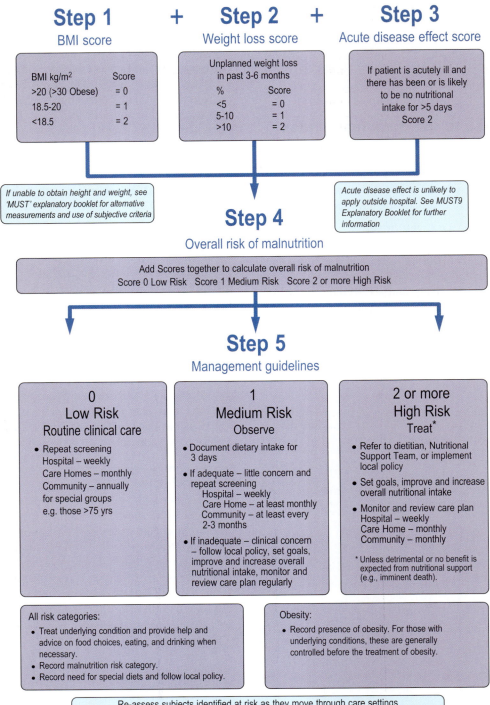

Fig. 32.9 **Malnutrition Universal Screening Tool (MUST) developed by the British Association for Enteral and Parenteral Nutrition.** Steps involved in nutritional assessment. (Reproduced with permission from http://www.Bapen.org.uk.) Refer to the BAPEN website for further information.

Other laboratory tests provide information complementing nutritional assessment

The measurement of hemoglobin may uncover iron deficiency. Evaluation of liver (Chapter 34) and kidney (Chapter 35) function; measurement of plasma sodium, potassium, chloride, bicarbonate, calcium, phosphate, and magnesium; and the assessment of iron metabolism all provide useful additional information. Assessing daily fluid intake and loss (Chapter 35) is essential in patients who are being considered for intravenous nutritional support.

OBESITY

Obesity has emerged as a major health problem worldwide

Worldwide obesity has increased by more than 70% since 1980. In the United States, 35.7% of adults and 16.9% of children are obese (US National Health and Nutrition Examination Survey 2009). The main causes of this increase seem to be the wide availability of high-calorie food and the decrease in physical activity both at work and during leisure time.

Genetic regulation of food intake and energy expenditure

Obesity is concordant in 74% of monozygotic twins and 32% of dizygotic twins. The current obesity epidemic has prompted a search for genes that control energy expenditure and food intake. Large population studies have been used to look for a relationship between changes in genes and body weight. There is a close relationship between the body mass of members of the same family, especially identical twins. Therefore it is estimated that 40%–70% of the differences in the predisposition to obesity can be explained by genetics.

Changes within two genes have been found to be associated with obesity: fat mass and obesity-associated protein (*FTO*) and melanocortin-4 receptor (*MC4R*), which binds melanocortins in the arcuate nucleus that control food intake. *FTO* is expressed in the arcuate nucleus in response to hunger and therefore is thought to have an effect on body mass via control of food intake. These effects have been shown in a study where participants who had variations in the *FTO* gene associated with obesity picked food with a higher energy content from a lunch buffet compared with those without these genetic variants. However, in the general population, variation in *FTO* and regions near *MCR4* genes only account for an increase in body mass of 0.39 kg/m² and 0.23 kg/m², respectively, so they cannot explain the current obesity epidemic. No genes associated with energy expenditure have been found to date.

Obesity is associated with an increased risk of medical and surgical problems

Obesity is associated with an increased risk of diseases in every system in the body (Table 32.6). In particular, it is a risk factor for type 2 diabetes mellitus (Chapter 31); the increased incidence of diabetes worldwide parallels that of obesity. Insulin resistance

Table 32.6 Health risks associated with obesity

System	Conditions associated with obesity
Cardiovascular	Coronary heart disease, phlebitis/venous ulceration, high blood pressure, high plasma cholesterol
Endocrine	Type 2 diabetes, polycystic ovary syndrome, infertility
Gastrointestinal	Nonalcoholic fatty liver disease, esophageal reflux, gallstones, esophageal cancer, hepatocellular cancer
Respiratory	Asthma, obstructive sleep apnea
Central nervous system	Idiopathic intracranial hypertension, stroke
Locomotor	Osteoarthritis, gout
Genitourinary	Cervical, endometrial, renal cancer, prostate cancer
Other	Breast cancer, cataracts, psoriasis, complications of pregnancy

is an important common denominator of obesity and diabetes. Obesity and insulin resistance carry an increased risk of cardiovascular disease.

Attempting weight loss to reverse the consequences of obesity

Losing weight increases life expectancy, decreases blood pressure, decreases visceral fat deposition, improves plasma lipid concentrations, increases insulin sensitivity and normalizes glycemia, improves clotting and platelet function, and enhances the quality of life.

To lose weight, one needs to change the balance between energy intake and expenditure - that is, between food intake and physical activity

Losing weight also involves many other factors, such as motivation, available time, and cost of and access to appropriate weight-reduction programs. Low-calorie diets contain approximately 1200–1300 kcal/day, and very-low-calorie diets contain around 800 kcal/day. Generally, a combination of **diet** and **exercise** plus **behavior interventions** such as goal-setting and relapse avoidance is more effective in inducing weight loss than diet alone. However, there are limited evidence-based interventions that can induce a weight loss greater than 5% of body weight and maintain this long term, other than **surgical treatments** (bariatric surgery).

MALNUTRITION

Malnutrition is a gradual decline in nutritional status, which leads to a decrease in functional capacity and to other complications

Protein energy malnutrition (PEM) is defined as poor nutritional status due to inadequate nutrient intake. Reduced food intake

CLINICAL BOX

A 46-YEAR-OLD MAN WITH HYPERTRIGLYCERIDEMIA AND FATTY LIVER: THE BENEFITS OF WEIGHT LOSS

Mr. C. is worried about his father's history of type 2 diabetes and cardiovascular disease. He decides to try to lose weight. He thinks carefully about where he goes wrong in his diet and realizes that evening snacking on chocolate cookies and sugary drinks is his main weakness. He decides the best option is not to buy any of these snacks at the supermarket so that he can avoid temptation. He also decides he will join a gym and attend a circuit class twice per week. Six months into this regimen, he has lost 7 kg and is feeling well and enjoying his new lifestyle. He returns to the doctor to have his blood levels rechecked. His liver function tests have returned to within normal limits. However, although his triglycerides are also lower, they still remain elevated, and his HDL-cholesterol is still low. His blood glucose is lower than before but is still classed as impaired fasting glucose. Mr. C. is upset that all the results have not normalized and feels that his efforts have been in vain.

Comment.

Mr. C. has done very well to lose 7 kg of weight. When a person with excess visceral fat loses weight, it is this visceral fat that is lost first; this is why Mr. C.'s liver function tests have improved - the liver is no longer "irritated" by fat deposits. However, obesity is only one component of risk; in Mr. C.'s case, his sex, age, ethnicity, and strong family history are risk factors that he cannot modify. That does not make lifestyle intervention futile in this case because it will be good for general health and well-being. Nevertheless, Mr. C. may still go on to develop type 2 diabetes in the next 10 years. However, being less obese and participating in regular exercise may delay the onset of diabetes compared with what it would have been otherwise. Also, if he does develop diabetes, it should be simpler to treat.

CLINICAL BOX

A 55-YEAR-OLD OBESE MAN WITH TYPE 2 DIABETES, CORONARY DISEASE, AND ARTHRITIS: COMPROMISED ABILITY TO EXERCISE PREVENTING THE LOSS OF WEIGHT

Mr. K. is a 55-year-old man with type 2 diabetes and coronary disease. He suffers from angina on effort and also from severe arthritic knee pains. When he initially presented to the outpatient clinic, his weight was 140 kg, and his height is 1.80 m (BMI 43). Within a year, he managed to lose 12 kg by dieting. He was prescribed a lipase inhibitor, which he tolerated well. However, his arthritis worsened, and he was increasingly less able to exercise. As a result, his weight increased again to 137 kg. He was referred to a surgeon and is now being considered for gastric banding surgery.

Comment.

This patient illustrates multiple problems associated with obesity and, in particular, the way a concomitant disease may interfere with weight-reduction programs. Weight loss is difficult to maintain in the longer term, with some people using exercise as a means of controlling weight. This patient lost weight initially, but the maintenance of lower body weight was further compromised by decreased mobility caused by arthritis.

leads to reductive adaptation, which includes a decrease in nutrient stores, changes in body composition, and more efficient use of fuels such as the use of ketone bodies by the brain (Chapter 31).

Malnutrition is one of the key issues faced by public health in the developing world and needs to be viewed from not only medical but also social and economic perspectives. Mortality in malnourished patients (BMI between 10 and 13) is four times higher compared with well-nourished people. The effects of malnutrition are summarized in Table 32.7. Worldwide, malnutrition contributes to 54% of the 11.6 million deaths annually among children below 5 years of age.

Maternal and child malnutrition is responsible for 35% of deaths in children younger than 5 years in Africa, Asia, and Latin America. The effects of maternal and child malnutrition include intrauterine growth restriction, stunting, and wasting. The most important nutritional deficiencies in these regions are deficiencies of vitamin A and zinc and, to lesser extent, iron and iodine (see Further Reading).

In the developed world, malnutrition is a problem in hospitalized patients who are unable to eat because of their primary problem - for instance, stroke or cancer. Gastrointestinal problems, particularly colon pathology and celiac disease (Chapter 30), or postoperative state are associated with specific nutritional problems. Malnutrition also affects a large group of older individuals.

In the United Kingdom, 25%–34% of people admitted to the hospital are at risk of malnutrition, and 20%–40% of critically ill patients have evidence of protein-energy malnutrition. Malnutrition is associated with increased morbidity and mortality, with longer hospital stays, and with an increased rate of complications. In addition to malnutrition, specific deficiencies such as those of vitamin D, iron, and vitamin C may occur.

Markers of malnutrition risk

A BMI of below 18.5 kg/m² suggests significant risk of malnutrition, and so does the unintentional loss of 10% of body weight within the preceding 3–6 months. In the course of acute illness, inability to eat for more than 5 days poses a risk.

There are two types of protein–calorie malnutrition: marasmus and kwashiorkor

Marasmus results from a prolonged inadequate intake of calories and protein. It is a chronic condition that develops

Table 32.7 Consequences of protein–calorie malnutrition

Decreased protein synthesis
Decreased activity of Na$^+$/K$^+$-ATPase
Decreased glucose transport
Fatty liver, liver necrosis, liver fibrosis
Depression, apathy, mood changes
Hypothermia
Compromised ventilation
Compromised immune system: impaired wound healing
Risk of wound breakdown
Decreased cardiac output
Decreased renal function
Loss of muscle strength
Anorexia

over months or years. It is characterized by loss of muscle tissue and subcutaneous fat with the preservation of the synthesis of visceral proteins such as albumin. There is a clear loss of weight.

Kwashiorkor is a more acute form of undernutrition, which may also occur with a background of marasmus. It also develops because of inadequate nutrient intake after trauma or infection. In kwashiorkor, in contrast to marasmus, visceral tissues are not spared: the hallmark of kwashiorkor is edema due to the low concentration of plasma albumin and the loss of oncotic pressure (Chapter 35). Edema may mask the weight loss. Complications of kwashiorkor are dehydration, hypoglycemia, hypothermia, electrolyte disturbances, and septicemia. These patients have impaired immunity and wound healing and thus are prone to infection.

The World Health Organization (WHO) classification of malnutrition is based on anthropometry and the presence of bilateral pitting edema. Another classification has been proposed by Collins and Yates. It distinguishes complicated from uncomplicated malnutrition assessing the severity of malnutrition on the basis of a decrease in weight for height, mid-arm circumference, presence of edema, and general level of alertness (See Further reading). Marasmus and kwashiorkor are terms rarely used in the hospital practice in developed countries; **malnutrition** and **complicated malnutrition** are probably more appropriate.

Refeeding syndrome develops as a consequence of inappropriate feeding of a malnourished person

The treatment of malnutrition in famine areas includes standard preparations such as Formula 100 therapeutic milk (F100). F100 is a liquid diet with an energy content of 100 kcal/100 mL.

It includes dried skimmed milk, oil, sugar, and a mix of vitamins and minerals (without iron). In areas of famine, community feeding programs use the so-called life-sustaining general rations (at least 2100 kcal; 8786 kJ/day) containing grains, legumes, and vegetable oil. During treatment, this needs to be combined with providing adequate water, sanitation, and basic health care.

It is important to take time to replete a starved person nutritionally. Too quick a replacement may be dangerous due to the possibility of a major shift of fluid and electrolytes between intracellular and extracellular compartments. This is known as the **refeeding syndrome,** and it is characterized by a severe decrease in concentrations of plasma magnesium, phosphate, and potassium (the latter because of the stimulation of insulin secretion). Also, if thiamine deficiency is present, carbohydrate feeding can precipitate **Wernicke–Korsakoff syndrome** (Chapter 7). Frequent simple meals at short intervals are recommended during famine relief, and in a hospital setting, gradual introduction of nutritional support and close monitoring are required.

Syndromes related to malnutrition

Frailty is a multisystem deterioration associated with age

Frailty affects the nervous, endocrine, musculoskeletal, and immunologic systems. It was found to affect 6.9% of American men and women older than 65 years. The presence of chronic disease increases the risk of frailty. Muscle wasting (sarcopenia) is its main feature: after the age of 50, there is a 1%–2% loss of muscle per year.

Other characteristics of the frailty syndrome are anorexia, weight loss, exhaustion, slowness of gait, low daily energy expenditure, and muscular weakness. Osteoporosis further contributes to the risk of falls. Frailty may also be associated with deficiencies of micronutrients, vitamins, and amino acids. On a cellular level, there is abnormal unfolding, misfolding, and aggregation of proteins as well as mitochondrial dysfunction. The elderly have higher levels of TNF-α and IL-6.

Cachexia is weight loss predominantly related to disease

Cachexia is particularly linked with cancer or sepsis. It causes predominant loss of muscle and might be life threatening. It is characterized by anorexia and muscle protein breakdown that occurs earlier than in common PEM due to increased muscle catabolism and reduced muscle protein synthesis. It is characterized by increased activity of proinflammatory cytokines such as TNF-α, interferon-γ, and interleukin-6. They stimulate the NF-κB pathway, which, among other effects, leads to increased protein degradation through the ubiquitin proteasome pathway. There is insulin resistance related to increased glucocorticoid secretion.

The hypothalamic effects in cachexia, also mediated by proinflammatory cytokines, lead to increased metabolic rate, lethargy, and anorexia. Commonly seen laboratory results include increased plasma C-reactive protein (CRP), reduced albumin, and anemia.

Nutritional support and micronutrient supplementation are important in the prevention of frailty. However, in the latter condition. probably the most effective prevention is the encouragement of physical exercise (see Further Reading).

Nutritional support

Nutritional support is required for a substantial number of hospitalized patients and ranges from simple assistance with meals, to enriched or special-consistency diets, to enteral nutrition and total parenteral nutrition (Fig. 32.10).

Enteral nutrition entails feeding a person through special tubes placed in the stomach or jejunum

Enteral nutrition is appropriate when there are difficulties with taking food orally but the gastrointestinal tract functions properly. Standard enteral feeds contain carbohydrate, protein, fat, water, electrolytes, vitamins, and minerals, including trace elements. Predigested feeds contain short peptides or free amino acids.

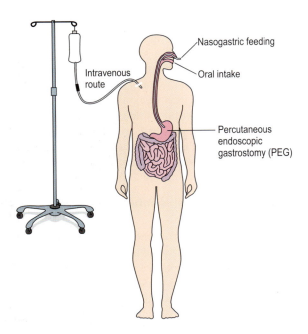

Fig. 32.10 **Routes of nutritional support.** The optimal route is oral intake. If oral intake is impossible, but the gastrointestinal (GI) tract is functional, enteral feeding is considered. This could be provided through the nasogastric or nasojejunal route. The alternative is using the percutaneous endoscopic gastrectomy (PEG), which provides direct access to the stomach. If the GI tract is nonfunctional, nutritional support can be provided by the intravenous route.

Total parenteral nutrition is appropriate when the gastrointestinal tract does not function because of, for instance, intestinal obstruction or when large parts of it have been surgically removed

Total parenteral nutrition (TPN) means intravenous feeding that covers all the nutritional requirements. Parenteral nutrition solutions contain fluids, glucose (dextrose), amino acids, and fats given as lipid emulsion (in the United States, derived from soybean oil, and in Europe also from fish oil, olive oil, and medium-chain triglycerides). Vitamins, minerals, and electrolytes are also included. Although total parenteral nutrition is life-saving in many instances, it is a treatment potentially associated with complications caused by intravenous-line infections (it requires strictly sterile procedures) as well as metabolic problems. For this reason, hospital TPN is managed by multidisciplinary teams that include specialist nurses, surgeons, gastroenterologists, dieticians, pharmacists, and laboratory medicine physicians.

The effectiveness of nutritional support using TPN depends on the cause of weight loss

Nutritional support is most effective in conditions where disease causes inability to take or absorb food or where a patient presents with a specific nutritional deficiency. Such conditions include the following:

■ Inability to eat due to oral mucositis
■ Obstruction of the GI tract
■ Radiation enteropathy
■ Short bowel syndrome resulting in malabsorption
■ Inflammatory bowel disease

Although nutritional support in patients with cachexia or sepsis tends to be less effective because of the presence of hypermetabolism, it is important in reducing muscle wasting and facilitating rehabilitation.

SUMMARY

■ Appropriate nutrition underpins health and well-being, and poor nutrition increases susceptibility to disease.
■ Food intake is controlled by the neuroendocrine system's response to signals generated in adipose tissue.
■ Genotype, food availability, state of health, and physical activity are factors that determine nutritional status.
■ Nutritional needs change during the life cycle.
■ The main categories of nutrients are carbohydrates, fats, proteins, and vitamins and minerals. Water balance is closely associated with nutrition.

ACTIVE LEARNING

1. Outline the processes that maintain energy homeostasis.
2. Describe the role of different classes of fatty acids in nutrition.
3. List the principles of a weight-reduction program.
4. Discuss instances when increased nutritional demand can precipitate malnutrition.
5. What diet would you recommend for a diabetic patient?

■ Assessment of nutritional status is an important part of a general clinical workup. It includes the assessment of current diet, dietary history, clinical examination, and a range of biochemical and hematologic tests.
■ Obesity has become a major health problem worldwide.
■ Malnutrition affects large areas of the developing world, and in the developed world, it is an issue among disadvantaged social groups and also in hospitalized persons.
■ Nutritional support includes graded assistance with nutrient intake, ranging from assistance with meals to total parenteral nutrition.

FURTHER READING

Black, R. E., Allen, L. H., Bhutta, Z. A., et al. (2008). Maternal and child malnutrition: Global and regional exposures and health consequences. *Lancetn, 371*, 243–260.
Collins, S., & Yates, R. (2003). The need to update the classification of acute malnutrition. *Lancet, 362*, 249.
Crowley, V. E. F. (2008). Overview of human obesity and central mechanisms regulating energy homeostasis, *Annals of Clinical Biochemistry, 45*, 245–255.
Dietary Reference Intakes: *Applications in dietary planning* (2003). Food and Nutrition Board, Institute of Medicine (IOM) of the National Academies.
Dietary Reference Values for food energy and nutrients for the United Kingdom (2003). *Report of the Panel on Dietary Reference Values of the Committee on Medical Aspects of Food Policy, Department of Health*. London: TSO.
Eckel, R. H. (2008). Nonsurgical management of obesity. *The New England Journal of Medicine, 358*, 1941–1950.
Gidden, F., & Shenkin, A. (2000). Laboratory support of the clinical nutrition service. *Clinical Chemistry and Laboratory Medicine, 38*, 693–714.
Management of severe malnutrition (1999). *A manual for physicians and other senior health workers*. Geneva: World Health Organization.
Mozzaffarian, D. (2016). Dietary and policy priorities for cardiovascular disease, diabetes, and obesity. A comprehensive review. *Circulation, 133*, 187–225.
Stemvinkel, P., et al. (2016). Nutrients and ageing. *Current Opinion in Clinical Nutrition and Metabolic Care, 19*, 19–25.
Vellas, B., Guigoz, Y., Garry, P. J., et al. (1999). The mini nutritional assessment (MNA) and its use in grading the nutritional state of elderly patients. *Nutrition, 15*, 116–122.

RELEVANT WEBSITES

University of Sydney - About glycemic Index: http://www.glycemicindex.com/about.php
National Academy of Sciences - Dietary Reference Intakes: https://cms.nationalacademies.org//hmd/~/media/Files/Infographics/2014/DRIs.pdf
Public Health England in association with the Welsh government, Food Standards Scotland, and the Food Standards Agency in Northern Ireland - The Eatwell Guide: http://www.nhs.uk/Livewell/Goodfood/Documents/The-Eatwell-Guide-2016.pdf
BAPEN - Introduction to malnutrition: http://www.bapen.org.uk/malnutrition-undernutrition/introduction-to-malnutrition
BAPEN - Malnutrition Universal Screening Tool (MUST): http://www.bapen.org.uk/pdfs/must/must_full.pdf
World Health Organization - Obesity: http://www.who.int/topics/obesity/en/
US Department of Agriculture - Scientific Report of the 2015 Dietary Guidelines Advisory Committee: https://health.gov/dietaryguidelines/2015-scientific-report/pdfs/scientific-report-of-the-2015-dietary-guidelines-advisory-committee.pdf
US Department of Agriculture - ChooseMyPlate.gov: https://www.choosemyplate.gov/

ABBREVIATIONS

AMPK	AMP-activated kinase
apoE	Apoprotein E
AUC	Area under the curve
BMI	Body mass index
BMR	Basal metabolic rate
CNS	Central nervous system
CRH	Corticoliberin
DEXA	Dual-energy X-ray absorptiometry
GABA	γ-aminobutyric acid
GI	Glycemic index
HDL	High-density lipoprotein
IL-6 and IL-8	Interleukins 6 and 8
JAK/STAT	Janus kinase/signal transducer and activator of transcription
MAPK	Mitogen-activated protein kinase
α-MSH	Melanocortin
MCH	Melanin-concentrating hormone
MCP-1	Monocyte chemoattractant protein-1
MET	Metabolic equivalent of task
NFκB	Nuclear factor κB
NPY	Neuropeptide Y
PDGF	Platelet-derived growth factor
PEM	Protein energy malnutrition
PI3K	Phosphatidyl-inositol 3′ kinase
POMC	Proopiomelanocortin
PPARα	Peroxisome proliferator-activated receptor-α
RER	Respiratory exchange rate
SREBP1c	Sterol regulatory element-binding protein 1c
SSB	Sugar-sweetened beverage
TNF-α	Tumor necrosis factor α
TPN	Total parenteral nutrition
TRH	Thyroliberin
VLDL	Very-low-density lipoprotein
VO$_2$	Oxygen consumption rate

Lipoprotein Metabolism and Atherogenesis

Marek H. Dominiczak

INTRODUCTION

Lipoproteins are particles found in plasma, composed of proteins and various classes of lipids. Their structure allows transport of hydrophobic lipids in the aqueous environment of the plasma. **Lipoproteins distribute triacylglycerols and cholesterol between the intestine, liver, and peripheral tissues.** Transport of triacylglycerols is linked to body fuel metabolism, whereas the transported cholesterol forms an extracellular pool available to cells. Abnormal lipoprotein metabolism is the principal factor in the development of **atherosclerosis,** a process that underpins **arteriosclerotic cardiovascular disease (ASCVD),** including coronary heart disease, stroke, and peripheral vascular disease.

Lipoproteins distribute triacylglycerols and cholesterol between the intestine and liver, on the one hand, and peripheral tissues, on the other

Cholesterol is also transported from the peripheral cells back to the liver.

Long-chain fatty acids can be esterified and stored as triacylglycerols in the adipose tissue (Chapter 13). Triacylglycerols present in food are digested and absorbed in the gastrointestinal tract and then reassembled in the enterocytes for tissue distribution.

Triacylglycerols are transported in plasma within lipoprotein particles, whereas short- and medium-chain fatty acids are transported bound to **albumin**. Triacylglycerols can also be synthesized endogenously, primarily in the liver.

Cholesterol is also transported from the periphery back to the liver. This is known as **reverse cholesterol transport**. Lipoproteins also transport fat-soluble vitamins such as vitamin A and vitamin E.

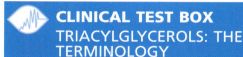

CLINICAL TEST BOX
TRIACYLGLYCEROLS: THE TERMINOLOGY

Triacylglycerols are esters of glycerol and fatty acids. They are synonymously called triglycerides, While many biochemistry textbooks employ the term "triacylglycerols", clinical literature uses "triglycerides". Here we will use the term "triacylglycerols" but when describing clinical context we will occasionally switch to "triglycerides" to famliarize the readers with both terms.

NATURE OF LIPOPROTEINS

Lipoproteins are clusters of hydrophilic, hydrophobic, and amphipathic molecules

Lipoprotein particles contain triacylglycerols, cholesterol, phospholipids, and proteins (known as apolipoproteins). Hydrophobic cholesteryl esters and triacylglycerols reside in the core of these particles, whereas the amphipathic phospholipids, as well as free cholesterol and apolipoproteins, form their outer layer (Fig. 33.1). Some apolipoproteins, such as apolipoprotein B (apoB), are embedded in the particle surface; others, such as apoC, are only loosely bound and can be exchanged between different lipoprotein classes.

Lipoproteins differ in size and density

We classify lipoproteins on the basis of either their density or their apolipoprotein content. Lipoproteins present in plasma form a continuum of size and density (Table 33.1). They are classified into chylomicrons, very-low-density lipoproteins (VLDL), intermediate-density lipoproteins (IDL; these are nearly identical with so-called remnant particles), low-density lipoproteins (LDL), and high-density lipoproteins (HDL). The VLDL and IDL are triacylglycerol rich, whereas the LDL are triacylglycerol poor and cholesterol rich. Decreasing triacylglycerol content increases particle density and decreases particle size. Thus density increases from chylomicrons through VLDL, IDL, LDL, to HDL.

Table 33.1 Lipoprotein classes

Particle	Density (kg/L)	Main component(s)	Apolipoproteins*	Diameter (nm)
Chylomicrons	0.95	TG	B48 (A, C, E)	75–1200
VLDL	0.95–1.006	TG	B100 (A, C, E)	30–80
IDL	1.006–1.019	TG and cholesterol	B100, E	25–35
LDL	1.019–1.063	Cholesterol	B100	18–25
HDL	1.063–1.210	Protein	AI, AII (C, E)	5–12

TG, triacylglycerol (triglyceride); VLDL, very-low-density lipoproteins; IDL, intermediate-density lipoproteins; HDL, high-density lipoproteins. When separated by electrophoresis, VLDL are called pre-β-lipoproteins, LDL are called β-lipoproteins, and HDL are called α-lipoproteins.
*The most abundant apoproteins present in a given lipoprotein particle are indicated first, with those that are exchanged with other particles in parentheses.

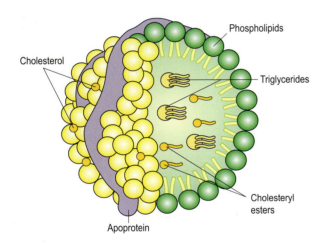

Fig. 33.1 **Lipoprotein particle.** A lipoprotein particle has a hydrophilic external surface and hydrophobic interior. The surface layer contains free cholesterol, phospholipids, and apolipoproteins. Cholesteryl esters and triacylglycerols are located in the hydrophobic particle core.

 ADVANCED CONCEPT BOX
SEPARATION OF LIPOPROTEINS BY ULTRACENTRIFUGATION

Clinical laboratories routinely use centrifuges to separate red blood cells from serum or plasma. These machines develop a moderate centrifugal force, 2000–3000 g. However, in the lipid, protein, and nucleic acid work, much larger centrifugal forces (40,000–100,000 g) are applied to plasma to separate particles and molecules. This technique is called ultracentrifugation. When centrifugal force is applied to a solution, particles heavier than the surrounding solvent sediment, and those lighter than the solvent float to the surface at a rate proportional to the centrifugal force and the particle density and size.

In a technique known in lipid biochemistry as **flotation ultracentrifugation,** the plasma is overlayered with a solution of defined density (e.g., 1.063 kg/L, the density of the VLDL). After several hours of centrifugation with the rotor speeds around 40,000 rev/min, the VLDL float to the surface and can be harvested. Solutions of different density can be used to separate other lipoproteins. Modifications of the ultracentrifugation technique, such as density gradient centrifugation, allow separation of plasma into several "bands" containing different lipoprotein fractions.

Apolipoproteins

Apolipoproteins are proteins present in lipoprotein particles; they fulfill structural and metabolic functions

Different apolipoproteins are designated by letters prefixed by the abbreviation "apo" (e.g., apoA, apoB, etc.). Apolipoproteins that are embedded into the surface of lipoprotein particles determine their interactions with cellular receptors. Others regulate activity of enzymes and other proteins involved in lipid transport and distribution. Each class of lipoproteins contains a characteristic set of apolipoproteins. The main apolipoproteins are listed in Table 33.2.

Apolipoproteins A (apoAI and apoAII) are present in the HDL particles. ApoAI is a small protein consisting of 243 amino acids. It is synthesized in the liver and in the intestine. The APOA1 gene is part of the APOA1/C3/A4/A5

complex. ApoA1 activates a cholesterol-esterifying enzyme, lecithin:cholesterol acyltransferase (LCAT). ApoAI binds to the scavenger receptor BI. It is a marker of HDL concentration in plasma.

ApoAII is also present primarily in the HDL. It is a 77–amino acid protein synthesized mostly in the liver. It inhibits lipoprotein lipase (LPL) and serves as a cofactor for LCAT and for the cholesterol ester transfer protein (CETP).

Apolipoprotein B exists in two common variants, apoB100 and apoB48. **ApoB100** is a large protein with a molecular mass of 513,000 kDa, comprising 4509 amino acids. It is synthesized in the liver. Apo B100 **is present in VLDL, IDL,**

Table 33.2 Structure and function of apolipoproteins

Apo	Genes	Examples of isoforms	Synthesis	Structure	Function	Lipoproteins	Lipoprotein metabolism pathway
AI	Chromosome 11, AI/C3/A4/A5 gene cluster	Six polymorphic isoforms Mutations: Apo AI Tangier AI Milano AI Marburg	Liver, intestine	243 AA, 28,000 Da	Structural in HDL LCAT activator	70% of HDL protein Most abundant protein in HDL Chylomicrons, VLDL	RCT, fuel distribution stage
AII	Chromosome 1		Liver, intestine	77 AA, 17,400 Da Mainly present as dimer (molecular mass above is that of the dimer)	Structural in HDL	20% of HDL protein Second most abundant after apoAI Chylomicrons, VLDL	RCT (main marker), fuel distribution stage
AIV	Chromosome 11, A1/C3/A4/A5 gene cluster	ApoAIV 360 (common) ApoAIV-1, ApoAIV-2	Liver, intestine		Metabolism of TG-rich particles Interacts with CII in LPL LCAT activator	Chylomicrons, HDL, free in plasma	Fuel distribution stage RCT
AV	Chromosome 11, A1/C3 A4/A5 gene cluster	Multiple variants	Liver		Chylomicron and VLDL assembly LPL activator	Chylomicrons, VLDL, HDL	Fuel distribution stage RCT
CIII	Chromosome 11, A1/C3 A4/A5 gene cluster	Variants with differing sialic acid content: CIII-0, CIII-1, CIII-2	Liver, intestine	79 AA, 8800 Da	LPL inhibitor. Masks or displaces apoE from LRP	Surface of TG-rich particles: chylomicrons, VLDL remnants, HDL	Fuel distribution stage RCT
CII	Chromosome 19		Liver, intestine	79 AA, 8900 Da	LPL activator: deficiency leads to gross hypertriglyceridemia	Chylomicrons, VLDL, HDL	Fuel distribution stage RCT
B100	Chromosome 2	More than 100 polymorphisms	Liver	4536 AA, 550,000 Da	Structural component of VLDL, IDL, LDL Ligand for LDL-receptor	VLDL, IDL, LDL One molecule per particle Marker of particle number	Fuel distribution stage Cholesterol distribution stage
B48	Chromosome 2		Intestine	2152 N-terminal AA of B100, 264,000 Da 8%–10% CHO	Structural component of chylomicrons and chylomicron remnants	Chylomicrons, chylomicron remnants	Fuel distribution stage
E	Chromosome19, E/C1/C2/C4 gene cluster	Three main isoforms: E2, E3, E4 Many variants	Liver, intestine, brain, kidney, spleen, adrenals, and other tissues	299 AA, 34,200 Da	Multifunction protein LDL-receptor ligand for LDL and chylomicron remnants. LRP ligand Modulates LPL, CETP, LCAT, HTGL. Antioxidant molecule Regulator of inflammatory response	Chylomicrons, VLDL remnants, HDL	Fuel distribution stage, RCT
(a)	Chromosome 6 linkage with plasminogen gene	Over 20 isoforms, dependent on number of kringle 4 repeats Kringle 4 region most variable	Liver	Variable molecular mass: 187,000– 800,000 Da pre-beta mobility High sialic acid content	HDL-2, LDL	Lp(a)	Role in fibrinolysis?

CHO, carbohydrates; AA, amino acids; RCT, reverse cholesterol transport; LRP, LDL-receptor-like protein; LPL, lipoprotein lipase; LCAT, lecithin:cholesterol acyltransferase; CETP, cholesteryl ester transfer protein; HTGL, hepatic triglyceride lipase.
See text for references.
Reproduced, with permission, from Dominiczak MH, Caslake MJ. Apolipoproteins: metabolic role and clinical biochemistry applications. Ann Clin Biochem 2011; 48: 498–515.

and LDL. It controls the metabolism of the LDL. Because there is only one molecule of apoB100 per each lipoprotein particle, the measurement of the apoB in plasma reflects the sum of the VLDL, IDL, and LDL. ApoB100 binds to the LDL (apoB/E) receptor. Mutation at its amino acid residue 3500 decreases its receptor binding and is the cause of a condition known as **familial defective apoB** (FDB).

ApoB48 is present in the chylomicrons. It is a truncated form of apoB100 synthesized from the same gene. A stop codon is introduced during editing of apoB100 mRNA ("B48" reflects that it comprises 48% of the apoB sequence, starting from the amino-terminal). It is synthesized by the enterocytes. Note that apoB48 does not bind to the LDL receptor. Its plasma concentration reflects the sum of chylomicrons and chylomicron remnants.

Apolipoprotein E is present in all lipoprotein classes. It has a molecular mass of 34,200 Da and comprises 299 amino acids. It binds to the LDL receptor with higher affinity than apoB100. It also binds to the LDL-receptor-related protein (LRP). ApoE stimulates the LPL, the hepatic triglyceride lipase (HTGL), and the LCAT. Its synthesis is controlled by three major alleles, ε2, ε3, and ε4, and it exists in three isoforms, E2, E3, and E4. The **E2 isoform** results from cysteine-for-arginine substitution at position 158 in E3 and has lower affinity to receptors. Thus in E2/E2 homozygotes, the uptake of the remnant particles is impaired and results in **familial dyslipidemia** (also known as type III hyperlipidemia).

In the HDL, apoE contributes to cholesterol removal from cells. In the brain, ApoE is synthesized by astrocytes and microglia: it affects growth and repair of central nervous system (CNS) cells. Individuals with E4 phenotype were shown to be at an increased risk of the sporadic form of **Alzheimer's disease**. ApoE also has antiinflammatory and antioxidant functions. ApoE phenotyping and genotyping is used in the diagnosis of familial dyslipidemia.

Apolipoproteins C (apoCI, apocii, and apoCIII) are enzyme activators and inhibitors, and they are extensively exchanged between different lipoprotein classes.

Apolipoprotein (a), or apo(a), possesses a protease domain and a number of repeating sequences of approximately 80–90 amino acids in length. They are stabilized by disulfide bridges into a triple-loop structure and are called kringles (the name of a Danish pastry of a similar shape). One of the kringles, kringle 4_2, is repeated 35 times within the apo(a) sequence; generally, the number of repeats determines the size of the lp(a) isoforms. Apo(a) is synthesized in the liver, and it binds to the LDL receptor. It is structurally related to plasminogen.

Apo(a) is a component of lipoprotein (a), lp(a). Lp(a) is an LDL-like particle where apo(a) is covalently bound to apoB100. Lp(a) is highly polymorphic - its molecular mass may vary from 187,000 to 800,000 Da. Its concentration in plasma is almost entirely genetically determined and is little influenced by lifestyle factors. Lp(a) is modestly associated with cardiovascular risk.

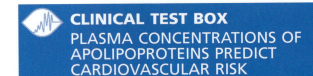

LIPOPROTEIN RECEPTORS

The LDL receptor is regulated by the intracellular cholesterol concentration

Cellular uptake of lipoproteins is mediated by membrane receptors. The key lipoprotein receptor is the LDL receptor, also known as the apoB/E receptor. As its name indicates, it can bind either apoB100 or apoE. It was discovered by Joseph Goldstein and Michael Brown, who jointly received the Nobel Prize for this work in 1985. Mature receptor protein contains 839 amino acids and spans the cell membrane. The receptor gene is located on chromosome 19, and its expression is regulated by the intracellular free-cholesterol concentration.

Scavenger receptors are nonspecific and nonregulated

Scavenger receptors are present on phagocytic cells such as macrophages. They are designated class A, class B, and CD36. Scavenger receptors can bind many different molecules. They do not bind intact LDL but readily bind LDL that has been acetylated or oxidized. Class B receptor binds HDL particles in the liver. Importantly, scavenger receptors are not subject to feedback regulation, and therefore they may overload a cell with their ligand.

ENZYMES AND LIPID TRANSFER PROTEINS

Two hydrolases, lipoprotein lipase (LPL) and hepatic triglyceride lipase (HTGL), remove triacylglycerols from lipoprotein particles. LPL is bound to heparan sulfate proteoglycans on the surface of vascular endothelial cells, and HTGL is associated with liver plasma membranes.

Lecithin:cholesterol acyltransferase (LCAT) associates with the HDL and esterifies cholesterol acquired by HDL from cells. Inside the cells, however, cholesterol is esterified by a different enzyme - the acyl-CoA: acyl-cholesterol transferase (ACAT). There are two isoforms of ACAT: ACAT1 present in macrophages and ACAT2 present in the intestine and liver.

Cholesterol ester transfer protein (CETP) facilitates the exchange of cholesteryl esters for triacylglycerols between the HDL and other lipoproteins.

PATHWAYS OF LIPOPROTEIN METABOLISM

Lipoproteins fulfill a dual function: distribution of triacylglycerols and cholesterol delivery to cells

Lipoproteins distribute triacylglycerols and cholesterol between intestine and liver, on the one hand, and peripheral tissues, on the other.

Triacylglycerols are transported toward the periphery for long-term storage in adipose tissue. Cholesterol, conversely, is moved in both directions (its transport from the peripheral tissues back to the liver is known as "reverse transport"). Cholesterol present in the lipoproteins forms an extracellular pool available to cells through the LDL receptor. Cholesterol delivered to the liver can be excreted in the bile.

Lipoprotein metabolism: The fuel distribution stage

In the fed state, triglycerides are delivered from the intestine to the periphery by chylomicrons; chylomicron remnants form after triacylglycerols are removed

After a fat-containing meal, triacylglycerols present in food are acted upon by pancreatic lipases and are absorbed *in the intestine* as monoacylglycerols, free fatty acids, and free glycerol (Chapter 30). Then the enterocyte-synthesized triacylglycerols, together with phospholipids and cholesterol, are assembled on the template of apoB48 into chylomicron particles. These are secreted into the lymph and reach plasma through the thoracic duct. They also acquire apoA, C, and E. Chylomicrons give plasma a milky appearance, and their half-life is less than 1 hour.

In the peripheral tissues, triacylglycerols are hydrolyzed by the LPL, and the fatty acids enter cells. Chylomicrons depleted of triacylglycerols become **chylomicron remnants.**

Triglycerides synthesized in the liver are transported to the periphery by the VLDL; this happens in both fed and fasting states

VLDL are assembled in the liver on apoB100 molecules in a process facilitated by the microsomal triglyceride transfer protein (MTP). After being secreted into plasma, VLDL acquire cholesteryl esters, apoC, and apoE from the HDL. Their apoB100 and apoE remain in conformations that do not allow binding to the LDL receptor. In the peripheral tissues, analogously to chylomicrons, VLDL triacylglycerols are hydrolyzed by the LPL. VLDL depleted of triglycerides become **VLDL remnants** (also known as IDL). The fuel distribution aspect of lipoprotein metabolism is illustrated in Fig. 33.2

Note that clinical laboratories measure the cholesterol content of lipoprotein particles as a marker of their concentration. Thus we infer the LDL concentration from the measurements of LDL-cholesterol (LDL-C). Similarly, we measure VLDL-C, IDL-C (or remnant cholesterol), and HDL-C.

Lipoprotein metabolism: The cholesterol delivery stage

Cholesterol present in the remnant particles and in the LDL is transported to the liver

Chylomicron and VLDL remnants are smaller and denser than their precursors. The remnant particles are relatively cholesterol rich. In the chylomicron remnants, the change in particle size uncovers the apoE, so they can bind to LRP and to the LDL receptor.

Similarly, in the VLDL remnants, apoE and apoB assume conformations that allow binding to the LDL receptor. The VLDL remnants are either taken up by the liver or depleted of remaining triacylglycerols by the HTGL, and instead of being taken up, they transform into LDL. The LDL are released to plasma and eventually are internalized by cells after binding to the LDL receptor. About 80% of LDL is taken up by the liver; the rest is taken by peripheral tissues.

After internalization, the LDL–receptor complex is digested by the lysosomal enzymes. The released free cholesterol is esterified within the cell, and the receptor protein recycles back to the membrane. The cholesterol distribution stage of lipoprotein metabolism is illustrated in (Fig. 33.3).

Plasma lipoprotein cholesterol forms an extracellular pool available to cells

Most cells can synthesize cholesterol for their own needs. The concentration of free cholesterol in cell membranes regulates the way a cell acquires cholesterol. Free cholesterol exerts negative feedback on cellular cholesterol synthesis. This is mediated by transcription factors known as sterol regulatory element-binding proteins (SREBP). SREBPs regulate the

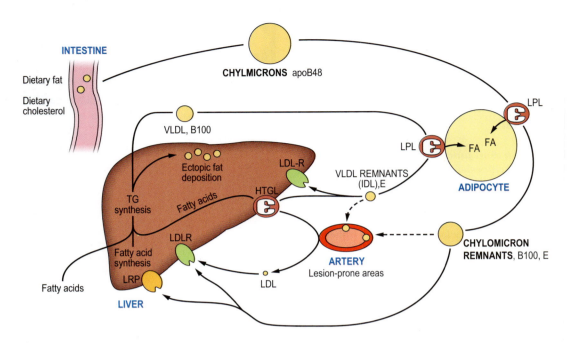

Fig. 33.2 **Lipoprotein metabolism: the fuel distribution stage.** The **fuel distribution stage** is linked to fatty acid metabolism and to the feed–fast cycle. In the **fed state,** chylomicrons transport triacylglycerols to the periphery, where the LPL hydrolyzes them, liberating the fatty acids into cells. Chylomicron remnants are metabolized in the liver after binding through the apoE, to the LDL receptor, and also to the LRP. VLDL particles transport fuel from the liver to peripheral tissues. The VLDL:VLDL-remnant pathway is active both in the fed and fasted states. VLDL are assembled in the liver and, analogously to chylomicrons, travel in plasma to the periphery. Offloading of triacylglycerols by LPL generates VLDL remnants, which return to the liver. Approximately 65% is taken up after binding to the LDL receptor, and the remaining ones are hydrolyzed by HTGL, yielding LDL particles. Apolipoproteins that drive metabolism of different particles are indicated. Those participating in enzyme activation have been omitted for clarity. Note that fatty acids contributing to liver triacylglycerol synthesis derive either from de novo synthesis, from free fatty acids delivered directly to the liver, bound to albumin, or from the internalized remnant particles. Excess availability of triacylglycerols in the liver can lead to ectopic lipid deposition (nonalcoholic fatty liver). Plasma triacylglycerol (triglyceride) concentration is the marker of the activity of the fuel distribution stage.

 ADVANCED CONCEPT BOX
VLDL ENRICHED WITH CHOLESTERYL ESTERS GIVE RISE TO SMALL-DENSE LDL PARTICLES

VLDL can enrich themselves in cholesteryl esters obtained from HDL in exchange for triglycerides. This process is facilitated by CETP. When these enriched particles are acted upon by HTGL, they yield small-dense LDL (sd-LDL), which are strongly atherogenic. Because only one molecule of apoB100 is present in each LDL particle, the presence of sd-LDL can manifest itself as **hyperapobetalipoproteinemia,** an increased plasma apoB100 concentration with relatively normal cholesterol. This condition is associated with increased CVD risk. sd-LDL could be responsible for an increased CVD risk in some patients with seemingly "normal" plasma lipid concentrations, as happens in diabetes mellitus.

transcription of genes coding for key enzymes in cholesterol synthesis - the 3-hydroxy-3-methylglutaryl coenzyme A synthase and HMG-CoA reductase - but also of the gene coding for the LDL receptor.

Cellular depletion of free cholesterol increases the SREBPs level, and consequently, both cholesterol synthesis and expression of the LDL receptor increase. Conversely, when a cell is replete in cholesterol, the SREBP pathway is inhibited, decreasing cholesterol synthesis and receptor expression (Fig. 33.3). This is discussed in more detail in Chapter 14. Thus the

cholesterol contained in plasma lipoproteins is linked to its cellular content by a precisely regulated system.

Reverse cholesterol transport

HDL particles remove cholesterol from cells

The HDL are assembled in the liver and the intestine. Their main apolipoproteins are apoAI and apoAII, but they also contain apoC and apoE. HDL acquire cholesterol from peripheral

CLINICAL BOX
DYSLIPIDEMIA IS COMMON IN DIABETES MELLITUS

Mr. B. is 67 years old, is overweight (BMI 28 kg/m²), and has type 2 diabetes and mild hypertension. When he visited the outpatient clinic, his cholesterol concentration was 6.9 mmol/L (265 mg/dL), triglycerides were 1.9 mmol/L (173 mg/dL), and HDL-C was 0.9 mmol/L (35 mg/dL). Fasting blood glucose was 8.5 mmol/L (153 mg/dL), and hemoglobin A_{1c} (HbA$_{1c}$) was 7.3% (56 mmol/mol) [desirable value below 6.7% (48 mmol/mol)]. He was being treated with diet and metformin, which improves insulin sensitivity. The patient was prescribed a statin in addition to metformin. Blood pressure was treated with an angiotensin-converting enzyme inhibitor (see Chapter 37).

Comment

The presence of diabetes mellitus carries a two to three times increased risk of coronary heart disease. This patient's diabetes was fairly well controlled (judged by the only mildly elevated HbA$_{1c}$ concentration), but his cholesterol level remained high, so he required lipid-lowering drug treatment. A low HDL-C concentration is relatively common in type 2 diabetes.

A frequent lipid pattern seen in diabetes is an increase in the plasma triglyceride concentration combined with a decrease in HDL-C. LDL metabolism remains relatively unaffected: patients often have a normal LDL-C concentration. However, because diabetic patients generate small-dense LDL, diabetic LDL, although not increased, may be more atherogenic than the nondiabetic particles. The combination of increased concentration of remnant particles (resulting in mild hypertriglyceridemia), increased sd-LDL, and low HDL is sometimes referred to as the "atherogenic triad."

cells and either transport it by a direct route to the liver or indirectly transfer it to triglyceride-rich particles, chylomicrons, VLDL, or LDL, where they follow the remnant/LDL route (see following discussion).

HDL take cholesterol out of cells

The HDL are formed as discoid, lipid-poor particles (pre-β-HDL) that contain mainly apoAI. They are partly constructed from the excess phospholipids shed from the VLDL during their hydrolysis by LPL. They accept cholesterol from cells through the action of a membrane ATP-binding cassette transporter A1 (ABCA1; Chapter 4). ABCA1 uses ATP as a source of energy and is rate-limiting for the efflux of free cholesterol to apoAI.

Transfer of cholesterol from HDL to triglyceride-rich particles is the principal route of cholesterol transport in humans

The free cholesterol acquired by the nascent HDL is esterified by LCAT. Cholesteryl esters move into the interior of the particle, which enlarges and becomes spherical - it is now designated HDL-3. Aided by the CETP, it transfers some of its cholesteryl esters to chylomicrons, VLDL, and remnant particles in exchange for triglycerides. Acquisition of triglycerides enlarges the particle further - it now becomes HDL-2. This exchange

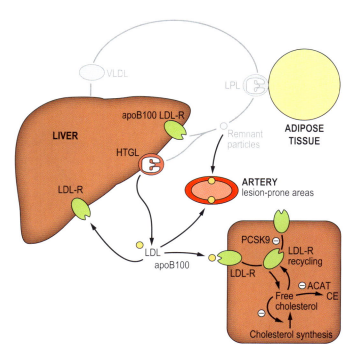

Fig. 33.3 **Lipoprotein metabolism: cholesterol distribution stage.** The LDL emerge after VLDL remnants that have been further depleted of triacylglycerols by the HTGL. The LDL bind to the LDL receptor and are taken up by cells in response to a decrease in intracellular free cholesterol. After internalization of the LDL-R complex, the free cholesterol is released and is esterified by ACAT. The receptor recycles to the membrane, a process that is inhibited by PCSK9. Intracellular cholesterol concentration regulates the activity of HMG-CoA reductase, the rate-limiting enzyme in cholesterol synthesis by negative feedback. It also controls the expression of LDL-R. The plasma total cholesterol and LDL-C are markers of the extracellular cholesterol pool. Note that the LDL (and the remnant particles) can deposit in the arterial intima in lesion-prone areas. This depends on the endothelial function and on LDL concentration. ACAT, Acyl-CoA: acyl-cholesterol transferase; LPL, lipoprotein lipase; LRP, LDL-receptor-related protein; HTGL, hepatic triglyceride lipase; CEs, cholesteryl esters; LDL-R, LDL-receptor; PCSK9, proprotein convertase subtilisin/kexin type 9 (discussed in more detail later).

route seems to be the principal pathway of reverse cholesterol transport in humans.

Cholesterol remaining in the HDL-2 can also be carried directly to the liver. There, HDL-2 binds to the scavenger receptor BI and transfers cholesterol to the cell membrane. The now redundant parts of the HDL "shell" become ready for the next cycle of cholesterol transport.

Reverse cholesterol transport is summarized in Fig. 33.4.

THE CONCEPT OF CARDIOVASCULAR RISK

Cardiovascular risk means the probability of an ASCVD event

Cardiovascular risk is the probability that a person will develop clinical ASCVD in a defined period in the future. The main cardiovascular risk factors are listed in Table 33.3.

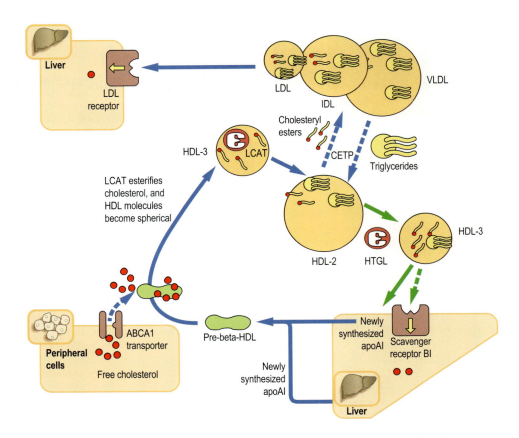

Fig. 33.4 **Reverse cholesterol transport.** HDL are assembled in the liver and intestine as discoid particles. They acquire cholesterol from cell membranes through the ABCA1 transporter. The LCAT associated with HDL esterifies the acquired cholesterol. Cholesteryl esters (CE) move to the inside of the particle, making it spherical (HDL-2). CETP facilitates the exchange of apolipoproteins and CEs between HDL and triglyceride-rich lipoproteins; as a result, the HDL-2 particles increase in size, becoming HDL-3. This exchange inserts CEs into the fuel distribution system and is the main route of reverse cholesterol transport in humans. HDL-3 particles bind to the scavenger receptor BI on the hepatocyte membrane and transfer CEs to the liver. When the transfer is completed, the size of the HDL particle decreases again. Some of the redundant surface material is released, forming apoAI-rich, lipid-poor pre-β-HDL, which reenter the cholesterol-removal cycle. Thus note the two routes of delivery of cholesterol to the liver: the HDL3 > HDL2 > VLDL/LDL > LDL receptor route and the HDL3 > HDL2 > HDL3 > scavenger receptor BI route. CEs, cholesteryl esters; LCAT, lecithin: cholesterol acyltransferase; CETP, cholesterol ester transfer protein; HTGL, hepatic triglyceride lipase.

CLINICAL BOX
RECURRENT PANCREATITIS AND SEVERE MIXED HYPERLIPIDEMIA: LIPOPROTEIN LIPASE DEFICIENCY

A 46-year-old man was referred to the lipid clinic with a history of recurrent pancreatitis and a markedly mixed hyperlipidemia with an elevated total cholesterol of 25.8 mmol/L (996 mg/dL) and triglycerides > 100 mmol/L (8850 mg/dL). He suffered from type 2 diabetes mellitus secondary to chronic pancreatitis.

Comment
Genetic testing was undertaken to screen for causes of hyperlipidemia, and the report revealed a heterozygous mutation in the lipoprotein lipase (*LPL*) gene, consistent with a diagnosis of **familial lipoprotein lipase deficiency (LPLD)**. LPLD is a very rare, inherited condition that disrupts the normal breakdown of fats in the body. Raised triglycerides are often present from childhood, but the condition may not be diagnosed until adulthood. Symptoms include recurrent attacks of acute pancreatitis and fat-filled spots known as "eruptive xanthomata." The extremely high cholesterol concentration in this patient is related to the large number of chylomicrons present, rather than to the LDL.

Cardiovascular risk is strongly related to plasma concentrations of total cholesterol and LDL-C. It is also inversely related to the plasma HDL-C.

Recent research makes it quite clear that the plasma concentration of triacylglycerols (triglycerides) also contributes to risk. There is now substantial evidence that postprandial lipemia may play a role in atherogenesis. Nonfasting plasma triglyceride concentration (reflecting an increase in atherogenic lipoprotein remnants) has been linked to the risk of ASCVD. Postprandial elevation of plasma triglycerides is particularly

CLINICAL BOX

PLASMA LIPID CONCENTRATIONS ARE AN ESSENTIAL COMPONENT OF CARDIOVASCULAR RISK ASSESSMENT

According to the US National Cholesterol Education Program Adult Treatment Panel III (ATP III), a desirable level of total cholesterol is below 5.2 mmol/L (200 mg/dL), and the optimal level of LDL-C is below 2.6 mmol/L (100 mg/dL). The risk steeply increases when total plasma cholesterol concentration increases above 5.2 mmol/L (200 mg/dL). More recently, an even lower LDL-C level of 1.8 (70 mg/dL) has been used as a cutoff point for treatment in persons with an elevated risk of ASCVD (see Further Reading).

It seems that there is no lower threshold of cholesterol concentration at which the risk would level out (in other words, the lower the cholesterol, the better).

HDL-C concentration below 1 mmol/L (40 g/dL) in men or 1.2 mmol/L (47 mg/dL) in women is regarded as low. Conversely, it seems that a concentration above 1.6 mmol/L (60 mg/dL) provides some protection against coronary disease. The principles of lipid testing in clinical practice are summarized in Fig. 33.5.

For current recommendations on statin treatment, see the Further Reading section. Note that the diagnostic cutoff points and recommended treatments change and are periodically updated by the relevant professional organizations. For current recommendations, consult the websites of organizations listed in the Relevant Websites section.

Table 33.3 The main and emerging cardiovascular risk factors

Risk factor	Comment
Male sex	Cardiovascular risk between sexes equalizes in postmenopausal women.
Age	In elderly people, age and gender alone may determine the high risk.
Smoking	
Hypertension	
High plasma total cholesterol	
High LDL-cholesterol	
Low plasma HDL-cholesterol	
Diabetes mellitus	CVD is the main cause of death in diabetes.
Impaired renal function	
Family history of premature ASCVD	Positive family history of premature CVD increases the calculated risk by a factor of 1.7–2.0.
High plasma apoB	
Low plasma apoA	Newer studies show that prediction of risk based on apolipoproteins is better than that based on cholesterol concentration.
High lp(a)	Refines risk assessment
High hsCRP/fibrinogen	Refine risk assessment
Low adiponectin	Important in obesity and diabetes
Central obesity	
Sedentary lifestyle	
Increased carotid intima-media thickness	
Social deprivation	
Autoimmune inflammatory conditions (rheumatoid arthritis, SLE, psoriasis)	

The highlighted risk factors are used in most CVD risk algorithms.

important in persons with diabetes mellitus and insulin resistance.

Whereas a decreased concentration of HDL-C is associated with an increased risk for cardiovascular disease (CVD), a high plasma concentration of HDL-C seems to be protective. The principles of lipid testing in clinical practice are summarized in Fig. 33.5.

Overall CVD risk is calculated using risk calculators

Lipid factors significantly contribute to the overall risk of atherosclerotic cardiovascular disease (ASCVD) but are not the only risk factors. Clinicians are primarily concerned with the overall risk so that appropriate preventive measures and treatments can be devised. To calculate the overall risk, they use algorithms based on data from large, long-term epidemiologic studies. The most widely used one was derived from the Framingham Study data generated in the United States. The algorithm is based on age, presence of diabetes, smoking, systolic blood pressure, and total cholesterol and HDL-C concentrations. It refers to a population aged 34–74 years without ASCVD at baseline. This algorithm does not take into account a family history of early cardiovascular disease.

In Europe, the Systematic Coronary Risk Evaluation (SCORE) and the Prospective Cardiovascular Munster Study (PROCAM) algorithms are used.

ATHEROSCLEROSIS

ASCVD is presently the most frequent cause of death in the world; ischemic heart disease and cerebrovascular disease are together responsible for 23.6% of all deaths worldwide (WHO 2011).

Atherogenesis is a process that leads to the narrowing, or a sudden complete occlusion, of the arterial lumen. The result is ASCVD. An occlusion may cause **myocardial**

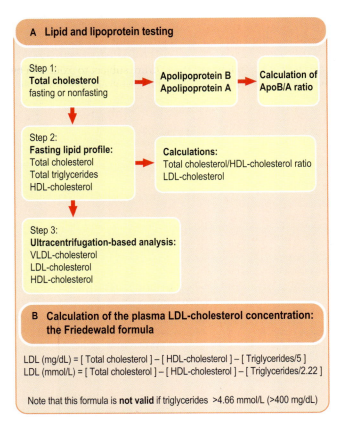

A   Lipid and lipoprotein testing

Step 1:
Total cholesterol
fasting or nonfasting

→ **Apolipoprotein B
Apolipoprotein A**

→ **Calculation of
ApoB/A ratio**

Step 2:
Fasting lipid profile:
Total cholesterol
Total triglycerides
HDL-cholesterol

→ **Calculations:**
Total cholesterol/HDL-cholesterol ratio
LDL-cholesterol

Step 3:
Ultracentrifugation-based analysis:
VLDL-cholesterol
LDL-cholesterol
HDL-cholesterol

**B   Calculation of the plasma LDL-cholesterol concentration:
the Friedewald formula**

LDL (mg/dL) = [Total cholesterol] − [HDL-cholesterol] − [Triglycerides/5]
LDL (mmol/L) = [Total cholesterol] − [HDL-cholesterol] − [Triglycerides/2.22]

Note that this formula is **not valid** if triglycerides >4.66 mmol/L (>400 mg/dL)

Fig. 33.5 **Laboratory diagnosis of dyslipidemias.** (A) The measurement of plasma lipids and apolipoproteins. (B) Calculation of plasma LDL-cholesterol concentration. Apo, apolipoprotein.

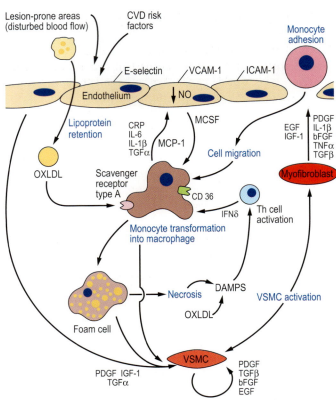

Fig. 33.6 **Atherogenesis.** Atherogenesis involves endothelial dysfunction; deposition of lipids in the arterial intima; migration and activation of inflammatory cells; continuing low-grade inflammatory reaction, migration, and activation (phenotypic switching) of VSMC; activation of both innate and adaptive immune systems; and thrombosis. Note the role of oxidized lipids in the formation of lipid-laden (foam) cells. Atherogenesis is mediated by cytokines, chemokines, and growth factors and adhesion molecules generated by endothelial cells, macrophages, T lymphocytes, and VSMC. Note the multiple activation paths that perpetuate the inflammatory response. See text for details. bFGF, basic fibroblast growth factor; CD36, cluster of differentiation 36; DAMP, damage associated molecular-pattern; IFNγ, interferon-γ; IGF-1, insulin-like growth factor 1; ICAM-1, intracellular cell-adhesion molecule 1; IL-1β, interleukin 1β; oxLDL, oxidized LDL; MCP-1, monocyte chemoattractant protein 1; NO, nitric oxide; PDGF, platelet-derived growth factor; TNFβ, tumor necrosis factor-β; TNFα, tumor necrosis factor-α; EGF, epidermal growth factor; TGFβ, transforming growth factor-β; VCAM-1, vascular cell-adhesion molecule 1.

infarction (if the blockage is in a coronary artery), **stroke** (blockage in an artery supplying the brain), or **peripheral vascular disease** (blockage in leg arteries; this leads to characteristic pain that occurs during walking, with fast relief on stopping, known as intermittent claudication). Atherogenesis involves lipid deposition in the subendothelial layer of the arterial wall (intima). This occurs on the background of endothelial damage, and it initiates inflammatory reaction (Chapters 42 and 43). Eventually, remodeling of the arterial wall takes place as a result of migration and proliferation of vascular smooth muscle cells (VSMC) and new vessel formation (angiogenesis). Thrombosis (Chapter 41) contributes to plaque maturation and destabilization. The term **atherothrombosis** is sometimes used to emphasize this. Fig. 33.6 outlines processes involved in atherogenesis.

Atherogenesis: The role of vascular endothelium

Normal endothelium has anticoagulant and antiadhesion properties

The lumen of a healthy artery is lined by a confluent layer of endothelial cells. The normal endothelial surface is strongly

antithrombotic and antiadhesive: it repels cells floating in plasma. The arterial wall itself consists of three layers: the subendothelial layer (the intima); the middle layer, the media, which contains VSMC; and the outer layer, the adventitia, composed of looser connective tissue and containing relevant nerves. Particles with a diameter greater than approximately 60–80 nm penetrate the endothelium either through junctions between the endothelial cells or by transgressing the cells themselves and then lodge in the intima.

Endothelium controls vasodilatation by secreting nitric oxide

Endothelium also controls vasodilatation and vasoconstriction and thus regulates blood flow. The most important vasodilatory substance is nitric oxide, also known as the endothelium-derived relaxing factor (EDRF). NO is synthesized from L-arginine by the endothelial NO synthase (eNOS). The activity of eNOS is controlled by the intracellular calcium concentration. The eNOS is constitutively (constantly) expressed in the endothelium, whereas another isoenzyme, inducible NOS (iNOS), is found in VSMC and in macrophages. NO signals via guanylate cyclase and cyclic GMP. A decrease in NO production contributes to arterial hypertension. **Glyceryl trinitrate,** a drug commonly used to relieve chest pain caused by inadequate oxygen supply to the heart muscle **(angina pectoris),** dilates coronary arteries by stimulating NO release.

Atherogenesis is initiated by endothelial damage

Endothelium can be functionally damaged over time by the presence of CVD risk factors such as hypercholesterolemia, hypertension, components of the cigarette smoke, and a high-saturated-fat diet and also by diabetes mellitus and obesity (Fig. 33.6). The effect is particularly evident in so-called **lesion-prone areas,** which are usually located either at branching points or curving sections of the arteries. The dynamics of blood flow in these areas damage the endothelial cells. **Endothelial dysfunction** precedes the formation of atherosclerotic lesions. Initially, the damage is functional rather than structural. The endothelium loses its cell-repellent quality. It becomes more permeable to lipoproteins, which deposit in the intima. It also admits inflammatory cells into the vascular wall. Normally, there is a balance between synthetic programs controlled by two sets of transcription factors acting as transcriptional integrators. Kruppel-like factors (KLF2, KLF4) control the antiatherogenic/antiinflammatory program, and NFκB controls the proinflammatory program. In the dysfunctional endothelium, the KLF factors become suppressed, and the NFκB predominates.

Dysfunctional endothelium increases expression of **cell-adhesion molecules** (CAMS) that include glycoproteins known as selectins and the vascular cell-adhesion molecule 1 (VCAM-1), which promotes adhesion of monocytes and T lymphocytes to endothelium. This process is further intensified by a decrease in NO production, which promotes vasoconstriction.

Atherogenesis: Contribution of retained lipoproteins

Dysfunctional endothelium facilitates entry and retention of lipoproteins in the intima

Retention of lipoproteins in the intima is the central event of atherogenesis. The atherogenecity of lipoprotein particles depends on their size. Small particles, such as the remnants and the LDL, enter the vascular wall when the endothelium is damaged. In the plasma, the LDL particles are protected against oxidation by antioxidants such as vitamin C and β-carotene. Once they lodge in the intima, this protection is removed. Fatty acids and phospholipids in the LDL are subject to oxidation by macrophages expressing a range of oxidizing enzymes, including lipoxygenases, myeloperoxidase, and NADPH oxidases. Oxidized LDL further stimulates expression of VCAM-1 and MCP-1 in the endothelium, maintaining the influx of cells into the intima; it is also mitogenic for macrophages. Oxidation of LDL also generates damage-associated molecular patterns (DAMP), small protein molecules that perpetuate inflammation.

Cellular basis of atherogenesis

Cells enter vascular intima

Adhering monocytes are stimulated by the monocyte chemoattractant protein 1 (MCP-1) to cross the endothelium and lodge in the intima. Monocytes also secrete matrix metalloproteinase 9 (MMP-9, a protease), which further facilitates their migration.

Generation of **inflammatory cytokines** and **adhesion molecules** also stimulates the exit of T leukocytes and neutrophils from plasma and their activation in the intima. Normally, migration of inflammatory cells into tissues is initiated by an antigen or trauma. Intriguingly, no specific antigen capable of initiating atherogenesis has been identified. Molecular mimicry could exist between such putative antigen(s) and the exogenous pathogens (Chapter 43). The antigen(s) could be infectious agents or molecules generated in the course of oxidation, or DAMPs generated during cell necrosis. For instance, the phosphorylcholine group found in oxidized LDL is also a component of the capsular polysaccharide of bacteria. Oxidized LDL remains a candidate antigen that could be responsible for the inflammatory reaction in atherogenesis.

Monocytes transform into resident macrophages

Monocytes transform into macrophages under the influence of inflammatory cytokines such as tumor necrosis factor-α (TNFα), granulocyte-macrophage colony-stimulating factor, and monocyte colony-stimulating factor 1 (MCSF-1), secreted by the endothelial cells and the VSMC, and interferon-γ secreted by T-helper cells. Macrophages themselves produce proinflammatory cytokines, interleukin 1β (IL-1β), IL-6, and TNFα, as well as a range of chemotactic cytokines (chemokines).

Oxidized lipoproteins are taken up by macrophages

Activated macrophages respond to cytokines secreted by the endothelium and the VSMC. They express several receptors, including scavenger receptors, CD36, and toll-like (pattern-recognition) receptors. Oxidized apoB100 binds to the scavenger receptors rather than to the LDL receptor. The recognition of molecules by scavenger receptors is part of the innate immune response (Chapter 43). In addition, DAMPs and oxidized apoB are taken up by the antigen-presenting cells, such as dendritic cells, and they activate T-helper cells present in atherosclerotic lesions, initiating the adaptive immune response. B cells also participate: circulating IgG and IgM-type antibodies against oxidized LDL have been identified in plasma.

Binding of these molecules to macrophage receptors activates the NFκB pathway and thus upregulates the cytokine, chemokine, and adhesion molecule response, enhancing and perpetuating inflammation. Because scavenger receptors are not feedback regulated by intracellular cholesterol concentration, the macrophages engorge themselves with oxidized lipids and take the appearance of **foam cells.** Conglomerates of such cells form **fatty streaks.** Foam cells continue to secrete proinflammatory cytokines.

Migration of vascular smooth muscle cells changes the structure of the vascular wall

Cytokines and growth factors secreted by endothelial cells and activated macrophages (platelet-derived growth factor [PDGF], epidermal growth factor [EGF], insulin-like growth factor 1 [IGF-1], and TGFβ) activate the VSMC in the arterial media. VSMC migrate into the intima and undergo phenotypic switching, transforming into myofibroblast-like cells. Transformed VSMC further perpetuate the inflammatory response by secreting IL-1, TNFα, and adhesion molecules. They also synthesize extracellular collagen, depositing it in the growing plaque, which forms the fibrous cap. All this disrupts the structure of the arterial wall: the newly formed plaque starts to protrude into the lumen of the artery, obstructing the flow of blood.

Finally, there is new vessel formation. The interplay of cells participating in atherogenesis and their secretory products is summarized in Fig. 33.6.

Inflammatory activity destabilizes the plaque, making it prone to rupture

Dying foam cells can be removed by efferocytosis (a phagocytic removal) or can undergo necrosis and release their lipids, which enlarge lipid pools within the intima. In the mature plaque (Fig. 33.7), the lipid pool is surrounded by foam cells, lymphocytes, and VSMC that have migrated into the intima. Macrophages continue to secrete cytokines, growth factors, adhesion molecules, and MMPs. This attracts T cells and facilitates their activation to effector cells. The plaque "cap" contains collagenous matrix synthesized by VSMC. Advanced lesions may also calcify.

An unstable plaque has fewer VSMC and contains an increased number of macrophages, which reside preferentially at plaque cap edges. The macrophages degrade the matrix of the plaque cap. In addition, lysosomal proteases (cathepsins) help degrade collagen and elastin. Activated T cells secrete IFNγ and proinflammatory cytokines that further induce macrophages to release MMPs and inhibit VSMC collagen synthesis, further weakening the plaque cap. VSMC present in the most vulnerable edge regions of the plaque may also undergo apoptosis.

ADVANCED CONCEPT BOX
A MINUTE INCREASE IN PLASMA CONCENTRATION OF C-REACTIVE PROTEIN REFLECTS CHRONIC LOW-GRADE INFLAMMATION ASSOCIATED WITH ATHEROGENESIS

C-reactive protein (CRP) is synthesized in the liver and also in the VSMC and the endothelial cells in response to stimulation by proinflammatory cytokines. The name refers to its binding to the capsular (C) polysaccharide of bacteria such as *Streptococcus pneumoniae*, by which it mediates their clearance.

Minute increases in the plasma concentration of CRP can be detected using a highly sensitive (hs) analytical method able to measure concentrations below 10 mg/L. They may reflect chronic low-grade inflammation in the vascular wall. Because the increase in hsCRP is independent of plasma LDL-C concentration, this measurement enhances cardiovascular risk assessment. It is suggested that CRP < 1 mg/dL signifies low CVD risk, whereas CRP > 3 mg/L is associated with high risk of coronary disease. Increased plasma concentrations of other proinflammatory molecules, such as IL-6 and serum amyloid A, have also been linked to coronary heart disease.

Atherogenesis: The role of thrombosis

Platelets stimulate thrombotic phenomena in the plaques

Initial adhesion of platelets to the vascular wall occurs through platelet glycoprotein receptors for von Willebrand factor and fibrinogen. Adhesion is further facilitated by β₃-integrins, transmembrane proteins that bind ligands such as collagen. Also, platelet binding to circulating cells leads to leukocyte activation.

Tissue factor, a transmembrane cytokine receptor and the primary physiologic trigger of the coagulation cascade (Chapter 41), may be expressed in the plaque VSMC and macrophages. Tissue factor complexes with coagulation factor VII (FVII), and this induces cell signaling through the protease-activated receptor 2 (PAR2), stimulating a range of events, including monocyte chemotaxis, VSMC migration and proliferation, angiogenesis, and apoptosis. Thrombin continues to be generated in the plaques. It activates monocytes, macrophages, endothelial cells, and platelets to secrete inflammatory mediators such as CD40 ligand (CD40L), a member of TNF family that, after binding to antigen-presenting cells, further amplifies secretion of MMPs, cytokines, and adhesion molecules. Formation of small thrombi contributes to plaque instability and accelerates its growth. Growth of the plaque is accelerated by cycles of plaque mini-ruptures and thrombosis. Newly formed vessels facilitate hemorrhages within the formed plaques.

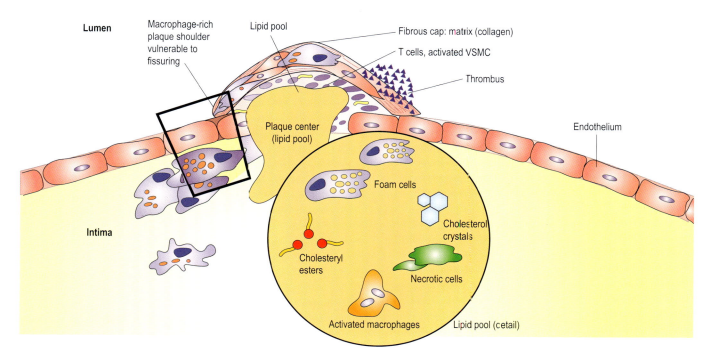

Fig. 33.7 **Atherosclerotic plaque. Mature atherosclerotic plaque.** The lipid center and fibrous cap are the main parts of the mature atherosclerotic plaque, which emerges from the structurally remodeled vascular wall. The plaque, which is cell-poor and collagen-rich, is relatively stable and grows slowly over the years. Conversely, the plaque, which is cell-rich and collagen-poor, becomes unstable and may rupture. The key process leading to plaque rupture is digestion of the collagenous matrix of the plaque cap. The synthesized fibrous cap provides a degree of protection of the plaque content from thrombosis. Rupture of the cap stimulates thrombus formation. The figure illustrates areas vulnerable to breakage and shows the obstructing thrombus formed at the site of rupture. Whereas stable fibrous plaques cause a slowly progressing angina, the disruption of an unstable, highly cellular plaque leads to acute clinical events such as a myocardial infarction. VSMC, vascular smooth muscle cell.

After a major rupture, a thrombus forming on the plaque surface may completely occlude the lumen of the affected artery, cutting off oxygen supply and causing tissue necrosis. This precipitates sudden, and sometimes catastrophic, clinical events.

 ADVANCED CONCEPT BOX
GENETICS OF ATHEROSCLEROSIS

Genes coding for the LDL receptors, apolipoproteins, and LRP6 are currently the only ones that have been directly linked with atherosclerotic disorders. Deep sequencing (sequencing a genome a large number of times to minimize the error rate) in patients of African descent identified two variants of the proprotein convertase subtilisin/kexin type 9 (**PCSK9, gene coding for a serine protease)** gene responsible for low lipid levels and a decreased risk of myocardial infarction.

The majority of cardiovascular diseases are **polygenic**. A current working hypothesis is that common variants, occurring with a frequency below 5%, are important in the pathophysiology of polygenic diseases. Associations between a disease and common variants across the entire genome are investigated using genome-wide association studies (GWAS).

DYSLIPIDEMIAS

Defects in lipoprotein metabolism lead to disorders known as dyslipidemias, synonymously but less accurately called hyperlipidemias. Their original, now outdated, classification into types I to V was based on the electrophoretic behavior of lipoproteins (Table 33.4). This classification has been superseded by the genetic one (Table 33.5). Another commonly used classification is phenotypic, which simply divides dyslipidemias into **hypercholesterolemia, hypertriglyceridemia, and mixed dyslipidemia.**

In the industrialized countries, approximately 30% of people have undesirably high plasma cholesterol concentrations. The most frequent dyslipidemia (known as the **common hypercholesterolemia**) is polygenic and is a result of the combined effect of genetic and environmental factors.

Obesity and diabetes lead to dyslipidemia caused by increased VLDL production. This can also be a result of **alcohol abuse;** however, in contrast to diabetes, alcohol, while raising VLDL, also raises the HDL concentration. Importantly, weight loss decreases VLDL secretion.

High dietary intake of saturated fats affects LDL concentration.

Familial hypercholesterolemia is a monogenic disorder caused by a mutation in the gene coding for the LDL receptor. Cellular uptake of remnant particles and the LDL is either impaired (heterozygous FH) or completely inhibited (very rare homozygous FH). Other mutations disrupt LDL-receptor recycling to the plasma membrane. Patients with FH have very high plasma cholesterol and LDL-C concentrations. The mode of inheritance of FH is autosomal dominant, so there usually is a prominent family history of early ASCVD disease (i.e., symptoms occurring in a man younger than 55 years of age or a woman younger than 65 years of age). Some patients develop lipid deposits on hand and knee tendons and particularly on the Achilles tendon: these are known as **xanthomata** and are diagnostic for the disorder. FH carries a high risk of early cardiovascular disease.

Table 33.4 Phenotypic classification of dyslipidemias

Dyslipidemia type (Fredrickson)	Increased electrophoretic fraction (lipoprotein type)	Increased cholesterol	Increased triglycerides
I	Chylomicrons	Yes	Yes
IIa	Beta (LDL)	Yes	No
IIb	Pre-beta and beta (VLDL and LDL)	Yes	Yes
III	"Broad beta" band (IDL)	Yes	Yes
IV	Pre-beta (VLDL)	No	Yes
V	Pre-beta (VLDL) plus chylomicrons	Yes	Yes

On electrophoresis, the α-lipoproteins (HDL) migrate farthest toward the anode ([+] electrode), followed by the pre-β-lipoproteins (VLDL) and the β-lipoproteins (LDL). The chylomicrons remain at the cathodic end, at the origin of the electrophoretic strip.
This classification has been developed by Fredrickson and adopted by the WHO; it is based on the electrophoretic separation of serum lipoproteins. It has been largely superseded by the genetic classification. Dyslipidemias are also simply classified as hypercholesterolemia, hypertriglyceridemia, or mixed dyslipidemia.

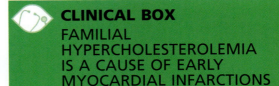

CLINICAL BOX
FAMILIAL HYPERCHOLESTEROLEMIA IS A CAUSE OF EARLY MYOCARDIAL INFARCTIONS

A 32-year-old man who smoked heavily developed sudden crushing chest pain. He was admitted to the emergency department. Myocardial infarction was confirmed by EKG changes and by high cardiac troponin concentration in plasma. On examination, the patient had tendon xanthomata on his hands and Achilles tendons. There was a strong family history of coronary heart disease (his father had a coronary bypass graft at the age of 40, and his paternal grandfather died of myocardial infarction in his early 50s). His cholesterol was 10.0 mmol/L (390 mg/dL), triglycerides were 2.0 mmol/L (182 mg/dL), and HDL-C 1.0 was mmol/L (38 mg/dL).

Comment

This patient has familial hypercholesterolemia (FH), an autosomal dominant disorder characterized by a decreased number of LDL receptors. FH carries a high risk of premature coronary disease, and heterozygotes may suffer heart attacks as early as the third or fourth decade of life. The frequency of FH homozygotes in Western populations is approximately 1:500. This patient was immediately given an intravenous thrombolytic treatment. Subsequently, he underwent coronary artery bypass grafting and was treated with lipid-lowering drugs. His cholesterol concentration decreased to 4.8 mmol/L (185 mg/dL) and triglyceride to 1.7 mmol/L, with HDL-C increasing to 1.1 mmol/L (42 mg/dL).

Table 33.5 The most important genetically determined dyslipidemias

Dyslipidemia	Frequency /inheritance	Defect	Plasma lipid pattern	Increased cardiovascula risk
Familial hypercholesterolemia	1:500 Autosomal dominant	LDL-receptor deficiency or functional impairment	Hypercholesterolemia or mixed hyperlipidemia (IIa or IIb)	Yes
Familial combined hyperlipidemia	1:50 Autosomal dominant	Overproduction of apoB100	Hypercholesterolemia or mixed hyperlipidemia (IIa or IIb) Characteristically variable patterns in different family members	Yes
Familial dysbetalipoproteinemia (type III hyperlipidemia)	1:5000 Autosomal recessive	Presence of APO E2/E2 genotype Defective remnant binding to LDL receptor	Mixed hyperlipidemia	Yes

Mixed hyperlipidemia: plasma cholesterol and plasma triglyceride concentration are both increased.

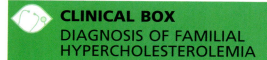

CLINICAL BOX
DIAGNOSIS OF FAMILIAL HYPERCHOLESTEROLEMIA

The Simon Broome criteria for the diagnosis of definite FH used in the UK are as follows:
- Plasma total cholesterol above 7.5 mmol/L (290 mg/dL) or LDL-cholesterol above 4.9 mmol/L (189 mg/dL) in an adult
- Total cholesterol above 6.7 mmol/L or 4.0 mmol/L (154 mg/dL) in a child under 16
  plus:
- Tendon xanthomata in a patient or first-degree relative (parent, sibling, child) or in a second-degree relative (grandparent, uncle, aunt)
  or:
- DNA-based evidence of an LDL receptor mutation, familial-defective apoB100

Comment
Currently, genetic screening to support the diagnosis of FH involves searching for mutations in the LDL-receptor gene; one is the sequence1637G>A, which results in the substitution of glycine by aspartic acid (Gly546Asp). It results in a reduced activity of the LDL receptor. Another mutation of the *APOB* gene, Arg-3527Gln, has been found in 5%–7% of FH patients, as well as a less frequent mutation of the *PCSK9* gene, Asp374Tyr.

Familial defective apolipoprotein B (FDB) is caused by a mutation of the apoB100 molecule that impairs its binding to the receptor. These patients also have high plasma cholesterol. Xanthomata seems to be rarer than in patients with FH.

Familial combined hyperlipidemia is characterized by an overproduction of apoB100 rather than the receptor impairment. There is increased production of VLDL and, consequently, increased generation of LDL. This dyslipidemia presents with variable plasma lipid patterns (either with hypercholesterolemia alone or hypercholesterolemia with hypertriglyceridemia). It is a relatively common cause of premature myocardial infarctions.

Familial dysbetalipoproteinemia, previously known as type III hyperlipidemia, is caused by a mutation in the apoE gene, yielding apoE isoform with low affinity for the LDL receptor. This leads to accumulation of remnant particles, and there is an increase in both plasma cholesterol and triglycerides. Characteristic palmar xanthomata are present. Familial dyslipidemia is associated with early coronary disease.

Lipoprotein lipase deficiency is very rare. It results in extremely high VLDL, chylomicrons, and plasma triglycerides. The latter may exceed 100 mmol/L (8850 mg/dL). Clinical signs include characteristic rash-like skin xanthomata. LPL deficiency is associated with the risk of pancreatitis (Chapter 30) precipitated by the very high triacylglycerol concentration. Affected patients often suffer repeated incidents of pancreatitis.

Mutations in the gene coding for apoB can also lead to low VLDL and, consequently, low LDL concentrations.

Abetalipoproteinemia is very rare and results from the mutation of the gene coding for the microsomal transfer protein (MTP), which is involved in the cellular assembly of VLDL.

Conditions associated with low HDL concentration

Low plasma HDL can result from mutations in genes coding for apoA1, ABCA1 transporter, and LCAT. Patients with apoAI deficiency present with low HDL-C accompanied by xanthelasma, corneal clouding, and arteriosclerosis. Heterozygotes occur in 1% of the population. They also develop amyloidosis.

Those with ABCA1 mutations, apart from low plasma HDL-C, have large, orange-colored tonsils and present with hepatosplenomegaly, peripheral neuropathy, and thrombocytopenia. The condition is known as **Tangier disease**.

LCAT deficiency is known as **fish-eye disease.** It is characterized by HDL deficiency and also by corneal clouding, nephropathy, and hemolytic anemia.

Conditions associated with high plasma HDL concentration

Deficiency of CETP leads to high HDL.

Fig. 33.8 shows how different abnormalities affect lipoprotein metabolism.

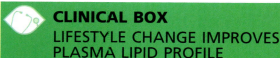

CLINICAL BOX
LIFESTYLE CHANGE IMPROVES PLASMA LIPID PROFILE

A 57-year-old man was referred to the lipid clinic because of hypertriglyceridemia. He was obese, drank 30 units of alcohol per week, and led a sedentary lifestyle.

Triglycerides were 6.0 mmol/L (545 mg/dL), cholesterol was 5.0 mmol/L (192 mg/dL), and HDL-C was 1.0 mmol/L (39 mg/dL).

After initial difficulties, he eventually managed to lose 7 kg of weight over 6 months, he cut drinking to below 20 units per week, and he started to exercise regularly. Twelve months later, his triglycerides were 2.5 mmol/L (227 mg/dL), cholesterol was 4.8 mmol/L (186 mg/dL), and HDL-C was 1.2 mmol/L (46 mg/dL).

Comment
Lifestyle change can result in appreciable improvements in the lipid profile. To achieve this, individuals need to become committed to changing their lifestyles and, in particular, to maintaining the change over a prolonged period of time.

Note: 1 unit of alcohol is one measure (60 mL) of liquor, one glass (170 mL) of wine, or a half-pint (284 mL) of beer.

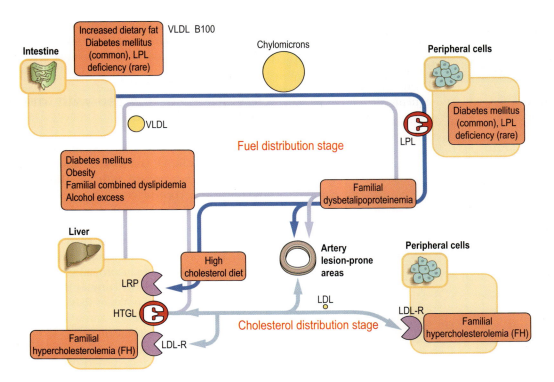
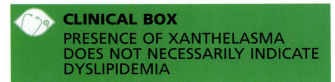

Fig. 33.8 **An overview of the abnormalities of lipoprotein metabolism. Conditions that primarily affect the fuel distribution stage.** Fuel transport is affected by excessive dietary intake of fats, obesity, and diabetes. LPL deficiency causes extreme elevation of chylomicrons and VLDL. Familial dysbetalipoproteinemia leads to an increased remnant concentration because of the impaired uptake caused by the mutation in apoE. **Conditions that primarily affect the cholesterol distribution stage.** Plasma LDL concentration can be increased due to increased generation (by HTGL-mediated digestion of VLDL remnants) or due to impaired cellular uptake or receptor binding. Most important is familial hypercholesterolemia (FH), where an impaired uptake is caused by mutations in the LDL receptor gene. This leads to gross elevation of plasma LDL concentrations. Remnant uptake is also impaired. **Conditions that affect both stages of lipoprotein metabolism.** Familial combined hyperlipidemia is due to increased apoB100 and thus increased production of VLDL. Excess VLDL causes a consequent increase in LDL generation. A high-fat diet also affects both stages of lipoprotein metabolism.

PRINCIPLES OF TREATMENT OF DYSLIPIDEMIAS

Management of dyslipidemias combines lifestyle measures and drug treatment

Effective cardiovascular prevention needs an approach that combines lifestyle modification (smoking cessation, diet, and regular exercise) with drug treatment of dyslipidemia, hypertension, and diabetes. Plasma LDL concentration can decrease by approximately 15% when a person consistently follows a low-cholesterol diet. When lifestyle measures fail to correct the abnormalities, one resorts to drug treatment. It is now accepted that the cholesterol concentration that should be achieved with treatment needs to be the lowest in people who are at the greatest risk of cardiovascular events, such as individuals with several risk factors or those who already have ASCVD, diabetes, or renal disease. There are several classes of drugs that lower plasma cholesterol concentration.

Statins inhibit HMG-CoA reductase

Statins, such as simvastatin, pravastatin, atorvastatin, and rosuvastatin, are competitive inhibitors of HMG-CoA reductase, the rate-limiting enzyme in cholesterol synthesis. They primarily lower plasma LDL. The inhibition of this enzyme results in a decrease in intracellular cholesterol concentration. This decrease (Chapter 14) increases the expression of LDL receptors on the cell membrane. This in turn leads to increased cellular uptake of LDL and, consequently, to a lower plasma cholesterol. Treatment with statins decreases plasma cholesterol concentration by 30%–60% and decreases the risk of future cardiovascular events by 20%–30%. Statins also seem to decrease inflammatory phenomena in the arterial wall.

Fibrates act through PPARα transcription factor

Derivatives of fibric acid (fibrates) are agonists of the transcription factor PPARα. They stimulate the LPL, decrease plasma triglyceride concentrations, and increase the concentration of HDL-C. Their effect on LDL and total cholesterol levels is less pronounced than that of the statins.

ADVANCED CONCEPT BOX
PEROXISOME PROLIFERATOR-ACTIVATED RECEPTORS CONTROL CARBOHYDRATE AND LIPID METABOLISM

Peroxisome proliferator-activated receptors (PPAR) belong to the superfamily of nuclear receptors that function as transcription factors. They regulate genes controlling carbohydrate and lipid homeostasis. PPARs form dimers with retinoid X receptor (RXR); the dimers subsequently bind to response elements in the promoter regions of target genes.

PPARα stimulates fatty acid catabolism, ketogenesis, and gluconeogenesis. It is also involved in the assembly of lipoproteins and in cholesterol metabolism. It increases the expression of LPL and of apoAI and apoAII, and it reduces the expression of the apoCIII gene.

PPARβ/δ is involved in the control of cell proliferation and differentiation and in fatty acid catabolism. PPARγ influences energy homeostasis and adipose tissue differentiation, and it improves insulin sensitivity. Actions of PPARα and PPARγ are antiinflammatory.

PPARs are important targets of drug action. The commonly used lipid-lowering drugs, derivatives of fibric acid (fibrates), activate PPARα. Thiazolidinediones, antidiabetic drugs, activate PPAR γ. See also Chapter 31.

Inhibitors of intestinal absorption bind bile acids and inhibit cholesterol transporter

Inhibitors of intestinal absorption of cholesterol include older drugs, the bile acid–binding resins, that are now rarely used. They decrease plasma cholesterol concentration by interrupting the recirculation of cholesterol from the intestine and increasing its excretion. A newer drug, ezetimibe, inhibits the intestinal cholesterol transporter, the Niemann–Pick C1-like 1 (NPC1L1) protein in the intestinal brush border, and lowers total cholesterol by approximately 20%.

Omega-3 fatty acids lower plasma triglyceride concentration

A substantial decrease in plasma triglyceride concentration can be achieved by treatment with omega-3 fatty acids, present in fish oil. Interestingly, fish oil preparations are also antiarrhythmic, particularly in patients who have already suffered myocardial infarction.

PCSK9 inhibitors are the newest class of cholesterol-lowering drugs

PCSK9 is a serine protease that binds to the LDL receptor. When the LDL binds to the receptor, PCSK9 channels the LDL:LDL receptor complex toward degradation rather than recycling.

PCSK9 inhibitors are monoclonal antibodies against proprotein convertase subtilisin/kexin type 9. They increase the availability of the LDL receptor and can decrease LDL-C by 50%–60%. Development of these antibodies followed the observation that people with rare gain-of-function mutations in the PCSK9 gene had hypercholesterolemia and suffered from premature ASCVD.

SUMMARY

- Lipoproteins transport hydrophobic lipids between organs and tissues.
- Chylomicrons mediate transport of dietary triacylglycerols.
- VLDL mediate the transport of endogenously synthesized triacylglycerols.
- Chylomicrons, VLDL, and remnant lipoproteins are part of the organism's fuel distribution network.
- LDL are cholesterol-rich lipoproteins generated from the VLDL remnants. Similar to the remnant particles, they are small enough to enter the arterial wall.
- HDL mediate reverse cholesterol transport (e.g., removal of cholesterol from the peripheral cells and its transport to the liver).
- Atherogenesis involves endothelial dysfunction, lipid deposition in the intima, and continuing low-grade inflammatory reaction in the arterial wall mediated by an array of cytokines, growth factors, and adhesion molecules. This leads to activation and proliferation of the arterial smooth muscle cells and to remodeling of the arterial wall.
- Atherosclerotic plaque disrupts the structure of the arterial wall and narrows the lumen of the affected artery. However, the immediate cause of myocardial infarction is not the slow growth of the plaque but its sudden rupture.

■ ASCVD includes coronary heart disease, stroke, and peripheral vascular disease. Assessment of cardiovascular risk involves measurements of several lipid parameters and identification other risk factors, such as hypertension, smoking, and the presence of diabetes. The intensity of treatment depends on the overall risk.

ACTIVE LEARNING

1. Compare the composition of VLDL and LDL.
2. What are the differences between the transport to the peripheral tissues of dietary triacylglycerols and the triacylg-lycerols synthesized in the liver?
3. Give examples of interactions between different cell types in atherogenesis.
4. How does an atherosclerotic plaque rupture?
5. In what way does endothelial dysfunction contribute to atherosclerosis?

FURTHER READING

A Report of the American College of Cardiology Foundation/American Heart Association Task Force on Practice Guidelines. (2010). 2010 ACCF/AHA Guideline for Assessment of Cardiovascular Risk in Asymptomatic Adults. *Journal of the American College of Cardiology*, 56.

Borissoff, J. I., Spronk, H. M. H., & ten Cate, H. (2011). The hemostatic system as a modulator of atherosclerosis. *The New England Journal of Medicine*, 364(18), 1746–1760.

Dominiczak, M. H. (2001). Risk factors for coronary disease: The time for a paradigm shift? *Clinical Chemistry and Laboratory Medicine*, 39, 907–919.

Dominiczak, M. H., & Caslake, M. J. (2011). Apolipoproteins: Metabolic role and clinical biochemistry applications. *Annals of Clinical Biochemistry*, 48, 498–515.

Durrington, P. (2003). Dyslipidaemia. *Lancet*, 362, 717–731.

Salisbury, D., & Bronas, U. (2014). Inflammation and Immune System. Contribution to the Etiology of Atherosclerosis. Mechanisms and Methods of Assessment. *Nursing Research*, 63, 375–385.

Tabas, I., García-Cardeña, G., & Owens, G. K. (2015). Recent insights into the cellular biology of atherosclerosis. *The Journal of Cell Biology*, 209, 13–22.

RELEVANT WEBSITES

Heart UK - Diagnostic Criteria for Familial Hypercholesterolemia Using Simon Broome Register: https://heartuk.org.uk/files/uploads/documents/HUK_AS04_Diagnostic.pdf

Framingham Heart Study: http://www.framinghamheartstudy.org/

European Society of Cardiology Clinical Practice Guidelines – Dyslipidaemias 2016 (Management of): http://www.escardio.org/Guidelines/Clinical-Practice-Guidelines/Dyslipidaemias-Management-of

Third Report of the National Cholesterol Education Program (NCEP) Expert Panel on Detection, Evaluation, and Treatment of High Blood Cholesterol in Adults (Adult Treatment Panel III) - Final Report: https://www.ncbi.nlm.nih.gov/pubmed/12485966

ACC/AHA Guideline on the Treatment of Blood Cholesterol to Reduce Atherosclerotic Cardiovascular Risk in Adults - A Report of the American College of Cardiology/American Heart Association Task Force on Practice Guidelines (Stone NJ, et al. 2013): https://www.nhlbi.nih.gov/health-pro/guidelines/in-develop/cholesterol-in-adults

National Cholesterol Education Program High Blood Cholesterol ATP III Guidelines At-A-Glance Quick Desk Reference: https://www.nhlbi.nih.gov/files/docs/guidelines/atglance.pdf

---

MORE CLINICAL CASES

Please refer to Appendix 2 for more cases relevant to this chapter.

ABBREVIATIONS

ACAT	Acyl-CoA: acyl-cholesterol transferase
apoAI/apoAII	Apolipoproteins A
apoB100/apoB48	Apolipoprotein B
apoCI/apoCII/apoCIII	Apolipoproteins C
apoB	Apolipoprotein B
ASCVD	Arteriosclerotic cardiovascular disease
CAMS	Cell-adhesion molecules
CD36	Cluster of differentiation 36
CETP	Cholesterol ester transfer protein
DAMPs	Damage-associated molecular patterns
EDRF	Endothelium-derived relaxing factor nitric oxide
EGF	Epidermal growth factor,
FVII	Factor VII
FH	Familial hypercholesterolemia
FDB	Familial defective apolipoprotein B
GWAS	Genome-wide association studies
HDL	High-density lipoprotein(s)
HTGL	Hepatic triglyceride lipase
IDL	Intermediate-density lipoprotein(s)
IL-1β	Interleukin 1β,
IL-6	Interleukin-6
IGF-1	Insulin-like growth factor 1
KLF	Kruppel-like factor (KLF2, KLF4)
LCAT	Lecithin:cholesterol acyltransferase
LDL	Low-density lipoprotein(s)
LPL	Lipoprotein lipase
MCP-1	Monocyte chemoattractant protein 1
MCSF-1	Monocyte colony-stimulating factor 1
MMP-9	Matrix metalloproteinase 9
MTP	Microsomal transfer protein
PAR2	Protease-activated receptor 2
PDGF	Platelet-derived growth factor
TG	Triacylglycerols (also triglycerides)
TGFβ	Tumor growth factor β
TNFα	Tumor necrosis factor-α
VCAM-1	Vascular cell adhesion molecule 1
VLDL	Very-low-density lipoprotein(s)
VSMC	Vascular smooth muscle cell(s)

Role of the Liver in Metabolism
Alan F. Jones

LEARNING OBJECTIVES

After reading this chapter, you should be able to:

- Discuss the role of the liver in carbohydrate metabolism and, in particular, its role in endogenous glucose production.
- Discuss the role of the liver in lipid metabolism.
- Outline changes in the hepatic protein synthesis that take place during the acute-phase reaction.
- Describe ubiquitin-mediated mechanisms of proteolysis.
- Describe the pathway of heme synthesis.
- Describe the metabolism of bilirubin and the main types of jaundice.
- Understand the basic mechanisms of hepatic drug metabolism and hepatotoxicity of drugs and alcohol.

INTRODUCTION

The liver has a central role in metabolism because of both its anatomic placement and its many biochemical functions. It receives venous blood from the intestine; thus all of the products of digestion, including drugs and other xenobiotics taken orally, reach it and may be further metabolized before entering the systemic circulation. The hepatic parenchymal cells, the hepatocytes, have an immensely broad range of synthetic and catabolic functions, which are summarized in Table 34.1.

This chapter describes the specialized metabolic functions of the liver and the abnormalities that occur in liver disease. The liver plays important roles in carbohydrate, lipid, and amino acid metabolism; in the synthesis and breakdown of plasma proteins; and in the storage of vitamins and metals. It also has the ability to metabolize, and so detoxify, an infinitely wide range of xenobiotics. The liver also has an excretory function, in which metabolic waste products are secreted into a branching system of ducts known as the biliary tree, which in turn drains into the duodenum; the biliary constituents are then excreted in feces.

The liver is the largest organ in the body and has a substantial reserve metabolic capacity

Mild liver disease may cause no symptoms and be evident only if biochemical changes consequent upon that disease are detected when a blood sample is analyzed in the clinical laboratory. However, the patient with liver disease of a severity sufficient to disrupt its normal metabolism can be critically unwell. The characteristic clinical sequelae of severe liver disease include a yellow pigmentation of the skin **(jaundice);** ready bruising and **profuse bleeding,** commonly from varicosities of the esophageal vasculature due to increased pressure in the portal circulation; abdominal distension due to the accumulation of fluid **(ascites);** and an altered consciousness level (**hepatic encephalopathy**; Fig. 34.1). This chapter describes the specialized metabolic functions of the liver and the abnormalities that occur in liver disease.

STRUCTURE OF THE LIVER

Structure of the liver facilitates exchange of metabolites between hepatocytes and plasma

The liver is the largest solid organ in the body and, in adults, weighs about 1500 g. Approximately 75% of its blood flow is supplied by the portal vein, which drains blood from the intestine. The systemic arterial circulation supplies the remainder of its blood by the hepatic artery. Blood leaving the liver enters the systemic venous system in the hepatic vein. The biliary component of the liver comprises the gallbladder and bile ducts.

Under the microscope, the substance of the liver is composed of a very large number of hepatocytes arranged in polyhedral lobules (Fig. 34.2). Portal tracts at the "corners" of these polyhedrons contain branches of the portal vein, hepatic artery, and interlobular bile ducts. Blood sinusoids arise from the terminal branches of the portal vein and interconnect and interweave through the hepatocytes before joining the central lobular vein, which in turn eventually flows into the hepatic vein.

Sinusoids are lined by two cell types. The first is **vascular endothelial cells,** which are loosely connected one with another, leaving numerous gaps. There is no basement membrane between the endothelial cells and the hepatocytes. **Kupffer cells,** the second type of sinusoidal cells, are mononuclear phagocytes; they are generally found in the gaps between endothelial cells.

These anatomical arrangements facilitate the exchange of metabolites between hepatocytes and plasma, allow the hepatocytes to receive an arterial supply, and permit the excretory products from hepatocyte metabolism destined for biliary excretion to enter the biliary ducts.

LIVER AND CARBOHYDRATE METABOLISM

The liver plays a central role in glucose metabolism, specifically in maintaining the circulating concentration of glucose

The function of the liver in glucose metabolism (see also Chapters 12 and 31) depends on its ability both to store a supply of glucose in a polymerized form as glycogen and also to synthesize glucose de novo from noncarbohydrate sources, principally amino acids derived from the catabolism of the body's proteins, through gluconeogenesis. Lipid cannot provide a substrate for gluconeogenesis. In the fasting state, when hepatic glycogen stores are exhausted, hepatic gluconeogenesis is critical to maintaining adequate blood-glucose concentrations as a fuel for those organs, principally the brain, that are obligatorily dependent on glucose as a source of energy.

Depending on metabolic conditions, the liver can either take up or produce glucose

The liver possesses glucose-6-phosphatase, which permits the release of free glucose to the blood. Although muscle stores more glycogen than the liver, it has no glucose-6-phosphatase and therefore cannot directly contribute glucose to the blood. The kidney both has the ability to synthesize glucose-6-phosphate de novo by gluconeogenesis and has glucose-6-phosphatase activity, but quantitatively, it contributes much less than the liver. Moreover, the kidneys do not store glycogen.

The adult human liver in the fasting state releases around 9 g of glucose each hour to the blood to maintain the blood-glucose concentration. The substrates for gluconeogenesis are derived from lactate released by glycolysis in the peripheral tissues and from hepatic deamination of amino acids (mainly

alanine) generated from the proteolysis of skeletal muscle (Chapter 31).

LIVER AND PROTEIN METABOLISM

Most plasma proteins are synthesized in the liver

Hepatocellular disease may alter protein synthesis both quantitatively and qualitatively. **Albumin** is the most abundant protein in the blood and is synthesized exclusively by the liver (Chapter 40). Low plasma albumin concentration occurs commonly in liver disease. It is, however, a poor index of hepatic synthetic function because in systemic illness (which often accompanies hepatic disease), there is an increased vascular endothelial permeability that allows the leakage of albumin into the interstitial space.

A better index of hepatocyte synthetic function is the production of the coagulation factors II, VII, IX, and X

All the coagulation factors undergo posttranslational γ-carboxylation of specific glutamyl residues, allowing them to bind calcium. As a group, their functional concentration can be readily assessed in the hematology laboratory by measuring the prothrombin time (PT; Chapter 41).

The liver also synthesizes most of the plasma α- and β-globulins. Their plasma concentrations change in hepatic disease and in systemic illness; in the latter case, these changes form part of the **acute-phase response.**

Response to an acute insult is associated with wide-ranging changes in liver protein synthesis

"Acute-phase response" is a term encompassing all the systemic changes that occur in response to infection or inflammation (Chapter 40). The liver synthesizes a number of acute-phase proteins, which have been defined as those whose plasma concentrations change by more than 25% within a week of the onset of an inflammatory or infective process. The production of these proteins is stimulated by proinflammatory cytokines released by macrophages, and of these, interleukin-1

Table 34.1 Functions of hepatic parenchymal cells and their disturbances in liver disease

Function	Plasma markers of impairment
Heme catabolism	↑Bilirubin
Carbohydrate metabolism	↓Glucose
Protein synthesis	↓Albumin Prolonged prothrombin time
Protein catabolism	↑Ammonia ↓Urea
Lipid metabolism	↑Triglycerides, ↑cholesterol
Drug metabolism	Altered biological half-time of a drug
Bile acid metabolism	↑Bile acids

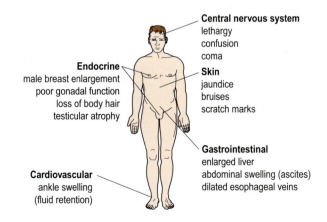

Central nervous system
lethargy
confusion
coma

Skin
jaundice
bruises
scratch marks

Endocrine
male breast enlargement
poor gonadal function
loss of body hair
testicular atrophy

Gastrointestinal
enlarged liver
abdominal swelling (ascites)
dilated esophageal veins

Cardiovascular
ankle swelling
(fluid retention)

Fig. 34.1 **Clinical features of severe liver disease.**

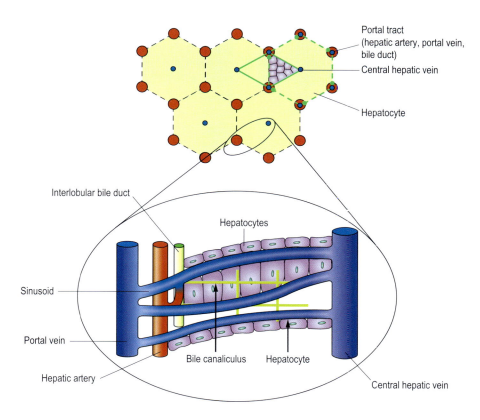

Fig. 34.2 **Structure of the liver.**

(IL-1), IL-6, and tumor necrosis factor (TNF) have a central role. The acute-phase proteins have a number of different functions. **Binding proteins,** opsonins such as C-reactive protein (CRP), bind to macromolecules released by damaged tissue or infective agents and promote their phagocytosis (Chapter 43). **Complement factors** also promote the phagocytosis of foreign molecules. **Protease inhibitors,** such as α_1-antitrypsin and α_1-antichymotrypsin, inhibit proteolytic enzymes. The latter two also stimulate fibroblast growth and the production of connective tissue required for the repair and resolution of the injury.

A substantial supply of amino acids is required as substrates for this increase in hepatic protein synthesis, and these amino acids are derived from the proteolysis of skeletal muscle. TNF and IL-1, again, are involved by stimulating the breakdown of specific intracellular proteins by the ubiquitin–proteasome system (see following discussion).

Protein degradation by the ubiquitin–proteasome system

Ubiquitin marks intracellular proteins for proteasomal degradation

Hepatic protein turnover is highly regulated, which allows metabolic pathways to adapt to changing physiologic circumstances. Mammalian cells possess several proteolytic systems.

Plasma proteins and membrane receptors are endocytosed and then hydrolyzed by acid proteases within the lysosomes. Intracellular proteins, on the other hand, are degraded within structures known as proteasomes by the so-called ubiquitin–proteasome system (UPS; Chapter 22). The discoverers of protein ubiquinylation were awarded the Nobel Prize in chemistry in 2003. The UPS is important in the activation of the NFκB proinflammatory pathway, and the function of UPS is modified by reactive oxygen species (Chapter 42).

Removal of nitrogen

The urea cycle is essential for the removal of nitrogen generated by amino acid metabolism

Catabolism of amino acids generates ammonia (NH_3) and ammonium ions (NH_4^+). Ammonia is toxic, particularly to the central nervous system (CNS). Most ammonia is detoxified at its site of formation, by amidation of glutamate to glutamine, which is mainly derived from muscle and is used as an energy source by the enterocytes. The remaining nitrogen enters the portal vein either as ammonia or as alanine, both of which are used by the liver for the synthesis of **urea** (Chapter 15).

Impaired clearance of ammonia causes brain damage

The urea cycle is the major route by which waste nitrogen is excreted; it is described in Chapter 15. In neonates, inherited defects of any of the enzymes of the urea cycle lead to **hyperammonemia,** which impairs the function of the brain, causing encephalopathy. Such problems arise within the first 48 h of life and inevitably are made worse by protein-rich foods such as milk.

HEME SYNTHESIS

Heme is a constituent of hemoglobin, myoglobin, and cytochromes

Heme is synthesized in most cells of the body. The liver is the main nonerythrocyte source of its synthesis. Heme is a por-phyrin, a cyclic compound that contains four pyrrole rings linked together by methenyl bridges. It is synthesized from glycine and succinyl-coenzyme A, which condense to form **5-aminolevulinate (5-ALA).** This reaction is catalyzed by 5-ALA synthase, located in mitochondria, and is rate limiting in heme synthesis. Subsequently, in the cytosol, two molecules of 5-ALA condense to form a molecule containing a pyrrole ring, **porphobilinogen (PBG).** Then four PBG molecules combine to form a linear tetrapyrrole compound, which cyclizes to yield uroporphyrinogen III and then coproporphyrinogen III. The final stages of the pathway occur again in the mito-chondria, where a series of decarboxylation and oxidation of side chains in uroporphyrinogen III yield protoporphyrin IX. At the final stage, iron (Fe^{2+}) is added by ferrochelatase to protoporphyrin IX to form heme. Heme controls the rate of its synthesis by feedback inhibition of 5-ALA synthase (Fig. 34.3).

✦ ADVANCED CONCEPT BOX
THE PORPHYRIAS

Defects in the heme synthetic pathway lead to rare disorders known as porphyrias. Different porphyrias are caused by deficien-cies of different enzymes in the biosynthetic pathway, starting from 5-ALA synthase and ending with ferrochelatase. Porphyrias are classified as hepatic or erythropoietic, depending on the primary organ affected.

Three porphyrias are known as **acute porphyrias** and can be a cause of emergency admissions to hospital with abdominal pain (which needs to be differentiated from various surgical causes). They also cause neuropsychiatric symptoms. **Acute intermittent porphyria (AIC)** is caused by the deficiency of hydroxymethylbilane synthase, an enzyme converting PBG to a linear tetrapyrrole; in this disorder, the concentrations of 5-ALA and PBG increase in the plasma and urine. **Hereditary copro-porphyria** is due to a defect in the conversion of coproporphy-rinogen III to protoporphyrinogen III (coprooxidase). The third acute porphyria is **variegate porphyria,** the clinical manifesta-tions of which are very similar to those of AIC.

Other porphyrias, such as porphyria cutanea tarda, present clinically as the sensitivity of skin to light **(photosensitivity),** which may cause disfiguration and scarring. Also, the pathway is inhibited by metallic lead at the stage of porphobilinogen synthase.

BILIRUBIN METABOLISM

Excess bilirubin causes jaundice

Bilirubin is the catabolic product of heme. About 75% of all bilirubin is derived from the breakdown of hemoglobin from senescent red blood cells, which are phagocytosed by mono-nuclear cells of the spleen, bone marrow, and liver (reticulo-endothelial cells). In normal adults, the daily load of bilirubin is 250–350 mg. The ring structure of heme is oxidatively cleaved to biliverdin by heme oxygenase, a P-450 cytochrome (see following discussion). Biliverdin is, in turn, enzymatically reduced to bilirubin (Fig. 34.4). The normal plasma concentra-tion of bilirubin is less than 21 μmol/L (1.2 mg/dL). Increased concentrations (more than 50 μmol/L, or 3 mg/dL) can be recognized clinically because at this concentration or more, bilirubin imparts a yellow color to the skin and conjunctivae known clinically as jaundice, or icterus. Jaundice is a clinically important sign to the presence of significant liver disease.

Bilirubin is metabolized by the hepatocytes and excreted in bile

Whereas biliverdin is water soluble, bilirubin, paradoxically, is not. Therefore it must be further metabolized before excretion (Fig. 34.5). Bilirubin produced by the catabolism of heme in the reticuloendothelial cells is transported in plasma bound to albumin. The hepatic uptake of bilirubin is mediated by a membrane carrier and may be competitively inhibited by other organic anions. The hydrophilicity of bilirubin is increased by esterification, usually known as conjugation, of one or both of its carboxylic acid side chains with glucuronic acid, xylose, or ribose. The glucuronide diester is the major conjugate, and its formation is catalyzed by the uridine diphosphate (UDP)-glucuronyl transferase. Conjugated bilirubin is water soluble and may be secreted by the hepatocyte into the biliary canaliculi. If this excretory process is impaired and the patient becomes jaundiced, some conjugated bilirubin may be excreted in the urine, which is then characteristically dark in color.

Conjugated bilirubin in the gut is catabolized by bacteria to form stercobilinogen, also known as fecal urobilinogen, which is colorless. Stercobilinogen is oxidized to stercobilin (otherwise known as fecal urobilin), which is colored; stercobilin is mainly responsible for the color of feces. Some stercobilin may be reabsorbed from the gut and can then be reexcreted by either the liver or the kidneys. If the biliary excretion of conjugated bilirubin is impaired by a disease that obstructs the flow of bile into the intestine (obstructive jaundice), no stercoblinogen/stercobilin is formed, and the feces is pale in color.

BILE ACIDS AND CHOLESTEROL METABOLISM

Bile acids are key elements in fat metabolism

Bile acids are synthesized in the hepatocytes and have a detergent-like effect in the intestinal lumen, solubilizing biliary

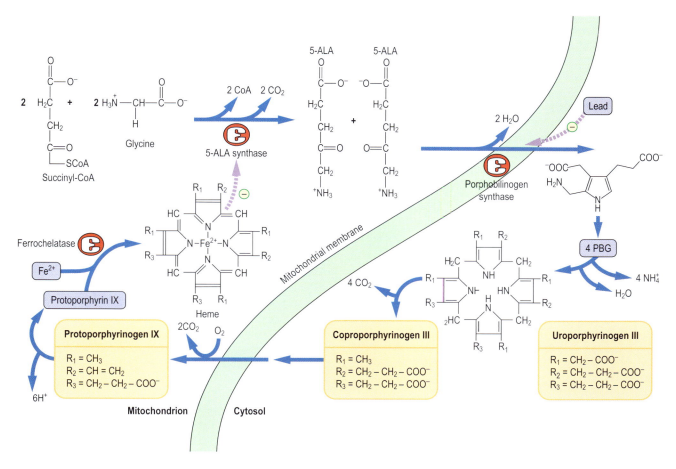

Fig. 34.3 **The pathway of heme synthesis.** Part of the pathway is located in the mitcchondria and part in the cytosol, as shown. ALA, 5-aminolevulinate; PBG, porphobilinogen. Hemoglobin is discussed in Chapter 5.

lipids and emulsifying dietary fat to facilitate its digestion. Bile acid metabolism is described in Chapter 14. Biliary excretion is also the only route by which cholesterol can be eliminated from the body.

DRUG METABOLISM

The low substrate specificity of some hepatic enzymes produces a wide-ranging capability for drug metabolism

Most drugs are metabolized in the liver. Among other effects, this hepatic metabolism usually increases the hydrophilicity of drugs and therefore their ability to be excreted by the kidneys or in bile. Generally, drug metabolites are less pharmacologically active than the parent drugs; however, some drugs are inactive when administered but are converted to their active forms as a result of liver metabolism (pro-drugs). The hepatic drug-metabolizing systems must be able to deal with an infinite range of molecules that could be encountered after ingestion or administration; this is achieved by the responsible enzymes involved having low substrate specificity.

Drug metabolism proceeds in two phases

Phase I is the addition of a polar group: the polarity of the drug is increased by its oxidation or hydroxylation, catalyzed by a family of microsomal enzymes known collectively as cytochrome P-450 oxidases.

Phase II is conjugation: cytoplasmic enzymes conjugate the functional groups introduced in the first-phase reactions, most often by glucuronidation or sulfation but also by acetylation and methylation.

Three of the 18 cytochrome P-450 gene families share the responsibility for drug metabolism

The human cytochrome P-450 (CYP) superfamily is made up of 18 families and 43 subfamilies containing 57 genes and 59 pseudogenes. The cytochrome P-450 enzymes are heme-containing proteins that colocalize with NADPH:cytochrome P-450 reductase. They are present in the endoplasmic reticulum. Most of the metabolic activities associated with the cytochrome P-450 superfamily takes place in the liver, but these enzymes are also present in the epithelium of the small intestine. The reaction sequence catalyzed by these enzymes is shown in Fig. 34.6. There are 18 cytochrome P-450 gene families, of which 3, designated *CYP1*, *CYP2*, and *CYP3*, are responsible for most of the phase I drug metabolism. Of these, CYP1A2, CYP3A4, CYP2B6, CYP2C9, CYP2C19, CYP2D6, and CYP2E1 are responsible for approximately 90% of drug metabolism. Of these, CYP3A4 is responsible for most metabolic transformations, but mounting evidence demonstrates that CYP2B6 plays a much larger role in human drug metabolism than was previously believed. Drugs are often administered in cocktails and clinically important drug–drug interactions (DDI) can occur when drugs that share a common CYP metabolic fate are coadministered. Many DDIs are well recognized.

Induction and competitive inhibition of cytochrome P-450 enzymes underpin mechanisms of drug interactions

Hepatic synthesis of cytochromes P-450 is induced by certain drugs and other xenobiotic agents that increase the rate of the phase I reactions. Conversely, drugs that form a relatively stable complex with a particular cytochrome P-450 inhibit the metabolism of other drugs that are normally substrates for that cytochrome. For instance, CYP1A2 metabolizes, among others, caffeine and theophylline. It can be inhibited by grapefruit juice, which contains a substance known as naringin,

or by the antibiotic ciprofloxacin. When a person takes any of the inhibitory substances, normal substrates for CYP1A2 are metabolized more slowly, and their plasma levels increase.

The dose of the immunosuppressant ciclosporin may need to be reduced by up to 75% if the patient also takes the antifungal drug ketoconazole (see Wilkinson in Further Reading) to avoid adverse clinical reactions.

The drugs that induce induction or repression of CYP3A enzymes often act through the nuclear receptor mechanism. They combine with nuclear receptors (i.e., in the case of CYP3A4, the pregnane X receptor [PXR]), which then form heterodimers with retinoid X receptors (Chapter 14). Such complexes upregulate CYP3 synthesis by binding to response elements in the gene promoter.

Cytochrome P-450 gene polymorphisms determine the response to many drugs

Allelic variation that affects the catalytic activity of a cytochrome P-450 also affects the pharmacologic activity of drugs. The best-described example of such polymorphism is that of the P-450 cytochrome CYP2D6, which was recognized initially in the 5%–10% of normal individuals who were noted to be slow to hydroxylate debrisoquine, a now little-used blood pressure–lowering drug. However, CYP2D6 also metabolizes

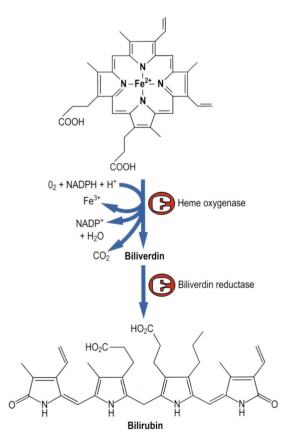

Fig. 34.4 **Degradation of heme to bilirubin.**

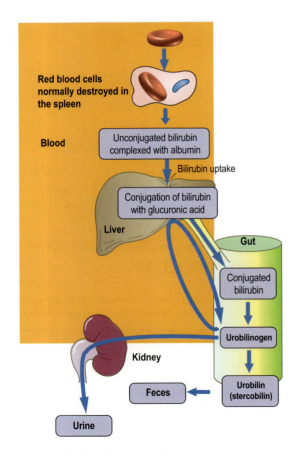

Fig. 34.5 **Normal bilirubin metabolism.**

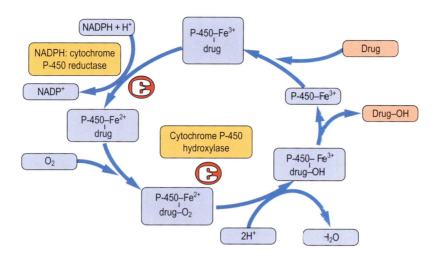

Fig. 34.6 **Role of the cytochrome P-450 system in the metabolism of drugs.**

a significant number of other commonly used drugs so that "debrisoquine polymorphism" remains clinically significant.

The antiplatelet drug clopidogrel is given together with aspirin in patients with coronary artery disease after a revascularization procedure. However, approximately 25% of patients experience a subtherapeutic antiplatelet response to clopidogrel. Clopidogrel is a prodrug that undergoes hepatic biotransformation by CYP2C19 into its active metabolite. Several studies have reported that carriers of the CYP2C19 variant allele exhibit a significantly lower capacity to transform clopidogrel to its active metabolite and are therefore at significantly higher risk of adverse cardiovascular events. Consequently, in the United States, the Food and Drug Administration (FDA) has recently changed clopidogrel prescribing information to highlight the impact of CYP2C19 genotype on the clinical response to clopidogrel.

Genotyping of cytochromes P-450 to identify gene-relevant polymorphisms may become more common in an attempt to personalize an individual's response to a particular drug.

Drug hepatotoxicity

Drugs that exert their toxic effects on the liver may do so through the hepatic production of a toxic metabolite

Drug-induced liver injury (DILI) may occur in all individuals exposed to a sufficient concentration of a particular drug. However, a drug may be toxic in some individuals at concentrations normally tolerated by most other patients. This phenomenon is known as idiosyncratic drug toxicity and may be due to a genetic or immunologic cause. The potential for DILI to be responsible for an individual's hepatic dysfunction may therefore not be obvious if it is not a recognized toxic effect of the drug, and the routine biochemical liver function tests are unhelpful.

The commonly used drug acetaminophen (paracetamol) is hepatotoxic in excess

Acetaminophen is widely used as a painkiller and is available without prescription. Taken in the usual therapeutic dose, it is eliminated by conjugation with glucuronic acid or sulfate, which are then excreted through the kidney. In acetaminophen overdose, the capacity of the normal conjugation pathways is overwhelmed, and acetaminophen is oxidized by a liver P-450 cytochrome CYP3A4 to N-acetyl benzoquinoneimine (NABQI). NABQI can cause a free radical–mediated peroxidation of membrane lipids and consequently lead to hepatocellular damage, which may be sufficiently serious to lead to fulminant hepatic failure and the patient's death. NABQI may be detoxified by conjugation with glutathione, but in acetaminophen overdose, glutathione stores also become exhausted, and hepatotoxicity ensues (Fig. 34.7). Therapeutically, a sulfhydryl compound, N-acetylcysteine (NAC), is routinely used as an antidote in acetaminophen poisoning. It promotes detoxification of NABQI by the glutathione pathway and also scavenges free radicals. The risk of hepatotoxicity can be reliably predicted from measurement of the plasma concentration of acetaminophen in relation to the time that has elapsed since the overdose, and NAC can be given to patients who are at risk of liver damage. Measurement of acetaminophen is one the toxicologic tests offered on an emergency basis by clinical laboratories.

ALCOHOL

Alcohol excess is a major cause of liver disease

Excess intake of ethyl alcohol (ethanol) is a common cause of liver disease. Ethanol may cause excessive fat deposition in the liver **(alcoholic steatosis),** and this may progress to **hepatitis**

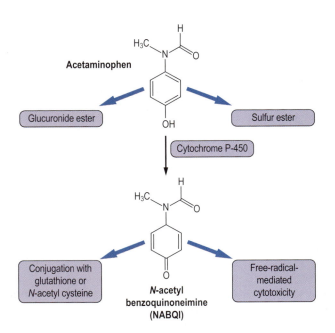

Fig. 34.7 **Metabolism of acetaminophen (paracetamol).**

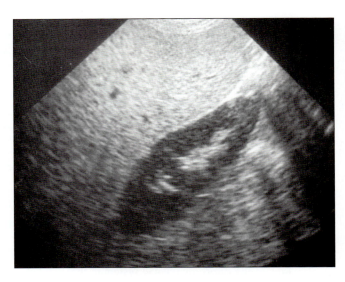

Fig. 34.8 **An ultrasound scan of a liver showing steatosis.** Courtesy Dr. A. Bannerjee, Heart of England NHS Foundation Trust UK.

and finally **fibrosis** (known as **cirrhosis**), which in turn leads to **liver failure.** There are more than 25,000 deaths associated with liver disease in the United States annually, and 40% of these are linked to alcoholic cirrhosis (see Donohue in Further Reading).

Ethanol is oxidized in the liver, mainly by alcohol dehydrogenase (ADH), to form acetaldehyde, which is in turn oxidized by aldehyde dehydrogenase (ALDH) to acetate. Nicotinamide adenine dinucleotide (NAD$^+$) is the cofactor for both these oxidations, being reduced to NADH. A P-450 cytochrome, CYP2E1, also contributes to ethanol oxidation but is quantitatively less important than the ADH–ALDH pathway. Liver damage in patients who abuse alcohol may arise from the toxicity of acetaldehyde, which forms Schiff base adducts with other macromolecules.

Ethanol oxidation alters the redox potential of the hepatocyte

Ethanol oxidation results in the increased ratio of NADH to NAD$^+$ within the hepatic parenchymal cells. Pyruvate is the end product of glycolysis, and this oxidative pathway also reduces NAD$^+$ to NADH. To permit glycolysis to continue unchecked, NADH is oxidized to NAD$^+$ via the mechanism of pyruvate reduction to lactate, with NADH being oxidized to NAD$^+$. The altered ratio of NADH/ NAD$^+$ after ethanol further promotes the reduction of pyruvate to lactate and creates the potential for the development of lactic acidosis. Because pyruvate is a substrate for hepatic gluconeogenesis, there is also a risk of hypoglycemia. The risk of hypoglycemia is further increased in alcoholics when, because of poor nutrition, they have low hepatic glycogen stores. Also, the shift in the NADH/ NAD$^+$ ratio inhibits β-oxidation of fatty acids and promotes triglyceride synthesis: excess triglycerides are deposited in the liver and secreted into the plasma as VLDL (see Clinical Box in Chapter 32, p. 477). Hepatic steatosis can be readily diagnosed by ultrasonography of the liver when one sees a uniform increased echogenicity (Fig. 34.8). It is often associated with an elevation in serum levels of the transaminase enzymes released by damaged hepatic parenchymal cells.

Ethanol consumption also affects the ubiquitin system of protein degradation (Chapter 22). Chronic alcohol consumption decreases proteasome activity. This can deregulate the hepatocyte signaling system by inhibiting the Janus kinase / signal transducer and activator of transcription (JAK/STAT) signaling pathway, which is involved in the acute-phase response, antiviral defense, and hepatic repair (Chapter 25). Inhibition of proteasome activity may also lead to increased apoptosis (Chapter 28), a feature of **alcoholic liver disease (ALD).** The ethanol-induced decrease in proteasome activity prevents the degradation of CYP2E1, which is involved in peroxidation reactions; this increases oxidative stress and may be another factor contributing to ALD.

Finally, the alcohol-induced decrease in proteasome activity may lead to the accumulation of protein in the liver, which in turn causes liver enlargement (hepatomegaly; common in ALD). Other ethanol-induced phenomena include increased secretion of chemokines (including IL-8 and monocyte-chemoattractant protein-1, MCP-1; Chapter 33) by hepatocytes, leading to liver infiltration by neutrophils.

Symptoms of alcohol intolerance are exploited to reinforce abstinence

Both ADH and ALDH are subject to genetic polymorphisms, which have been investigated as a potential inherited basis of susceptibility to alcoholism and ALD. Possession of the ALDH2^2 allele, which encodes an enzyme with reduced catalytic activity, leads to increased plasma concentrations of acetaldehyde after the ingestion of alcohol. This causes the individual to experience unpleasant flushing and sweating, which discourages alcohol abuse. Disulfiram, a drug that inhibits ALDH, also causes these symptoms when alcohol is taken and may be given to reinforce abstinence from alcohol.

PHARMACOGENOMICS

The response to any particular drug is influenced by the drug's kinetic properties (pharmacokinetics) and its effects (pharmacodynamics)

An individual's response to a drug can be influenced by genes that code for drug-metabolizing enzymes, receptors, and transporters. Any variability in these genes may lead to interindividual differences in response to that drug.

The effectiveness and safety of drug therapy, particularly in elderly patients or those with renal or hepatic diseases as comorbidities, and in patients whose metabolic capacity is diminished, is currently a major problem. Approximately 3% of US hospital admissions are linked to drug–drug interactions, and a Dutch study reported values as high as 8.4%. In the United States, there are 2 million cases of adverse drug reactions annually, including 100,000 deaths. Combined with the fact that most drugs are effective in only 25%–60% of patients to whom they are prescribed, this makes research into individual response to drugs absolutely essential.

Pharmacogenomics studies the effects of genetic heterogeneity on drug responsiveness

Because the liver plays a central role in drug metabolism, the pharmacogenomics of some hepatic drug-metabolizing enzymes, specifically the cytochrome P-450 oxidases, is clinically very relevant. CYP2D6 is responsible for the metabolism of more than 100 pharmaceuticals, and a polymorphism of this enzyme is responsible for the long-established variation in the metabolism of debrisoquine, mentioned earlier. Patients are classified as ultra-rapid, extensive, intermediate, and poor metabolizers of debrisoquine. There is one CYP2D6 genetic locus, and individuals may have two, one, or no functional alleles corresponding to extensive, intermediate, and poor metabolizers, respectively; gene multiplication can lead to three functional alleles and the ultra-rapid metabolizer phenotype. Seventy five CYP2D6 allelic variants have been identified, and pharmacogenetic techniques can identify the metabolizer phenotype, thereby predicting clinical response to treatment. Although debrisoquine is now obsolete, the CYP2D6 polymorphism is relevant for some drugs used in cardiac and psychiatric practice. For instance, poor metabolizers are more likely than other individuals to experience drug toxicity, and they are less likely to gain benefit from the analgesic codeine, a prodrug that is metabolized by CYP2D6 to morphine, the active drug. A polymorphism of CYP2C19, again leading to extensive and poor metabolizer phenotypes, affects the metabolism of the proton-pump inhibitor drugs used in gastroesophageal reflux disease and the effectiveness of treatment (Chapter 4).

BIOCHEMICAL TESTS OF LIVER FUNCTION

Clinical laboratories offer a panel of measurements on plasma or serum specimens (Table 34.2). This group of tests is usually, and incorrectly, described as liver "function" tests. Although plasma activities of liver enzymes are markers of liver disease, they do not exactly reflect the function of the liver. Prothrombin synthesis, assessed by prothrombin time (PT), is a better indicator of liver synthetic function.

The tests commonly include measurements of the following:

- Bilirubin
- Albumin
- Aspartate aminotransferase (AST) and alanine aminotransferase (ALT)
- Alkaline phosphatase (ALP)
- γ-Glutamyl transpeptidase (GGT)

Transaminases

AST and ALT are involved in the interconversion of amino and keto acids and are required for metabolism of proteins and carbohydrates (Chapter 15). Both are located in the

Table 34.2 Laboratory tests used in differential diagnosis of jaundice			
Test	Prehepatic	Intrahepatic	Posthepatic
Bilirubin	Increased	Increased	Increased
Conjugated bilirubin	Absent	Increased	Increased
AST and ALT	Normal	Increased	Normal
ALP	Normal	Normal	Increased
Urine bilirubin	Absent	Present	Present
Urine urobilinogen	Present	Present	Absent

Reference ranges for liver function tests:
AST (aspartate aminotransferase), men 15–40 U/L, women 13–35 U/L;
ALT (alanine aminotransferase), men 10–40 U/L, women 7–35 U/L; ALP
(alkaline phosphatase), 50–140 U/L: ALP is physiologically elevated in
children and adolescents; bilirubin 3-16 μmol/L (0.18–0.94 mg/dL); GGT
(γ-glutamyl transpeptidase men < 90 U/L, women < 50 U/L.

mitochondria; ALT is also found in the cytoplasm. Serum activity of ALT and AST increases in liver disease (ALT is the more sensitive measurement due to its cytoplasmic location).

Prothrombin time

In liver disease, the synthetic functions of the hepatocytes are likely to be affected, and so the patient would be expected to have a prolonged prothrombin time (Chapter 41) and low serum albumin concentration.

Alkaline phosphatase

ALP is synthesized both by the biliary tract and by bone, and in pregnancy by the placenta, but these tissues contain different ALP isoenzymes. The origin of the ALP may be determined from the isoenzyme pattern. Alternatively, the plasma activity of another enzyme, such as γ-glutamyl transpeptidase (GGT), which also originates in the biliary tract, may be measured and used to confirm the hepatic origin for a raised serum ALP activity.

CLASSIFICATION OF LIVER DISORDERS

Hepatocellular disease

Inflammatory disease of the liver is termed **hepatitis** and may be of short (acute) or long (chronic) duration. Viral infections,

CLINICAL BOX
A SEEMINGLY HEALTHY 45-YEAR-OLD MAN WITH ABNORMAL TRANSAMINASES

A 45-year-old businessman had a routine medical examination, at which he was found to have a slightly enlarged liver. Tests revealed bilirubin 15 μmol/L (0.9 mg/dL), AST 434 U/L, ALT 198 U/L, ALP 300 U/L, GGT 950 U/L, and albumin 40 g/L (4 g/dL). He seemed perfectly well.

Comment
The patient has asymptomatic liver disease. The biochemical tests show evidence of hepatocellular damage. This may be due to excess alcohol intake, in which case there may also be enlarged red blood cells (macrocytosis) and an increased serum uric acid concentration. Patients may deny alcohol abuse. **Nonalcoholic fatty liver disease** (NAFLD) is increasingly recognized as a cause of isolated abnormalities in serum transaminase concentrations. NAFLD occurs in 40% of patients with the so-called metabolic syndrome, in which central overweight due to the accumulation of visceral fat leads to insulin resistance, hypertension, dyslipidemia, and hepatic steatosis. The latter may lead to cirrhosis, as may alcohol-induced liver disease. The risk of fibrosis can be calculated from a variety of laboratory parameters, and those at highest risk may have a specialized liver scan to identify fibrotic changes noninvasively. However, biopsy of the liver may be necessary for diagnosis. Other causes, such as chronic viral infection of the liver or an autoimmune active chronic hepatitis, can be detected by blood tests. For reference ranges, see Table 35.2.

particularly hepatitis A and E, are common infectious causes of acute hepatitis, whereas alcohol and acetaminophen are the most common toxicologic causes, and metabolic syndrome is now a very common cause. Chronic hepatitis, defined as inflammation persisting for more than 6 months, may also be due to the hepatitis B and C viruses, alcohol, and immunologic diseases, in which the body produces antibodies against its own tissues (autoimmune diseases; Chapter 43). **Cirrhosis** is the result of chronic hepatitis and is characterized microscopically by fibrosis of the hepatic lobules. The term "**hepatic failure**" denotes a clinical condition in which the biochemical function of the liver is severely, and potentially fatally, compromised.

Cholestatic disease

Cholestasis is the clinical term for **biliary obstruction,** which may occur in the small bile ducts in the liver itself or in the larger extrahepatic ducts. Biochemical tests cannot distinguish between these two possibilities, which generally have radically different causes; imaging techniques such as ultrasound are more helpful.

Jaundice

Jaundice can be pre-, post, or intrahepatic

Jaundice is clinically obvious when plasma bilirubin concentrations exceed 50 μmol/L (3 mg/dL). Hyperbilirubinemia is the result of an imbalance between its production and excretion. The causes of jaundice (Table 34.3) are conventionally classified as follows:

- **Prehepatic:** increased production or impaired hepatic uptake of bilirubin (Fig. 34.9)
- **Intrahepatic:** impaired hepatic metabolism or secretion of bilirubin (Fig. 34.10)
- **Posthepatic:** obstruction to biliary excretion (Fig. 34.11 and Box on p. 519)

Prehepatic hyperbilirubinemia results from excess production of bilirubin caused by hemolysis or a genetic abnormality in the hepatic uptake of unconjugated bilirubin

Hemolysis is usually the result of immune disease, the presence of structurally abnormal red cells, or the breakdown of extravasated blood. Intravascular hemolysis results in the release of hemoglobin into the plasma, where it is either oxidized to methemoglobin (Chapter 5) or complexed with haptoglobin. More commonly, red cells are hemolyzed extravascularly, within phagocytes, and hemoglobin is converted to bilirubin, which is **unconjugated.** Unconjugated and conjugated bilirubin can be distinguished in the laboratory as so-called indirect and direct bilirubin.

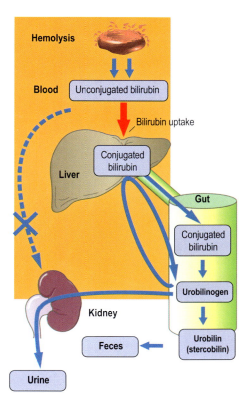

Fig. 34.9 **Prehepatic (hemolytic) jaundice.** There is an increased concentration of plasma total bilirubin due to excess of the unconjugated fraction (see also Table 34.2). There is an increase in urine bilirubin because unconjugated bilirubin is insoluble in water. Urine urobilinogen is increased.

Table 34.3 Causes of jaundice

Type	Cause	Clinical example	Frequency
Prehepatic	Hemolysis	Autoimmune	Uncommon
		Abnormal hemoglobin	Depends on region
Intrahepatic	Infection	Hepatitis A, B, C	Common/very common
	Chemical/drug	Acetaminophen	Common
		Alcohol	Common
	Genetic errors:	Gilbert's syndrome	1 in 20
	bilirubin	Crigler–Najjar syndrome	Very rare
	metabolism	Dubin–Johnson syndrome	Very rare
		Rotor's syndrome	Very rare
	Genetic errors: synthesis of	Wilson's disease	1 in 200,000
	specific proteins	α_1-antitrypsin	1 in 1000 with genotype
	Autoimmune	Chronic active hepatitis	Uncommon/rare
	Neonatal	Physiologic	Very common
Posthepatic	Intrahepatic bile ducts blockage	Drugs	Common
		Primary biliary cirrhosis	Uncommon
		Cholangitis	Common
	Extrahepatic bile ducts blockage	Gallstones	Very common
		Pancreatic tumor	Uncommon
		Cholangiocarcinoma	Rare

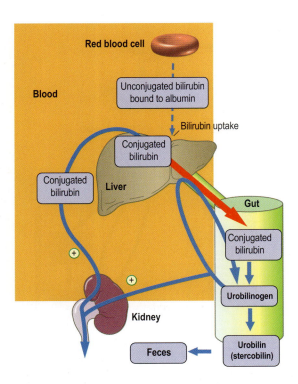

Fig. 34.10 **Intrahepatic jaundice.** Bilirubin in plasma is increased due to an increase in the conjugated fraction. Increased serum enzyme activities signify hepatocyte damage (see also Table 34.2). Increased urine urobilinogen.

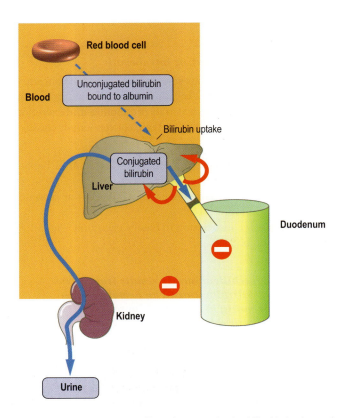

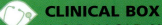

Fig. 34.11 **Posthepatic jaundice.** Plasma and urine bilirubin is elevated due to an increase in the conjugated fraction. Obstruction of the bile duct does not allow passage of bile to the gut. Stools are characteristically pale in color, and urobilinogen is absent from urine (see also Table 34.2).

Intrahepatic jaundice reflects a generalized hepatocyte dysfunction

In this condition, hyperbilirubinemia is usually accompanied by other abnormalities in biochemical markers of hepatocellular function.

In neonates, transient jaundice is common, particularly in premature infants, and is due to immaturity of the enzymes involved in bilirubin conjugation. Unconjugated bilirubin is toxic to the immature brain and causes a condition known as **kernicterus.** If plasma bilirubin concentrations are judged to be too high, phototherapy with blue-white light, which isomerizes bilirubin to more soluble pigments that might be excreted with bile, or exchange blood transfusion to remove the excess bilirubin, is necessary to avoid kernicterus.

Posthepatic jaundice is caused by obstruction of the biliary tree

In this posthepatic jaundice, the plasma bilirubin is conjugated, and other biliary metabolites, such as bile acids, accumulate in the plasma. The clinical features are pale-colored stools, caused by the absence of fecal bilirubin and urobilin, and dark urine as a result of the presence of water-soluble conjugated bilirubin. In complete obstruction, urobilinogen and urobilin are absent from urine because there can be no intestinal conversion of bilirubin to urobilinogen/urobilin, and hence no renal excretion of reabsorbed urobilinogen/urobilin.

CLINICAL BOX
A 65-YEAR-OLD MAN WITH JAUNDICE AND NO ABDOMINAL SYMPTOMS: THE SIGNIFICANCE OF ADULT JAUNDICE

A 65-year-old man was admitted to the hospital because of jaundice. There was no abdominal pain, but he had noticed dark urine and pale stools. Liver function tests showed bilirubin 230 μmol/L (13.5 mg/dL), AST 32 U/L, and ALP 550 U/L. Dipstick urine testing revealed the presence of bilirubin, but no urobilin.

Comment
The patient had a history typical of obstructive jaundice. The increased ALP and normal AST concentrations were consistent with this, and the absence of urobilin in the urine indicated that the biliary tract was obstructed. It was important to carry out liver imaging tests to find the site of the obstruction; the absence of pain suggested that gallstones were not the cause. Ultrasound showed dilatation of the common bile duct, and a computed tomography scan showed a solid mass in the pancreas with probable metastatic deposits in the liver and paraaortic lymph nodes. This is pancreatic cancer, and because the tumor may arise in the body of the pancreas and not initially obstruct biliary drainage, it can be clinically inapparent and metastasize before symptoms develop. For reference ranges, see Table 34.2.

GENOMICS OF LIVER DISEASE

Several hepatic diseases arise due to single-gene disorders. Genetic techniques can identify individuals with a propensity to develop a disease or confirm the diagnosis in affected persons.

Hereditary hemochromatosis is a genetically determined disorder of iron metabolism

Hemochromatosis is the most common inherited disease in Northern Europeans. Although several mutations can lead to the hemochromatosis clinical phenotype, the most frequently seen mutation is in the HFE gene leading to a p.Cys282Tyr substitution. This mutation is present in about 10% of Northern Europeans, and so 1 in 100 would be homozygous and may develop iron overload. Other factors, both environmental and genetic, play a role in determining whether or not HFE homozygotes actually develop clinical hemochromatosis. Mutations in the HFE gene and some others can impair the synthesis of hepcidin, which in turn leads to the excessive expression of ferroportin at the cell surface of intestinal cells and macrophages, increased iron egress. Increased plasma iron is deposited in hepatic, pancreatic, endocrine, and cardiac cells, causing parenchymal damage because iron catalyzes the production of reactive oxygen species. Patients can develop multiorgan dysfunction, including cirrhosis of the liver.

Wilson's disease is a condition associated with liver and CNS damage; it results from abnormal tissue copper disposition

Wilson's disease is a monogenic, autosomal recessive inherited condition. The causative gene *ATP7B* encodes a copper-transporting P-type ATPase. More than 500 ATP7B mutations have now been identified. Wilson's disease is a condition associated with damage to both the liver and the CNS.

The widely cited prevalence figure of 1 : 30,000 for Wilson's disease with a heterozygous *ATP7B* mutation carrier frequency of 1 : 90 was estimated before the identification of *ATP7B* as the causative gene. More recent studies suggest a considerably higher prevalence of 1 : 1500–1 : 3000 based on measurements of **plasma ceruloplasmin**, a copper-containing plasma protein.

Increased intracellular copper levels lead to oxidative stress and free-radical formation as well as mitochondrial dysfunction arising independently of oxidative stress. The combined effects results in cell death in hepatic and brain tissue as well as other organs.

Deficiency of α₁-antitrypsin presents in infancy as liver disease or in adulthood as lung disease

α_1-Antitrypsin is a member of the serpin family of serine protease inhibitors, and contrary to its name, its predominant target is macrophage-derived elastase. Genetic **deficiency of α₁-antitrypsin** presents in infancy as liver disease or in adulthood as lung disease caused by elastase-mediated tissue destruction - early-onset lung disease and liver cirrhosis.

Several isoforms of α_1-antitrypsin exist as a result of allelic variation of the AA1T gene: the normal isoform is known as M, and the two common defective isoforms as S and Z; the null allele produces no α_1-antitrypsin.

More than 90 allelic variants of the AA1T gene at the so-called proteinase inhibitor (Pi) locus have been described, the majority of which do not affect plasma levels or activity of AA1T. Phenotypic variants in AA1T were initially described by their relative mobility on electrophoresis, with the most common variant, M, having medium mobility. The Z and S variants are most frequently associated with AA1T deficiency, and both are due to point mutations that can also be detected by polymerase chain reaction (PCR) assays.

Liver cancer is associated with particularly high plasma concentrations of α-fetoprotein

α-Fetoprotein (AFP) and albumin have considerable sequence homology and appear to have evolved by reduplication of a single ancestral gene. In the fetus, AFP appears to serve physiologic functions similar to those performed by albumin in the adult; furthermore, by the end of the first year of life, AFP in the plasma is entirely replaced by albumin. During hepatic regeneration and proliferation, AFP is again synthesized; thus high plasma concentrations of AFP are observed in liver cancer.

There are a number of genetic disorders that impair bilirubin conjugation or secretion

Gilbert's syndrome affects up to 5% of the population and causes a mild unconjugated hyperbilirubinemia that is harmless and asymptomatic. It is caused by a dinucleotide polymorphism in the TATA box promoter of the bilirubin UDP-glucuronyl transferase gene that impairs the hepatic uptake of unconjugated bilirubin.

Other inherited diseases of bilirubin metabolism are rare. **Crigler–Najjar syndrome,** which is the result of a complete absence or marked reduction in bilirubin conjugation, causes severe unconjugated hyperbilirubinemia that presents at birth; when the enzyme is completely absent, the condition is fatal. **Dubin–Johnson** and **Rotor's syndromes** impair biliary secretion of conjugated bilirubin and therefore cause conjugated hyperbilirubinemia, which is usually mild.

SUMMARY

- The liver plays a central role in human metabolism.
- It is extensively involved in the synthesis and catabolism of carbohydrates, lipids, and proteins.
- It synthesizes an array of acute-phase proteins in response to inflammation and infection, and laboratory measurements of such proteins are clinically useful in monitoring disease progress.
- It is involved in the metabolism of bilirubin derived from the catabolism of heme.
- Disease processes often cause the patient to present with jaundice due to hyperbilirubinemia.
- The liver has a central role in the detoxification of drugs.
- Its biochemical function is assessed in clinical practice using a panel of blood tests called liver function tests, abnormalities of which can point to disease affecting the hepatocellular or biliary systems.

ACTIVE LEARNING

1. Discuss how the anatomic position and structure of the liver allow it to absorb and metabolize lipids, proteins, and carbohydrates, as well as xenobiotics, from the intestine before releasing such molecules or their derivatives to the systemic circulation.
2. Describe the function of the liver in protein synthesis and in the systemic response to inflammation.
3. Outline how the liver processes bilirubin, and describe the biochemical causes of hyperbilirubinemia (jaundice) and its classification.
4. How does the liver metabolize drugs?
5. Discuss biochemical tests used by the clinical laboratory in the investigation of liver disease.

FURTHER READING

Agrawal, S., Dhiman, R. K., & Limdi, J. K. (2016). Evaluation of abnormal liver function tests. *Postgraduate Medical Journal, 92,* 223–234.

Bandmann, O., Weiss, K. H., & Kaler, S. G. (2015). Wilson's disease and other neurological copper disorders. *The Lancet. Neurology, 14,* 103–113.

Bernal, W., Jalan, R., Quaglia, A., et al. (2015). Acute on chronic liver failure. *Lancet, 386,* 1576–1578.

Donohue, T. M., Cederbaum, A. I., & French, S. W. (2007). Role of the proteasome in ethanol-induced liver pathology. *Alcoholism, Clinical and Experimental Research, 31,* 1446–1459.

Haque, T., Sasolomi, E., & Hayashi, P. H. (2016). Drug induced liver injury: Pattern recognition and future directions. *Gut and Liver, 10,* 27–36.

Leise, M. D., Poterucha, J. J., & Talwalkar, J. A. (2014). Drug-induced liver injury. *Mayo Clinic Proceedings. Mayo Clinic, 89,* 95–106.

National Collaborating Centre for Women's and Children's Health (UK) (2010). *Neonatal Jaundice.* NICE Clinical Guidelines, no. 98. London: RCOG Press.

Powell, L. W., Seckington, R. C., & Deugnier, Y. (2016). Haemochromatosis. *Lancet, 388,* 706–716.

Puy, H., & Gouya, L. (2010). Deybach J-C: Porphyrias. *Lancet, 375,* 924–937.

Schuckit, M. A. (2009). Alcohol-use disorders. *Lancet, 373,* 492–501.

Wijnen, P. A. H. M., Op den Buijsch, R. A. M., Drent, M., et al. (2007). Review article: The prevalence and clinical relevance of cytochrome P-450 polymorphisms. *Alimentary Pharmacology and Therapeutics, 26*(Suppl. 2), 211–219.

Wilkinson, G. R. (2005). Drug metabolism and variability among patients in drug response. *The New England Journal of Medicine, 352,* 2211–2221.

Woreta, T. A., & Alqahtani, S. A. (2014). Evaluation of abnormal liver tests. *The Medical Clinics of North America, 98,* 1–16.

RELEVANT WEBSITES

MedlinePlus - Liver Diseases: https://medlineplus.gov/liverdiseases.html
Lab Tests Online - Liver Disease: https://www.labtestsonline.org/understanding/conditions/liver-disease/
Lab Tests Online - Liver Function Tests: labtestsonline.org.uk/understanding/analytes/liver-panel/
PharmGKB - The Pharmacogenomics Knowledgebase: https://www.pharmgkb.org/

MORE CLINICAL CASES

Please refer to Appendix 2 for more cases relevant to this chapter.

ABBREVIATIONS

ADH	Alcohol dehydrogenase
AFP	α-fetoprotein
AIC	Acute intermittent porphyria
5-ALA	5-aminolevulinate
ALD	Alcoholic liver disease
ALDH	Aldehyde dehydrogenase
ALP	Alkaline phosphatase
ALT	Alanine aminotransferase
AST	Aspartate aminotransferase
CNS	Central nervous system

CRP	C-reactive protein	NAD⁺	Nicotinamide adenine dinucleotide
DDI	Drug–drug interaction		
DILI	Drug-induced liver injury	NAFLD	Nonalcoholic fatty liver disease
GGT	γ-glutamyl transpeptidase	NFκB, NF-κB	Nuclear factor kappa-light-chain-enhancer of activated B cells
IL-1, IL-6, IL-8	Interleukins		
JAK/STAT	Janus kinase/signal transducer and activator of transcription	PBG	Porphobilinogen
MCP-1	Monocyte-chemoattractant protein-1	PT	Pprothrombin time
		PXR	Pregnane X receptor
NABQI	N-acetyl benzoquinoneimine	TNF	Tumor necrosis factor
NAC	N-acetylcysteine	UPS	Ubiquitin–proteasome system

CHAPTER
35
Water and Electrolytes Homeostasis
Marek H. Dominiczak and Mirosława Szczepańska-Konkel

LEARNING OBJECTIVES

After reading this chapter, you should be able to:

■ Describe the body water compartments in the adult and the composition of the main body fluids.

■ Explain the role of albumin in the movement of water between plasma and interstitial space, including the consequences of proteinuria.

■ Describe how osmolality changes induce movement of water between the extracellular and intracellular space.

■ Explain why sodium/potassium ATPase is essential for cell ion transport.

■ Describe factors affecting plasma potassium concentration, and describe the clinical consequences of hyperkalemia and hypokalemia.

■ Discuss the links between sodium and water homeostasis.

■ Describe the assessment of a dehydrated patient.

INTRODUCTION

Water and electrolytes are constantly exchanged with the environment

Water is essential for survival and, in an adult person, accounts for approximately 60% of the body weight. This changes with age: it is about 75% in the newborn and decreases to below 50% in the elderly. Water content is highest in the brain tissue (about 90%) and lowest in the adipose tissue (10%).

Stability of subcellular structures and activities of enzymes depend on adequate hydration, and the maintenance of ion gradients and electrical potential across membranes is essential for muscle contraction, nerve conduction, and secretory processes (Chapter 4).

Because both water deficiency and water excess impair the function of organs and tissues, the intake and loss of water are subject to complex regulation. Water and electrolyte disorders are common in clinical practice.

BODY WATER COMPARTMENTS

Approximately two-thirds of total body water is in the **intracellular fluid (ICF)**, and one-third remains in the extracellular **fluid (ECF)**. ECF consists of interstitial fluid and lymph (15% body weight), plasma (3% body weight), and the so-called

transcellular fluids, which include gastrointestinal fluid, urine, and cerebrospinal fluid (Fig. 35.1). Two barriers are important for the understanding of water and electrolyte movements between different compartments: the **wall of the capillary blood** vessel and the **cell membrane**.

The body exchanges water with the environment

The main source of water is oral intake, and the main source of its loss is urine excretion. Water is also lost through the lungs, sweat, and feces: this is known as "insensible loss" and in normal circumstances amounts to approximately 500 mL daily (Fig. 35.2). In a steady state, the intake of water equals its loss. Insensible loss can increase substantially in high temperatures, during intensive exercise, and also as a result of fever. Checking the patient's fluid balance is one of the essential daily routines on medical and surgical wards.

CLINICAL TEST BOX
CONCENTRATION OF IONS IN PLASMA AND SERUM

All physiologic phenomena occur in plasma, and therefore discussion of physiologic or pathologic conditions relates to plasma concentrations of ions. However, the concentration of most ions is measured after the sampled blood has been allowed to clot (i.e., using serum). Thus, in the discussion of laboratory results, we often mention serum values (Chapter 40).

The capillary vessel wall separates plasma and the interstitial fluid

The capillary wall separates plasma from the interstitial fluid and is freely permeable to water and electrolytes but not to proteins. Ions and low-molecular-weight molecules are present in similar concentrations in the ECF and plasma, but protein concentration is four to five times higher in plasma. The total concentration of cations in plasma is about 150 mmol/L, of which sodium constitutes approximately 140 mmol/L and potassium 4 mmol/L. The most abundant plasma anions are chloride and bicarbonate, with average concentrations of 100 mmol/L and 25 mmol/L, respectively (Fig. 35.3). In clinical practice, the rest of the anions are, for the purposes of electrolyte balance, considered together, constituting the so-called anion gap (AG), which is calculated as follows:

$$AG = (Na^+ + K^+) - (Cl^- + HCO_3^-)$$

The anion gap (in a healthy person, approximately 10 mmol/L) includes mostly negatively charged albumin and phosphate

523

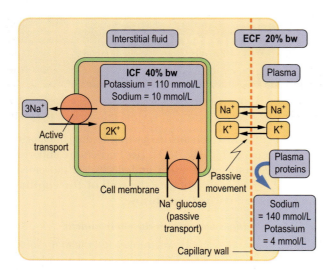

Fig. 35.1 **Distribution of body water, sodium, and potassium.** The main body water compartments are the intracellular fluid (ICF) and the extracellular fluid (ECF). ECF includes interstitial fluid and plasma. The gradient of sodium and potassium concentrations between ICF and ECF is maintained across cell membranes by the Na⁺/K⁺-ATPase. Sodium is a major contributor to the osmolality in the ECF and a determinant of the distribution of water between ECF and ICF. Distribution of water between plasma and interstitial fluid is determined by the oncotic pressure exerted by plasma proteins. bw, body weight.

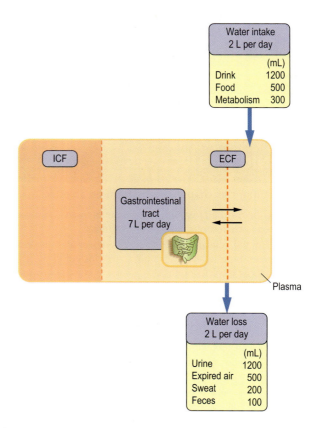

Fig. 35.2 **Daily water balance in an adult person.** Water is obtained from the diet and from oxidative metabolism, and it is lost through the kidneys, skin, lungs, and intestine. Note how much water enters and leaves the gastrointestinal tract daily; this explains why severe diarrhea quickly leads to dehydration. See also Chapter 30.

anion but also sulfate and organic anions such as lactate, citrate, pyruvate, acetoacetate, and β-hydroxybutyrate. It may increase several-fold when its constituent anions accumulate - for example, in renal failure, diabetic ketoacidosis, or some cases of poisoning (e.g., with ethylene glycol or methanol). Calculating the anion gap focuses physician's thinking on these conditions.

To get a better insight into behavior of abnormal constituents, a calculation of AG adjusted for albumin and lactate concentration has been suggested (see papers by Hawfield and DuBose and by Kellum in Further Reading).

The plasma membrane separates the intracellular and extracellular fluid

The main cation in the ICF is potassium, present in a concentration of about 110 mmol/L. This is almost 30-fold greater than its concentration in the ECF and in plasma (4 mmol/L). The concentration of sodium is only 10 mmol/L. The main anions in the ICF are proteins and phosphate (Fig. 35.3).

Ion movements and transport systems

Water diffuses freely across most cell membranes, but the movement of ions and neutral molecules is restricted; Na⁺/K⁺-ATPase maintains the sodium and potassium gradients across the cell membrane

Small molecules are transported across cell membranes by **specific transport proteins, ion pumps, and ion channels**.

The most important of them is the sodium–potassium ATPase (Na⁺/K⁺- ATPase), also referred to as the sodium–potassium pump (Fig. 35.4). This enzyme uses ATP to transport sodium and potassium against their concentration gradients. It hydrolyzes one ATP molecule, and the released energy drives the transfer of three sodium ions from the cell to the outside and two potassium ions from the outside into the cell (Fig. 35.5). The Na⁺/K⁺-ATPase is the major determinant of cytoplasmic sodium concentration. It maintains concentration gradients and electrical potential across membranes (it is electrogenic). Gradients created by the Na⁺/K⁺-ATPase enable other (passive) transport processes in the cell, where sodium is transported along the created concentration gradient. It also has an important role in regulating cell volume and calcium levels through the Na⁺/H⁺ and Na⁺/Ca²⁺ exchangers.

The Na⁺/K⁺-ATPase is subject to regulation by a number of hormones, including aldosterone

The Na⁺/K⁺-ATPase has three subunits. The structure of the enzyme includes the α-catalytic subunit, which possesses the Na-, K-, and ATP-binding sites and also several phosphorylation sites. The β-subunit stabilizes the enzyme's conformation, and

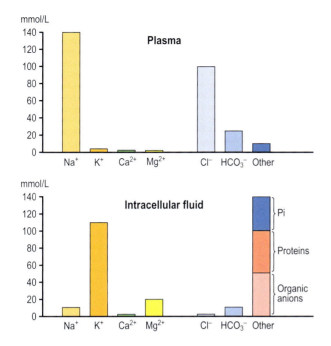

Fig. 35.3 **Ions present in the plasma and in the intracellular fluid.** The most important ions in plasma are sodium, potassium, calcium, chloride, phosphate, and bicarbonate. Sodium chloride, in a concentration close to 0.9% (thus "physiologic saline"), is the main ionic component of the extracellular fluid. Glucose and urea also contribute to plasma osmolality. Their contribution is normally small because they are present in plasma in relatively low molar concentrations (about 5 mmol/L each). However, when glucose concentration increases in diabetes, its contribution to osmolality becomes significant. Plasma urea increases in renal failure, but because it freely crosses cell membranes, it does not contribute to water movement between ECF and ICF. Potassium is the main intracellular cation, and the main anions are phosphates and proteins. There is also a substantial amount of magnesium in cells.

the γ-subunit plays a minor regulatory role in some tissues. Na$^+$/K$^+$-ATPase is activated by sodium and ATP. Half-maximal activation of the enzyme by intracellular sodium occurs at sodium concentration of 10 mM, which is often above the steady-state concentration. Accordingly, small changes in the cytoplasmic sodium can have large effects on its activity. Another requirement for continuous adaptation is changes in dietary sodium and potassium.

Short-term regulation involves either direct effects on the kinetic properties of the enzyme or its translocation between the plasma membrane and intracellular sites. Some hormones appear to alter the Na$^+$/K$^+$-ATPase activity by changing the enzyme's affinity for sodium; for instance, angiotensin II and insulin increase the affinity. Peptide hormones such as vasopressin and PTH that act through G-protein-coupled receptors and adenylyl cyclase, which generates cAMP. cAMP, in turn, activates protein kinase A (PKA). PTH, angiotensin II, norepinephrine, and dopamine trigger G-protein-mediated activation of phospholipase C, which in turn activates protein kinase C (PKC). Both PKA and PKC affect Na$^+$/K$^+$-ATPase by serine phosphorylation of its α-subunit.

Importantly, **digoxin**, the cardiac glycoside used in the treatment of heart failure and atrial fibrillation, inhibits the Na$^+$/K$^+$-ATPase. This slows conduction and increases the so-called refractory period. The resulting increased intracellular Na$^+$ concentration leads to a decreased extrusion of calcium, which in turn causes the positive inotropic effect associated with the drug.

The electrochemical gradient drives the passive movement of electrolytes through ion channels

For most cells, the membrane potential ranges from 50 to 90 mV, being negative inside the cell. The electrochemical gradient is

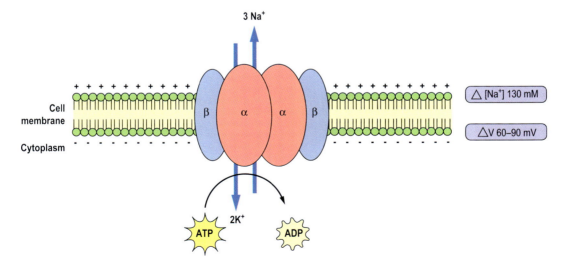

Fig. 35.4 **Na$^+$/K$^+$-ATPase (the sodium–potassium pump) generates transmembrane potential and ion concentration gradients across the cell membrane.** The transmembrane difference in sodium concentration (ΔNa$^+$) and transmembrane voltage difference (ΔV) are shown on the right. For each molecule of hydrolyzed ATP, the **Na$^+$/K$^+$-ATPase** moves two potassium ions into the cell and three sodium ions out of the cell. The enzyme consists of two main subunits - the catalytic subunit (α), which contains phosphorylation sites, and the structural subunit (β). The third (γ) subunit plays a minor regulatory role in some tissues.

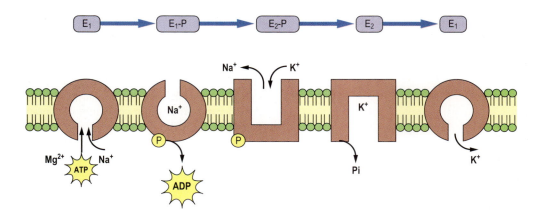

Fig. 35.5 **Catalytic function of the Na⁺/K⁺-ATPase.** The catalytic subunit of the Na⁺/K⁺-ATPase can be phosphorylated (E_1-P and E_2-P) and dephosphorylated (E_1 and E_2), and the phosphorylation status changes its conformation and affinity toward substrates. The E_1 form exhibits high affinity toward ATP, magnesium, and sodium and low affinity toward potassium, whereas the E_2 form has a high affinity for potassium and low affinity for sodium. After the release of ADP, there is conformational change from E_1-P to E_2-P. This facilitates extracellular delivery of sodium and the binding of extracellular potassium. The latter process induces dephosphorylation of E_2-P and potassium release into the intracellular compartment.

the source of energy for transport of many substances. Sodium enters the cell along its concentration gradient, cotransporting other molecules passively. The SGLT transporters, for instance, cotransport sodium and glucose. Other sodium cotransporters transport amino acids and phosphate (Chapter 30).

Membrane depolarization activates voltage-dependent Ca^{2+} channels. This causes an increase in intracellular calcium concentration (Chapter 4). The role of ion gradients in nerve transmission is described in Chapter 26. Because water follows the movement of sodium, the ion gradient generated by the Na⁺/K⁺-ATPase is critical for water absorption in the intestine and for its reabsorption in kidneys. Impairment of this function is linked to the pathophysiology of chronic diarrhea and hypertension, respectively.

Cells protect themselves against changes in volume

An increase in the intracellular concentration of sodium stimulates the Na⁺/K⁺-ATPase, which extrudes sodium from the cell. This is followed by extrusion of water and protects the cell from volume changes. Another protective mechanism is the **intracellular generation of osmotically active substances** (osmolytes) such as glutamate, taurine, myoinositol, or sorbitol. This is particularly important in the brain, where the potential for volume expansion is limited by the skull, and in the renal medulla, which can be exposed to hyperosmotic environment.

The role of osmotic pressure in fluid shifts between ECF and ICF

Osmolality depends on the concentration of molecules in water

Osmotic pressure is proportional to the molal concentration of a solution. One millimole of a substance dissolved in 1 kg H_2O at 38°C exerts an osmotic pressure of approximately 19 mmHg.

Normally the average concentration of all osmotically active substances in the ECF and ICF is identical, 290 mmol/kg H_2O.

Differences in osmolality drive movement of water between ICF and ECF

A primary change in the concentration of osmotically active ions in either ECF or ICF creates a gradient of osmotic pressure, which leads to the movement of water. **In order to equalize osmotic pressures, water always moves from a compartment with lower osmolality (lower concentration of dissolved molecules) to the one with higher osmolality** (Fig. 35.6).

Sodium is the most important determinant of ECF osmolality. The other important molecule is glucose, although at its normal plasma concentration (5.0 mmol/L; 90 mg/dL), it does not contribute much to total plasma osmolality. However, when its concentration increases in diabetes, it makes a significant contribution, causes water shifts, and leads to osmotic symptoms such as polyuria (Chapter 31).

Balance between the oncotic and hydrostatic pressures is fundamental for the circulation of substrates and nutrients

Proteins, particularly albumin, exert osmotic pressure in the plasma (about 3.32 kPa; 25 mmHg). This is known as the **oncotic pressure,** and it retains water in the vascular bed. It is balanced by the **hydrostatic pressure,** which forces fluid out of the capillaries. In the arterial part of the capillaries, the hydrostatic pressure prevails over the oncotic pressure, thus pushing out water and low-molecular-weight compounds, including nutrients, into the extravascular space. In contrast, in the venous part of capillaries, oncotic pressure prevails, and fluid is drawn back into the vascular lumen (Fig. 35.7). A reduction in plasma oncotic pressure, caused by low plasma albumin concentration, results in the movement of fluid into the extravascular space: this is observable as **edema.**

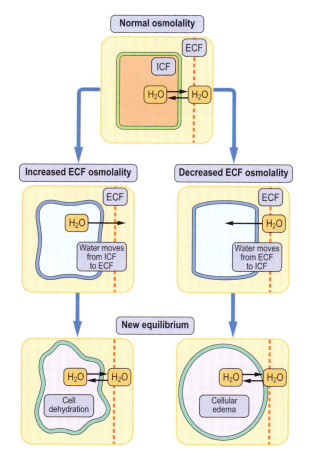

Fig. 35.6 **Water redistribution caused by changes in osmolality.** Osmotic pressure controls the movement of water between compartments. An increase in ECF osmolality draws water from the cells and leads to cellular dehydration. Conversely, when ECF osmolality decreases, water moves into the cells, and this may cause cell edema. The arrows indicate direction of water movement. ECF, extracellular fluid; ICF, intracellular fluid.

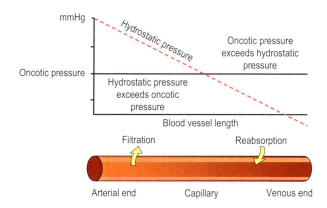

Fig. 35.7 **Oncotic and hydrostatic pressures determine the movement of fluid between plasma and interstitial fluid.**

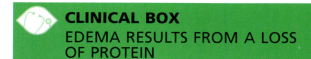

CLINICAL BOX
EDEMA RESULTS FROM A LOSS OF PROTEIN

An 8-year-old girl was referred to a nephrologist after it had been noticed that her face was puffy and her ankles became swollen over a period of about 2 weeks. Dipstick test for urine protein yielded a strongly positive (++++) result, and measurement in a 24-h collection showed protein excretion of 7.00 g/day. The reference value for urinary protein excretion is less than 0.15g/day.

Comment
The cause of the proteinuria was damage to the renal filtration barrier. Renal biopsy showed the so-called minimal change disease, with the urinary protein loss causing, in turn, hypoalbuminemia and a decrease in the plasma oncotic pressure. This led to edema. The condition went into remission after treatment with a glucocorticoid.

ROLE OF THE KIDNEYS IN WATER AND ELECTROLYTE BALANCE

The kidneys play a key role in the regulation of volume and composition of ECF due to their ability to regulate excretion of ions and water. They are also essential for maintaining the acid–base balance (Chapter 36). Most of the metabolic processes in the kidneys are aerobic, and consequently, their oxygen consumption is high: it approximately equals that of the cardiac muscle, and is three times greater than that of the brain. Such a high metabolic activity is required to maintain tubular reabsorption: about 70% of the oxygen consumed by the kidney is used to support active sodium transport, which in turn determines reabsorption of glucose and amino acids.

Each kidney consists of approximately 1 million nephrons composed of glomerulus and an excretory tubule (Fig. 35.8). The segments of each tubule (starting from the glomerular end) are known as the **proximal tubule**, the **loop of Henle**, the **distal tubule**, and the **collecting duct.**

The structure positioned between the glomerulus and distal tubule known as the **juxtaglomerular apparatus** includes the cells of the macula densa that serve as **sodium sensors** and site of **renin** secretion.

Sodium transport systems in the renal tubules

Sodium reabsorption occurs along the nephron, with the exception of the descending limb of the loop of Henle (Fig. 35.7). **Approximately 80% of the filtrate is reabsorbed in the proximal tubule.** The driving force for the reabsorption of sodium and other solutes is the electrochemical gradient generated by the Na^+/K^+-ATPase in the basolateral membrane

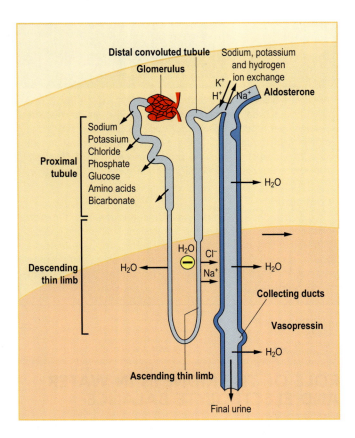

Fig. 35.8 **The nephron and its major transport sites.** Approximately 80% of filtered sodium is actively reabsorbed in the proximal tubule, where molecules such as amino acids and phosphate are also reabsorbed. Sodium and chloride ions are reabsorbed also in the ascending limb of the loop of Henle. A different mechanism operates in the distal tubule, where sodium reabsorption is stimulated by **aldosterone** and is coupled with the secretion of hydrogen and potassium ions. Aldosterone causes sodium retention and an increase in potassium excretion. Water enters cells passively with the reabsorbed sodium. Water reabsorption regulated by vasopressin takes place in the collecting duct.

of tubular cells. Sodium is reabsorbed through specific ion channels located on the luminal membrane, in exchange for the hydrogen ion, and in cotransport with glucose, amino acids, phosphate, and other anions. **The movement of sodium leads to reabsorption of water.** The entry of sodium into tubular cells is passive. This is possible because the Na$^+$/K$^+$-ATPase maintains low sodium concentration in the cytoplasm.

In the thin ascending limb of the loop of Henle, the sodium ions move into the cell via sodium–potassium–chloride cotransporter (known as NKCC2), which can be inhibited by **frusemide.** In this segment, potassium ions are secreted into the lumen by the ATP-sensitive rectifier potassium channel.

In the distal tubule, the reabsorption of sodium ions involves sodium–chloride cotransporter (NCC), which is **thiazide**-sensitive.

In the collecting duct, the sodium ions are reabsorbed by **amiloride**-sensitive sodium channel (ENaC). Aldosterone stimulates both ENaC expression and the activity of the Na$^+$/K$^+$-ATPase (Fig. 35.8). The pharmacologic antagonist of aldosterone is the diuretic **spironolactone**.

Inhibitors of sodium reabsorption - for example, thiazide diuretics (hydrochlorothiazide), loop diuretics (e.g., frusemide), amiloride, and spironolactone - are extensively used in clinical practice.

CLINICAL TEST BOX
URINE

Under normal conditions, the kidneys form 1–2 liters of urine per day. Urine composition is summarized in Table 35.1. Urine volume can vary from 0.5 L to more than 10.0 L of urine daily. The minimum volume necessary to remove the products of metabolism (mainly nitrogen, excreted as urea) is approximately 0.5 L/24 h. The osmolality of the glomerular filtrate is about 300 mmol/L. The osmolality of urine varies from about 50–1200 mmol/L.

Urine Analysis Provides Clinically Important Information

Urine analysis (urinalysis) in clinical laboratories includes testing for the presence of protein, glucose, ketone bodies, bilirubin, and urobilinogen and for traces of blood. Measuring urinary osmolality assesses the concentrating capacity of the kidney. The urine is also tested for the presence of leukocytes and various crystals and deposits. Specialist investigations include detailed analysis of urinary amino acids, hormones, and other metabolites.

The adult kidney filters around 180 g of glucose per day. Practically all of it is reabsorbed in the kidney tubules; 90% of it is reabsorbed in the proximal tubule by a low-affinity, high-capacity SGLT2 transporter. There is also another transporter, a high-affinity, low-capacity SGLT1, which is predominant in the brush border of the small intestine but is also present in the proximal tubule. The normal urine glucose concentration is equal to or below 0.8 mmol/L (15 mg/dL).

Only traces of protein are normally detectable in the urine. This increases when the glomeruli are damaged: significant proteinuria is an important sign of **renal disease.** Even a minimal amount of albumin in the urine (microalbuminuria) predicts the development of diabetic nephropathy (Chapter 31). Larger proteins such as immunoglobulins appear in the urine when the damage is more extensive: the immunoglobulin light chains (the Bence Jones protein) are present in urine in **multiple myeloma** (Chapter 40). In **hemolytic anemia,** urine may contain free hemoglobin and urobilinogen. The presence of myoglobin is a marker of muscle damage **(rhabdomyolysis).** Measurement of urine glucose and ketones is important in the assessment of glycemic control in **diabetic** patients (Chapter 31). Measurements of urobilinogen and bilirubin help to assess **liver function** (Chapter 34).

CLINICAL BOX
DIURETICS ARE USED FOR TREATMENT OF EDEMA, CARDIAC FAILURE, AND HYPERTENSION

Diuretics are drugs that stimulate water and sodium excretion. **Thiazide diuretics** (e.g., bendrofluazide) decrease sodium reabsorption in the distal tubules by blocking sodium and chloride cotransport. **Loop diuretics,** such as frusemide, inhibit sodium reabsorption in the ascending loop of Henle. **Spironolactone,** a potassium-sparing diuretic, is a competitive inhibitor of aldosterone: it inhibits sodium–potassium exchange in the distal tubules and decreases potassium excretion. An osmotic diuresis may be induced by the administration of the sugar alcohol **mannitol.**

The net effect of treatment with diuretics is increased urine volume and loss of sodium and water. Diuretics are important in the treatment of edema associated with circulatory problems such as heart failure, in which impaired cardiac function may lead to a severe breathlessness caused by pulmonary edema. They are also essential in the treatment of hypertension.

CLINICAL BOX
INHERITED NEPHRON TRANSPORT DISORDERS

Gitelman's syndrome is a result of inactivating mutations in the gene encoding the thiazide-sensitive sodium–chloride cotransporter (gene *SLC12A3*). It is an autosomal recessive disorder. Homozygous individuals are generally normotensive. The biochemical abnormalities include hypochloremic metabolic alkalosis, hypokalemia, hypocalciuria, and sometimes hypomagnesemia.

Bartter's syndrome is a group of inherited defects in ion transport along the thick ascending limb of the loop of Henle. The neonatal Bartter's syndrome is linked to a mutation in the furosemide-sensitive sodium–potassium–chloride cotransporter gene (*SLC12A2*) or the thick ascending limb potassium channel gene (*ROMK/KCNJ1*). The classic Bartter's syndrome results from chloride channel gene (*CLCNKB*) mutation. Clinical symptoms include polyuria and polydipsia, and there is also hypokalemia and alkalosis.

CLINICAL TEST BOX
ASSESSMENT OF RENAL FUNCTION

Serum Creatinine and Urea Are First-Line Tests in the Diagnosis of Renal Disease
Renal clearance is the volume of plasma (in milliliters) that the kidney clears of a given substance every minute. The glomerular filtration rate (GFR; mL/min) is the most important characteristic describing kidney function. GFR can be estimated by measuring the clearance of a polysaccharide inulin which is neither secreted nor reabsorbed in the renal tubules. Urine excretion rate (V; mL/min) is calculated by dividing the urine volume by the collection time. The amount of inulin filtered from plasma (i.e., its plasma concentration, P_{in}, multiplied by GFR) equals the amount recovered in the urine (i.e., its urinary concentration, U_{in}, multiplied by the urine formation rate, V):

$$P_{in} \times GFR = U_{in} \times V \qquad (1)$$

From this, we calculate the GFR:

$$GFR = U_{in} \times V / P_{in} \qquad (2)$$

The average GFR is 120 mL/min in men and 100 mL/min in women. The renal clearance of inulin is equal to the GFR. However, administering inulin intravenously every time one wants to assess the GFR is impractical. In clinical practice, we use the creatinine clearance instead.

Creatinine Is Derived From Skeletal Muscle Phosphocreatine (Fig. 35.9)
Although some creatinine is reabsorbed in the renal tubules, this is compensated by an equivalent tubular secretion, and thus the clearance of creatinine is similar to that of inulin (i.e., is a good approximation of the GFR). To calculate creatinine clearance, one needs a sample of blood and also urine collected over 24 h. The concentrations of creatinine in serum (P_{Cre}) and urine (U_{Cre}) are measured first. The creatinine clearance is then calculated according to the formula:

$$\text{Creatinine clearance} = U_{Cre} \times V / P_{Cre}$$

Estimated GFR
In current practice, the estimated GFR (eGFR) values are calculated from serum creatinine concentration using formulas that include factors such as age, gender, weight, and race. eGFR is used for classification, screening, and monitoring of chronic kidney disease.

In Clinical Practice, Serum Urea and Creatinine Are First-Line Tests in the Diagnosis of Renal Failure (Fig. 35.9)
An increase in serum creatinine concentration reflects the decrease in GFR. Serum concentration of creatinine is 20–80 mmol/L (0.28–0.90 mg/dL). An increase in serum creatinine concentration reflects the decrease in GFR: serum creatinine concentration doubles when the GFR decreases by 50%. Another test used to assess kidney function is the measurement of serum **urea** concentration. However, because urea is the end product of protein catabolism, its level in plasma is also dependent on factors such as the dietary protein intake and the rate of tissue breakdown.

Renal failure leads to a decrease in urine volume and creatinine clearance and to an increase in serum urea and creatinine.

Note that some laboratories express urea concentration as blood urea nitrogen (BUN).

To convert urea (mg/dL) to BUN (mg/dL), multiply by 0.467.
To convert urea (mmol/L) to BUN (mmol/L), multiply by 1.0.
To convert urea (mmol/L) to BUN (mg/dL), multiply by 2.8.

Serum Cystatin C Concentration Is Another Marker of the GFR
Cystatin C is a 122-amino acid, 13-kDa protein belonging to the family of cysteine proteinase inhibitors. It is expressed in all nucleated cells and is produced at a constant rate. Cystatin C is freely filtered through the glomerulus. It is not secreted by the tubules, and although it is reabsorbed, it is subsequently catabolized and therefore does not return to plasma. Its serum concentration is not significantly affected by age, and therefore it is a preferential marker of GFR in children. However, factors such as the inflammatory phenomena may affect serum cystatin C concentration.

Table 35.1 Daily excretion of nitrogen compounds and main ions in urine (mmol/24 h)

Urea	Uric acid	Creatinine	Ammonia
250–500	1–5	7–15	30–50
Sodium	**Potassium**	**Chloride**	**Phosphate**
100–250	30–100	150–250	15–40

Urea is a major contributor to urine nitrogen excretion. It is the final product of protein catabolism in humans. Daily urea excretion also reflects nutritional status and strongly depends on protein intake.
Uric acid excretion depends mainly on endogenous purine degradation, but it might be elevated on a purine-rich diet.
Creatinine is derived from the skeletal muscle phosphocreatine.
At metabolic steady state, urinary excretion of *nitrogen* compounds strictly depends on kidney function.
In *renal failure*, urine output falls, and this leads to an increase in plasma urea and creatinine concentrations.
Urinary excretion of sodium, potassium, and chloride reflects their intake. Excessive sodium intake or impaired elimination might lead to hypertension.
Ammonia is generated in the kidney by deamination of glutamine, and glutamate and is excreted as the ammonium ion. Daily excretion of ammonia and phosphate depends on hydrogen ion excretion in urine (Chapter 36).
Approximate values in an average adult person are given.

CLINICAL BOX
A 25-YEAR-OLD MAN ADMITTED AFTER A MOTORCYCLE ACCIDENT: ACUTE RENAL FAILURE

A 25-year-old man was admitted to the hospital unconscious after a motorcycle accident. He had evidence of shock with hypotension and tachycardia, a fractured skull, and multiple injuries to his limbs. Despite treatment with intravenous colloid and blood, he showed persistent oliguria (urine output 5–10 mL/h; oliguria is < 20 mL/h).

On the third day, his serum creatinine concentration had risen to 300 µmol/L (3.9 mg/dL), and his urea concentration was 21.9 mmol/L (132 mg/dL). BUN was 21.9 mmol/L (61.3 mg/dL). eGFR was 22 mL/min/1.73 m². Reference values are as follows:
1. **Serum creatinine:** 20–80 µmol/L (0.23–0.90 mg/dL)
2. **Serum urea:** 2.5–6.5 mmol/L (16.2–39 mg/dL)
3. **Blood urea nitrogen (BUN):** 2.5–6.5 mmol/L (7.5–18.2 mg/dL)
4. **eGFR:** see Appendix 1

Comment
This young man developed acute renal failure due to acute tubular necrosis as a consequence of hypovolemic shock. He subsequently underwent emergency hemofiltration. Renal function started to recover after 2 weeks with an initial increase in urine volume, the so-called diuretic phase.

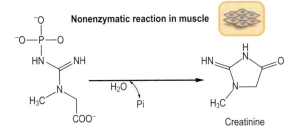

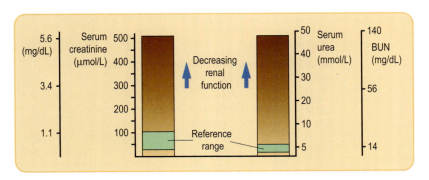

Fig. 35.9 **Serum urea and creatinine concentrations.** The upper panel shows the conversion of muscle phosphocreatine to creatinine. Loss of 50% of nephrons results in an approximate doubling of serum creatinine concentration. Note that in the United States, blood urea nitrogen (BUN) measurement is used instead of serum urea. To convert urea (mmol/L) to BUN (mg/dl), multiply by 2.8. To convert creatinine from umol/l to mg/dL, multiply by 0.0113.

A 37-year-old woman with a 12-year history of type 1 diabetes came for a routine visit to the diabetic clinic. Her glycemic control was poor, and glycated hemoglobin (HbA$_{1c}$) was 9% (75 mmol/mol). Blood pressure was mildly raised at 145/88 mmHg. A quantitative measurement of albumin in urine revealed protein concentration of 5 mg/mmol creatinine, indicating microalbuminuria. Reference values are as follows:

1. **HbA$_{1c}$:** desirable value on treatment below 7% (53 mmol/mol).
2. **Urine microalbumin:** less than 3.5 mg/mmol creatinine.

Comment
This patient had mildly impaired renal function and raised blood pressure as a result of glomerular damage from diabetes. The presence of microalbuminuria predicts future overt diabetic nephropathy.

REGULATION OF WATER AND ELECTROLYTE BALANCE

Renin, angiotensin, and aldosterone

The Renin–angiotensin system controls blood pressure and the vascular tone

Renin is a protease produced principally in the juxtaglomerular apparatus of the kidney; it is released in response to a decreased renal perfusion pressure (decreased delivery of Na$^+$ to the cluster of cells in the renal tubule known as macula densa). Renin secretion is regulated by pathways involving G-protein-coupled receptors, adenylate cyclase, PKA, and cAMP-responsive binding protein (CREB). CREB, a transcription factor, recruits its coactivators and binds to cAMP-responsive element in the renin gene promoter, initiating transcription. Renin secretion is also stimulated by norepinephrine and prostaglandin E$_2$.

Renin cleaves a 10–amino acid peptide, angiotensin I, from the circulating glycoprotein angiotensinogen. Angiotensin I in turn becomes a substrate for peptidyl-dipeptidase A **(angiotensin-converting enzyme [ACE])**, which removes two amino acids, producing **angiotensin II**. Another form of angiotensin, angiotensin 1–9, is formed by an isoform of ACE (ACE2) and is subsequently degraded to angiotensin 1–7. The latter can also be formed from angiotensin II by endopeptidases. The renin–angiotensin system is illustrated in Fig. 35.10.

Angiotensin receptors are important in the pathogenesis of cardiovascular disease

Angiotensin II binds to receptors on the tubular and renal vascular cells. It constricts vascular smooth muscle, thereby increasing blood pressure and reducing renal blood flow and glomerular filtration rate. It also promotes aldosterone release and vascular smooth muscle proliferation through the activation of AT1 receptors that signal through G-proteins and phospholipase C. Generally, **AT1 receptor activation** has effects that promote cardiovascular disease: stimulation of inflammatory phenomena, deposition of extracellular matrix, generation of reactive oxygen species (ROS), and prothrombotic effects. These actions are counteracted by the stimulation of the AT2 receptors, which causes vasodilatation through stimulation of NO production, promotes sodium loss, and inhibits vascular smooth muscle cell proliferation. The actions of angiotensin (1–7), which acts through the so-called MAS receptor (it may also bind to AT1 and AT2), also seem to be cardioprotective. Drugs that inhibit ACE are now extensively used in the treatment of **hypertension** and **heart failure**.

A 65-year-old man with a previous anterior myocardial infarction presented with increasing fatigue, shortness of breath, and ankle edema. Physical examination showed mild tachycardia and a raised jugular venous pressure. An echocardiogram demonstrated impaired systolic function of the left ventricle. The patient's serum measurements revealed sodium 140 mmol/L, potassium 3.5 mmol/L, protein 34 (normal 35–45) g/dL, creatinine 80 μmol/L (0.90 mg/dL), urea 7.5 mmol/L (45 mg/dL), and BUN 7.5 mmol/l (21 mg/dL).

Comment
This man presents with symptoms and signs of cardiac failure. The impaired function of the left ventricle leads to a decreased blood flow through the kidney, activation of the renin–angiotensin system, and stimulation of aldosterone secretion. Aldosterone causes an increased renal reabsorption of sodium and water retention, thereby increasing extracellular fluid volume and edema.
Reference values are as follows:
Sodium: 135–145 mmol/L
Potassium: 3.5–5.0 mmol/L
Bicarbonate: 20–25 mmol/L
Urea: 2.5–6.5 mmol/L (16.2–39 mg/dL)
Blood urea nitrogen (BUN): 2.5–6.5 mmol/L (7.5–18.2 mg/dL)

Aldosterone regulates sodium and potassium homeostasis

Aldosterone is a mineralocorticosteroid hormone produced in the adrenal cortex (Chapter 14). It regulates extracellular volume and vascular tone and controls renal transport of sodium and potassium. It binds to the cytosolic receptor in the epithelial cells, principally in the renal collecting ducts. Aldosterone regulates the Na$^+$/K$^-$-ATPase in both the long and short term. It also regulates transporters such as the Na$^+$/H$^+$ exchanger type 3 in the proximal tubule, the

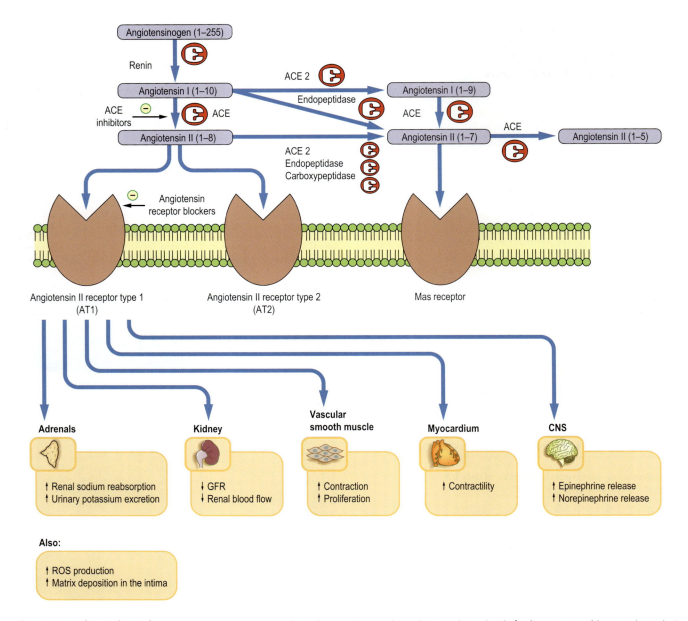

Fig. 35.10 **Renin–angiotensin system.** Renin converts angiotensinogen into angiotensin I. Angiotensin I is further converted into angiotensin II by the angiotensin-converting enzyme (ACE). It also yields other angiotensin peptides. Cellular actions of angiotensins are mediated by angiotensin receptors type 1 (AT1), type 2 (AT2), and MAS receptors that bind angiotensin (1–7). The renin–angiotensin system is a target for two major classes of hypotensive drugs: ACE blockers (e.g., ramipril, enalapril) and AT1-receptor antagonists (e.g., losartan). ACE blockers are also extensively used in the treatment of heart failure. VSMC, vascular smooth muscle cells; CNS, central nervous system; ROS, reactive oxygen species. AT1 receptor is blocked by e.g. losartan and AT2 receptor by saralasin.

 CLINICAL BOX
ARTERIAL HYPERTENSION IS A COMMON DISEASE

Hypertension is inappropriately increased arterial blood pressure. The desirable level of systolic blood pressure is below 140 mmHg and diastolic pressure 90 mmHg (optimal values are lower still, below 120/80 mmHg). According to the World Health Organization, the number of people with hypertension worldwide increased from 600 million in 1980 to 1 billion in 2008. Arterial hypertension has been classified as "essential" (primary) or "secondary." A cause of essential hypertension has not yet been identified, although it is known to involve multiple genetic and environmental factors, including neural, endocrine, and metabolic components. A sodium-rich diet is a recognized factor in the development of hypertension.

Hypertension is associated with an increased risk of stroke and myocardial infarction. Drugs used in the treatment of hypertension include diuretics, drugs blocking adrenoreceptors, inhibitors of the angiotensin-converting enzyme, and the antagonists of angiotensin AT1 receptors.

Na$^+$/Cl$^-$ cotransporter in the distal tubule, and the epithelial sodium channel in the renal collecting duct. The overall result is **increased sodium reabsorption** and **increased excretion of potassium and hydrogen ions**.

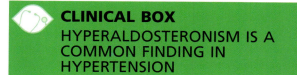

CLINICAL BOX
HYPERALDOSTERONISM IS A COMMON FINDING IN HYPERTENSION

Primary hyperaldosteronism occurs as a result of abnormal adrenal activity and is rare. It may be a result of a single adrenal tumor, adenoma **(Conn's syndrome)**. The more common secondary hyperaldosteronism is due to an increased secretion of renin. **Pheochromocytomas** are catecholamine-secreting tumors that cause hypertension in about 0.1% of hypertensive patients. It is important to correctly diagnose pheochromocytoma because it can be surgically removed (See also Chapter 26).

The natriuretic peptides

Natriuretic peptides promote sodium excretion and decrease the blood pressure. They are important markers of heart failure

A family of peptides known as the natriuretic peptides is involved in the regulation of fluid volume. The two main ones are the **atrial natriuretic peptide** (ANP) and the **brain natriuretic peptide** (BNP). ANP is synthesized predominantly in the cardiac atria as a 126–amino acid propeptide (pro-ANP). It is then cleaved into a smaller 98–amino acid N-terminal peptide and the biologically active 28–amino acid ANP. BNP is synthesized in the cardiac ventricles as a 108–amino acid propeptide and is cleaved into a 76–amino acid N-terminal peptide and a biologically active 32–amino acid BNP. BNP 32 was isolated from the porcine brain, thus the name. All natriuretic peptides have a ring-type structure due to the presence of a disulfide bond.

Natriuretic peptides increase sodium excretion and decrease the blood pressure. ANP and BNP are secreted in response to atrial stretch and to ventricular volume overload. They bind to G-protein-linked receptors: the A-type receptors are located predominantly in the endothelial cells and the B-type receptors in the brain. The signaling pathway includes two guanyl cyclases, one of them being stimulated by NO. The generated cGMP acts on PKC and on phosphodiesterases, regulating cAMP synthesis.

Vasopressin and aquaporins

Vasopressin regulates water reabsorption by the kidneys

The posterior pituitary hormone vasopressin (also known as the **antidiuretic hormone** [ADH]) controls the reabsorption

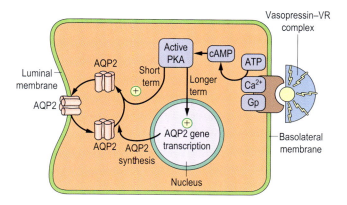

Fig. 35.11 **Vasopressin regulates water reabsorption in the collecting duct.** Vasopressin controls the aquaporin 2 (AQP2) water channel. Vasopressin binds to its receptor (VR), and through G-proteins, (Gp) stimulates the production of cAMP, which, in turn, activates protein kinase A (PKA). PKA phosphorylates cytoplasmic AQP2 and induces its translocation to the cell membrane, increasing capacity for water transport. Vasopressin also regulates expression of the *AQP2* gene.

CLINICAL TEST BOX
DIAGNOSTIC USE OF THE BRAIN NATRIURETIC PEPTIDE (BNP) PROPEPTIDES

The BNP propeptides are present in plasma in equimolar amounts to the active species. Thus, proBNP (1–76) reaches higher levels in cardiac failure than BNP 32. Similarly, proANP (1–98) has a longer half-life in plasma than biologically active 1–28 ANP and therefore is present in the circulation in higher concentrations. It is the propeptides that are measured in clinical laboratories.

The concentrations of ANP and BNP are increased in heart failure. These measurements are particularly useful for excluding heart failure in patients who present with nonspecific symptoms such as shortness of breath.

of water in the collecting ducts of the kidney by regulation of the membrane water channels, **aquaporins**.

Vasopressin controls water reabsorption in the collecting ducts of the kidney. It is synthesized in the hypothalamus and is transported along axons to the posterior pituitary. It is stored there before being further processed and released. It binds to a receptor located on the membranes of tubular cells in the renal collecting ducts (Fig. 35.11). The receptor is coupled to G-proteins and activates PKA. The PKA in turn phosphorylates aquaporin 2 (AQP2), stimulating its translocation to the cell membrane, thus increasing water reabsorption in the collecting duct. Suppression of vasopressin secretion results in the production of diluted urine. Failure to suppress vasopressin adequately results in the inability to dilute urine below the osmolality of plasma.

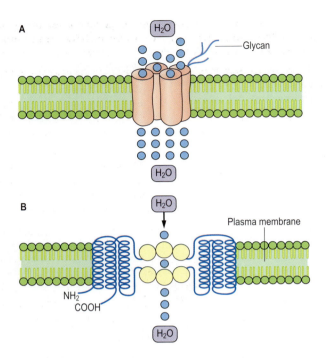

Fig. 35.12 **Aquaporin water channel.** (A) Aquaporin 1 is a multisubunit water channel. (B) Each of the two monomers has two tandem repeat structures, each consisting of three membrane-spanning regions and connecting loops embedded in the membrane.

Aquaporins are membrane channel proteins which transport water

The aquaporin water channel is illustrated in Fig. 35.12. AQP2 and AQP3 are present in the collecting ducts of the kidney and are regulated by vasopressin. AQP1 is expressed in the proximal tubules and in the descending loop of Henle and is not under vasopressin control.

Defects in vasopressin secretion and defective aquaporins cause diabetes insipidus

Vasopressin deficiency causes the condition known as **diabetes insipidus.** Mutations in the vasopressin receptor and *AQP2* gene lead to different types of **nephrogenic diabetes insipidus.** In both conditions, large amounts of dilute urine are excreted, leading to dehydration.

A synthetic analogue of vasopressin, **desmopressin**, is used in the treatment of diabetes insipidus.

Excessive secretion of vasopressin could be due to intracranial disease and also occurs after a major trauma, infection, or surgery and in malignant disease. Defective suppression of vasopressin is known as known as the **syndrome of inappropriate antidiuretic hormone secretion (SIADH)** and leads to water retention.

Vasopressin antagonists such as tolvaptan can be used as adjuncts in the treatment of severe hyponatremia.

Integration of water and sodium homeostasis

Handling of sodium and water is subject to integrated control by aldosterone and vasopressin

Normally, despite variations in fluid intake, plasma osmolality is maintained within narrow limits (280–295 mmol/kg H_2O). Vasopressin regulates osmolality by adjusting the volume of body water, responding to both osmotic and volume signals. Hypothalamic osmoreceptors respond to very small (approximately 1%) increases in plasma osmolality, stimulating both vasopressin secretion and thirst. Vasopressin release is also stimulated by a larger than 10% decrease in the circulating volume.

Water deficit (dehydration) decreases plasma volume, renal blood flow, and GFR

When there is water deficit **(dehydration)**, the decrease in renal blood flow stimulates the renin–angiotensin–aldosterone system. This results in the suppression of urinary sodium excretion and in water retention. In parallel, an increase in the plasma osmolality caused by water deficit stimulates vasopressin, with a consequent decrease in the urine volume. Thus the **overall response to water deficit is sodium and water retention** (Fig. 35.13).

Water excess increases plasma volume, renal blood flow, and GFR

When there is water excess, production of renin is suppressed. A low concentration of aldosterone allows urinary sodium loss. Plasma osmolality decreases. This is sensed by the osmoreceptors, which suppress vasopressin. Suppression of vasopressin secretion leads to the urinary loss of water. Thirst is also suppressed, decreasing water intake. **Thus the overall response to water excess is increased loss of sodium and water in urine.**

Plasma sodium concentration

Disorders of plasma sodium concentration are closely linked to dehydration and overhydration

The plasma sodium concentration is 135–145 mmol/l (mEq/L). Disorders of sodium concentration are clinically important and are closely associated with water balance, in a way sometimes not easy to disentangle. Water and sodium losses are frequently concomitant, and whether they will result in hypo- or hypernatremia depends on the relative degree of sodium and water loss.

Clinical abnormalities that develop after excessive fluid loss depend on the ionic composition of the lost fluid

For instance, **sweat** contains less sodium than extracellular fluid; therefore excessive sweating leads to a predominant loss of water and "concentrates" sodium in the extracellular fluid,

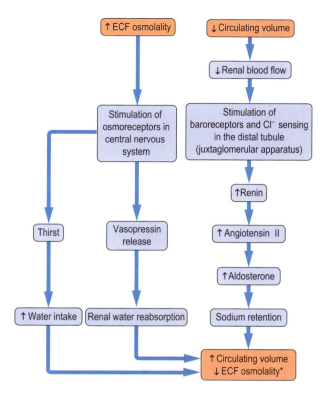

Fig. 35.13 **Water and sodium metabolism are closely interrelated.** An increase in ECF osmolality stimulates secretion of vasopressin and leads to increased renal water reabsorption. This "dilutes" the ECF and leads to a decrease in osmolality. This response is reinforced by the stimulation of thirst. A decrease in the plasma volume also leads to water retention through stimulation of the pressure-sensitive receptors (baroreceptors) in the juxtaglomerular apparatus. This activates the renin–angiotensin system and secretion of aldosterone. The result is increased sodium reabsorption. *Osmolality will decrease if the degree of water retention is relatively greater than that of sodium retention.

Table 35.2 Electrolyte content of the body fluids

	Sodium (mmol/L)	Potassium (mmol/L)	Bicarbonate (mmol/L)	Chloride (mmol/L)
Plasma	140	4	25	100
Gastric juice				
Small intestinal fluid	140	10	Variable	70
Feces in diarrhea	50–140	30–70	20–80	Variable
Bile, pleural, and peritoneal fluids	140	5	40	100
Sweat	12	10	—	12

Loss of fluid that has an electrolyte content similar to that of plasma leads to dehydration with normal serum electrolyte concentrations. However, when the sodium content of the lost fluid is less than that of plasma (e.g., sweat), dehydration may be accompanied by hypernatremia. Overhydration is usually accompanied by hyponatremia. Adapted with permission from Dominiczak MH, editor: Seminars in Clinical Biochemistry, ed. 2, Glasgow, 1997, Glasgow University.

causing hypernatremia. Conversely, the sodium content of the **intestinal fluid** is similar to that of plasma but contains considerable amounts of potassium. Thus its loss, such as happens in severe diarrhea, would result in dehydration and hypokalemia, but plasma sodium concentration would usually remain close to normal (Table 35.2).

A decreased sodium concentration (**hyponatremia**) usually indicates that the extracellular fluid is being "diluted" (due to an excess of water). Hyponatremia can be caused by an excessive intake of water, as in compulsive water drinking, or (most frequently) by water retention, as happens in SIADH. It may also be caused by a large loss of sodium in chronic diarrhea and vomiting or (rarely) by aldosterone deficiency in Addison's disease. Hyponatremia observed in athletes during intense exercise results from supplementing water during a dehydrating exercise in the form of hypotonic drinks, thus "diluting" the ECF.

 CLINICAL BOX
POOR ORAL FLUID INTAKE LEADS TO DEHYDRATION

An 80-year-old man had been admitted to the hospital after being found lying on the floor at home after suffering acute stroke. He had poor tissue turgor, dry mouth, and tachycardia, and he was hypotensive. Serum measurements revealed the following: sodium 150 mmol/L, potassium 5.2 mmol/L, bicarbonate 35 mmol/L, urea 19 mmol/L (90.3 mg/dL), BUN 19.0 mmol/L (42 mg/dL), and creatinine 110 µmol/L (1.13 mg/dL).

Reference values are as follows:
Sodium: 135–145 mmol/L
Potassium: 3.5–5.0 mmol/L
Bicarbonate: 20–25 mmol/L
Urea: 2.5–6.5 mmol/L (16.2–39 mg/dL),
Blood urea nitrogen (BUN): 2.5–6.5 mmol/L (7.5–18.2 mg/dL)
Creatinine: 20–80 µmol/L (0.28–0.90 mg/dL)

Comment
This patient presents with dehydration, indicated by the high sodium and urea values and mildly elevated creatinine. He was treated with intravenous fluids, predominantly in the form of 5% dextrose, to replace the water deficit.

Hypernatremia is most commonly associated with dehydration

An increased sodium concentration **(hypernatremia)** means that the extracellular fluid is being "concentrated" (due to water loss). Hypernatremia is most commonly associated with dehydration due to decreased intake of water (as in sick elderly persons unable to drink enough) or excess loss of water, such as in diarrhea, vomiting, or diabetes (osmotic diuresis is the cause in diabetes). It can also be caused by excessive administration of sodium salts (e.g., sodium bicarbonate infused during resuscitation).

Both severe hypernatremia and hyponatremia cause neurologic symptoms

In hyponatremia, the symptoms are predominantly related to hypoosmolality and consequent brain swelling. Sodium does not cross the blood–brain barrier, and thus hyponatremia and hypoosmolality cause ingress of fluid into the brain. Chronic hypernatremia can also lead to encephalopathy. Importantly, a quick correction of hyponatremia and hypernatremia can exacerbate neurologic symptoms; therefore it is crucial that the therapy proceeds at an appropriate pace (see Further Reading).

Plasma potassium concentration

Disorders of plasma potassium concentration carry the risk of cardiac arrhythmias

The normal plasma concentration of potassium is 3.5–5.0 mmol/L (mEq/; Fig. 35.14). Because its intracellular concentration is much higher, a relatively minor shift of potassium between the ECF and ICF results in major changes in its serum concentration. Both high and low concentrations of potassium **(hyperkalemia** and **hypokalemia**, respectively) affect the cardiac muscle, cause arrhythmias, and can be life-threatening.

On the EKG, hyperkalemia leads to the loss of P-waves, characteristic tall peaked T-waves, and widened QRS complexes. Hypokalemia, on the other hand, may prolong the PR intervals, cause peaked P-waves, flatten the T-waves, and cause prominent U-waves.

Monitoring plasma potassium concentration is fundamentally important

Plasma potassium concentration below 2.5 mmol/L or 3 above 6.0 mmol/L is dangerous (Fig. 35.14). The most common cause of severe hyperkalemia is renal failure; in this condition, the nonfunctioning kidney cannot excrete enough potassium in the urine. On the other hand, low serum potassium usually results from losses, either renal or gastrointestinal. Diarrhea is an important cause. Hyperaldosteronism also leads to hypokalemia. Normally, the kidneys account for more than 90% of the body potassium loss; thus treatment with diuretics is an important cause of both hypo- and hyperkalemia (this depends on the type of diuretic used). Similarly, poorly controlled

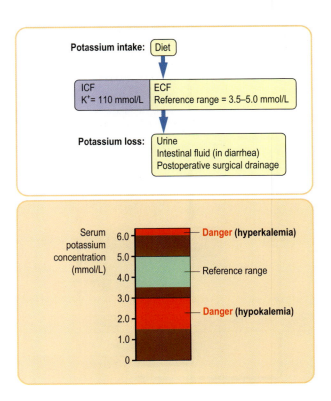

Fig. 35.14 Potassium balance. Serum potassium concentration is maintained within narrow limits. Both low (hypokalemia) and high (hyperkalemia) concentrations are dangerous because potassium affects the contractility of heart muscle. Generally, serum potassium concentrations above 6.0 mmol/L and below 2.5 mmol/L are regarded as emergencies. The upper panel shows main sources of potassium loss.

diabetes can present with either hypokalemia or, more rarely, hyperkalemia (Chapter 31).

Note that changes in the plasma potassium concentration are also associated with acid–base disorders: alkalosis leads to hypokalemia and acidosis to hyperkalemia (Chapter 36).

Assessment of water and electrolyte status in clinical practice

To assess water and electrolyte balance in a patient, the following measurements are required in addition to the physical examination and medical history:

- **Serum electrolyte concentrations:** sodium, potassium, chloride, and bicarbonate concentrations
- **Serum urea (blood urea nitrogen) and creatinine**
- **Urine volume, osmolality, and sodium concentration**
- **Serum osmolality**
- **Fluid balance chart:** a daily record of fluid intake and loss

ACTIVE LEARNING

1. Comment on the role of Na⁺/K⁺-ATPase in maintaining the ion gradients across cell membranes.
2. Explain the role of the renin–angiotensin system in the maintenance of sodium and water balance.
3. Describe the water movements between ECF and ICF that take place in water deprivation.
4. Why does a low concentration of albumin in plasma lead to edema?
5. What are the most common causes of hyperkalemia?
6. What water and electrolyte disorders would you expect in chronic diarrhea?

SUMMARY

■ Both a deficit of body water (dehydration) and its excess (overhydration) cause potentially serious clinical problems. Therefore assessment of water and electrolyte balance is an important part of clinical examination.

■ Body water balance is closely linked to the balance of dissolved ions (electrolytes), the most important of which are sodium and potassium.

■ Na⁺/K⁺-ATPase is essential for maintenance of ion gradients between the cell and its surroundings, electrical potential, and the performance of the cellular ion transport system. It also controls cell hydration and its volume.

■ Movement of water between the ECF and ICF is controlled by osmotic gradients.

■ Movement of water between the lumen of a blood vessel and the interstitial fluid is controlled by the osmotic and hydrostatic pressures.

■ Main regulators of water and electrolyte balance are vasopressin (water) and aldosterone (sodium and potassium).

■ The renin–angiotensin–aldosterone system is the principal regulator of blood pressure and vascular tone.

■ Measurements of natriuretic peptides help diagnose cardiac failure.

FURTHER READING

Adrogue, H. J., & Madias, N. E. (2000). Hyponatremia. *The New England Journal of Medicine, 342*, 1581–1589.

Ellison, D. H., & Berl, T. (2007). The syndrome of inappropriate antidiuresis. *The New England Journal of Medicine, 356*, 2064–2072.

Frost, P. (2015). Intravenous fluid therapy in adult inpatients. *BMJ (Clinical Research Ed.), 350*, g7620.

James, P. A., Oparil, S., Carter, B. L., et al. (2014). 2014 evidence-based guideline for the management of high blood pressure in adults: Report from the panel members appointed to the eighth joint national committee (JNC 8). *JAMA: The Journal of the American Medical Association, 311*, 507–520.

Richards, A. M., & Troughton, R. W. (2012). Use of natriuretic peptides to guide and monitor heart failure therapy. *Clinical Chemistry, 58*, 62–71.

Schmieder, R. E., Hilgers, K. F., Schlaich, M. P., et al. (2007). Renin-angiotensin system and cardiovascular risk. *Lancet, 369*, 1208–1219.

Schrier, R. W. (2006). Body water homeostasis: Clinical disorders of urinary dilution and concentration. *Journal of the American Society of Nephrology, 17*, 1820–1832.

Sterns, R. H. (2015). Disorders of plasma sodium–causes, consequences, and correction. *The New England Journal of Medicine, 372*, 55–65.

Verbalis, J. G., Goldsmith, S. R., Greenberg, A., et al. (2013). Diagnosis, evaluation, and treatment of hyponatremia: expert panel recommendations. *The American Journal of Medicine, 126*, S5–S41.

Verkman, A. S. (2012). Aquaporins in clinical medicine. *Annual Review of Medicine, 63*, 303–316.

RELEVANT WEBSITES

Medline Plus - Water and Electrolyte Balance: http://www.nlm.nih.gov/medlineplus/fluidandelectrolytebalance.html

British Consensus Guidelines on Intravenous Fluid Therapy for Adult Surgical Patients 2011: http://www.bapen.org.uk/pdfs/bapen_pubs/giftasup.pdf

MORE CLINICAL CASES

Please refer to Appendix 2 for more cases relevant to this chapter.

ABBREVIATIONS

ACE	Angiotensin-converting enzyme
ADH	Antidiuretic hormone, vasopressin
AG	Anion gap
ANP	Atrial natriuretic peptide
AQP	Aquaporin
AT1, AT2	Angiotensin receptors
BNP	Brain natriuretic peptide
BUN	Blood urea nitrogen
bw	Body weight
CNS	Central nervous system
CREB	cAMP-responsive binding protein, transcription factor
ECF	Extracellular fluid
eGFR	Estimated glomerular filtration rate
ENaC	Amiloride-sensitive calcium channel
GFR	Glomerular filtration rate
ICF	Intracellular fluid
MAS	Angiotensin 1–7 receptor
NCC	Sodium–chloride co-transporter
NKCC2	Sodium–potassium–chloride co-transporter
PKA	Protein kinase A
PKC	Protein kinase C
PTH	Parathyroid hormone
ROS	Reactive oxygen species
SIADH	Syndrome of inappropriate antidiuretic hormone expression
VSMC	Vascular smooth muscle cells

The Lung and the Regulation of Hydrogen Ion Concentration (Acid–Base Balance)

Marek H. Dominiczak and Mirosława Szczepańska-Konkel

INTRODUCTION

Metabolism generates acids

Cellular metabolism generates carbon dioxide. Carbon dioxide dissolves in water, forming carbonic acid, which in turn dissociates releasing hydrogen ion. It is called a volatile acid. There are other acids derived from sources other than CO_2, and these are known as nonvolatile; by definition, they cannot be removed through the lungs and must be excreted via the kidney. The net production of nonvolatile acids is around 50 mmol/24 h.

Lactic acid is produced during anaerobic glycolysis, and its concentration in plasma is the hallmark of hypoxia. Keto acids (acetoacetic and β-hydroxybutyric acid) are important in diabetes (Chapter 31). Metabolism of sulfur-containing amino acids and phosphorus-containing compounds generates inorganic acids.

In spite of the amount of hydrogen ion produced, its blood concentration (often expressed as a negative logarithm of the concentration, the pH) is remarkably constant: it remains between 35 and 45 nmol/L (pH 7.35–7.45). Maintenance of stable pH is essential because it affects ionization of proteins (Chapter 2) and, consequently, the conformation of proteins, which in turn affects the activity of enzymes and other biologically active molecules such as ion channels. A decrease in pH increases sympathetic tone and may lead to cardiac dysrhythmias. Also, pH and partial pressure of carbon dioxide (pCO_2) affect the shape of the hemoglobin saturation curve, and thus tissue oxygenation (Chapter 5).

Maintaining the acid–base balance involves the lungs, erythrocytes, and the kidneys

Maintaining the acid–base balance involves the lungs, erythrocytes, and the kidneys (Fig. 36.1). The lungs control the exchange of carbon dioxide and oxygen between the blood and the atmosphere, the erythrocytes transport these gases between the lungs and tissues, and the kidneys control plasma bicarbonate synthesis and the excretion of the hydrogen ion.

Clinical relevance

Understanding acid–base balance has a general relevance to medical practice because its abnormalities underline many disorders across clinical specialties.

BODY BUFFER SYSTEMS: RESPIRATORY AND METABOLIC COMPONENTS OF THE ACID–BASE BALANCE

Blood and tissues contain buffer systems that minimize changes in hydrogen ion concentration

The main buffer system that neutralizes hydrogen ions released from cells is the **bicarbonate buffer.** Another important one is **hemoglobin.** Within cells, the hydrogen ion is neutralized by intracellular buffers, mainly **proteins** and **phosphates** (Table 36.1 and Chapter 2).

Bicarbonate buffer remains at equilibrium with atmospheric air

The key concept is that the bicarbonate buffer is an open system. This means that it has much greater buffering potential than the "closed-system" buffers. The CO_2 produced in the course of metabolism diffuses through cell membranes and dissolves in plasma. Its plasma solubility coefficient is 0.23 if pCO_2 is measured in kPa (0.03 if pCO_2 is measured in mmHg; 1 kPa = 7.5 mmHg or 1 mmHg = 0.133 kPa). Thus at the normal pCO_2 of 5.3 kPa (40 mmHg), the concentration of dissolved CO_2 (dCO_2) is

$$dCO_2 \, (mmol/L) = 5.3 \, kPa \times 0.23 = 1.2 \, mmol/L$$

The CO_2 equilibrates with carbonic acid H_2CO_3 in plasma in the course of a slow, nonenzymatic reaction. Normally, H_2CO_3 concentration is very low, about 0.0017 mmol/L. The key point is that because of the equilibrium between H_2CO_3

539

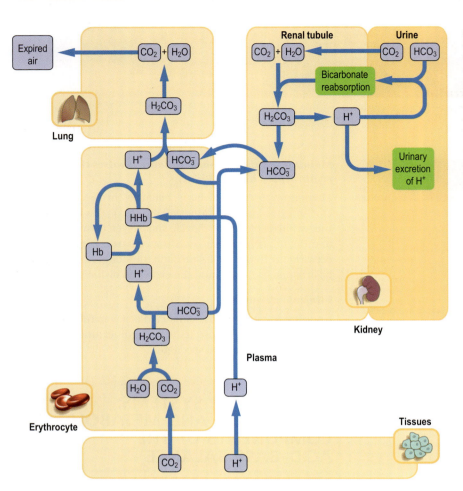

Fig. 36.1 **Acid–base balance.** The lungs, kidneys, and erythrocytes contribute to the maintenance of the acid–base balance. The lungs control the gas exchange with the atmospheric air. CO_2 generated in tissues is transported in plasma as bicarbonate; the erythrocyte hemoglobin contributes to CO_2 transport. Hemoglobin buffers the hydrogen ion derived from carbonic acid. The kidneys reabsorb filtered bicarbonate in the proximal tubules and generate new bicarbonate in the distal tubules, where there is a net secretion of hydrogen ion. Hb, hemoglobin.

Table 36.1 Principal buffers in the human body

Buffer	Acid	Conjugate base	Site of main buffering action
Hemoglobin	HHb	Hb^-	Erythrocytes
Proteins	HProt	$Prot^-$	Intracellular fluid
Phosphate buffer	$H_2PO_4^-$	HPO_4^{2-}	Intracellular fluid
Bicarbonate	$CO_2 \rightarrow H_2CO_3$	HCO_3^-	Extracellular fluid

See Chapter 2 for the principles of buffering action. The Brønsted–Lowry definition of an acid is "a molecular species that has a tendency to lose a hydrogen ion, forming a conjugate base."

and dissolved CO_2 (theoretically all dissolved CO_2 could eventually convert into H_2CO_3), this component of the bicarbonate buffer can be taken as equal to the sum of the H_2CO_3 and the dissolved CO_2. The equation describing the behavior of the bicarbonate buffer is the **Henderson–Hasselbalch equation** (see also Chapter 2). It expresses the relationship between pH and the components of the buffer:

$$pH = pK + \log([\text{bicarbonate}]/pCO_2 \times 0.23)$$

The equation demonstrates that blood pH is determined by the ratio between the concentration of plasma bicarbonate (the **"base" component** of the buffer) and the concentration of dissolved CO_2 (the **"acid" component,** because it converts to carbonic acid). Normally, at pCO_2 of 5.3 kPa and dissolved CO_2 concentration of 1.2 mmol/L, the plasma bicarbonate concentration is about 24 mmol/L. The pK of the bicarbonate buffer is 6.1. Let's insert the actual concentrations of buffer components into the preceding equation:

$$pH = 6.1 + \log(24/1.2) = 7.40$$

Thus the normal concentration of bicarbonate and normal partial pressure of CO_2 correspond to pH 7.40 (hydrogen ion concentration 40 nmol/L). The bicarbonate buffer minimizes changes in hydrogen ion concentration when acid is added to the blood.

When the H^+ concentration in the system increases, the bicarbonate component of the buffer accepts (H^+), forming carbonic acid, which is subsequently converted into CO_2 and H_2O in the reaction catalyzed by **carbonic anhydrase:**

$$H^+ + HCO_3^- \rightleftharpoons H_2CO_3 \rightleftharpoons CO_2 + H_2O$$

At the first stage, the bicarbonate concentration decreases and pCO_2 increases. However, because the CO_2 is eliminated through the lungs, the bicarbonate/pCO_2 ratio is subsequently brought back toward normal.

Conversely, when the H⁺ concentration decreases, the carbonic acid component of the buffer will dissociate to supply H⁺:

$$H_2CO_3 \rightarrow H^+ + HCO_3^-$$

The ventilation rate will decrease, retaining CO_2 to increase the pCO_2, thus normalizing the bicarbonate/pCO_2 ratio:

$$CO_2 + H_2O \rightarrow H_2CO_3$$

Looking at the Henderson–Hasselbalch equation, we see that its denominator (pCO_2) is controlled by the lungs. For this reason, it is called the **"respiratory component of the acid–base balance."** Conversely, plasma bicarbonate concentration is controlled by the kidneys and erythrocytes, and consequently, it is called the **"metabolic component of the acid–base balance"** (Fig. 36.2).

Bicarbonate is generated in erythrocytes and renal tubules

Erythrocytes and renal tubular cells contain a zinc-containing enzyme, carbonic anhydrase (CA), that converts dissolved CO_2 into carbonic acid. Carbonic acid dissociates, yielding hydrogen and bicarbonate ions:

$$CO_2 + H_2O \xrightleftharpoons{CA} H_2CO_3 \rightleftharpoons H^+ + HCO_3^-$$

The kidneys regulate bicarbonate reabsorption and synthesis, and **the erythrocytes** adjust bicarbonate concentration in response to changes in pCO_2.

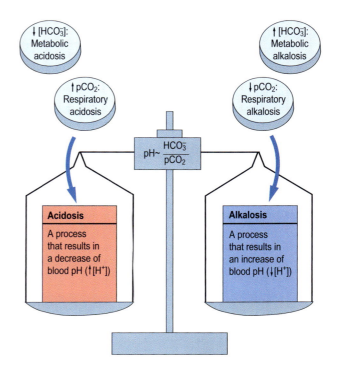

Fig. 36.3 **Disorders of the acid–base balance.** A primary increase in pCO_2 or a decrease in plasma bicarbonate concentration can lead to acidosis. A decrease in pCO_2 or an increase in plasma bicarbonate can lead to alkalosis. If the primary change is in pCO_2, the disorder is called respiratory, and if the primary change is in plasma bicarbonate, it is called metabolic.

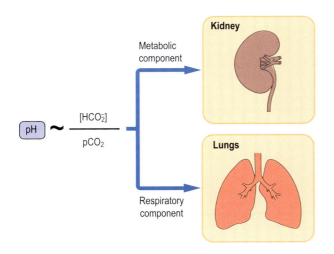

Fig. 36.2 **The bicarbonate buffer.** Blood pH depends on the ratio of plasma bicarbonate to the partial pressure of carbon dioxide (pCO_2). The pCO_2 is the respiratory component of acid–base balance, and bicarbonate concentration is the metabolic component.

Respiratory and metabolic components of the acid–base balance are interlinked

The respiratory and metabolic components of the acid–base balance are closely interdependent: one tends to compensate for the changes in the other. When the primary disorder is respiratory - for instance, severe **chronic obstructive airway disease (COAD)** - and leads to accumulation of CO_2, there is a compensatory increase in bicarbonate reabsorption by the kidney. Conversely, a decrease in pCO_2 - resulting, for instance, from **hyperventilation in an asthmatic attack** - leads to increased renal bicarbonate excretion.

When the primary problem is metabolic (e.g., **diabetic ketoacidosis**), a decrease in bicarbonate concentration stimulates the respiratory center to increase ventilation rate. The CO_2 is removed, and plasma pCO_2 decreases. Clinically, this can be observed as hyperventilation. Conversely, an increase in plasma bicarbonate leads to a decrease in the ventilation rate and to CO_2 retention. Thus the compensatory change always tends to normalize the bicarbonate/pCO_2 ratio, helping to bring the pH toward normal (Fig. 36.3).

Intracellular buffering

Inside cells, hydrogen ion is buffered by proteins and phosphates

The two main intracellular buffers are proteins and phosphates, and the buffering is governed by the $HPO_4^{2-}/H_2PO_4^-$ and protein/protein-H ratios. Hemoglobin is an important extracellular protein buffer.

It is practically important that when an excess of hydrogen ion is present in the plasma, it enters cells in exchange for potassium ion. This increases plasma potassium concentration. Conversely, when there is a decrease in plasma hydrogen ion, and thus bicarbonate excess, hydrogen ion will be supplied from cells. It will enter plasma in exchange for potassium, decreasing plasma potassium. Thus low blood pH (acidemia) is generally associated with hyperkalemia, and high blood pH (alkalemia) is associated with hypokalemia (Fig. 36.4).

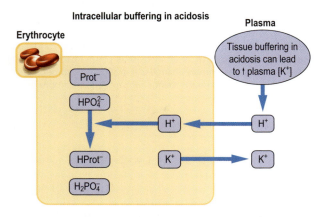

Intracellular buffering in acidosis

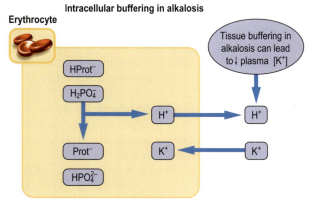

Intracellular buffering in alkalosis

Fig. 36.4 **Intracellular buffers: proteins and phosphates. Potassium–hydrogen ion exchange.** Intracellular buffers are primarily proteins and phosphates. However, the hydrogen ion enters cells in exchange for potassium. Therefore an accumulation of the hydrogen ion in the plasma (acidemia) and the consequent entry of excess of hydrogen ion into cells increase plasma potassium concentration. Conversely, a deficit of hydrogen ion in plasma (alkalemia) may lead to a low plasma potassium concentration. Prot, protein.

CLINICAL TEST BOX
LABORATORY ASSESSMENT OF ACID–BASE BALANCE

The "blood gas measurement" is an important first-line laboratory investigation. In patients with respiratory failure, it is also an essential guide to oxygen therapy and assisted ventilation.

Measurements are performed on a sample of arterial blood, usually taken from the radial artery. The jargon term "blood gases" means the measurements of **pO₂, pCO₂, and pH** (or hydrogen ion concentration), from which the concentration of **bicarbonate** is calculated using the Henderson–Hasselbalch equation. Several other indices are also computed; they include the total amount of buffers in the blood (the **buffer base**) and the difference between the desired (normal) amount of buffers in the blood and the actual amount (**base excess**). Reference values for pH, pCO₂, and O₂ are given in Table 36.2.

Table 36.2 Reference ranges for blood gas results

A. Reference ranges*		
	Arterial	**Venous**
[H⁺]	35–45 mmol/L	
pH	7.35–7.45	
pCO₂	4.6–6.0 kPa (35–45 mmHg)	4.8–6.7 kPa (36–50 mmHg)
pO₂	10.5–13.5 kPa (79–101 mmHg)	4.0–6.7 kPa (30–50 mmHg)
Bicarbonate	23–30 mmol/L	22–29 mmol/L
B. Comparison of conventional and SI units of hydrogen ion concentration		
Conventional units: pH	**SI units: [H⁺] nmol/L**	
6.8	160	
7.1	80	
7.4	40	
7.7	20	

*The measured values in "blood gases" are pH, pCO₂, and pO₂; the bicarbonate concentration is calculated from pH and pCO₂ values; pH below 7.0 or above 7.7 is life threatening. (Adapted with permission from Hutchinson AS. In Dominiczak MH, editor. Seminars in clinical biochemistry, Glasgow, 1997, Glasgow University Press.)

LUNGS: THE GAS EXCHANGE

The lungs supply oxygen necessary for tissue metabolism and remove the generated CO_2

Approximately 10,000 L of air passes through the lungs of an average person each day.

The airways are "tubes" of progressively decreasing diameter. They consist of the trachea, large and small bronchi, and even smaller bronchioles (Fig. 36.5). At the end of the bronchioles, there are pulmonary alveoli - structures lined with endothelium and covered with a film of surfactant, the main component of which is dipalmitoyl phosphatidylcholine. Surfactant decreases the surface tension of the alveoli. The gas exchange takes place in the alveoli.

The respiratory center in the brainstem controls respiration rate

Ventilation rate is influenced by partial pressures of oxygen (pO_2) and carbon dioxide (pCO_2). The respiratory center in the brainstem has chemoreceptors sensitive to pCO_2 and to pH. Under normal circumstances, the stimulus for ventilation is the increase in pCO_2 or decrease in pH and not the pO_2. However, if the pO_2 falls and hypoxia develops, the pO_2 begins to control the ventilation rate through a set of receptors located in the carotid bodies in the aortic arch. It becomes the dominant

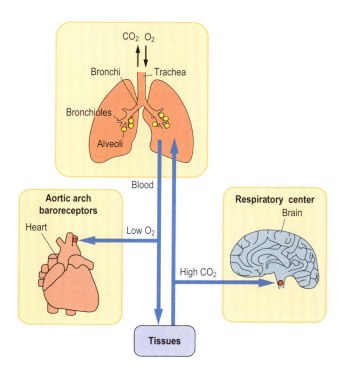

Fig. 36.5 **Control of the respiratory rate by pCO_2 and pO_2.** Lung ventilation and lung perfusion are main factors controlling gas exchange. pCO_2 regulates the ventilation rate through central chemoreceptors in the brainstem. However, at low pO_2, the ventilation rate is controlled by pO_2-sensitive peripheral receptors in the carotid bodies and in the aortic arch.

mechanism at pO_2 below 8 kPa (60 mmHg). This is known as the **hypoxic drive** (Fig. 36.5).

Ventilation and lung perfusion together determine gas exchange

The pulmonary arteries carry deoxygenated blood from the periphery, through the right ventricle, to the pulmonary alveoli. After oxygenation, the blood flows through pulmonary veins to the left atrium. In the alveolar capillaries, the blood accepts oxygen, which diffuses through the alveolar wall from the inspired air; at the same time, the CO_2 diffuses from the blood into the alveoli and is expired.

The diffusion rate of gases is determined by the difference in partial pressures between alveolar air and blood. Table 36.3 shows the pO_2 and pCO_2 in the lungs. Compared with the atmospheric air, pCO_2 in the alveolar air is slightly higher and pO_2 slightly lower (this is due to the water vapor pressure). Carbon dioxide is much more soluble in water than oxygen

---

CLINICAL BOX
A WOMAN PRESENTING WITH SHORTNESS OF BREATH: RESPIRATORY ACIDOSIS

A 56-year-old woman was admitted to a general ward with increasing breathlessness. She had smoked 20 cigarettes a day for the previous 25 years and reported frequent attacks of "winter bronchitis." Blood gas measurements revealed a pO_2 of 6 kPa (45 mmHg), pCO_2 of 8.4 kPa (53 mmHg), and pH 7.35 (hydrogen ion concentration 51 nmol/L); bicarbonate concentration was 35 mmol.

Comment

This patient presented with an exacerbation of **chronic obstructive airway disease** (COAD) and respiratory acidosis. Her pCO_2 was high, and therefore her ventilation was dependent on the hypoxic drive. Her bicarbonate concentration was also increased as a result of metabolic compensation of respiratory acidosis. One must be careful when treating such patients with high concentrations of oxygen because the increased pO_2 may remove the hypoxic drive and cause respiratory depression. Monitoring of arterial pO_2 and pCO_2 on oxygen treatment is mandatory. This patient was successfully treated with 28% oxygen (for reference ranges, refer to Table 36.2).

Table 36.3 Partial pressures of oxygen and carbon dioxide in atmospheric air, lung alveoli, and the blood, kPa (mmHg)

	Dry air	Alveoli	Systemic arteries	Tissue
pO_2	21.2 (39)	13.7 (98)	12.0 (90)	5.3 (40)
pCO_2	<0.13 (0.1)	5.3 (40)	5.3 (40)	6.0 (45)
Water vapor		6.3 (47)		

Partial-pressure gradients determine the diffusion of gases through the alveolar/blood barrier (1 kPa = 7.5 mmHg).

and equilibrates with blood more rapidly. Therefore when problems develop, one first notices a decrease in blood pO_2 (hypoxia). An increase in pCO_2 (hypercapnia) occurs later and usually indicates a more severe problem. The other factor determining gas exchange is the rate at which the blood flows through the lungs (the perfusion rate). Normally, the alveolar ventilation rate is approximately 4 L/min and the perfusion 5 L/min (the ratio of ventilation to perfusion [Va/Q] is 0.8).

Different combinations of disturbed ventilation and perfusion may occur

When some lung alveoli collapse and are unable to exchange gases, parts of the lung may be well perfused but poorly ventilated. As a result, blood pO_2 decreases because there is less diffusion of oxygen from the alveolar air. The presence of oxygen-poor blood in the arterial circulation is known as the **"shunt" condition**. Conversely, when ventilation is adequate but perfusion is poor, gas exchange cannot take place; in such cases, part of the lung behaves as if it had no alveoli at all, forming the **"physiologic dead space."** The Clinical Box below shows the examples of conditions related to poor ventilation, poor perfusion, and the combination of both.

Handling of carbon dioxide by erythrocytes

Erythrocytes transport CO_2 to the lungs in a "fixed" form - as bicarbonate

Human metabolism produces CO_2 at a rate of 200–800 mL/min. The CO_2 dissolves in water and generates carbonic acid, which in turn dissociates into hydrogen and bicarbonate ions. Thus CO_2 generates large number of hydrogen ions:

$$CO_2 + H_2O \rightleftharpoons H_2CO_3 \rightleftharpoons H^+ + HCO_3^-$$

In plasma, this reaction is nonenzymatic and proceeds slowly, generating only minute amounts of carbonic acid, which remains in equilibrium with a large amount of dissolved CO_2. However, the same reaction in the erythrocytes is catalyzed by carbonic anhydrase, which "fixes" CO_2 as bicarbonate. The generated hydrogen ion is buffered by hemoglobin.

The bicarbonate ion then moves to plasma in exchange for chloride ion (the "chloride shift"; Fig. 36.6). As much as 70%

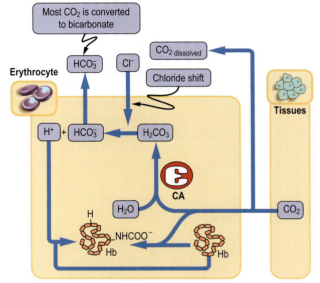

Removal of CO_2 from tissues

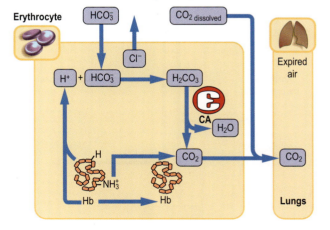

Excretion of CO_2 with expired air

Fig. 36.6 **CO_2 transport by the erythrocytes.** Erythrocyte carbonic anhydrase converts approximately 70% of the CO_2 produced in tissues into bicarbonate for transport to the lungs: approximately 20% of the total amount is transported bound to hemoglobin, as carbamates ($NHCOO^-$), and the rest as dissolved gas in the plasma. CA, carbonic anhydrase.

CLINICAL BOX
DISORDERS OF LUNG VENTILATION AND PERFUSION

- **Rib-cage deformities** impair ventilation by limiting lung movement.
- **Chest trauma** may decrease ventilation as a result of lung collapse.
- **Pulmonary emphysema** may destroy the alveoli.
- **Inadequate synthesis of surfactant** causes the collapse of alveoli and impairment of ventilation (this is known as the respiratory distress syndrome).
- **Obstruction of the bronchi** by inhaled objects or narrowing by a growing tumor impairs ventilation.
- **Constriction of the bronchi** in asthma impairs ventilation.
- **Impaired elasticity of the lung** or dysfunction of the diaphragm and intercostal muscles of the chest wall reduces ventilation.
- **Fluid present in the alveoli** (pulmonary edema) impairs ventilation by affecting diffusion of gases.
- **Defects in neural control** impair ventilation by affecting lung movement.
- **Circulatory problems** such as shock and heart failure compromise lung perfusion.

of all CO_2 produced in tissues becomes bicarbonate; approximately 20% is carried linked to hemoglobin as carbamino groups, and only 10% remains dissolved in plasma.

In the lungs, higher pO_2 facilitates dissociation of CO_2 from hemoglobin. This is known as the **Haldane effect.** The hemoglobin releases the hydrogen ion, which reacts with bicarbonate, forming carbonic acid, which, in turn, yields CO_2 and H_2O.

BICARBONATE HANDLING BY THE KIDNEYS

Similarly to the erythrocytes, proximal and distal renal tubular cells contain carbonic anhydrase.

Normally, bicarbonate filtered through the glomerulus is reabsorbed in the proximal tubule, and the urine is almost bicarbonate-free. The surfaces of the renal tubular cells facing the lumen are impermeable to bicarbonate. Filtered bicarbonate combines in the lumen with hydrogen ion secreted by the cells. The formed carbonic acid is converted to CO_2 and H_2O by carbonic anhydrase located on the luminal membrane. CO_2 diffuses into cells, and there the intracellular carbonic anhydrase converts it back into carbonic acid, which dissociates into hydrogen and bicarbonate ions. Bicarbonate is returned to plasma, and the hydrogen ion is secreted into the lumen of the tubule to trap more filtered bicarbonate. Note that in this process, hydrogen ion is used exclusively to aid **bicarbonate reabsorption**, and there is **no net hydrogen ion excretion** (Fig. 36.7).

Distal tubules generate new bicarbonate and excrete hydrogen

As bicarbonate is being generated in the distal tubule, there is both a net loss of hydrogen ions from the body and a net gain of bicarbonate. The process is as follows: CO_2 diffuses from the lumen into cells, where intracellular carbonic anhydrase converts it into carbonic acid, which dissociates into hydrogen ion and bicarbonate. Bicarbonate is then transported to the plasma and **hydrogen ion secreted into the tubule lumen.** Because no bicarbonate is present in the lumen of the distal tubule (all has been reabsorbed in the proximal tubule), the **hydrogen ion is buffered (trapped) by phosphate ions** present in the filtrate and by ammonia synthesized in the renal tubules. It is subsequently excreted in the urine (Fig. 36.8).

Ammonia generated by glutaminase reaction participates in the excretion of hydrogen ion

Ammonia is generated in a reaction catalyzed by glutaminase, which transforms glutamine into glutamic acid. Ammonia diffuses across the luminal membrane, allowing hydrogen ion to be trapped inside the tubule as the ammonium ion (NH_4^+), to which the membrane is impermeable.

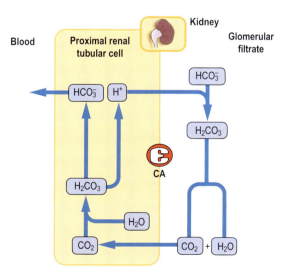

Fig. 36.7 **Bicarbonate reabsorption in the kidney.** Bicarbonate reabsorption takes place in the proximal tubule. There is no net excretion of hydrogen ion. CA, carbonic anhydrase.

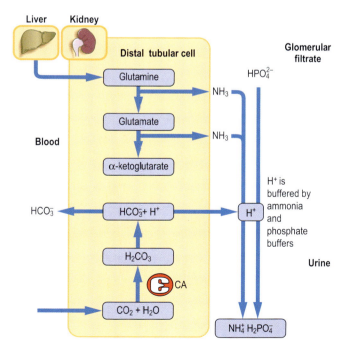

Fig. 36.8 **Hydrogen ion excretion by the kidney.** Excretion of the hydrogen ion takes place in the distal tubules. Hydrogen ion reacts with ammonia, forming the ammonium ion. Hydrogen ion is also buffered in the tubule lumen by phosphate. Approximately 50 mmol of hydrogen ion is excreted daily. CA, carbonic anhydrase.

DISORDERS OF THE ACID–BASE BALANCE

Classification of the acid–base disorders

The two principal disturbances of the acid–base balance are **acidosis** and **alkalosis**. Each is further divided into respiratory and metabolic types. Acidosis is a process that leads to the accumulation of hydrogen ion. Alkalosis causes a decrease in hydrogen ion concentration. Acidosis and alkalosis result in acidemia and alkalemia, respectively.

There are four main disorders of acid–base balance

Further classification takes on account respiratory and metabolic components. If the primary cause is the change in pCO_2, acidosis or alkalosis is called **respiratory,** and if it is bicarbonate concentration, acidosis or alkalosis is called **metabolic.** Thus there are four main disorders of acid–base balance: **respiratory acidosis, metabolic acidosis, respiratory alkalosis,** and **metabolic alkalosis** (Fig. 36.3). However, mixed disorders can also develop; we consider them later.

> ### CLINICAL BOX
> ### ESSENTIAL DEFINITIONS
>
> An **acid**, according to the Brønsted–Lowry definition, is "a molecular species that has a tendency to lose a hydrogen ion, forming a conjugate base."
> **Acidemia** is an increased concentration of hydrogen ion in blood.
> **Alkalemia** is a decreased concentration of hydrogen ion in blood.
> **Acidosis** is the process that leads to accumulation of hydrogen ion.
> **Alkalosis** is the process that decreases the amount of hydrogen ion.

The lungs and kidneys work in a concerted way to minimize changes in plasma pH

Acidosis is characterized by a decreased ratio of plasma bicarbonate to pCO_2, and alkalosis is characterized by an increased ratio. Referring to the Henderson–Hasselbalch equation, whenever a problem occurs, compensating mechanisms are triggered to bring hydrogen ion concentration back toward normal through normalization of the bicarbonate/pCO_2 ratio.

Thus when the respiratory acidosis causes an increase in pCO_2, more bicarbonate will be generated in the kidney, increasing its plasma concentration. Conversely, when diabetic ketoacidosis causes depletion of plasma bicarbonate, ventilation rate increases, and pCO_2 decreases. Note that the respiratory compensation can occur within minutes, but metabolic compensation takes hours to days to develop fully (Table 36.4).

Acidosis

Respiratory acidosis occurs most often in lung disease and results from decreased ventilation

The most common cause is the chronic obstructive airways disease (COAD). A severe asthmatic attack can also result in respiratory acidosis because of bronchial constriction. Respiratory acidosis often accompanies hypoxia (respiratory failure); in such a case, an increase in pCO_2 often parallels the decrease in pO_2 (Table 36.5).

Metabolic acidosis results from excessive production or inefficient metabolism or excretion, of nonvolatile acids

A classic example of metabolic acidosis is diabetic ketoacidosis, when acetoacetic acid and β-hydroxybutyric acid (keto acids) accumulate in the plasma (Chapter 31). Acidosis may also develop during extreme exercise as a result of the accumulation of lactic acid; in normal circumstances, lactate would be quickly metabolized on cessation of exercise. However, when a large amount is generated during hypoxia - for instance, in circulatory shock - severe lactic acidosis may become life-threatening.

Table 36.4 Respiratory and metabolic compensation in the acid–base disorders

Acid–base disorder	Primary change	Compensatory change	Timescale of compensatory change
Metabolic acidosis	↓ Plasma bicarbonate	↓ pCO_2 (hyperventilation)	Minutes/hours
Metabolic alkalosis	↑ Plasma bicarbonate	↑ pCO_2 (hypoventilation)	Minutes/hours
Respiratory acidosis	↑ pCO_2	↑ Renal bicarbonate generation ↑ Plasma bicarbonate	Days
Respiratory alkalosis	↓ pCO_2	↓ Renal bicarbonate reabsorption ↓ Plasma bicarbonate	Days

Respiratory and metabolic compensation in the acid–base disorders minimizes changes in the blood pH. A change in the respiratory component leads to metabolic compensation, and a change in the metabolic component stimulates respiratory compensation.

Table 36.5 Causes of acid–base disorders

Metabolic acidosis	Respiratory acidosis	Metabolic alkalosis	Respiratory alkalosis
Diabetes mellitus (ketoacidosis)	Chronic obstructive airways disease	Vomiting (loss of hydrogen ion)	Hyperventilation (anxiety, fever)
Lactic acidosis (lactic acid)	Severe asthma	Nasogastric suction (loss of hydrogen ion)	Lung diseases associated with hyperventilation
Renal failure (inorganic acids)	Cardiac arrest	Hypokalemia	Anemia
Severe diarrhea (loss of bicarbonate)	Depression of respiratory center (drugs, e.g., opiates)	Intravenous administration of bicarbonate (e.g., after cardiac arrest)	Salicylate poisoning
Surgical drainage of intestine (loss of bicarbonate)	Failure of respiratory muscles (e.g., poliomyelitis, multiple sclerosis)		
Renal loss of bicarbonate (renal tubular acidosis type 2 - rare)	Chest deformities		
Defective hydrogen ion excretion (renal tubular acidosis type 1 - rare)	Airway obstruction		

Respiratory acidosis is common and is caused primarily by diseases of the lung that affect gas exchange. *Respiratory alkalosis* is rarer and is caused by hyperventilation, which decreases pCO_2. *Metabolic acidosis* is common and results from either overproduction or retention of nonvolatile acids in the circulation. *Metabolic alkalosis* is rarer - its most common causes are vomiting and gastric suction, both causing loss of hydrogen ion from the stomach.

Metabolic acidosis can also develop in renal failure where excretion of nonvolatile acids is impaired. Renal failure develops when the perfusion of the kidneys is inadequate (e.g., in trauma, shock, or dehydration) or as a result of intrinsic kidney disease such as glomerulonephritis.

In the diagnosis and treatment of metabolic acidoses caused by the accumulation of acids, the interpretation of plasma electrolyte concentrations, particularly the anion gap (AG), is important (Chapter 35).

Conventionally, AG is calculated as

$$AG = [Na^+ + K^+] - [Cl^- + HCO_3^{2-}]$$

However, major components of the AG are negatively charged albumin and phosphate anion.

Because albumin concentration may change substantially in critically ill people, a correction of the calculated AG for albumin, phosphate, and possibly lactate has been suggested (see Kellum in Further Reading).

Primary loss of bicarbonate may also be a cause of metabolic acidosis. This happens when bicarbonate present in the intestinal fluid is lost as a result of severe diarrhea or postoperative surgical drainage.

Rare renal tubular acidoses are characterized by impaired bicarbonate reabsorption and hydrogen ion secretion

Defects in renal handling of bicarbonate and hydrogen ion lead to a group of disorders known as renal tubular acidoses (RTA). The proximal (type 2) RTA is caused by impaired reabsorption of bicarbonate, and the distal (type 1) RTA by impaired hydrogen ion excretion. Proximal RTA is usually accompanied by other defects in proximal transport mechanisms; this is known as the **Fanconi syndrome**.

Alkalosis

Alkalosis is rarer than acidosis

A mild respiratory alkalosis may be a consequence of hyperventilation caused by exercise, anxiety attack, or fever. It also occurs in pregnancy. Metabolic alkalosis is often associated with low serum potassium concentration as a result of cellular buffering (see previous discussion). Thus **alkalosis can cause hypokalemia, and conversely, hypokalemia** (Chapter 35)

A MAN WITH CHRONIC VOMITING: METABOLIC ALKALOSIS

A 47-year-old man came to the outpatient clinic with a history of intermittent profuse vomiting and loss of weight. He had tachycardia, reduced tissue turgor, and hypotension. His blood pH was 7.55 (hydrogen ion concentration 28 nmol/L), and pCO_2 was 6.4 kPa (48 mmHg). His bicarbonate concentration was 35 mmol/L, and there was also hyponatremia and hypokalemia.

Comment
This patient presents with metabolic alkalosis caused by the loss of hydrogen ion through vomiting. Investigations showed gastric outlet obstruction due to scarring from chronic peptic ulceration. He subsequently underwent surgery for pyloric stenosis, with a good outcome. Note the increased pCO_2 as a result of respiratory compensation for metabolic alkalosis. Reference ranges are given in Table 36.2.

may lead to alkalosis. Severe metabolic alkalosis may also occur as a result of the loss of hydrogen ion from the stomach during vomiting or as a result of nasogastric suction after surgery. Lastly, it may occur when too much bicarbonate is given intravenously - for instance, during resuscitation in cardiac arrest (Table 36.5).

Mixed acid–base disorders

More than one acid–base disorder can exist in a patient. The result is a mixed acid–base disorder, which can sometimes be quite difficult to diagnose (Table 36.6).

SUMMARY

- Maintenance of the hydrogen ion concentration is vital for survival.
- Acid–base balance is regulated by the concerted action of the lungs and kidneys. Erythrocytes play a key role in the transport of carbon dioxide in the blood.
- The main buffers in the blood are hemoglobin and bicarbonate. The bicarbonate buffer system communicates with atmospheric air.
- The main intracellular buffers are proteins and phosphate.
- Acid–base disorders are acidosis and alkalosis, and each of them can be either metabolic or respiratory.
- Measurement of pH, pCO_2 and bicarbonate, and pO_2, known as "blood gas analysis," is an investigation frequently required in emergencies.

Table 36.6 Comparison of simple and mixed disorders of acid–base balance

A. Mixed metabolic and respiratory acidosis

Condition	pH	pCO_2	Plasma bicarbonate
Metabolic acidosis	↓	↓ (Respiratory compensation)	↓ (Primary change)
Respiratory acidosis	↓	↑ (Primary change)	↑ (Metabolic compensation)
Mixed respiratory and metabolic acidosis	↓↓	↑ (Respiratory acidosis)	↓ (Metabolic acidosis)

B. Mixed metabolic and respiratory alkalosis (rare)

Disorder	pH	pCO_2	Plasma bicarbonate
Metabolic alkalosis	↑	↑ (Respiratory compensation)	↑ (Primary change)
Respiratory alkalosis	↑	↓ (Primary change)	↓ (Metabolic compensation)
Mixed respiratory and metabolic alkalosis	↑↑	↓ (Respiratory alkalosis)	↑ (Metabolic acidosis)

Mixed acid–base disorders result in a greater change in blood pH than simple disorders; they may pose diagnostic difficulties.

RESPIRATORY AND METABOLIC DISORDERS OF ACID–BASE BALANCE CAN OCCUR TOGETHER: CARDIAC ARREST

During resuscitation of a 60-year-old man from a cardiorespiratory arrest, blood gas analysis revealed pH 7.00 (hydrogen ion concentration 100 nmol/L) and pCO_2 7.5 kPa (52 mmHg). His bicarbonate concentration was 11 mmol/L. pO_2 was 12.1 kPa (91 mmHg) during treatment with 48% oxygen.

Comment
This patient presents with a mixed disorder: a respiratory acidosis caused by lack of ventilation and metabolic acidosis caused by the hypoxia. The acidosis was caused by an accumulation of lactic acid: the measured lactate concentration was 7.0 mmol/L (reference range is 0.7–1.8 mmol/L [6–16 mg/dL]). Two acid–base disorders may occur in one patient - another example would be a patient with emphysema causing respiratory acidosis who is admitted with developing diabetic ketoacidosis. The result is usually a more severe change in pH than would have resulted from one of these disorders.

ACTIVE LEARNING

1. Describe how the bicarbonate buffer copes with an addition of an acid to the system.
2. Compare bicarbonate handling by the proximal and distal tubules of the kidney.
3. Outline the role of ventilation in acid–base disorders.
4. Which disorders of the acid–base balance may be associated with gastrointestinal surgery?
5. Discuss the association between acid–base disorders and plasma potassium concentration.

FURTHER READING

Corey, H. E. (2005). Bench-to-bedside review: Fundamental principles of acid–base balance. *Critical Care: The Official Journal of the Critical Care Forum, 9,* 184–192.

Edwards, S. L. (2008). Pathophysiology of acid base balance: The theory practice relationship. *Intensive and Critical Care Nursing, 24,* 28–40.

Kamel, K. S., & Halperin, M. L. (2015). Acid–base problems in diabetic ketoacidosis. *The New England Journal of Medicine, 372,* 546–554.

Kellum, J. A. (2007). Disorders of acid–base balance. *Critical Care Medicine, 35,* 2630–2636.

RELEVANT WEBSITES

Acid–base balance disorders: http://www.els.net

ABBREVIATIONS

CA	Carbonic anhydrase
COAD	Chronic obstructive airway disease
Hb	Hemoglobin
pCO_2	Partial pressure of carbon dioxide
pO_2	Partial pressure of oxygen
Prot	Protein
RTA	Renal tubular acidosis
Va/Q	The ratio of ventilation to perfusion

Muscle: Energy Metabolism, Contraction, and Exercise

John W. Baynes and Matthew C. Kostek

LEARNING OBJECTIVES

After reading this chapter, you should be able to:

- Describe muscle structure and its function in mechanical force production, including differences among skeletal, cardiac, and smooth muscle types that are related to their physiologic functions.
- Describe the structure and protein composition of the sarcomere, the sliding-filament model of muscle contraction, and the source of the banding pattern in striated muscle.
- Describe the sequence of events in excitation–contraction coupling, including the roles of membrane depolarization, the sarcoplasmic reticulum, and calcium triggering.
- Identify the key sites of energy utilization during muscle contraction, the role of creatine phosphate in skeletal muscle, and the impact of skeletal muscle fiber type on substrate utilization and muscle function.
- Describe the changes in skeletal muscle mass and metabolism with age, in response to acute and prolonged exercise, and in diseases such as sarcopenia, metabolic syndrome, and wasting conditions.

INTRODUCTION

There are three types of muscle: skeletal, cardiac, and smooth muscle - each with a unique physiologic role

All muscles function to convert chemical energy to mechanical energy, but the various types of muscle differ in their mechanism of initiation of contraction, rate of force development, duration of contraction, ability to adapt to their environment, and substrate utilization. Muscle accounts for about 40% of total body mass, and muscle metabolism is a major determinant of whole-body metabolic rate in both the basal and active state. Changes in skeletal muscle metabolism occur with physical activity and are directly related to the required force output and duration of activity. These factors also affect the muscle's relative utilization of glucose and fatty acids for fuel. Besides locomotion, skeletal muscle is also a source of body heat, provides amino acids for hepatic gluconeogenesis during fasting, and is a major site of glucose and triglyceride uptake after a meal. Because of its critical role in the regulation of systemic fuel flux and metabolism, loss of muscle mass has a profound effect on overall metabolism. Advancing age, sepsis, and wasting diseases, such as HIV/AIDS and cancer, are conditions associated with loss of muscle mass, and this loss is associated with increased morbidity and mortality.

The primary focus of this chapter is skeletal muscle, supplemented by discussion of similarities and differences in skeletal, cardiac, and smooth muscle structure, function, and metabolism. The chapter begins with a discussion of the mechanism of muscle contraction, proceeds to the signaling that initiates the contractile process, examines the energy metabolism essential for contraction, and then discusses recent advances in the understanding of muscle in regenerative medicine and the prescription of exercise as medicine.

MUSCLE STRUCTURE

The sarcomere: The functional contractile unit of muscle

A common characteristic of cardiac myocytes, smooth muscle cells, and skeletal myofibers is that their cytoplasm is packed full of contractile protein. The contractile protein is organized in linear arrays of sarcomere units in skeletal myofibers and cardiac myocytes, giving these muscles a striated appearance, thus the term **striated muscle.** Contractile protein in **smooth muscle** cells is not organized into a sarcomeric structure, and this tissue is described as nonstriated muscle. Skeletal muscle's hierarchic structure (Fig. 37.1) consists of bundles (**fasciculi**) of elongated, multinucleated fiber cells (**myofibers**). The myofiber cells contain bundles of **myofibrils**, which are in turn composed of myofilament proteins, primarily myosin and actin, that form the sarcomere (Table 37.1). Electron microscopic analysis of muscle reveals a repeating pattern of light- and dark-staining regions in the myofibril (Fig. 37.2). These regions are known as the I (isotropic)- and A (anisotropic)-bands, respectively. At the center of the I-band is a discrete, darker-staining Z-line, whereas the center of the A-band has a lighter-staining H-zone with a central M-line. The contractile unit, the **sarcomere,** is centered on the M-line, extending from one Z-line to the next. Smooth muscle, in contrast, lacks a defined Z-line. This molecular structural difference between striated and smooth muscle helps explain the functional differences as related to muscle contraction. Striated muscle

CLINICAL BOX
MUSCULAR DYSTROPHIES

A young boy was brought to the clinic because his mother had noticed that he walked with a waddling gait. Physical evaluation confirmed muscle weakness especially in the legs, although his calf muscles were large and firm. There was a 20-fold elevation in serum creatine (phospho)kinase (CK) activity, identified as the MM (muscle) isozyme. Histology revealed muscle loss, some necrosis, and increased connective tissue and fat volume in muscle. A tentative diagnosis of Duchenne muscular dystrophy (DMD) was confirmed by immunoelectrophoretic (Western blot) analysis showing the lack of the cytoskeletal protein dystrophin in muscle.

Comment

Although there are many forms of muscular dystrophy, some genetic and some acquired, DMD is the most common genetic dystrophy and is lethal. **Dystrophin** is a high-molecular-weight cytoskeletal protein that reinforces the plasma membrane of the muscle cell and mediates interactions with the extracellular matrix. In its absence, the plasma membrane of muscle cells shears during the contractile process, leading to muscle cell death.

The dystrophin gene is located on the X chromosome and is nearly 2.5×10^6 base pairs in length. Spontaneous mutations in this gene are relatively common, with the frequency of DMD being approximately 1 in 3500 male births. DMD is a progressive myodegenerative disease, commonly leading to confinement to a wheelchair by puberty, with death by age 30 years from respiratory or cardiac failure. Dystrophin is completely absent in DMD patients, although a variant of the disease, known as Becker muscular dystrophy, has milder symptoms and is characterized by expression of an altered dystrophin protein and survival into the fifth decade. Although there is currently no treatment for DMD, gene therapy still holds some promise, and newer technologies that utilize "exon skipping" are allowing cells to skip over mutated exons and thereby translate a slightly smaller, but still functional, protein product. The smaller dystrophin protein produces Becker-like symptoms in animal experiments and thus could translate to a doubling of human life-span if the results are reproducible in humans.

generally contracts (shortens its cellular length) in a straight line, whereas smooth muscle contraction causes a circumferential cellular contraction. The circumferential contraction is ideally suited to the function of smooth muscle, to surround hollow structures in the body (e.g., arteries, veins, intestine, stomach), and contract or relax to modify their diameter.

The thick and thin filaments

Actin and myosin account for more than 75% of muscle protein

The sarcomere may shorten by as much as 70% in length during muscle contraction (see Fig. 37.2). The components effecting the contraction are the thick and thin filaments. **The thick filament is composed of myosin and titin protein, and the thin filament is mainly made up of actin, with associated proteins tropomyosin and troponins.** The thin filament also has some interaction with titin. Thick and thin filaments extend in opposite directions from both sides of the M- and Z-lines, respectively, and overlap and slide past one another during the contractile process (see Fig. 37.2). The M- and Z-lines are, in effect, base plates for anchoring the myosin and actin filaments. In striated muscle, thick and thin filaments intercalate during contraction, causing the H-zone (myosin only) and I-bands (actin only) to shrink. In smooth muscle, thick and thin filaments are anchored at structures called dense bodies that are further anchored by intermediate filaments. Although all three muscle types contain the same proteins (Table 37.2), each muscle type expresses tissue-specific isoforms; the cardiac actin and troponins, for example, differ slightly from those in skeletal muscle.

Sarcomere proteins

Myosin

Interaction between actin and myosin during muscle contraction is dependent on cytoplasmic Ca++ concentration

Myosin is one of the largest proteins in the body, with a molecular mass of approximately 500 kDa, and accounts for more than half of muscle protein. Under the electron microscope, myosin appears as an elongated protein with two globular heads. It is the primary component of the thick filament in muscle. Each myosin molecule is made up of two heavy chains (~200 kDa) and four light chains (~20 kDa). The heavy chain can be subdivided into the helical tail and globular head regions; the four light chains are bound to the globular heads. Structural analysis by limited proteolysis indicates that there are two flexible hinge regions in the myosin molecule (Fig. 37.3): one where the globular head attaches to the helical region and the other farther into the helical region. The myosin filaments are associated through their helical regions and extend outward from the M-line toward the Z-line of each myofibril (see Figs. 37.2 and 37.3). The hinge regions allow the myosin heads to interact with actin and provide the flexibility needed for reversible interactions and conformational changes during muscle contraction.

There are several features of myosin that are essential for muscle contraction:

- The myosin globular heads have binding sites for ATP and its hydrolysis products, ADP and phosphate (Pi).
- The myosin globular heads have a Ca^{2+}-dependent ATPase activity.
- Myosin binds reversibly to actin as a function of Ca^{2+}, ATP, and ADP + Pi concentrations.

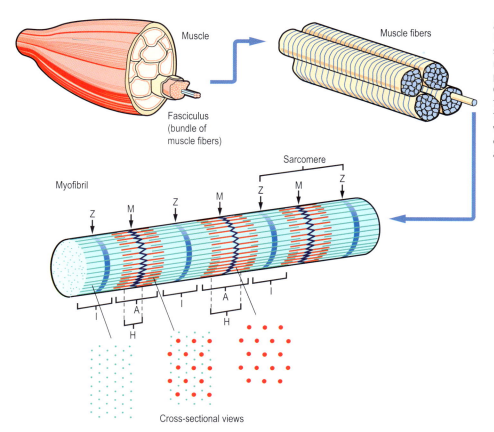

Fig. 37.1 **Hierarchic structure of muscle.** Hierarchic structure of skeletal muscle, showing an exploded view of fasciculi, myofibers, myofibrils, and myofilament proteins and the location of the I-band (thin actin filaments extending from the Z-line) and the A-band (thick myosin filaments extending from the M-line), with darker-staining regions of the A-band corresponding to the region of overlap of actin and myosin filaments.

Table 37.1 The structural elements of skeletal muscle arranged in descending order of size

Microscopic unit	Fasciculus: bundle of muscle cells
Cellular unit	Myofiber cell: long, multinucleated cell
Subcellular unit	Myofibril: composed of myofilament proteins
Functional unit	Sarcomere: contractile unit, repeating unit of the myofibril
Myofilament components	Proteins: primarily actin and myosin

- The binding of calcium and hydrolysis of ATP lead to major changes in the conformation of the myosin molecule and its interaction with actin.
- **Myosin-ATPase** activity, myosin–actin interactions, and conformational changes are integrated into the **sliding-filament model** of muscle contraction (discussed later in the chapter). They also explain the development of **rigor mortis.** The increase in Ca^{2+} in the muscle cytoplasm (sarcoplasm) and decrease in ATP after death lead to tight binding between myosin and actin, forming rigid muscle tissue.

Actin

Actin is composed of 42 kDa subunits, known as **G-actin** (globular), which polymerize into a filamentous array **(F-actin).** Two polymer chains coil around one another to form the F-actin myofilament (see Fig. 37.3). F-actin is the major component of the thin filament and interacts with myosin in the actomyosin complex. The F-actin chains extend in opposite directions from the Z-line, overlapping with the myosin chains extending from the M-line. Each myosin-containing thick filament is surrounded by six actin-molecule-containing thin filaments. Each thin filament interacts with three myosin-containing thick filaments (see Fig. 37.1 for a cross-sectional view).

Tropomyosin and troponins

Troponins modulate the interaction between actin and myosin

Calcium activation of muscle contraction in striated muscle involves thin-filament-associated proteins tropomyosin and the troponins. **Tropomyosin** is a fibrous protein that extends along the grooves of F-actin, with each molecule contacting about seven G-actin subunits. Tropomyosin has a role in stabilizing F-actin and coordinating conformational changes among actin subunits during contraction. In the absence of Ca^{2+}, tropomyosin blocks the myosin-binding site on actin.

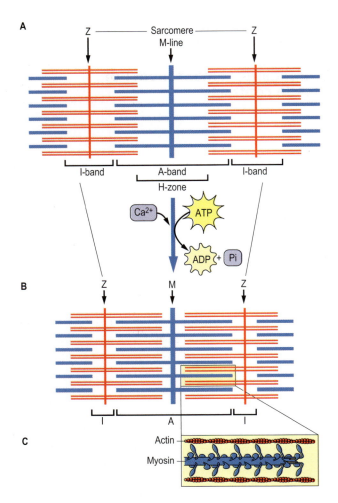

Fig. 37.2 **Schematic structure of the sarcomere, indicating the distribution of actin and myosin in the A- and I-bands.** (A) Relaxed sarcomere. (B) Contracted sarcomere. (C) Magnification of contracted sarcomere, illustrating the polarity of the arrays of myosin molecules. Increased overlap of actin and myosin filaments during contraction, accompanied by a decrease in the length of the H-zones and I-bands, illustrates the sliding-filament model of muscle contraction.

Table 37.2 Muscle proteins and their functions

Protein	Function
Myosin	Ca²⁺-dependent ATPase activity
C-protein	Assembly of myosin into thick filaments
M-protein	Binding of myosin filaments to M-line
Actin	G-actin polymerizes to filamentous F-actin
tropomyosin	Stabilization and propagation of conformational changes of F-actin
troponins-C, I and T	Modulation of actin–myosin interactions
α- and β-actinins	Stabilization of F-actin and anchoring to Z-line
nebulin	Possible role in determining length of F-actin filaments
titin	Control of resting tension and length of the sarcomere
desmin	Organization of myofibrils in muscle cells
dystrophin	Reinforcement of cytoskeleton and muscle cell plasma membrane

Actin and myosin account for more than 90% of muscle proteins, but several associated proteins are required for assembly and function of the actomyosin complex.

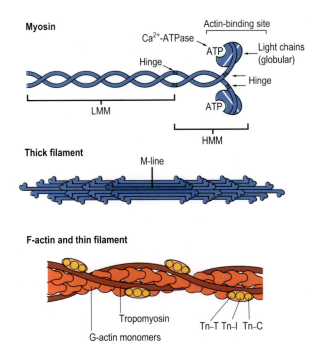

Fig. 37.3 **Polymerization of myosin and actin into thick and thin filaments.** Tn-C, calcium-binding troponin; Tn-I, troponin inhibitory subunit; Tn-T, tropomyosin-binding troponin; LMM, light meromyosin; HMM, heavy meromyosin.

A complex of **troponin** proteins is bound to tropomyosin: Tn-T (tropomyosin-binding), Tn-C (calcium-binding), and Tn-I (inhibitory subunit). Calcium binding to Tn-C, a calmodulin-like protein, induces changes in Tn-I that shift the interaction between tropomyosin and actin, exposing the myosin-binding site on F-actin and permitting actin–myosin interactions. For a description of the diagnostic use of cardiac troponin measurements, see the box at end of this chapter.

Titin

Titin modulates the passive tension of muscle

Titin is the largest protein in the human body, with more than 34,000 amino acids and a mass of 3800 kDa. Structurally, titin spans half the length of the sarcomere, with its N-terminus anchored to the Z-line and its C-terminus anchored to the thick filament at the M-line. Titin has an elastic, extensible **PEVK domain** (rich in Pro, Glu, Val, and Lys) that contributes to passive myocardial and skeletal muscle tension and a kinase domain that participates in intracellular signaling. Depending on the skeletal muscle, titin may account for more than half of the passive tension of the muscle and contributes a spring-like property to the sarcomere - when a muscle is stretched, potential energy is stored in the PEVK domain, which re-coils during relaxation. Mutations in one region of titin may cause a genetic disease of the heart (e.g., hypertrophic cardiomyopathy), whereas a mutation elsewhere in the gene causes a disease of skeletal muscle only (e.g., limb girdle muscular dystrophy).

THE CONTRACTILE PROCESS

The sliding-filament model of muscle contraction

The sliding-filament model describes how a series of chemical and structural changes in the actomyosin complex can induce sarcomere shortening

The contractile response depends on reversible, Ca^{2+}-dependent **cross-bridge** formation between the myosin head and its binding site on actin. A conformational change in the hinge regions of myosin occurs after cross-bridge formation, providing the **power stroke** for muscle contraction (Fig. 37.4). This conformational change, the relaxation of the high-energy form of myosin, is accompanied by dissociation of ADP and Pi. After the stroke is completed, the binding and hydrolysis of ATP restore the high-energy conformation. The stability of the contracted state is maintained by multiple and continuous Ca^{2+}-dependent actin–myosin interactions so slippage is minimized until calcium is removed from the sarcoplasm, allowing dissociation of the actomyosin complex and muscle relaxation.

Higher myosin-ATPase activity increases cross-bridge cycling, which allows for an increased rate of contraction. Different myosin isoforms have varying levels of ATPase activity, with fast muscles having higher rates of myosin-ATPase activity. Isoforms of actin and myosin are also found in the cytoskeleton of nonmuscle cells, where they have roles in diverse processes such as cell migration, vesicle transport during endocytosis and exocytosis, maintenance or changing of cell shape, and anchorage of intracellular proteins to the plasma membrane.

Excitation–contraction coupling: Muscle membrane depolarization

T tubules transmit electrochemical signals for efficient muscle contraction

Skeletal muscle contraction is initiated by neuronal stimulation at the neuromuscular endplate. As described previously (see Fig. 4.4), this stimulus leads to depolarization of the electrochemical gradient across the muscle plasma membrane (sarcolemma). The depolarization, caused by an influx of Na^+, propagates rapidly along the **sarcolemma membrane** and signals a voltage-gated calcium release from the **sarcoplasmic reticulum** (SR), a membrane-bound, calcium-sequestering compartment inside the muscle cell. The influx of Ca^{2+} from the SR to the sarcoplasm initiates cross-bridge formation and excitation–contraction coupling (see Fig. 37.4). In striated muscle, depolarization is transmitted into the muscle fiber by invaginations of the plasma membrane, called **transverse tubules** (T tubules; Fig. 37.5). The transmission of depolarization through the highly branched T-tubule network, which interacts closely with the SR, leads to rapid, concerted release

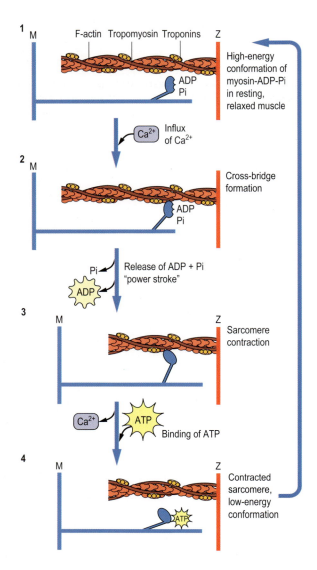

Fig. 37.4 Proposed stages in muscle contraction, according to the sliding-filament model. (1) In resting, relaxed muscle, calcium concentration is ~10^7 mol/L. The head group of myosin chains contains bound ADP and Pi and is extended from the axis of the myosin helix in a high-energy conformation. Although the myosin–ADP–Pi complex has a high affinity for actin, binding of myosin to actin is inhibited by tropomyosin, which blocks the myosin-binding site on actin at low calcium concentrations. (2) When muscle is stimulated, calcium enters the sarcoplasm through voltage-gated calcium channels (Chapter 4). Calcium binding to Tn-C causes a conformational change in Tn-I, which is transmitted through Tn-T to tropomyosin. Movement of tropomyosin exposes the myosin-binding site on actin. Myosin–ADP–Pi binds to actin, forming a cross-bridge. (3) Release of Pi, then ADP, from myosin during the interaction with actin is accompanied by a major conformational change in myosin, producing the "power stroke," which moves the actin chain about 10 nm (100 Å) in the direction opposite the myosin chain, increasing their overlap and causing muscle contraction. (4) The uptake of calcium from the sarcoplasm and binding of ATP to myosin leads to dissociation of the actomyosin cross-bridge. The ATP is hydrolyzed, and the free energy of hydrolysis of ATP is conserved as the high-energy conformation of myosin, setting the stage for continued muscle contraction in response to the next surge in Ca^{2+} concentration in the sarcoplasm.

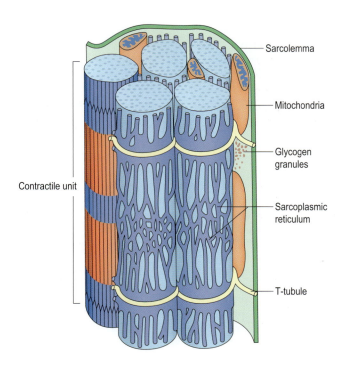

Fig. 37.5 Side view of the transverse tubular network in skeletal muscle cells. Transverse tubules are invaginations of the sarcolemma, which are connected to the sarcoplasmic reticulum (SR) by protein channels. The SR is a continuous, tubular compartment in close association with the myofibrils. The transverse tubules are extensions of the sarcolemma around the Z-line. They transmit the depolarizing nerve impulse to terminal regions of the SR, coordinating calcium release and contraction of the myofibril.

of calcium from the SR into the sarcoplasm. In order for depolarization to occur again, sodium must be actively pumped out of the cytosol by Na^+/K^+-ATPase pumps located in the sarcolemma. The rate of muscle repolarization is affected by both the rate and density of these pumps. Higher levels of Na^+/K^+-ATPase activity are found in fast-contracting muscles, and increased Na^+/K^+-ATPase pump density is an important adaptation to exercise.

Skeletal, cardiac, and smooth muscle differ in their mechanism of neural stimulation and have different structural adaptations for propagating the depolarization. Skeletal muscle contraction is volitional, and fibers are innervated by motor nerve endplates that originate in the spinal cord; acetylcholine functions as the neurotransmitter (see Chapter 26). The **neuromuscular junction** is a special structural feature of skeletal muscle that is not found in cardiac or smooth muscle. Each individual fiber is innervated by only one motor nerve, and all the fibers innervated by one nerve are defined as a **motor unit.** Motor unit control and synchronization is the basis for coordinated whole-muscle contraction. Skeletal muscle cramping is a nonvoluntary muscle contraction resulting from alterations in neuromuscular control and/or from electrolyte imbalances after excessive fluid loss, typically during intense exercise in hot, humid conditions.

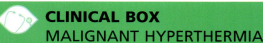

Cardiac muscle is striated and contracts rhythmically under involuntary control. The general mechanism of contraction of heart muscle is similar to that in skeletal muscle; however, the sarcoplasmic reticulum is less developed in the heart, and the transverse tubule network is more developed. The heart is more dependent on, and actually requires, extracellular calcium for its contractile response (see Fig. 4.4); the influx of extracellular calcium enhances Ca^{2+} release from the SR. Lacking direct neural contact, cardiac myocytes propagate depolarization from a single node, the SA node, throughout the myocardium. The depolarization is passed cell to cell along membrane structures called **intercalated disks.** These disks are specialized forms of cell junctions, ion channels that allow passage ions between cells, which in this case allow the depolarization wave to pass from cell to cell uninterrupted. Cardiac muscle cells thus act as a functional syncytium, whereas in skeletal muscle, each cell must receive nerve input to contract. Cardiac muscle is also more responsive to hormonal regulation. For example, cAMP-dependent protein kinases phosphorylate transport proteins and Tn-I, mediating changes in the force of contraction in response to epinephrine.

Smooth muscle can respond to both neural and circulating factors. Unlike skeletal muscle, neural input to smooth muscle innervates bundles of smooth muscle cells that cause both phasic (rhythmic) and tonic (sustained) contractions of the tissue. Smooth muscle can also be induced to depolarize by ligand–receptor interactions at the sarcolemma. This is called pharmacomechanical coupling and is the basis for many drugs that target smooth muscle contraction or relaxation. **Nitric oxide donors,** such as amyl nitrite and nitroglycerin, used for the treatment of angina, relax vascular smooth muscles, increasing the flow of blood to cardiac muscle.

Excitation–contraction coupling: The calcium trigger

The calcium content of the sarcoplasm is normally very low, 10^{-7} mol/L or less, but increases rapidly by more than 100-fold in response to neural stimulation. The sarcoplasmic reticulum, a specialized organelle derived from the smooth endoplasmic reticulum, is rich in a Ca^{2+}-binding protein, **calsequestrin,** and serves as the site of calcium sequestration inside the cell. In striated muscle, T-tubule depolarization opens the Ca^{2+} channels in the SR (see Fig. 37.5). **The influx of Ca^{2+} into the sarcoplasm triggers both actin–myosin interactions and myosin-ATPase activity, leading to muscle contraction.** Troponins are not expressed in smooth muscle. In this case, calcium triggers contraction by binding to calmodulin and activating myosin light chain kinase, which then phosphorylates myosin. Myosin phosphorylation enhances myosin–actin interaction.

Increased intracellular calcium activates more cross-bridges and causes sarcomere shortening through activation of myosin-ATPase. Thus higher calcium levels increase muscle contractile

CLINICAL BOX
MALIGNANT HYPERTHERMIA

About 1 in 150,000 patients treated with halothane (gaseous halocarbon) anesthesia or muscle relaxants responds with excessive skeletal muscle rigidity and severe hyperthermia with a rapid onset, up to 2°C (4°F) within 1 h.

Unless treated rapidly, cardiac abnormalities may be life-threatening; mortality from this condition exceeds 10%. This genetic disease results from the excessive or prolonged release of Ca^{2+} from the sarcoplasmic reticulum (SR), most commonly the result of mutations in the gene(s) that code for the Ca^{2+}-release channels within the SR. Excessive release of Ca^{2+} leads to a prolonged increase in sarcoplasmic Ca^{2+} concentration.

Muscle rigidity results from Ca^{2+}-dependent consumption of ATP, and hyperthermia results from increased metabolism to replenish the ATP. As muscle metabolism becomes anaerobic, lacticacidemia and acidosis may also develop. Treatment of malignant hyperthermia includes use of muscle relaxants (e.g., dantrolene, an inhibitor of the ryanodine-sensitive Ca^{2+}-channel) to inhibit Ca^{2+} release from the SR. Supportive therapy involves cooling, administration of oxygen, correction of blood pH and electrolyte imbalances, and also the treatment of cardiac abnormalities.

force until saturation is reached. Calcium-channel blockers used for the treatment of **hypertension**, such as nifedipine, inhibit the flow of Ca^{2+} into the SR, thereby limiting the force of contraction of cardiac myocytes. Whereas muscle contraction is triggered by increased calcium, muscle relaxation is dependent on calcium being actively pumped back into the SR. The rate of muscle relaxation is directly related to SR Ca^{2+}-ATPase activity. The SR is rich in Ca^{2+}-ATPase, which maintains cytosolic calcium in the sarcoplasm at submicromolar ($\sim 10^{-7}$ mol/L) concentrations. As intracellular calcium levels decrease, the number of active cross-bridges also decreases, and muscle contractile force declines.

MUSCLE ENERGY METABOLISM

Energy resources in the muscle cell

Muscle is the primary site of **glucose disposal** (uptake from the circulation) in the body and is thus a natural target for treatment of the hyperglycemia of diabetes. The glucose transporter GLUT-4 is moved to the cell surface not only in response to insulin or pharmaceuticals but also in response to cellular energy status and by muscle contractions. The glucose that enters the muscle cell is trapped as glucose-6-phosphate and is routed to glycogenesis or glycolysis. Because of the lack of a glucose-6-phosphate transporter and glucose-6-phosphatase activity, muscle glucose is not available to replenish blood glucose, as occurs after glycogenolysis or gluconeogenesis in liver.

In this context, exercise draws glucose from the blood and, in effect, counters hyperglycemia in diabetes - exercise, in this context, is good medicine. The muscle content and activity of hexokinase also increase with exercise, both acutely (~3 h after one session) and chronically (after several weeks of training).

ATP is used for muscle contraction

Three ATPases are required for muscle contraction: Na^+/K^+-ATPase, Ca^{2+}-ATPase, and myosin-ATPase. Decreased ATP availability or inhibition of any of these ATPases will cause a decrease in muscle-force production. However, the intracellular concentration of ATP does not change dramatically during exercise. Actively contracting muscle relies on the rapid resynthesis of ATP from ADP. Energy systems that synthesize ATP for muscle contraction include the creatine phosphate shuttle, anaerobic glycolysis from plasma glucose or glycogen, and aerobic metabolism of glucose and fatty acids via oxidative phosphorylation. The energy systems that synthesize ATP are not equivalent and directly affect the amount and duration of power output from the contracting muscle.

Short-duration, high-power output contractions

Creatine phosphate is a high-energy phosphate buffer used for rapid regeneration of ATP in muscle

A metabolic reality for skeletal muscle is that high force output can only be maintained for a short period of time. Contractions at or near maximal power levels depend on high myosin-ATPase activity and rapid ATP resynthesis by substrate-level phosphorylation using the high-energy compound creatine phosphate (creatine-P). Creatine is synthesized from arginine and glycine and is phosphorylated reversibly to creatine-P by the enzyme **creatine (phospho)kinase** (**CK or CPK**; Fig. 37.6). CK is a dimeric protein and exists as three isozymes: the MM (skeletal muscle), BB (brain), and MB isoforms. The MB isoform is enriched in cardiac tissue.

The level of creatine-P in resting muscle is several-fold higher than that of ATP (Table 37.3). Thus ATP concentration remains relatively constant during the initial stages of exercise. It is replenished not only by the action of CK but also by adenylate kinase **(myokinase)** as follows:

$$\text{Creatine (Cr) phosphokinase: CrP + ADP} \rightarrow \text{Cr + ATP}$$

$$\text{Adenylate kinase: 2 ADP} \rightleftharpoons \text{ATP + AMP}$$

Creatine phosphate stores decline rapidly during the first minute of high-power-output muscle contraction. As creatine phosphate stores are depleted, the muscle becomes unable to sustain the high force output, and contractile force rapidly declines. At this point, muscle glycogenolysis becomes a major

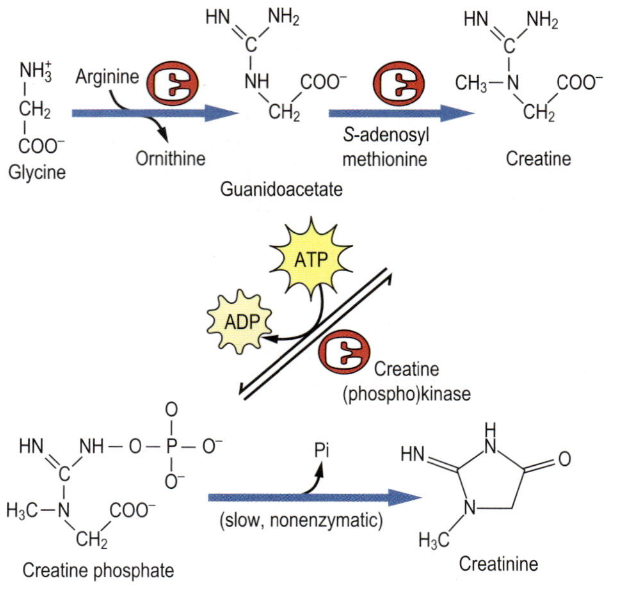

Fig. 37.6 **Synthesis and degradation of creatine phosphate (creatine-P).** Creatine is synthesized from glycine and arginine precursors. Creatine-P is unstable and undergoes slow, spontaneous degradation to Pi and creatinine, the cyclic anhydride form of creatine, which is excreted from the muscle cell into plasma and then into urine.

Table 37.3 Changes in energy resources in working muscle: Concentrations of energy metabolites in human leg muscle during bicycle exercise

Metabolite	Metabolite concentration (mmol/kg dry weight)		
	Resting	3 min	8 min
ATP	27	26	19
Creatine-P	78	27	7
Creatine	37	88	115
Lactate	5	8	13
Glycogen	408	350	282

These experiments were conducted during ischemic exercise, which exacerbates the decline in ATP concentration. They illustrate the rapid decline in creatine-P and the increase in lactate from anaerobic glycolysis of muscle glycogen.
Data are adapted from Timmons, J. A., et al. (1998). Substrate availability limits human skeletal muscle oxidative ATP regeneration at the onset of ischemic exercise. Journal of Clinical Investigation, 101, *79–85.*

source of energy. Calcium entry into muscle, in addition to its role in activation of myosin-ATPase-dependent contraction, also leads to the formation of a Ca^{2+}–calmodulin complex, which activates phosphorylase kinase, catalyzing the conversion of phosphorylase *b* to phosphorylase *a*. AMP also allosterically activates muscle phosphorylase and phosphofructokinase-1, accelerating glycolysis from muscle glycogen (see Chapter 12).

A further decline in force occurs as pyruvate and lactate gradually accumulate in the contracting muscle, resulting in a decrease in muscle pH. Force will then decline to a level that can be maintained by the aerobic metabolism of fatty acids. Maximal aerobic power is about 20% of the initial maximal power output, and about 50%–60% of maximal aerobic power can be sustained for long periods of time.

Low-intensity, long-duration contractions

Fatty acids are the major source of energy in muscle during prolonged exercise

The availability and utilization of oxygen in working muscle are major limitations for maintaining continuous physical activity. Long-duration contractile activity requires adequate oxygen delivery and the capacity for the muscle to utilize the oxygen delivered. Oxygen delivery to muscle is affected by the red blood cell and hemoglobin concentrations in blood, the number of capillaries within the muscle, and heart pump capacity. Highly oxidative muscle has a higher capillary density than glycolytic muscle, and muscle capillary density increases with endurance exercise training. Muscle oxygen utilization is also directly related to the number and size of muscle mitochondria. Muscles subjected to continual contractile activity, such as postural muscles, have more mitochondria than infrequently contracted muscle. A standard observation in muscle subjected to increased contractile demands is an elevation in oxidative enzyme activity.

At rest or at low intensities of physical work, oxygen is readily available, and the aerobic oxidation of lipid predominates as the main source of ATP synthesis. However, at higher work intensities, oxygen availability for lipid catabolism can become limiting, and subsequently, the muscle work rate decreases. During the first 15–30 min of exercise, there is a gradual shift from glycogenolysis and glycolysis to aerobic metabolism of fatty acids. Perhaps this is an evolutionary response to deal with the fact that lactate, produced by glycolysis, is more acidic and less diffusible than CO_2. As exercise continues, epinephrine contributes to activation of hepatic gluconeogenesis, providing an exogenous source of glucose for muscle. Lipids gradually become the major source of energy in muscle during long-term, lower-intensity exercise when oxygen is not limiting.

Long-term muscle performance (stamina) depends on levels of muscle glycogen

Fats burn in the flame of carbohydrates; glycogen is required for efficient metabolism of lipids in muscle

Marathon runners typically "hit the wall" when muscle glycogen reaches a critically low level. Glycogen is the storage form of glucose in skeletal muscle, and its muscle concentration can be manipulated by diet - for example, by **carbohydrate loading** before a marathon run. Fatigue, which can be defined as an inability to maintain the desired power output, occurs when the rate of ATP utilization exceeds its rate of synthesis. For efficient ATP synthesis, there is a continuing, but poorly understood, requirement for a basal level of glycogen metabolism, even when glucose is available from plasma and when fats are the primary source of muscle energy. Carbohydrate metabolism is important as a source of pyruvate, which is converted to oxaloacetate by the anaplerotic pyruvate carboxylase reaction. Oxaloacetate is required to maintain the activity of the TCA cycle, for condensation with acetyl-CoA derived from fats. To some extent, muscle glycogen can be spared and performance time increased during long-term, vigorous physical activity by increasing the availability of circulating glucose, either by gluconeogenesis or by carbohydrate ingestion (e.g., bread or Gatorade®). Increased utilization of fatty acids during early stages of exercise is an important training adaptation to regular vigorous physical activity - it serves to spare glycogen stores.

Muscle consists of two types of striated muscle cells: Fast-glycolytic and slow-oxidative fibers

Striated muscle cells are generally classified by their physiologic contractile properties (fast versus slow) and primary type of metabolism (oxidative versus glycolytic). The muscle type is closely related to muscle function in skeletal muscle, and this comparison can easily be seen with muscles whose contraction is for infrequent-burst activities versus muscles used continuously for maintaining posture (antigravity). The coloring of the two striated muscle types readily distinguishes them. **Fast-glycolytic muscle** used for burst activity is white in appearance (like chicken breast - chickens squawk a lot, but cannot fly far!) because of less blood flow, lower mitochondrial density, and decreased myoglobin content compared with slow-twitch oxidative muscle, which is red. Fast-glycolytic fibers also have increased glycogen stores and lower fat content; they rely on glycogen and anaerobic glycolysis for short bursts of contraction when additional muscle force is required, such as in the fight-or-flight stress response. In contrast, **slow-oxidative fibers** in postural muscles (and in goose breast - geese are migratory birds) are well perfused with blood and rich in mitochondria and myoglobin. This muscle type has the ability to sustain low-intensity contractions for long periods. Slow muscle uses fatty acid oxidation for ATP synthesis, which requires mitochondria. Cardiac muscle, which is continuously contracting, has many contractile and metabolic characteristics that are similar to those of slow-oxidative skeletal muscle. Cardiac muscle is well perfused with blood, is rich in mitochondria, and relies largely on oxidative metabolism of circulating fatty acids. Goose breast, which powers long, migratory flights, is a fairly fatty and dark meat compared with chicken breast, and it has many characteristics of cardiac muscle.

CLINICAL BOX
MUSCLE-WASTING SYNDROMES

Many patients with conditions that include HIV/AIDS and colon and other cancers experience severe body weight loss, a condition known as **cachexia.** Patients with cachexia are frequently unable to tolerate radiation or chemotherapy and have higher morbidity and mortality. The loss of body weight is often independent of caloric intake and is not just akin to starvation; appetite stimulants alone are often not effective. The weight loss in cachexia is associated with the loss of both muscle and adipose tissue. Fast-glycolytic muscle fibers undergo more protein loss than slow-oxidative muscle fibers. This preferential loss of fast-glycolytic fibers with wasting is the opposite of what is seen in muscle with extended periods of disuse (disuse atrophy). Slow-oxidative fibers atrophy preferentially during muscle disuse.

Although the exact mechanisms inducing wasting are not certain, prime candidates with many wasting syndromes involve systemic inflammatory signaling by cytokines, such as TNF-α and IL-6. Inflammatory signaling induced by the disease process can activate muscle protein degradation, inhibit muscle protein synthesis, and induce adipose tissue lipolysis. Maintaining or preventing severe body weight loss in many disease states can improve patient treatment options, survival rates, and quality of life. Anabolic agents, such as testosterone, have proven beneficial in maintaining muscle mass in HIV/AIDS patients and are widely used clinically. With other wasting diseases, research in animal models has demonstrated that inhibition of inflammatory signaling can inhibit wasting. Further research is necessary before this approach is widely applied to human populations.

ADVANCED CONCEPT BOX
SARCOPENIA

Sarcopenia, the loss of skeletal muscle mass, develops gradually in humans after the fifth decade of life and can lead to frailty and loss of functional capacity. Besides the basic erosion of quality of life, loss of skeletal muscle mass also increases the risk of mortality and morbidity. The cause of sarcopenia appears to be related to gradual decreases in physical activity and loss of regenerative capacity. Muscle fiber innervation by spinal motor neurons is critical to both development and maintenance of muscle fibers (cells). Spinal motor neurons decrease in number with advancing age, possibly because of cumulative oxidative damage to these postmitotic cells. The loss of motor neurons appears to cause the substantial (>40%) loss in the muscle fiber number, which is the primary determinant of **age-dependent sarcopenia,** and is accompanied by an increase in motor unit size and a decrease in fine motor skill. Sarcopenia has also been linked to age-induced systemic changes to the endocrine, cardiovascular, and immune systems, whose functions are all critical for the maintenance of skeletal muscle mass.

Comment
The scientific evidence is clear that most older individuals can increase muscle strength and mass with a regular resistance exercise program. Pharmaceutical treatments have also been examined for individuals who cannot regularly exercise. Currently there is no treatment for spinal motor neuron loss. Pharmaceutical treatments targeting muscle have had varying degrees of success and are usually limited by side effects. The treatments include endocrine interventions with male or female sex hormone replacement therapy as well as growth hormone therapy. Anti-inflammatory medication is also employed to allow individuals to participate in physical activity programs. One of the best defenses against sarcopenia is regular exercise in order to maintain muscle mass during middle age.

CLINICAL TEST BOX
ASSAY OF CREATINE TO ASSESS RENAL FUNCTION AND URINE DILUTION

Because creatine phosphate concentration is relatively constant per unit muscle mass, the production of creatinine (Fig. 37.6) is relatively constant during the day. Creatinine is eliminated in urine at a relatively constant amount per hour, primarily by glomerular filtration and to a lesser extent by tubular secretion. Because its concentration in urine varies with the dilution of the urine, levels of metabolites in random urine samples are often normalized to the urinary concentration of creatinine. Otherwise, a 24-h collection would be required to assess daily excretion of a metabolite. Normal creatinine concentration in plasma is about 20–80 mmol/L (0.23–0.90 mg/dL). Increases in plasma creatinine concentration are commonly used as an indicator of renal failure. The albumin:creatinine ratio in a random urine sample, an indicator of protein filtration selectivity of the glomerulus, is used as a measure of the microalbuminuria to assess the progression of diabetic nephropathy (see also Chapter 31).

TISSUE ENGINEERING AND REPLACEMENT OF MUSCLE

As the field of tissue engineering research, muscle tissue is at the forefront of experiments to grow an organ outside the human body. The biochemical plasticity and proliferative capacity of muscle make this possible. Muscle is derived from proliferating cells that originate in the mesenchyme germ layer in the developing embryo. These cells are "determined" into the muscle lineage, hence becoming myoblasts. Myoblasts exit the cell cycle and differentiate (fusing together) into a mature multinucleated muscle cell. This proliferation and differentiation process can be reproduced ex vivo.

Skeletal muscle cells are terminally differentiated, but skeletal muscle contains a small population (<5% of myonuclei) of undifferentiated myoblast-like satellite cells. Satellite cell proliferation and differentiation are essential for postnatal

Myocardial infarction (MI) is the result of blockage of blood flow to the heart. Tissue damage results in leakage of intracellular enzymes into blood (Fig. 37.7). Among these are glycolytic enzymes, such as LDH; however, measurements of myoglobin, total plasma CK, and CK-MB isozymes are more commonly used for diagnosis and management of MI. Myoglobin, a small protein (17 kDa), rises rapidly in plasma within 2 h following MI. Although it is sensitive, it lacks specificity for heart tissue. It is cleared rapidly by renal filtration and returns to normal within 1 day. Because plasma myoglobin also increases following skeletal muscle trauma, it would not be useful for diagnosis of MI (e.g., following an automobile accident). Total plasma CK and the CK-MB isozyme begin to rise within 3–10 h following an MI and reach a peak value of up to 25 times normal after 12–30 h; they may remain elevated for 3–5 days. Total CK may also increase as a result of skeletal muscle damage, but the measurement of CK-MB provides specificity for cardiac damage.

Comment

Enzyme-linked immunosorbent assays (ELISA) for the myocardial troponins are now recommended for use in the diagnosis and management of MI. These assays depend on the presence of unique isoforms of troponin subunits in the adult heart. Plasma Tn-T concentration increases within a few hours after a heart attack, peaks at up to 300 times normal plasma concentration, and may remain elevated for 1–2 weeks. An assay for a specific isoform in an adult heart, Tn-T$_2$, is essentially 100% sensitive for a diagnosis of MI and yields fewer than 5% false-positive results. Significant increases in plasma Tn-T$_2$ are detectable even in patients with unstable angina and transient episodes of ischemia in the heart. Troponins are commonly used as a component of an algorithm to differentiate high-risk from low-risk patients in terms of the need for immediate invasive intervention. The recent definition of myocardial infarction is based on observed serum troponin concentrations.

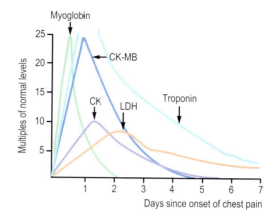

Fig. 37.7 **Serum enzyme changes after myocardial infarction (MI).** Various marker enzymes increase in plasma after MI. These are still used for the diagnosis of MI, but the currently recommended test is the measurement of serum troponin concentration. CK, creatine phosphokinase; CK-MB, cardiac isozyme of CK; LDH, lactate dehydrogenase. (Adapted from Pettigrew, A. R., Pacanis, A. [1997]. Diagnosis of myocardial infarction. In M. H. Dominiczak [ed.], *Seminars in clinical biochemistry*, Glasgow: University of Glasgow Computer Publishing Unit.)

is not surprising considering that skeletal muscles are highly specialized for their anatomical location and function. Muscle grafting surgeries, for example, using donor muscle for the hand have shown that morphological and biochemical differences must be taken into account when selecting muscle tissue for transplantation within the body to a new anatomical location. Because muscle is highly adaptive *(plastic fantastic)*, it is likely that skeletal muscle will be one of the first tissues (along with skin) to be completely engineered ex vivo for in vivo transplantation.

Terminally differentiated myoblasts in the heart (cardiac myocytes) remain single or binucleated throughout life. The heart, in contrast to skeletal muscle, has very limited regenerative capacity due to a lack of satellite cells, so the effects of myocardial infarction are long-lasting. Myoblasts of smooth muscle differentiate into their mature smooth muscle cells (SMC). But SMCs, unlike heart and skeletal muscle, are not terminally differentiated. SMC phenotype also varies based on the cell's location and function. SMCs are found throughout the body in the vascular wall and retain the ability to proliferate (e.g., in response to hypertension or during angiogenesis).

muscle growth and repair (e.g., in response to exercise) and for regeneration after damage. Skeletal muscle is one of the few human tissues that can largely regenerate itself after extensive injury. After injury or tissue loss, satellite cells proliferate and recapitulate the developmental (differentiation) process in adult tissue. A critical component in this process (ex vivo or in vivo) is the muscle extracellular matrix (ECM). An ECM with the correct three-dimensional structure directs myoblast or satellite cells to differentiate into that organ structure and shape. Then the biochemical plasticity of muscle allows adaptation to its environment both mechanically (myosin-ATPase) and metabolically (ATP production pathways). Recent studies in animals and humans demonstrate the ability of skeletal muscle to regenerate into a functional form only when the biochemical and mechanical stresses of physical therapy or exercise are applied to the muscle while it is regenerating. This

EFFECT OF EXERCISE

Strength or resistance training increases muscle mass

A change in daily use of skeletal muscle has a profound effect upon its functional capacity. Both an increase and a decrease in daily activity level can change muscle structure, force-production capacity, and fatigability. From a biochemical point of view, these changes are caused primarily by changes in tissue perfusion and metabolic enzymes, and thus the muscle's ability to take up glucose, utilize fat as an energy source, and generate ATP. The amount and intensity of daily physical activity occur on a continuum, and muscle adaptation to this occurs in response to the specific stress placed upon it. For the sake of simplicity, and because this is how most research studies are designed, we can separate increased use (exercise training) into two categories: strength and aerobic training. The primary purpose of strength training, also called resistance training, is to increase the ability of a specific muscle, or group of muscles, to produce force. This is typically conducted through a small number of repetitions of one exercise movement against a resistance that only allows the muscle to contract through a full range of motion a very limited number of times (e.g., six to eight repetitions of a bicep curl). In contrast, the primary purpose of aerobic training, also called endurance training, is to increase endurance and decrease fatigue during prolonged, lower-intensity physical activity (e.g., running or walking). This is achieved through a high number of repetitions of muscle contractions at a low resistance. Each muscle contraction in strength training might be 75%–90% of the maximal voluntary force production of that muscle, whereas in an aerobic training session, it might be 15%–20%. The biochemical changes in response to these types of exercise are distinct.

Strength training has minimal effects on muscle biochemistry. The increase in force-production capacity that occurs with strength training is the result of increased cell size (i.e., hypertrophy). The hypertrophy of individual muscle cells occurs as a result of an increase in structural and sarcomeric proteins. With more myofibrils and sarcomeres (the contractile units of muscle) comes an increase in force-production capability. When glycolytic enzymes are examined and normalized to the increased cell size, there is no change with strength training. When mitochondrial enzyme activity is normalized to the increased cell size of strength training, there is usually a slight decrease, suggesting that although force-production capacity increases, ATP-production capacity (at least based on the size of the cell) has slightly decreased. In terms of contraction speed and sarcomere cross-bridge cycling, this is primarily determined by myosin-ATPase activity, which remains relatively unchanged in response to resistance training.

Endurance, or aerobic, training increases the oxidative metabolic capacity of muscle

In response to aerobic training, the primary biochemical change is an increase in capacity to metabolize fat, supported by increases in mitochondrial number, size, and enzymes. All muscle fiber types (fast and slow) will increase their concentration and activity of citrate synthase and cytochrome-*c* by two- to threefold, resulting in increased ATP production at a given workload (i.e., exercise intensity) so that muscle can then rely more on fat oxidation and less on anaerobic metabolism. The shift toward aerobic metabolism delays muscle fatigue; there are only minor effects on glycolytic enzymes in response to aerobic training, and the effects on cell size due to aerobic training are also minimal. Small shifts in myosin-ATPase

composition may also occur, leading to a slower muscle phenotype (slower cross-bridge formation during contraction), due to aerobic training. Increases in glucose utilization as a result of increased expression of GLUT-4 and hexokinase also develop more in response to aerobic training, as opposed to strength training, but it is easy to see, considering the amount of skeletal muscle in the body, how blood glucose is decreased in a person with diabetes by an exercise program. It should also be noted that nearly all of these adaptations will occur in reverse in response to any form of de-training, whether that is due to the cessation of an exercise program or bed rest due to injury or disease. Decreased use of muscle causes it to become much less metabolically efficient; unfortunately, this de-adaptation becomes apparent within a few days after cessation of exercise. Other factors induced by endurance training include changes in cardiac output, increases in capillary density, and increases in glycogen stores. Of critical importance to health and medicine are the continuum within which these adaptations occur and the fact that small changes may impact many chronic diseases, including diabetes, atherosclerosis, and cancer cachexia. Further, as changes occur relative to the original status of the muscle, older sedentary persons will see responses in muscle biochemistry comparable to those observed in younger persons. Thus, regardless of age, sedentary individuals who start even a moderate exercise program are likely to see substantial biochemical adaptations and health benefits. Much research is still ongoing in these areas in an attempt to understand the molecular genetic and signaling pathways that bring about these responses and how they might be modified after injury or disease.

SUMMARY

■ Muscle is the major consumer of fuels and ATP in the body. Glycogenolysis, blood glucose uptake for muscle, glycolysis, and lipid metabolism are essential for optimal muscle activity. Reliance on these energy-producing pathways varies with muscle type and its prior contractile activity.

■ Skeletal, cardiac, and smooth muscle have a common actomyosin contractile complex but differ in innervation, contractile protein arrangement, calcium regulation of contraction, and propagation of depolarization from cell to cell.

■ The sarcomere is the fundamental contraction unit of striated muscle.

■ Contraction is described by a "sliding-filament" model in which hydrolysis of ATP is catalyzed by an influx of Ca^{2+} into the sarcoplasm and is coupled with changes in the conformation of myosin. Relaxation of the high-energy conformation of myosin during interaction with actin produces a "power stroke," resulting in

ACTIVE LEARNING

1. When chickens are frightened, they squawk a lot, may jump high, and fly for short distances, but they are unable to take flight and fly for great distances, either normally or to escape danger. In contrast, geese have the ability to fly for great distances during semiannual migrations. Compare the types of muscle fibers and energy sources in the breast of chicken and geese, and explain how the differences in fiber type are compatible with the flying capacity of these birds.

2. Discuss the impact of muscle glycogen phosphorylase deficiency (McArdle's disease) and carnitine or carnitine palmitoyl transferase I deficiency on muscle performance during short- and long-duration exercise.

3. Review the merits of blood doping, carbohydrate loading, and creatine supplementation to enhance performance during marathon events.

increased overlap of the actin–myosin filaments and shortening of the sarcomere.

- The ATP produced in muscle drives the maintenance of ion gradients, restoration of intracellular calcium levels, and continuation of the contractile process.

- Fast-glycolytic muscle relies largely on glycogen and anaerobic glycolysis for short, high-intensity bursts of muscle activity.

- Slow-oxidative muscle is an aerobic tissue; at rest, it uses fats as its primary source of energy. During the initial phases of exercise, it relies on glycogenolysis and glycolysis but then gradually shifts to fat metabolism for long-term energy production.

- Enzymes and proteins are released from muscle in response to damage. Measurements of plasma CK-MB activity and troponin concentration are used as biomarkers of damage to cardiac muscle and are commonly used in the diagnosis and treatment of myocardial infarction.

- Exercise is good medicine; it increases insulin sensitivity and glucose disposal and assists in maintenance of muscle mass and function during aging.

FURTHER READING

Aguirre, L. E., & Villareal, D. T. (2015). Physical exercise as therapy for frailty. *Nestlé Nutrition Workshop Series, 83,* 83–92.

Bodor, G. S. (2016). Biochemical markers of myocardial damage. *Electronic Journal of the International Federation of Clinical Chemistry and Laboratory Medicine, 27,* 95–111.

Bowen, T. S., Schuler, G., & Adams, V. (2015). Skeletal muscle wasting in cachexia and sarcopenia: Molecular pathophysiology and impact of exercise training. *Journal of Cachexia, Sarcopenia and Muscle, 6,* 197–207.

Cooke, R. (2004). The sliding filament model: 1972–2004. *Journal of General Physiology, 123,* 643–656.

Madeddu, C., Mantovani, G., Gramignano, G., et al. (2015). Muscle wasting as main evidence of energy impairment in cancer cachexia: Future therapeutic approaches. *Future Oncology, 11,* 2697–2710.

Marzetti, E., Calvani, R., Tosato, M., et al. (2017). Physical activity and exercise as countermeasures to physical frailty and sarcopenia. *Aging Clinical and Experimental Research, 29,* 35–42.

Mondello, C., Cardia, L., & Ventura-Spagnolo, E. (2017). Immunohistochemical detection of early myocardial infarction: A systematic review. *International Journal of Legal Medicine, 131,* 411–421.

Sicari, B. M., Rubin, J. P., Dearth, C. L., et al. (2014). An acellular biologic scaffold promotes skeletal muscle formation in mice and humans with volumetric muscle loss. *Science Translational Medicine, 6,* 234ra58.

RELEVANT WEBSITES

Muscular dystrophies:
http://www.muscular-dystrophy.org/conditions
http://www.mirm.pitt.edu/tissue-engineering/regenerative-medicine-improves-strength-and-function-in-severe-muscle-injuries/
Animations:
https://www.youtube.com/watch?v=1cRCRaxon6g
https://www.youtube.com/watch?v=7O_ZHyPeIIA&t=17s
https://www.youtube.com/watch?v=e3Nq-P1ww5E

MORE CLINICAL CASES

Please refer to Appendix 2 for more cases relevant to this chapter.

ABBREVIATIONS

CK/CPK	Creatine (phospho)kinase
SR	Sarcoplasmic reticulum
T-tubule	Transverse tubule

Bone Metabolism and Calcium Homeostasis

Marek H. Dominiczak

INTRODUCTION

Bone, apart from its structural and protective function, is metabolically active and serves as a reservoir of calcium. The skeleton contains 99% of the calcium present in the body in the form of hydroxyapatite. The remainder is distributed in the soft tissues, teeth, and the extracellular fluid (ECF).

Many cell functions depend on the control of cytoplasmic and extracellular calcium concentration. This includes neural transmission, cellular secretion, muscle contraction, cell proliferation, permeability of cell membranes, and blood clotting. Plasma concentration of calcium is kept within a narrow range.

Disorders of bone metabolism are very common; for instance, about 40% of white postmenopausal women are affected by osteoporosis, and vitamin D deficiency is thought to affect around 1 billion people worldwide.

CELLULAR ROLE OF CALCIUM

Entry of calcium into cytoplasm is an important biological signal

There is an approximately 10,000-fold difference between Ca^{2+} concentration in the cytoplasm (low Ca^{2+}) and the ECF (high Ca^{2+}). Calcium is pumped out of the cell, and inside the cell, it is compartmentalized into the endoplasmic reticulum (ER) and mitochondria. In the ER, its concentration is close to that in the ECF. Entry of calcium from the ECF or from ER into the cytoplasm is one of the fundamental cellular signals.

Opening of calcium channels in the cell membrane and the ER is part of the signaling pathway tracking from phospholipase C, an enzyme that in turn can be activated by G proteins linked to membrane receptors for polypeptide hormones. Phospholipase C hydrolyzes phosphatidyinositol 4,5- bisphosphate (PIP_2) to inositol 1, 4,5- bisphosphate (PIP_3) and diacylglycerol (DAG). PIP_3 stimulates the influx of Ca^{2+} across plasma membrane Ca^{2+} and its release from ER stores to the cytoplasm. Depletion of ER stores also activates calcium channels known as store-operated (CRAC) channels, which replenish them.

Entry of Ca^{2+} into cytoplasm contributes to the activation of PKC by DAG and further dissemination of signals (for more detail, see Chapter 25).

BONE STRUCTURE AND BONE REMODELING

Bone is a specialized connective tissue that, along with cartilage, forms the skeletal system

There are two types of bone: the thick, densely calcified external bone (cortical, or compact, bone) and a thinner, honeycomb network of calcified tissue (trabecular bone). The main components of bone matrix are **collagen and hydroxyapatite**. Type 1 collagen constitutes 90% of all bone protein (Chapter 19). Crystals containing hydroxyapatite ($Ca_{10}[PO_4]_6[OH]_2$) are found on, within, and between the collagen fibers. Collagen fibers orientate so that they have the greatest density per unit volume and are packed in layers, giving bone its lamellar microscopic structure. Posttranslational modifications of collagen result in the formation of intra- and intermolecular crosslinks.

Noncalcified organic matrix within bone, the **osteoid**, becomes mineralized through two mechanisms. Within the extracellular space of the bone, plasma membrane–derived matrix vesicles act as a focus for deposition of calcium phosphate. Crystallization eventually obliterates the vesicle membrane, leaving clustered hydroxyapatite crystals. Within this environment, the bone-forming cells **(osteoblasts)** secrete matrix proteins that rapidly mineralize and combine with matrix vesicle–derived crystals. Pyrophosphate present in the matrix inhibits this process, but the alkaline phosphatase secreted by the osteoblasts destroys it, allowing mineralization to proceed. Mineralization is highly dependent on an adequate supply of calcium and phosphate. Deprivation of either calcium or phosphate results in an increase in the nonmineralized osteoid, resulting in the clinical condition known in adults as **osteomalacia** and in children, before the fusion of the growth plate, as **rickets** (see the following discussion).

Bone growth

Bone formation starts with the differentiation of mesenchymal cells into either chondroblasts or osteoblasts. Chondrocytes synthesize matrix proteins containing type II collagen and proteoglycans, forming cartilage. Chondrocytes subsequently enlarge and become the central cells of the growing bone (the **growth plate, or epiphyseal plate**). They attract blood vessels and chondroclasts that digest the matrix. The chondrocytes subsequently undergo apoptosis, and the matrix they had synthesized is colonized by osteoblasts, which commence bone formation. Eventually the entire growth plate becomes bone, and the growth stops.

Several signaling pathways are relevant to bone growth

The signaling pathway underlying chondrocyte maturation is known as the hedgehog pathway and includes growing cartilage also secretes the parathyroid hormone–related protein (PTHrP), which acts on receptors common with the parathyroid hormone (PTH; see the following discussion) and maintains chondrocyte proliferation by regulating the hedgehog pathway.

Chondrocyte proliferation is also controlled by several fibroblast growth factors (FGF).

Another signaling pathway that is important in skeletal development is the Wnt/β-catenin pathway. This signaling cascade involves several secreted glycoproteins that bind to a membrane receptor called Frizzled. The key downstream molecules in the Wnt pathway are β-catenin and a protein kinase mTOR (compare Chapter 31). The LDL-receptor-related protein 5 (LRP5; Chapter 33) serves as a coreceptor that, together with Frizzled, activates the Wnt pathway.

Bone remodeling

Bone constantly changes its structure through remodeling

Mechanical load stimulates bone formation. Calcium is ex changed between bone and the ECF as a result of constant bone remodeling - that is, coupled processes of bone formation by the **osteoblasts** and bone resorption by the **osteoclasts** (Fig. 38.1).

Osteoblasts are bone-forming cells

Osteoblasts are derived from mesenchyme. Mature osteoblasts synthesize type 1 collagen and a range of other matrix proteins, such as osteocalcin, growth-related proteins, cell-attachment proteins, and proteoglycans. Osteoblasts are controlled by several autocrine growth factors and cytokines

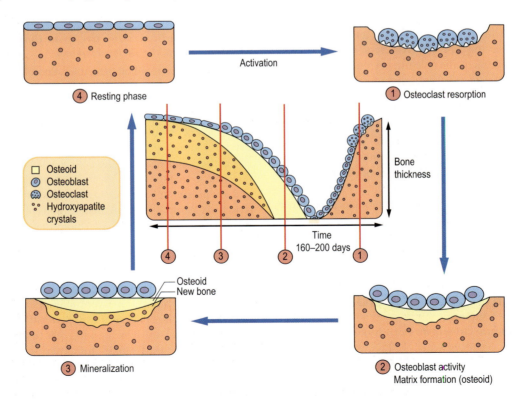

Fig. 38.1 **Maintaining bone mass: the bone remodeling cycle.** Resorption and formation of bone by osteoclasts and osteoblasts is coupled. The processes numbered 1–4 are set in a timeline in the central panel. Note that resorption takes less time than new bone formation.

that include the TGF-β, insulin-like growth factors (IGF-1 and IGF-2), osteoblast-stimulating factor 1 (OSF-1), and platelet-derived growth factor (PDGF) as well as the bone morphogenetic proteins (BMP) belonging to the TGF-β superfamily.

Osteoclasts are bone-resorbing cells

Osteoclasts derive from pluripotent hematopoietic mononuclear cells in the bone marrow.

Maturation of osteoclasts from their progenitor cells is directed by growth factors, particularly monocyte-colony stimulating factor (M-CSF).

RANK prepares the osteoclast to resorb bone

Osteoclasts possess a membrane receptor structurally related to the tumor necrosis factor (TNF) receptor, called **receptor activator of nuclear factor NFκB (RANK)**. Its ligand is the TNF-related cytokine called **RANK ligand (RANKL)** produced by the osteoblasts. The RANKL can also bind to a decoy receptor named **osteoprotegerin (OPG),** a protein that also belongs to the TNF receptor superfamily. This decreases its binding to RANK.

RANK signaling involves recruitment of adaptor molecules known as TNF receptor–associated cytoplasmic factors (TRAF), which bind to the cytoplasmic domains of RANK. The signal then spreads to groups of different kinases, one of the branches involving the phosphatidylinositol-3-kinase (PI3K), Akt kinase, and mTOR kinase. Other branches of the pathway involve c-Jun terminal kinase (JNK), stress-activated protein kinase (p38), extracellular signal–regulated kinase (ERK), and the NFκB kinase (IKK). Kinase activation in turn leads to activation of an array of transcription factors, including NFκB and AP-1. (Fig. 38.2; compare Chapter 28).

The end result is the induction of genes coding for tartrate-resistant acid phosphatase, cathepsin K, calcitonin, and the β2 integrin, which directly control bone resorption. Resorption of bone by activated osteoclasts also involves cathepsins and colla-genases, which generate collagen fragments and hydroxyproline.

Local factors and PTH contribute to osteoclast activation

Osteoclasts are controlled by both local factors and systemic hormones. Cytokines such as interleukin-1 (IL-1), tumor necrosis factor (TNF), transforming growth factor-β (TGF-β), and interferon-α (INF-α) control the osteoclasts acting through RANKL and OPG. PTH activates osteoclasts indirectly via osteoblasts and calcitonin. Estrogens exert their resorption-inhibiting effect through reduction of osteoclast numbers. They also induce OPG synthesis.

BONE MARKERS

Resorption of bone generates **collagen fragments** and other breakdown products, such as hydroxyproline, and calcium from the bone matrix. Different collagen fragments appear in serum and urine during collagen formation and during its degradation and can serve as markers of bone metabolism (Fig. 38.3).

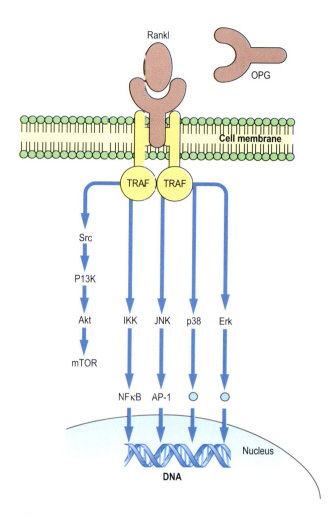

Fig. 38.2 **RANKL signaling pathway.** RANK signals through adaptor proteins, tumor necrosis factor receptor–associated factors (TRAF). Signaling pathways then involve a number of kinases and, eventually, a range of transcription factors. Compare the insulin signaling cascade in Chapter 31. RANKL, RANK ligand; OPG, osteoprotegerin; PI3K, phosphatidylinositol-3-kinase; Akt, Akt kinase; JNK, c-Jun terminal kinase, p38 stress-activated kinase; ERK, extracellular signal–regulated kinase; IKK, NFκB kinase.

Thus **carboxy-terminal procollagen I extension peptide** and **amino-terminal procollagen extension peptides** (PINP, P1CP) are cleaved from the procollagen I molecule and increase in concentration during collagen formation, thus serving as markers of bone formation. Proteins secreted by osteoblasts, such as **osteocalcin**, and **bone-specific alkaline phosphatase** also reflect bone formation.

Conversely, during collagen degradation, **amino-terminal and carboxy-terminal telopeptides** (NTX and CTX), as well as the **pyridinium crosslinks** (pyridinoline [PYD] and deoxypyridinoline [DPD]), are released. They serve as bone resorption markers. Enzymes such as tartrate-resistant acid phosphatase, cathepsins K, and a group of enzymes known as metalloproteinases are also markers of bone resorption.

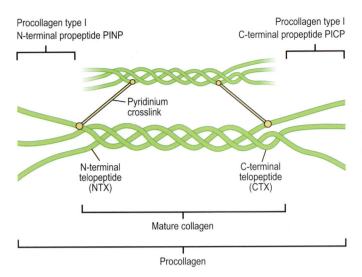

Fig. 38.3 **Fragments of procollagen and mature collagen type I used as bone markers.** Pyridinium crosslinks can be of pyridinoline (PYD) or deoxypyridinoline (DPD). The procollagen peptides PINP and PICP serve as markers of bone formation. NTX, CTX, and pyridinium crosslinks are markers of collagen degradation (bone resorption).

Hydroxyproline present in collagen is a result of post-translational hydroxylation of proline. Both formation and resorption of bone contribute to its release from collagen.

CALCIUM HOMEOSTASIS

Calcium in plasma

Calcium is present in the circulation in three forms

The plasma calcium concentration is maintained within narrow limits, between 2.20 and 2.60 mmol/L (8.8–10.4 mg/dL). Calcium is present in the circulation in three forms. The **ionized Ca²⁺** is the most important, physiologically active form, comprising 50% of the total plasma calcium. The majority of the remaining calcium is **protein bound,** mainly to negatively charged **albumin** (40%), and the rest is complexed to compounds such as citrate and phosphate (10%).

If plasma protein concentration increases as a result of, for instance, dehydration, protein-bound calcium and total serum calcium increase. Conversely, when plasma protein concentration is reduced (e.g., in liver disease, nephrotic syndrome, or malnutrition), the protein-bound calcium fraction is reduced, thus decreasing the total calcium concentration, although ionized calcium remains constant. In many acute and chronic illnesses, albumin concentration decreases; this consequently decreases the total calcium concentration but does not affect the ionized fraction. Therefore clinical laboratories report the **"adjusted calcium"** concentration, mathematically extrapolating the measured calcium value to an albumin concentration of 40 g/L (4 g/dL).

$$\text{Adjusted Ca}^{2+} = \text{measured Ca}^{2+}\,(\text{mmol/L}) + 0.02(40 - \text{albumin}\,[\text{g/L}])$$

$$\text{Adjusted Ca}^{2+} = \text{measured Ca}^{2+}\,(\text{mg/dL}) + 0.8(4.0 - \text{albumin}\,[\text{g/dL}])$$

Parathyroid hormone (PTH)

PTH is the main regulator of calcium homeostasis

PTH is an 84–amino acid, single-chain peptide secreted by the chief cells of the parathyroid glands. The full-length PTH(1–84) is metabolized into a biologically active amino-terminal fragment, PTH(1–34), and an inactive carboxy-terminal fragment, PTH(35–84; Fig. 38.4).

A decrease in plasma calcium concentration is sensed by a calcium-sensing, G protein–coupled receptor (CaSR) present in the chief cells of the parathyroid gland and in the kidney tubule. In the parathyroid gland, it leads to the secretion of PTH.

PTH binds to a specific receptor and acts through cyclic adenosine monophosphate (cAMP)

PTH secretion is stimulated by a decrease in extracellular ionized calcium concentration or by an increase in serum phosphate. **PTH mobilizes calcium from several sources**. It stimulates osteoclast-mediated bone resorption, renal reabsorption of calcium, and calcium absorption in the small intestine mediated by calcitriol. It increases the activity of renal 1-hydroxylase and thus the production of 1, 25OHD₃. Conversely, an increase in plasma calcium decreases PTH secretion.

Severe chronic magnesium deficiency can inhibit PTH release from secretory vesicles, and a low concentration of calcitriol interferes with its synthesis.

Calcitonin

Calcitonin inhibits bone resorption

Calcitonin is another hormone regulating the calcium balance. It is a 32–amino acid peptide secreted primarily by the parafollicular C cells of the thyroid gland. The main effect of calcitonin is inhibition of bone resorption, reducing the release of calcium and phosphate from bone (Fig. 38.5). Its secretion is regulated by plasma calcium through the CaSR: an increase in serum calcium results in a proportional increase in calcitonin, and a decrease elicits a corresponding calcitonin reduction.

Vitamin D

Vitamin D is synthesized in the skin by ultraviolet (UV) radiation

Vitamin D₂ (ergocalciferol) is synthesized in the skin by UV radiation of ergosterol, and **vitamin D₃ (cholecalciferol)** is synthesized in the skin by UV irradiation of

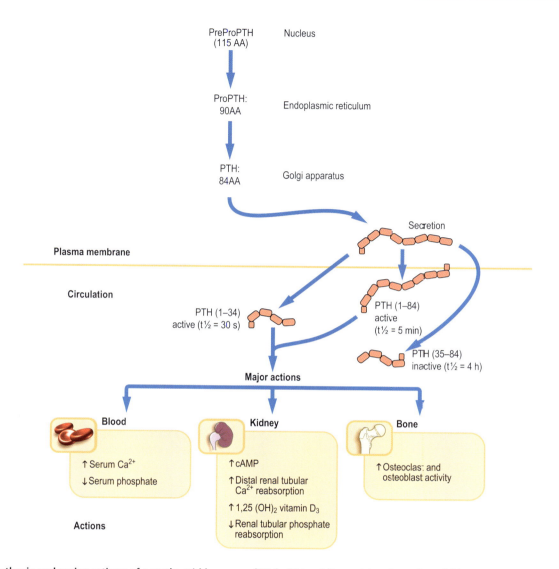

Fig. 38.4 **Synthesis and major actions of parathyroid hormone (PTH).** PTH mobilizes calcium from all available sources and decreases its renal excretion. AA, amino acids.

CLINICAL BOX
A WOMAN WITH SEVERE RIGHT-SIDED FLANK PAIN: PRIMARY HYPERPARATHYROIDISM

A 52-year-old woman presented to the emergency department with severe right-sided flank pain. Further questioning revealed a history of recent depression, generalized weakness, recurrent indigestion, and aches in both hands. Blood was detected on urine testing, and radiography revealed the presence of kidney stones. The pain settled with opiate analgesia. Serum adjusted calcium was 3.20 mmol/L (12.8 mg/dL; normal range 2.2–2.6 mmol/L, 8.8–10.4 mg/dL), serum phosphate was 0.65 mmol/L (2.0 mg/dL; normal range 0.7–1.4 mmol/L, 2.2–5.6 mg/dL), and PTH was 16.9 pmol/L (169 pg/mL; normal range 1.1–6.9 pmol/L, 11–69 pg/mL).

Comment
Most patients with primary hyperparathyroidism are identified when asymptomatic hypercalcemia is discovered on routine biochemical testing. Primary hyperparathyroidism classically affects the skeleton, kidneys, and gastrointestinal tract, resulting in the well-recognized triad of complaints described as "bones, stones, and abdominal groans." Kidney stone disease is now the most common presenting complaint.

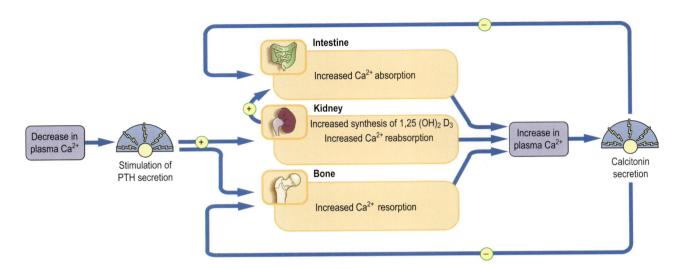

Fig. 38.5 Major hormones influencing calcium homeostasis. A decrease in plasma ionized calcium stimulates the release of PTH. This promotes Ca^{2+} reabsorption in the kidney, its resorption from bone, and its absorption from the gut mediated by increased production of $1,25(OH)_2D_3$. As a result, plasma calcium increases. Conversely, an increase in plasma ionized calcium stimulates the release of calcitonin, which inhibits reabsorption of calcium in the kidney and osteoclast-mediated bone resorption.

7-dehydrocholesterol. Vitamin D_3 and its hydroxylated metabolites are transported in the plasma bound to a specific globulin, vitamin D–binding protein (DBP). Cholecalciferol is also found in the diet, where its absorption is linked to the absorption of fats. Absorbed vitamin D is transported to the liver in **chylomicrons** and is released to the liver, where it is hydroxylated at the 25-position by a hydroxylase designated CYP2R1, forming **calcidiol** (25-hydroxycholecalciferol; $25[OH]D_3$).

Calcidiol is the storage form of vitamin D

Calcidiol is the major form of the vitamin found in the liver and in the circulation. It is bound to DBP in both compartments. The rate of hydroxylation is regulated by its hepatic content, and its levels in the circulationreflect the size of hepatic stores. A significant proportion of calcidiol is subject to enterohepatic circulation, being excreted in the bile and reabsorbed in the small bowel. Thus disturbed enterohepatic circulation can cause vitamin D deficiency.

Calcitriol is the most potent form of vitamin D

In the renal tubules, calcidiol (25OHD3) is further hydroxylated at the 1-position by a hydroxylase designated CYP27B1to form calcitriol ($1\alpha,25$-dihydroxycholecalciferol; $1,25[OH]2D3$). The vitamin D–DBP complex is excreted by the tubule and reabsorbed by receptors known as megalin and cubilin. This reaction also takes place in the placenta. **Calcitriol** is the most potent of the vitamin D metabolites. The 1α-hydroxylase is stimulated by PTH, by low plasma concentrations of calcium or phosphate, and by calcitonin as well as by estrogens and by vitamin D deficiency. It is feedback inhibited by calcitriol, hypercalcemia, high phosphate concentration, and low PTH.

Calcitriol increases the absorption of calcium and phosphate from the gut

Calcitriol is a hormone. It is transported in plasma bound to DBP. In the intestinal epithelium, analogously to other steroid hormones, it binds to a cytoplasmic receptor (Chapters 14 and 23). The receptor forms heterodimers with the retinoid X receptor (RXR), and this complex transfers to the nucleus, where it induces gene expression. Vitamin D upregulates gut Ca^{2+} channel TRPV6, the intracellular transporter calbindin D, and the calcium pump PMCA1b, increasing the transport of Ca^{2+} from enterocytes to plasma.

Renal tubules, cartilage, intestine, and placenta contain yet another hydroxylase, the 24-hydroxylase (CYP24A1), which produces the inactive 24,25-dihydroxycholecalciferol ($24,25[OH]2D3$). Vitamin D metabolism is summarized in Fig. 38.6.

Calcitriol, together with PTH, stimulates bone resorption by osteoclasts. This increases plasma concentrations of calcium and phosphate. Calcitriol deficiency disrupts the mineralization of newly formed osteoid as a result of decreased calcium and phosphate availability and reduced osteoblast function, leading to the development of **rickets** in children and **osteomalacia** in adults.

Intestinal absorption and renal excretion of calcium

Calcium is absorbed in the small intestine and is excreted in urine and feces

Calcium absorption in the proximal small intestine is also regulated by its quantity in the diet and by two cellular calcium transport processes: the active, saturable transcellular absorption

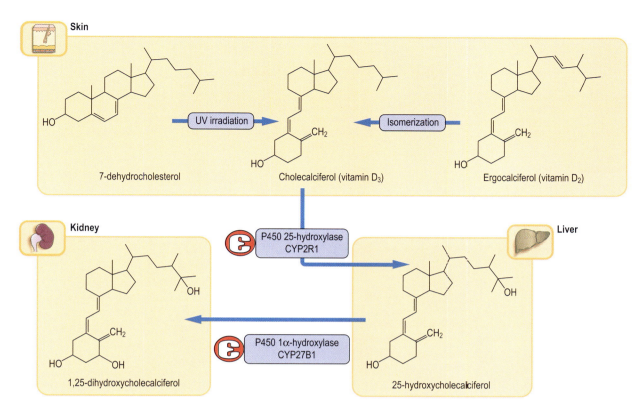

Fig. 38.6 **Vitamin D metabolism.** Vitamin D is mainly synthesized in response to the action of sunlight on the skin; a smaller component comes from the diet. Normal liver and kidney function are essential to the formation of the active form $1,25(OH)_2D_3$ (calcitriol). Plasma calcium concentration controls the level of $1,25(OH)_2D_3$ through PTH. Note that hydroxylases involved in vitamin D metabolism belong to the cytochrome P450 superfamily. $1,25(OH)_2D_3$, 1,25-Dihydroxycholecalciferol, calcitriol; 25-hydroxycholecalciferol, calcidiol, $25(OH)D_3$.

stimulated by $1,25(OH)2D3$ and the nonsaturable paracellular absorption controlled by the concentration of calcium in the intestinal lumen relative to the plasma.

In a normal adult following a Western diet, calcium intake and its deposition in bone are matched by the excretion in urine and feces. During growth, a child is in positive calcium balance, whereas an elderly person may be in negative calcium balance. Changes in calcium absorption reflect alterations in dietary calcium intake, its intestinal availability, and vitamin D metabolism.

Calcium is excreted through the kidney

PTH promotes calcium reabsorption acting on the proximal renal tubules. In hypercalcemia, renal calcium filtration is increased, and tubular reabsorption is inhibited.

Hypocalcemia is associated with a reduction in urinary excretion, mainly as a result of decreased amounts of filtered calcium. Calcium reabsorption is reduced in hypoparathyroidism.

Several other hormones affect bone metabolism and calcium homeostasis

Thyroid hormone stimulates bone resorption. Adrenal and gonadal steroids, particularly estrogens in women and testosterone in men, stimulate osteoblasts and inhibit osteoclast function. They also increase intestinal calcium absorption and decrease renal calcium

and phosphate excretion. Growth hormone promotes skeletal growth. Its effects are mediated by IGF-1 and IGF-2 acting on cells of the osteoblast lineage. Growth hormone increases urinary excretion of calcium and decreases urinary excretion of phosphate.

The central nervous system is probably also involved in bone homeostasis. Leptin, an adipokine that regulates adipose tissue mass (Chapter 32), has been shown to inhibit bone formation. However, mutations in the leptin signaling pathway have no effect on bone mass; this suggests that it is a central effect, probably mediated by the sympathetic nervous system.

DISORDERS OF CALCIUM METABOLISM

Hypercalcemia

Hypercalcemia is most commonly caused by primary hyperparathyroidism or by malignancy

In practice, 90% of cases of hypercalcemia are due to either primary hyperparathyroidism or malignancy. There is a wide individual variation in the development of symptoms and signs of hypercalcemia (Fig. 38.7). The measurement of PTH makes it possible to discriminate between primary hyperparathyroidism

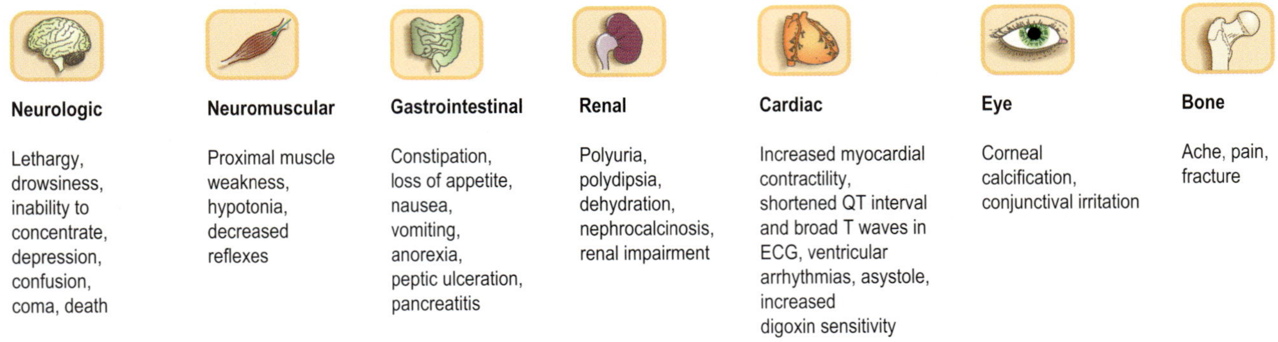

Neurologic	Neuromuscular	Gastrointestinal	Renal	Cardiac	Eye	Bone
Lethargy, drowsiness, inability to concentrate, depression, confusion, coma, death	Proximal muscle weakness, hypotonia, decreased reflexes	Constipation, loss of appetite, nausea, vomiting, anorexia, peptic ulceration, pancreatitis	Polyuria, polydipsia, dehydration, nephrocalcinosis, renal impairment	Increased myocardial contractility, shortened QT interval and broad T waves in ECG, ventricular arrhythmias, asystole, increased digoxin sensitivity	Corneal calcification, conjunctival irritation	Ache, pain, fracture

Fig. 38.7 **Symptoms and signs of hypercalcemia.** The severity of symptoms is associated with the degree of hypercalcemia.

CLINICAL BOX
A 60-YEAR-OLD WOMAN WITH ACHES AND PAINS IN HER BONES: OSTEOMALACIA

A 60-year-old woman who had become increasingly infirm and housebound was referred to the metabolic outpatient clinic. She had experienced gradual onset of diffuse aches and pains throughout her skeleton but especially around the hips. She was having difficulty walking, experienced generalized weakness, and recently developed sudden severe pain in her ribs and pelvis. Radiography detected fractured ribs. Adjusted serum calcium was 2.1 mmol/L (8.4 mg/dL; normal range 2.2–2.6 mmol/L, 8.8–10.4 mg/dL), serum phosphate was 0.56 mmol/L (1.7 mg/dL; normal range 0.7–1.4 mmol/L, 2.2–4.3 mg/dL), alkaline phosphatase was 300 IU/L (normal range 50–260 IU/L), and PTH was 12.6 pmol/L (normal range 1.1–6.9 pmol/L, 11–69 pg/mL).

Comment
In severe forms of osteomalacia, biochemical abnormalities are commonly seen, including low serum–adjusted calcium, low serum phosphate, increased alkaline phosphatase, and increased PTH(1–84). Patients may have diffuse bone pain or more specific pain related to a fracture, lateral bowing of the lower limbs, and a distinctive waddling gait. Ethnic groups with dark skin are particularly at risk in countries with low average sunlight because the majority of vitamin D in the body comes from synthesis by the action of UV light on 7-dehydrocholesterol. This may be exacerbated by traditional clothing that provides little skin exposure and also by a diet that is high in phytates (unleavened bread) and low in calcium and vitamin D.

and nonparathyroid causes of hypercalcemia, particularly malignancy. In primary hyperparathyroidism, we see an increased PTH in the presence of hypercalcemia, whereas in nonparathyroid causes of hypercalcemia, PTH is undetectable.

Primary hyperparathyroidism is common

Primary hyperparathyroidism is a relatively common endocrine disease, characterized by hypercalcemia associated with an increased concentration of PTH. Its incidence is 1:500 to 1:1000. In 80%–85% of patients, the cause is a solitary parathyroid gland adenoma.

Secondary hyperparathyroidism occurs when other organs involved in calcium mobilization are affected by disease, causing hypocalcemia, which in turn stimulates PTH release. Thus kidney and liver disease, which disrupt vitamin D metabolism, and bowel disease, which may impair calcium absorption, all cause secondary hyperparathyroidism.

Hypercalcemia occurs in advanced malignant disease and is usually a poor prognostic sign

PTHrP, mentioned previously in the context of bone formation, can also be produced by tumors and is the most common cause of hypercalcemia of malignancy (HCM). The amino-terminal portion of PTHrP possesses PTH-like activity. Production of PTHrP is common in breast, lung, and kidney tumors and other solid tumors.

Another type of hypercalcemia associated with malignancy results from increased osteoclastic bone resorption, where compounds produced by the primary tumor or by metastases, such as prostaglandins, and growth factors, including IL-1, TNF-α, lymphotoxin, and TGF, alter the RANKL/OPG balance and stimulate osteoclasts.

Hypercalcemia can also be caused by overtreatment with vitamin D

Vitamin D toxicity is the third most common cause of hypercalcemia. Vitamin D excess causes enhanced calcium absorption and bone reabsorption, leading to hypercalcemia and metastatic calcium deposition. The symptoms are anorexia, weight loss, and polyuria. There is also a tendency to develop kidney stones because of the hypercalciuria secondary to hypercalcemia.

Hypocalcemia

Hypocalcemia is common in clinical practice

Changes in plasma-ionized calcium can result from pH changes. Alkalemia (Chapter 36) increases binding of calcium to proteins, decreasing the ionized calcium. Clinical signs of hypocalcemia are mostly due to neuromuscular irritability. In some cases,

Table 38.1 Causes of hypocalcemia

Hypoparathyroid	Nonparathyroid	Parathyroid hormone resistance
Postoperative	Vitamin D deficiency	Pseudohypoparathyroidism
Idiopathic	Vitamin D malabsorption	Hypomagnesemia
Neck irradiation	Vitamin D resistance	
Anticonvulsant therapy	Renal disease	
	Hypophosphatemia	

Table 38.2 Causes of vitamin D deficiency

Cause of deficiency	Comment
Reduced exposure to sunlight	Common in institutionalized elderly persons and persons wearing clothing allowing limited skin exposure to sunlight
Poor dietary intake	Diets such as strict vegetarian diet, which have inadequate vitamin D content Premature infants: breastfeeding without vitamin D supplementation
Malabsorption of vitamin D	Celiac disease, Crohn's disease, pancreatic insufficiency, inadequate bile salt secretion, nontropical sprue
Liver disease	Deficient 25-hydroxylation
Renal failure	Deficient 1-hydroxylation Fanconi syndrome or renal tubular acidosis
Vitamin D resistance	Mutation in *CYP27B1* gene or *VDR* gene Very rare

the irritability may be demonstrated by eliciting specific clinical signs. **Chvostek's sign** is the observed twitching of the muscles around the mouth (circumoral muscles) in response to tapping the facial nerve, and **Trousseau's sign** is the typical contraction of the hand in response to reduced blood flow in the arm induced by inflation of a blood pressure cuff. Numbness, tingling, cramps, tetany, and even seizures may occur. Causes of hypocalcemia can be divided into those associated with low PTH(1–84) and rare cases in which there is PTH resistance. If hypocalcemia is primary, the decreased serum calcium causes secondary hyperparathyroidism. The most common cause of hypoparathyroidism is a complication of neck surgery.

Pseudohypoparathyroidism is characterized by hypocalcemia, hyperphosphatemia, and increased concentrations of PTH(1–84). The classic form of pseudohypoparathyroidism is due to end-organ resistance to PTH, caused by a genetic defect resulting in an abnormal regulatory G-protein subunit. Confirmation of the diagnosis is made by demonstrating a lack of increase in plasma or urinary cAMP in response to PTH infusion.

Hypocalcemia may result from abnormal vitamin D metabolism

Vitamin D deficiency, acquired or inherited disorders of its metabolism, and vitamin D resistance may occur. The main causes of hypocalcemia are listed in Table 38.1, and the most common causes of vitamin D deficiency are shown in Table 38.2.

Rickets

The original description of rickets dates back to the 17th century. Rickets develops in children before the closure of the growth plate. It results in growth retardation and bone deformities such as bow legs and rib-cage deformities such as "funnel chest" and Harrison sulcus, the formation of the "rickety rosary" around costochondral junctions. Conversely, adult osteomalacia is characterized by bone pain and muscle weakness.

The principal cause of rickets is vitamin D deficiency. Low calcium intake or a combination of the two can also be a cause. Phosphate wasting also underlies a group of inherited disorders resulting in rickets (Table 38.3). The peak prevalence of rickets is between 6 and 18 months of age.

Rickets can also develop as a result of phosphate deficiency

There are several abnormalities associated with renal phosphate wasting and consequent rickets, the most common being X-linked hypophosphatemic rickets (Table 38.3). Hypophosphatemic rickets results from the inhibition of renal Na/P cotransporter. A relatively recently discovered peptide, fibroblast growth factor 23 (FGF23), seems to play a key role in the development of these disorders. FGF 23 is a 251–amino acid peptide produced in bone. It binds to the FGF receptor, and its signaling requires the coreceptor function of membrane proteins

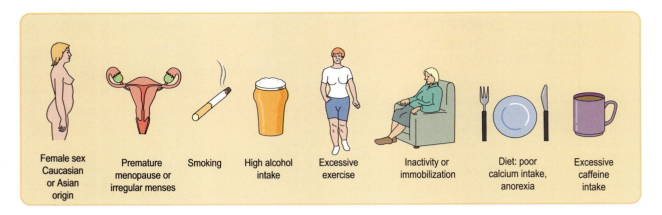

Fig. 38.8 **Risk factors and secondary causes of osteoporosis.**

Table 38.3 Rickets and osteomalacia associated with hypophosphatemia	
Disorder	**Cause**
X-linked hypophosphatemic rickets/osteomalacia	Frequency 1: 20,000 Most frequent cause of vitamin D–resistant hypophosphatemic rickets Mutation in the *Phex* gene Overexpression of *FGF23*
Autosomal dominant hypophosphatemic rickets/osteomalacia	Rare mutations in *FGF23* gene
Autosomal recessive hypophosphatemic rickets/osteomalacia	Mutation in dentin matrix protein (DMP) Overexpression of *FGF23*

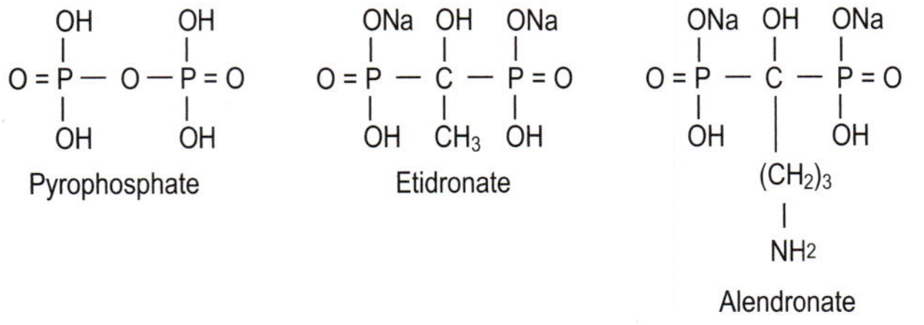

Fig. 38.9 **Structural formulae of pyrophosphate and bisphospho-nates.** The P-C-P bonds of the biphosphonates resist enzymatic cleavage. The potency of these drugs is determined by the chemical sequence attached to the carbon molecule.

called alpha-Klotho. It suppresses the expression of sodium phosphate cotransporters in the proximal tubules. It also reduces serum calcitriol synthesis. Thus it stimulates renal phosphate excretion and decreases its intestinal absorption, leading to hypophosphatemia.

Enhanced phosphate reabsorption may result in ectopic calcification

Calcification of soft tissues (calcinosis) occurs in an inherited disorder where there is enhanced renal phosphate reabsorption leading to hyperphosphatemia. It may involve, among others, mutations in the *klotho* gene.

Osteoporosis

Osteoporosis is a common age-related disease of bone

Osteoporosis is defined as a reduction of bone mineral density with an increased susceptibility to fractures. Bone density decreases from a peak achieved by the age of 30 years in men and women. The rate of bone loss accelerates in women after the loss of estrogen at menopause. Progressive loss of bone is a result of uncoupling of bone turnover, with a relative **increase of bone resorption** or **decrease in bone formation**. A number of factors have been recognized as contributing to an increased risk of osteoporosis (Fig. 38.8).

Paget's disease of bone is characterized by areas of accelerated bone turnover

Paget's disease of bone is characterized by increased focal osteoclastic activity. It is characterized by typical "punched-out" lesions of bones visible on X-ray. It seems that there is an increased sensitivity of osteoclast to calcitriol and RANKL. A common biochemical abnormality in this disease is increased plasma alkaline phosphatase. As a result of increased collagen breakdown by osteoclasts, there is an increased plasma and urine concentration of hydroxyproline and collagen fragments. Paget's disease affects 1%–2% of white adults older than 55 years. The first choice for treating Paget's disease is the bisphosphonates, which exert antiosteoclastic activity (see Fig. 38.9).

SUMMARY

- Bone is a metabolically active tissue that undergoes constant remodeling.

CLINICAL BOX
A 62-YEAR-OLD WOMAN ADMITTED AFTER A FALL: OSTEOPOROSIS

A 62-year-old woman was admitted to the hospital after a fall in her bathroom because of sudden onset of severe pain between the shoulder blades. Radiography detected a wedge fracture of two thoracic vertebrae with reduced bone density. Bone density assessment using dual-energy X-ray absorptiometry (DEXA) scan showed severely reduced density in the femur and spine. She had experienced menopause after a hysterectomy at age 41 years but had been unable to tolerate hormone-replacement therapy (HRT). Biochemical investigations were all within normal limits.

Comment
Symptoms of osteoporosis develop at a late stage of the disease and are often caused by fractures. Hip, vertebral, and wrist fractures are common in patients with osteoporosis.

ACTIVE LEARNING

1. Describe the RANK–RANKL signaling system.
2. Discuss factors that regulate osteoblast function.
3. Describe the forms of calcium present in plasma. Which form is biologically active?
4. Discuss feedback mechanisms that maintain the plasma calcium concentration.

■ Major cell types involved in the remodeling process are osteoblasts and osteoclasts.
■ Bone metabolism is closely linked to calcium homeostasis, which involves the parathyroid gland, the intestine, the liver, and the kidney.
■ The main controllers of calcium balance are PTH, vitamin D, and calcitonin.
■ Both hypercalcemia and hypocalcemia lead to clinical symptoms.
■ The main causes of hypercalcemia are primary hyperparathyroidism, malignancy, and vitamin D excess.
■ Osteoporosis, a decrease in bone density leading to bone fractures, is a major health problem.

FURTHER READING

Fraser, W. D. (2009). Hyperparathyroidism. *Lancet, 374,* 145–158.
Hlaing, T. T., & Compston, J. E. (2014). Biochemical markers of bone turnover-uses and limitations. *Ann Clin Biochem, 51,* 189–202.
Rachner, T. D., Khosla, S., & Hofbauer, L. (2011). Osteoporosis: Now and the future. *Lancet, 377,* 1276–1287.
Ralston, S. H., Langston, A. L., & Reid, I. R. (2008). Pathogenesis and management of Paget's disease of bone. *Lancet, 372,* 155–163.
Richards, J. B., Rivadeneira, F., Pastinen, T. M., et al. (2008). Bone mineral density, osteoporosis, and osteoporotic fractures: A genome-wide association study. *Lancet, 371,* 1505–1512.
Saito, T., & Fukumoto, S. (2009). Fibroblast growth factor 23 (FGF23) and disorders of phosphate metabolism. *Int J Pediatr Endocrinol,* doi:10.1155/2009/496514.
Walsh, M. C., & Choi, Y. (2014). Biology of RANKL-RANKL-OPG system in immunity, bone and beyond. *Front Immunol, 5,* 511.

ABBREVIATIONS

AP-1	Activator protein-1
cAMP	Cyclic adenosine monophosphate
BMP	Bone morphogenetic proteins that belong to the TGF-β superfamily
CTX	Carboxy-terminal telopeptide
$1,25(OH)_2D_3$, calcitriol	1 25-dihydroxycholecalciferol
DMP	Dentin matrix protein
ECF	Extracellular fluid
ER	Endoplasmic reticulum
ERK	Extracellular signal–regulated kinase
FGFs	Fibroblast growth factors
IGF-1/IGF-2	Insulin-like growth factors
Ihh	Indian hedgehog, a signaling protein
IKK	NFκB kinase
IL-1	Interleukin-1
INF-α	Interferon-α
JNK	C-Jun terminal kinase
LRP5	LDL-receptor-related protein 5
M-CSF	Monocyte-colony stimulating factor
mTOR	Mechanistic target of rapamycin
NFAT2	Transcription factor: nuclear factor of activated T cells-2
NFκB	Nuclear factor kappa-light-chain-enhancer of activated B cell
NTX	Amino-terminal and telopeptide
OSF-1	Osteoblast-stimulating factor 1
OPG	Osteoprotegerin
PDGF	Platelet-derived growth factor
PI3K	Phosphatidylinositol-3-kinase
P1NP	Procollagen type 1N-terminal propeptide
P1CP	Procollagen type 1 C-terminal peptide
PIP_2	Phosphatidylinositol 4,5- bisphosphate,
PIP_3	Inositol 1, 4,5- bisphosphate PTH, parathyroid hormone
PKC	Protein kinase C
p38	Stress-activated protein kinase
p62	Nucleoporin
RANK	Receptor activator of nuclear factor NFκB

RANKL	RANK ligand
TNF	Tumor necrosis factor
TRAFs	TNF receptor–associated cytoplasmic factors
TGF-β	Transforming growth factor-β

| Wnt | A signaling pathway related to cell growth and proliferation; Describes a family of proteins. The pathway abbreviation relates to "Wingless-related integration site" |

Neurochemistry

Hanna Bielarczyk and Andrzej Szutowicz

INTRODUCTION

The brain is, in many ways, a chemist's delight. This is so because it illustrates various general principles of biology applied to a highly specialized tissue that ultimately regulates all the other tissues of the body. This chapter highlights the differences between the **central nervous system (CNS)** - that is, the brain and spinal cord - and the **peripheral nervous system (PNS),** which is outside the dura (the thick fibrous covering that contains the cerebrospinal fluid [CSF]).

BRAIN AND PERIPHERAL NERVE

The distinction between brain and peripheral nerve essentially reflects the division between the CNS and the PNS, with a convenient dividing line being the confines of the dura, within which watertight compartment is the CSF, partially produced (about one-third of the total volume) through the action of the blood–brain barrier. **Myelin** insulates the axons of nerves; the chemical composition of CNS myelin is quite distinct from that of PNS myelin, not least because the two forms are produced by two different types of cells: the oligodendrocytes within the CNS and the Schwann cells within

the PNS. The distinction between the functions of the CNS and those of the PNS is fundamental to differential diagnosis in neurology. A typical example is the difference between the demyelination of the CNS that occurs in **multiple sclerosis** and the demyelination of the PNS that occurs in **Guillain–Barré syndrome.**

The blood–brain barrier

The term blood–brain barrier (BBB) is a slight misnomer in that the "barrier" is not absolute but relative: its permeability depends on the size of the molecule in question

Initially, experiments based on the use of a dye (Evans blue) bound to albumin showed that over a period of hours, an animal progressively turned blue in all tissues, with the notable exception of the brain, which remained white. It subsequently became clear that 1 molecule in 200 of serum albumin passed normally into the CSF, which is analogous to lymph. It also became obvious that for any given protein, the ratio of its concentrations in CSF and serum was a linear function of the molecular radius of the molecules in solution. About 15% of the CSF protein pool is synthesized within the brain (prostaglandin D synthase, cystatin C, transthyretin). In degenerative or inflammatory conditions, pathologic proteins are released from damaged cells (tau, S-100; Table 39.1) or synthesized by infiltrating lymphocytes (immunoglobulins). Some of them are used in clinical practice as laboratory markers of various pathologies of the nervous system. Proteins are large polyanionic particles, and this, due to the existing concentration gradient, creates an anion deficit in CSF compared with plasma. It is replenished by increased Cl^- anion concentration in the CSF (about 120 mmol/L compared with 100 mmol/L in plasma; the phenomenon is known as Donnan's equilibrium). Conversely, the glucose concentration in CSF is two-thirds of that in plasma due to its avid utilization by neurons and other brain cells. Glucose is transported into the brain by GLUT1 insulin-independent transporters present on endothelial cells and adjacent astroglial endfoots constituting the BBB. There is an inverse correlation between average glycemia and GLUT1 density in the BBB.

There are six sources of the CSF

Under normal and pathologic conditions, proteins pass from external cells and tissues into the CSF, and their degree of

Table 39.1 Protein markers of CNS cells and relevant brain pathologies

Cell	Protein	Pathology
Neuron	Neuron-specific enolase	Brain death
Astrocyte	GFAP	Plaque (or scar)
Oligodendrocyte	Myelin basic protein	De/remyelination
Microglia	Ferritin	Stroke
Choroid plexi	Asialotransferrin	CSF leak (rhinorrhea)

GFAP, glial fibrillary acidic protein.

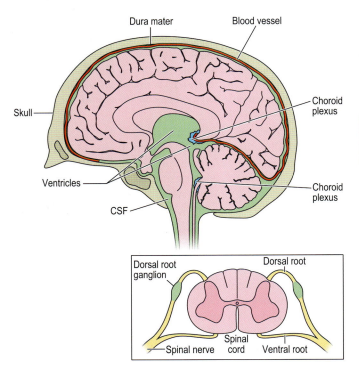

Fig. 39.1 **Main sources of cerebrospinal fluid (CSF).** The main source of the CSF is the choroid plexus situated in the lateral ventricles. Other interfaces between blood and brain tissue include the brain capillaries and the capillaries of the dorsal root ganglia in the spinal cord. A contribution to the composition of the CSF also comes from direct sources, the cells in the brain parenchyma. The anatomy is simplified for clarity.

filtration and/or rate of local synthesis vary. The total quantity of the CSF therefore constitutes the algebraic sum of these six sources (Fig. 39.1).

■ **The blood–brain barrier** (the parenchymal capillaries) gives rise to about one-third of the volume of CSF and is known as the source of interstitial fluid.
■ **The blood–CSF barrier** provides the bulk of CSF (almost all of the remaining two-thirds), termed choroidal fluid

because it is principally provided by the choroid plexuses (capillary tufts) situated in the lateral ventricles and, to a lesser degree, the plexuses situated in the third and fourth ventricles.

■ **The dorsal root ganglia** contain capillaries that have a much greater degree of permeability.
■ **The brain parenchyma of the CNS** produces a number of brain-specific proteins. These include prostaglandin synthase (formerly called β-trace protein) and transthyretin (formerly called prealbumin).
■ **The circulating CSF cells**, mainly lymphocytes within the CNS, synthesize local antibodies. However, in the CNS, there is a strong presence of immune suppressor cells. Because of this, in brain infections such as **meningitis,** steroids are given in addition to antibiotics to suppress the potentially devastating effects, within this confined space, of inflammation associated with the intrathecal immune response.
■ **The meninges** represent a sixth source of CSF under pathologic conditions; they can give rise to a dramatic increase in the concentrations of CSF proteins.

✦ ADVANCED CONCEPT BOX
DIFFERENTIAL DIAGNOSIS OF NASAL DISCHARGE (RHINORRHEA)

In clinical practice, it is essential to distinguish CSF rhinorrhea from local nasal secretions caused by, say, influenza infection. The ear, nose, and throat (ENT) surgeon must know whether the fluid present is CSF because any leak must be surgically repaired, lest it remain a chronic potential source of meningitis as a result of the migration of nasal flora into the subarachnoid space. One characteristic and useful marker protein in the CSF is **asialotransferrin,** which is transferrin lacking sialic acid. In the systemic circulation, this absence of sialic acid gives a molecular signal for the protein to be recycled, and it is thus immediately removed from the systemic circulation by all reticuloendothelial cells. The brain has no true reticuloendothelial cells along the path of CSF flow, and hence asialotransferrin is present in quite high concentrations. The aqueous humor of the anterior chamber of the eye also produces the characteristic asialotransferrin, and the same asialotransferrin can also be found in the perilymph of the semicircular canals in the inner ear.

CELLS OF THE NERVOUS SYSTEM

About 10% of the cells of the human nervous system are large neurons. They present diverse morphologic features concerning cell bodies, axons, and dendrites, as well as neurotransmitter and functional phenotypes. A human neuron's body size may vary from 10 to 100 μm. They form axons, from a few micrometers to 1 m long, ending with nerve terminals (outward signaling). They also extend multiple dendritic branches that collect outside signals from nerve terminals of other neurons. Each human brain neuron forms thousands of bidirectional connections with other ones, constituting sophisticated networks.

The three major types of glial cells in the nervous system (each constitute about 30%) are **astrocytes**, which also make up part of the blood–brain barrier and thereby avidly take up glucose and provide energy substrates (lactate) and neurotransmitter precursors (glutamine) to neurons; **oligodendrocytes,** which generate myelin sheets and are principally composed of fat and serve to insulate the axons; and **microglia**, which are essentially resident macrophages (scavengers).

These different cell types are associated with predominant protein molecules that are important in various brain pathologies (Table 39.1). Other minor constituents of the nervous system include the ependymal cells, which are ciliated cells secreting brain-specific proteins such as prostaglandin synthase. The brain endothelial cells, unlike other tissue capillaries, have tight junctions that bind them together; this feature is also believed to contribute to the blood–brain barrier, although it is the basement membrane that is the major source of molecular sieving of the different-sized proteins.

Neurons

The significant features of neurons are their length, their many interconnections, and the fact that they do not divide postpartum

There is an archetypal notion of the electrical activity of the nervous system - in particular, of the electrical activity of neurons. However, three other biological features of neurons are particularly worthy of note: their **length**, their **prolific interconnections**, and the fact that **they do not divide postpartum**.

Because of their great length, neurons depend on an efficient system of axonal transport

Some axons of motor and sensory neurons can typically be up to 1 m long; thus the nucleus, the source of information for the synthesis of proteins and neurotransmitters, is typically quite remote from the synaptic terminal, the site of synthesis and release of those transmitters. Because of this extensive length, a crucial requirement is the neuron's ability to transport materials both from the nucleus/perikaryon toward the synapse (anterograde transport) and from the synapse to the nucleus (retrograde transport). The **anterograde transport** is conducted through neurofilaments built of three types of subunits and provides packages of different proteins and mitochondria necessary for nerve terminal function. **Retrograde transport** takes place through a neurotubular system consisting of

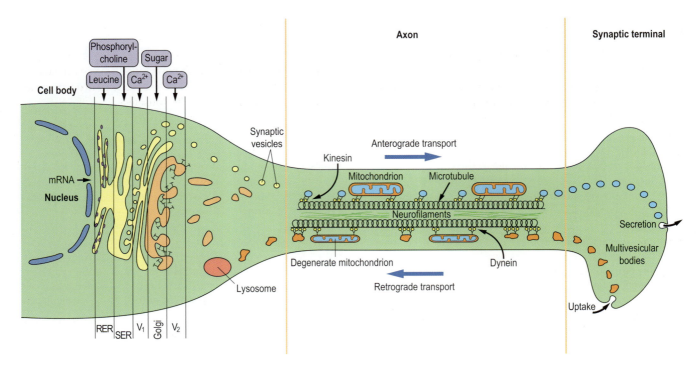

Fig. 39.2 **Functional structure of a neuron.** Within the cell body, there is specialized movement through the Golgi stack by the components required to form synaptic vesicles (V1, V2). In the axon, there is fast axonal transport along microtubules via the motile proteins, kinesin (anterograde transport) or dynein (retrograde transport). RER, rough endoplasmic reticulum; SER, smooth endoplasmic reticulum.

α- and β-tubulin subunits stabilized by nonphosphorylated tau peptides. It removes impaired particles and transfers signaling peptides released from postsynaptic neurons, such as nerve growth factor and brain-derived neurotrophic factor. Neurons have evolved special characteristics to deal with the separation of these two functions (Fig. 39.2).

The normal "resting" movement within the axon is mediated by separate **molecular "motors"** (motile proteins): **kinesin** in the case of anterograde transport and **dynein** in retrograde transport. The materials being transported in each direction are also rather different, and the different components of axonal structure shown in Fig. 39.2 possess the capacity for different speeds of transportation. During growth, a separate form of transport (toward the synapse) occurs that takes place at the rate of about 1 mm/day; this flow constitutes bulk movement of the building blocks such as the filamentous proteins.

Neurotransmission is an energy-demanding process

The brain constitutes 2% of body mass, yet under resting conditions, it responsible for 20% of the overall glucose consumption. **Glucose is almost exclusively the energy substrate for the brain.** The final product of glycolysis, pyruvate, is transported from the cytoplasmic to the mitochondrial compartment, where pyruvate dehydrogenase complex converts it to acetyl-CoA, feeding the tricarboxylic acid (TCA) cycle, coupled to the electron transport chain (ETC). This generates the entire energy pool in the brain. Astrocytes utilize glucose, releasing significant amounts of lactate to the extracellular compartment, which serves as complementary energy source for the neurons. However, neither exogenous nor endogenous lactate can fully replace glucose as the principal energy source. In fact ^{13}F-deoxyglucose uptake is used as a marker of energy metabolism of specific brain areas, using functional diagnostic tests (positron emission tomography / magnetic resonance imaging [PET/MRI]) to detect neurodegenerative alterations and their influence on specific brain functions. The brain does not utilize fatty acids for energy production. Under ketogenic conditions (starvation, high-fat diet), it may utilize β-hydroxybutyrate derived from circulation.

Neurons generate 60%–80% of brain energy, which is necessary for the restoration of their plasma membrane potentials. A relatively stable high rate of glucose provision is secured by the high-affinity transporter GLUT3, expressed only in neurons.

A small fraction of the mitochondrial acetyl-CoA in neurons is utilized for the synthesis of *N*-acetyl-L-aspartate (NAA), which reaches a concentration as high as 10 mmol/L in the brain. More than 95% of NAA is located in neurons. Therefore the level of NAA, determined by MRI, is considered to be a marker of the metabolic competency of the brain neurons.

Large amounts of energy are required to maintain the resting plasma membrane potentials of the neurons, which are subject to continuous (10- to 60-Hz frequency) **depolarization cycles** known as **action potentials**. To meet these demands, more than 70% of brain energy is produced and utilized by neurons.

Neuroglial structures

Astrocytes and oligodendrocytes comprise the neuroglial structures

In the cortex, or gray matter, one typically finds a protoplasmic astrocyte with one set of processes surrounding the endothelial cells, thereby helping to "filter" materials from the blood, and a separate set of processes surrounding the neurons, which are thereby being "fed" selected substances that have been extracted from the blood for passage to the neurons.

In the white matter, the astrocytes have a rather more fibrous appearance and have more of a structural role. When there is injury to the CNS, astrocytes can play a major part in the reaction, synthesizing large amounts of the **glial fibrillary acidic protein (GFAP)**. This is the cellular equivalent of scar tissue and is found in diseases such as **multiple sclerosis**, in which it is the major constituent of the characteristic plaques. Astrocytes are not present in the PNS.

The **oligodendrocytes** present in the CNS can wrap around as many as 20 axons, forming the myelin sheath that insulates these neuronal processes from one another and stops cross-talk between neurons. There is also intense oligodendrocyte mito-chondrial activity at the nodes of Ranvier, which are parallel to the sites of depolarization within the underlying axon. In the PNS, the Schwann cells form the myelin and typically wrap around only a single axon.

SYNAPTIC TRANSMISSION

One of the unique chemical characteristics of the brain is the massively high density of synapses between different neurons

Thus a locally acting neurohormone is released by one axon onto many other cell bodies. On the receiving end, a given cell body will typically receive myriad cellular products via its profusely branched dendritic tree: each branch can be smoth-ered in **synapses.** The "neurotransmitter" (neurohormone) is released by the axon's nerve terminals of the first neuron onto the dendrite of the second neuron or a non-neuronal cell. This is mediated by a neurotransmitter **receptor** on the respondent cell. There are two groups of neurotransmitter receptors: metabotropic and ionotropic. Binding neurotrans-mitter with metabotropic receptor (e.g., muscarinic, metabo-tropic glutamate receptor [mGluR]) activates a **second messenger,** such as a cyclic nucleotide, which may stimulate protein phosphorylation. Typically, **G proteins** are found just under the neurotransmitter receptor protein spanning the cell membrane, where they act to "couple" the first messenger (e.g., norepinephrine) to a second messenger (e.g., cyclic AMP [cAMP]; Chapter 25). Other neurotransmitter receptors are coupled with **ion channels** (e.g., nicotinic, NMDA). The binding of neurotransmitter agonists opens those channels to Na^+, resulting in its influx into postsynaptic cells evoking their depolarization (action potential) and influx of Ca^{2+}. It brings about fusion of neurotransmitter-loaded synaptic vesicles with presynaptic plasma membranes triggering its quantal release. Binding neurotransmitter with postsynaptic membrane recep-tors activates proper reaction of recipient neuron or other target cells (e.g., endocrine cells, muscles).

Neurotransmitters are normally inactivated after their actions on the target cell. Hydrolysis of acetylcholine in the synaptic cleft by plasma membrane–bound acetylcholinesterase is one of the major mechanisms by which this is achieved. Neurotransmitter (glutamate) may also be taken up from the synaptic cleft by postsynaptic neurons or adjacent astrocytes, followed by its intracellular neutralization. They may be taken back by their own presynaptic terminals (as are catecholamines) to be inactivated by mitochondrial monoamine oxidase. The best-studied example is that of the enzyme acetylcholinesterase. There can also be regulation at the level of the second mes-senger, such as cAMP, which is broken down by the enzyme phosphodiesterase. Phosphodiesterase is inhibited by caffeine and other methylxanthines, thereby mimicking many of the effects of adrenergic neurotransmission.

Synaptic transmission involves the recycling of membrane components

In addition to the release of a specific neurohormone, there is also an extensive system for recycling of membrane con-stituents associated with this process. The synaptic vesicles contain a very high concentration of the relevant neurotrans-mitter, which is bounded by a membrane (Chapter 26). During synaptic release of the transmitter, there is fusion of the synaptic vesicle membrane (containing the neurotransmitter) with the presynaptic membrane. This increase in total membrane mass is redressed by invagination of the lateral aspects of the nerve terminals, where an inward puckering movement of the membrane is effected by contractile movements of the protein clathrin. There then follows a form of pinocytosis of the excess membrane, which is transported in retrograde fashion toward the nucleus, to be digested in lysosomes.

Types of synapse

Because of the multitude of different synaptic inputs to a given neuron, the final algebraic summation results in a "decision" at the level of the axon hillock (the site of origin of the axon from the cell body) as to whether to transmit an action potential down the axon as an all-or-nothing phenomenon. However, even before this decision is made, the input of a particular neurotransmitter can essentially be classified as **excitatory** or **inhibitory.**

In addition to the relatively short-term decisions concerning action potentials (Chapter 26), there is longer-term modulation of the resting membrane potential, moving it either closer to (excitation) or further from (inhibition) the critical membrane potential, which is the level at which the resting membrane potential will finally trigger an action potential at the axon hillock. Many drugs, in addition to the short-term effect, have a longer-term effect on modulation, which partially explains their addictive effect; this can be seen with alcohol or the opioid drugs. There are also long-term effects during treatment with various drugs (e.g., those used to treat endogenous depression), such that it may be weeks before any beneficial effects are seen.

Cholinergic transmission

The best-studied neurotransmitter is acetylcholine

Acetylcholine (ACh) is synthesized in the cytoplasmic compartment of cholinergic nerve terminals from acetyl-CoA and choline by **choline acetyltransferase** (ChAT). The specific vesicular ACh transporter (VAChT) loads transmitter into synaptic vesicles. Both proteins are expressed exclusively in the cholinergic neurons. Acetyl-CoA is synthesized from pyruvate derived from glycolysis, whereas choline is taken up from the extracellular compartment by the high-affinity choline uptake system driven by plasma membrane potential.

As a model system, this transmitter can have two rather different effects, depending on its site of origin within the nervous system (i.e., central or peripheral). The effects originally demonstrated by experiments with **nicotine** are characteristic of the nicotinic receptors, whereas those demonstrated with **muscarine** characterize the muscarinic receptors. The nicotinic type of transmission is exerted by motor neurons located in the brainstem and anterior horns of the medulla oblongata. Another group of central cholinergic neurons located in the brain septum plays a key role in the basic and higher cognitive functions through activation of postsynaptic muscarinic receptors. There is a complex picture of the agonists and antagonists associated with the regional actions of ACh (Fig. 39.3). The classic antagonist of the muscarinic effect is **atropine,** and the best-studied blocker for the nicotinic receptor is the poisonous snake venom α-**bungarotoxin**. ACh synthesis and the functional competence of cholinergic neurons strongly depend on the provision of acetyl-CoA by **pyruvate dehydrogenase**. Several encephalopathies caused by ACh deficits are accompanied by marked inhibition/inactivation of this enzyme. Inhibition of metabolic flux through the pyruvate dehydrogenase step occurs in several brain pathologies, such as hypoxia, thiamine pyrophosphate deficit, excitotoxic neuronal injury, aluminum or zinc overload, Alzheimer's disease, and inherited deficits of this enzyme.

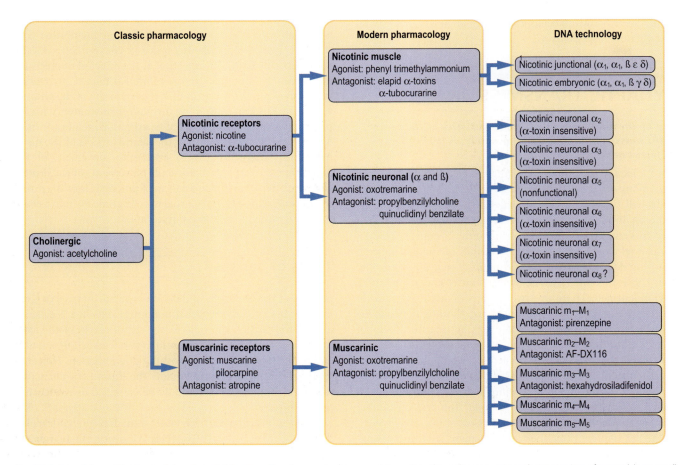

Fig. 39.3 **Agonists and antagonists of acetylcholine.** Development of nomenclature describing the agonists and antagonists of central (neuronal) and peripheral (muscle) actions of acetylcholine.

Vascular dementia and **Alzheimer's disease** (AD) are the most common neurodegenerative brain pathologies in aging human populations. Neurons impaired by several neurotoxic signals, such as hypoxia, hypoglycemia, or glutamate excitotoxicity, activate aberrant proteolysis of amyloid precursor protein (APP), yielding excessive production of the amyloid-β peptide (1–42). About 30% of neurons and all stimulated astrocytes express excess of APP. Therefore it accumulates preferentially in certain brain regions responsible for memory formation and cognitive functions. Its presence in the brains of AD patients may be visualized with Pittsburgh compound B and other tracing ligands using PET/MRI techniques. Degenerating neurons release several structural proteins, including **tau peptides**. Their levels increase in CSF, thus being a diagnostic marker for these conditions. Despite increased synthesis, levels of amyloid-β in the CSF decrease due to its facilitated aggregation and intraneuronal accumulation.

In AD amyloid-β(1–42) oligomers, in combination with other neurotoxic factors, cause preferential impairment of cholinergic neurons in the brain septum, yielding progressive loss of cognitive function, which leads to dementia. In the early stages of this disease, the inhibitors of acetylcholinesterase with M_2 receptor agonist properties improve cognitive function but have no effect on disease progression. The antagonists of glutamatergic NMDA receptors are employed to reduce the excitotoxic effects of excessive activation of glutamatergic neurons.

In **myasthenia gravis,** autoantibodies are formed against the nicotinic receptor. However, by blocking the hydrolysis of ACh, for example, by means of the drug edrophonium (which inhibits acetylcholinesterase), the concentration of ACh can be effectively increased.

Peripheral cholinergic neurons are located in parasympathetic ganglia and innervate all visceral tissues. They dilate the blood vessels of the gastrointestinal tract and enhance salivation and peristalsis. They also constrict the airways, control heart function, constrict the pupils and regulate lens accommodation, and stimulate sexual arousal and genital erection.

In **Wernicke–Korsakoff** encephalopathy, the activities of complexes of pyruvate dehydrogenase and ketoglutarate dehydrogenase are inhibited due to the deficit of their cofactor thiamine pyrophosphate (Chapter 7). It inhibits acetyl-CoA synthesis and its utilization by TCA cycle. Therefore general energy deficits appear, which impair not only central cognitive functions but also the peripheral motor terminal functions of smooth and striated muscle.

Catecholamine transmission

Catecholamines, **epinephrine** and **norepinephrine**, are synthesized from L-tyrosine in the sequence of reactions catalyzed by tyrosine hydroxylase/L-aromatic amino acid decarboxylase (AADC), then dopamine β-hydroxylase/AADC

CLINICAL BOX
A 25-YEAR OLD MAN WITH PERSISTENT DIARRHEA, VOMITING, AND LOSS OF SENSATION IN HIS LEGS

A 25-year old man of Asian origin (a migrant construction worker) was admitted to the hospital emergency unit with persistent vomiting, heavy diarrhea, edema, and loss of sensation in his legs. He had no past medical history and was discharged, after short observation, with the diagnosis of a gastrointestinal upset and was given dietary recommendations. After 4 days, the patient came back to the emergency unit with intensifying dyspnea, then collapsed. Blood pressure was 60/40 mmHg. He was hypothermic (33°C) and had atrial fibrillation and severe edema. He was anuric. There were no changes on chest X-ray. Computed tomography (CT) of the abdomen showed slight pancreatic edema. Exploratory laparotomy was inconclusive. Laboratory tests displayed severe lactic acidosis (blood pH 6.90, lactic acid 20 mmol/L). Ethanol, methanol, acetone, and drugs tests were not detected. The patient died 12 h after admission without final diagnosis.

Postmortem tests on collected blood samples revealed an extremely low level of thiamine in his blood. The majority of his Asian colleagues from the workplace were later found to have asymptomatic thiamine deficiency.

This condition most probably resulted from a frugal diet based on polished rice without supplementation with essential nutrients. In developed countries, high-risk groups for thiamine deficiency are alcoholics, drug abusers, and also low-income elderly/disabled people (see Chapter 7).

and phentolamine-N-methyltransferase, yielding dopamine, norepinephrine, and epinephrine, respectively. Dopamine is a precursor of norepinephrine and epinephrine (Chapter 26).

Dopamine is a transmitter in the dopaminergic neurons located in several brain areas, including the *substantia nigra*, that are involved in reward-driven learning, regulation of mood, attention, learning, and prolactin release through different classes of dopamine receptors (D1–5). Disturbances of dopamine metabolism are associated with several CNS pathologies, including **Parkinson's disease, schizophrenia,** and **restless legs syndrome.** To overcome dopamine deficits in some of these diseases, L-DOPA, its precursor, is administered because it easily crosses the blood–brain barrier. Dopamine is given to patients in **shock and with heart failure** to elevate cardiac output and increase blood pressure and renal filtration. Several drugs, including **amphetamines, cocaine, and nicotine**, exert their behavioral and addictive effects through excessive stimulation of the release and the increase of dopamine level in the synaptic cleft. They also stimulate serotoninergic and norepinephrinergic transmission in the brain.

Norepinephrine and epinephrine are synthesized in the brain and peripheral sympathetic ganglia by respective groups of neurons acting as neurotransmitters. Conversely, catecholamines released from chromaffin cells into the circulation exert endocrine effects. In the brain, they exert regulatory functions in decision-making processes. Peripherally, they increase blood pressure (they cause vasoconstriction and increase the rate and force of cardiac muscle contraction), cause bronchial and pupil dilatation, inhibit peristalsis, increase sweating and renin secretion, and promote ejaculation. **Their actions are mediated through two separate receptors: α-adrenergic receptor, blocked by phentolamine, and β-adrenergic receptor, blocked by propranolol.** The latter drug was commonly used by cardiologists (other β-blockers are the mainstay of treatment for coronary heart disease), but neurologists also use it as part of the treatment of Parkinson's disease. Many adrenergic effects are mediated by cAMP (Chapter 26).

The action of catecholamines is terminated by their reuptake and degradation to aldehydes by mitochondrial **monoamine oxidases** and subsequent methylation by **catechol-O-methyltransferase** to homovanillic or vanillylmandelic acids, which are excreted with urine. Excess of these compounds in urine may indicate the presence of adrenal medullar tumor, **pheochromocytoma.**

Glutamate: Glutamatergic transmission

Depending on the brain region, 50–80% of the neuronal population is glutamatergic

The mean L-glutamate level in the brain is in the range of 5–10 mmol/L. It is synthesized from α-ketoglutarate by glutamate dehydrogenase and aminotransferases or from glutamine by phosphate-activated glutaminase. The L-glutamate/glutamate–zinc complex is taken up by synaptic vesicles of glutamatergic presynaptic nerve terminals, where it reaches concentrations exceeding 100 mmol/L. Glutamate-Zn is released upon depolarization, transiently reaching high concentrations in the synaptic clefts. Its binding to different classes of receptors, including NMDA (the principal one), causes depolarization/activation of postsynaptic recipient neurons. Glutamatergic receptor stimulation is subject to multiple regulatory mechanisms that play an important role in synaptic plasticity, termed **long-term potentiation**. This phenomenon takes place in the hippocampus and in the different regions of brain cortex, and it is involved in learning, memory formation, and other cognitive functions.

Glutamate is quickly taken up from the synaptic space by specific transporters expressed mainly on the adjacent astroglial cells. There, glutamine synthetase converts glutamate to glutamine, which is subsequently transported back to glutamatergic neurons.

Excessive glutamate release or its impaired uptake, which takes place in ischemia, hypoglycemia, and exposure to neurotoxic xenobiotics, among other conditions, may cause its excessive accumulation in the extracellular synaptic space. This in turn causes prolonged depolarization of the postsynaptic cells yielding a rise in intracellular Ca^{2+}, free oxygen, nitrosyl, and synthesis of fatty acid radicals. In consequence, excitotoxic functional and structural damage of neurons takes place. **Epilepsy** is the pathologic condition caused by excessive glutamate release by pathologically stimulated glutamatergic neurons and/or the deficiency of inhibitory GABAergic transmission (see the following discussion). Zinc, coreleased with glutamate, is also taken up by postsynaptic neurons through several transporting entities (voltage-gated Ca-channels, ZnT1). An excessive accumulation of zinc under neurodegenerative conditions may inhibit multiple energy-producing enzymes (pyruvate and ketoglutarate dehydrogenase complexes, aconitase, isocitrate dehydrogenase, respiratory chain complex I, and others), aggravating glutamate excitotoxicity.

γ-Aminobutyric acid (GABA): GABA-ergic transmission

GABA is the chief inhibitory neurotransmitter in the brain

The inhibitory effect of GABA on postsynaptic neurons results from binding to specific $GABA_A$ receptors. GABA concentration remains in the range of 4–6 mmol/L. It is the ligand for gated chloride channels. Their opening upon GABA binding causes the flow of Cl^- ions into the neuron, causing its hyperpolarization and inhibition of transmitter function. GABA is synthesized by the L-glutamate decarboxylase present in the cytoplasm of GABA-ergic neurons. GABA action is terminated mainly through its uptake by presynaptic terminals through high-affinity GABA transporter. GABA may then be either loaded again into vesicles or metabolized to succinate - a TCA cycle intermediate. Several $GABA_A$ receptor agonists and GABA uptake or GABA-transaminase inhibitors are used as sedatives, tranquilizers, or anxiolytic drugs. The most common groups include **barbiturates, benzodiazepines, chloral hydrate, and valproate.** Ethanol also acts as the $GABA_A$ receptor agonist.

ION CHANNELS

Even at rest, the neuron is working to pump ions along ionic gradients

The "resting" neuron is, nevertheless, continually pumping sodium out of the cell and potassium in, through ion channels. During an action potential, there is a momentary reversal of these ionic movements: sodium enters the cell, and potassium then leaves, effectively repolarizing the resting membrane (Chapter 26). Mutations of sodium channels can occur at different sites and give rise to **hyperkalemic periodic paralysis.** The negative ion chloride moves through separate channels, which are implicated in specific pathologic states, such as **myotonia.**

Calcium ions have an important role in the synchronization of neuronal activity

The movement of calcium ions within cells often provides a trigger for the cells to synchronize an activity such as synaptic release of neurotransmitter; this synchronization also has a prominent role in the sarcoplasmic reticulum of muscle (Chapter 37). Within the CNS, **Lambert–Eaton syndrome** is a disease that affects predominantly the P/Q subtype of calcium channels, in an example of **molecular mimicry.** The patient may have a primary oat cell carcinoma of the lung; the immune system responds by making antibodies against the malignant cells. However, the malignant cells and the calcium channels possess a common epitope, the effect of which is that the immune response causes the release of neurotransmitter to be blocked at the presynaptic site. This is analogous to, but nevertheless can be clearly distinguished from, the condition in **myasthenia gravis,** in which the block is postsynaptic.

It is also worth noting that blockade of the presynaptic release of neurotransmitter may be usefully exploited by therapeutic application of **botulinum toxin** (a protein derived from anaerobic bacteria), which contains enzymes to hydrolyze the presynaptic proteins involved in the release of neurotransmitters. This toxin is used in special cases of spasticity, such as **torticollis,** in which the patient can be relieved of the excessive contractures of the neck muscles, which turn the head chronically to one side and thus cause pain and distraction if untreated.

MECHANISM OF VISION

The mechanism by which the human eye can detect a single photon of light provides a fascinating example of the chemical processes underlying neuronal function

The mechanism of vision involves both trapping of photons and the transducer effect, whereby the energy of light is converted into a chemical form, which is then ultimately transmuted into an action potential by a retinal ganglion neuron. A number of the intermediates are as yet not precisely known, but the underlying hypothesis is that the receptor protein, **rhodopsin,** is coupled to the G protein. There are several sequence homologies of rhodopsin with the adrenergic β-receptor and with the muscarinic ACh receptor. The main steps (Fig. 39.4) take place in the following order:

- *Cis*-retinal is converted to *trans*-retinal.
- Rhodopsin becomes activated.
- The level of cGMP decreases.
- Na^+ entry into the cell is blocked.
- The rod cell hyperpolarizes.
- There is release of glutamate (or aspartate).
- An action potential depolarizes the adjacent bipolar cell.
- This depolarizes the associated ganglion neuron to send an action potential out of the eye.

CLINICAL BOX
AN 18-YEAR-OLD MAN WITH WEAKNESS OF ARMS AND LEGS: FAMILIAL PERIODIC PARALYSIS

An 18-year-old male awoke in the night with intense weakness of the proximal muscles of his arms and legs. Before retiring, he had consumed a meal of pasta and cake. His brother and father had previously been similarly affected. He was taken to the emergency room of the local hospital, where the weak limbs were noted to be hypotonic, with depressed tendon reflexes. Serum concentration of potassium was reduced at 2.9 mmol/L (normal 3.5–5.3). By the next day, he had fully recovered, and serum potassium had risen spontaneously to normal levels. A further attack of paralysis was induced by an infusion of intravenous glucose, thus confirming a diagnosis of familial periodic paralysis.

Comment

Hypokalemic periodic paralysis is inherited as a Mendelian dominant trait and results from a mutation in the gene encoding the **L-type calcium channel**. Genetic diseases that affect ion-channel function are called **channelopathies** (see also Chapter 4).

Both hypokalemic and hyperkalemic types of the disorder exist. Different molecular lesions in the sodium-channel pores can give rise to hyperkalemic periodic paralysis. As the name suggests, the patient has intermittent muscle weakness, during which time the serum potassium concentration is increased. This is caused by an imbalance of cationic movements in which sodium enters the cell and potassium leaves it. In these patients, the abnormal flux of sodium into the muscle is not correctly regulated with its counterflux of potassium ions.

CLINICAL BOX
A WOMAN WITH PROGRESSIVE BLURRED VISION, DYSPHAGIA, AND LIMB WEAKNESS: BOTULISM

Twenty-four hours after eating home-preserved vegetables, a healthy young woman experienced the progressive onset of blurred vision, severe vomiting, dysphagia, and advancing limb weakness starting in the shoulders. Her doctor admitted her to the hospital, and electrophysiological studies confirmed the clinical diagnosis of botulism. Trivalent antiserum, made from inactivated toxin, was administered immediately, and with the help of assisted ventilation, the patient recovered within a few weeks.

Comment

The vegetables contained the exotoxin of the anaerobe *Clostridium botulinum*, which had not been destroyed during the preservation process. The toxin hydrolyzes the presynaptic proteins involved in the release of neurotransmitter, and thus the blockade is similar to the functional lesion in Lambert–Eaton myasthenic syndrome; however, in botulism the blockade can be lethal, especially at the level of the phrenic nerve, which is essential for respiratory lung movement.

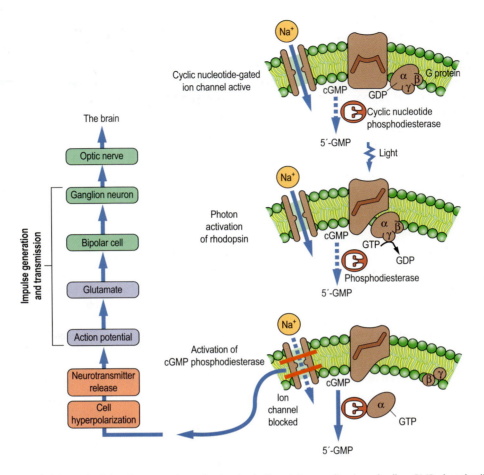

Fig. 39.4 **The mechanism of vision.** The light photons activate rhodopsin via G protein–coupling in rod cells. cGMP phosphodiesterase is activated and hydrolyzes cGMP (second messenger), thereby blocking the entry of sodium and causing hyperpolarization of the cell. Compare the chemistry of vitamin A and the activities of the G protein–coupled receptors. Dotted lines indicate an inactive process.

SUMMARY

■ The nervous system contains a number of distinct cells, forming diverse but tightly interacting structural, metabolic, and functional compartments.

■ The specialized functions of the nervous system are assured by the expression and strict compartmentalization of specific proteins, metabolites, and signaling compounds in different cellular loci.

■ Neurotransmission is a basic function of the nervous system. Neurotransmitters in the brain are synthesized and released into synaptic clefts from axonal terminals of specific groups of neurons (glutamatergic, GABA-ergic, catecholaminergic, cholinergic, etc.).

■ Anterograde and retrograde axonal transport warrants bidirectional movements of organelles and proteins maintaining intraneuronal signaling and integrity.

ACTIVE LEARNING

1. G proteins are widely used throughout the body as "coupling" agents between the first extracellular messenger and the second intracellular messenger. Discuss some of the roles for which the G protein has been adapted among various cell types.
2. Mitochondria play an important role in providing for the metabolic requirements at the nodes of Ranvier, along the considerable length of the axon. Discuss the role of the two molecular motors in recycling the mitochondria required to support this function.
3. Chloride is an important anion that forms part of the complex movements with cations such as sodium and potassium during depolarization. Discuss the consequences of congenital abnormalities in chloride transport.
4. Describe the reactions that occur in the process of vision.
5. Give an example of molecular mimicry.

- Maintenance of neurotransmission requires large amounts of energy, which is assured by effective glucose transport through the blood–brain barrier and high rates of glycolysis and tricarboxylic acid cycling.
- Neurons receive metabolic support from astroglial and microglial cells and structural support from oligodendroglial cells.
- The blood–brain barrier is diverse in anatomic origin and is not absolute but relative (specifically based on molecular size of the transferred molecules). There are also proteins of intrathecal origin, including antibodies, produced under certain pathologic conditions by infiltrating lymphocytes.

FURTHER READING

Barry, D. M., Millecamps, S., Julien, J. P., et al. (2007). New movements in neurofilament transport, turnover and disease. *Experimental Cell Research, 313,* 2110–2120.

Bettens, K., Sleegers, K., & Van Broeckhoven, C. (2013). Genetic insights in Alzheimer's disease. *The Lancet. Neurology, 12,* 92–104.

Bos, J. L., Rehmann, H., & Wittinghofer, A. (2007). GEFs and GAPs: Critical elements in the control of small G proteins. *Cell, 129,* 865–877.

Cannon, S. C. (2007). Physiologic principles underlying ion channelopathies. *Neurotherapeutics, 4,* 174–183.

de Leon, M. J., Mosconi, L., Blennow, K., et al. (2007). Imaging and CSF studies in the preclinical diagnosis of Alzheimer's disease. *Annals of the New York Academy of Sciences, 1097,* 114–145.

George, D. R., Whitehouse, P. J., D'Alton, S., et al. (2012). Through the amyloid gateway. *Lancet, 380,* 1986–1987.

Honig, L. S. (2012). Translational research in neurology: Dementia. *Archives of Neurology, 69,* 969–977.

Stein-Streilein, J., & Taylor, A. W. (2007). An eye's view of T regulatory cells. *Journal of Leukocyte Biology, 81,* 593–598.

ABBREVIATIONS

Ach	Acetylcholine
AMPA	α-amino-3-hydroxy-5-methyl-4-isoxazolepropionic acid
APP	Amyloid precursor protein
BBB	Blood–brain barrier
ChAT	Choline acetyltransferase
CNS	Central nervous system
CSF	Cerebrospinal fluid
ETC	Electron transport chain
GABA	γ-aminobutyric acid
GFAP	Glial fibrillary acidic protein
IgG	Immunoglobulin G
NAA	N-acetyl-L-aspartate
NMDA	N-methyl-D-aspartate
PET/MRI	Positron emission tomography–magnetic resonance imaging
PNS	Peripheral nervous system
TCA	Tricarboxylic acid cycle
VAChT	Acetylcholine transporter

Blood and Plasma Proteins

Marek H. Dominiczak

LEARNING OBJECTIVES

After reading this chapter, you should be able to:

- ■ Describe major components of blood.
- ■ Explain the difference between plasma and serum.
- ■ Discuss the roles of plasma proteins and their broad classification.
- ■ Identify diseases associated with a deficiency of specific proteins.
- ■ Discuss the structure and function of the immunoglobulins.
- ■ Explain the pathologic significance of monoclonal gammopathies.
- ■ Define the acute-phase response and the change it induces in the concentrations of circulating plasma proteins.
- ■ Understand the concept of a biomarker

INTRODUCTION

Plasma is an important "window" on metabolism

Blood delivers essential nutrients to tissues and removes waste products. It also serves as a route of communication and long-range signals by, for instance, transporting hormones from sites of secretion to their target tissues. Blood is a suspension of cellular elements in a solution containing a wide range of molecules, from small-molecular-weight metabolites to large multi-subunit proteins. There are several classes of cellular elements. Components of blood participate in the body's defense against external insult, in wound healing, and in tissue repair. Also, blood is easily sampled and therefore is by far the most common material for biochemical testing. Most of the diagnostic laboratory tests in biochemistry, hematology, and immunology are performed using blood, plasma, or serum.

Chemical measurements require serum or plasma

The formed elements of blood are suspended in an aqueous solution: the plasma. Plasma is the supernatant obtained after centrifugation of a blood sample collected into a test tube containing an **anticoagulant**. Several anticoagulants are used in laboratory practice, the most common being lithium heparinate and ethylenediaminetetraacetic acid (EDTA). Heparinate prevents clotting by binding to thrombin. EDTA and citrate

bind Ca^{2+} and Mg^{2+} ions, thus blocking the calcium- and magnesium-dependent enzymes in the clotting cascade (Chapter 41). Citrate is used as an anticoagulant for coagulation tests and also when blood is collected for transfusion. Potassium fluoride inhibits glycolysis and is used in samples taken for the measurement of plasma glucose.

Serum is the supernatant obtained after a blood sample has been allowed to clot spontaneously. During clotting, fibrinogen is converted to fibrin. Therefore a major difference between plasma and serum is the **absence of fibrinogen** in serum.

Throughout this book, when we describe physiologic or pathologic mechanisms, we refer to plasma; for example, we would say "albumin binds many drugs present in *plasma*." We mention serum when we refer to the results of laboratory tests specifically performed on serum; for example, we would say "patient's *serum* albumin was 40 mg/dL."

Clinical laboratories perform a large number of biochemical analyses on body fluids to provide answers to specific clinical questions

Most of the specimens received by clinical laboratories are blood and urine samples. Whereas some measurements are performed on whole blood, serum or plasma is preferred for most analyses of metabolites and ions. The process from a request for analysis to receipt of a result involves many steps. Throughout the process, constant checking and quality assurance are performed to ensure that the produced results are analytically and clinically valid.

Hospital laboratories rely on automation, robotics, and information technology

A laboratory in a large hospital can easily perform several million tests a year.

Application of these technologies allows clinical laboratories to perform large numbers of analyses while being able to customize or modify requested test profiles as well as prioritize tests required urgently (see Appendix 1).

FORMED ELEMENTS OF BLOOD

Hematopoiesis

The very early hematopoiesis (the primitive hemopoiesis) during embryonic development starts in the yolk sac. Later,

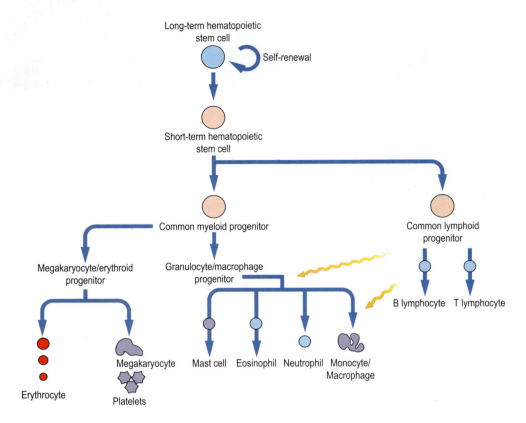

Fig. 40.1 **Overview of hematopoiesis.** The figure shows the main pathways of hematopoiesis from the pluripotent stem cell, through the common progenitor cells, to committed lineages for different cell types. The long-term hematopoietic stem cell has the ability to self-renew, providing long-term population of these nondifferentiated cells. For clarity, precursor cells downstream from committed megakaryocyte/erythroid progenitor, granulocyte/macrophage progenitor, and common lymphoid progenitor cells have been omitted. The reader is referred to hematology textbooks for more details. Based on Orkin et al. (see Further Reading).

the definitive hemopoiesis takes place in the peri-aortic site known as aorta-gonad-mesonephros, then subsequently in the placenta, fetal liver, and, after birth, primarily in the bone marrow. All formed elements of blood have a common precursor: the **hematopoietic stem cell.** These cells migrate to the sites of hemopoiesis and reside in bone marrow niches, microenvironments that regulate these cells. Stem cell niches in the bone marrow are usually located in the trabecular bone area in endosteum (i.e., at an interface between bone marrow and the bone) (Chapter 38). In addition to the hematopoietic stem cells and other types of progenitor cells, the niche contains mesenchymal stromal cells, macrophages, sympathetic nerve cells, and endothelial cells. The osteoblasts are in the vicinity. It is also close to bone marrow sinusoids. The niche provides a complex environment of cytokines and growth factors that regulate the stem cell. Interactions with osteoblasts also take place, and it is thought that osteoblasts influence the development of so-called restricted progenitors, cells developing down the line from the stem cell. Fig. 40.1 shows the main pathways of hematopoiesis, from the pluripotent stem cells through the common progenitor cells to committed lineages of particular cell types. There are three major cell lineages among blood

cells: **the red blood cells (erythrocytes), the white blood cells (leukocytes),** and **the blood platelets (thrombocytes).**

Erythrocytes do not possess nuclei and intracellular organelles

Erythrocytes are cellular remnants, containing specific proteins and ions that can be present in high concentrations. They are the end product of erythropoiesis in the bone marrow, which is under the control of the hormone erythropoietin produced by the kidney (Fig. 40.2). Hemoglobin is synthesized in the erythrocyte precursor cells (erythroblasts and reticulocytes) under a tight control dictated by the concentration of heme (Chapter 34). The main functions of erythrocytes are the transport of oxygen and the removal of carbon dioxide and hydrogen ions (Chapters 5 and 36). Erythrocytes are not capable of protein synthesis and repair; as a result, they have a finite life span of approximately 120 days before being trapped and broken down in the spleen.

Leukocytes protect the body from infection

Most leukocytes are produced in the bone marrow; some are produced in the thymus, and others mature within several

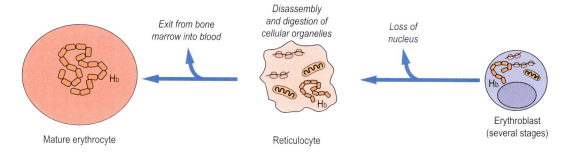

Fig. 40.2 **Simplified scheme of the formation of erythrocytes.** In an average day, 10^{11} erythrocytes are formed. Hemoglobin is synthesized in the erythrocyte and reticulocyte before the loss of ribosomes and mitochondria. The presence of an increased number of reticulocytes in the blood commonly indicates stimulation of erythropoiesis.

Leukocyte group	Subgroup	Function
Granulocytes	Neutrophils	Destroy small organisms
	Basophils	Secrete histamine, mediate inflammatory response, and secrete platelet-activating factor
	Eosinophils	Destroy parasites and participate in allergic reaction
Lymphocytes	B lymphocytes	Synthesize antibodies
	T lymphocytes	Participate in the specific immune response
Monocytes	Macrophages	Destroy invading organisms

Fig. 40.3 **Leukocytes.** Classification and functions of leukocytes. Mature B lymphocytes are known as plasma cells. See also Chapter 43 and Table 43.1.

different tissues (Fig. 40.3; Chapter 43). Leukocytes control their own development by secreting signal peptides that act on bone marrow stem cells. Leukocytes can migrate out of the bloodstream into surrounding tissues.

Thrombocytes are fragments derived from megakaryocytes

Megakaryocytes reside in the bone marrow. They yield blood platelets and are essential for blood clotting (Chapter 41).

PLASMA PROTEINS

Plasma proteins can be broadly classified into two groups: **albumin** and the heterogeneous **globulins**. The main component of the latter is the **immunoglobulins** produced by plasma cells of the bone marrow.

Albumin serves as an osmotic regulator and is a major transport protein

Albumin accounts for approximately 50% of protein in human plasma. It has no known enzymatic or hormonal activity. Its molecular weight is about 66 kDa, and it has a highly polar nature. At pH 7.4, it is an anion with 20 negative charges per molecule; this gives it a high capacity for nonselective binding of many ligands. It is also critical for maintaining the colloid osmotic pressure of the plasma. Its normal concentration is 35–45 g/L, and its half-life is about 20 days.

The rate of albumin synthesis (14–15 g daily) depends on nutritional status, and the rate of its synthesis is vulnerable to an inadequate supply of amino acids. Although its concentration does reflect nutritional status in the longer term, in hospitalized patients, the short-term changes in its concentration are much more often due to changes in hydration (Chapter 35).

Albumin is not essential for human survival, and a rare congenital defect where it is completely absent (**analbuminemia**) has been described.

Albumin transports fatty acids, bilirubin, and drugs

Albumin binds (and thus solubilizes) a range of hydrophobic molecules, such as long-chain fatty acids, sterols, and various foreign compounds (xenobiotics), which include drugs and their metabolites. The albumin molecule possesses numerous fatty acid–binding sites with variable affinities.

It binds unconjugated bilirubin (Chapter 34) and many drugs, including salicylates, barbiturates, sulfonamides, penicillin, and warfarin. These interactions are weak, and therefore the **bound molecules (ligands) may be displaced** by other substances competing for the common binding site.

Proteins that transport metal ions

A number of plasma proteins other than albumin have the ability to bind other molecules with high affinity and specificity. This helps control the distribution of molecules, such as steroid hormones, and their availability to tissues. Protein binding

Table 40.1 Transport proteins and their ligands

Proteins	Ligands
Cation binding	
Albumin	Divalent and trivalent cations (e.g., Cu^{2+}, Fe^{3+})
Ceruloplasmin	Cu^{2+}
Transferrin	Fe^{3+}
Hormone binding	
Thyroid-binding globulin (TBG)	Thyroxine (T4), triiodothyronine (T3)
Cortisol-binding globulin (CBG)	Cortisol
Sex hormone–binding globulin (SHBG)	Androgens (testosterone), estrogens (estradiol)
Hemoglobin/protoporphyrin binding	
Albumin	Heme, bilirubin, biliverdin
Haptoglobin	Hemoglobin dimers
Fatty acid binding	
Albumin	Nonesterified fatty acids, steroids

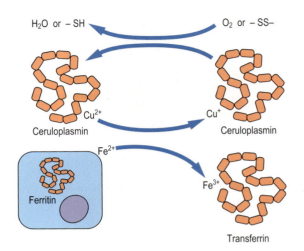

Fig. 40.4 **Plasma ferroxidase activity of ceruloplasmin.** Oxidation of Fe^{2+} by ceruloplasmin permits the binding and transport of iron by plasma transferrin. The cupric ion (Cu^{2+}) bound to ceruloplasmin is regenerated by reaction with oxygen or with oxidized thiol groups.

may also render a toxic substance less harmful. Major binding proteins and their ligands are shown in Table 40.1.

Transferrin transports iron

The binding of ferric ions (Fe^{3+}) to transferrin protects against the toxic effects of these ions. During an inflammatory reaction, the iron–transferrin complex is degraded by the reticuloendothelial system without a corresponding increase in the synthesis of either of its components; this results in low plasma concentrations of transferrin and iron (Chapter 7).

Ferritin is the major iron storage protein found in almost all cells of the body

Ferritin acts as the reserve of iron in the liver and bone marrow. The concentration of ferritin in plasma is proportional to the amount of stored iron. The measurement of plasma ferritin is one of the best markers of iron deficiency.

Ceruloplasmin is the major transport protein for copper

Ceruloplasmin transports copper from the liver to peripheral tissues and is essential for the regulation of oxidation–reduction reactions, transport, and utilization of iron (Fig. 40.4; see also Chapter 7).

Immunoglobulins

Immunoglobulins are proteins produced in response to foreign substances (antigens)

Immunoglobulins (antibodies) are secreted by the B lymphocytes (Chapter 43). They have defined specificity for foreign substances

ADVANCED CONCEPT BOX
HEMOLYSIS AND FREE HEMOGLOBIN

When erythrocytes are hemolyzed, hemoglobin is released into the plasma, where it dissociates into dimers that bind to **haptoglobin.** The hemoglobin–haptoglobin complex is metabolized in the liver and reticuloendothelial system more rapidly than haptoglobin alone. When excessive hemolysis occurs, plasma haptoglobin concentration decreases. Thus it serves as a **marker of hemolysis.** If hemoglobin breaks down into heme and globin, the free heme is bound by **hemopexin.** Unlike haptoglobin, which is an acute-phase protein, hemopexin is not affected by the acute-phase response. The heme–hemopexin complex is taken up by the liver cells, where iron binds to ferritin. A third complex, called **methemalbumin,** can form between oxidized heme and albumin. These mechanisms have evolved to prevent major losses of iron and to complex the free heme, which is toxic to many tissues.

that stimulate their synthesis. Not all foreign substances entering the body can elicit this response, however; those that do are called **immunogens,** whereas any agent that can be bound by an antibody is termed an **antigen.** Immunoglobulins form a uniquely diverse group of molecules, recognizing and reacting with a wide range of specific antigenic structures **(epitopes)** and giving rise to a series of effects that result in the eventual elimination of the presenting antigen. Some immunoglobulins have additional effector functions; for example, IgG is involved in complement activation.

Immunoglobulins share a common Y-shaped structure of two heavy and two light chains

An immunoglobulin is a Y-shaped molecule containing two identical units termed heavy (H) chains and two identical, but smaller, units termed light (L) chains. Several H chains exist, and the nature of the H chain determines the class of immunoglobulin: IgG, IgA, IgM, IgD, and IgE are characterized by α, γ, δ, µ, and ε heavy chains, respectively. L chains are of only two types, κ and λ. Each polypeptide chain within the immunoglobulin is characterized by a series of globular regions, which have considerable sequence homology and, in evolutionary terms, are probably derived from a protogene duplication.

The N-terminal domains of both H and L chains contain a region of variable amino acid sequence (the V region); together, these regions determine antigenic specificity. Both H and L chains are required for full antibody activity because the physically opposed V regions in the L and H chains form a functional pocket into which the epitope fits; this is termed the antibody recognition region (Fab'$_2$). The domain immediately adjacent to the V region is much less variable in both H and L chains. The remainder of the H chain consists of a further constant region (Fc region) consisting of a hinge region and two additional domains. The constant region is responsible for immunoglobulin functions other than epitope recognition,

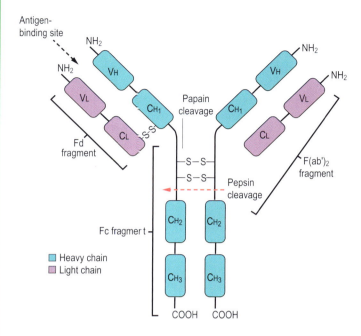

The immunoglobulin G molecule

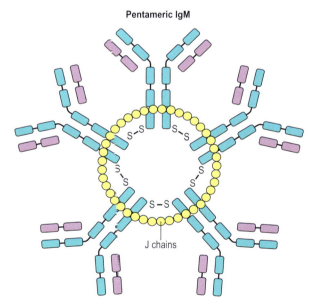

Pentameric IgM

Fig. 40.5 **The structure of immunoglobulins.** Diagrammatic representation of the basic structure of a monomeric immunoglobulin and that of pentameric immunoglobulin (IgM). V, variable region; C, constant region; H, heavy chain; L, light chain; J chain, joining chain; F(ab')$_2$, fragment generated by pepsin cleavage of the molecule; Fc, Fd, fragments generated by papain proteolysis.

such as complement activation (Chapter 43). The basic structure of immunoglobulins is depicted in Fig. 40.5. When antigen binds to the immunoglobulin, conformational changes are transmitted through the hinge region of the antibody to the Fc region, which is then said to have become activated.

Major classes of immunoglobulins

IgG, the most abundant immunoglobulin, protects tissue spaces and freely crosses the placenta

IgG, with an overall molecular mass of 160 kDa, consists of the basic 2H2L immunoglobulin subunit joined by a variable number of disulfide bonds. The γH chains have several antigenic and structural differences, allowing classification of IgG into a number of subclasses according to the type of H chain present; however, functional differences between the subclasses are minor.

IgG circulates in high concentrations in the plasma, accounting for 75% of immunoglobulin present in adults, and has a half-life of 22 days. It is present in all extracellular fluids and appears to eliminate small, soluble, antigenic proteins through aggregation and enhanced phagocytosis by the reticuloendothelial system. From weeks 18–20 of pregnancy, IgG is actively transported across the placenta and provides humoral immunity for the fetus and neonate before maturation of the immune system.

IgA is found in secretions and presents an antiseptic barrier that protects mucosal surfaces

IgA has an H chain similar to the γ chain of IgG, and α chains possess an extra 18 amino acids at the C-terminus. The extra peptide sequence enables the binding of a "joining," or J, chain. This short, 129-residue acidic glycopeptide, synthesized by plasma cells, allows dimerization of secretory IgA. IgA is often found in noncovalent association with the so-called secretory component, a highly glycosylated 71kDa polypeptide, synthesized by mucosal cells and capable of protecting IgA against proteolytic degradation.

IgA represents 7%–15% of plasma immunoglobulins and has a half-life of 6 days. It is found, in particular, in the dimerized form in **parotid, bronchial**, and **intestinal** secretions. It is a major component of **colostrum** (the first milk from the mother's breasts after the birth of a child). IgA appears to function as the primary immunologic barrier against pathogenic invasion of mucous membranes. It promotes phagocytosis, causes eosinophilic degranulation, and activates complement via the alternative pathway.

IgM is confined to the intravascular space and helps eliminate circulating antigens and microorganisms

Immunoglobulins belonging to IgM class are polyvalent, with a high molecular mass. The basic form of IgM is similar to that of IgA, having the extra H-chain domain that allows for J-chain binding, and is thus capable of polymerization. It normally circulates as a pentamer, with a molecular mass of 971 kDa, linked by disulfide bonds and the J chain (Fig. 40.5).

IgM accounts for 5%–10% of plasma immunoglobulins and has a half-life of 5 days. With its polymeric nature and high molecular mass, most IgM is confined to the intravascular space, although lesser amounts may be found in secretions, usually in association with a secretory component. It is the first antibody to be synthesized after an antigenic challenge.

Minor classes of immunoglobulins

IgD is the surface receptor in B lymphocytes

IgD was only discovered in 1965 and differs from the standard immunoglobulin structure chiefly in its high carbohydrate content of numerous oligosaccharide units, resulting in an increased molecular mass of 190 kDa. Its δ chains are characterized by having only a single interconnecting disulfide bridge and an elongated hinge region that is particularly susceptible to proteolysis.

IgD serves as an antigen receptor on peripheral B lymphocytes and is also present in a secretory form. It is present on B cells in the upper respiratory tract and probably contributes to protection against airborne antigens. IgD accounts for less than 0.5% of the circulating plasma immunoglobulin mass.

IgE binds antigens and promotes release of vasoactive amines from mast cells

IgE is similar to IgM in its unit structure. It has ε heavy chains, but J-chain binding and polymerization do not occur. The extended H chain helps explain its high molecular mass of approximately 200 kDa. It is present only in trace amounts in plasma.

IgE has a high affinity for binding sites on mast cells and basophils. Antigenic binding at Fab_2 region induces crosslinking of the high-affinity receptor, granulation of the cell, and release of vasoactive amines. By this mechanism, IgE plays a major part in allergy/atopy and mediates antiparasitic immunity.

Monoclonal immunoglobulin synthesis is a result of benign or malignant transformation of B cells

Monoclonal immunoglobulins result from the proliferation of a single B-cell clone. On gel electrophoresis, monoclonal immunoglobulin forms a single band in the γ region (the **paraprotein band**; Fig. 40.6). Monoclonal immunoglobulins are associated with malignant pathologies such as **myeloma** and **Waldenström's macroglobulinemia** and also with more benign transformations that are known as **monoclonal gammopathies of uncertain significance** (MGUS).

THE ACUTE-PHASE RESPONSE

The acute-phase response is a nonspecific response to tissue injury or infection

The acute-phase reaction is a systemic response to stresses such as infection trauma, surgery, cancer, or immunologic disorders. It is set off by, for instance, bacterial toxins stimulating secretion of proinflammatory cytokines such as TNFα, IL1, and IL6. These in turn elicit a range of responses, including the stimulation of hypothalamic–pituitary–adrenal axis with

Normal serum

A

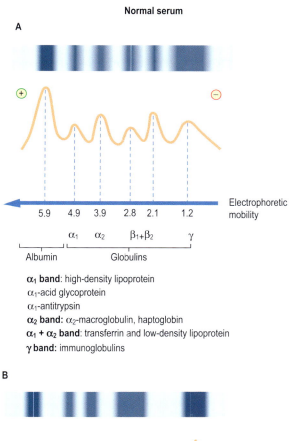

5.9 4.9 3.9 2.8 2.1 1.2

Electrophoretic mobility

α₁ α₂ β₁+β₂ γ

Albumin   Globulins

α₁ band: high-density lipoprotein
α₁-acid glycoprotein
α₁-antitrypsin
α₂ band: α₂-macroglobulin, haptoglobin
α₁ + α₂ band: transferrin and low-density lipoprotein
γ band: immunoglobulins

B

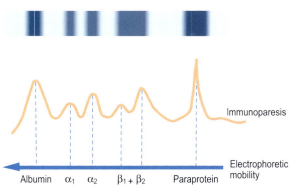

Immunoparesis

Albumin α₁ α₂ β₁ + β₂ Paraprotein

Electrophoretic mobility

Fig. 40.6 **Comparison of gel electrophoretic appearance of normal serum and that containing monoclonal immunoglobulins.** The scanning-pattern peaks (solid line) represent the relative concentrations of the separated proteins. (A) Normal serum. (B) Monoclonal gammopathy: a strongly stained band is present in the γ-globulin region on electrophoresis, and there is an associated reduction of staining in the remainder of the γ-region (immunoparesis).

the rise of cortisol concentration and also stimulation of catecholamine and nitric oxide secretion. There is also activation of complement and the coagulation system. Secretion of growth factors leads to activation of neutrophils, monocytes, and fibroblasts. Central to the acute-phase response is a major shift in the pattern of liver protein synthesis. The synthesis of a number of proteins, including albumin, transthyretin, (prealbumin), and transferrin, decreases (they are known as the negative acute-phase reactants; Fig. 40.7), whereas the

synthesis of others increases. Among the proteins that increase in concentration (the positive acute-phase reactants) are C-reactive protein; haptoglobin (the free hemoglobin–binding globulin); ceruloplasmin (copper-binding globulin); fibrinogen; α1-globulins, including α1-antitrypsin (proteinase inhibitor); and α2 macroglobulin, which binds proteolytic enzymes (see also Chapter 34).

Synthesis of these proteins requires amino acids obtained primarily from increased muscle catabolism. Thus the acute-phase reaction contributes to a negative nitrogen balance (Chapter 32).

Albumin is a negative acute-phase reactant. Therefore note that a decreased plasma albumin concentration observed acutely in a patient may be a result of an infection, rather than a marker of nutritional status.

C-reactive protein (CRP) is a major component of the acute-phase response and a marker of bacterial infection

CRP is synthesized in the liver and is constructed of five polypeptide subunits. It has a molecular mass of around 130 kDa. It is present in only minute quantities (<1 mg/L in normal serum). It promotes phagocytosis, participates in opsonization, and facilitates activation of the complement via the classic pathway (Chapter 43). Measurement of CRP concentration in plasma is an essential laboratory test in the diagnosis and monitoring of infection and sepsis (Fig. 40.8).

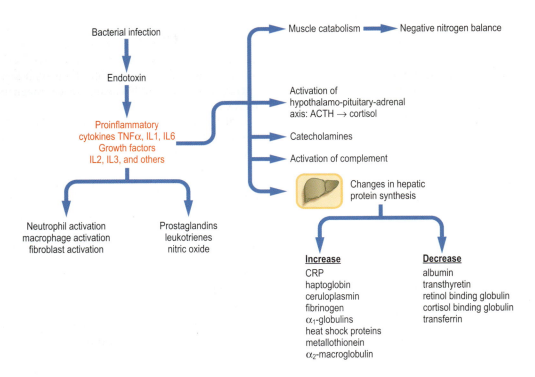

Fig. 40.7 **Acute-phase response. Development and resultant shift in the pattern of liver protein synthesis.** Note the initial role of proinflammatory cytokines in triggering the acute-phase response.

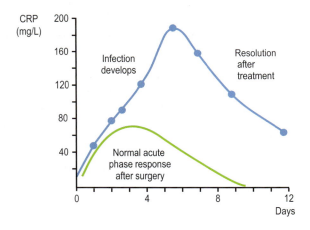

Fig. 40.8 **C-reactive protein (CRP) and the postoperative acute-phase reaction.** The concentration of CRP increases as part of the acute-phase response to surgical trauma, and a further increase may be observed if recovery is complicated by infection.

High-sensitivity CRP assay is used in the assessment of cardiovascular risk

An assay for CRP, which is approximately 100 times more sensitive than the conventional method, detects minimal fluctuations in the concentration of this protein. Very small increases in CRP concentration (in infection-free individuals) seem to reflect a state of **chronic low-grade inflammation**

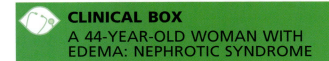

CLINICAL BOX
A 44-YEAR-OLD WOMAN WITH EDEMA: NEPHROTIC SYNDROME

A 44-year-old woman was admitted to the hospital because of weakness, anorexia, recurrent infections, bilateral leg edema, and breathlessness. Her plasma albumin concentration was 19 g/L (normal range 36–52 g/L), and her urinary protein excretion was 10 g/24 h (normal value ≤ 0.15 g/24 h). There was microscopic hematuria. Renal biopsy confirmed the diagnosis of membranoproliferative glomerulonephritis.

Comment

This woman had the classic triad of nephrotic syndrome: hypoalbuminemia, proteinuria, and edema. The nephritis resulted in damage to the glomerular basement membrane, with resultant leak of albumin. In nephrotic syndrome, the continued loss of albumin exceeds the synthetic capacity of the liver, resulting in hypoalbuminemia; consequently, the capillary osmotic pressure is significantly reduced. This leads to both peripheral (leg) edema and pulmonary edema (breathlessness). With increasing glomerular damage, proteins of larger molecular mass, such as immunoglobulins and complement, are lost in the urine.

associated, for instance, with an increased risk of cardiovascular disease (Chapter 33). Other inflammatory conditions, such as inflammatory bowel disease, type 2 diabetes, and metabolic syndrome, have also been associated with these minute increases in serum CRP concentration.

CLINICAL BOX
A WOMAN ADMITTED AFTER A TRAFFIC ACCIDENT: ACUTE-PHASE RESPONSE

A 45-year-old woman suffered severe lower limb injuries in a traffic accident. After admission to the hospital, biochemical profiling revealed slightly decreased concentrations of total serum protein (58 g/L; normal 60–80 g/L) and serum albumin (38 g/L; normal 36–52 g/L). Serum electrophoresis revealed an increase in the α1 and α2 protein fractions. Four days after her operation, the patient's condition deteriorated, and she developed an increased temperature, sweating, and confusion. An acute infection was diagnosed, and treatment with appropriate antibiotics was commenced. CRP concentrations peaked 5 days after the operation.

Comment

Increased concentrations of α1 and α2 proteins (which include α1-antitrypsin, α1-acid glycoprotein, and haptoglobin), together with a decrease in serum albumin concentration, suggest an acute-phase response. This response is also associated with an increase in CRP, the erythrocyte sedimentation rate (ESR), and plasma viscosity. The patient's response to treatment of infection is associated with a decrease in plasma CRP concentration.

BIOMARKERS

A biomarker is a substance or a characteristic that is measured as an indicator of normal or pathologic processes

Biomarkers, once established, are used for screening, risk assessment, and diagnosis and for monitoring treatments and side effects. The process of discovery of new biomarkers is driven by the application of -omic technologies: genomics, transcriptomics, proteomics, and metabolomics (Chapter 24).

Metabolomics explores patterns of small molecules

Metabolomics is the study of all metabolites generated in the organism, including metabolites of drugs, food-derived compounds, and substances generated by the microbial flora. The Human Metabolome Database (version 3.6) contains 43,003 metabolite entries and includes 5701 protein sequences (see Relevant Websites section). An additional database, the Small Molecule Pathway Database (SMPDB), contains individual compounds and extensive descriptions of metabolic pathways.

Exploration of metabolites is a process located downstream from genomics and transcriptomics - the study of genes and their expression, respectively (Chapter 24). Metabolomic methodologies allow exploration of entire pathways, producing **patterns of metabolite concentrations**. They provide a dynamic picture of any given condition. The drawback is that such picture can be confounded by compounds derived from ingested food or by metabolites of drugs and other foreign substances **(xenobiotics).** Therefore the key process is the comparison of metabolite patterns between the reference and affected populations using techniques such as mass spectrometry linked with gas chromatography (GC-MS) or liquid chromatography (LC-MS). Individual metabolites can subsequently be identified using nuclear magnetic resonance (NMR).

Validation of biomarkers requires studies on large cohorts. Required population sizes usually exceed the capabilities of a single study. Therefore **meta-analysis** (comparison of different studies) is extensively used. A meta-analysis may simply be a comparison of several published studies, may involve a combined analysis of group data from different studies, or may be an analysis of individual participants' data from different studies pooled into one "new," very large group, the most laborious but also the most reliable method.

SUMMARY

- Erythrocytes, leukocytes, and platelets constitute the formed elements of blood derived from the hematopoietic stem cell. They are suspended in plasma and have several specialized functions, such as transport of oxygen, destruction of external agents, and blood clotting.
- Most biochemical tests are done on plasma. To obtain plasma, blood must be taken into a test tube containing an anticoagulant. Plasma allowed to clot yields serum.
- Plasma contains many proteins broadly classified into albumin and globulins. Albumin functions as a determinant of the osmotic pressure and a major transport protein. Other binding proteins bind specific ligands; for example, ceruloplasmin binds Cu^{2+}, and thyroxine-binding globulin (TBG) binds thyroid hormones.
- Immunoglobulins participate in the defense against antigens. Several classes of immunoglobulin exist and perform different protective functions.

ACTIVE LEARNING

1. Compare and contrast plasma and serum, and discuss the different types of blood samples taken for laboratory tests.
2. Discuss the transport role of serum albumin.
3. Describe the core structure of immunoglobulins and the different roles played in immunity by the different classes of immunoglobulins.
4. How does the acute-phase reaction affect the results of blood tests?
5. Characterize Wilson's disease.
6. What happens to hemoglobin when erythrocytes become disrupted?

■ Changes in the concentration of plasma proteins provide important clinical information. A characteristic pattern of suppressed and stimulated liver protein synthesis indicates the acute-phase response.
■ Serum and urine protein electrophoresis is used for identifying the presence of monoclonal immunoglobulins.

FURTHER READING

Gilstrap, L. G., & Wang, T. J. (2012). Biomarkers and cardiovascular risk assessment for primary prevention: An update. *Clinical Chemistry, 58,* 72–82.

Gruys, E., Toussaint, M. J. M., Niewold, T. A., et al. (2005). Acute phase reaction and acute phase proteins. *Journal of Zhejiang University. Science, 6B,* 1045–1056. doi:10.1631/jzus.2005.B1045.

Morrison, S. J., & Scadden, D. T. (2014). The bone marrow niche for haematopoietic stem cells. *Nature, 505,* 327–334. doi:10.1038/nature12984.

(2011). Nature Outlook: Multiple myeloma. *Nature, 480,* 833–858.

Orkin, S. H., & Zon, L. (2008). Hematopoiesis: An evolving paradigm for stem cell biology. *Cell, 132,* 631–644.

Pavlou, M. P., Diamandis, E. P., & Blasutig, I. M. (2013). The long journey of cancer biomarkers from the bench to the clinic. *Clinical Chemistry, 59,* 147–157.

Suhre, K., Shin, S.-Y., Petersen, A.-K., et al. (2011). Human metabolic individuality in biomedical and pharmaceutical research. *Nature, 477,* 54–60.

Zimmermann, M. A., Selzman, C. H., & Cothren, C. (2003). Diagnostic implications of C-reactive protein. *Archives of Surgery, 138,* 220–224.

RELEVANT WEBSITES

HMDB (Human Metabolome Database), Version 3.6: http://www.hmdb.ca/
The Metabolomics Innovation Centre - SMPDB (Small Molecule Pathway Database), Version 2.0: http://www.smpdb.ca

ABBREVIATIONS

CBG	Cortisol-binding globulin
CRP	C-reactive protein
EDTA	Ethylenediaminetetraacetic acid
ESR	Erythrocyte sedimentation rate
GC-MS	Gas chromatography linked with mass spectrometry
HMDB	Human Metabolome Database
Ig	Immunoglobulin (IgG, IgA, IgM, IgD, and IgE)
IL	Interleukin (IL-1, IL-6, etc.)
LC-MS	Liquid chromatography linked with mass spectrometry
NMR	Nuclear magnetic resonance
SHBG	Sex hormone–binding globulin
SMPDB	Small Molecule Pathway Database
T3	Triiodothyronine
T4	Thyroxine
TBG	Thyroxine-binding globulin
TNFα	Tumor necrosis factor α

41

Hemostasis and Thrombosis

Catherine N. Bagot

INTRODUCTION

Circulation of the blood within the cardiovascular system is essential for the transportation of gases, nutrients, minerals, metabolic products, and hormones between different organs. It is also essential that blood should not leak excessively from blood vessels when they are injured by the traumas of daily life. Animal evolution has therefore resulted in the development of an efficient but complex series of hemodynamic, cellular, and biochemical mechanisms that limit such blood loss by forming platelet–fibrin plugs at sites of vessel injury (**hemostasis**). Genetic disorders that result in loss of individual protein functions, and therefore in excessive bleeding (e.g., hemophilia), have played an important part in the identification of many of the biochemical mechanisms in hemostasis.

It is also essential that these hemostatic mechanisms are appropriately controlled by inhibitory mechanisms; otherwise, an exaggerated platelet–fibrin plug may produce local occlusion of a major blood vessel (artery or vein) at its site of origin **(thrombosis)** or may break off and block a blood vessel downstream **(embolism).**

Arterial thrombosis is the major cause of heart attacks, stroke, and nontraumatic limb amputations in developed countries (atherothrombosis is discussed in Chapter 33). Venous thrombosis and embolism are also major causes of death and disability. The clinical use of **antithrombotic drugs** (antiplatelet, anticoagulant, and thrombolytic agents) is now widespread in developed countries and requires an understanding of how they interfere with hemostatic mechanisms to exert their antithrombotic effects.

HEMOSTASIS

Hemostasis means "the arrest of bleeding"

After tissue injury that ruptures smaller vessels (including everyday trauma, injections, surgical incisions, and tooth extractions), a series of interactions between the vessel wall and the circulating blood normally occurs, resulting in cessation of blood loss from injured vessels within a few minutes (hemostasis). Hemostasis results from effective sealing of the ruptured vessels by a hemostatic plug composed of **blood platelets** and **fibrin.** Fibrin is derived from circulating fibrinogen, whereas platelets are small cell fragments that circulate in the blood and have an important role in the initiation of hemostasis.

Hemostasis requires the coordinated function of blood vessels, platelets, coagulation factors, and the fibrinolytic system

Fig. 41.1 provides an overview of hemostatic mechanisms and illustrates some of the interactions among blood vessels, platelets, and the coagulation system in hemostasis; each of these components of hemostasis also interacts with the **fibrinolytic system.** The initial response of small blood vessels to injury is arteriolar vasoconstriction, which temporarily reduces local blood flow. Flow reduction transiently reduces blood loss and may also promote the formation of the platelet–fibrin plug. Activation of blood platelets is followed by their adhesion to the vessel wall at the site of injury and their subsequent aggregation to each other, building up an occlusive platelet mass that forms the **initial (primary) hemostatic plug**. This platelet plug is friable, and unless it is subsequently stabilized by fibrin, it will be washed away by local blood pressure when vasoconstriction reverses.

Vascular injury also activates coagulation factors, which interact sequentially to form **thrombin,** which converts circulating soluble plasma fibrinogen to insoluble, crosslinked fibrin. This forms the subsequent **(secondary) hemostatic plug**, which is relatively resistant to dispersal by blood flow, or fibrinolysis. There are two pathways of the activation of coagulation factors: the **extrinsic pathway,** which is initiated by the exposure of the flowing blood to tissue factor, released from subendothelial tissue, and the **intrinsic pathway,** which

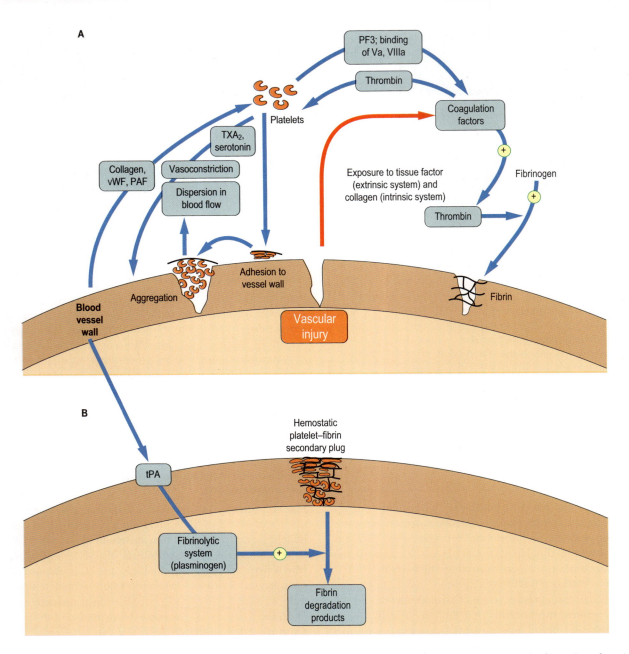

Fig. 41.1 **Overview of hemostatic mechanisms.** (A) Vascular injury sets in motion a series of events culminating in the formation of a primary plug of platelets. This can be dispersed by blood flowing through the vessel, unless the plug is stabilized. (B) The primary plug is stabilized by a network of fibrin formed from crosslinked fibrinogen. The secondary plug is stable and is degraded only when the fibrinolytic system has been activated. PAF, platelet-activating factor; PS, phosphatidylserine; tPA, tissue-type plasminogen activator; TXA_2, thromboxane A_2; Va, activated coagulation factor V; VIIIa, activated coagulation factor VIII; vWF, von Willebrand factor. Reproduced from Dominiczak MH. Medical Biochemistry Flash Cards. London: Elsevier, 2012.

has an important amplification role in generating thrombin and fibrin.

The lysis of fibrin is as important to health as its formation

Hemostasis is a continuous process throughout life and would result in excessive fibrin formation and vascular occlusion if

unchecked. Evolution has therefore produced a **fibrinolytic system**; this is activated by local fibrin formation, resulting in local generation of **plasmin,** an enzyme that digests fibrin plugs (in parallel with tissue-repair processes), thus maintaining vascular patency. Digestion of fibrin results in generation of circulating **fibrin degradation products (FDP).** These are detectable in the plasma of healthy individuals at low

Table 41.1 Congenital and acquired causes of excessive bleeding

	Congenital	Acquired
Vessel wall	**Disorders of collagen synthesis** (Ehlers–Danlos syndrome)	Vitamin C deficiency (scurvy) Corticosteroid excess
Platelets	**Disorders of adhesion** vWF deficiency (von Willebrand disease) Platelet GPIb-IX deficiency (Bernard–Soulier syndrome) **Disorders of aggregation** Platelet GPIIb-IIIa deficiency (Glanzmann's thrombasthenia) **Disorders of storage granules** (i.e., storage pool disorders affecting alpha granules, dense granules, or both) **Disorders of platelet secretion and signal transduction** (e.g., defects in platelet–agonist interactions, abnormalities in arachidonic acid pathway)	Antiplatelet drugs (e.g., aspirin, dipyridamole, clopidogrel) Defective formation of platelets Excessive destruction of platelets

Coagulation	**Coagulation factor deficiencies**
	(hemophilias):
	    factor VIII
	    factor IX
	    factor XI
	    fibrinogen (etc.)
		Vitamin K deficiency
		(factors II, VII, IX, X)
		Parenteral anticoagulants
		(e.g., unfractionated heparin [UFH], low-molecular-weight heparin [LMWH])
		Oral anticoagulants
		(vitamin K antagonists, e.g., warfarin; direct thrombin inhibitors, e.g., dabigatran; direct Xa inhibitors, e.g., rivaroxaban) liver disease
		Disseminated intravascular coagulation (DIC)

Fibrinolysis	Antiplasmin deficiency PAI-1 deficiency	Fibrinolytic drugs (e.g., tPA, urokinase, streptokinase)

GPIb-IX, gpiib-IIIa, glycoprotein receptors Ib-IX and IIb-IIIa; PAI-1, plasminogen activator inhibitor type 1; tPA, tissue plasminogen activator.

concentration, which illustrates that fibrin formation and lysis are continuing processes in health.

Excessive bleeding may result from defects in each of the components of hemostasis, which may be caused by disease (congenital or acquired) or by antithrombotic drugs (Table 41.1). The vascular, platelet, coagulation, and fibrinolytic components of hemostasis will now be discussed in turn.

THE VESSEL WALL

Vascular injury plays a key role in initiating local formation of the platelet–fibrin plug and in its subsequent removal by the fibrinolytic system

All blood vessels are lined by a flat sheet of endothelial cells, which have important roles in the interchange of chemicals, cells, and microbes between the blood and the body tissues. Endothelial cells in the smallest blood vessels (capillaries) are supported by a thin layer of connective tissue, rich in collagen fibers, called the **intima.** In veins, a thin layer (the **media**) of contractile smooth muscle cells allows some venoconstriction; for example, superficial veins under the skin constrict

in response to surface cooling. In arteries and arterioles, a well-developed muscle layer allows powerful vasoconstriction, including the vasoconstriction after local injury that forms part of the hemostatic response. Larger vessels also have a supportive connective tissue outer layer (the **adventitia**) (see also Chapter 33).

Normal endothelium has an antithrombotic surface

Intact normal endothelium does not initiate or support platelet adhesion or blood coagulation. Its surface is antithrombotic. This thrombo-resistance is partly due to endothelial production of two potent vasodilators and inhibitors of platelet function: prostacyclin (prostaglandin I_2 [PGI_2]) and nitric oxide, otherwise known as endothelium-derived relaxing factor (EDRF).

Endothelial damage exposes blood to tissue factor and to collagen

The vasoconstriction that occurs after vascular injury is partly mediated by two platelet activation products: serotonin (5-hydroxytryptamine, Chapter 26), and thromboxane A_2 (TXA_2), a product of platelet prostaglandin metabolism. The endothelial cell damage also exposes flowing blood to

ADVANCED CONCEPT BOX
PROSTACYCLIN AND NITRIC OXIDE: BIOCHEMICAL MEDIATORS OF VASOCONSTRICTION AND VASODILATATION

The diameters of arteries and arterioles throughout the body continuously alter to regulate blood flow according to local and general metabolic and cardiovascular requirements. Control mechanisms include neurogenic (sympathetic/adrenergic; Chapter 26) and myogenic pathways and local biochemical mediators, including prostacyclin (PGI_2) and nitric oxide.

Prostacyclin is the major arachidonic acid metabolite formed by vascular cells. It is a potent vasodilator and also a potent inhibitor of platelet aggregation. It has a short half-life in platelet-rich plasma of approximately 3 min.

Nitric oxide is also a potent vasodilator formed by vascular endothelial cells, also with a short half-life. It was initially termed endothelium-derived relaxing factor (EDRF). In common with prostacyclin, its generation by endothelial cells is enhanced by many compounds and also by blood flow and shear stress (the tangential force applied to the cells by the flow of blood). In the normal circulation, nitric oxide appears to have a key role in flow-mediated vasodilatation. It is synthesized by two distinct forms of endothelial nitric oxide synthase (eNOS): constitutive and inducible. Constitutive eNOS rapidly provides relatively small amounts of nitric oxide for short periods, related to vascular flow regulation. The beneficial effects of nitrate drugs in hypertension and angina may partly reflect their effects on this pathway. Inducible eNOS is stimulated by cytokines in inflammatory reactions and releases large amounts of nitric oxide for long periods. Its suppression by glucocorticoids may partly account for their antiinflammatory effects.

Both prostacyclin and nitric oxide appear to exert their vasodilator actions by diffusing locally from endothelial cells to vascular smooth muscle cells, where they stimulate guanylate cyclase, resulting in increased formation of cyclic guanosine 3'5'-monophosphate (cGMP) and relaxation of vascular smooth muscle via alteration of the intracellular calcium concentration (Chapter 25).

ADVANCED CONCEPT BOX
THROMBOXANE A₂ AND ASPIRIN

It has already been noted that prostacyclin, PGI_2, the major arachidonic acid metabolite formed by vascular cells, is a potent vasodilator and inhibitor of platelet aggregation. In contrast, the major arachidonic acid metabolite formed by platelets is **thromboxane A₂ (TXA_2)**, which is a potent vasoconstrictor and stimulates platelet aggregation. In common with prostacyclin, TXA_2 has a short half-life. In the late 1970s, Salvador Moncada and John Vane contrasted the effects of PGI_2 and TXA_2 on blood vessels and platelets and hypothesized that a balance between these two compounds was important in the regulation of hemostasis and thrombosis.

Congenital deficiencies of cyclooxygenase or thromboxane synthase (the enzymes involved in TXA_2 synthesis) result in a mild bleeding tendency. Ingestion of even low doses of **acetyl-salicylic acid (aspirin)** irreversibly acetylates cyclooxygenase and suppresses TXA_2 synthesis and platelet aggregation for several days, resulting in an antithrombotic effect and a mild bleeding tendency. Bleeding is especially likely from the stomach as a result of the formation of stomach ulcers secondary to the inhibition of cytoprotective gastric mucosal prostaglandins by aspirin. Although in persons at high risk of arterial thrombosis (e.g., previous myocardial infarction) this bleeding tendency is outweighed by a reduction in risk of thrombosis, aspirin is contraindicated in individuals with a history of bleeding disorders or existing stomach or duodenal ulcers.

Collagen plays a key role in the structure and hemostatic function of small blood vessels

Because collagen plays a key role in the structure and hemostatic function of small blood vessels, vascular causes of excessive bleeding include congenital or acquired deficiencies of collagen synthesis (Table 41.1). Congenital disorders include the rare **Ehlers–Danlos syndrome**. Acquired disorders include the relatively common vitamin C deficiency, scurvy (Chapter 7), and excessive exogenous or endogenous corticosteroids.

PLATELETS AND PLATELET-RELATED BLEEDING DISORDERS

Blood platelets form the initial hemostatic plug in small vessels and the initial thrombus in arteries and veins

Platelets are circulating, anuclear microcells of mean diameter 2–3 μm. They are fragments of bone marrow megakaryocytes and circulate for approximately 10 days in the blood. The concentration of platelets in normal blood is $150–400 \times 10^9$/L.

Congenital defects in platelet adhesion/aggregation can cause lifelong excessive bleeding

A simple screening test - measurement of the skin bleeding time (reference range, 2–9 min) - can frequently detect

---

subendothelial tissue factor, which activates the extrinsic pathway of blood coagulation (Fig. 41.1). In addition, after a vascular injury that disrupts the endothelial cell lining, flowing blood is exposed to subendothelial collagen, which activates the intrinsic pathway of blood coagulation.

Exposure of flowing blood to collagen as a result of endothelial damage also stimulates platelet activation

Platelets bind to collagen via von Willebrand factor (vWF), which is released from the endothelial cells. vWF in turn binds both to collagen fibers and to platelets (via a platelet-membrane glycoprotein receptor, GPIb-IX). Platelet-activating factor (PAF) from the vessel wall may also activate platelets in hemostasis (Fig. 41.1).

ADVANCED CONCEPT BOX
PLATELET ACTIVATION EXPOSES GLYCOPROTEIN RECEPTORS

Platelets can be activated by several chemical agents, including adenosine diphosphate (ADP; released by platelets, erythrocytes, and endothelial cells), epinephrine, collagen, thrombin, and PAF; by infection (e.g., HIV, *Helicobacter pylori*); and by high physical shear stresses. Most of the chemical agents appear to act by binding to specific receptors on the platelet surface membrane. After receptor stimulation, several pathways of platelet activation can be initiated, resulting in several phenomena:

- **Change in platelet shape** from a disk to a sphere with extended pseudopodia, which facilitates aggregation and coagulant activity
- **Release of several compounds involved in hemostasis** from intracellular granules (e.g., ADP, serotonin, fibronectin, and vWF)
- **Aggregation**, via exposure of GPIb-IX membrane receptor and linking by vWF (under high shear conditions) and via exposure of another membrane glycoprotein receptor, GPIIb-IIIa, and linking by fibrinogen (under low shear conditions)
- **Adhesion to the vessel wall** via exposure of the GPIb-IX membrane receptor, through which vWF binds platelets to subendothelial collagen.

Finally, stimulation of the platelet-membrane receptor triggers the activation of platelet-membrane phospholipases, which hydrolyze membrane phospholipids, releasing arachidonic acid. Arachidonic acid is metabolized by cyclooxygenase and thromboxane synthase to TXA_2, a potent but labile (half-life approximately 30 s) mediator of platelet activation and vasoconstriction.

congenital defects of platelet adhesion/aggregation, in which the time is characteristically prolonged. The most common such defect is **von Willebrand disease** (Table 41.1), a group of both autosomal dominant and autosomal recessive disorders that result in either quantitative or qualitative defects of vWF multimers. These multimers are composed of subunits (molecular weight 220–240 kDa) that are released from storage granules known as the Weibel–Palade bodies in endothelial cells and alpha granules in platelets. Not only does vWF have an important role in platelet hemostatic function, but it also transports coagulation factor VIII in the circulation and delivers it to sites of vascular injury. Hence, plasma concentrations of factor VIII may also be low in von Willebrand disease. Treatment of this disease is to increase the low plasma vWF activity, usually by means of either desmopressin (a synthetic analogue of vasopressin [Chapter 35], which releases vWF from endothelial cells into plasma) or administration of vWF concentrates derived from human plasma.

Less common congenital platelet-related bleeding disorders include **GPIb-IX deficiency** (Bernard–Soulier syndrome), **GPIIb-IIIa deficiency** (Glanzmann's thrombasthenia), and **fibrinogen deficiency** (fibrinogen bridges GPIIb-IIIa receptors of adjacent platelets).

Acquired disorders may be caused by defective formation and excessive destruction or consumption of platelets

Acquired disorders of platelets include a low platelet count **(thrombocytopenia),** which may be the result of either defective formation of platelets by bone marrow megakaryocytes (e.g., in myelodysplasia or acute myeloid leukemia), excessive destruction of platelets (e.g., by antiplatelet antibodies), and excessive consumption of platelets (e.g., in disseminated intravascular coagulation [DIC]) or by sequestration in an enlarged spleen.

Antiplatelet drugs are used in the prevention or treatment of arterial thrombosis

Antiplatelet drugs are used in the prevention or treatment of arterial thrombosis; their sites of action are illustrated in Fig. 41.2. Aspirin inhibits cyclooxygenase and hence reduces the formation of TXA_2. Because it also has the effect of reducing the formation of PGI_2, which itself has antiplatelet activity, agents acting more specifically as thromboxane synthase inhibitors (e.g., picotamide) or thromboxane receptor antagonists, such as ifetroban, have also been investigated as potential antiplatelet agents. However, these do not appear to be more effective than aspirin. Dipyridamole acts by both reducing the availability of ADP and inhibiting thromboxane synthase, and ticlopidine, clopidogrel, and prasugrel inhibit the ADP receptor. Ticagrelor also inhibits the ADP receptor, but its effect is reversible, unlike the other ADP receptor inhibitors, making its use potentially preferable in patients at increased bleeding risk. These drugs have antithrombotic effects similar to those of aspirin, but they cause less gastric bleeding because they do not interfere with the synthesis of prostaglandins in the stomach. GPIIb-IIIa antagonists (e.g., tirofiban or abciximab) can also be used in acute coronary thrombosis. Each of these antiplatelet drugs adds to the antithrombotic efficacy of aspirin but also increases the risk of bleeding when used in combination.

COAGULATION

Blood coagulation factors interact to form the secondary, fibrin-rich hemostatic plug in small vessels and the secondary fibrin thrombus in arteries and veins

Plasma coagulation factors are identified by Roman numerals; they are listed in Table 41.2, together with some of their properties. Tissue factor was formerly known as factor III, calcium ion as factor IV; factor VI does not exist.

The coagulation cascade

Fig. 41.3 illustrates the currently accepted scheme of blood coagulation. Since the early 1960s, this has been accepted as a "waterfall" or "cascade" sequence of interactive proenzyme-to-enzyme conversions, with each enzyme activating the next proenzyme in the sequence(s). **Activated factor enzymes are designated by the letter "a" - for example, factor XIa.** Although the process of blood coagulation is complex

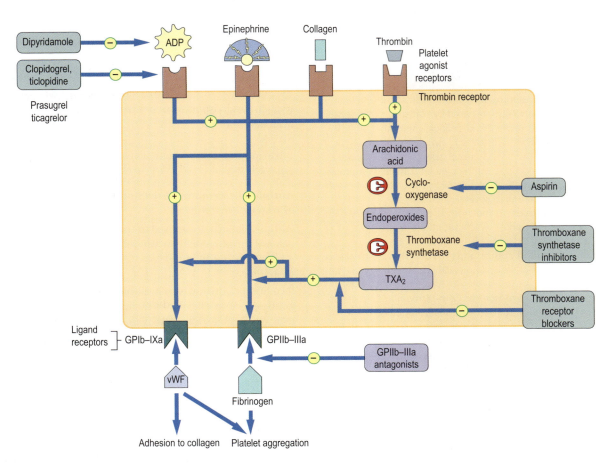

Fig. 41.2 **Pathways of platelet activation and mechanisms of action of antiplatelet drugs.** Normally, stimulation of platelet agonist receptors results in exposure of platelet ligand receptors, through the platelet prostaglandin (cyclooxygenase) pathway and other routes. Ligand receptors bind vWF and fibrinogen, and this results in platelet adhesion/aggregation. The antiplatelet drugs block this process at various stages. vWF, von Willebrand factor; TXA_2, thromboxane A_2.

ADVANCED CONCEPT BOX
PLATELET MEMBRANE RECEPTORS: THEIR LIGANDS, vWF, AND FIBRINOGEN

Platelets have a key role in hemostasis and thrombosis through adhesion to the vessel wall and subsequent aggregation to form a platelet-rich hemostatic plug or thrombus. These processes involve exposure of specific membrane glycoprotein receptors after platelet activation by several compounds.

Platelet receptor GPIb-IX plays a key part in the adhesion of platelets to subendothelium. It binds vWF, which also interacts with specific subendothelial receptors, including those on subendothelial collagen. Congenital deficiencies of GPIb-IX (Bernard–Soulier syndrome) or, more commonly, of vWF result in a bleeding tendency.

Another receptor, **GPIIb-IIIa,** has a key role in platelet aggregation. After platelet activation, hundreds of thousands of GPIIb-IIIa receptors can be exposed in a single platelet. These receptors interact predominantly with fibrinogen but also with vWF, which bind platelets together, forming a hemostatic or thrombotic plug. Congenital deficiency of GPIIb-IIIa (the rare Glanzmann's thrombasthenia) causes a severe bleeding disorder; in contrast, deficiencies of either fibrinogen or vWF cause a milder bleeding disorder because these two ligands can substitute for each other. GPIIb-IIIa inhibitors (e.g., tirofiban, abciximab) have been developed for patients undergoing angioplasty for coronary artery disease to prevent further coronary events.

Table 41.2 Coagulation factors and their properties

Factor	Synonyms	Molecular weight (Da)	Plasma concentration (mg/dL)
I	Fibrinogen	340,000	200–400
II	Prothrombin	70,000	10
III	Tissue factor (thromboplastin)	44,000	0
IV	*Calcium ion	40	9–10
V	Proaccelerin, labile factor	330,000	1
VII	Serum prothrombin conversion accelerator (SPCA), stable factor	48,000	0.05
VIII		220,000	0.01
von Willebrand factor (vWF)		$(250,000)n$	1
IX	Christmas factor	55,000	0.3
X	Stuart–Power factor	59,000	1
XI	Plasma thromboplastin antecedent (PTA)	160,000	0.5
XII	Hageman factor	80,000	3
XIII	Fibrin-stabilizing factor (FSF)	32,000	1–2
Prekallikrein	Fletcher factor	85,000	5
High-molecular-weight kininogen (HMWK)	Fitzgerald, Flaujeac, or Williams factor; contact activation cofactor	120,000	6

n *indicates number of subunits.*
*To convert calcium ion to mmol/L, divide by 0.2495

hence, three tests of coagulation are performed in clinical laboratories on citrated platelet-poor plasma:

- Activated partial thromboplastin time (APTT), testing the intrinsic pathway
- Prothrombin time (PT), testing the extrinsic pathway
- Thrombin clotting time (TCT), testing the final common pathway.

Platelet-poor plasma is used in these tests because the platelet count influences clotting-time results. To obtain platelet-poor plasma, blood is collected in tubes containing citrate anticoagulant to sequester calcium ions reversibly, and the blood is centrifuged at 2000 *g* for 15 min. The coagulation time tests are initiated by adding calcium and appropriate initiating agents.

However, these tests have their limitations in describing the in vivo phenotype of a patient's blood to coagulate effectively. The so-called global assays of coagulation have therefore been developed, and they are thought to better reflect an individual's ability to clot. These include **thromboelastography** and **thrombin generation**

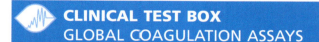

CLINICAL TEST BOX
GLOBAL COAGULATION ASSAYS

Thromboelastography (TEG) and **rotational thromboelastometry (ROTEM)** assess the ability of whole blood to clot in response to a mechanical stimulus, allowing an assessment of all aspects of hemostasis: platelet function, fibrin crosslinking, and fibrinolysis.

Thrombin generation assay is a global coagulation assay thought better able to assess an individual's ability to coagulate than standard coagulation assays. Tests such as the PT and APTT described earlier measure only 5% of the total thrombin generated - that is, at the time of first clot generation.

Thrombin is central to the coagulation cascade in that it converts fibrinogen to fibrin and also has numerous positive and negative feedback roles. The measurement of thrombin generation enables quantification over time of all thrombin generated in a plasma sample by its ability to "cut" either a chromophore or fluorochrome and measure the resultant chromogenic or fluorescent activity.

Despite promising results from ROTEM and thrombin generation, both assays are limited by numerous preanalytical and analytical variables, making comparisons between laboratories difficult. There is still no reliable standardization of these assays with robust internal or external quality control. For this reason, both remain research tools.

and nonlinear, traditionally, the scheme has been divided into three parts:

- The intrinsic pathway,
- The extrinsic pathway, and
- The final common pathway.

The status of the intrinsic, extrinsic, and final common pathway is assessed by specific laboratory tests

The three components of the coagulation system are distinguished on the basis of the nature of the initiating factor and its corresponding test in the clinical hemostasis laboratory;

Congenital deficiencies of coagulation factors (I–XIII) result in excessive bleeding

Congenital deficiencies of coagulation factors (I–XIII) result in excessive bleeding, which illustrates their physiologic importance in hemostasis. The exception is factor XII deficiency, which does not increase the bleeding tendency, despite prolonging blood clotting times in vitro; the same is true for its

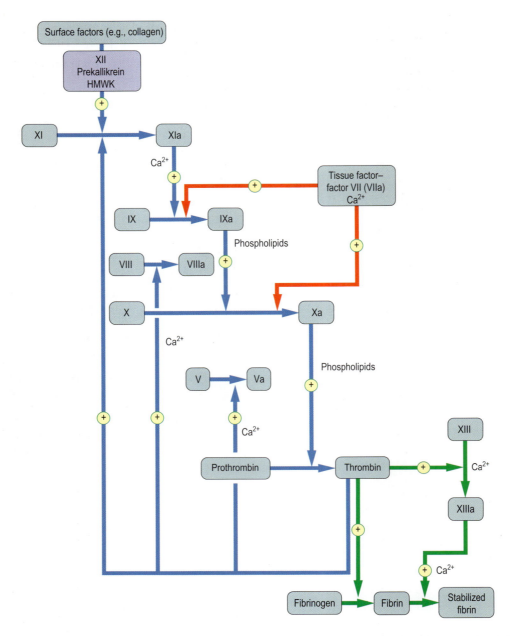

Fig. 41.3 **Blood coagulation: activation of coagulation factors.** After the initiation of blood coagulation, the coagulation factor proenzymes are sequentially activated; activated factor enzymes are designated by the letter "a.". Intrinsic pathway: blue arrows; extrinsic pathway, red arrows; common pathway: green arrows. HMWK, high-molecular-weight kininogen. Reproduced from Dominiczak MH. Medical Biochemistry Flash Cards. London: Elsevier, 2012.

cofactors, prekallikrein or high-molecular-weight kininogen (HMWK). A possible explanation for this is given in later in the chapter.

Activated partial thromboplastin time (APTT) assesses the intrinsic pathway

The term "intrinsic" implies that no extrinsic factor, such as tissue factor or thrombin, is added to the blood, besides a contact with nonendothelial "surface." The clinical test of this pathway is the APTT, also known as the kaolin–cephalin clotting time (KCCT), because kaolin (microparticulated clay) is added as a standard "surface," and cephalin (brain phospholipid extract) is used as a substitute for platelet phospholipid. The reference range of the APTT is about 30–40 s; prolongations are observed in deficiencies of factors XII (or its cofactors, prekallikrein or HMWK), XI, IX (or its cofactor, factor VIII), X (or its cofactor, factor V), or prothrombin (factor II; Tables 41.1 and 41.2).

The test is used to exclude the common congenital hemophilias (deficiencies of factors VIII, IX, or XI) and to monitor unfractionated heparin treatment. Hemophilias caused by factor VIII or IX deficiency occur in approximately 1 in 5000 and 1 in 30,000 males, respectively; inheritance is X-linked recessive, transmitted by carrier females. Treatment is usually with recombinant factor VIII or IX concentrates.

CLINICAL BOX
A BOY WITH EXTENSIVE BRUISING: CLASSIC HEMOPHILIA (CONGENITAL FACTOR VIII DEFICIENCY)

A 3-year-old boy was admitted from the emergency room of his local hospital because of extensive bruising after a fall down a few stairs. A routine coagulation screen test showed a greatly prolonged APTT of more than 150 s (normal range 30–40 s). Assay of coagulation factor VIII showed a very low level; the vWF level was normal. His mother recollected a family history of excessive bleeding, which had affected her brother and father.

Comment
Because of this typical history of an X-linked recessive bleeding disorder, a low coagulation factor VIII level, and a normal vWF level, the diagnosis of congenital factor VIII deficiency was made. The family was referred to the local hemophilia center and counseled about the risks of further affected sons and carrier daughters. The child was treated with intravenous recombinant factor VIII concentrate for the present bleed and prophylactically to prevent further bleeding episodes in the future.

Prothrombin time assesses the extrinsic pathway

The term "extrinsic" refers to the effect of tissue factor, which (after combining with coagulation factor VII) greatly accelerates coagulation by activating both factor IX and factor X (Fig. 41.3). Tissue factor is a polypeptide that is expressed in all cells other than endothelial cells. The clinical test of this pathway is the **prothrombin time (PT)**, in which tissue factor is added to plasma. The reference range is approximately 10–15 s; prolongations are observed in deficiencies of factors VII, X, V, or II. In clinical practice, the test is used to diagnose both the rare congenital defects of these factors and, much more commonly, acquired bleeding disorders resulting from the following:

- **Vitamin K deficiency** (e.g., in malabsorption or obstructive jaundice; see also Chapter 7), which reduces hepatic synthesis of factors II, VII, IX, and X. Treatment is by oral or intravenous administration of vitamin K.
- **Administration of oral vitamin K antagonists** (e.g., warfarin), which reduce hepatic synthesis of these factors.

Excessive bleeding in patients taking warfarin can be treated by stopping the drug, giving vitamin K, or replacing factors II, VII, IX, and X with either prothrombin complex concentrates containing only the relevant factors (e.g., Beriplex) or fresh frozen plasma.

- **Liver disease**, which reduces hepatic synthesis of all coagulation factors, including those that affect the PT. For example, the prothrombin time is a prognostic marker of liver failure after acetaminophen (paracetamol) overdose (Chapter 34). Treatment is by replacing coagulation factors with fresh frozen plasma.

CLINICAL TEST BOX
MONITORING ORAL ANTICOAGULANT THERAPY

Oral anticoagulant therapy with **vitamin K antagonists** (e.g., **warfarin**) is given long term to patients at risk of thrombosis within the chambers of the heart (e.g., patients with atrial fibrillation or heart valve prostheses, which may embolize to the brain, causing a stroke).

Monitoring of an internationally standardized prothrombin time (i.e., the **International Normalized Ratio [INR]**) every few weeks is essential to minimize the risk not only of thromboembolism but also of excessive bleeding. Up to 1% of the adult population in developed countries now receives long-term anticoagulants; hence traditional monitoring by doctors and nurses (taking blood samples, sending them to the laboratory, getting results, and giving dosage instructions to patients) has created an unsustainable workload.

In recent years, near-patient or point-of-care INR testing has become available for warfarin monitoring, with a finger prick capillary sample being drawn into a portable INR analyzer. With this technique, some patients can self-monitor and occasionally self-manage their warfarin dosage, similar to blood glucose self-management by persons with diabetes. Computerized algorithms for dosing warfarin have also been developed to assist healthcare workers to alter dosing accurately. Direct oral anticoagulants (e.g., dabigatran, rivaroxaban, apixaban, edoxaban) for patients with atrial fibrillation are now available, which require no monitoring of anticoagulation levels.

Thrombin clotting time assesses the final common pathway

The term "final common pathway" refers to the conversion of prothrombin to thrombin via Xa, with Va acting as a cofactor

This in turn allows the conversion of fibrinogen to fibrin. This final stage of fibrin production in the common pathway is tested clinically by the **thrombin clotting time (TCT)**, in which exogenous thrombin is added to the plasma. The reference range of values is approximately 10–15 s; prolongations are observed in fibrinogen deficiency and in the presence of inhibitors (e.g., heparin, dabigatran, fibrin degradation products). Fibrinogen deficiency may be congenital or due to acquired consumption of fibrinogen in DIC or may occur after administration of fibrinolytic drugs (see following discussion). Treatment is with cryoprecipitate or fibrinogen concentrates.

Several assays assess platelet function

Apart from assessing platelet number, size, and morphology through complete blood count (CBC) analysis and blood film review, platelet function can also be assessed in other ways.

One method of platelet function assessment is the **Platelet Function Analyzer** (PFA-100, Siemens). Whole blood is passed over a cartridge containing an aperture coated with a combination of two platelet agonists: collagen/epinephrine or collagen/ADP. The time to aperture closure as a result of platelet aggregation is measured. It cannot define specific disorders, but an abnormal result is suggestive of a platelet disorder and can be used as a screening test.

Light-transmission aggregometry (LTA) is considered the gold standard for investigating specific disorders of platelet function. Platelet-rich plasma is exposed to various platelet agonists (e.g., collagen, ADP, and epinephrine), and light transmission is monitored to produce standard curves. The pattern of curves obtained with a combination of agonists can help determine which platelet-function defect is present.

The production and release of platelet nucleotides (i.e., ATP and ADP) can be measured to assess nucleotide production and nucleotide release from granules. Flow-cytometry analysis of various **platelet receptors** can also be performed.

Such an array of tests should mean that platelet function disorders should be easy to diagnose. However, preanalytical and analytical variables mean that results can often be unreliable, and the results are often difficult to interpret.

Thrombin

Thrombin converts circulating fibrinogen to fibrin and activates factor XIII, which crosslinks the fibrin, forming a clot

It is currently believed that activation of blood coagulation is usually initiated by vascular injury, causing exposure of flowing blood to tissue factor, which results in activation of factors VII and IX (Fig. 41.3). Subsequently, activation of factors X and II (prothrombin) occurs preferentially at sites of vascular injury, alongside activated platelets: the latter provide procoagulant activity as a result of exposure of negatively charged platelet surface membrane phospholipids, such as phosphatidylserine, and high-affinity binding sites for several activated coagulation factors, allowing the formation of the prothrombinase complex (Va, Xa, and II) and tenase complex (VIIIa, IXa, and Xa), which both greatly enhance the production

of thrombin. As a result of these biochemical interactions, thrombin and fibrin formation are efficiently localized at sites of vascular injury.

Thrombin has a central role in hemostasis

Not only does thrombin convert circulating fibrinogen to fibrin at sites of vascular injury, producing the secondary, fibrin-rich hemostatic plug; it also activates factor XIII, a transglutaminase, which crosslinks fibrin, rendering it resistant to dispersion by local blood pressure or by fibrinolysis (Figs. 41.1 and 41.3). Furthermore, thrombin stimulates its own generation in a positive feedback cycle in three ways:

- **It catalyzes activation of factor XI.** This may explain why congenital deficiencies of factor XII, prekallikrein, or HMWK are not associated with excessive bleeding (Fig. 41.3).
- **It catalyzes activation of factors VIII and V.**
- **It activates platelets** (Fig. 41.2).

Thrombin inhibitors have been developed as anticoagulant drugs

Now that the central role of thrombin in hemostasis and thrombosis has been recognized, a number of **direct thrombin inhibitors (DTI)** have been developed as anticoagulant drugs. Dabigatran, an oral DTI, has been demonstrated in large randomized controlled clinical trials to be as effective as warfarin in the treatment and secondary prevention of venous thrombosis and in the prevention of stroke in patients with atrial fibrillation. It has a license in the United Kingdom for both of these indications. The major advantage of this drug for these indications is that dose monitoring is not required. Dabigatran is the first of the direct oral anticoagulants to have an effective antidote, idarucizumab, a monoclonal antibody that can reverse the anticoagulant effect of dabigatran within minutes.

Argatroban is another oral DTI and is an effective alternative to heparin when the latter is contraindicated after an episode of heparin-induced thrombocytopenia (HIT). It has a UK license for this indication. Bivalirudin, a derivative of hirudin, originally obtained from the medicinal leech *Hirudo medicinalis*, is a parenteral DTI that has been shown to be effective for the treatment of acute coronary syndromes. It is also an alternative to heparin for patients with acute coronary syndromes who have HIT.

This central role of thrombin is also the rationale for the intensive research that is now being performed to refine the thrombin generation assay and apply it to both bleeding and thrombotic clinical pathologies.

Coagulation inhibitors are essential to prevent excessive thrombin formation and thrombosis

Three systems of naturally occurring coagulation inhibitors have been identified (Fig. 41.4 and Table 41.3):

- **Antithrombin:** This is a protein synthesized in the liver. Its activity is catalyzed by the antithrombotic drug heparin

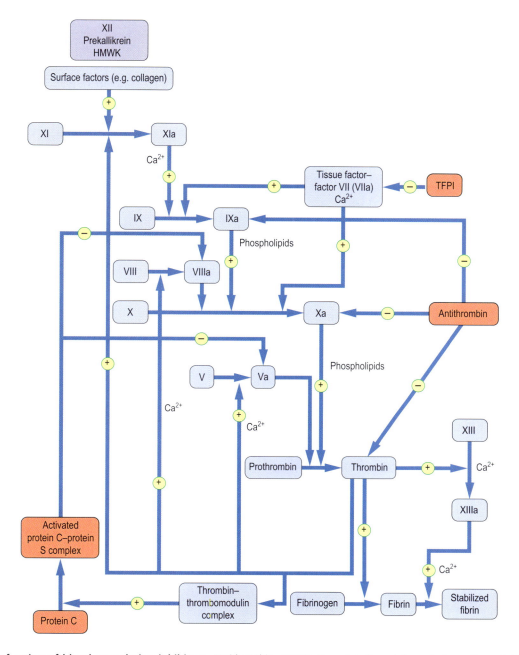

Fig. 41.4 **Sites of action of blood coagulation inhibitors.** Antithrombin, protein C, protein S, and tissue factor pathway inhibitor (TFPI). See text for details.

(unfractionated and low-molecular-weight heparins) and by heparin-like endogenous glycosaminoglycans (GAG) that are present on the surface of vascular endothelial cells. It inactivates not only thrombin but also factors IXa and Xa (Fig. 41.3). As a result, congenital antithrombin deficiency results in a significantly increased risk of venous thromboembolism.

■ **Heparins** are referred to as indirect Xa inhibitors due to their augmentation of antithrombin activity. Heparins are used in both treatment and prevention of acute venous

thrombosis, usually in the form of a low-molecular-weight heparin (LMWH), such as enoxaparin or dalteparin. They are usually replaced by oral anticoagulants, such as warfarin, for longer-term anticoagulation. LMWHs also play a role in the management of acute arterial thrombosis as it pertains to acute coronary syndromes (e.g., enoxaparin or fondaparinux).

■ **Direct Xa inhibitors** have now been developed as anticoagulants. Rivaroxaban, apixaban, and edoxaban have been shown to be effective alternatives to warfarin for

Table 41.3 Properties of coagulation inhibitors

Inhibitor (synonym)	Molecular weight	Plasma concentration (mg/dL)
Antithrombin (antithrombin III)	65,000	18–30
Protein C	56,000	0.4
Protein S	69,000	2.5
Tissue factor pathway inhibitor (TFPI) (lipoprotein-associated coagulation inhibitor [LACI])	32,000	0.1

CLINICAL BOX
A 40-YEAR-OLD MAN WITH PAIN AND LEG SWELLING: ANTITHROMBIN DEFICIENCY

A 40-year-old man was admitted from the emergency room of his local hospital because of acute pain and swelling of his left leg 10 days after recent major surgery. Ultrasound imaging of the leg confirmed occlusion of the left femoral vein by thrombus.

Comment
He was prescribed anticoagulant therapy with low-molecular-weight heparin at standard doses. The patient volunteered a strong family history of "clots in the legs" at a young age. He was commenced on warfarin and LMWH, the latter being discontinued when his INR was > 2. He was followed up at the anticoagulation and specialist thrombophilia clinic for long-term management.

the treatment and prevention of venous thrombosis and for the prevention of stroke in patients with atrial fibrillation. All these medications are in an oral form, and no monitoring of their anticoagulation effect is required. A modified recombinant derivative of factor Xa, is currently under investigation as a potential antidote for all of these drugs.

■ **Protein C and its cofactor, protein S:** These are vitamin K–dependent proteins, synthesized in the liver. When thrombin is generated, it binds to **thrombomodulin** (molecular weight 74 kDa), which is present on the surface of vascular endothelial cells. The thrombin–thrombomodulin complex activates protein C, which forms a complex with its cofactor, protein S. This complex selectively degrades factors Va and VIIIa by limited proteolysis (Fig. 41.3). Hence, this pathway forms a negative feedback upon thrombin generation. Congenital deficiencies of protein C or protein S result in an increased risk of venous thromboembolism. A further cause of increased risk of venous thromboembolism is a **mutation in coagulation factor V (factor V Leiden)**, which confers resistance to its inactivation by activated protein C. This mutation is common, occurring in approximately 5% of the population in Western countries.

■ **Tissue factor pathway inhibitor (TFPI):** This protein is synthesized in endothelium and the liver; it circulates bound to lipoproteins. It inhibits the tissue factor–VIIa complex (Fig. 41.3). However, deficiency of TFPI does not appear to increase the risk of thrombosis.

FIBRINOLYSIS

The fibrinolytic system acts to limit excessive formation of fibrin through plasmin-mediated fibrinolysis

The coagulation system acts to form fibrin; the fibrinolytic system acts to limit excessive formation of fibrin (both intra- and extravascular) through **plasmin-mediated fibrinolysis**. Circulating plasminogen binds to fibrin via lysine-binding sites;

it is converted to active plasmin by plasminogen activators. **Tissue-type plasminogen activator** (tPA) is synthesized by endothelial cells; it normally circulates in plasma in low basal concentrations (5 ng/mL), but it is released into plasma by stimuli that include venous occlusion, exercise, and epinephrine. Together with plasminogen, it binds strongly to fibrin, which stimulates its activity (the K_m for plasminogen decreases from 65 to 0.15 µmol/L in the presence of fibrin), thereby localizing plasmin activity to fibrin deposits.

CLINICAL TEST BOX
MEASUREMENT OF FIBRIN D-DIMER IN THE DIAGNOSIS OF SUSPECTED DEEP VEIN THROMBOSIS

Fibrin D-dimer (a degradation product of crosslinked fibrin and a marker of fibrin turnover) is normally present in blood at concentrations of < 250 µg/L. In **deep vein thrombosis of the leg (DVT)**, deposition of a large mass of cross-linked fibrin within the leg veins, followed by partial lysis by the body's fibrinolytic system, increases fibrin turnover, and blood D-dimer levels are elevated. Many patients arrive at emergency departments with a swollen and/or painful leg, which may be due to a DVT.

Rapid immunoassays for blood D-dimer can be performed in the emergency department and are now widely used as an adjunct to clinical diagnosis. About one-third of patients with clinically suspected DVT have normal D-dimer levels, which in combination with a low clinical probability score usually excludes the diagnosis and may allow early discharge of such patients without the need for further investigation or treatment. In patients with raised D-dimer levels, heparin treatment is started, and imaging of the leg is performed (usually by ultrasound) to confirm the presence and extent of a DVT.

Plasmin inhibitors prevent excessive fibrinolytic activity

Excessive tPA activity in plasma is normally prevented by an excess of its major inhibitor, **plasminogen-activator inhibitor type 1 (PAI-1)**, which is synthesized by both endothelial cells and hepatocytes. **Urokinase-type plasminogen activator (uPA)** circulates in plasma both as an active single-chain precursor form (scuPA, pro-urokinase) and as a more active two-chain form (tcuPA, urokinase). One activator of scuPA is surface-activated coagulation factor XII, which therefore links the coagulation and fibrinolytic systems. Major components of the fibrinolytic system are listed in Table 41.4 and illustrated in Fig. 41.5. Excessive formation of plasmin is normally prevented by

- binding of 50% of plasminogen to histidine-rich glycoprotein (HRG), and
- rapid inactivation of free plasmin by its major inhibitor, α_2-antiplasmin.

The physiologic importance of PAI-1 and α_2-antiplasmin is illustrated by the increased bleeding tendency that is

CLINICAL BOX
ANTITHROMBOTIC TREATMENT IN ACUTE CORONARY SYNDROME

Occlusion of a coronary artery by a thrombus causes the features of acute coronary syndrome, which include electrocardiographic and biochemical changes. **Myocardial infarction** refers to the permanent death of the part of the heart muscle that is supplied by that artery. In acute coronary syndromes, including myocardial infarction, the patient typically experiences **severe chest pain.**

Aspirin and heparin are usually given in acute myocardial infarction and other acute coronary syndromes to inhibit the platelet and fibrin components of the developing coronary artery thrombus. Some patients may require the addition of clopidogrel and/or ADP receptor antagonists and/or GPIIb-IIIa inhibitors.

Many patients with evolving acute myocardial infarction are candidates for **thrombolytic treatment** with a plasminogen activator drug, given intravenously. Prompt thrombolysis dissolves the coronary artery thrombus, reduces the size of the infarct, and reduces the risk of complications, including death and heart failure. However, in recent years, direct removal of the thrombus **(percutaneous coronary intervention [PCI])** is undertaken instead of thrombolytic therapy because it appears to give favorable outcomes in thrombolysis and does not increase the risk of bleeding, for example, into the brain. Patients undergoing PCI should, in addition, receive a GPIIb-IIIa inhibitor.

Table 41.4 The components of fibrinolytic system

Component (synonym)	Molecular weight (Da)	Plasma concentration (mg/dL)
Plasminogen	92,000	0.2
Tissue-type plasminogen activator (tPA)	65,000	5 (basal)
Urokinase-type plasminogen activator type 1 (uPA)	51,600	20
Plasminogen activator inhibitor type 1 (PAI-1)	48,000	200
Antiplasmin (α_2-antiplasmin)	70,000	700

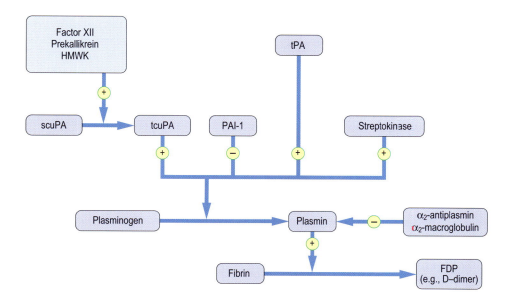

Fig. 41.5 **The fibrinolytic system.** Plasminogen can be activated to plasmin by tcuPA (urokinase), tPA, or streptokinase. tcuPA and tPA are inhibited by plasminogen activator inhibitor type 1 (PAI-1). Plasmin is inhibited by α2-antiplasmin and α2-macroglobulin. Plasmin degrades fibrin to fibrin degradation products (FDP). HMWK, high-molecular-weight kininogen; scuPA, single-chain plasminogen activator (pro-urokinase); tcuPA, two-chain urokinase-type plasminogen activator (urokinase); tPA, tissue-type plasminogen activator. Reproduced from Dominiczak MH. Medical Biochemistry Flash Cards. London: Elsevier, 2012.

associated with the rare cases of their congenital deficiencies (Table 41.1); the excessive plasma plasmin activity that results from these deficiencies has the effect of lysing hemostatic plugs.

SUMMARY

- Hemostasis constitutes a number of processes that guard the body against blood loss.
- Injury to the blood vessel wall sets in motion complex phenomena that involve blood platelets (activation, adhesion, aggregation) and a cascade of coagulation factors, classified into intrinsic, extrinsic, and final common pathways.
- The integrity of these three systems may be tested by simple laboratory tests. Global coagulation assays such as thrombin generation and thromboelastography, currently used in research, may be more effective in assessing an individual's coagulation phenotype.
- Deficiencies of factors participating in the coagulation cascade and/or disordered platelet function result in bleeding disorders.
- Eventually, blood clots are degraded by the fibrinolytic system. The process of fibrinolysis prevents thrombotic phenomena, and there is normally a balance between hemostasis and thrombosis.
- Aspirin and heparin are used in patients with acute myocardial infarction or other acute coronary syndromes.
- Aspirin (or other antiplatelet agents) is also used to reduce the risk of recurrent myocardial infarction and stroke.
- Anticoagulant drugs (e.g., heparin, warfarin, rivaroxaban) are used in the treatment of acute venous thrombosis or embolism.
- Anticoagulant drugs (e.g., warfarin, dabigatran, rivaroxaban) are used long term to prevent

thromboembolism arising from the heart (atrial fibrillation, heart valve prostheses).

FURTHER READING

Kearon, C., et al. (2016). Antithrombotic therapy for VTE disease 2016. *Chest, 149*, 315–352.

Key, N. S., Marris, M., O'Shaugnessy, D., et al. (Eds.), (2009). *Practical hemostasis and thrombosis* (3rd ed.). Oxford: Wiley.

Ozaki, Y., (Ed.). (2011). State of the art 2011. *Journal of Thrombosis and Haemostasis, 9*(Suppl.s1), 1–395.

Holbrook, A., Schulman, S., Witt, D. M., Vandvik, P. O., Fish, J., Kovacs, M. J., et al. Evidence-based management of anticoagulant therapy: Antithrombotic therapy and prevention of thrombosis (9th ed.). American College of Chest Physicians Evidence-Based Clinical Practice Guidelines 2012. *Chest, 141*(Suppl. 2), e152S–e184S.

Wright, I. S. (1962). The nomenclature of blood clotting factors. *Canadian Medical Association Journal, 86*, 373–374.

RELEVANT WEBSITES

Practical-Haemostasis.com - A Practical Guide to Laboratory Haemostasis: http://www.practical-haemostasis.com/

BSH Guidelines - Haemostasis and Thrombosis: http://www.b-s-h.org.uk/guidelines/?status=Guideline&category=Haemostasis+and+Thrombosis&p=1&search=#guideline-filters__select__status

International Society on Thrombosis and Haemostasis: http://www.isth.org

ABBREVIATIONS

AHF	Antihemophilic factor
APTT	Activated partial thromboplastin time
cGMP	Cyclic guanosine 3′5′-monophosphate
DIC	Disseminated intravascular coagulation
DTI	Direct thrombin inhibitor
DVT	Deep vein thrombosis
EDRF	Endothelium-derived relaxing factor, nitric oxide
eNOS	Endothelial nitric oxide synthase
FDPs	Fibrin degradation products
FSF	Fibrin-stabilizing factor
GAGs	Glycosaminoglycans
GPIb-IX, GPIIb-IIIa	Platelet membrane glycoprotein receptors
HIT	Heparin-induced thrombocytopenia
HMWK	High-molecular-weight kininogen
HRG	Histidine-rich glycoprotein
INR	International Normalized Ratio
KCCT	Kaolin–cephalin clotting time, APTT
LACI	Lipoprotein-associated coagulation inhibitor
LMWH	Low-molecular-weight heparin
LTA	Light transmission aggregometry
PAF	Platelet-activating factor
PAI-1	Plasminogen activator inhibitor type 1
PCI	Percutaneous coronary intervention
PGI$_2$	Prostaglandin I$_2$

ACTIVE LEARNING

1. When a patient presents with excessive bleeding from multiple sites, what laboratory tests are available to identify the likely cause of the hemostatic defect?
2. When a patient presents with a painful, swollen leg, possibly due to acute deep venous thrombosis (DVT), what laboratory tests can be performed to help the clinician
   - establish or exclude this diagnosis?
   - monitor anticoagulant treatment after the diagnosis has been confirmed?
3. When a patient presents with acute coronary artery thrombosis (evolving to myocardial infarction), what antithrombotic drugs should be urgently considered to reduce the risk of complications?

PTA	Plasma thromboplastin antecedent	TEG	Thromboelastography
PT	Prothrombin time	tPA	Tissue-type plasminogen activator
ROTEM	Rotational thromboelastometry	TXA_2	Thromboxane A_2
SPCA	Serum prothrombin conversion accelerator	UFH	Unfractionated heparin
TCT	Thrombin clotting time	uPA	Urinary-type plasminogen activator
TFPI	Tissue factor pathway inhibitor	vWF	von Willebrand factor

42 Oxidative Stress and Inflammation

John W. Baynes

INTRODUCTION

At body temperature, oxygen is a relatively sluggish oxidant

The element oxygen (O_2) is essential for the life of aerobic organisms. Although it is highly reactive in combustion reactions at high temperature, oxygen is relatively inert at body temperature; it has a high activation energy for oxidation reactions. This is fortunate; otherwise, we might spontaneously combust. About 90% of our O_2 usage is committed to oxidative phosphorylation. Enzymes that use O_2 for hydroxylation and oxygenation reactions consume another 10%, and a residual fraction, <1%, is converted to **reactive oxygen species (ROS)**, such as superoxide and hydrogen peroxide, which are reactive forms of oxygen. ROS are important in metabolism - some enzymes use H_2O_2 as a substrate. ROS also play a role in the regulation of metabolism and in immunologic defenses against infection. However, ROS are also a source of chronic damage to tissue biomolecules. One of the risks of harnessing O_2 as a substrate for energy metabolism is that we may, and do, get burned. For this reason, we have a range of antioxidant defenses that protect us against ROS.

This chapter will deal with the biochemistry of reactive oxygen, the mechanisms of formation and detoxification of ROS, and their role in human health and disease.

THE INERTNESS OF OXYGEN

In most textbooks, oxygen is shown as a diatomic molecule with two bonds between the oxygen atoms. This is an attractive presentation from the viewpoint of electron dot structures and electron pairing to form chemical bonds, but it is incorrect. In fact, at body temperature, O_2 is a biradical, a molecule with two unpaired electrons (Fig. 42.1). These electrons have parallel spins and are unpaired. Because most organic oxidation reactions (e.g., the oxidation of an alkane to an alcohol or an aldehyde to an acid) are two-electron oxidation reactions, O_2 is generally not very reactive in these reactions. In fact, it is completely stable, even in the presence of a strong reducing agent such as H_2. When enough heat (activation energy) is applied, one of the unpaired electrons flips to form an electron pair, which then participates in the combustion reaction. Once started, the combustion provides the heat needed to propagate the reaction, sometimes explosively.

Oxygen is activated by transition metal ions, such as iron or copper, in the active site of metalloenzymes

Metabolic reactions are conducted at body temperature, far below the temperature required to activate free oxygen. In biological redox reactions involving O_2, the oxygen is always activated by redox active metal ions, such as iron and copper; these metals also have unpaired electrons and form reactive metal–oxo complexes. All enzymes that use O_2 in vivo are metalloenzymes, as are the oxygen binding proteins, hemoglobin and myoglobin, which contain iron in the form of heme (Chapter 5). These metal ions provide one electron at a time to oxygen, activating O_2 for metabolism. Because iron and copper, and sometimes manganese and other ions, activate oxygen, these redox-active metal ions are kept at very low (submicromolar) free concentrations in vivo. Normally, they are tightly sequestered (compartmentalized) in storage or transport proteins, and they are locally activated at the active sites of enzymes, where oxidation chemistry can be contained and focused on a specific substrate. Free redox-active metal ions are dangerous in biological systems because, in free form, they activate O_2, and ROS formed in these reactions cause oxidative damage to biomolecules. Damage to proteins is often site specific, occurring

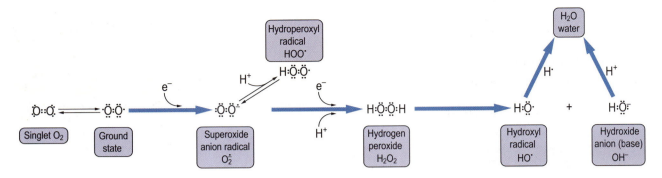

Fig. 42.1 **Structure of oxygen and reactive oxygen species (ROS).** Oxygen is shown at the far left as the incorrect double-bonded diatomic form. This form, known as singlet oxygen, exists to a significant extent only at high temperature or in response to irradiation. The diradical is the natural, ground-state form of O_2 at body temperature. ROS are partially reduced, reactive forms of oxygen. The first reduction product is the anion radical, superoxide ($O_2^•$), which is in equilibrium with the weak acid, hydroperoxyl radical (pK_a, ~4.5). Reduction of superoxide yields hydroperoxide O_2^{-2} in the form of H_2O_2. Reduction of H_2O_2 causes a hemolytic cleavage reaction that releases hydroxyl radical ($OH^•$) and hydroxide ion (OH^-). Water is the end product of complete reduction of O_2.

at sites of metal binding to proteins, indicating that metal–oxo complexes participate in ROS-mediated damage in vivo.

> ### CLINICAL BOX
> ### IRON OVERLOAD INCREASES RISK FOR DIABETES AND CARDIOMYOPATHY
>
> Patients with hematologic disorders such as hereditary hemochromatosis, thalassemias, and sickle cell disease, or who receive frequent blood transfusions, gradually develop **iron overload,** a condition that increases the risk for development of cardiomyopathy and diabetes. The heart and β cells are rich in mitochondria. The development of secondary disease in iron overload is considered the result of iron-mediated enhancement of mitochondrial ROS production in these tissues. Mutations in the mitochondrial genome may lead to progressive mitochondrial dysfunction, compromising cardiac and β-cell function.

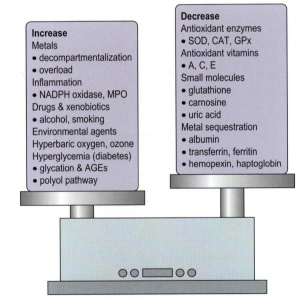

Fig. 42.2 **Oxidative stress: an imbalance between prooxidant and antioxidant systems.** As described in this chapter, numerous factors contribute to the enhancement and inhibition of oxidative stress. AGE, advanced glycation end product; CAT, catalase; GPx, glutathione peroxidase; MPO, myeloperoxidase; SOD, superoxide dismutase.

REACTIVE OXYGEN SPECIES AND OXIDATIVE STRESS

ROS are reactive, strongly oxidizing forms of oxygen

Oxidative stress is defined as a condition in which the rate of generation of ROS exceeds our ability to protect ourselves against them, resulting in an increase in oxidative damage to biomolecules (Fig. 42.2). Oxidative stress is a characteristic feature of inflammatory diseases in which cells of the immune system produce ROS in response to challenge. Oxidative stress may be localized, for instance, in the joints in arthritis or in the vascular wall in atherosclerosis, or can be systemic, for example, in systemic lupus erythematosus (SLE) or diabetes.

Among the ROS, **H_2O_2** is present at the highest concentration in blood and tissues, albeit at micromolar or lower concentrations. H_2O_2 is relatively stable; it can be stored in the laboratory or medicine cabinet for years but decomposes in the presence of redox-active metal ions. The **hydroxyl radical** ($OH^•$) is the most reactive and damaging species; its half-life, measured in

A   Fenton reaction

$$Fe^{2+} + H_2O_2 \longrightarrow Fe^{3+} + OH^{\bullet} + OH^-$$

B   Haber–Weiss reaction

$$O_2^{\bullet -} + H_2O_2 \longrightarrow O_2 + OH^{\bullet} + OH^-$$

C   Metal-catalyzed Haber–Weiss reactions

Fig. 42.3 **Formation of ROS by the Fenton and Haber–Weiss reactions.** (A) Fenton first described the oxidizing (bleaching) power of solutions of Fe^{2+} and H_2O_2. This reaction generates the strong oxidant $OH^{\bullet}$. Cu^+ catalyzes the same reaction. (B) The Haber–Weiss reaction describes the production of $OH^{\bullet}$ from $O_2^{\bullet}$ and H_2O_2. (C) Under physiologic conditions, the Haber–Weiss reaction is catalyzed by redox-active metal ions.

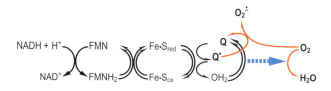

Fig. 42.4 **Formation of superoxide by mitochondria**. The mitochondrion is considered the major source of ROS in nucleated cells - this is where most oxidative metabolism occurs. After the oxidation of NADH (Complex I) or $FADH_2$ (Complex II), the electron transport chain catalyzes single-electron redox reactions. The semiquinone radical, an intermediate in the reduction of Q to QH_2 (Chapter 8), is sensitive to oxidation by molecular oxygen and is considered a major source of superoxide radicals in the cell.

nanoseconds, is diffusion limited (i.e., determined by the time to collision with a target biomolecule). **Superoxide** ($O_2^{\bullet}$) is intermediate in stability and may actually serve as either an oxidizing or a reducing agent, forming H_2O_2 or O_2, respectively. At physiologic pH, the **hydroperoxyl radical** (HOO$^{\bullet}$, $pK_a < 4.5$), the protonated form of superoxide (see Fig. 42.1), represents only a small fraction of total $O_2^{\bullet}$ (about 0.1%), but this radical is intermediate in reactivity, between $O_2^{\bullet}$ and $OH^{\bullet}$. HOO$^{\bullet}$ and H_2O_2 are small, uncharged molecules and readily diffuse through cell membranes.

ROS are formed by three major mechanisms in vivo: by reaction of oxygen with decompartmentalized metal ions (Fig. 42.3), as a side reaction of mitochondrial electron transport (Fig. 42.4), or by normal enzymatic reactions, such as formation of H_2O_2 by fatty acid oxidases in the peroxisome (Chapter 11). Secondary ROS are also formed by enzymatic reactions; for example, myeloperoxidase in the macrophage catalyzes the reaction of H_2O_2 with Cl^- to produce another ROS, hypochlorous acid (HOCl).

ADVANCED CONCEPT BOX
RADIOTHERAPY: MEDICAL APPLICATION OF REACTIVE OXYGEN

Radiation therapy uses a focused beam of high-energy electrons or γ-rays from an X-ray or cobalt-60 source to destroy tumor tissue. The radiation produces a flux of hydroxyl radicals (from water) and organic radicals at the site of the tumor. The localized oxidative stress causes damage to all biomolecules in the tumor cell, but the damage to DNA is critical - it prevents tumor cell replication, inhibiting tumor growth. Irradiation is also used as a method of sterilization of food, destroying the DNA of viral or bacterial contaminants or insect infestations and preserving food products during long-term storage.

Exposure to ionizing radiation from nuclear explosions or accidents, or breathing or ingestion of radioactive elements, such as radon gas or strontium-90, also causes oxidative damage to DNA. Cells that survive the damage may have mutations in DNA that eventually lead to the development of cancers. Leukemias are particularly prominent because of the rapid division of bone marrow cells.

CLINICAL BOX
TOXICITY OF HYPEROXIA

Supplemental oxygen therapy may be used for the treatment of patients with hypoxemia, patients with respiratory distress, or patients who have been exposed to carbon monoxide. Under normobaric conditions, the fraction of oxygen in air can be increased to nearly 100% using a facial mask or nasal cannula. However, patients develop chest pain, cough, and alveolar damage within a few hours of exposure to 100% oxygen. Edema gradually develops and compromises pulmonary function. The damage results from overproduction of ROS in the lung. Rats can be protected from oxygen toxicity by gradually increasing the oxygen tension over a period of several days. During this time, antioxidant enzymes, such as superoxide dismutase, are induced in the lung and provide increased protection against oxygen toxicity.

The lung is not the only tissue affected by hyperoxia. Premature infants, especially those with acute respiratory distress syndrome (ARDS), often require supplemental oxygen for survival. During the 1950s, it was recognized that the high oxygen tension used in incubators for premature infants increased the risk for blindness, resulting from retinopathy of prematurity (retrolental fibroplasia).

REACTIVE NITROGEN SPECIES (RNS) AND NITROSATIVE STRESS

Peroxynitrite is a strongly oxidizing reactive nitrogen species

Nitric oxide synthases (NOS) catalyze the production of the free radical nitric oxide (NO$^{\bullet}$) from the amino acid L-arginine.

CLINICAL BOX
ISCHEMIA/REPERFUSION INJURY: A PATIENT WITH MYOCARDIAL INFARCTION

A patient suffered a severe myocardial infarction, which was treated with tissue plasminogen activator, a clot-dissolving (thrombolytic) enzyme. During the days after hospitalization, the patient experienced palpitations, or irregular rapid heartbeat, associated with weakness and faintness. The patient was treated with antiarrhythmic agents.

Comment
Ischemia, meaning limited blood flow, is a condition in which a tissue is deprived of oxygen and nutrients. Damage to heart tissue during a myocardial infarction occurs not during the hypoxic or ischemic phase but during reoxygenation of the tissue. This type of damage also occurs after transplantation and cardiovascular surgery. ROS are thought to play a major role in reperfusion injury. When cells are deprived of oxygen, they must rely on anaerobic glycolysis and glycogen stores for ATP synthesis. NADH and lactate accumulate, and all the components of the mitochondrial electron transport system are saturated with electrons (reduced) because the electrons cannot be transferred to oxygen. The mitochondrial membrane potential is increased (hyperpolarized), and when oxygen is reintroduced, great quantities of ROS are rapidly produced, overwhelming antioxidant defenses. ROS flood throughout the cell, damaging membrane lipids, DNA, and other vital cellular constituents, leading to necrosis. Antioxidant supplements and drugs are being evaluated for use during recovery from myocardial infarction and stroke, during surgery, and for the protection of tissues before transplantation.

There are three isoforms of NOS: nNOS in neuronal tissue, where NO$^{\bullet}$ serves a neurotransmitter function; iNOS in the immune system, where it is involved in regulation of the immune response; and eNOS in endothelial cells, where NO$^{\bullet}$, known as endothelium-derived relaxation factor (EDRF), has a role in the regulation of vascular tone.

In a side reaction at sites of inflammation, NO$^{\bullet}$ reacts with $O_2^{\bullet}$ to form the strong oxidant and RNS peroxynitrite (ONOO$^-$). Like ROS, which produce oxidative stress, RNS produce nitrosative stress by reaction with biomolecules. ONOOH has many of the strong oxidizing properties of OH$^{\bullet}$ but has a longer biological half-life. It is also a potent nitrating agent, producing nitrotyrosine in proteins, nitrated phospholipids in membranes, and nucleotides in DNA. Simultaneous production of NO$^{\bullet}$ and $O_2^{\bullet}$, with the concomitant increase in ONOO$^-$ and a decrease in NO$^{\bullet}$, is thought to limit vasodilatation and exacerbate hypoxia and oxidative stress in the vascular wall during ischemia-reperfusion injury, setting the stage for vascular disease. ONOOH degrades, in part, by homolytic cleavage to produce two very reactive species, OH$^{\bullet}$ and NO$_2^{\bullet}$. NO$_2^{\bullet}$ is also formed by eosinophil peroxidase or myeloperoxidase-catalyzed oxidation of NO$^{\bullet}$ by H_2O_2.

THE NATURE OF OXYGEN RADICAL DAMAGE

The hydroxyl radical is the most reactive and damaging ROS

The reaction of ROS with biomolecules produces characteristic products, described as biomarkers of oxidative stress. These compounds may be formed either directly in the oxidation reaction with the ROS or by secondary reactions between oxidation products and other biomolecules. The hydroxyl radical reacts with biomolecules primarily by hydrogen abstraction and addition reactions. One of the most sensitive sites of free radical damage are cell membranes, which are rich in readily oxidized polyunsaturated fatty acids (PUFA). Peroxidative damage to the plasma membrane affects the integrity and function of the membrane, compromising the cell's ability to maintain ion gradients and membrane phospholipid asymmetry. As shown in Fig. 42.5, when OH$^{\bullet}$ abstracts a hydrogen atom from a PUFA, it initiates a chain of lipid peroxidation reaction, producing secondary oxidation products, lipid peroxides, and lipid peroxyl radicals. The lipid oxidation products formed in this reaction degrade to form reactive carbonyl compounds, such as **malondialdehyde** (MDA) and **hydroxynonenal** (HNE). These compounds react with proteins to form adducts and crosslinks, known as **advanced lipoxidation end products (ALE)**. MDA and HNE adducts to lysine residues are increased in lipoproteins in plasma and the vascular wall in atherosclerosis and in amyloid plaque in Alzheimer's disease, implicating oxidative stress and damage in the pathogenesis of these diseases.

Hydroxyl radicals also react by addition to phenylalanine, tyrosine, and nucleic acid bases to form hydroxylated derivatives and crosslinks (Fig. 42.6). Other ROS and RNS leave tell-tale tracks, such as nitro- and chlorotyrosine, formed from ONOOH and HOCl, respectively, and methionine sulfoxide, formed by reaction of H_2O_2 or HOCl with methionine residues in proteins (see Fig. 42.6). Nitrotyrosine, like ALEs, is increased in atherosclerotic and Alzheimer's plaques.

ROS also react with carbohydrates to form reactive carbonyl compounds that react with protein to form **adducts and crosslinks, known as advanced glycation end products (AGE)**. AGEs are increased in tissue proteins in diabetes as a result of hyperglycemia and oxidative stress, and the increase in chemical modification of proteins by AGEs and ALEs is implicated in the development of diabetic vascular, renal, and retinal complications (see Chapter 31).

ANTIOXIDANT DEFENSES

There are several levels of protection against oxidative damage

ROS damage to lipids and proteins is repaired largely by degradation and resynthesis. Oxidized proteins, for example, are

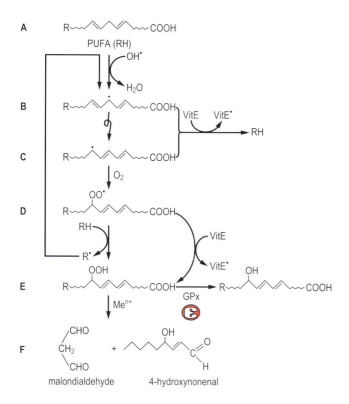

Fig. 42.5 Pathway of lipid peroxidation. OH• attacks PUFA (A), forming a carbon-centered lipid radical (B). The radical rearranges to form a conjugated dienyl radical (C). This radical reacts with ambient O_2, forming a hydroperoxyl radical (D), which then abstracts a hydrogen from a neighboring lipid, forming a lipid peroxide (E) and regenerating R• (B), initiating a cyclic chain reaction. This reaction continues until the supply of PUFA is exhausted, unless a termination reaction occurs. Vitamin E (discussed later in the chapter) is the major chain-terminating antioxidant in membranes; it reduces both the conjugated dienyl and the hydroperoxyl radicals, quenching the chain or cycle of lipid peroxidation reactions. Lipid peroxides may also be reduced by glutathione peroxidase (GPx), forming inert lipid alcohols. Otherwise, they decompose to form a range of **"reactive carbonyl species,"** such as malondialdehyde and hydroxynonenal (F), which react with protein to form advanced lipoxidation end products (ALE), which are biomarkers of oxidative stress. The reaction scheme shown here for PUFA also occurs with intact phospholipids and cholesterol esters in lipoproteins and cell membranes.

preferred targets for proteasomal degradation, and damaged DNA is repaired by a number of excision-repair mechanisms. The process is not perfect. Some proteins, such as collagens and crystallins, turn over slowly, so damage accumulates, and function may be impaired (e.g., age-dependent browning and precipitation of lens proteins (leading to cataracts), crosslinking of collagen and elastin, and loss of elasticity or changes in permeability of the vascular wall and renal basement membrane; see Chapter 29). The association between chronic inflammation and cancer indicates that chronic exposure to ROS causes cumulative damage to the genome in the form of nonlethal mutations in DNA.

Our first line of defense against oxidative damage is sequestration or chelation of redox-active metal ions

Endogenous chelators include a number of metal-binding proteins that sequester iron and copper in inactive form, such as transferrin and ferritin, the transport and storage forms of iron. The plasma protein haptoglobin binds to hemoglobin from ruptured red cells and delivers the hemoglobin molecule to the liver for catabolism. Plasma hemopexin binds heme, the lipid-soluble form of iron, which catalyzes ROS formation in lipid environments; it delivers the heme to the liver for

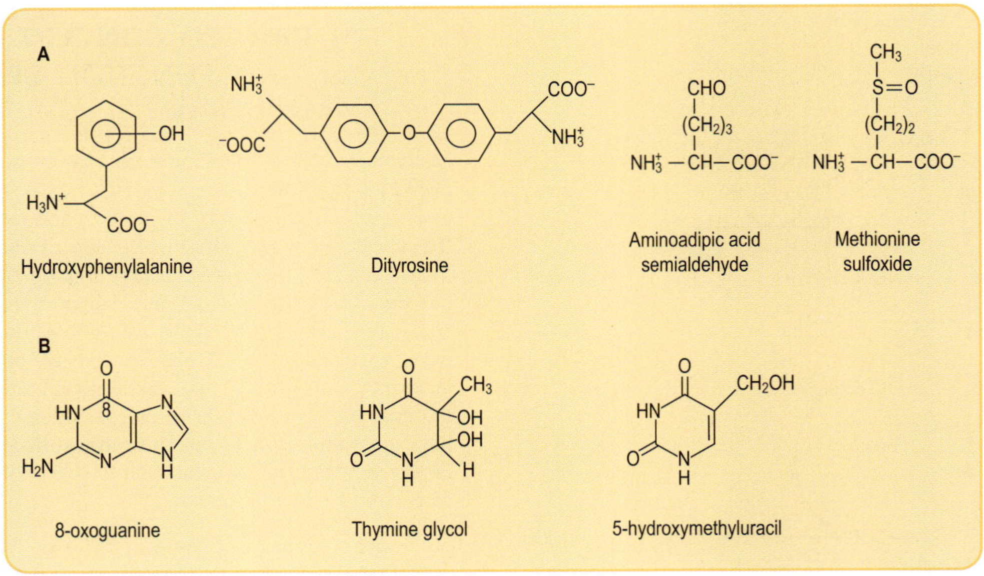

Fig. 42.6 **Products of hydroxyl radical damage to biomolecules.** (A) Amino acid oxidation products: *o*-, *m*- and *p*-tyrosine and dityrosine from phenylalanine; amino adipic acid semialdehyde from lysine; methionine sulfoxide. Other products include chlorotyrosine (from HOCl), nitrotyrosine (from ONOO⁻ and NO₂•), dihydroxyphenylalanine produced by hydroxylation of tyrosine, and aliphatic amino acid hydroperoxides, such as leucine hydroperoxide. (B) Nucleic acid oxidation products: 8-oxoguanine, thymine glycol, 5-hydroxymethyluracil, and others. 8-Oxoguanine is the most commonly measured indicator of DNA damage.

ADVANCED CONCEPT BOX
SELENIUM, AN ANTIOXIDANT MICRONUTRIENT

Selenocysteine is an unusual amino acid found in only 25 proteins in the human proteome. It is encoded by UGA, which is normally a STOP codon, under the direction of a SElenoCysteine Insertion Sequence (SECIS), a 50-nucleotide stem-loop structure in the mRNA. The 25-member selenoproteome includes five glutathione peroxidase isozymes, three thioredoxin reductases, methionine sulfoxide reductase (one of three enzymes that reduce methionine sulfoxide back to methionine), and three iodothyronine deiodinases. Selenium is essential for life, in part because of severe hypothyroidism and oxidative stress in its absence. Selenium deficiency in adults is associated with cardiomyopathy in Keshan disease, with osteoarthropathy (cartilage degeneration) in Kashin–Beck disease, and with symptoms of hypothyroidism, including chronic fatigue and goiter.

ADVANCED CONCEPT BOX
THE ANTIOXIDANT RESPONSE ELEMENT

Cells adapt to oxidative stress by induction of antioxidant enzymes. Many of these are controlled by the **antioxidant response element** (ARE), also known as the electrophile response element. The central regulator of the ARE is the transcription factor Nrf2, which is retained in an inactive form in the cytoplasmic compartment by binding to a cysteine-rich protein, Keap1. Under normal conditions, Keap1 directs ubiquitination and proteasomal degradation of Nrf2. During oxidative stress, modification of the sulfhydryl groups of Keap1 by nucleophiles, such as the lipid peroxidation products hydroxynonenal and acrolein, causes dissociation of Nrf2 from Keap1. Nrf2 then translocates to the nucleus and activates ARE-dependent genes. Keap1 also reacts with exogenous nucleophiles, including carcinogens that would otherwise react with DNA.

ARE-dependent enzymes include catalase (CAT), superoxide dismutase (SOD), and enzymes that catalyze the oxidation and conjugation of carcinogens and oxidants for excretion. One of these enzymes, hepatic glutathione *S*-transferase, catalyzes conjugation with GSH. The conjugates are then excreted in urine as **mercapturic acid,** which is an *S*-substituted *N*-acetyl-cysteine derivative.

CLINICAL BOX
A 36-YEAR-OLD MAN ADMITTED AFTER AN AUTOMOBILE ACCIDENT: RHABDOMYOLYSIS

A 36-year-old man presented to the emergency room after an automobile accident the previous evening. He had heavy bruising on his upper body and legs as a result of the impact. X-rays of his pelvis and hip showed no fractures and there was no evidence of head trauma - a good air bag! His creatine kinase (CK) level was >30,000 U/L (55–170 U/L), mostly the MM isozyme, suggesting that the accident was not the result of loss of control following a myocardial infarction. His plasma troponin T was also normal. Urine was tea-brown in color and yielded a positive urine dipstick for blood; however, no red cells were detected in urine. Creatinine was 150 umol/L(1.69 mg/dL), reference value 44-80 umol/Ll(0.50-0.90 mg/dL) Plasma potassium was 5.5 mmol/L (3.5 − 5.3 mmol/L).

Comment: The elevated level of the muscle isozyme, creatine kinase, and tea-colored urine is consistent with a diagnosis of rhabdomyolysis, the breakdown of striated muscle (from the Greek *rhabdos* = rod) as a result of crush syndrome (a compression of muscle and following reperfusion). This is a serious condition resulting from the breakdown of skeletal muscle and release of muscle cytoplasmic proteins, including myoglobin, into plasma. Since the dipstick test does not distinguish hemoglobin from myoglobin, the absence of red blood cells in urine suggests that the pigment is not hemoglobin. The breakdown of muscle releases potassium. A high potassium may also reflect compromised renal tubular function, confirmed by elevated plasma creatinine concentration.

Rhabdomyolysis may be caused by crush injury, extended immobilization, extreme physical exercise, genetic disease such as McArdle's Disease (muscle phosphorylase deficiency; Chapter 37), and some drugs, such as statins. Myoglobin is a low-molecular-weight protein that is filtered through the glomerulus and partially resorbed in renal tubules, resulting in myoglobinuria. Under acidic conditions, the heme group of myoglobin induces oxidative stress and renal tubular damage. The patient was treated with intravenous fluids, and his renal function returned to normal before he was discharged.

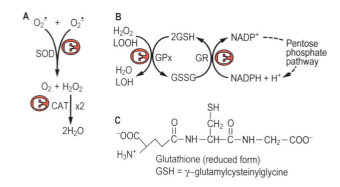

Fig. 42.7 **Enzymatic defenses against ROS.** (A) Superoxide dismutase (SOD) and catalase (CAT) are dismutases, catalyzing simultaneous oxidation and reduction of two separate substrate molecules; both are highly specific for their substrates, $O_2^{\bullet}$ and H_2O_2, respectively. (B) Glutathione peroxidase (GPx) reduces H_2O_2 and lipid peroxides (LOOH), using GSH as a cosubstrate. The GSH is recycled by glutathione reductase (GR) using NADPH from the pentose phosphate pathway. (C) Structure of GSH.

SOD: an MnSOD isozyme, which is found in mitochondria, and CuZnSOD isozyme, which is widely distributed throughout the cell. An extracellular secreted glycoprotein isoform of CuZnSOD (EC-SOD) binds to proteoglycans in the vascular wall and is thought to protect against $O_2^{\bullet}$ and $ONOO^-$ injury. CAT, which inactivates H_2O_2, is found largely in peroxisomes, the major site of H_2O_2 generation in the cell.

GPx is widely distributed in the cytosol, in mitochondria, and in the nucleus. It reduces H_2O_2 and lipid hydroperoxides to water and a lipid alcohol, respectively, using reduced glutathione (GSH) as a cosubstrate. GSH is a tripeptide (γ-glutamyl-cysteinyl-glycine; Fig. 42.7) that is present at a 1- to 5-mM concentration in all cells. The GSH is recycled by an NADPH-dependent enzyme, GSH reductase. The NADPH, provided by the pentose phosphate pathway, maintains a GSH:GSSG ratio of about 100:1 in the cell. GPx is actually a family of selenium-containing isozymes; a phospholipid hydroperoxide glutathione peroxidase will reduce lipid hydroperoxides in phospholipids in lipoproteins and membranes, whereas other isozymes are specific for free fatty acid or cholesterol ester hydroperoxides. There is also an isoform of GPx in intestinal epithelial cells, which is thought to have a role in detoxification of dietary hydroperoxides (e.g., in fried foods).

Vitamin C is the outstanding antioxidant in biological systems

Three antioxidant vitamins, A, C, and E, provide the third line of defense against oxidative damage. These vitamins, primarily vitamin C (ascorbate; Fig. 42.8) in the aqueous phase and vitamin E (α- and γ-tocopherol; Fig. 42.9) in the lipid phase, act as chain-breaking antioxidants (see Fig. 42.5). They act as reducing agents, donating a hydrogen atom (H·) and quenching organic radicals formed by reaction of ROS with biomolecules. The vitamin C and E radicals produced in this reaction are unreactive, resonance-stabilized species;

catabolism. Albumin, the major plasma protein, has a strong binding site for copper and effectively inhibits copper-catalyzed oxidation reactions in plasma. Carnosine (β-alanyl-L-histidine) and related peptides are present in muscle and brain at millimolar concentrations; they are potent copper chelators and may have a role in intracellular antioxidant protection.

Despite these manifold and potent metal chelation systems, ROS are formed continuously in the body, both by enzymes and by spontaneous metal-catalyzed reactions. In these cases, there is a group of enzymes that act to detoxify ROS and their precursors. These include **superoxide dismutase (SOD), catalase (CAT),** and **glutathione peroxidase (GPx**; Fig. 42.7). SOD converts $O_2^{\bullet}$ to the less toxic H_2O_2. There are two classes of

they do not propagate radical damage and are enzymatically recycled (e.g., by dehydroascorbate reductase; see Fig. 42.8). Vitamin C reduces superoxide and lipid peroxyl radicals but also has a special role in reduction and recycling of vitamin E. In response to severe oxidative stress, vitamin C recycles vitamin E so that vitamin E is maintained at constant concentration in the lipid phase until all the vitamin C is consumed (see Fig. 42.9). These antioxidants work together to inhibit lipid peroxidation reactions in plasma lipoproteins and membranes. Vitamin A (carotene; Chapter 7) is also a lipophilic antioxidant. Although best understood for its role in vision, it is a potent singlet oxygen scavenger and protects against damage from sunlight in the retina and skin.

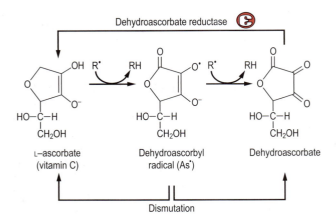

Fig. 42.8 Antioxidant activity of ascorbate. Vitamin C exists as the enolate anion at physiologic pH. The enolate anion spontaneously reduces superoxide, organic (R•) and vitamin E radicals, forming a dehydroascorbyl radical (As•). Dehydroascorbyl radical may dismutate to ascorbate and dehydroascorbate. Dehydroascorbate is recycled by dehydroascorbate reductase, a GSH-dependent enzyme present in all cells.

Glutathionylation of proteins - protection against ROS under stress

Despite the multiplicity of defensive mechanisms, there is always some evidence of ongoing oxidative damage in tissues. Under physiologic conditions, when proteins are exposed to O_2, their sulfhydryl groups gradually oxidize to form disulfides, either intramolecularly or intermolecularly with other proteins. This is multistep process. First, a protein sulfhydryl group is oxidized to a **sulfenic acid** (PrSOH) by an ROS, such as H_2O_2 or HOCl, then the sulfenic acid reacts with another PrSH to form a crosslinked protein PrS-SPr. These crosslinking reactions may be reversed by glutathione to form oxidized glutathione and regenerate the native protein with free sulfhydryl groups. The reaction sequence is

$$PrSH + ROS \rightarrow PrSOH$$

$$PrSOH + PrSH \rightarrow PrS\text{-}SPr + H_2O$$

$$PrS\text{-}SPr + 2\,GSH \rightarrow 2\,PrSH + 2\,GSSG$$

During oxidative stress, there is a significant increase in S-glutathionylated proteins (PrS-SG) in the cell. In this case, the reaction sequence is

$$PrSH + ROS \rightarrow PrSOH$$

$$PrSOH + GSH \rightarrow PrS\text{-}SG + H_2O$$

$$PrS\text{-}SG + GSH \rightarrow PrSH + GSSG$$

S-glutathionylation is reversed by nonenzymatic reduction by GSH or by enzymes using thiol protein cofactors (**thioredoxin**, glutaredoxin). This pathway inhibits the formation of crosslinked protein aggregates, such as **Heinz bodies,** which are hemoglobin precipitates that develop in red cells in glucose-6-phosphate dehydrogenase deficiency, characterized by decreased levels of GSH (Chapter 9). S-glutathionylation is thought to have a dual role, not only in protecting cysteine

Fig. 42.9 Antioxidant activity of vitamin E. The term vitamin E refers to a family of tocopherol and tocotrienol isomers with potent lipophilic antioxidant and membrane-stabilizing activity. Tocopherols reduce lipid hydroperoxyl radicals and also inactivate singlet oxygen. α-Tocopherol is the most effective form in humans and the major form of vitamin E in the diet. It consists of a chromanol ring structure with a polyisoprenoid side chain, which helps anchor the vitamin in membranes; the isoprene units are unsaturated in tocotrienol. The α, β, γ, and δ isomers differ in the pattern of methyl groups on the benzene ring (see Fig. 11.3). The major commercial form of vitamin E is α-tocopherol acetate, which is more stable than free tocopherol during storage. The tocopheryl radical, the major product formed during antioxidant action of vitamin E, is recycled by ascorbate. Tocopheryl quinone is also formed in small quantities.

against irreversible oxidation to the sulfinic or sulfonic acid during oxidative and/or nitrosative stress but also in modulating cellular metabolism (redox regulation). Target proteins include a wide range of enzymes with active site or regulatory –SH groups, such as glyceraldehyde-3-phosphate dehydrogenase in glycolysis and protein kinases in signaling cascades, as well as chaperones and transport proteins. S-glutathionylation appears to limit irreversible oxidation of thiol groups to sulfonic acids and sulfones and protect proteins from ubiquitin-mediated proteasomal degradation during oxidative stress.

CLINICAL TEST BOX
PEROXIDASE ACTIVITY FOR DETECTION OF OCCULT BLOOD

Peroxidases, such as the glutathione peroxidase (GPx), are enzymes that catalyze the oxidation of a substrate using H_2O_2. Hemoglobin and heme have a pseudoperoxidase activity in vitro. In the guaiac-based test for occult fecal blood, a stool sample is applied to a small card containing guaiac acid. Hemoglobin in a stool specimen oxidizes phenolic compounds in guaiac acid to quinones. A positive test is indicated by a blue stain along the edge of the fecal smear. Incompletely digested hemoglobin and myoglobin from animal meat and some plant peroxidases may cause false positives. Similar peroxidase-dependent assays are used to identify bloodstains at crime scenes.

THE BENEFICIAL EFFECTS OF REACTIVE OXYGEN SPECIES

ROS are essential for many metabolic and signaling pathways

Although this chapter has focused thus far on the dangerous aspects of reactive oxygen, it is worth closing with some recognition of the beneficial effects of ROS. Among these are the regulatory functions of NO, the role of ROS in activation of the ARE, the requirement for ROS in the bactericidal activity of macrophages (Fig. 42.11), and the use of ROS as substrates for enzymes (e.g., H_2O_2 for the hemeperoxidases involved in iodination of thyroid hormone). There is also increasing evidence that ROS, particularly H_2O_2, are important signaling molecules involved in the regulation of metabolism. The tissue concentration of H_2O_2 is estimated to be in the submicromolar range; estimates vary widely, from 1 to 700 nmol/L. However, significant changes in H_2O_2 concentration occur in response to cytokines, growth factors, and biomechanical stimulation. The fact that these signaling events are inhibited by peroxide scavengers or by overexpression of catalase implicates H_2O_2 in the signaling cascade. Insulin signaling, for example, appears to

ADVANCED CONCEPT BOX
THE GLYOXALASE PATHWAY: A SPECIAL ROLE FOR GLUTATHIONE

A small fraction of triose phosphates produced during metabolism spontaneously degrades to **methylglyoxal** (MGO), a reactive dicarbonyl sugar. MGO is also formed during metabolism of glycine and threonine and as a product of nonenzymatic oxidation of carbohydrates and lipids - it is a significant precursor of advanced glycation and lipoxidation end products (AGE/ALEs; see Chapters 29 and 31). MGO reacts primarily with arginine residues in proteins but also with lysine, histidine, and cysteine, leading to enzyme inactivation and protein crosslinking.

MGO is inactivated by enzymes of the glyoxalase pathway, a GSH-dependent system found in all cells in the body. The glyoxalase pathway (Fig. 42.10) consists of two enzymes that catalyze an internal redox reaction in which carbon-1 of MGO is oxidized from an aldehyde to a carboxylic acid group, and carbon-2 is reduced from a ketone to a secondary alcohol. The end product, D-lactate, does not react with proteins; D-lactate is distinct from L-lactate, the product of glycolysis, but may be converted into L-lactate for further metabolism.

Levels of MGO and D-lactate are increased in the blood of diabetic patients because levels of glucose and glycolytic intermediates, including triose phosphates, are increased intracellularly in diabetes. The glyoxalase system also inactivates glyoxal and other dicarbonyl sugars produced during nonenzymatic oxidation of carbohydrates and lipids. Glyoxalase inhibitors are being evaluated for chemotherapy because cancer cells appear to be more sensitive to glyoxalase inhibitors, perhaps because of their increased reliance on glycolysis.

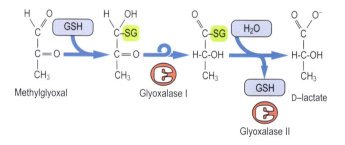

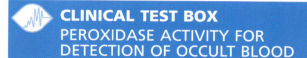

Fig. 42.10 **The glyoxalase system.** Glyoxalase I catalyzes the formation of a thiohemiacetal adduct between GSH and MGO and its rearrangement to a thioester. Glyoxalase II catalyzes the hydrolysis of the thioester, forming D-lactate and regenerating GSH. Unlike GPx, this pathway does not consume GSH.

involve H_2O_2 as part of the mechanism for reversible inactivation of some protein tyrosine phosphatases at the same time that protein tyrosine kinases are activated through the insulin receptor (Chapter 31). As the evidence for the signaling role of H_2O_2 has become convincing, there is increasing interest in research on the regulatory role of superoxide.

ADVANCED CONCEPT BOX
THE RESPIRATORY BURST IN MACROPHAGES

As outlined in Fig. 42.11, macrophages launch a sequence of ROS-producing reactions during the burst of oxygen consumption accompanying phagocytosis. **NADPH oxidase** in the macrophage plasma membrane is activated to produce $O_2^{\bullet}$, which is then converted to H_2O_2 by superoxide dismutase. The H_2O_2 is used by another macrophage enzyme, myeloperoxidase (MPO), to oxidize chloride ion, ubiquitous in body fluids, to hypochlorous acid (HOCl). H_2O_2 and HOCl mediate bactericidal activity by oxidation and chlorination of microbial lipids, proteins, and DNA. The macrophage has a high intracellular concentration of antioxidants, especially ascorbate, to protect itself during ROS production, but its relatively short life span, 2–4 months, suggests that it is not immune to oxidative damage.

The consumption of O_2 by NADPH oxidase is responsible for the "**respiratory burst**," the sharp increase in O_2 consumption for production of ROS, that accompanies phagocytosis. One of the end products of this reaction sequence, HOCl, is also the active oxidizer in chlorine-containing laundry bleaches. Intravenous infusion of dilute HOCl solutions was actually used for the treatment of bacterial sepsis in battlefield hospitals during World War I, before the advent of penicillin and other antibiotics. **Chronic granulomatous disease** (CGD) is an inherited disease resulting from a genetic defect in NADPH oxidase. The inability to produce superoxide leads to chronic life-threatening bacterial and fungal infections.

ADVANCED CONCEPT BOX
ANTIOXIDANT DEFENSES IN THE RED BLOOD CELL (RBC)

The RBC does not use oxygen for metabolism, nor is it involved in phagocytosis. However, because of the high O_2 tension in arterial blood and the heme iron content of RBCs, ROS are formed continuously in the RBC. Hb spontaneously produces superoxide ($O_2^{\bullet}$) in a minor side reaction associated with binding of O_2. The occasional reduction of O_2 to $O_2^{\bullet-}$ is accompanied by oxidation of normal (ferro) Hb to methemoglobin (ferrihemoglobin), a rust-brown protein that does not bind or transport O_2. **Methemoglobin** may release heme, which reacts with $O_2^{\bullet-}$ and H_2O_2 in Fenton-type reactions to produce hydroxyl radical ($OH^{\bullet}$) and reactive iron-oxo species. These ROS initiate lipid peroxidation reactions that can lead to loss of membrane integrity and cell death.

The RBC is well fortified with antioxidant defenses to protect itself against oxidative stress. These include catalase (CAT), superoxide dismutase (SOD), and glutathione peroxidase (GPx) as well as methemoglobin reductase activity that reduces methemoglobin back to normal ferrihemoglobin. Normally, less than 1% of Hb is present as methemoglobin. However, persons with congenital **methemoglobinemia,** resulting from methemoglobin reductase deficiency, typically have a dark and cyanotic appearance. Treatment with large doses of ascorbate (vitamin C) is used to reduce their methemoglobin to functional hemoglobin.

GSH, present at ~2 mmol/L in the RBC, not only supports antioxidant defenses but also is an important sulfhydryl buffer, maintaining –SH groups in hemoglobin and enzymes in the reduced state.

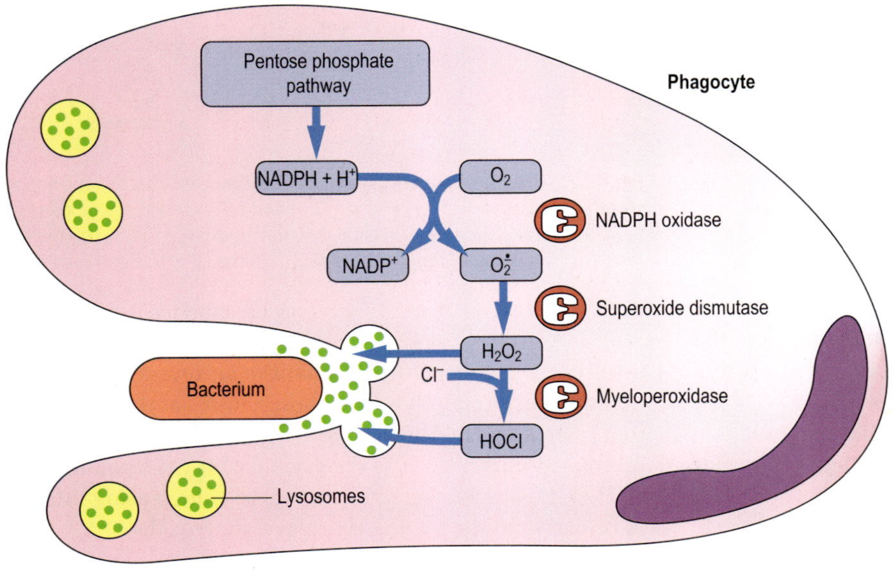

Fig. 42.11 **Generation and release of ROS during phagocytosis.** A cascade of reactions generating ROS is initiated during phagocytosis to kill invading organisms. Hydrolytic enzymes are also released from lysosomes to assist in degradation of microbial debris.

ACTIVE LEARNING

1. Review the evidence that atherosclerosis is an inflammatory disease resulting from overproduction of ROS in the vascular wall.
2. Discuss the evidence that hyperglycemia induces a state of oxidative stress that leads to renal and vascular complications in diabetes.
3. Review the data on the use of antioxidants in therapy for atherosclerosis and diabetes. Based on these studies, how strong is the evidence that the chronic pathology in these diseases is the result of increased oxidative stress?
4. Discuss recent advances in the use of antioxidants for organ and tissue protection during surgery and transplantation.

SUMMARY

- Reactive oxygen species (ROS) are the sparks produced by oxidative metabolism, and oxidative stress may be viewed as the price we pay for using oxygen for metabolism.
- ROS and RNS, such as superoxide, peroxide, hydroxyl radical, and peroxynitrite, are reactive, toxic, and sometimes difficult to contain, but their production is important for regulation of metabolism, turnover of biomolecules, and protection against microbial infection.
- ROS and RNS cause oxidative damage to all classes of biomolecules: proteins, lipids, and DNA.
- There are a number of protective antioxidant mechanisms, including sequestration of redox-active metal ions; enzymatic inactivation of major ROS; inactivation of organic radicals by small molecules, such as GSH and vitamins; and when all else fails, repair and/or turnover and, in extremis, apoptosis.
- Biomarkers of oxidative stress are readily detected in tissues in inflammation, and oxidative stress is increasingly implicated in the pathogenesis of age-related chronic disease.
- Despite their damaging actions, ROS are also essential for the normal functions of the immune system and for many enzymes and cell-signaling pathways.

FURTHER READING

Ahmed, S. M., Luo, L., Namani, A., et al. (2017). Nrf2 signaling pathway: Pivotal roles in inflammation. *Biochimica et Biophysica Acta, 1863*(2), 585–597.

Forman, H. J. (2016). Redox signaling: An evolution from free radicals to aging. *Free Radical Biology and Medicine, 97*, 398–407.

Halliwell, B., & Gutteridge, J. M. C. (2015). *Free radicals in biology and medicine* (5th ed.). Oxford, UK: Oxford University Press.

Koekkoek, W. A., & van Zanten, A. R. (2016). Antioxidant vitamins and trace elements in critical illness. *Nutrition in Clinical Practice, 31*, 457–474.

Speckmann, B., Steinbrenner, H., Grune, T., et al. (2016). Peroxynitrite: From interception to signaling. *Archives of Biochemistry and Biophysics, 595*, 153–160.

Wang, P., & Wang, Z. Y. (2017). Metal ions influx is a double edged sword for the pathogenesis of Alzheimer's disease. *Ageing Research Reviews, 35*, 265–290.

RELEVANT WEBSITES

Antioxidants and cancer: http://www.cancer.gov/cancertopics/factsheet/antioxidantsprevention

Oxidative stress and disease: http://www.oxidativestressresource.org/

Reactive oxygen species: http://www.biotek.com/resources/articles/reactive-oxygen-species.html

Virtual Free Radical School: http://www.sfrbm.org/sections/education/frs-presentations

ABBREVIATIONS

A1AT	Alpha-1 antitrypsin
AGE	Advanced glycation end-product
ALE	Advanced lipoxidation end-product
ARE	Antioxidant response element
CAT	Catalase
CGD	Chronic granulomatous disease
EDRF	Endothelial-derived relaxation factor
GPx	Glutathione peroxidase
HNE	Hydroxynonenal
MDA	Malondialdehyde
MGO	Methylglyoxal
MetSO	Methionine sulfoxide
MPO	Myeloperoxidase
NOS	Nitric oxide synthase
PUFA	Polyunsaturated fatty acid
RBC	Red blood cell
RNS	Reactive nitrogen species
ROS	Reactive oxygen species
SECIS	Selenocysteine insertion sequence
SLE	Systemic lupus erythematosus
SOD	Superoxide dismutase

The Immune Response: Innate and Adaptive Immunity

J. Alastair Gracie and Georgia Perona-Wright

LEARNING OBJECTIVES

After reading this chapter, you should be able to:

- Discuss the basis of the innate and adaptive immune responses, and describe the similarities and differences between them.
- Describe the cellular and humoral components of both innate and adaptive immunity, and explain their individual functions.
- Compare and contrast antigen recognition by the cells of both the innate and adaptive immune responses.
- Describe the characteristic features of an inflammatory response.
- Outline the functions of the key cytokines, chemokines, and adhesion molecules used by the immune system.
- Describe the main function of T-cell subsets that characterize the adaptive immune response.
- Describe the basis of antibody diversity.
- Discuss the consequence of aberrant immune responses that may result in immunodeficiency, hypersensitivity, or autoimmunity.

INTRODUCTION

The immune system has evolved to provide a coordinated response to protect the host from infection, both preventing invasion and eradicating pathogens as quickly as possible.

The immune system includes multiple layers of defense against pathogens, from the structural barriers that deter entry, to the cells and signals that destroy unwanted microbes, to the intricate mechanisms that enhance the defenses if the pathogen returns. A key feature of the immune system is its ability to recognize a pathogen and mount an exactly appropriate response.

The importance of a healthy and effective immune system can be seen in individuals who have one of the many **immunodeficiency states.** These patients present with a range of conditions, from minor recurring infections to life-threatening illnesses, depending on the severity of the immunodeficiency. Inappropriate responses can result in disease, including conditions such as **autoimmunity** or **hypersensitivity.** The

following sections will explain how the different parts of the immune system work together to protect against infection and discuss the benefits and risks for us as the host.

THREE LAYERS OF IMMUNE PROTECTION

The first line of defense is the anatomical and physiologic barriers of the body

The importance of protection against infection is such that any gaps in defense can be catastrophic. The immune system therefore uses multiple layers of defense, each reinforcing the others. The first line of defense is the physicochemical **barriers** of the body, such as the skin and mucosal epithelia and their associated secreted products (e.g., sweat, mucus, and acid). These anatomic and physiologic defenses are often referred to as natural or constitutive defenses because they are present and active even before any pathogen is encountered.

The second line of defense is innate immunity

If a pathogen successfully breaches the body's barriers, the immune system's **immediate** response to infection is called **innate immunity.** Key to innate immunity is the immune system's **ability to distinguish *self* from *non-self* -** that is, to identify a pathogen as something foreign that should not be present. Innate immunity is often also called nonspecific because the particular features of the individual pathogen matter less than the generic fact that it is a foreign pathogen. Some components of the same anatomical and physiologic defense system are also part of the innate immune system; for example, saliva contains enzymes such as lysozyme, which can damage bacterial cell walls. Lysozyme is constitutively present in saliva, and as such, it is a physiologic defense against infection. However, the concentration of lysozyme in salvia dramatically increases when the presence of a pathogen is detected, and this *response* is an example of innate immunity.

The third level of defense is the adaptive immune response

The innate immune system is able to defeat the great majority of infectious agents. For pathogens that evade innate immunity, additional highly specific, targeted defenses are essential. The activation of these targeted defenses constitutes the **adaptive immune response.** The adaptive immune response takes time to develop, but once active, it is powerful and highly effective. Its key features are that it is specific to an individual pathogen, being triggered by the recognition of unique components of the microbe, and that it is variable, with the cells and molecules selected to combat the pathogen being chosen in response to the specific infection under way. **Different pathogens elicit different adaptive immune responses.** Adaptive immunity also has the exclusive ability to **remember** any previous encounters with the same pathogen and to respond more quickly and more powerfully in subsequent interactions. Such immune memory is the basis of **vaccination,** which we discuss later in the chapter.

THE INNATE IMMUNE RESPONSE

When activated, the innate response can present as an inflammatory response

Innate immunity is the body's immediate response to an infection. It is a nonspecific response, meaning that the same response is mounted to a large number of different pathogens. When activated, the innate response is often seen as an **inflammatory response.** Inflammation is the body's response to injury or tissue damage. Its purpose is to limit, and then repair, the damage brought about by any injurious agent. It involves the interaction of the microvasculature, circulating blood cells, other immune cells in the tissues, and their secreted effector molecules. Endothelial activation, increased vascular permeability, and vasodilation allow the normally circulating leukocytes to migrate into tissue where, along with other tissue resident immune cells, they mount an effective and rapid response to try to eliminate the pathogen (Table 43.1). This will often include the release of toxic mediators and **phagocytosis,** a process first described more than 100 years ago by Mechnikov, who observed cells "eating" the pathogens. The vasodilation, cell activation, and accumulation of fluid in the tissues means that inflammation often presents clinically as **redness, swelling, heat, and pain.**

Table 43.1 Cells involved in inflammation

	Circulating	Tissue based
Polymorphonuclear leukocytes		
Neutrophil	Yes	Migrate as required
Eosinophil	Yes	Migrate as required
Basophil	Yes	Migrate as required
Mast cell		Yes
Mononuclear phagocytes	Monocyte	Macrophage
Lymphocytes (primarily part of adaptive response)	Yes	Migrate as required
Endothelial cells		Yes

Cells of the innate response

Neutrophils and monocytes are recruited to sites of infection

One of the key functions of inflammation is to allow phagocytes to enter the infected tissue. Neutrophils and monocytes, precursors of macrophages, are normally found circulating in the bloodstream and are recruited to sites of infection by the process of extravasation. Receptors on the phagocyte interact with ligands on vascular endothelium, and the cells attach, arrest, and move from the circulation to the infected tissue. Neutrophils are the most abundant leukocytes in the bloodstream, numbering 4000–10,000/mm^3. This increases rapidly during infection through recruitment from the bone marrow, and numbers often reach 20,000/mm^3. **Neutrophils are generally the first cells to respond to infection**, phagocytosing microbes in the circulation and moving rapidly into infected tissue. They are short-lived (normally a few hours to days) and die rapidly by apoptosis after reaching the tissue and exerting their effect (Table 43.1).

Monocytes transform into macrophages, which are the "trash can" of the immune response

Monocytes are found in much lower numbers within the blood, 500–1000/mm^3, and in contrast with neutrophils, they are longer lived. Similar to neutrophils, they can also migrate into tissue, and on doing so differentiate into macrophages. Macrophages have a number of key functions, including phagocytosis of infecting microbes, antigen presentation, and general removal of dying or damaged host cells. Indeed, the macrophage has often been termed the "trash can" of the immune response. Most organs of the body and connective tissue have **resident macrophages,** whose job it is to survey their environment for signs of infection. Incoming monocytes help to increase the number of macrophages in infected tissues. Both sets of macrophages respond to infection with the release of numerous cytokines and chemokines, secreted signals that initiate the inflammatory response (Table 43.1).

Neutrophils and macrophages use their receptors to recognize attacking microbes

To mount an efficient response to infection, neutrophils and macrophages must realize that the body is under attack. They do so through a number of **germline-encoded cell-surface and intracellular receptors** that, unlike the receptors used by cells of the adaptive immune response, are not produced by somatic recombination of their genes (Table 43.2). As a result, the response elicited by such receptors is amnesic, meaning that the cells will respond similarly on reinfection. The receptors involved in microbial recognition, often termed **pattern-recognition receptors (PRR)**, identify structures that are shared by various microbes and are generally not present on host cells, such as nucleic acids, lipids, sugars, proteins, or a combination of molecules. Often the structures recognized by these receptors, called **pathogen-associated molecular**

Table 43.2 Comparison of antigen receptors of innate and adaptive immunity

Receptor characteristic	Innate immunity	Adaptive immunity
Triggers an immediate response	Yes	No
Germline encoded	Yes	No
Specificity same across lineage	Yes	No
Broad spectrum of recognition	Yes	No
Encoded by multiple gene segments	No	Yes
Gene rearrangement occurs	No	Yes
Each receptor has unique specificity	No	Yes

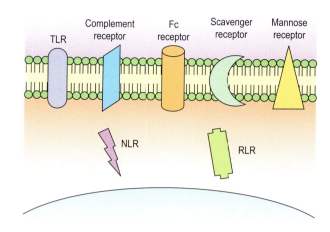

Fig. 43.1 **Phagocytes utilize numerous receptors to detect pathogens.** Cells of the innate immune system express numerous receptor types, both on the cell membrane and intracellularly, to detect pathogens and initiate an effective immune response. TLR, toll-like receptor; NLR, Nod-like receptor; RLR, Rig-1-like receptor. See text for details.

patterns **(PAMP)**, are conserved structural features required by the pathogen for survival or infectivity. They are typically shared by particular microbial families.

There are several main categories of pattern recognition receptors, classified according to location and function

The first is mannose-binding lectin (MBL), which is actually not a cell-associated molecule but rather a free circulating plasma protein; on recognizing and binding to the pathogen PAMP, MBL can activate the complement cascade via the lectin pathway (Fig. 43.1). Other mannose and scavenger receptors are cell-surface receptors. Mannose receptors belong to a larger family called **C-type lectin receptors (CLR)**, which, as their name suggests, detect carbohydrate moieties on pathogens. Both mannose and scavenger receptors allow direct microbial recognition by phagocytes. The remaining types of PRRs are either surface-bound receptors that promote the phagocytic function of the cell, or membrane-bound signaling receptors that are found either on the outer cell membrane, in the endosomes, or within the cell cytoplasm.

PRRs are used by innate immune cells to trigger many of their functions

One of the best-characterized signaling PRR families is the evolutionary conserved **toll-like receptor (TLR) system** in mammals, named after a homologous receptor system used by the *Drosophila* fruit fly for protection from infection. In humans, there are 10 expressed TLR genes (13 in mice), their products forming homo- or heterodimers with other family members, thus increasing the repertoire for recognition. TLR4, for example, has been shown to be the receptor recognizing lipopolysaccharide (LPS) found on the surface of Gram-negative bacteria such as *Escherichia coli* but not present on mammalian

cells. The effect of pathogen components binding to TLRs on innate immune cells is TLR activation, which initiates signaling into the immune cell and the increased expression of a large number of target genes. The genes involved depend on the pattern of TLRs engaged, but common outcomes include increased production of inflammatory mediators such as cytokines and chemokines, enhanced phagocytosis (internalization and killing of the pathogen), upregulation of costimulatory molecules on the cell surface, cell migration, and in the case of macrophages, increased processing and presentation of pathogen antigens to activate an adaptive immune response. Table 43.3 summarizes TLR function and cellular distribution. TLRs can be expressed either on the **external cell membrane** or on **intracellular vesicles** and function primarily to recognize extracellular pathogens. Certain intracellular TLRs (TLR 3/7/9) can detect viral RNAs and DNAs, but even these TLRs interact primarily with products from the extracellular pathogen that have entered the cell by the endocytic pathway.

NOD-like receptors are located in the cytoplasm

In contrast to TLRs, other pattern recognition receptors are located within the **cytoplasm**. These include the more recently described **NOD-like receptors** (NLR), which act as **intracellular sensors,** ultimately triggering the NFκB pathway. The outcome of NLR signaling results in similar responses to those activated by TLR engagement, including increased phagocytosis and the production of cytokines and chemokines. In the presence of certain pathogenic stimuli, TLRs and NLRs cooperate, activating a cytoplasmic multiprotein complex called the **inflammasome.** Inflammasome activation results in caspase-1 activation, leading to the processing and release of mature

Table 43.3 Toll-like receptor (TLR) ligands and cellular distribution			
TLR	**Cellular expression**	**Ligands**	**Pathogen species**
TLR1-TLR2 heterodimer	Monocytes, DCs	Zymosin	Fungi
TLR2-TLR6 heterodimer	NK cells Eosinophils Basophils	Lipoproteins Lipoteichoic acid β-glucans Lipomannans	Bacteria Gram-positive bacteria Bacteria and fungi Mycobacteria
TLR3	NK cells	Double-stranded RNA	Viruses
TLR4	Macrophages, DCs, eosinophils, mast cells	LPS	Gram-negative bacteria
TLR5	Gut epithelium	Flagellin	Bacteria
TLR7	DCs, NK cells, eosinophils, B cells	Single-stranded RNA	Viruses
TLR8	NK cells	Single-stranded RNA	Viruses
TLR9	DCs, NK cells, eosinophils, B cells, basophils	Unmethylated CpG (DNA)	Bacteria
TLR10	DCs, NK cells, eosinophils, B cells	Unknown	Bacteria

DC, dendritic cell, the main type of antigen-presenting cell; LPS, lipopolysaccharide; CpG, cytosine-guanine dinucleotide; NK cells, natural killer cells.

forms of proinflammatory cytokines, including IL-1 and IL-18. Another family of intracellular signaling PRRs is the RIG-1-like receptors (RLR), which detect viral RNAs and stimulate antiviral responses through the production of type I interferons (Fig. 43.1).

Inflammatory mediators contribute to the immune response

Innate immune cells such as neutrophils and macrophages function both to cause direct killing of the invading pathogen, largely through phagocytosis, and to activate other immune cells to amplify the defense response. Both neutrophils and macrophages, when activated through PRRs, synthesize and secrete a wide variety of different soluble chemical substances termed **inflammatory mediators**. Some are directly toxic to the pathogen, whereas others (cytokines) function to recruit and activate other immune cells. During inflammation, the liver also releases a number of these mediators into the blood, including acute-phase reactants such as C-reactive protein (CRP) and components of the complement system described later in this chapter.

Cytokines

Cytokines are soluble mediators of inflammatory and immune responses

Cytokines are produced by a variety of cell types, including those of the innate and adaptive immune responses. Covering a large number and different families, cytokines are small (usually less than 20 kDa) peptides or glycoproteins active at concentrations between 10^{-9} and 10^{-15} mol/L. In general, macrophages are often their main producers during innate responses, and T cells are the main producers during adaptive responses. Many cell types other than those of the immune system, including fibroblasts, epithelial cells, and adipocytes, can also secrete cytokines. All cytokines exert their effects by interacting with specific receptors on the surfaces of their target cells. The majority exert their effect on neighboring cells (paracrine action) or on the same cells that produced them (autocrine action). A few, however, signal to cells more distant from their site of production (endocrine action). The cytokine network displays both redundancy and pleiotropy, with several having overlapping effects and the ability to act on numerous cell types. Cytokines have been grouped into subfamilies, based on structure and function, as discussed briefly in the following list. Cytokine receptors are not restricted to cells of the immune system, being found widespread on disparate cell types. For more detail on cytokine signaling, see Chapter 25.

Cytokines may be classified into families by their principal effect:

- **Colony-stimulating factors:** As the name suggests, these are involved in the development and differentiation of immune cells from bone marrow precursors.
- **Interferons (IFN):** Whereas IFN-α and IFN-β have a role in inhibiting viral replication, IFN-γ regulates immune responses. The latter is made primarily by T cells and activates macrophages.
- **Interleukins (IL):** Currently, there are in excess of 30 interleukins recognized, participating in both innate and

adaptive immune responses. They are made by a number of immune (and other) cell types; as the name suggests, the principal function is communication between leukocytes.

- **Tumor necrosis factor (TNF) family:** This is a mixed collection of cytokines whose effects range from promoting inflammation (TNF-α and TNF-β) to stimulating osteoclasts and bone resorption (osteoprotegerin).
- **Chemokines:** These are a family of cytokines that bring about chemokinesis - cell movement in response to chemical stimuli. Interest has increased dramatically in the receptors for these mediators because some appear to act as coreceptors for infection (in particular, HIV infection of CD4+ T lymphocytes).

Cytokines in the innate immune response

Macrophages that are activated by direct interaction with pathogens are major producers of a number of cytokines that amplify inflammation. These include TNF-α, which increases vasodilation, and IL-1, IL-6, and IL-8, which recruit additional neutrophils and monocytes into the infected tissue. Several cytokines released by activated macrophages also promote the activation of the adaptive immune system.

The complement system

Activated complement proteins contribute to pathogen killing

The innate immune system is very effective in eradicating infections. Phagocytosis is one major mechanism of pathogen destruction, but other pathways also contribute. The complement system plays an important role in antimicrobial host defense. The complement system is a series of proteins, present in the blood, whose activation leads to the destruction of bacterial cell walls and consequent death of the pathogen. Certain complement proteins exist in soluble form, whereas others are membrane-bound. They are activated in a series of sequential steps. **There are three pathways of complement activation.** During the innate response, and in the absence of antibody, the alternative and lectin pathways activate complement. In both of these pathways, early complement proteins are activated by directly binding to structural components of the invading pathogen. For example, lipopolysaccharide found on Gram-negative bacterial cell walls triggers the alternative pathway, and mannose and other carbohydrates found in the cell walls of fungi, bacteria, and viruses trigger the lectin pathway. Later in the immune response, antibody produced during the adaptive response can bind microbial antigens and activate complement via the third pathway, called the **classic pathway.**

The **"classic activation pathway"** comprises complement components C1q, C1r, C1s, C4, and C2. Sequential activation of these components leads to the activation of the pivotal and critically important C3 component, which is an absolute requirement for full complement activation. Once this is achieved,

the terminal membrane attack complex, which comprises the components C5, C6, C7, C8, and C9, is activated. This complex eventually generates the polymeric ring structure that inserts into the cell membrane of bacteria and is responsible for cell lysis.

The classical pathway is triggered by C1q binding an IgG or IgM that is already bound to its specific antigen (see the following discussion).

In all cases, the sequential activation of complement proteins proceeds as a cascade, in which activated proteins activate subsequent members by proteolytic cleavage. It is an auto-amplifying response, rapidly producing a number of effector molecules involved in the elimination of the microbial infection, as shown in Fig. 43.2. The three activation pathways converge to produce a common outcome, whereby the late components combine with each other to form a multimolecular complex, called the **membrane attack complex,** that assembles on the surface of infecting organisms and breaches the integrity of the pathogen by insertion into their membranes. The cleavage fragments produced as a result of the cascade of complement activation also have multiple biological activities, which include enhancing phagocytosis through **opsonization,** increasing the recruitment of inflammatory cells through **chemotaxis,** and stimulating the degranulation of immune cells (**anaphylatoxin** activity).

Adhesion molecules

Adhesion molecules mediate adhesion between cells

Cellular interactions during an immune response are dependent on the expression of the molecules and ligands that mediate adhesion between cells or between cells and the extracellular matrix. These are termed "adhesion molecules." They are found on a wide variety of cell types, not only cells of the immune system but also, for instance, on vascular endothelium. A major determinant of their expression is the prevailing cytokine environment and the surrounding connective tissue matrix. Typically, they are **transmembrane glycoproteins.** They deliver intracellular signals, and during immune responses, they are primarily involved in promoting cell–cell interactions and cell migration. The migration includes the movement of innate cells from blood to tissue during infection as well as aiding lymphocytes to enter and leave lymph nodes as they circulate, looking for activation signals resulting from antigen presentation in these peripheral organs. Adhesion molecules involved in immunity are grouped into major families:

- **Integrins:** These are heterodimeric proteins expressed on leukocytes, such as lymphocyte function-associated antigen 1 (LFA-1) or the macrophage adhesion molecule 1 (MAC-1).
- **Immunoglobulin supergene family adhesion molecules:** These are often expressed on endothelial cells - for example, intercellular adhesion molecule 1 (ICAM-1; CD54) or platelet/cell adhesion molecule 1 (PECAM-1; CD31).

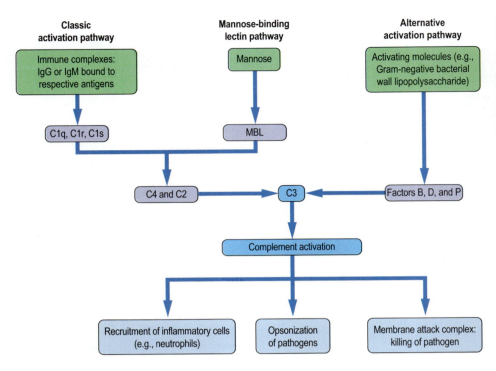

Fig. 43.2 **Complement cascade.** Activating stimuli include surfaces that trigger complement activation and to which the activated component can attach itself. Activation of complement recruits innate cells during the early phase of an immune response. The polymeric structure (the membrane attack complex) generated as a result of complement activation can insert itself into the activating surface (e.g., the bacterial cell wall), breaching its integrity and causing osmotic lysis. Note that activation of the classic pathway is triggered by C1q binding an IgG or IgM that is already bound to its specific antigen. The alternative pathway includes three proteins known as factor B, factor D (a serine protease), and factor P (properdin), which contribute to the activation of the C3 component. MBL, mannose-binding lectin.

- **Selectins:** These are expressed on leukocytes and endothelial cells (e.g., L-selectin or P-selectin).
- **Mucin-like vascular addressins:** These are often found on leukocytes and endothelium. They bind selectins.

DENDRITIC CELLS LINK THE INNATE AND ADAPTIVE IMMUNE RESPONSES

Antigen-presenting cells (APC) are specialized cells that display microbial antigens on their surface to initiate the adaptive immune response through activation of T cells

Dendritic cells (DC) are the major APC and are found in tissues throughout the body. The skin and different organs each have resident populations of such cells. Like macrophages, DCs have cell-surface and internal receptors, including TLRs, that allow them to interact with pathogens in the infected tissue; however, whereas macrophages respond to pathogens locally by increasing phagocytosis and producing cytokines, DCs engulf the pathogen and migrate out of the tissue and into the lymphatic circulation, then enter specialized secondary lymphoid organs such as lymph nodes. On uptake of antigen, APCs can process and reexpress it, in the context of specialized structures on the cell surface, to allow **presentation to the T cell**. Dendritic cells are termed **"professional APCs"** because, in addition to being able to present the antigen, they also possess a number of other cell-surface molecules (e.g., CD80, CD86, and CD40), which provide additional signals to the T cell. These additional signals are called "costimulation" and are required

by a naïve T cell for complete activation. In addition, DCs may release certain cytokines (e.g., IL-12) that influence T-cell activation and differentiation (see the following discussion). Macrophages and B cells are also capable of presenting antigens to T cells and hence can be considered APCs, but DCs are unique in their ability to migrate from infected tissues to the lymph nodes where naïve T cells are located, and hence DCs are the key to the initiation of the adaptive immune response.

ADAPTIVE IMMUNE RESPONSE

Specificity of the response is achieved through unique receptors that recognize antigen

Adaptive immune responses are essential when our innate defenses are unsuccessful. The adaptive response is slower than the innate, but it is highly specific and very effective. The two major cell types in the adaptive immune system are **T cells** and **B cells**, collectively called **lymphocytes**, and these cells are the foot soldiers of the immune defenses. The adaptive response begins when the lymphocytes recognize components of the infectious agent. The components of the infectious agents are called **antigens**, and **the binding of antigens to receptors on lymphocytes triggers an adaptive response.** Receptors on B cells and T cells differ and recognize quite different forms of antigen.

T and B lymphocytes have distinct cell-surface markers that can assist in assigning their identification

The effector cells primarily involved in the adaptive immune response are the T and B lymphocytes. In total, lymphocytes

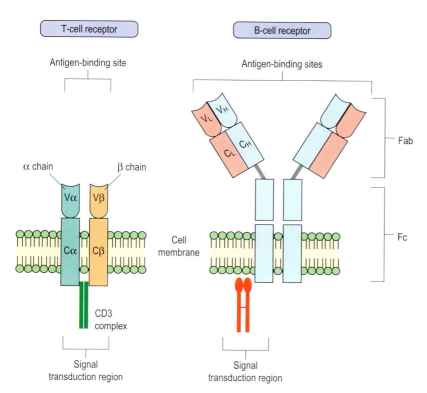

Fig. 43.3 **Similarity in structure of T- and B-cell antigen receptors.** The receptors used by T cells and B cells to detect antigen share structural similarity. V, variable regions; C, constant regions.

are present in the peripheral blood at $1.3–4.0 \times 10^9/L$; of these, approximately 50%–70% are T cells, and 10%–20% are B cells.

Identification of T- and B-cell lineages is possible by using either flow cytometry to identify their receptor expression or through functional studies. The surface markers on lymphocytes (and other immune cells) are classified according to the **cluster of differentiation (CD) system**. For example, T cells are positive for either CD4 or CD8, whereas B cells are CD19 positive. The distinction between T and B cells is most easily made with reference to their antigen-recognition receptors (Fig. 43.3).

B and T lymphocytes are activated by recognition of antigen and through costimulatory molecules

The antigen-recognition receptors on T cells and B cells are structurally different. Within each type of lymphocyte, however, there is great diversity in the precise shape of the antigen-recognition receptor on each cell: the overall structure is conserved, but there is intense variability in the contact sites that interact with the pathogen component. This diversity provides the exquisite specificity of the adaptive immune response. Each antigen is recognized by only one, or very few, T cells and B cells. When it encounters its one specific antigen, and on the receipt of additional costimulatory signals, the lymphocyte becomes activated and begins to proliferate and differentiate. For T cells, this occurs when DCs arrive in the lymph node, carrying antigens from the infected tissues. The antigens are displayed on the DC surface in the context of

surface structures called **major histocompatibility complex (MHC) molecules.** Macrophages and B cells also express MHC molecules. The part of the T cells that interacts with the antigen presented in MHC is called the **T-cell receptor (TCR).** The B-cell antigen-recognition receptor is named the **B-cell receptor (BCR),** and it is a surface immunoglobulin also termed surface Ig (sIg).

Molecules involved in antigen recognition

Antigen is recognized by specific receptors on T and B cells

The ability to recognize the enormous number of possible antigenic configurations is achieved by differences in the amino acid sequences of these receptors, which give rise to differences in their shape or conformation. The antigen and its specific receptor have a "hand-in-glove" relationship. Both T- and B-cell antigen receptors show marked variability in the sequence of amino acids that come into contact with the antigen, whereas other parts of these molecules are relatively constant with regard to their amino acid sequences.

Unlike the antigen receptors found on innate cells, which are germline encoded, the receptors found on the T and B cells are generated by random recombination of receptor genes during cell maturation. These antigen-recognition receptors are clonally distributed. As a result, each clone will exhibit unique specificity for a particular antigen, thus generating the enormous pool of cells capable of responding to all antigens.

As mentioned previously, T and B cells differ in how they recognize what is "foreign." The sIg antigen receptor found on B cells is capable of recognizing intact macromolecules (proteins, polysaccharides, lipids, etc.), whereas T-cell receptors recognize small peptides of proteins previously processed and presented by the APC.

Although the number of T- and B-cell clones, each recognizing different antigens, is enormous, the engagement by appropriate antigen will generally induce a similar response, that is, **signal transduction**. This may lead to full cell activation, resulting in antibody production for B cells; for T cells, it results in the proliferation and promotion of the cellular adaptive immune response.

Another group of surface receptors on T and B cells binds to the costimulatory molecules on APCs

After exposure to antigen, the interaction between T cells and DCs also allows CD28 on T cells to bind CD80 and CD86 on the APC and for CD40 ligand (CD40L) on the T cell to bind CD40 on the APC. Both signals, antigen and costimulation, are essential for full activation of a lymphocyte. B cells receive their costimulation from activated T cells: the sIg antigen receptor on the B cell recognizes free antigen, and CD40 on the B cell binds CD40L on a neighboring T cell, resulting in B-cell activation. Without costimulation, T and B cells would not be fully activated after exposure to antigen and could instead become **anergic** (i.e., permanently nonresponsive).

The T-cell antigen receptor

The T-cell antigen receptor is termed the T-cell receptor (TCR), and it is complexed with CD3

The TCR is a heterodimer made up of two nonidentical polypeptide chains termed α and β (see Fig. 43.3), held together by covalent and noncovalent bonds. In addition, a small, unique T-cell population found primarily within the gut expresses alternative TCRs, their chains being termed γ and δ. Each chain of the TCR comprises two domains - one **constant** and one **variable** amino acid sequence. The antigen-binding site of the TCR is in the cleft formed by the adjoining single N-terminal variable domains of the constituent α (Vα) or β (Vβ) chains. Structurally, the TCR resembles the binding portion of an immunoglobulin molecule, the antigen receptor

found on B cells, but it is quite distinct, being the result of different gene products. The effector function of the antigen-receptor chains is signal transduction. An additional protein complex, called CD3, binds to the TCR and facilitates TCR signaling.

Major histocompatibility complex

The MHC proteins are the display units that present antigen in a way that T cells can recognize against a background of self

As indicated previously, for an immune response to be initiated, antigen cannot simply bind to the nearest T cell but must be "formally" presented to the immune system. This occurs when APCs express processed antigenic peptides bound within grooves of MHC molecules on their cell surface. The MHC class I and II molecules also provide a mechanism for distinguishing antigens that originate from within cells (e.g., viruses) from those that arise from the extracellular environment (e.g., many bacterial antigens). **MHC class I presents intracellular antigens to CD8+ cytotoxic T cells, and MHC class II presents extracellular antigens to CD4+ helper T cells.** CD8+ cytotoxic T cells are highly trained assassins that, once activated, kill infected cells and the pathogens within them. CD4+ helper T cells provide appropriate "help" (costimulation and cytokines) to a number of other immune cell types, to enhance their function. For example, antibody production from fully activated B cells requires CD40L and cytokines from CD4+ T cells.

The MHC complex of genes is grouped into three regions, termed class I, II, and III

The MHC complex of genes is found on the short arm of chromosome 6 and is grouped into three regions, termed class I, II, and III (Fig. 43.4). The **polygenic and polymorphic nature of the MHC** is key to the success of the adaptive immune response. By this, we mean that there are various different MHC class I and II genes, and for any one gene, multiple variants or alleles exist. Class I and II molecules are directly involved in immune recognition and cellular interactions, whereas class III molecules are involved in the inflammatory response by coding for soluble mediators, including complement components of the innate immune response and TNF.

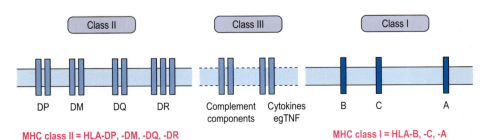

Fig. 43.4 Genetic organization of the MHC and expressed products. Genes of the MHC in humans are located on chromosome 6. The gene products are the human leukocyte antigens (HLA). Class II gene products include complement components and cytokines.

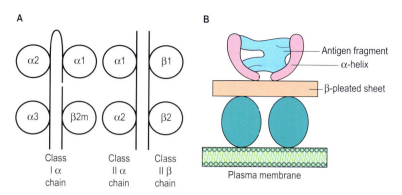

Fig. 43.5 **Class I and II MHC (HLA) structure.** (A) Schematic structures of class I and class II MHC molecules. In class I molecules, β2-microglobulin (β2m) is one of the four domains. (B) The protein conformation and folding of the MHC molecules shape the binding groove for antigenic peptides.

MHC class I genes are organized into several loci, the most important of which are termed HLA-A, HLA-B, and HLA-C

MHC alleles are transmitted and expressed in Mendelian codominant fashion. Owing to their closeness on the chromosome, they are inherited *en bloc* as parts of a haplotype and are expressed on the surface of all nucleated cells. The α-chains they encode have three domains, one of which is structurally similar to those found in immunoglobulin molecules, but the other two show significant differences. The α-chains combine with β2-microglobulin to give rise to a functional class I molecule

MHC class II genes are HLA-DR, HLA-DQ, HLA-DM, and HLA-DP

The class II subregion genes, termed HLA-DR, HLA-DQ, HLA-DM, and HLA-DP, are organized into α- and β-loci, giving rise to α- and β-polypeptide chains, respectively. Both chains are of approximately the same molecular weight and combine to form a heterodimer with a tertiary structure similar to a class I molecule, with a peptide groove into which the processed antigenic fragment is inserted during antigen presentation (Fig. 43.5). Unlike class I expression, class II is far more restricted, being expressed mainly on APCs, such as DCs, macrophages, and B cells.

Many (currently in excess of 1000) allelic variants can be identified in each of the MHC class II loci associated with antigen presentation. There are six major loci, each having between 10 and 60 functionally recognizable alleles. Each parent passes on to the offspring one set or haplotype on each chromosome, so it is easy to appreciate that the likelihood of another individual in the same species having an identical set of MHC molecules is remote.

The B-cell antigen receptor

The B-cell antigen receptor (BCR) is a membrane form of the immunoglobulin molecules found circulating in serum

Immunoglobulins are Y-shaped molecules made up of four polypeptide chains (Chapter 40, Fig. 40.5) - a pair of heavy chains, each with an approximate molecular weight of 150 kDa, and a pair of light chains, each with an approximate molecular weight 23 kDa. Their structure is based on domains with constant and variable sequences of amino acids in both the heavy and the light chains. It is the variably sequenced amino-terminal domains of both the heavy and the light chains that form a pocket that constitutes the antigen-binding site; the "fragment antigen-binding" (**Fab**) portion sits at the end of the arms. The remaining relatively constant amino acid sequence domains of the chains are termed **constant heavy (CH)** or **constant light (CL)** and form the stem of the Y-shaped molecule ("fragment constant," or **Fc portion**). The Fc portions of antibodies have a number of functions, including binding complement components and binding to Fc receptors on leukocytes, including macrophages, natural killer (NK) cells, neutrophils, mast cells, and B cells; for the BCR, the Fc portion of the sIg molecule is the signaling component of the receptor.

There is an almost infinite range of possibilities for antibody specificities

The B-cell receptor and T-cell receptor repertoires, which each have likely in excess of 10^{11} different specificities, occur as a result of a combination process of the various genes involved in making the molecule. For the BCR, the variable region of a light chain is the product of two different genes (V = variable, and J = joining). This product in turn combines with the gene product for the constant (C) region, giving the complete transcribed and translated light-chain protein. For the heavy chain, the level of complexity is increased with the addition of the D (diversity) gene product, forming part of the variable area in addition to V and J gene segments. Again, these will combine to the C region segments, but for heavy chains, multiple C-gene products make up the completed protein. Multiple copies of each of the gene segments in germline DNA, used randomly, as well as polymorphisms between individuals, result in the almost infinite number of possible antibody specificities. Mature B cells also have the capacity to accumulate small point mutations in the DNA encoding the heavy and light chains of immunoglobulin, termed **somatic hypermutations,** which add further variation to the range of specificities available.

The process of generating diversity in T-cell receptors is very similar and also results from the combination of multiple gene segments. Each B cell and T cell that develops in the body generates its BCR or TCR independently, and the large number of different receptors generated means at least one is likely to recognize any pathogen that we may encounter.

Thymic education and self-tolerance help distinguish between self and non-self

The risk in using random gene combination to produce antigen-recognition receptors is that the process is just as likely to produce TCRs and BCRs that recognize **self** antigens as it is to produce functional receptors that recognize **non-self**, or foreign antigens. The **ability to distinguish between self and non-self** is crucial for successful adaptive responses. The immune system achieves this through the complicated processes of **thymic education** and **self-tolerance.** Thymic education and selection ensure that any T cells that are capable of recognizing self antigens are deleted before entering the circulation. Because B-cell activation requires T-cell help, the absence of self-reactive T cells also reduces the likelihood of activated, self-reactive B cells. Failure of this process can result in inappropriate activation of the immune response by self-antigens, leading to **autoimmune diseases** such as **rheumatoid arthritis** and **systemic lupus erythematosus.**

The adaptive immune response needs time to develop and remembers what it sees

When an adaptive immune response is first initiated, relatively few cells and components are likely to be available that have the right specificity for any one antigen. There is a delay while the activation and consequent proliferation of these cells increase the number of specific cells to a level that can ensure elimination of the antigen, or at least reduce the antigen to a level that would be manageable by the innate immune response. This delay is typically 7 to 10 days long during the first encounter with a particular pathogen, but the adaptive immune response employs a mechanism to remember a specific encounter, and if the same foreign antigen is encountered again, it can be dealt with more quickly and effectively. This process is called **immunologic memory.** Thus in comparison to innate immunity, the adaptive response exhibits both **specificity** for and **memory** of the foreign or non-self antigen.

The adaptive response is an integrated response

The cells and molecules of adaptive immunity that eradicate a pathogen include **CD4$^+$ helper T cells**, **CD8$^+$ cytotoxic T cells**, and the **antibodies** produced by **activated B cells.** The adaptive immune response is thus mediated by cellular and humoral elements, T cells being considered responsible for cellular immunity and B cells for humoral immunity. It is important to consider the adaptive response as being an integrated response, not occurring in isolation. For example, many T-cell functions affect how efficiently B cells respond. Similarly, B cells can in turn activate T cells. The integrated response includes innate immunity too. For example, macrophages increase their rate of phagocytosis in response to cytokines released by T cells. Microbes can become coated with antibodies in a process termed **opsonization,** which makes phagocytosis by neutrophils and macrophages more efficient.

Atypical lymphocytes

A population of atypical lymphocytes is termed **"natural killer" (NK) cells**, so called because they demonstrate the ability to kill neoplastic or virally infected cells without apparent prior exposure or sensitization. They are generally considered to be part of the innate response.

Lymphoid tissues

The immune system is unusual in body systems in that cells are mobile and must patrol the whole body. Much of the action during an immune response takes place in the infected tissue, whether that be the skin, gut, lung, or other area, but there are specific lymphoid tissues that are unique to the immune system.

Primary (central) lymphoid tissues

All immune cells are derived from hematopoietic stem cells resident, in adults, in the bone marrow. Lymphocytes originating from these bone marrow–derived hematopoietic stem cells undergo early development and differentiation in one of two **primary lymphoid organs,** the bone marrow or the thymus.

Maturation of most B cells occurs within the bone marrow

One of the earliest steps in B-cell development is the rearrangement of the progenitor B cells' immunoglobulin genes. This is an antigen-independent process achieved by interacting with stromal cells within the bone marrow. The resulting immature B cells express **surface IgM** as an antigen receptor. If they interact too strongly with environmental antigens at this stage, they are removed by a process of negative selection, thus reducing the chance of autoreactivity. After their exit into the periphery, B cells will express both **surface IgM and IgD** and can be activated by antigen engagement. Activated B cells proliferate, some becoming **antibody-secreting plasma cells** and others **long-lived memory cells.**

T-lymphocyte progenitors travel to the thymus, where they develop into T lymphocytes

The thymus is a multilobed structure found in the midline of the body just above the heart. At the macroscopic level, there is an outer cortex and an inner medullary area within each lobule. T-cell development progresses in the thymus as the immature T cells migrate from the cortex to the medulla. The immature T cells interact with thymic epithelia and DCs and, in doing so, undergo the processes of **positive and negative selection** that constitute the "thymic education of T cells." During positive selection, the T cells are assessed for their ability to interact with MHC molecules, and only successful T cells receive survival signals. In negative selection, cells that show excessive reactivity to self-antigens receive death signals, causing their deletion while still within the thymus. This removes **autoreactive** cells, which, if released into the periphery, could potentially induce autoimmunity. The development of both early T and B cells in the primary lymphoid tissues is independent of extrinsic antigen stimulation.

Secondary lymphoid tissues

The secondary lymphoid organs comprise **lymph nodes, spleen, and the mucosa-associated lymphoid tissues (MALT).** These tissues are functionally organized throughout the body and have a degree of compartmentalization in common, with areas specific for T cells or B cells, and areas of overlap where they interact and respond to antigen. It is in secondary lymphoid organs that adaptive immune reactions begin. For example, on exiting the thymus, naïve T cells recirculate via the bloodstream and enter the lymph nodes by appropriate upregulation of adhesion molecules and chemokine receptors, which allows them to localize in the T-cell areas of the tissue. Naïve T cells move from lymph node to lymph node, scanning all arriving DCs, checking for the presence of one specific antigen.

Within the lymph node, the T-cell area is the paracortex, and the B-cell areas are the follicular areas of the medulla

Secondary lymphoid organs contain two types of follicular structures: the unstimulated primary follicle and stimulated secondary follicles that are characterized by the presence of germinal centers. Secondary lymphoid organs contain two types of follicular structures: the unstimulated primary follicle and stimulated secondary follicles that are characterized by the presence of germinal centers. Lymph, which drains from the tissues to the lymph nodes, carries DCs and free antigens, and the antigen-loaded DCs hope to activate the rare T cells with appropriate specificity. On activation, the T cell will again alter chemokine receptor expression and leave the lymph node to recirculate back to the site of infection, where it can induce an effector response. Similarly, B cells within the lymph node can sample the free antigen being delivered via the lymph and, after receiving costimulation from CD4$^+$ T helper cells, will proliferate, complete maturation, and become antibody-secreting plasma cells.

The spleen contains nonlymphoid tissue (the red pulp) as well as lymphoid areas, the white pulp

Within the white pulp, follicular B-cell areas are evident, and the T-cell areas lie between them in the interfollicular space. The spleen is the location for the presentation of blood-borne antigens to cells of the adaptive immune response.

MALT comprises the lymphoid elements adjacent to the mucosal surfaces

MALT is found at the entrance to the respiratory tract and gut and includes the **tonsils** and **adenoids**. Further down the digestive tract, unencapsulated aggregates of lymphoid cells referred to as **Peyer's patches** are found, overlaid by specialized areas of epithelium for sampling the antigenic environment. Similar to the lymph nodes and spleen, these tissues are important for initial antigen sampling and presentation, in particular for antigens that enter the body through a breach of the epithelium or via the gut.

Elimination of pathogens by the adaptive immune response

On binding to the antigen, lymphocytes differentiate into progeny with either an effector or a memory function

On successful recognition of antigen, the activated lymphocyte undergoes repeated division or proliferation. Differentiation follows, which can lead to either the development of an **effector function** or the generation of **memory** for response to subsequent exposure of the same microbe (antigen).

Clonal selection creates clones of identical cells with unique antigen specificity

Clonal selection is the process whereby the immune response creates clones of identical lymphocytes, with each clone having the unique antigen specificity of the founding, activated cell. With this clonal repertoire, the antigen determines which specific lymphocytes will be activated. The process of antigen drainage and lymphocyte recirculation to the peripheral lymphoid tissue ensures that **antigen is inspected by many lymphocytes** and can select for proliferation and differentiation of all cells that bear a **specific antigen receptor**. Clonal selection ensures not only an adequate number of effector cells to deal with the threat at the time of initial stimulation but also a suitable number of part-primed memory cells that are able to complete their activation more rapidly on subsequent antigen exposure. Fig. 43.6 shows key events in effector and memory formation for B cells. Note that T cells also undergo a similar process, resulting in proliferating clones of primed effector cells and memory cells being generated for subsequent responses.

Immunologic memory distinguishes the adaptive immune response from the innate response

Exactly how immunologic memory is generated is still the subject of much research. On reexposure to the same antigen, the adaptive immune response, due to the reactivation of long-lived memory cells, mounts a more rapid and more effective response compared with the primary response. **The long-lasting protection offered by vaccination is a result of immunologic memory.** There are clear differences between the way naïve and memory lymphocytes respond to antigen.

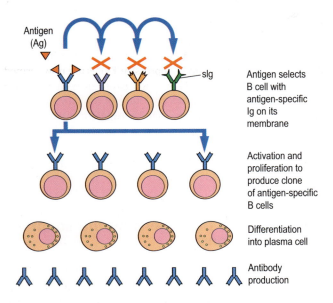

Antigen
(Ag)

sIg

Antigen selects
B cell with
antigen-specific
Ig on its
membrane

Activation and
proliferation to
produce clone
of antigen-specific
B cells

Differentiation
into plasma cell

Antibody
production

Fig. 43.6 **Clonal selection in B cells.** Antigen-specific surface immunoglobulin on the B-cell membrane has a shape reciprocal to the antigen. Antigen–immunoglobulin binding leads to activation and proliferation to produce a clone of antigen-specific B cells. Each member of the specifically activated clone then undergoes differentiation into a plasma cell, which produces and secretes large quantities of a single homogeneous immunoglobulin, with specificity identical to the sIg that triggered the response. sIg, surface immunoglobulin.

For example, naïve and effector cells are relatively short-lived, but memory lymphocytes persist for years and, as a result, often give lifelong protection after initial exposure. Additionally, there are more memory cells specific for the same antigen compared with naïve cells.

Effector T cells

Distinct populations of T cells exist. All T cells, once they have left the thymus, express either CD4 or CD8 on their surface. This phenotypic distinction also has major consequences for effector function: CD4$^+$ T cells are often called **T helper cells (T$_H$)**, whereas CD8$^+$ cells are **cytotoxic T lymphocytes (CTL)**. T$_H$ cells can be further subdivided. They were originally divided into T$_H$1 and T$_H$2 cells, but there are now recognized to be many such functional subsets. There is much current interest in T$_H$17 cells and T follicular helper cells (T$_{FH}$), for example. T$_H$17 cells are so named due to their release of the cytokine IL-17, and T$_{FH}$ cells are a subset found within lymph nodes that interact with B cells and regulate antibody production. T cells are also involved in enhancing the activity of other adaptive and innate immune cells, for example, by activating macrophages. They achieve this by direct cell–cell contact and by the secretion of cytokines. Different cytokines promote the function of different effector cells. The different subsets of T cells are described schematically in Fig. 43.7.

T helper cell subsets: T$_H$1/T$_H$2, T$_H$17, T$_{FH}$, and T regulatory (Treg)

The effector functions of CD4$^+$ T cells are largely in "helping" other immune responses. We have said previously that T cells need to be presented with antigen in the context of MHC on the surface of an APC; **for CD4$^+$ T cells, this is done by MHC II molecules**. Costimulatory signals are also important. Once activated, the T helper cell differentiates, proliferates, and performs different effector functions, restricted by the type of T$_H$ cell that it has become. The T$_H$ subset is

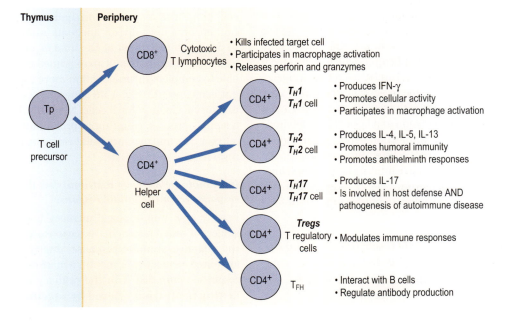

Thymus | Periphery

CD8$^+$ — Cytotoxic T lymphocytes
• Kills infected target cell
• Participates in macrophage activation
• Releases perforin and granzymes

Tp — T cell precursor

CD4$^+$ — Helper cell

CD4$^+$ — *T$_H$1* T$_H$1 cell
• Produces IFN-γ
• Promotes cellular activity
• Participates in macrophage activation

CD4$^+$ — *T$_H$2* T$_H$2 cell
• Produces IL-4, IL-5, IL-13
• Promotes humoral immunity
• Promotes antihelminth responses

CD4$^+$ — *T$_H$17* T$_H$17 cell
• Produces IL-17
• Is involved in host defense AND pathogenesis of autoimmune disease

CD4$^+$ — *Tregs* T regulatory cells
• Modulates immune responses

CD4$^+$ — T$_{FH}$
• Interact with B cells
• Regulate antibody production

Fig. 43.7 **Functional T-cell subsets.** T-cell precursor cells within the thymus develop into cells with different effector functions. T$_{FH}$, T follicular helper cells.

determined by cytokines secreted by the DC at the time of T-cell activation.

T_H1/T_H2 cells

The subdivision into T_H1 and T_H2 subsets was originally made on the basis of their apparent function. T_H1 cells appeared to function as promoting cellular responses: once activated, T_H1 release IFN-γ, which promotes macrophage activity. In addition, they may release TNF-α, which, through endothelial activation and subsequent upregulation of adhesion molecules and chemokines, would promote further leukocyte recruitment. In addition, T_H1 cells provide help to B cells, enhancing antibody production.

T_H2 cells help cellular responses in a different way. They too appear to help B cells make antibodies, although different antibody types - for example, IL-4 released by T_H2 cells encourages B cells to produce IgE. T_H2 cells also preferentially stimulate eosinophil-driven inflammation through their production of IL-5. Together, IgE and eosinophils promote the major antihelminth responses. By releasing IL-4, IL-5, and IL-13, T_H2 cells limit the T_H1 activation of macrophages, and similarly, T_H1 products will inhibit T_H2 responses when required. Therefore the effector functions of T_H cells appear to be determined by the cytokine environment they produce, which is in turn directed by the nature of the invading pathogen. The expression of distinct transcription factors appears to be crucial in driving either T_H1 or T_H2 development, with the transcription factor T-bet responsible for characteristic gene expression by T_H1 cells and the transcription factor GATA-3 responsible for that by the T_H2 subset.

T_H17 cells

The T_H17 cell was originally identified in animal models of a number of autoimmune diseases, including multiple sclerosis, rheumatoid arthritis, and inflammatory bowel disease. Understanding the potential role of this subset, particularly in human disease, has been a major research focus. It is known that in the presence of IL-6 and TGF-β, but the absence of IL-4 and IL-12, CD4$^+$ T_H cells will develop into T_H17 cells. They can also require IL-21, itself a T-cell product, and IL-23, produced by APCs. T_H17 cells make IL-22 in addition to IL-17, and these cytokines can be useful in driving antifungal and some antibacterial immune responses. Both IL-17 and IL-22 act on the stromal and epithelial cells of infected tissue, promoting local production of chemokines such as IL-8, which, in turn, recruit innate effector cells such as neutrophils. This again shows the close interaction between innate and adaptive responses for effective immunity.

T follicular helper (T_{FH})

This subset of CD4+ T_H cells is resident within the lymph nodes and appears to have a role in the removal of most pathogens. T_{FH} cells provide help to B cells, promoting germinal center reactions, and are crucial for the varied antibody responses that can develop. Research is currently ongoing to tease apart the distinct roles of differing T_H cell subsets.

T regulatory cells (Treg)

Originally, cells that can limit a cell-mediated response were identified as "suppressor cells," but early controversy in the field disputed these findings, and suppressive T cells are now termed T regulatory cells (Treg). This appears to be a heterogeneous group. The most studied is a CD4$^+$ T cell that appears to be able to control the action of other immune cells through a combination of soluble mediator release (e.g., IL-10 and TGF-β) and direct cell–cell contact. Many of these cells express the transcription factor FOXP3, which is often used as a defining marker of T regulatory cells. As discussed earlier, the thymus plays an important role in deleting autoreactive T cells, but this process is not 100% efficient, and T regulatory cells play an important role in the process of **peripheral tolerance** - that is, the suppression of potentially self-reactive T cells present in the circulation that, if allowed, would cause autoimmunity. The use of Tregs in clinical applications to treat or prevent autoimmune disease is currently under investigation. The potential of the Treg cells may also be applicable to induce tolerance to transplanted organs.

CD8$^+$ cytotoxic T cells (CTL) kill infected cells

In addition to CD4$^+$ T_H cells, the other major population of T cells is known as cytotoxic T cells (CTL). CTLs express CD8 rather than CD4, which enhances the interaction of CTLs with MHC class I molecules. The role of CD8$^+$ T cells is **primarily to kill infected cells** (e.g., cells infected by viruses) because by doing this, they also destroy the intracellular pathogens. CD8$^+$ T cells recognize their target cells as infected by the antigenic peptides of the pathogen displayed in MHC I on the surface of the infected cell. Like CD4$^+$ T cells, CD8$^+$ T cells must be activated by antigen presentation and costimulation on an APC to become effector cells. It is likely that, initially, naïve CD8$^+$ cells also require help from CD4$^+$ T cells, most probably in the form of IL-2 secreted by the T_H cell. Once activated, effector CTLs are drawn into sites of infection. If they encounter virally infected cells displaying the right antigenic peptide, they will bind tightly to the infected cell using adhesion molecules and kill primarily by the calcium-dependent release of serine proteases known as **granzymes** into the target cell, through holes created in the target cell membrane by **perforins.** Both granzymes and perforins are released from granules present in activated CD8$^+$ T cells. The result of delivery of granzymes to the infected cell is the activation of caspase-driven apoptosis (Chapter 28). Apoptotic cells and associated debris are subsequently removed by innate phagocytic cells such as macrophages - the "trash can."

The adaptive humoral immune response

Humoral immune responses are characterized by the release of antibodies from fully matured plasma cells

The adaptive immune response is summarized in Fig. 43.8. Humoral or antibody-mediated specific immunity is directed at **extracellular infection,** especially bacteria and their

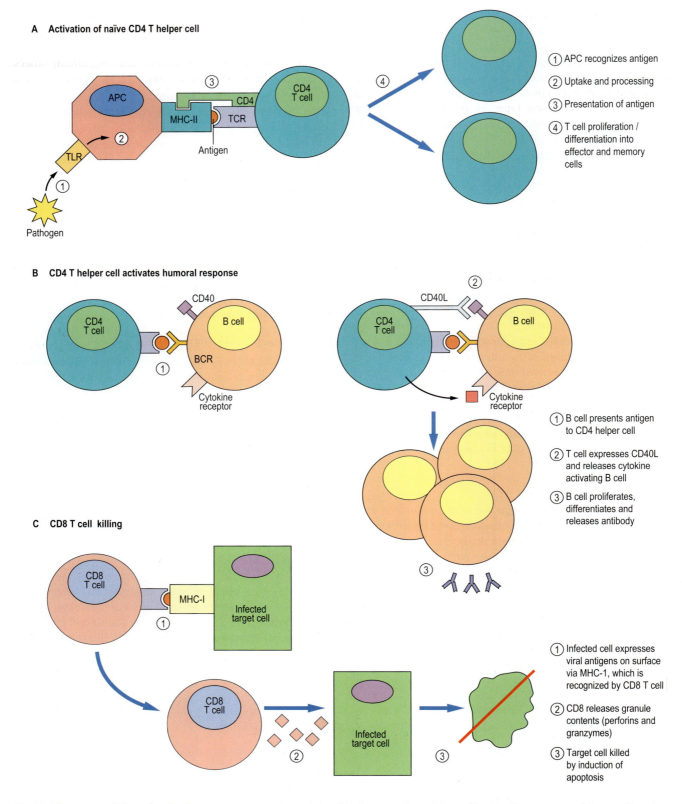

A Activation of naïve CD4 T helper cell

① APC recognizes antigen

② Uptake and processing

③ Presentation of antigen

④ T cell proliferation / differentiation into effector and memory cells

B CD4 T helper cell activates humoral response

① B cell presents antigen to CD4 helper cell

② T cell expresses CD40L and releases cytokine activating B cell

③ B cell proliferates, differentiates and releases antibody

C CD8 T cell killing

① Infected cell expresses viral antigens on surface via MHC-1, which is recognized by CD8 T cell

② CD8 releases granule contents (perforins and granzymes)

③ Target cell killed by induction of apoptosis

Fig. 43.8 **Summary of the adaptive immune response.** Interrelationships between the cellular and humoral components of the specific immune response. APCs activate naïve CD4⁺ T cells, which in turn can activate B cells. Cytotoxic T cells kill infected target cells. APC, antigen-presenting cell; BCR, B-cell receptor; CD40L, CD40 ligand; TLR, toll-like receptor; TCR, T-cell receptor.

products; extracellular parasites; and also at the extracellular phase of viral infection. Antibodies also play a major role in the immunopathogenesis of many autoimmune or aberrant responses resulting in hypersensitivity. The humoral immune response is characterized by the release of antibodies from fully matured plasma cells of the B-lymphocyte lineage. As antibodies recognize many types of molecules, including polysaccharides and lipids, this response is particularly effective against extracellular pathogens. The antibody binding to structural surface components of microbes helps prevent the harmful effects of their toxins in a process termed **neutralization.** However, simple antibody binding, in most situations, will not guarantee elimination of the antigen. To promote the response, the non-antigen-binding fragment of the molecule (Fc portion) is able to activate further components of the innate system, through complement activation or by binding to receptors on phagocytes. The diversity of effector functions of antibodies is achieved by the genetic recombinations of the heavy- and light-chain genes, as described previously.

B-cell subsets are involved in the humoral immune response

Similar to the cellular response, which is mediated by a number of T-cell subsets, the humoral response uses distinct B-cell subsets. As noted earlier, T cells interact with B cells both directly and indirectly via cell-surface receptors and cytokines, respectively. This happens to such a degree that effective B-cell responses are often described as being T-cell dependent. The B cells termed **B2** are found in the follicles of the secondary lymphoid organs. They typically respond to protein antigens and produce the high-affinity antibodies typical of effective humoral responses. Within the marginal zone of the spleen, there is another population of B cells, which typically responds to polysaccharide antigens delivered via the bloodstream. They tend to secrete IgM but can class-switch to produce IgG. Another population, termed **B1**, which express similar receptors, accounts for around 5% of all B cells and is found in mucosal tissue and the peritoneum. They express surface IgM as their antigen receptor and little surface IgD (the pattern opposite to that of the classical B2 follicular B cells). B1 cells predominantly show an IgM response, typically to nonprotein antigens, undergo little somatic hypermutation, and exhibit little memory development.

Antibodies illustrate the capability of the immune system for diversity

For T-cell-dependent responses, reexposure to antigen will induce a secondary antibody response. The higher levels of the produced antibody will have increased affinity and avidity for the particular antigen as a result of the processes of heavy-chain class switching and affinity maturation. The normal human immune system is capable of producing a limitless number of highly specific antibodies with the ability to recognize any and all non-self elements with which it comes

into contact. Failure of effective immune response control can result in the production of antibodies against self-antigens, termed **"autoantibodies,"** and these are characteristic of a number of **autoimmune diseases,** including, among others, **systemic lupus erythematosus (SLE)** and **rheumatoid arthritis (RA)**.

The terms antibody, gamma globulin, and immunoglobulin are synonymous

Five classes of immunoglobulin are recognized - IgG, IgA, IgM, IgD, and IgE - with subclasses being recognized for IgG (IgG1, 2, 3, and 4) and for IgA (1 and 2). When studied at the individual molecular level, no other proteins show such amino acid sequence variation between individual members of the same class or subclass. This is most evident in the N-terminal domains of both heavy and light chains that are responsible for the antigen-recognition portion of the molecule. Antibodies are capable of discriminating between the molecules that characterize the outer capsular coverings of differing bacterial species, which may vary by a single amino acid or a monosaccharide residue. This is a consequence of the dimensions of the area recognized by the antibody molecule being 10–20 Å (10^{-10}m) and thus being capable of being influenced by the alteration in three-dimensional conformation brought about by the change of a single residue.

Antibodies are good examples of how function is intimately related to structure

Antibodies (immunoglobulins) are Y-shaped molecules (Chapter 40, Fig. 40.5). The ends of the arms interact specifically with the pathogen (antigen), and the stem provides additional effector functionality. This secondary or effector function endows the antibody with an ability to initiate immune responses that help eliminate the pathogen to which it is directed. An example of this is the activation of complement. The effector functions of antibodies are summarized in Table 43.4.

Activation of the complement system is one of the most important antibody functions

Activation of the complement system (see Fig. 43.2) is one of the most important antibody effector functions in the adaptive immune response. This is achieved by using a set of components termed the **classic activation pathway** (see previous discussion). This pathway is triggered by complement component C1q binding an IgG or IgM that is already bound to its specific antigen.

Two other pathways of activation exist, both constituting parts of the nonspecific immune response; they are probably older in evolutionary terms and have been described earlier in the chapter.

Fig. 43.8 shows the interrelationships between the cellular and humoral components of the adaptive immune response.

Table 43.4 The effector functions of antibodies

Type	Functions
IgG	Neutralization Opsonization for neutrophils and macrophages Passive immunity for fetus via transplacental passage Complement activation via classic pathway Antibody-dependent, cell-mediated cytotoxicity Natural killer function: cell killing of antibody-bound cells achieved by the receptors for the Fc portion Major isotype used in a secondary antibody response
IgA	Defense of mucosal surfaces; the most predominant immunoglobulin produced by MALT Neutralization
IgM	Neutralization Most effective classic complement pathway activator Predominant isotype in primary antibody responses
IgD	Possible role in signal transduction and B-cell maturation Significance of circulating IgD is undefined
IgE	Major role is defense of mucosal surfaces against multicellular microorganisms

Table 43.5 The consequences of failure of the immune system

Autoimmunity	Inappropriate response to self-antigens through the breakdown of self-tolerance can lead to autoimmune conditions.
	Examples: Rheumatoid arthritis, SLE, type 1 diabetes mellitus
Hypersensitivity	Inappropriate reaction or overreaction to pathogen or antigen can often result in a response that does more harm to the body than the actual cause.
	Examples: Hay fever in response to pollen, anaphylactic response to foodstuffs (e.g., peanuts).
Immunodeficiency	Ineffective immune response to infection can cause immunodeficiency. This can often be hereditary or induced by infection or drug treatment.
	Primary immunodeficiency is an intrinsic defect of one or more components of the immune response (e.g., impaired production of antibody).
	Examples: X-linked agammaglobulinemia, which presents as very low B cell numbers and serum immunoglobulin.
	Severe combined immunodeficiency (SCID) occurs when the thymus fails to develop, and no T cells are present.
	Secondary immunodeficiency can develop after infection (e.g., AIDS, where the virus infects CD4 T cells) or as response to certain drugs (e.g., steroids, which can impair immune cell function).

VACCINATION

Vaccination has probably been the single most beneficial application developed to harness the immune response

The process of vaccination illustrates well the interactions of the humoral and cellular arms of the adaptive immune response and the features that characterize it best: **specificity and memory**. On first encounter with antigen, lymphocytes with the receptors specific for that antigen are activated and undergo activation, proliferation, and differentiation into effector cells, a process that may take up to 14 days to complete (Fig. 43.8). As part of this process, a population of cells semi-primed for that specific antigen also develops (memory cells). On subsequent exposure, the response is more rapid in view of the partly activated state of the memory cells. It is also more effective as a consequence of the maturation, selection, and differentiation of the lymphocytes that has already taken place.

The primary challenge elicits a predominantly IgM response. On subsequent challenge, "help" from appropriate CD4+ T cells induces isotype switching in the B cell to a predominantly IgG response. This offers a heightened and more effective response, resulting in the removal of infecting pathogen.

FAILURE OF THE IMMUNE RESPONSE

Autoimmunity is normally prevented by thymic education; a breakdown in the processes may lead to autoimmune disease

Although the immune system's activities are mostly beneficial, there are several situations in which they can have deleterious effects. These are best considered as aberrations of the quality, quantity, or direction of the response (summarized in Table 43.5).

One particular aspect of these disorders, that of **autoimmunity** (self-reactivity), is avoided by the processes of central tolerance (during thymic education) and peripheral tolerance, which induces clonal deletion and anergy. The self-reactive clones are eliminated or rendered impotent either through deletion within the thymus or by being controlled by T regulatory cells in the periphery. These mechanisms can be seen as a multilayered fail-safe strategy. Should these processes break down or be circumvented, the resulting state of self-reactivity and the inflammatory damage constitute autoimmune disease.

The form of autoimmune disease is determined by the target antigen and immune response that develop. At its simplest, reactions against ubiquitous antigens lead to what are termed non-organ-specific autoimmune diseases. Conversely, reactions to unique components of individual tissues, organs, or systems lead to organ-specific disease. The former is best exemplified by conditions such as **systemic lupus erythematosus (SLE),** in which the apparent target antigens are components common to all nuclei. Damage is seen in several tissues, including the skin, joints, kidneys, and nervous system. Aberrant responses to self-tissues have been identified for almost every body system, organ, and tissue type within the body.

When there is too much of a good thing: hypersensitivity

The accompanying Clinical Box presents an example of **Type I hypersensitivity.** In this case, an inappropriate and excessive response to a normally innocuous foodstuff resulted in a life-threatening condition. The immune response did not evolve with the intention of causing harm to the host, but this is an example of the many conditions caused by such a response. Given the term *hypersensitivity*, it encompasses several responses, each with differing mechanisms but all of which result in damage to the host. Broadly, there are four types, named Type I–IV, where types I–III are mediated by inappropriate antibody responses, and Type IV is considered a T-cell-driven response.

CLINICAL BOX
A YOUNG MAN WHO DEVELOPED SUDDEN STRIDOR AND WIDESPREAD NETTLE RASH: ANAPHYLACTIC SHOCK

A young man was brought into the emergency room in a state of shock with stridor (a high-pitched sound on inspiration) and widespread urticaria (nettle rash). A companion told the admitting medic that the patient had developed difficulties in breathing shortly after eating a snack. Allergy to peanuts was suspected, and a diagnosis of **anaphylaxis** was made. An intramuscular injection of epinephrine was given promptly as well as treatment with intravenous antihistamine, corticosteroid, and cardiorespiratory support. The man recovered.

Comment
Although the physiologic role of the IgE response is considered to be protection against parasite infestation, this response is seen to be subverted in those who experience **atopic diseases** and **anaphylaxis.**

The major fraction of IgE is bound via Fc receptors to mast cells in the tissues. When antigen binds and crosslinks its specific IgE on the mast cells, it triggers their degranulation and release of preformed mediators (principally histamine). When the **mast cell degranulation** is localized to one site, it usually gives rise to only localized reactions, such as allergic rhinitis and asthma. If the degree of sensitization with the antigen-specific IgE and/or the antigenic burden is greater, systemic degranulation can occur, with consequent **anaphylactic shock.** Significant vasodilatation takes place, reducing the blood pressure. This is accompanied by large increases in vessel wall permeability, leading to substantial swelling, which particularly affects the skin and other loose connective tissue, such as that in the larynx. Smooth muscle spasm also occurs, leading to bronchoconstriction with consequent respiratory difficulty and wheezing. These features are accompanied by increased secretory activity of seromucous glands in the respiratory and gastrointestinal tract as well as itching of the skin.

When the response doesn't develop correctly: immunodeficiency

Another example in the accompanying Clinical Box illustrates the interrelationship and dependency of the different components of the immune system. Without an intact immune system, even the slightest fault can have severe effects and prevent protective responses developing against infective agents. These examples where the host does not always mount the required or wanted response, summarized in Table 43.5, are the focus of the disciplines of clinical immunology and immunopathology. More information can be found in the books cited in the Further Reading section.

CLINICAL BOX
A 2-YEAR-OLD WITH RECURRENT INFECTIONS: IMMUNODEFICIENCY STATE

A 2-year-old child presented with a history of recurrent *Candida albicans* and chest infections. Investigations revealed a decreased number of neutrophils, IgG, and IgA. Assessments of lymphocyte proliferative response showed decreased expression of CD40L (CD154) on T cells. A diagnosis of **X-linked hyper-IgM** syndrome was made, and treatment with intravenous immunoglobulin was commenced.

Comment
Immunodeficiency states are classified as either primary or secondary. **Primary immunodeficiencies** are inherited conditions, and with more than 100 different conditions described, they can affect all parts of the immune system, both innate and adaptive. **Secondary immunodeficiencies** are often the consequence of infection (e.g., HIV) or other underlying conditions or environmental factors (e.g., malnutrition).

T-cell help is required for effective B-cell responses. Particular interactions are required for the switch of isotype from the IgM response that is typical of a primary antibody response to the more mature IgG and/or IgA isotypes seen during secondary antibody responses produced to subsequent antigenic challenges. CD40L on the T cell is required to interact with the CD40 on B cells, giving "help" to achieve this. In its absence, antibody production is limited to IgM, and the affected individual is immunocompromised because of the lack of the other important isotypes so critical to the integrity of the immune response. The issue of infection more typically associated with cellular problems suggests that the T-cell defect has functional consequences for this arm of the immune response.

HARNESSING THE POWER OF ANTIBODIES FOR IMMUNOTHERAPY

In recent years, there has been great interest in trying to manipulate immune responses when they are, at least in part, contributing to the medical condition or pathology with which a patient presents. The **use of monoclonal antibodies** offers potential for such an approach. As discussed previously, antibodies have unique specificity against their antigen, and this property has been used in an attempt to specifically target cells and molecules within the human body. One of the best examples has been the development of several monoclonal antibodies against TNFα. Generally considered to be a proinflammatory molecule, TNFα plays a key role in the immunopathology of several conditions, including rheumatoid arthritis. Successfully neutralizing the pro-inflammatory effects of TNFα has resulted in remarkable clinical improvement in patients suffering from this condition. Another example from the field of oncology is the use of a monoclonal antibody specifically designed to target B cells (anti-CD20 antibody) to successfully treat patients diagnosed with chronic lymphocytic leukemia. Many other examples exist, and pharmaceutical companies are currently spending vast sums of money and expending much effort in the hope of developing the "magic bullets" that will become the treatment of choice for many medical conditions in the years ahead.

SUMMARY

- The integrated immune response to non-self or altered-self elements (antigens) is made up of a number of components. Some of these show unique specificity for the particular stimulating antigen(s) and comprise the specific or adaptive immune response, whereas others recognize pathogen signatures and comprise the nonspecific or innate immune response.
- The innate response represents the first-line response and is present in all eukaryotes. The cells and soluble mediators involved are primarily those associated with the processes of inflammation and vascular activation.
- The adaptive response is more refined and usually invoked only in the face of either failure or continued stimulation of the innate response. The cells responsible for the adaptive immune response are the T and B lymphocytes. The specificity they show for the inciting antigen is achieved via the use of specific antigen receptors, expressed on the cell surface after clonal expansion.
- T cells recognize processed antigen via their antigen receptors, interacting with antigen presented by MHC-bearing cells. This leads to the secretion of additional cytokines and the generation of effector functions such as T-cell help and T-cell-mediated cytotoxicity, brought about by the T helper and T cytotoxic subsets, respectively. A distinct CD4+ subset of T cells, termed "T regulatory cells," functions to control adaptive responses and in part prevent autoreactivity by the immune response.
- B cells recognize native antigen and secrete antibodies, which can bind directly to the antigen.

- Both T and B cells and their products are able to recruit and utilize components of the innate response in a more effective and targeted manner, with the aim of eliminating or eradicating the antigen.
- In addition to demonstrating specificity, the adaptive immune response also demonstrates another critically important characteristic not seen with the innate response: memory after its encounter with antigen. The benefit of this is that on subsequent contact with the same antigen, a heightened and more efficient response will lead to a quicker removal of the causative agent, hopefully with less tissue damage than on the first encounter.

FURTHER READING

Abbas, A. K., Lichtman, A. H., & Pillai, S. (2015). *Cellular and molecular immunology* (8th ed.). London: Elsevier.
Chapel, H., Heaney, M., Misbah, S., et al. (2014). *Essentials of clinical immunology* (6th ed.). Oxford: Blackwell.
Helbert, M. (2017). *Immunology for medical students* (3rd ed.). London: Elsevier.
Kumar, H., Kawai, T., & Akira, S. (2011). Pathogen recognition by the innate immune system. *International Reviews of Immunology, 30*, 16–34.
Murphy, K. (2017). *Janeway's immunobiology* (9th ed.). New York: Garland.
Sallusto, F. (2016). Heterogeneity of human CD4+ T cells against microbes. *Annual Review of Immunology, 34*, 317–334.

ABBREVIATIONS

APC	Antigen-presenting cell
BCR	B-cell receptor
CD	Cluster of differentiation system cell surface molecules
CD4+	T helper cells (T$_H$)
CD8+	Cytotoxic T lymphocyte (CTL)
CD40L	CD40 ligand
CLR	C-type lectin receptors
CpG	Cystine-guanine dinucleotide
CRP	C-reactive protein

CD40L	CD40 ligand	LFA-1	Lymphocyte function–associated antigen 1
C_H	Constant heavy, fragment antigen-binding sequence domains	LPS	Lipopolysaccharide
C_L	Constant light, fragment antigen-binding sequence domains	MAC-1	Macrophage adhesion molecule 1
		MALT	Mucosa-associated lymphoid tissues
C1q, C1r, C1s, and C2–C9	Complement components	MBL	Mannose-binding lectin
		MHC	Major histocompatibility complex
		NK	Natural killer cells
CTL	Cytotoxic T lymphocytes (CD8$^+$ cells)	NLR	NOD-like receptor
DC	Dendritic cell	PAMP	Pathogen-associated molecular pattern
Fc	"Fragment constant" of immunoglobulin molecule	PECAM-1	Platelet/cell-adhesion molecule 1 (CD31)
		PRR	Pattern-recognition receptors
FOXP3	Transcription factor	RA	Rheumatoid arthritis
HIV	Human immunodeficiency virus	RLR	RIG-1-like receptor
HLA	Human leukocyte antigen	sIg	Surface Ig
HLA-DR, HLA-DQ, HLA-DM and HLA-DP	MHC class II genes	SLE	Systemic lupus erythematosus
		TCR	T-cell receptor
		T_H	T helper cells (CD4$^+$ T cells)
ICAM-1	Intercellular adhesion molecule 1 (CD54)	TGFβ	Transforming growth factor β
IFN	Interferon (IFN-α, IFN-β, and IFNγ)	TLR	Toll-like receptor
Ig	Immunoglobulin (IgG, IgA, IgM, IgD, and IgE)	TNF	Tumor necrosis factor
		Tregs	T regulatory cells, suppressive T cells
IL	Interleukin (IL-1 -IL-23)	T_{FH}	T follicular helper cells

Selected Clinical Laboratory Reference Ranges

Yee Ping Teoh and Marek H. Dominiczak

REFERENCE RANGES

Reference ranges are values of a given substance (analyte) obtained in a reference population (usually a group of healthy individuals)

Reference values represent the physiologic quantities of a substance to be expected in healthy persons. The term "reference range" is preferred over "normal range" because although the reference population can be clearly defined, no clear definition exists for what is "normal" in a clinical sense.

Deviation above or below the reference range may be associated with a disease process, and the severity of the disease process may be associated with the magnitude of the deviation. The ideal reference population is one that is appropriate for the individual's age, sex, and ethnicity. The reference range may also vary with the instrument and assay procedure used for the measurement.

Distribution of values within the reference population

When data from a large cohort of healthy subjects fit a Gaussian distribution, the reference limits are defined as two standard deviations above and below the mean

This constitutes the central 95% interval of the distribution. However, many analyte distributions are non-Gaussian, and these values are usually mathematically transformed (e.g., logarithmic, reciprocal, exponential transformation) to yield a Gaussian distribution.

Interpretation of laboratory results in individual persons

The interpretation of results of laboratory tests is based on comparison with reference values

If a value falls outside the reference interval, it signifies that - with a probability of 95% - the result is different from the reference population. Note that this does not necessarily mean that it is abnormal: by definition, 5% of individuals in a reference population (1 in 20 subjects) will have results outside the reference range. However, the further the result is from the reference range, the greater is the probability that it is associated with pathology.

Clinical decision limits

In some cases, instead of reference values, clinical decision limits are the basis for interpretation

Clinical decision limits are used in the interpretation of tests such as plasma glucose, lipids, and cardiac troponin measurements. These limits, or cut-off points, are usually derived from epidemiologic studies linking the levels of an analyte with the risk of a particular condition.

The use of cut-off points gives a "yes" or "no" answer to the presence of particular condition or risk, but by definition, it does not address the severity of the condition.

Significant change in serial results

There are many factors that will affect the changes in an individual's serial laboratory results. These repeated results are seldofm identical due to contributions from biological variability, analytical imprecision, and changes in the individual's clinical condition. These factors determine the magnitude of change that must occur before the difference is considered medically significant.

Final notes and cautions when using reference intervals

The reference values given in this chapter are taken from the UK Pathology Harmonization Reference Ranges and from the National Health Service (NHS) Greater Glasgow and Clyde Clinical Biochemistry Service (UK) test menu.

In the tables that follow, we have included the tests that will be helpful in the interpretation of information presented in the **Clinical Boxes** throughout this book. The reader is referred to Further Reading for comprehensive lists of tests offered in clinical laboratories.

The reference intervals are given in SI and conventional units wherever possible, with the factor for converting from SI to conventional units.

- **To convert from an SI unit to a conventional unit**, multiply by the conversion factor.
- **To convert from a conventional unit to an SI unit**, divide by the conversion factor.
- Unless indicated, the ranges given are for serum/plasma concentrations.

These values are given **for guidance only** and to enable the reader to simulate a clinical situation when reading Clinical Boxes. Remember that reference ranges may differ in different laboratories. Therefore before interpreting laboratory tests in a clinical situation, **always verify these with the local laboratory.** Laboratories usually provide their reference ranges together with results.

Finally, precisely as the Clinical Boxes aim to illustrate, **laboratory tests should always be interpreted in the context of medical history and physical examination**.

Table A1.1 Blood gases

Analytes	SI units	Conversion factor (SI to conventional units)	Conventional units
H^+ ion activity / arterial pH	35–45 nmol/L	Negative logarithm of the H^+ ion activity	7.35–7.45
Arterial oxygen partial pressure (PaO_2)	12–15 kPa	7.5	79–101 mmHg
Arterial carbon dioxide partial pressure ($PaCO_2$)	4.6–6.0 kPa	7.5	34–45 mmHg
Bicarbonate	21–29 mmol/L		22–29 mEq/L
Carboxyhemoglobin	0.1%–3.0%		—
Oxygen saturation	>97%		—

Table A1.2 Serum electrolytes and markers of renal function

Analytes	SI units	Conversion factor (SI to conventional units)	Conventional units
Sodium	133–146 mmol/L	1.0	133–146 mEq/L
Potassium	3.5–5.3 mmol/L	1.0	3.5–5.3 mEq/L
Chloride	95–108 mmol/L	1.0	95–108 mEq/L
Bicarbonate	21–29 mmol/L	1.0	21–29 mEq/L
Anion gap $[(Na^+ + K^+) - (HCO_3^- + Cl^-)]$	12–16 mmol/l	1.0	12–16 mEq/L
Urea*	2.5–7.8 mmol/L	6.02	15.2–47.0 mg/dL
Creatinine	44–80 µmol/L	0.0113	0.50–0.90 mg/dL
Calcium (adjusted for serum albumin)	2.20–2.60 mmol/L	4.0	8.8–10.4 mg/dL
Phosphate	0.8–1.5 mmol/L	3.1	2.5–4.7 mg/dL
Magnesium	0.7–1.0 mmol/L	2.43	1.7–2.4 mg/dL
Serum osmolality	270–295 mmol/kg	1.0	270–295 mOsm/kg

*Note that in the United States, blood urea nitrogen (BUN) measurement is used instead of serum urea. The conversion is as follows: urea (mmol/L) × 2.8 = BUN (mg/dL).

Table A1.3 The staging of chronic kidney disease

Stage	Description	eGFR (mL/min/1.73 m^2)
1	Normal kidney function but urine findings or structural abnormalities of the kidney*	≥90
2	Slightly decreased GFR	60–89
3	Moderate decrease in GFR	30–59
4	Severe decrease in GFR	15–29
5	End-stage kidney failure or dialysis	<15

The severity of chronic kidney disease is categorized in six stages. The eGFRs used in this classification have been derived from the abbreviated MDRD GFR equation.

*Proteinuria, albuminuria, hematuria lasting for at least 3 months and/or structural abnormalities.

Reference: KDOQI Clinical Practice Guidelines for Chronic Kidney Disease: Evaluation, Classification, and Stratification (see Further Reading for details).

Table A1.4 Serum proteins and liver function tests

Analytes	SI units	Conversion factor (SI to conventional units)	Conventional units
Serum proteins			
Total protein	60–80 g/L	0.1	6–8 g/dL
Albumin	35–50 g/L	0.1	3.5–5.0 g/dL
Globulins [Globulins] = [total protein] –[albumin]	20–35 g/L	0.1	2.0–3.5 g/dL
C-reactive protein (CRP)	<10 mg/L	—	<1 mg/dL
Liver function tests			
Bilirubin	3–16 umol/L	0.06	0.18–0.94 mg/dL
Alkaline phosphatase adults	50–140 U/L	—	—
Alanine aminotransferase (ALT)	Men 10–40 U/L Women 7–35 U/L	—	—
Aspartate aminotransferase (AST)	Men 15–40 U/L Women 13–35 U/L	—	—
γ-Glutamyl transferase (GGT)	Men < 90 U/L Women < 50 U/L	—	—

Table A1.5 Selected hormones

Analyte	SI units	Conversion factor (SI to conventional units)	Conventional units
Thyroid-stimulating hormone (TSH)	0.35–4.5 mU/L		—
Free T4	9–21 pmol/L	0.08	0.7–1.6 ng/dL
Free T3	2.6–6.5 pmol/L	65	162–422 pg/dL
Cortisol (plasma):			
at 08:00 h	240–600 nmol/L	0.036	8.6–21.6 µg/dL
at 24:00 h	<50 nmol/L		<1.8 µg/dL
Follicle-stimulating hormone (FSH):			
Men	1–10 U/L	0.22	0.2–2.2 ng/mL
Women: early follicular phase	3–10 U/L	0.22	0.7–2.2 ng/mL
Women: postmenopausal	30–150 U/L		6.7–33 ng/mL
Luteinizing hormone:			
Men	1–9 U/L	0.11	0.1–1.0 ug/L
Women: early follicular phase	2–9 U/L	0.11	0.2–1.0 ug/L
Women: postmenopausal	20–65 U/L		2.2–7.15 ug/L
Progesterone (midluteal phase)			
Consistent with ovulation	>30 nmol/L	0.33	>9.3 ng/mL
Probable ovulatory cycle	15–30 nmol/L		4.7–9.3 ng/mL
Anovulatory cycle	<15 nmol/L		<3 ng/mL
Testosterone			
Men	10–30 nmol/L		290–860 ng/dL
Women	0.3–1.9 nmol/L		10–90 ng/dL
Prolactin			
Women	<630 mU/L		<25 ng/mL
Men	<400 mU/L		<16 ng/mL
hCG Cut-off point for detection of pregnancy	> 5 U/L		
Androstenedione	<5.5 nmol/L		<158 ng/mL
Dehydroepiandrosterone sulphate (DHAS) women	(2.0–12.5 µmol/L)		74–463 ug/dL
17-hydroxyprogesterone	<6.0 nmol/L		<200 ng/dL
Insulin-like growth factor (IGF-1)	72–259 µg/L		
Parathyroid hormone	1.1–6.9 pmol/L	9.16	11–69 pg/mL
Calcitonin			
Men	0.0–7.5 ng/L		0–7.5 pg/mL
Women	0.0–5.1 ng/L		0–5.1 pg/mL

Note that many hormones are unstable, and collection details are critical; please refer to local laboratory guidance. Hormone reference ranges are also method dependent; again, please refer to local laboratory ranges (if available).

Table A1.6 Serum tumor markers

Analyte/test interpretation	SI units	Conversion factor (SI to conventional units)	Conventional units
CA 125	<35 kU/L		<35 U/mL
CA 19-9	<37 kU/L		<37 U/mL
CA 15-3	<33 kU/L		<33 U/mL
Carcinoembryonic antigen (CEA)			
Nonsmokers	0.0–3.0 ug/L		0.0–3.0 ng/mL
Smokers	0.0–5.0 ug/L		0.0–5.0 ng/mL
Prostate-specific antigen (PSA)	0.0–4.0 ug/L		0.0–4.0 ng/mL
Thyroglobulin Assay is affected by the presence of thyroglobulin antibodies	1.3–31.8 ug/L		1.3–31.8 ng/mL

Table A1.7 Diagnostic criteria for diabetes mellitus and glucose intolerance

Condition	Diagnostic criteria (mmol/L)	Diagnostic criteria (mg/dL)
Normal range	4–6 mmol/L	72–109 mg/dL
Normal fasting plasma glucose	Below 6.1 mmol/L	Below 110 mg/dL
Impaired fasting glucose (IFG)	(ADA) Equal or above 5.6 but below 7.0 (WHO) Equal or above 6.1 but below 7.0	Equal or above 100 but below 126
Impaired glucose tolerance (IGT)	Plasma glucose during OGTT, 2 h after 75-g load 7.8 or above, but below 11.1	Plasma glucose during OGTT, 2 h after 75-g load 140 or above, but below 200
Prediabetes	(ADA) HbA$_{1c}$ 5.7%–6.4% (39–46 mmol/mol)	
Diabetes mellitus*		
ADA Criterion 1	Random plasma glucose 11.1 or above†	Random plasma glucose 200 or above†
ADA Criterion 2	Fasting plasma glucose 7.0 or above	Fasting plasma glucose 126 or above
ADA Criterion 3	2-h value during 75-g OGTT 11.1 or above	2-h value during 75-g OGTT 200 or above
ADA Criterion 4	HbA$_{1c}$ equal to or above 48 mmol/mol (6.5%)	

*If one of the criteria is fulfilled, diagnosis is provisional. Diagnosis needs to be confirmed the next day using a different criterion.
†If accompanied by symptoms (polyuria, polydipsia, unexplained weight loss).

Table A1.8 Diagnostic criteria for diabetes mellitus in pregnancy

Overt diabetes in pregnancy	mmol/L	Conversion factor (SI to conventional units)	mg/dL
Fasting	≥7.0 mmol/L	18.0	≥126 mg/dL
OGTT 2 h post glucose load	≥11.1 mmol/L		≥200
Gestational diabetes (75-g OGTT)			
Fasting	≥5.1		≥92
OGTT 1 h post glucose load	≥10.0		≥180
OGTT 2 h post glucose load	≥8.5		≥153

Table A1.9 Equivalent units of measurement for glycated hemoglobin (HbA₁c) measured using the traditional (DCCT) method and the newer reference method (IFCC)

DCCT units %	IFCC units (mmol/mol)
5	31
6	42
7	53
10	86

Formula to convert the conventional (DCCT) HbA₁c values to IFCC (SI) units

$HbA_{1c} \ (mmol/mol) = [HbA_{1c}(\%) - 2.15] \times 10.929$.

http://www.diabetes.org.uk/Professionals/Publications-reports-and-resources/Changes-to-HbA1c-values/

Notes

1. Criteria for the diagnosis of diabetes mellitus and glucose intolerance have been developed by several national and international bodies. Here we quote the widely accepted ones, developed by the American Diabetes Association (ADA) and the World Health Organization (WHO). These criteria are the same with the exception of the cut-off point for the diagnosis of impaired fasting glucose. Where the criteria differ, the source of recommendation is marked in the table.
2. Criteria for the diagnosis of overt diabetes in pregnancy are set lower than in nonpregnant persons. Interpretation of OGTT in pregnancy involves fasting glucose concentration and both 1-h and 2-h post–75-g glucose load values, whereas in nonpregnant persons, interpretation is based on the fasting and 2-h post-load values only.

HbA1c standardisation for laboratory professionals http://www.diabetesinscotland.org.uk/publications/hba1c_lab_leaflet_0509.pdf (Accessed Aug 2017).

Table A1.10 Cardiac troponin in the diagnosis of myocardial infarction

Analyte	SI units	Conversion factor (SI to conventional units)	Conventional units
Troponin* (method dependent; upper values are 99th percentile for healthy population; these values are for guidance only)			
Troponin T (highly sensitive method)	0–14 ng/L		0–0.014 ug/L
Troponin I (highly sensitive method)	0–40 ng/L		0–0.040 ug/L

*Troponin has replaced the MB fraction of creatine kinase (CK-MB) as the most useful biomarker for myocardial ischemia. Troponins T and I are released within 3–6 h after an event and will remain elevated for up to 2 weeks. The Third Universal Definition of Myocardial Infarction (2012) defines the criteria for acute myocardial infarction as the detection of a rise and/or fall of cardiac biomarker values (preferably cardiac troponin) with at least one value above the 99th percentile upper reference limit (URL) and with at least one of the following:

- Ischemic symptoms
- ECG changes of new ischemia (new ST-T changes or new left bundle branch block, LBBB)
- Development of pathologic Q waves in the EKG
- Imaging evidence of new loss of viable myocardium or new regional wall motion abnormality
- Identification of an intracoronary thrombus by angiography or autopsy

Additional information is available at https://www.escardio.org/Guidelines/Clinical-Practice-Guidelines/Third-Universal-Definition-of-Myocardial-Infarction

Table A1.11 Lipids

Analyte	SI units	Conversion factor (SI to conventional units)	Conventional units
Lipoprotein (a)	0–300 mg/L	10	0–30 mg/dL
Cholesterol (desirable concentration)*	< 5.18 mmol/L	38.6	<200 mg/dL
Triglycerides*	<1.7 mmol/L	88.4	<150 mg/dL
HDL cholesterol*	Low < 1.0 High >1.6	38.6	<40 mg/dL >60 mg/dL
LDL cholesterol[†]		38.6	
Treatment cut-off if low ASCVD risk	>4.9 mmol/L		>190 mg/dL
Treatment cut-off if high ASCVD risk	1.8 mmol/L		>70 mg/dL
Apolipoprotein A-1		100	
Men	0.94–1.78 g/L		94–178 mg/dL
Women	1.01–1.99 g/L		101–199 mg/dL
Apolipoprotein B			
Men	0.55–1.40 g/L		55–140 mg/dL
Women	0.55–1.25 g/L		55–125 mg/dL

*These values are given as an illustration of ASCVD risk-directed cut-off points. These values were recommended in 2001 by **ATP III (National Cholesterol Education Program Adult Treatment Panel 3, USA).**

[†] **The 2013 ACC/AHA Guideline on the Treatment of Blood Cholesterol to Reduce Atherosclerotic Cardiovascular Risk in Adults** provides recommendations on the use of drug treatment to lower the risk of atherosclerotic cardiovascular disease (ASCVD). These guidelines are directed primarily by the individual's overall risk and LDL-cholesterol. The recommendations suggest the use of statins in the following:
• Persons with clinical ASCVD
• Persons with LDL-cholesterol > 4.9 mmol/L (190 mg/dL)
• Persons without clinical ASCVD but with diabetes aged 40 to 75 years and LDL-cholesterol 1.8–4.9 mmol/L (70–189 mg/dL)
• Persons without clinical ASCVD or diabetes but with LDL-cholesterol 1.8–4.9 mmol/L (70–189 mg/dL) and estimated 10-year ASCVD risk > 7.5%.
Additional information on the 2013 ACC/AHA guideline is available at http://circ.ahajournals.org/content/circulationaha/early/2013/11/11/01.cir.0000437738.63853.7a.full.pdf (accessed April 2017).

Table A1.12 Miscellaneous tests

Analyte	SI units	Conversion factor (SI to conventional units)	Conventional units
Amylase	*		0–100 U/L
Urate:			
Men	0.2–0.5 mmol/L	16.8	5.0–8.0 mg/dL
Women	0.1–0.4 mmol/L		2.5–6.2 mg/dL
Lactate	0.7–1.8 mmol/L	9.0	6–16 mg/dL
Creatine kinase:			
Men	55–170 U/L		
Women	30–135 U/L		

Table A1.13 Urine analysis

Analyte	SI units	Conversion factor (SI to conventional units)	Conventional units
Urine microalbumin	<20 mg/L		
Urine albumin/creatinine ratio (ACR):			
Men			<2.5 mg/mmol creatinine
Women			<3.5 mg/mmol creatinine
Urine microalbumin excretion rate (AER)			<20 ug/min
Urine osmolality	50–1200 mmol/kg	1.0	50–1200 mOsm/kg
24-h urinary free cortisol	<250 nmol/24 h		<9 μg/dL

Table A1.14 Hematology tests

Analyte/test	SI units	Conventional units
Hemoglobin:		
Men	130–180 g/L	13.0–18.0 g/dL
Women	120–160 g/L	12.0–16.0 g/dL
Hematocrit	41%–46%	41–46 mL/dL
Erythrocytes cell count:		
Men	$4.4–5.9 \times 10^{12}$/L	$4.4–5.9 \times 10^{6}$/mm^3
Women	$3.8–5.2 \times 10^{12}$/L	$3.8–5.2 \times 10^{6}$/mm^3
Mean corpuscular volume (MCV)	80–96 fL	80–96 μm^3
Leukocytes, total	$4.0–11.0 \times 10^{9}$/L	4000–11,000/mm^3
Leukocytes, differential count:		
Neutrophils	$2.0–7.5 \times 10^{9}$/L	45%–74%
Lymphocytes	$1.3–4.0 \times 10^{9}$/L	16%–45%
Monocytes	$0.2–0.8 \times 10^{9}$/L	4.0%–10%
Eosinophils	$0.04–0.40 \times 10^{9}$/L	0.0%–7.0%
Basophils	$0.01–0.10 \times 10^{9}$/L	0.0%–2.0%
Platelets	$150–400 \times 10^{9}$/L	150,000–400,000/mm^3
Reticulocytes	$25–75 \times 10^{9}$/L	0.5%–1.5% of erythrocytes
Erythrocyte sedimentation rate (ESR)	2–10 mm/h	
Activated partial thromboplastin time (APTT)	30–40 sec	
Prothrombin time (PT)	10–15 sec	
Thrombin clotting time (TCT)	10–15 sec	
Skin bleeding time	2.0–9.0 min	
D-dimer	<0.25 g/L	

Table A1.15 Tests related to iron metabolism and investigation of anemia

Analyte	SI units	Conversion factor (SI to conventional units)	Conventional units
Ferritin (serum)	14–200 ug/L	0.445	14–200 ng/mL
Transferrin saturation	<55%		
Vitamin B$_{12}$ (serum)	138–780 pmol/L	1.36	187–1060 pg/mL
Folate (serum)	12–33 nmol/L	0.442	5.3–14.6 ng/mL

ABBREVIATIONS

AHA	American heart association
APTT	Activated partial thromboplastin time
ASCVD	Atherosclerotic cardiovascular disease
ATP III	National cholesterol education program adult treatment panel III
CEA	Carcinoembryonic antigen
CK-MB	MB fraction of creatine kinase
DCCT	Diabetic control and complications trial
ESR	Erythrocyte sedimentation rate
GFR	Glomerular filtration rate
HbA$_{1c}$	Hemoglobin A$_{1c}$, glycated hemoglobin
hCG	Human chorionic gonadotrophin
IFCC	International Federation of Clinical Chemistry and Laboratory Medicine
LBBB	Left bundle branch block
MCV	Mean corpuscular volume
MDRD	Modification of diet in renal disease study
OGTT	Oral glucose tolerance test
PSA	Prostate-specific antigen
PT	Prothrombin time
TCT	Thrombin clotting time
URL	Upper reference limit
WHO	World Health Organization

FURTHER READING

ACC/AHA Guideline on the Treatment of Blood Cholesterol to Reduce Atherosclerotic Cardiovascular Risk in Adults. (2013). A report of the

American College of Cardiology/American Heart Association Task Force on Practice Guidelines. *Circulation*. https://doi.org/10.1161/01.cir.0000437738.63853.7a.

American Diabetes Association. Position statement. (2012). Diagnosis and Classification of Diabetes mellitus. *Diabetes Care, 35*(Suppl1), S64–S71.

Bakerman, S. (2002). *Bakerman's ABC of interpretive laboratory data* (4th ed.). Scottsdale, AZ.

Burtis, C. A., Ashwood, E. R., & Bruns, D. E. (2012). *Tietz textbook of clinical chemistry and molecular diagnostics* (5th ed.). Philadelphia: Saunders.

Dominiczak, M. H. (Ed.). (1997). *Seminars in clinical biochemistry*. Glasgow: University of Glasgow.

National Kidney Foundation. Kidney Disease Outcomes Quality Initiative (2002). Clinical practice Guidelines for Chronic Kidney Disease: Evaluation, Classification and Stratification. *American Journal of Kidney Diseases, 39*(Suppl. 1), S1–S266.

Thygensen, et al. (2012). Expert consensus document, third universal definition of myocardial infarction. *European Heart Journal, 33*, 2551–2567.

RELEVANT WEBSITES

American Diabetes Association - Standards of Medical Care in Diabetes (2012): http://care.diabetesjournals.org/content/35/Supplement_1/S11

American Diabetes Association - Standards of Medical Care in Diabetes (2017): http://professional.diabetes.org/sites/professional.diabetes.org/files/media/dc_40_s1_final.pdf

European Society of Cardiology - Third Universal Definition of Myocardial Infarction, ESC Clinical Practice Guidelines: https://www.escardio.org/Guidelines/Clinical-Practice-Guidelines/Third-Universal-Definition-of-Myocardial-Infarction

Lab Tests Online: labtestsonline.org.uk/

Lab Tests Online - reference ranges: http://labtestsonline.org.uk/understanding/features/ref-ranges/

National Cholesterol Education Program ATP III Guidelines At-a-Glance Quick Desk Reference: http://www.nhlbi.nih.gov/guidelines/cholesterol/atglance.pdf

More Clinical Cases

Susan Johnston

CHAPTER 7 VITAMINS AND MINERALS

Joint pain and abnormal liver function tests: Hereditary hemochromatosis

A 52-year-old man visited his primary care physician complaining of joint pain. He was found to have abnormal liver function tests (raised alanine aminotransferase [ALT] and aspartate aminotransferase [AST]). Further investigation into his non-specific hepatitis found a very high ferritin concentration of > 2000 µg/L or > 2000 ng/mL (reference interval 14–200 µg/L; 14–200 ng/mL) and a fasting transferrin saturation of 93% (<55%).

Comment

A serum transferrin saturation of > 55% and a serum ferritin of > 200 µg/L in premenopausal women or > 300 µg/L in men and postmenopausal women suggests primary iron overload due to hemochromatosis. A raised serum ferritin in isolation may be due to inflammatory conditions and alcoholic liver disease. Gene testing confirmed the diagnosis of **hereditary hemochromatosis** in this patient, who was found to be homozygous for the most common mutation in the *HFE* gene (C282Y). He had gross iron overload and end-organ iron toxicity. He was treated by venesection to remove excess iron stores, and family screening was advised for first-degree relatives.

CHAPTER 14 BIOSYNTHESIS OF CHOLESTEROL AND STEROIDS

Hirsutism and irregular periods: Nonclassical congenital adrenal hyperplasia

A 37-year-old woman attended her primary care physician with hirsutism, weight gain, irregular periods, and secondary infertility. A hormone profile revealed raised concentrations of steroids: testosterone 2.5 nmol/L (reference interval 0.3–1.9 nmol/L), or 72 ng/dL (10–90 ng/dL); androstenedione 9.2 nmol/L (reference interval < 5.5 nmol/L), or 264 ng/dL (<158 ng/dL); and 17-hydroxyprogesterone 17.5 nmol/L (reference interval < 6.0 nmol/L), or 583 ng/dL (<200 ng/

dL). She was referred to a consultant endocrinologist for further investigation of her steroid excess.

Comment

A Synacthen test was performed in view of the patient's raised 17-hydroxyprogesterone. Synacthen, or synthetic adrenocorticotropic hormone (ACTH), is a hormone that stimulates the adrenal glands. Synacthen is injected, and 17-hydroxyprogesterone is measured 1 h later to assess how the adrenals have responded. In this case, an exaggerated rise in **17-hydroxyprogesterone** confirmed the diagnosis of **nonclassical congenital adrenal hyperplasia** due to partial deficiency of the 21-hydroxylase enzyme. Female patients who are not pursuing fertility are treated with an oral contraceptive to improve hirsutism. This woman desired fertility and was treated with glucocorticoids to suppress steroid synthesis to normalize ovulatory function.

A 72-year-old woman with hypersecretion of androgens: Leydig cell tumor

A 72-year-old woman presented with male-pattern baldness, hirsutism, and a deepening of the voice. She was found to have a markedly raised testosterone of 12 nmol/L (0.3–1.9 nmol/L), or 346 ng/dL (10–90 ng/dL), and androstenedione of 18.2 nmol/L (<5.5 nmol/L), or 521 ng/dL (<158 ng/dL). Dehydroepiandrosterone sulphate (DHAS) was 2.5 µmol/L (2.0–12.5 µmol/L), or 93 µg/dL (74–463 µg/dL). A computerized tomography (CT) scan of the adrenal glands and the ovaries was unremarkable.

Comment

Based on these findings, a provisional diagnosis of a testosterone-producing tumor was made. The measurement of androstenedione and DHAS can help distinguish the source of the excess testosterone. In ovarian tumors, androstenedione is the predominant androgen. DHAS is associated with adrenal tumors. Her ovaries were removed surgically, and histology confirmed the presence of a small (18-mm) steroid cell tumor in the right ovary, also known as a **Leydig cell tumor**. Leydig cell tumors are very rare steroid cell tumors that usually give rise to a high testosterone concentration. The tumors are characteristically small and can be hard to identify by imaging. After removal of the ovaries, her testosterone fell to 1.1 nmol/L (32 ng/dL), confirming that the ovary was the source of the testosterone.

A 30-year-old man with gynecomastia: Klinefelter's syndrome

A 30-year-old man with learning difficulties presented to his primary care physician with gynecomastia (an abnormal increase in breast tissue) and was referred to endocrinology for investigation. On examination, he was found to have prepubertal testes, and biochemical investigations found a subnormal testosterone 0.9 nmol/L (10–30 U/L), or 26 ng/dL (290–860 U/L) and raised follicle-stimulating hormone (FSH) of 27.2 U/L or 6.0 ng/mL (1–10 U/L; 0.2–2.2 ng/mL).

Comment

The subnormal testosterone and raised FSH are consistent with primary testicular failure. Chromosomal analysis was performed, and the patient was found to have hypogonadism secondary to **Klinefelter's syndrome.** Klinefelter's syndrome is a genetic condition that only affects males. Affected males have an extra copy of the X chromosome (XXY). Males with Klinefelter's syndrome have small testes that do not produce enough testosterone before birth and during puberty. This lack of testosterone means that during puberty, the normal male sexual characteristics do not develop fully. There is reduced facial and pubic hair, and gynecomastia often develops due to an imbalance between testosterone and estrogen. Treatment includes testosterone replacement.

CHAPTER 27 BIOCHEMICAL ENDOCRINOLOGY

A 71-year-old woman with hypothyroidism and seizure: Myxoedema coma

A 71-year-old woman was discovered by her husband having a seizure, which self-terminated after 20 min. She had a further seizure in the emergency room. She had a past medical history of hypothyroidism, and her thyroxine replacement had recently been stopped because she was thought to be overtreated. Her blood results found her to be profoundly hypothyroid, with a thyroid-stimulating hormone (TSH) of 52.8 mU/L (0.35–5.0 mU/L) and a free thyroxine (fT4) of < 5.0 pmol/L (9–21 pmol/L), or < 0.4 ng/dL (0.7–1.6 ng/dL).

Comment

This woman was moved to the intensive care unit for treatment of **myxoedema coma secondary to profound hypothyroidism.** Myxoedema coma is a rare complication of hypothyroidism that typically presents in elderly women in the winter months and is associated with a high mortality rate. The pathogenesis is not clear, but factors that predispose to its development include drugs and systemic illness (e.g., pneumonia). Clinical manifestations include reduced level of consciousness, sometimes associated with seizures; hypothermia; and other features of hypothyroidism. Myxoedema coma is a medical emergency and requires a multifaceted approach to treatment that includes intravenous thyroxine or triiodothyronine, glucocorticoids (there is impaired adrenal reserve in profound hypothyroidism), fluid replacement, and airway management.

A 28-year-old woman with headache and blurred vision: Acromegaly

A 28-year-old woman presented to the emergency room with a progressive headache and blurred vision. A magnetic resonance imaging (MRI) scan showed a large pituitary tumor. Visual field testing revealed partial blindness caused by compression of the optic chiasm by the tumor. On examination, it was noted that she had a protruding jaw, and further questioning revealed that she had noticed an increase in her foot and hand size over the preceding few years. She had an insulin-like growth factor (IGF-1) result of 994 µg/L, or 994 ng/mL (72–259 µg/L) and failed to suppress growth hormone in response to an oral glucose tolerance test.

Comment

This woman has **acromegaly** as a result of prolonged excessive secretion of growth hormone by the pituitary gland. Growth hormone stimulates the liver to produce IGF-1, which in turn causes growth of muscle, bone, and cartilage. Clinical features include large hands and feet and prominent facial features, such as protruding jaw and brow; enlarged lips, tongue, and nose; and widely spaced teeth. This patient had surgical excision of the tumor, and postoperatively, her visual fields were full, and her symptoms improved. Her postoperative IGF-1 was 139 µg/L (139 ng/mL).

A 32-year-woman with an elevated prolactin: Macroprolactin

A 32-year-old woman attended her physician with complaints of weight gain and no periods for several months. She was taking amisulpride, an antipsychotic drug, for schizophrenia. Routine blood tests excluded premature ovarian failure, hypothyroidism, and pregnancy. She was found to have a prolactin result of > 25,000 mU/L (<630 mU/L), or >1000 ng/mL (<25 ng/mL), and she was referred to an endocrinologist for review.

Comment

Drugs, such as antipsychotics, can cause elevations in prolactin of several thousand; however, drugs are unlikely to increase prolactin to > 25,000 mU/L (>1000 ng/mL). The sample was treated with polyethylene glycol (PEG) and tested **positive for the presence of macroprolactin.** Macroprolactin is a high-molecular-weight form of prolactin (prolactin bound to immunoglobulin G antibody) that interferes with prolactin measurement. It is biologically inactive, and its detection is of no clinical significance. Hyperprolactinemia attributable to macroprolactin is a frequent cause of misdiagnosis of patients. Macroprolactin should be considered if signs and symptoms of hyperprolactinemia are absent in the presence of an elevated prolactin.

Pituitary hCG production can result in a positive pregnancy test in postmenopausal women

A 53-year-old postmenopausal woman had her human chorionic gonadotrophin (hCG) level measured as part of a presurgical assessment. The hCG level was detectable at 9 U/L, or 9 mIU/mL (> 5 U/L is the cut-off for detection of pregnancy), and the clinician queried whether this could be gestational trophoblastic disease.

Comment

This woman was postmenopausal, with a follicle-stimulating hormone (FSH) of 85 U/L, or 18.7 ng/mL, and luteinizing hormone (LH) of 52 U/L, or 3.7 μg/mL (FSH values > 25 U/L: 5.5 ng/mL with prolonged amenorrhoea are indicative of menopause). A more probable cause of the raised hCG is the production of hCG by the pituitary. In menopausal females, production of estrogen decreases, which in turn decreases the production of gonadotrophin-releasing hormone (GNRH) by the hypothalamus. LH and FSH production increase to stimulate GNRH. Under this hyperstimulation, the pituitary may secrete an hCG-like molecule. Pituitary hCG is the cause of increased serum hCG results in nonpregnant women, most notably in the peri- and postmenopausal periods.

Primary hypothyroidism can cause an increased prolactin

A 32-year-old woman attended her primary care physician complaining of irregular periods. Laboratory workup found a slightly raised prolactin level of 713 mU/L (<630 mU/L), or 28 ng/mL (<25 ng/mL). Gonadotrophin levels and testosterone were normal, and she was not taking any medications. Thyroid function tests (TFT) were consistent with primary hypothyroidism. Thyroid-stimulating hormone (TSH) was 20.8 mU/L (0.35–5.0 mU/L), and free thyroxine (fT4) was 9.9 pmol/L (9–21 pmol/L), or 0.77 ng/dL (0.7–1.6 ng/dL).

Comment

Prolactin is a hormone secreted by the lactotroph cells of the anterior pituitary gland. Its secretion is under the negative control of dopamine from the hypothalamus. Causes of a slightly raised prolactin include stress and drugs that act as dopamine receptor blockers (e.g., antipsychotics). In this case, the raised prolactin was found to be secondary to primary hypothyroidism. The loss of thyroxine feedback inhibition in primary hypothyroidism causes overproduction of thyrotropin-releasing hormone (TRH) from the hypothalamus. TRH has a weak stimulatory effect on the lactotroph cells of the anterior pituitary, resulting in mild to moderate increases in prolactin.

Incidental finding of a prolactin-secreting tumor

An 87-year-old man presented to the emergency room following a fall resulting in a head injury. A CT scan showed no bony injury, but it did reveal a large pituitary mass measuring 3 cm. He was referred to endocrinology to assess pituitary function. Laboratory workup found a grossly elevated prolactin of 132,000 mU/L (<400 mU/L), or 5280 ng/m/l (<16 ng/mL), with normal pituitary-adrenal and pituitary-thyroid function.

Comment

These findings are consistent with a **prolactin-secreting tumor**, or prolactinoma. Prolactinomas are benign pituitary tumors producing prolactin. They are the most common type of pituitary tumors and are classified according to their size: macroprolactinomas are > 3 mm, and microprolactinomas are <3 mm. Symptoms are caused by too much prolactin in the blood or by the pressure of the tumor on surrounding tissue. The patient's visual fields were normal, confirming that the tumor was not compressing the adjacent optic nerve. This patient was treated with a drug that inhibits the release of prolactin by stimulating dopamine receptors in the hypothalamus.

CHAPTER 33 LIPOPROTEIN METABOLISM AND ATHEROGENESIS

Recurrent pancreatitis and severe mixed hyperlipidemia: Lipoprotein lipase deficiency

A 46-year-old man was referred to the lipid clinic with a history of recurrent pancreatitis and a markedly mixed hyperlipidemia with an elevated total cholesterol of 25.8 mmol/L (<5.18 mmol/L desirable), or 996 mg/dL (<200 mg/dL desirable), and triglycerides of > 100 mmol/L (<1.7 mmol/L), or 8850 mg/dL (<150 mg/dL desirable). He suffered from type 2 diabetes mellitus secondary to chronic pancreatitis.

Comment

Genetic testing was undertaken to screen for causes of hyperlipidemia, and the report revealed a heterozygous mutation in the lipoprotein lipase (*LPL*) gene, consistent with a diagnosis of **familial lipoprotein lipase deficiency (LPLD).** LPLD is a rare inherited condition that disrupts the normal breakdown of fats in the body. Raised triglycerides are often present from childhood, but the condition may not be diagnosed until adulthood. Symptoms include recurrent attacks of acute pancreatitis and fat-filled spots known as eruptive xanthomata. Genetic counseling was advised for this patient, and first-degree relatives had their lipid levels checked.

CHAPTER 34 ROLE OF THE LIVER IN METABOLISM

Glandular fever can cause abnormal liver function tests

An 18-year-old female presented with weight gain, lethargy, and swollen lymph glands. She was found to have a raised aspartate aminotransferase (AST) of 373 U/L (13–35 U/L) and alanine aminotransferase (ALT) of 699 U/L (7–35 U/L).

Comment

The clinical findings together with deranged liver function tests (LFT) led to the presumed diagnosis of **glandular fever,** or infectious mononucleosis. Glandular fever is a viral infection caused by the Epstein-Barr virus, a member of the herpes virus family. It is most common in teenagers and young adults. A full blood count and film found a high white blood cell count and a higher-than-usual number of atypical lymphocytes, consistent with the diagnosis of glandular fever. The **Monospot test** (or heterophile antibody test) was positive in the second week of the illness. The patient felt well after 2-3 weeks, her LFTs returned to normal, and the Monospot test was negative after the infection resolved.

CHAPTER 35 WATER AND ELECTROLYTE HOMEOSTASIS

A case of lithium-induced diabetes insipidus

A 70-year-old woman was admitted following a 6-week history of worsening confusion. History from her carers revealed that she was on long-term lithium therapy for bipolar disorder and that she was drinking more than usual and passing urine frequently. On admission, her serum sodium concentration was 163 mmol/L, or 163 mEq/L (133–146 mmol/L), and she was passing more than 4 L of urine per day. Her serum osmolality was 346 mmol/Kg (270–295 mmol/kg or mOsm/kg), and her urine osmolality was 195 mmol/Kg.

Comment

This woman has **nephrogenic diabetes insipidus secondary to long-term lithium therapy.** Diabetes insipidus is defined as the passage of large volumes (>3 L/24 h) of dilute urine (urine osmolality < 300 mmol/kg). Diabetes mellitus and renal failure must be excluded as the cause of the large urine output. Nephrogenic diabetes insipidus is due to renal resistance to vasopressin. Chronic lithium use can damage the cells of the kidney so that they no longer respond to vasopressin.

A 42-year-old man with a long history of hypertension: Primary aldosteronism

A 42-year-old man was feeling generally unwell and attended his primary care physician. He was found to have a low potassium of 2.8 mmol/L, or 2.8 mEq/L (3.5–5.3 mmol/L), and a high blood pressure (180/100 mmHg). He had no significant medical history and was on no medications. Antihypertensive medication was prescribed, and his blood pressure was well controlled. Daily potassium supplementation was required to keep his potassium in the normal range. He was referred to a blood pressure clinic for investigation of hypertension and persistent hypokalemia.

Comment

The patient was found to have a **raised aldosterone** level and a completely **suppressed renin** concentration. A CT scan identified a 1.2-cm left-sided adrenal adenoma. A diagnosis of **primary aldosteronism (Conn's syndrome)** was suspected, but further investigations were required for confirmation. Results of a **saline suppression test** were consistent with an adrenal adenoma producing aldosterone - the aldosterone failed to suppress despite being given a salt load. **Adrenal vein sampling** was performed to confirm the locality; there was evidence of significant aldosterone production from the left adrenal vein. The patient was treated with spironolactone (an aldosterone antagonist), and his blood pressure returned to normal.

CHAPTER 37 MUSCLE: ENERGY METABOLISM AND CONTRACTION EXERCISE

Rhabdomyolysis as a consequence of muscle ischemia

A 96-year-old man presented to the emergency room after a fall the previous evening. He had been unable to get back up and was found lying on the floor by his son the following morning. He had bruising on his arms and knees consistent with a fall. X-rays of his pelvis and hip showed no fractures, and there was no evidence of head trauma. His creatine kinase (CK) level was found to be > 30,000 U/L (55–170 U/L) and he had mild renal impairment and a raised C-reactive protein (CRP) of 198 mg/L, or 19.8 mg/dL (<10 mg/L; < 1.0 mg/dL).

Comment

The elevated level of the muscle enzyme creatine kinase is consistent with a diagnosis of **rhabdomyolysis.** This is a serious condition resulting from the breakdown of skeletal muscle and is likely to be the result of muscle ischemia following prolonged immobilization in this case. Breakdown products of the muscle cells are released into the bloodstream and can cause kidney damage. The patient was treated with intravenous fluids and antibiotics. His kidney function, CRP, and CK all returned to normal before he was discharged home.

Index

Page numbers followed by "*f*" indicate figures, "*t*" indicate tables, and "*b*" indicate boxes.